D1261519

VOLUME ONE

PEDIATRIC OTOLARYNGOLOGY

SECOND EDITION

EDITED BY:

CHARLES D. BLUESTONE, M.D.

Professor of Otolaryngology
University of Pittsburgh
School of Medicine
Director, Department of Otolaryngology
Children's Hospital of Pittsburgh

AND

SYLVAN E. STOOL, M.D.

Professor of Otolaryngology and Pediatrics
University of Pittsburgh
School of Medicine
Director of Education, Department of Otolaryngology
Children's Hospital of Pittsburgh

MARY D. SCHEETZ, M.L.S.

Associate Editor
Department of Otolaryngology
Children's Hospital of Pittsburgh

1990
W.B. SAUNDERS COMPANY
Harcourt Brace Jovanovich, Inc.
Philadelphia ▪ London ▪ Toronto ▪ Montreal ▪ Sydney ▪ Tokyo

W. B. SAUNDERS COMPANY
Harcourt Brace Jovanovich, Inc.

The Curtis Center
Independence Square West
Philadelphia, PA 19106

Library of Congress Cataloging-in-Publication Data

Pediatric otolaryngology / [edited by] Charles D. Bluestone,
Sylvan E. Stool.—2nd ed.
     p.   cm.

Includes bibliographies and index.

ISBN 0–7216–2120–1.—ISBN 0–7216–2923–7 (v. 1).
—ISBN 0-7216-2924-5 (v. 2)

1. Pediatric otolaryngology.   I. Bluestone, Charles D.,
1932–

II. Stool, Sylvan E., 1925–

[DNLM: 1. Otorhinolaryngologic Diseases—in infancy &
childhood. WV 100 P3703]

RF47.C4P38   1990   618.92′09751—dc19

DNLM/DLC   88–39226

Editor: Tom Mackey
Developmental Editor: David Kilmer
Designer: Liz Schweber
Cover Designer: Paul Fry
Production Manager: Bill Preston
Manuscript Editor: W. B. Saunders Staff
Illustrator: Arlette Ramphal
Illustration Coordinator: Lisa Lambert
Indexer: Alexandra Nickerson

Pediatric Otolaryngology, Second Edition

VOLUME 1 ISBN 0–7216–2923–7
VOLUME 2 ISBN 0–7216–2924–5
(SET) ISBN 0–7216–2120–1

© 1990 by W. B. Saunders Company. Copyright under the Uniform Copyright Convention. Simultaneously published in Canada. All rights reserved. This book is protected by copyright. No part of it may be reproduced, stored in a retrieval system, or transmitted in any form or by any means, electronic, mechanical, photocopying, recording, or otherwise, without written permission from the publisher. Made in the United States of America. Library of Congress catalog card number 88–39226.

Last digit is the print number: 9   8   7   6   5   4   3   2   1

Dedication

To our wives and children

PATSY, MARK, and JIMMY BLUESTONE

JUNE, EVELYN, DANIEL, LAURA, and KAREN STOOL

CONTRIBUTORS

JOHN C. ADKINS, M.D.

Clinical Assistant Professor of Pediatric Surgery, University of Pittsburgh School of Medicine. Active Staff, Children's Hospital of Pittsburgh, Forbes Health System, Pittsburgh, Pennsylvania.

Congenital Malformations of the Esophagus

WILLIAM A. ALONSO, M.D., F.A.C.S.

Associate Professor of Surgery, Division of Otolaryngology–Head and Neck Surgery, University of South Florida College of Medicine. Chairman, Department of Otolaryngology–Head and Neck Surgery, St. Josephs Hospital of Tampa. Consultant, Head and Neck Surgery, U.S. Veterans Hospital. Consultant, Head and Neck Surgery, U.S. Air Force Regional Hospital MacDill, Tampa, Florida.

Injuries of the Lower Respiratory Tract

BYRON J. BAILEY, M.D.

Wiess Professor and Chairman, Department of Otolaryngology, University of Texas Medical Branch. Clinical Staff, John Sealy Hospital, Galveston, Texas.

Methods of Examination

THOMAS J. BALKANY, M.D., F.A.C.S., F.A.A.P.

Director of Research, Colorado Otologic Research Center. Adjunct Professor, University of Northern Colorado. Clinical Assistant Professor, Department of Otolaryngology–Head and Neck Surgery, University of Colorado School of Medicine. Clinical Staff, University Hospital, Porter Memorial Hospital, Swedish Medical Center, Littleton Hospital, and Children's Hospital, Denver, Colorado.

Injuries of the Neck

JANUSZ BARDACH, M.D.

Professor of Plastic Surgery, University of Iowa College of Medicine. Chairman, Division of Plastic and Reconstructive Surgery of the Head and Neck, Department of Otolaryngology–Head and Neck Surgery. Professor, Division of Plastic Surgery, Department of Surgery. Director, Cleft Palate Surgical Research Laboratory, University of Iowa Hospitals and Clinics, Iowa City, Iowa.

Pediatric Plastic and Reconstructive Surgery of the Head and Neck

WALTER M. BELENKY, M.D.

Chief, Department of Pediatric Otolaryngology, Children's Hospital of Michigan. Clinical Associate Professor, Department of Otolaryngology, Wayne State University School of Medicine, Detroit, Michigan.

Nasal Obstruction and Rhinorrhea

LaVONNE BERGSTROM, M.D., F.A.C.S., F.A.A.P.

Professor, Department of Surgery–Head and Neck Surgery, University of California, Los Angeles, School of Medicine. Professor, Department of Surgery, University of California at Los Angeles Medical Center, Los Angeles, California.

Diseases of the External Ear; Diseases of the Labyrinthine Capsule

FRED H. BESS, Ph.D.

Professor and Chairman, Department of Hearing and Speech Sciences, Vanderbilt University School of Medicine, Nashville, Tennessee.

Amplification Selection for Hearing-Impaired Children

F. OWEN BLACK, M.D.

Senior Scientist, R. S. Dow Neurological Sciences Institute. Chief, Department of Neuro-otology, Good Samaritan Hospital and Medical Center, Portland, Oregon.

Tinnitus in Children

CHARLES D. BLUESTONE, M.D.

Professor of Otolaryngology, University of Pittsburgh School of Medicine. Director, Department of Pediatric Otolaryngology, Children's Hospital of Pittsburgh, Pittsburgh, Pennsylvania.

Methods of Examination: Clinical Examination; Otitis Media, Atelectasis, and Eustachian Tube Dysfunction; Intratemporal Complications and Sequelae of Otitis Media; Intracranial Suppurative Complications of Otitis Media and Mastoiditis; Burns and Acquired Strictures of the Esophagus

LINDA BOND, M.S.

Coordinator, Audiology Department, Clinical Research Center, Children's Hospital of Pittsburgh, Pittsburgh, Pennsylvania.

Perilymphatic Fistulas in Infants and Children

SIDNEY N. BUSIS, M.D.

Clinical Professor of Otolaryngology, University of Pittsburgh School of Medicine. Senior Staff, Eye and Ear Hospital, Children's Hospital, and Montefiore Hospital, Pittsburgh, Pennsylvania.

Vertigo

THOMAS C. CALCATERRA, M.D.

Professor, Division of Head and Neck Surgery, University of California, Los Angeles, School of Medicine, Los Angeles, California.

Orbital Swellings

VINCENT G. CARUSO, M.D.

Assistant Clinical Professor of Otolaryngology, Columbia University College of Physicians and Surgeons. Assistant Attending Physician, Presbyterian Hospital, New York. Attending Medical Staff, Southampton Hospital, Southampton, New York.

Embryology and Anatomy

WERNER D. CHASIN, M.D.

Chairman and Professor, Department of Otolaryngology, Tufts University School of Medicine. Otolaryngologist-in-Chief, Tufts–New England Medical Center, Boston, Massachusetts.

Otalgia

M. MICHAEL COHEN, Jr., D.M.D., Ph.D.

Professor of Oral Pathology, Faculty of Dentistry, and Professor of Pediatrics, Faculty of Medicine, Dalhousie University, Halifax, Nova Scotia, Canada.

Craniofacial Anomalies and Syndromes

SEYMOUR R. COHEN, M.S., M.D.

Clinical Professor of Surgery (Otolaryngology and Head and Neck Surgery), University of Southern California School of Medicine, Los Angeles, California.

Difficulty with Swallowing

GEORGE H. CONNER, M.D.

Professor and Chief, Division of Otolaryngology–Head and Neck Surgery, The Milton S. Hershey Medical Center of The Pennsylvania State University, Hershey, Pennsylvania.

Idiopathic Conditions of the Mouth and Pharynx

ROBIN T. COTTON, M.D.

Professor, Department of Otolaryngology and Maxillofacial Surgery, University of Cincinnati College of Medicine. Director, Department of Otolaryngology and Maxillofacial Surgery, Children's Hospital Medical Center, Cincinnati, Ohio.

Stridor and Airway Obstruction; Congenital Malformations of the Larynx; Management and Prevention of Subglottic Stenosis in Infants and Children; Velopharyngeal Insufficiency

WILLIAM N. CRAIG, Ph.D.

Superintendent, Western Pennsylvania School for the Deaf, Pittsburgh, Pennsylvania.

Education of the Deaf

WILLIAM S. CRYSDALE, M.D., F.R.C.S.(C.)

Associate Professor, Department of Otolaryngology, University of Toronto. Otolaryngologist-in-Chief, Hospital for Sick Children. Attending Staff, Wellesley Hospital. Consultant Staff, Hugh Macmillan Medical Centre, Toronto, Ontario, Canada.

Malformations and Syndromes

MARVIN C. CULBERTSON, Jr., M.D.

Clinical Professor, Department of Otolaryngology–Head and Neck Surgery, University of Texas, Southwestern Medical Center at Dallas. Senior Otolaryngologist, Children's Medical Center and St. Paul Hospital Medical Center, Dallas, Texas.

Epistaxis

MICHAEL J. CUNNINGHAM, M.D.

Instructor in Otolaryngology, Harvard Medical School. Assistant Surgeon in Otolaryngology, Massachusetts Eye and Ear Infirmary, Boston, Massachusetts.

Tumors of the Neck

RICHARD F. CURLEE, Ph.D.

Professor, Speech and Hearing Sciences, University of Arizona, Tucson, Arizona.

Disorders of Phonology, Phonation, and Fluency

HUGH D. CURTIN, M.D.

Associate Professor, Department of Radiology, University of Pittsburgh School of Medicine. Director of Radiology, Eye and Ear Hospital, Pittsburgh, Pennsylvania.

Methods of Examination: Radiologic Aspects

TIMOTHY W. DEAKERS, M.D., Ph.D.

Assistant Professor of Pediatrics, Children's Hospital of Los Angeles, Los Angeles, California.

Intensive Care of Respiratory Tract Disorders

DOUGLAS D. DEDO, M.D.

Clinical Assistant Professor of Otolaryngology–Head and Neck Surgery, University of Volunteer Staff, Jackson Memorial Hospital, Miami, Florida.

Neurogenic Diseases of the Larynx

HERBERT H. DEDO, M.D.

Professor and Vice Chairman, Department of Otolaryngology, University of California, San Francisco, Medical Center. Active Staff, Children's Hospital of San Francisco and San Francisco General Hospital Medical Center. Consulting Staff, Letterman Drug Medical Center, San Francisco, California.

Neurogenic Diseases of the Larynx

JOHN D. DURRANT, Ph.D.

Professor of Otolaryngology and Communication, University of Pittsburgh School of Medicine. Director of Audiology, Eye and Ear Hospital of Pittsburgh, Pittsburgh, Pennsylvania.

Physiology of the Ear

ROLAND D. EAVEY, M.D., F.A.A.D., F.A.C.S.

Assistant Professor of Otolaryngology, Harvard Medical School. Director of E.N.T. Pediatric Services, Massachusetts Eye and Ear Infirmary, Boston, Massachusetts.

Tracheotomy

BARBARA ESSES, M.D.

Resident in Otolaryngology–Head and Neck Surgery, University of Colorado School of Medicine, Denver, Colorado.

Injuries of the Neck

ABRAHAM EVIATAR, M.D.

Professor of Otolaryngology, Albert Einstein College of Medicine. Chief, Division of Otolaryngology, Albert Einstein Hospital of the Montefiore Medical Center, Bronx, New York.

The Neurovestibular Testing of Infants and Children

LYDIA EVIATAR, M.D.

Associate Professor of Pediatrics and Neurology, State University of New York at Stony Brook. Chief of Pediatric Neurology, The Schneider Children's Hospital of Long Island Jewish Medical Center, Stony Brook, New York.

The Neurovestibular Testing of Infants and Children

DAVID N. F. FAIRBANKS, M.D.

Clinical Professor of Otolaryngology–Head and Neck Surgery, George Washington University School of Medicine and Health Sciences. Active Staff, Sibley Memorial Hospital, Washington, D.C.

Embryology and Anatomy

PHILIP FIREMAN, M.D.

Professor of Pediatrics, University of Pittsburgh School of Medicine. Director, Allergy, Immunology, and Rheumatology, Children's Hospital of Pittsburgh, Pittsburgh, Pennsylvania.

Allergic Rhinitis

THOMAS J. FRIA, Ph.D.

Sea Girt, New Jersey.

The Assessment of Hearing and Middle-Ear Function in Children

JACOB FRIEDBERG, M.D., F.R.C.S.(C.), F.A.A.P.

Assistant Professor, Department of Otolaryngology, University of Toronto Faculty of Medicine. Consultant in Otolaryngology, Hospital for Sick Children, Mount Sinai Hospital, Sunnybrook Medical Centre, Bloorview Children's Hospital, and Women's College Hospital, Toronto, Ontario, Canada.

Hoarseness

ANTONIO G. GALVIS, M.D.

Associate Professor of Clinical Pediatrics, University of Southern California School of Medicine. Associate Director, Division of Pediatric Intensive Care, Children's Hospital of Los Angeles, Los Angeles, California.

Intensive Care of Respiratory Tract Disorders

CARLOS GONZALEZ, M.D., F.A.C.S., Major, Marine Corps, U.S. Army.

Assistant Professor of Surgery and Pediatrics, Uniformed Services University of the Health Sciences. Staff, Otolaryngology–Head and Neck Surgery, Walter Reed Army Medical Center, Washington, D.C.

Tumors of the Mouth and Pharynx

JACK L. GLUCKMAN, M.D., F.A.C.S., F.C.S.(S.A.).

Professor of Otolaryngology and Associate Dean for Clinical Affairs, University of Cincinnati College of Medicine. Clinical Staff, University Hospital Veterans Administration Hospital, and Children's Hospital, Cincinnati, Ohio.

Inflammatory Disease of the Mouth and Pharynx

E. RICHARD GRAVISS, M.D.

Professor of Radiology and Associate Professor of Pediatrics, St. Louis University School of Medicine. Director of Diagnostic Imaging, Cardinal Glennon Children's Hospital. Chief of Pediatric Radiology, University Hospital and St. Louis University Medical Center, St. Louis, Missouri.

Methods of Examination

KENNETH M. GRUNDFAST, M.D., F.A.C.S., F.A.A.P.

Associate Professor, Division of Otolaryngology, George Washington University School of Medicine. Chairman, Department of Otolaryngology, Children's National Medical Center, Washington, D.C.

Hearing Loss

DAVID J. HALL, D.D.S., M.S.

Clinical Associate Professor of Orthodontics, University of North Carolina School of Dentistry, Chapel Hill, North Carolina.

Orthodontic Problems in Children

STEVEN D. HANDLER, M.D.

Associate Professor of Otolaryngology and Human Communication, University of Pennsylvania School of Medicine. Associate Director (Otolaryngology and Human Communication), Children's Hospital of Philadelphia, Philadelphia, Pennsylvania.

Methods of Examination

DONALD B. HAWKINS, M.D.

Associate Professor and Chief of Pediatric Otolaryngology, University of Southern California School of Medicine. Clinical Staff, Los Angeles County–University of Southern California Medical Center, Los Angeles, California.

Noninfectious Disorders of the Lower Respiratory Tract

GERALD B. HEALY, M.D.

Professor of Otology and Laryngology, Harvard Medical School. Adjunct Professor of Otolaryngology, Boston University School of Medicine. Otolaryngologist-in-Chief, Children's Hospital, Boston, Massachusetts.

Methods of Examination

ARTHUR S. HENGERER, M.D.

Professor of Surgery (Otolaryngology) and Chairman, Division of Otolaryngology, University of Rochester School of Medicine and Dentistry. Otolaryngologist-in-Chief, Strong Memorial Hospital. Consulting Staff, Rochester General Hospital and Genesee Hospital. Director, ENT, Monroe Community Hospital, Rochester, New York.

Congenital Malformations of the Nose and Paranasal Sinuses; Complications of Nasal and Sinus Infections

SETH HETHERINGTON, M.D.

Assistant Professor of Pediactrics, Albany Medical College of Union University. Attending Pediatrician, Albany Medical Center Hospital, Albany, New York.

Infections of the Lower Respiratory Tract

LAUREN D. HOLINGER, M.D.

Head, Division of Pediatric Otolaryngology, Children's Memorial Hospital, Chicago, Illinois.

Foreign Bodies of the Larynx, Trachea, and Bronchi

ANDREW J. HOTALING, M.D.

Clinical Assistant Professor of Otolaryngology, Wayne State University of Medicine. Associate Chief, Department of Otolaryngology, Children's Hospital of Michigan. Attending Staff, St. John's Hospital, Detroit, Michigan.

Cough

DENNIS J. HURWITZ, M.D.

Clinical Associate Professor of Surgery (Plastic), University of Pittsburgh School of Medicine, Pittsburgh, Pennsylvania.

Principles and Methods of Management

GLENN C. ISAACSON, M.D.

Assistant Instructor of Otolaryngology, University of Pittsburgh School of Medicine. Responsible Surgeon and Fellow, Department of Pediatric Otolaryngology, Children's Hospital of Pittsburgh, Pittsburgh, Pennsylvania.

Phylogenetic Aspects and Embryology

BRUCE W. JAFEK, M.D., F.A.C.S.

Professor and Chairman, Department of Otolaryngology–Head and Neck Surgery, University of Colorado School of Medicine. Clinical Staff, University Hospital, Denver General Hospital, Veterans Administration Hospital, Children's Hospital, and Rose Medical Center, Denver, Colorado.

Injuries of the Neck

JOHN K. JONES, M.D.

Clinical Assistant Professor, Department of Otorhinolaryngology and Communication Science, Baylor College of Medicine. Staff, Texas Children's Hospital, Methodist Hospital, Houston, Texas.

Methods of Examination

COLLIN S. KARMODY, M.D.

Professor of Otolaryngology, Tufts University School of Medicine. Senior Surgon, New England Medical Center, Boston, Massachusetts.

Developmental Anomalies of the Neck

MARGARET A. KENNA, M.D.

Assistant Professor of Surgery (Otolaryngology) and Pediatrics, Yale University School of Medicine, New Haven, Connecticut.

Embryology and Developmental Anatomy of the Ear; Sore Throat in Children: Diagnosis and Management

JEROME O. KLEIN, M.D.

Professor of Pediatrics, Boston University School of Medicine. Director, Division of Pediatric Infectious Diseases, Maxwell Finland Laboratory for Infectious Disease, Boston City Hospital, Boston, Massachusetts.

Methods of Examination: Clinical Examination; Otitis Media, Atelectasis, and Eustachian Tube Dysfunction; Intratemporal Complications and Sequelae of Otitis Media; Intracranial Suppurative Complications of Otitis Media and Mastoiditis

MARTHA L. LEPOW, M.D.

Professor of Pediatrics, Albany Medical College of Union University. Attending Pediatrician, Albany Medical Center. Consulting Pediatrician, St. Peter's Hospital, Albany, New York.

Infections of the Lower Respiratory Tract

DAVID J. LILLY, Ph.D.

Adjunct Associate Professor, Portland State University. Director of Audiology, Good Samaritan Hospital and Medical Center, Portland, Oregon.

Tinnitus in Children

JOSÉ A. LIMA, M.D.

Clinical Assistant Professor of Otolaryngology–Head and Neck Surgery, St. Louis University School of Medicine. Staff Physician, St. Anthony's Medical Center, Cardinal Glennon Children's Hospital, University Hospital, St. John's Mercy Hospital, St. Mary's Health Center, and Deaconess Hospital, St. Louis, Missouri.

Methods of Examination

JOHN M. LORE, Jr., M.D.

Professor and Chairman, Department of Otolaryngology–Head and Neck Surgery, State University of New York at Buffalo School of Medicine. University Chief of Otolaryngology, Sister's Hospital, Buffalo, New York.

Tumors of the Nose, Paranasal Sinuses, and Nasopharynx

FRANK E. LUCENTE, M.D.

Chairman, Department of Otolaryngology, New York Medical College. Chairman and Attending Physician, Department of Otolaryngology–Head and Neck Surgery, New York Eye and Ear Infirmary, New York, New York.

Facial Pain and Headache

RODNEY P. LUSK, M.D.

Assistant Professor, Washington University School of Medicine. Assistant Professor of Otolaryngology and Director of Pediatric Otolaryngology, Children's Hospital, St. Louis, Missouri.

Neck Masses

BRUCE R. MADDERN, M.D.

Responsible Surgeon and Instructor of Otolaryngology, University of Pittsburgh School of Medicine. Fellow, Department of Pediatric Otolaryngology, Children's Hospital of Pittsburgh, Pittsburgh, Pennsylvania.

Snoring and Obstructive Sleep Apnea Syndrome

ROBERT H. MAISEL, M.D.

Associate Professor of Otolaryngology, University of Minnesota Medical School. Chief Otolaryngologist, Hennipen County Medical Center, Minneapolis, Minnesota.

Injuries of the Mouth, Pharynx, and Esophagus

SCOTT C. MANNING, M.D.

Assistant Professor, Department of Otorhinolaryngology, University of Texas Southwestern Medical Center. Clinical Staff, Parkland Memorial Hospital, Children's Medical Center, and St. Paul Hospital, Dallas, Texas.

Epistaxis; Foreign Bodies of the Pharynx and Esophagus

WILLIAM A. MARASOVICH, D.D.S., M.D.

ENT Resident, Geisinger Medical Center, Danville, Pennsylvania.

Craniofacial Anomalies and Syndromes; Postnatal Craniofacial Growth and Development

FRANK I. MARLOWE, M.D.

Professor and Chief, Division of Otolaryngology and Head and Neck Surgery, Medical College of Pennsylvania. Chief, Division of Otolaryngology and Head and Neck Surgery, Presbyterian Medical Center of Philadelphia. Consultant, Otolaryngology and Maxillofacial Surgery, Naval Regional Medical Center, Philadelphia, Pennsylvania.

Injuries of the Nose, Facial Bones, and Paranasal Sinuses

ROBERT H. MATHOG, M.D.

Professor and Chairman, Department of Otolaryngology, Wayne State University School of Medicine. Chief of Otolaryngology, Harper-Grace Hospitals and Detroit Receiving Hospital. Staff Physician, Children's Hospital of Michigan and Hutzel Hospital. Consulting Physician, Veterans Administration Medical Center (Allen Park), Detroit, Michigan.

Injuries of the Mouth, Pharynx, and Esophagus

MARK MAY, M.D., F.A.C.S.

Clinical Professor, Department of Otolaryngology–Head and Neck Surgery, University of Pittsburgh School of Medicine. Director, Facial Paralysis Center, Shadyside Hospital, Pittsburgh, Pennsylvania. Adjunct Professor, Cleveland Clinic, Cleveland, Ohio.

Facial Paralysis in Children

TIMOTHY P. McBRIDE, M.D.

Assistant Professor of Otolaryngology, University of Pittsburgh School of Medicine. Staff Otolaryngologist, Department of Pediatric Otolaryngology, Children's Hospital of Pittsburgh, Pittsburgh, Pennsylvania.

Nasal Physiology

BETTY JANE McWILLIAMS, Ph.D.

Professor of Communication Disorders and Director, Cleft Palate–Craniofacial Center, University of Pittsburgh School of Medicine, Pittsburgh, Pennsylvania.

Multiple Speech Disorders (Cleft Palate and Cerebral Palsy Speech)

ARLEN D. MEYERS, M.D., M.B.A.

Associate Professor of Otolaryngology–Head and Neck Surgery, University of Colorado School of Medicine. Attending Otolaryngologist, Children's Hospital of Denver and University Hospital. Chief, Division of Otolaryngology, Veterans Administration Medical Center, Denver, Colorado.

Aspiration

GEORGE A. MODRECK, M.A., C.C.C.-A.

Clinical Audiologist, Department of Audiology, Children's Hospital of Pittsburgh, Pittsburgh, Pennsylvania.

Perilymphatic Fistulas in Infants and Children

EUGENE N. MYERS, M.D., F.A.C.S.

Professor, Department of Otolaryngology, University of Pittsburgh School of Medicine. Chairman, Department of Otolaryngology, Eye and Ear Hospital of Pittsburgh, Pittsburgh, Pennsylvania.

Tumors of the Neck

JULIE A. NEWBURG, M.D.

Attending Staff, Baptist Medical Center, Easley, and St. Francis Hospital, Greenville, South Carolina.

Congenital Malformations of the Nose and Paranasal Sinuses

ROBERT J. NOZZA, Ph.D.

Assistant Professor, Department of Otolaryngology, University of Pittsburgh School of Medicine. Director, The Audiology Center, Department of Pediatric Otolaryngology, Children's Hospital of Pittsburgh, Pittsburgh, Pennsylvania.

The Assessment of Hearing and Middle-Ear Function in Children

MICHAEL J. PAINTER, M.D.

Associate Professor of Pediatrics and Neurology, University of Pittsburgh School of Medicine. Chief, Division of Child Neurology, Children's Hospital of Pittsburgh. Active Staff, Magee Women's Hospital, Pittsburgh, Pennsylvania.

Neurologic Disorders of the Mouth, Pharynx, and Esophagus

JACK L. PARADISE, M.D.

Professor of Pediatrics, University of Pittsburgh School of Medicine. Medical Director, Ambulatory Care Center, Children's Hospital of Pittsburgh, Pittsburgh, Pennsylvania.

Primary Care of Infants and Children with Cleft Palate; Tonsillectomy and Adenoidectomy

SIMON C. PARISIER, M.D.

Clinical Professor of Otolaryngology, New York Hospital, Cornell University Medical Center. Chairman, Department of Otolaryngology–Head and Neck Surgery, Manhattan Eye, Ear, and Throat Hospital, New York, New York.

Injuries of the Ear and Temporal Bone

JAMES L. PARKIN, M.D., M.S.

Professor of Surgery and Chairman, Division of Otolaryngology–Head and Neck Surgery, University of Utah School of Medicine. Clinical Staff, University Hospital, Veterans Administration Hospital, Primary Children's Hospital, and Holy Cross Hospital, Salt Lake City, Utah.

Congenital Malformations of the Mouth and Pharynx

DAVID S. PARSONS, M.D.

Chief Resident in Otolaryngology–Head and Neck Surgery, University of Colorado School of Medicine, Denver, Colorado.

Injuries of the Neck

ROBERT L. PINCUS, M.D.

Assistant Professor of Otolaryngology, New York Medical College, Valhalla. Director, Department of Otolaryngology, Lincoln Hospital. Attending Physician, Department of Otolaryngology, New York Eye and Ear Infirmary, New York, New York.

Facial Pain and Headache

WILLIAM P. POTSIC, M.D.

Associate Professor of Otorhinolaryngology and Human Communication, University of Pennsylvania School of Medicine. Director of Otolaryngology and Human Communication, Children's Hospital of Philadelphia, Philadelphia, Pennsylvania.

Methods of Examination

SETH M. PRANSKY, M.D., F.A.A.P.

Assistant Clinical Professor, University of California, San Diego, School of Medicine. Attending Physician and Staff, Children's Hospital and Health Center and Mercy Hospital, San Diego, California.

Tumors of the Larynx, Trachea, and Bronchi

DANIEL D. RABUZZI, M.D.

Clinical Professor of Otolaryngology and Communication Sciences, State University of New York, Health Science Center at Syracuse. Attending Surgeon, St. Joseph's Hospital and Crouse-Irving Memorial Hospital, Syracuse, New York.

Complications of Nasal and Sinus Infections

ROBERT RAPP, D.D.S., M.S., F.R.C.D.(C.)

Professor of Pediatric Dentistry for Research, Department of Pediatric Dentistry, School of Dental Medicine, University of Pittsburgh. Active Staff, Dental Clinic, Children's Hospital of Pittsburgh, Pittsburgh, Pennsylvania.

Dental and Gingival Disorders

JAMES S. REILLY, M.D.

Associate Professor of Surgery (Otolaryngology–Head and Neck Surgery), University of Alabama at Birmingham. Otolaryngologist-in-Chief, Children's Hospital of Alabama. Attending Surgeon, University Hospital, Birmingham, Alabama.

Perilymphatic Fistulas in Infants and Children; Stridor and Airway Obstruction; Congenital Malformations of the Larynx

MARK A. RICHARDSON, M.D.

Associate Professor of Otolaryngology–Head and Neck Surgery, University of Washington School of Medicine. Chief, Division of Otolaryngology, Children's Hospital and Medical Center, Seattle, Washington.

The Neck: Embryology and Anatomy

KEITH H. RIDING, M.D., F.R.C.S.(C.)

Clinical Associate Professor, University of British Columbia. Director, Department of Otolaryngology, Children's Hospital, Vancouver, British Columbia, Canada.

Burns and Acquired Strictures of the Esophagus

STEWART R. ROOD, Ph.D., M.P.H.

Associate Professor, Department of Otolaryngology, University of Pittsburgh School of Medicine. Coordinator of Medical Education and Administrative Coordinator, Department of Otolaryngology, Eye and Ear Hospital of Pittsburgh, Pittsburgh, Pennsylvania.

Anatomy and Physiology of Speech

ROBERT J. RUBEN, M.D.

Professor and Chairman, Department of Otolaryngology, Albert Einstein College of Medicine. Chairman, Department of Otorhinolaryngology, Montefiore Medical Center, Bronx Municipal Hospital, and North Central Bronx Hospital, Bronx, New York.

Diseases of the Inner Ear and Sensorineural Deafness

ISAMU SANDO, M.D., D.Med.Sc.

Professor of Otolaryngology and Pathology, Department of Otolaryngology, University of Pittsburgh School of Medicine. Director, Division of Otolaryngology, Department of Otolaryngology, Eye and Ear Hospital of Pittsburgh, Pittsburgh, Pennsylvania.

Congenital Anomalies of the External and Middle Ear

EBERHARDT K. SAUERLAND, M.D., Ph.D.

Adjunct Professor of Anatomy, University of Texas Medical Branch, Galveston, Texas.

Embryology and Anatomy

GARY L. SCHECHTER, M.D.

Professor and Chairman, Department of Otolaryngology–Head and Neck Surgery, Eastern Virginia Medical School. Chief, Pediatric Otolaryngology, Children's Hospital of the Kings Daughters. Director, Otolaryngology–Head and Neck Surgery, Sentara Norfolk General Hospital, Norfolk, Virginia.

Physiology of the Mouth, Pharynx, and Esophagus

JOYCE A. SCHILD, M.D.

Professor in Otolaryngology–Head and Neck Surgery, University of Illinois College of Medicine at Chicago. Attending Staff, University of Illinois Hospital. Affiliated Attending Staff, Children's Memorial Hospital, Chicago, Illinois.

Congenital Malformations of the Trachea and Bronchi

MELVIN D. SCHLOSS, M.D.

Associate Professor of Otolaryngology, McGill University. Director, Division of Otolaryngology, Montreal Children's Hospital, Montreal, Quebec, Canada.

Otorrhea

DANIEL M. SCHWARTZ, Ph.D.

Associate Professor, Department of Otorhinolaryngology and Human Communication, University of Pennsylvania School of Medicine. Director, Speech and Hearing Center, University of Pennsylvania Medical Center, Philadelphia, Pennsylvania.

Amplification Selection for Hearing-Impaired Children

ELLEN R. SCHWARTZ, M.A., C.C.C.-S.P.

Private practice, Philadelphia, Pennsylvania. Consultant, Department of Human Development, Bryn Mawr College, Bryn Mawr, Pennsylvania.

Early Identification of Speech and Language Disorders

M. WILLIAM SCHWARTZ, M.D.

Professor of Pediatrics, Children's Hospital of Philadelphia and University of Pennsylvania School of Medicine. Senior Physician, Children's Hospital. Chief of Newborn Services, Hospital of the University of Pennsylvania, Philadelphia, Pennsylvania.

Oropharyngeal Manifestations of Systemic Disease

ROBERT W. SEIBERT, M.D.

Associate Professor, Department of Otolaryngology and Maxillofacial Surgery, University of Arkansas Medical Sciences. Chief, Otolaryngology Section, Arkansas Children's Hospital, Little Rock, Arkansas.

Diseases of the Salivary Glands

ALLAN B. SEID, M.D., F.A.C.S., F.A.A.P.

Associate Clinical Professor of Surgery, University of California, San Diego, School of Medicine. Attending Physician, Children's Hospital and Health Center, San Diego, California.

Tumors of the Larynx, Trachea, and Bronchi

ROBERT S. SHAPIRO, M.D., F.R.C.S.(C.)

Associate Professor, Department of Otolaryngology, McGill University. Attending Otolaryngologist, Montreal Children's Hospital, Montreal, Quebec, Canada.

Foreign Bodies of the Nose

RALPH L. SHELTON, Ph.D.

Professor, Department of Speech and Hearing Sciences, University of Arizona College of Medicine, Tucson, Arizona.

Disorders of Phonology, Phonation, and Fluency

YOSHIHIRO SHIBAHARA, M.D., D.Med.Sc.

Assistant Professor, Department of Otolaryngology, Tohoku University School of Medicine, Sendai, Japan.

Congenital Anomalies of the External and Middle Ear

WILLIAM K. SIEBER, M.D.

Clinical Professor of Surgery, University of Pittsburgh School of Medicine. Active Staff, Children's Hospital of Pittsburgh, Pittsburgh, Pennsylvania.

Functional Abnormalities of the Esophagus

BONNIE M. SIMON, M.A., C.C.C.-S.P.

Private practice. Consultant, United Cerebral Palsy Association, Philadelphia, Pennsylvania.

Early Identification of Speech and Language Disorders

JOHN F. STANIEVICH, M.D.

Clinical Assistant Professor, Department of Otolaryngology, State University of New York at Buffalo School of Medicine. Co-Director, Department of Pediatric Otolaryngology, Children's Hospital of Buffalo, Buffalo, New York.

Cervical Adenopathy; Tumors of the Nose, Paranasal Sinuses, and Nasopharynx

SYLVAN E. STOOL, M.D.

Professor of Pediatrics and Otolaryngology, University of Pittsburgh School of Medicine. Director of Education, Department of Pediatric Otolaryngology, Children's Hospital of Pittsburgh, Pittsburgh, Pennsylvania.

Phylogenetic Aspects and Embryology; Postnatal Craniofacial Growth and Development; Craniofacial Anomalies and Syndromes; Foreign Bodies of the Pharynx and Esophagus; Tracheotomy

JOHN R. STRAM, M.D.

Assistant Clinical Professor, Department of Otolaryngology, Boston University School of Medicine, Boston, Massachusetts.

Tumors of the Ear and Temporal Bone

CHESTER L. STRUNK, M.D.

Assistant Professor, Department of Otolaryngology, University of Texas Medical Branch. Clinical Staff, John Sealy Hospital, Galveston, Texas.

Methods of Examination

I. DAVID TODRES, M.D.

Associate Professor of Anesthesia (Pediatrics), Harvard Medical School. Director, Neonatal and Pediatric Intensive Care Units, Massachusetts General Hospital, Boston, Massachusetts.

Respiratory Disorders of the Newborn

JOHN A. TUCKER, M.D.

Professor of Pediatric Otolaryngology, Temple University School of Medicine. Professor of Otolaryngology, Hahnemann University. Chairman, Division of Otolaryngology–Head and Neck Surgery and Chief of Pediatric Otolaryngology, Albert Einstein Medical Center. Staff Physician, St. Christopher's Hospital for Children and Hahnemann University Hospital, Philadelphia, Pennsylvania.

Development of the Human Air and Food Passages

ELLEN R. WALD, M.D.

Professor of Pediatrics, University of Pittsburgh School of Medicine and Children's Hospital of Pittsburgh, Pittsburgh, Pennsylvania.

Rhinitis and Acute and Chronic Sinusitis

DONALD W. WARREN, D.D.S., M.S., Ph.D.

Kenan Professor, Department of Dental Ecology and Dental Research Center, School of Dentistry. Research Professor, Division of Otolaryngology, University of North Carolina at Chapel Hill School of Medicine. Director, Oral, Facial and Communicative Disorders Program, University of North Carolina and North Carolina Memorial Hospital, Chapel Hill, North Carolina.

Orthodontic Problems in Children

LINTON A. WHITAKER, M.D.

Professor of Surgery (Plastic), University of Pennsylvania School of Medicine. Chief of Plastic Surgery, Hospital of the University of Pennsylvania and Children's Hospital of Philadelphia, Philadelphia, Pennsylvania.

Principles and Methods of Management

RAYMOND P. WOOD, II, M.D.

Associate Professor and Vice-Chairman, Department of Otolaryngology, University of Colorado Health Sciences Center, Denver, Colorado.

Congenital Anomalies of the External and Middle Ear

ROBERT E. WOOD, Ph.D., M.D.

Professor of Pediatrics, University of North Carolina at Chapel Hill School of Medicine. Attending Pediatrician, North Carolina Memorial Hospital, Chapel Hill, North Carolina.

Physiology of the Larynx, Airways, and Lungs

GEORGE H. ZALZAL, M.D.

Assistant Professor of Otolaryngology and Pediatrics, George Washington University and Children's Hospital National Medical Center. Attending Staff, Children's Hospital National Medical Center, Washington, D.C.

Velopharyngeal Insufficiency

PREFACE

Just as otolaryngology has grown into an important and broad specialty, so has increasing interest in its various subspecialties proportionately expanded. Diseases and disorders of the head and neck and of the air and food passages are the most common conditions encountered by health care professionals who care for children. Therefore, interest in pediatric otolaryngology has progressively increased during the past decade, which has resulted in an information explosion. As clinicians and teachers, we have been aware of a need for a comprehensive text that would embody the principles of otolaryngology and pediatrics. We undertook the task of writing and editing the first edition of this book to fill this perceived need. Since the areas covered by such a text cannot be adequately written by only one or two pediatric otolaryngologists, we selected the most knowledgeable and experienced authors for the chapters, and since the field is so diverse, we asked specialists not only in medicine, but in other disciplines as well, to contribute their expertise.

For this second edition, we have asked most of the original authors to again contribute chapters, but to completely update the content. In addition, we have invited other authors to submit new chapters on subjects not included in the first edition. We have also included chapters on topics not adequately covered in the first text, such as Subglottic Stenosis, Perilymphatic Fistulae, and Snoring and Sleep Apnea Syndrome.

It is the hope of the editors and publishers that this textbook will provide as complete a coverage of the field of pediatric otolaryngology as possible, with an authoritative, discriminating, precise, and concise presentation of what is currently known about diseases of the ear, nose, and throat in infants and children. The text is geared to medical students and to house staff officers in otolaryngology, pediatrics, and primary medicine, as well as to the practicing otolaryngologist, pediatrician, generalist, and other health professionals. It is not the intent of the editors that this book should compete with existing texts in pediatrics or otolaryngology, but rather that it should provide a single reference source oriented to pediatric otolaryngology. With this concept in mind, there has been no attempt to provide extensive details of surgical techniques that have been covered adequately in other texts and atlases. The emphasis is on concepts of surgical management rather than on explicit descriptions of techniques. At the end of each chapter, there are, in addition to the bibliography, selected references, which are annotated. Included are the references that are considered to have the best descriptions of surgical procedures that are applicable to children.

We believe that the text is unique in that we have combined the problem-oriented approach with an authoritative, comprehensive presentation of what is currently known about diseases and disorders of the head and neck and air and food passages in childhood. This has been accomplished by including several chapters early in each section that present the differential diagnoses of the common presenting signs and symptoms. The reader can then turn to the comprehensive review of the condition in the appropriate chapter. The length of these chapters varies considerably, since we have attempted to emphasize the conditions that are most common in children. Otitis media and its related conditions have been extensively covered in this text, since this disease is the most common condition encountered in children by otolaryngologists and primary care physicians.

It is the hope of the editors of this text that the health care of infants and children will be improved by those physicians who increase their knowledge by using this book as a reference.

CHARLES D. BLUESTONE

SYLVAN E. STOOL

ACKNOWLEDGMENTS

In a work of this scope, the editors and contributors receive help from many sources. It is difficult to acknowledge each of these adequately. We wish to acknowledge Sandra K. Arjona, M.L.S., for the organization of the first edition. For this edition, we thank Mary D. Scheetz, M.L.S., for her dedication and commitment to the coordination and collation of the manuscripts. They orchestrated this all-encompassing, arduous, and mammoth task with efficiency, skill, and a great sense of humor.

Artwork provides visual emphasis to the text. Jon Coulter created many excellent illustrations, and Robert Coulter provided valuable photographic support. We have been delighted with their contributions. Additional high-quality photography has been provided by Norman Rabinovitz and others of Children's Hospital of Pittsburgh.

A number of colleagues have been most helpful in reviewing chapters and in providing advice. In particular, Jack L. Paradise, M.D., participated in the early planning for the book. In Pittsburgh, members of the Departments of Pediatrics, Infectious Disease, Neurosurgery, and Radiology have been most accommodating.

In any effort as time-consuming as this, the authors' families and colleagues must provide support—and ours have made this task easier by their understanding and encouragement throughout.

CONTENTS

PEDIATRIC OTOLARYNGOLOGY

Section *I*

CRANIOFACIAL GROWTH, DEVELOPMENT, AND MALFORMATIONS

Chapter 1

PHYLOGENETIC ASPECTS AND EMBRYOLOGY

Sylvan E. Stool, M.D.   Glenn C. Isaacson, M.D.

It is appropriate that the first chapter of a text on pediatric otolaryngology be devoted to the broad subject of the development of the craniofacial complex. This is the major region involved in diseases of the ears, nose, and throat and serves as the entryway to the air and food passages. The more we know about the embryology, growth, and development of the face and about the various factors involved in normal variations and anomalies of this region, the better will be our understanding of the many otorhinolaryngologic disorders affecting infants and children.

The first region that the clinician and, indeed, the layperson usually inspect on encountering another person is the face. Usually, an impression of the face and an evaluation of the facial type and facial expression are made instantly. Following this, the general body type and posture are noted, and the degree of interpersonal communication is ascertained. DeMyer (1975) states,

> One glance at the patient's face may settle the diagnostic issue, an Augenblick, or eyeblink diagnosis, in which the clinician immediately knows what syndrome the patient has. I am neither describing nor advocating a hasty, careless snap judgment, I am merely pointing out that the clinician, utilizing the pattern recognition attributes of his own brain, sometimes can diagnose abnormal faces with the speed and certainty with which he distinguishes the faces of family and friends.

The clinician may decide, on the basis of certain facial features, that the patient has a recognizable syndrome that identifies him or her with a group of similar patients more than it does with his or her own family. Therefore, the face and the cranial configuration contribute immeasurably to the total, or *gestalt*, diagnosis.

Any observer can appreciate that there is great variation in the appearance of the normal face. In addition, there are certain characteristics that we associate with facial types almost on an instinctive basis. These variations and expectations in facial types can be appreciated by examining Figure 1–1, which is a sketch of a group of white children from the same grammar school class. The variations in facial configuration are obvious: There are round, oval, and triangular faces. Individual characteristics of the eyes and the nose also show tremendous variation. A diagnosis of an abnormality that is based on facial configuration may be very difficult to make unless the observer knows the hereditary background of the individual, although there are some abnormalities, such as Down syndrome, that are expresssed in similar facial features regardless of the child's origin. Thus, although we recognize great variations in facial type as being normal, we also instinctively recognize other features as being abnormal in a particular individual, based on our ability to assess facial patterns in the contexts of age, race, and hereditary background.

The human craniofacial complex is the result of at least 500 million years of progressive development. These structures, which developed in the anterior portion of an ancestral organism, were designed to obtain and maintain first contact with the environment. The pattern that developed in the invertebrates was continued in the vertebrates, and, according to Krogman (1974), there can be no doubt that the craniofacial complex from its beginning was a multistructured, highly integrated, diversely systematized center for almost every life need of the organism. In the development of the craniofacial complex in the human embryo and the fetus, the form and functions that have evolved over many millions of years take shape in fantastically rapid sequence. Those structures that required many millions of years of natural selection to evolve may form in minutes or hours in a human. This is especially true in the embryonic stages of development and is the reason that any interference with these processes in the early embryonic stages may have catastrophic consequences in the developing human. The embryogenesis of the craniofacial complex is indeed an amazing phenomenon; form and function must relate to one another with an almost unbelievable precision and at exactly the right points in time. In order to appreciate the structures and the physiology that the physician interested in diseases of the ears, nose, and throat so frequently sees go awry, we begin this text with a very abbreviated review of the normal development of the human head.

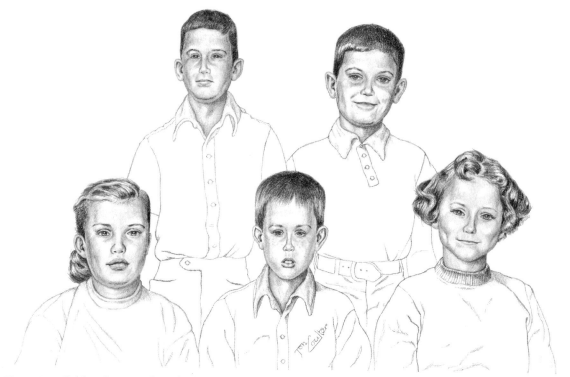

Figure 1–1. Children from a sixth grade class. Note the variation of facial types, even though all are the same age and race.

Although this text is organized into sections on the basis of organ systems and although each section has a discussion of the most important embryologic and developmental anatomy of that particular organ system, of necessity there is some duplication and lack of continuity in this method of presentation. Therefore, this section will be primarily concerned with the cranium, base of the skull, face, and eyes and will concentrate on the broad concepts involved in the development of these structures.

The subject of embryology is a complex one, running the gamut from descriptive chronology of events that transpire during prenatal life to details of genetic types and mutations and how they affect the individual proteins and nucleic acids that are part of the molecular biology of the embryo (Moore, 1977). A complete survey of even a portion of the aspects of the subcellular structure is beyond the scope of this text; however, since many of the advances in embryology of interest to the physician involved with craniofacial anomalies will undoubtedly occur because of a better understanding of subcellular events, it is important to mention these, if only briefly. A general overview of the structure of the human face will be presented first, followed by a discussion of the cellular and subcellular mechanisms that lead to the facial configuration. This method of presentation parallels the way in which the clinician usually views patients with anomalies of this region.

PLAN OF THE HUMAN FACE

In humans, the assumption of an upright posture has been associated with a number of anatomic devel-

opments, as can be appreciated from an examination of Figure 1–2A and B (Enlow, 1975). With the enlargements of the brain, especially of the frontal region, and the concomitant rotation of the eyes to the midline, there has been a relative decrease in the intraorbital distance in humans compared with that in lower mammals. This has resulted in a smaller region at the root of the nose and a shortening of the muzzle, or snout. Thus, humans have close-set eyes and short, narrow noses that do not interfere with binocular vision.

The growth of the frontal lobes and other evolutionary changes have resulted in flexure of the cranial base, as illustrated in Figure 1–2C, making the face appear to hang from the base of the skull. Other less obvious changes have occurred, such as rotation of the olfactory bulbs and nerves, so that the nasal region in humans has a vertical orientation and most of its important functional components are housed within the face. This placement of the face within the flexure of the cranial base may be of some clinical significance, as any condition that affects the cranial base may have some secondary effects on the airway and, ultimately, on the speech mechanisms, which are discussed in Chapter 91.

PRENATAL DEVELOPMENT OF THE FACE

The development of the face from midembryonic through midfetal life is illustrated in Figure 1–3. The embryo at about 3 to 4 weeks of age is illustrated in Figure 1–3A. At this stage, the embryo does not have

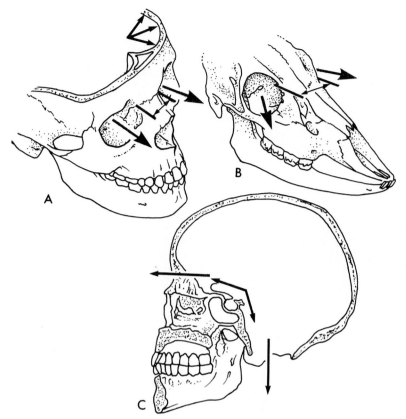

Figure 1–2. A, Plan of the human face demonstrating an enlargement of the frontal lobes in the human and rotation of the orbit, resulting in a narrow nasal root, in contrast to *(B)* that of a lower animal. C, Flexure of the cranial base results in an alteration of facial orientation. (Modified from Enlow, 1975.)

a face, the head is composed of a brain covered with a membrane, and the anterior neuropore (AN) is still present. The eyes, which are represented by optic vesicles, are on the lateral aspects of the head, as is seen in fish, and the future mouth is represented by a stomadeum (S). It is only in the latter part of this period of embryonic growth that nasal pits develop. At the embryonic age of 5 to 6 weeks, as is illustrated in Figure 1–3B, the general shape of the face has begun to develop. The frontonasal process is prominent, the nasal pits (NP) are forming laterally, and, with the increase in size of the first and second branchial arches (1st BA, 2nd BA), there is a suggestion of a mouth. In the subsequent weeks of embryonic life, as illustrated in Figure 1–3C, the structures that we associate with the human face—jaws, nose, eyes, ears, and mouth—will take on human configurations.

During this period of rapid growth and expansion, there is also tremendous *differential* growth. Thus, the development of a human baby is not merely the enlargement or rearrangement of a previous form, but, by differential growth, the development of a new configuration. This is a concept that has been difficult for students to comprehend, perhaps because of the tendency to illustrate different stages of embryonic development with drawings of equal size. These illustrating techniques have been used because minute structures are difficult to demonstrate without magnification, but it is important to try to view human

embryologic development in perspective in order to appreciate both its similarities to phylogenetic development and its unique course in humans.

The embryonic period ends at about eight weeks, when the embryo has achieved sufficient size and form so that facial characteristics can be recognized and photographed at actual size, as shown in Figure 1–3D. At this stage of late embryonic or early fetal development, the facial features are characterized by the appearance of hypertelorism; during subsequent growth, it will appear as though the eyes are moving closer together. This is not happening, however; the eyes continue to move farther apart, but the remainder of the face is growing at a much more rapid rate, and thus it appears that the eyes are moving closer together; hypertelorism is actually decreasing as a result of differential development. These observations may be of importance in understanding some of the craniofacial syndromes in which hypertelorism is a prominent feature.

The continued rapid growth and change in configuration, not only of the face but also of the extremities and body during the next few months, are illustrated in Figure 1–3E. The fetus has facial features that are easily recognized and associated with the human. The ears, nasal alae, and lips are well-developed, and the head constitutes a large portion of the body mass—a relationship that will exist at birth and gradually change during extrauterine life.

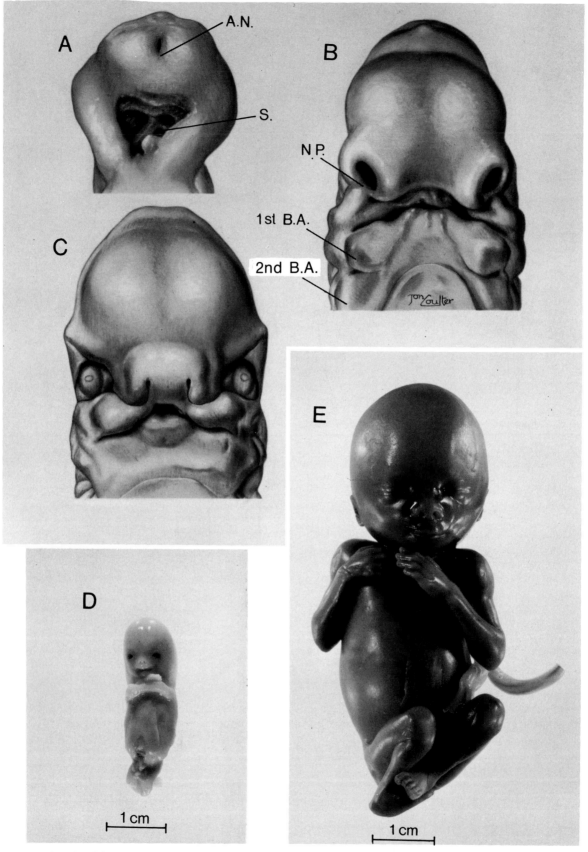

Figure 1–3. Prenatal facial development. *A*, An embryo of 3 to 4 weeks. A.N., anterior neuropore; S., stomadeum. *B*, An embryo of 5 to 6 weeks. N.P., nasal pit; 1st B.A., first branchial arch; 2nd B.A., second branchial arch. *C*, An embryo of 7 to 8 weeks. *D*, A fetus of 8 to 9 weeks. *E*, A fetus of 3 to 4 months. (Fetal specimens are from the Krause Collection, the Cleft Palate Center, University of Pittsburgh.)

The concept of differential growth is vital to the comprehension of both prenatal and postnatal development. Although this concept is difficult to grasp when the student must view development of structures of different ages magnified to the same size and when illustrations are in two dimensions, it is important to visualize the process in three dimensions *and* in the fourth dimension—time.

FORMATION OF THE CRANIOFACIAL COMPLEX

The structures and the factors that form the craniofacial complex have been the subject of investigation by embryologists for many years, and their study has involved use of a number of sophisticated, time-consuming techniques (Stewart, 1976). Among the most interesting studies has been the research of Johnston (1975) into the development and migration of cells in the neural crest. These cells are initially composed of ectoderm found at the junction of the neural plate and surface ectoderm; Figure 1–4A shows the neural crest cells forming around the anterior neuropore. It has been shown that the face of the amphibian, as well as of mammals, develops as a consequence of massive cell migrations and the interactions of loosely organized embryonic tissue. In most of the body, this embryonic tissue is derived from mesoderm; however, in the craniofacial complex, neural crest cells give rise to a large variety of connective and nervous tissues of the skull, face, and branchial arches. Therefore, this ectodermal tissue constitutes the majority of the pluripotential tissue of the face. The sequence of events after the initial formation of the neural crest cells is illustrated in Figure 1–4B. The differentiation, proliferation, and migration of those cells are critical in the formation of the face.

Migration occurs at different rates. For instance, the cells that form the frontonasal process are derived from the forebrain fold, and their migration is relatively short as they pass into the nasal region. However, the cells that form the mesenchyme of the maxillary processes have a considerably longer distance to migrate, since they must move into the branchial arches, where they surround the corelike mesodermal muscle plates (Krogman, 1974). In Figure 1–4C, the ultimate distribution of neural crest cells from the frontonasal process and from the branchial arches is illustrated. Since this mesenchymal tissue contributes the majority of the soft tissues and bone to the face, failure of proliferation or migration may be responsible for a number of abnormalities, such as orofacial clefts (Stark, 1977). An illustration of a severe facial abnormality secondary to failure of migration is illustrated in Figure 1–4D. Less severe clefts of the lip and the palate or both may also develop. In some cases, such as with severe holoprosencephaly, not only are mesodermal tissues involved but there are central nervous system abnormalities as well (DeMyer, 1975).

DIVISIONS OF THE HUMAN FACE

From the foregoing, it can be seen that the human face may be divided embryologically, as illustrated in Figure 1–4C. The median facial structures arise from the frontonasal processes, and the lateral structures arise from the branchial arches. This dual embryonic origin provides a basis for dividing the face into three *vertical* segments. The central segment, primarily the frontonasal process, includes the nose and the central portion of the upper lip. The two lateral segments that arise from the branchial arches may be called the otomaxillomandibular segments. For convenience of description, the face can also be divided into three almost equal *horizontal* planes. The upper, or frontal horizontal segment derives solely from the frontonasal process. The middle, or maxillary, segment derives from the maxillary process of the first branchial arch, and the prolabium comes from the frontonasal process. The third horizontal segment, the lower, or mandibular, segment, comes from the mandibular process of the first branchial arch (DeMyer, 1975).

PRENATAL CRANIOFACIAL SKELETAL COMPONENTS

The craniofacial skeleton provides support and protection for the human's most vital functions. Conceptually, it is a region with two divisions: that which is involved with the central nervous system—the *neurocranium*—and that which is involved with respiration and mastication—the *visceral cranium*. It consists of four components: the cranial base, cranial vault, nasomaxillary complex, and mandible.

The skeletal structures originate spontaneously from two types of bone. One type of bone is first formed in cartilage, and the other is derived from membrane. In general, the bones of the skull that represent the earliest phylogenetic structures are first formed as cartilage, which subsequently ossifies, and the more recently developed craniofacial structures are derived from membranous bone.

The components and structures of the fetal craniofacial complex are illustrated in Figures 1–5 through 1–8. Figure 1–5 is a parasagittal section through the cranial base and the facial structures. The cranial base is cartilaginous and provides a floor for the calvaria and a roof for the face. The nasal space and nasopharynx are part of the airway system. Although the airway is not functional in the fetus, alterations of the cranial base during fetal life may affect its subsequent development. Figure 1–6A and B shows the cartilaginous continuity of the cranial base and nasal septum as well as the arrangement of the fetal facial bones and teeth around the cartilaginous nasal capsule. The nasal septum is attached to the cranial base and the palate and, thus, constitutes a large portion of the skeletal structure in the fetal midface. Although there is much difference of opinion of this subject, growth of cranio-

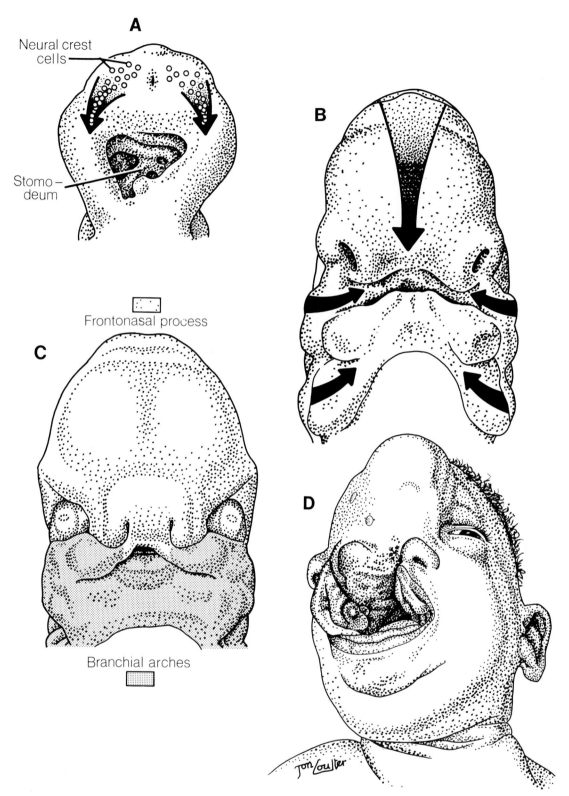

Figure 1–4. Formation of the craniofacial complex. *A*, An embryo of 3 to 4 weeks showing development and beginning migration of neural crest cells. *B*, Migration of neural crest cells to the forebrain and the branchial arches. *C*, Contributions to the face of the frontonasal process and branchial arches. *D*, Deformity caused by failure of neural crest cell migration.

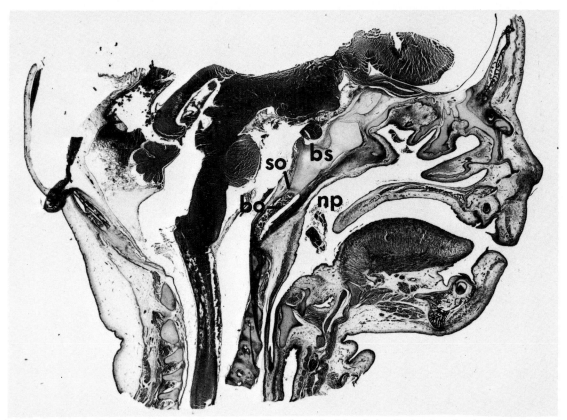

Figure 1–5. Photomicrograph of a parasagittal section of a 15-week-old fetal head. bo, Basiocciput; bs, basisphenoid cartilage; np, nasopharynx; so, sphenooccipital synchrondrosis. (From the Krause Collection, the Cleft Palate Center, University of Pittsburgh.)

Figure 1–6. A, Coronal section of a 15-week-old fetal head. B, Sagittal section of a 15-week-old fetal head. dt, Deciduous tooth germ; m, maxillary bone center; np, nasopharynx; s, nasal septum.

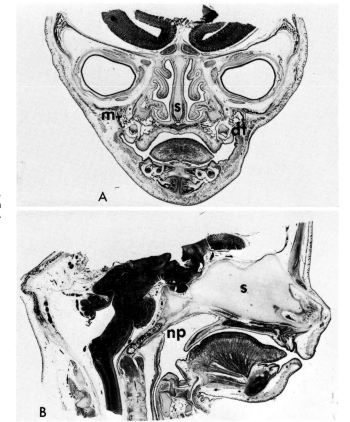

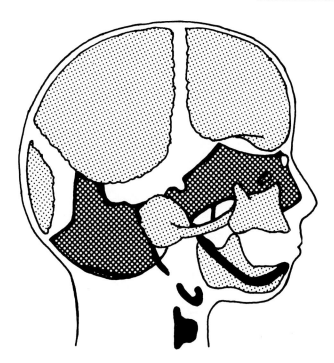

Figure 1–7. Schematic illustration of the components of the fetal craniofacial complex of membranous origin (light stipple) and cartilaginous origin (dark stipple). The cartilage of branchial arch origin is indicated in black. (Redrawn from Stewart, 1976.)

 Cartilaginous bone

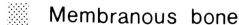 Membranous bone

facial cartilage is considered by some to be of prime importance in facial development (Latham, 1976).

As previously mentioned, the craniofacial skeletal complex is composed of bones of different embryonic origins. Figure 1–7 shows the bones of cartilaginous origin (dark stipple) and those of membranous origin (light stipple); cartilage that is of branchial arch origin is indicated by solid black. In general, the base of the skull and the sphenoid, petrosal, and ethmoid bones are of cartilaginous origin. The growth of the cartilage of the cranial base will be primarily at the cartilaginous synchondroses until cartilage is replaced by bone; thereafter, growth is at the periosteal margins. Most of the cranial and facial bones are membranous, and growth takes place primarily at the margins of these bones. The major facial bones are formed from multiple ossification centers, which subsequently produce single bones in later fetal life. The importance of understanding the dual embryonic origin of the skeleton is that many diseases that affect the craniofacial complex may be manifested because of their influence on particular types of bone; for example, achondroplasia, which affects bones of cartilaginous origin, usually results in a characteristic alteration of facial configuration. The formation of membranous and endochondral bones and remodeling of bone are discussed and illustrated in Chapter 2.

The sequential development of the fetal skeleton has been studied extensively by radiographic methods (Kier, 1971). However, it is anticipated that newer developments such as magnetic resonance imaging

(MRI) will provide better visualization of the relationship of the various tissues and improve our understanding of craniofacial morphogenesis (Maue-Dickson and Trefler, 1977; Prewitt, 1976; Isaacson, 1986). Figure 1–8 illustrates the definition of the structures that may be obtained by this technique. In addition, ultrasonography is a method of *in vivo* study that has achieved wide clinical use.

DEVELOPMENT OF CRANIOFACIAL ARTERIES, MUSCLES, AND NERVES

Figure 1–9 illustrates the development of the cranium, arteries, nerves, and muscles during embryonic and early fetal life. The characteristics of these structures will be discussed in their respective sections, since their growth and development are interrelated.

Arteries

Figure 1–9A shows that the early arterial supply to the head consists primarily of the dorsal aorta and an arch with a small branch coming from it, which is the primitive internal carotid artery. The future musculature consists of mesenchymal tissue in the first and second branchial arches, which are just beginning to form. As the head begins to grow and the embryo starts to develop a face, the internal carotid artery

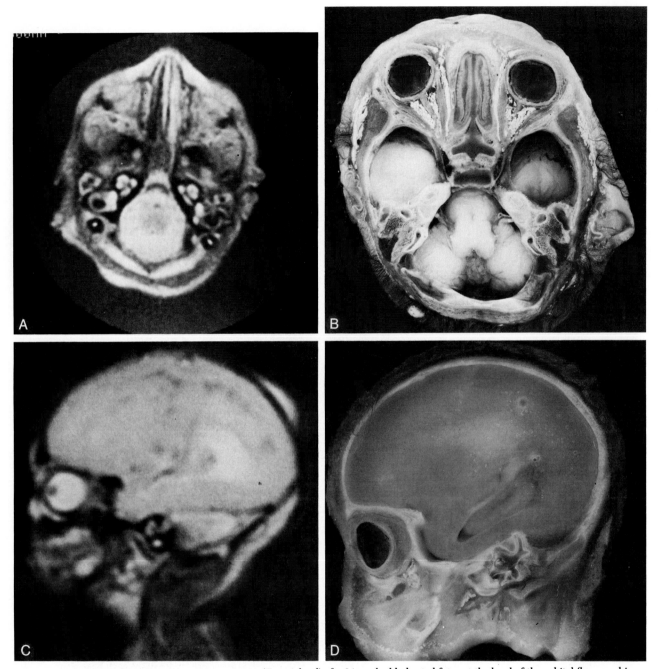

Figure 1–8. A, Transverse magnetic resonance image (T$_2$-weighted) of a 24-week-old aborted fetus at the level of the orbital floors and inner and middle ears. B, Transverse section through the fetal head at the level of the orbits (28 weeks of gestation). C, Sagittal magnetic resonance image of the fetal head (T$_2$-weighted). D, Sagittal section of the fetal head (24 weeks of gestation). (B, From Isaacson, G., Mintz, M. C., and Crelin, E. S.: Atlas of Fetal Sectional Anatomy. New York, Springer-Verlag, 1986. C, From Isaacson, G., and Mintz, M. C.: Magnetic resonance image of the fetal temporal bone. Laryngoscope 96:1343–1346, 1986. D, Reprinted with permission from Prenatal visualization of the inner ear, by G. Isaacson and M. C. Mintz. Journal of Ultrasound in Medicine, Vol. 5, pp. 409–410. Copyright 1986 by the American Institute of Ultrasound in Medicine.)

increases in both size and length, and the aortic arches begin to develop. Each of the branchial arches contains not only an artery but also a nerve and a core of mesodermal tissue. Figure 1–9B shows an embryo of about 6 weeks, when the first and second aortic arches and their arteries have formed. As the face continues to develop, these vessels will ultimately disappear. It must be appreciated that at this stage the embryo is still very small and these vessels are correspondingly

tiny. In fact, the vessels themselves are responding to the needs of the tissue surrounding them, and with further growth their anastomosis will ultimately come from another source. The internal carotid artery at this stage has increased in size, and the facial muscles are beginning to develop in a laminar fashion. One group of muscles develops a lamina that grows posteriorly, and the other group of muscles comes from a lamina that extends anteriorly.

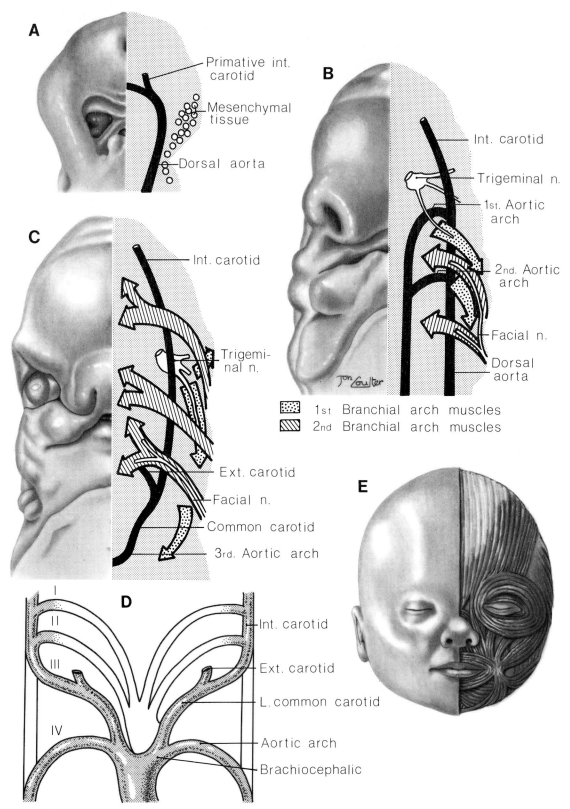

Figure 1–9. Development of the craniofacial arteries, muscles, and nerves. *A,* A 3- to 4-week-old embryo. *B,* A 5- to 6-week-old embryo. *C,* A 7- to 8-week-old embryo. *D,* The fate of the aortic arches (shaded vessels persist). (After Avery, 1974.) *E,* Distribution of the facial musculature in the 15-week-old fetus. (After Gasser, 1961.)

The nerves are beginning to develop as outgrowths of the central nervous system. The skull base forms and foramina exist where bone forms *around* any preexisting soft tissue (blood vessels or nerves). The fifth cranial nerve (trigeminal), which will ultimately supply sensation to the face, is really a combination of three nerves with ophthalmic, mandibular, and maxillary divisions and a division to the muscles of mastication. The seventh cranial nerve, which is the nerve supply to the second branchial arch, has also begun its development.

By the time the embryo has facial characteristics that appear more human (Fig. 1–9C), the blood supply to the face and cranium has developed the pattern that will persist into fetal and postnatal life. The third aortic arch is connected to the embryonic dorsal aorta. This arch becomes a common carotid artery, from which the external carotid artery develops to provide the major blood supply for the face. In general, these vessels have a recognizable pattern, but there is tremendous variation in their sites of origin and in the anastomosis between the internal and external carotid arteries. Figure 1–9D illustrates the formation of the arterial supply. Note the disappearance of the first and second aortic arches, the persistence of the third arch, which becomes the common carotid, and the disappearance of the dorsal aorta between the third and fourth arches, which on the left will become the aorta.

Muscles

By the end of embryonic life, the facial musculature has become rather well-developed and has migrated extensively superiorly into the craniofacial region. Figure 1–9E shows the muscles contributed by the various laminae (Gasser, 1961). The first branchial arch contributes the muscles that lie beneath the musculature of the second branchial arch and, in general, have a different orientation. These muscles include the temporal, masseter, pterygoid, mylohyoid, and anterior belly of the digastric, as well as the tensor muscle of the velum palatini and the tensor muscle of the tympanum.

Nerves

The nerve supply to the muscles of the face has been described by Gasser (1961) and is discussed in detail by him in May's book (1986) on the facial nerve. These cranial nerves are mixed nerves, having autonomic, sensory and motor components. By the time the fetus has reached 37 mm crown–rump length, all of the peripheral branches of the facial nerve are identifiable.

MOLECULAR BIOLOGY AND MORPHOGENESIS

As one traces human development back through the fetal and the embryonic periods in an attempt to understand the errors that produce disease, it becomes clear that many of the answers lie deeper—at the level of the cell and its genetic machinery. In one simple organism, it is possible to follow the developmental course of each cell of the embryo at the 500-cell stage and discover its role in determining the structure of the mature creature (Darnell et al., 1986). But what controls the internal order of these cells and directs them as the organism develops into a complete animal? This is a fundamental question addressed by the discipline of molecular biology (Watson et al., 1987).

Geneticists have long postulated that some chemical substance within the cell must contain the information that permits accurate transmission of traits from generation to generation. The key role of proteins, and specifically of the biochemically active proteins called enzymes, in the synthetic processes that produce intracellular structure was realized in the first half of this century. At the same time, it was thought that chromosomes must somehow carry the information to guide these processes, as these chromosomes were seen to divide, multiply, and segregate under the microscope during cellular reproduction. Still, it was not until deoxyribonucleic acid (DNA), a major component of chromosomes, was isolated and its structure defined that a molecule could be said to contain genetic information.

DNA is a colorless, gooey, acid substance composed of enormously long chains of four simple molecules, adenine, thymine, guanine, cytosine, known as nucleotide bases. Each base is linked to the sugar deoxyribose and a phosphate group to form a complete nucleotide. The DNA molecule is made up of two complementary chains of nucleotides wrapped about each other in a helical fashion and held together by weak molecular attractions between the nucleotide bases. Adenine is paired with thymine, and cytosine with guanine. The strands may be separated by enzymes within the cell or by heating in the laboratory, but they re-form quickly, like two halves of a complex jigsaw puzzle (Fig. 1–10). Within this long array of linked bases is hidden the information to create life.

A three-nucleotide set composed of four possible bases (i.e., 32 possible combinations) is called a codon and is capable of designating one of the 20 different amino acids that form the building blocks of proteins (e.g., CGA = arginine). The "central dogma" of molecular biology states that DNA molecules form a template for constructing corresponding proteins. Since DNA cannot be transported from the nucleus to the cytoplasm, where protein synthesis takes place, an intermediary template molecule called ribonucleic acid (RNA) is formed in the nucleus and journeys across the nuclear membrane. From the RNA "impression" of DNA, the codon information determines how amino acids will line up to form proteins. In short:

$$\text{DNA} \xrightarrow[\text{(transcription)}]{\text{codes for}} \text{RNA} \xrightarrow[\text{(translation)}]{\text{codes for}} \text{protein}$$

Proteins thus constructed fold up into unique, tiny

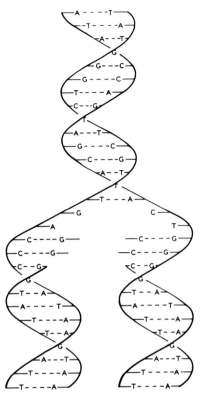

Figure 1–10. Replication of DNA, resulting in two identical daughter molecules, each composed of one parental strand and one newly synthesized strand. (From Thompson, M. W.: Thompson & Thompson Genetics in Medicine, 4th ed. Philadelphia, W. B. Saunders Co., 1986.)

electrical environments capable of stacking on one another, transporting oxygen, and assembling or pulling apart other molecules. The type, concentration, and arrangement of these proteins determine whether a cell will become part of a muscle or a hair, whether it will absorb glucose or kill bacteria.

The portion of a DNA molecule capable of coding for a protein is thus the molecular biologic equivalent of a gene. It is well-known, however, that there is a great diversity in the genetic make-up of individuals and that some diseases are caused by "bad" genes. Each of these observations requires that mutation be reflected by changes at the molecular level—and it is. For many years, the hemoglobin molecule stood as the model gene product. Its amino acid sequence is known, and the interactions of the electrically charged groups on these amino acids explain why the molecule folds into its unique configuration and why oxygen binds reversibly within its electrical microenvironment. Further, an alteration in a single nucleotide base in the DNA segment that codes for hemoglobin causes the substitution of an incorrect amino acid and disrupts both the structure and the function of the hemoglobin molecule, causing the disease sickle cell anemia. However, as the human genome was explored further, things became less cut and dry.

Unlike the simple genetic material of bacteria, human DNA has more functions than merely carrying the code to construct individual proteins. Contained

on the three billion base-pair–long human genome are areas involved in the regulation of genes—turning transcription off and on and thus controlling the generation of their gene products. There are often multiple copies of a gene, each identical or with minor variations, and there are large areas that code for old burnt-out forms of a protein or for nothing at all. To explore this immense warehouse of phylogeny, there must be a way of reducing the information to an approachable size so as to probe its meaning. The advances in molecular biology over the last 15 years have focused on these issues.

Bacteria make special enzymes designed to guard against the invasion of foreign DNAs, called restriction endonucleases. These enzymes chop up DNA into tiny pieces, and they do so at specific sites determined by short nucleotide sequences (e.g., G[chop]AATTC for one eyzyme from *Escherichia coli*). There are now over one hundred known restriction endonucleases capable of chopping at different sites. When mixed with a long DNA molecule, they can reduce it to workable-sized bits of several hundred bases.

Many probes are available to explore the cut-up DNA sequences. Among the most useful are those based on DNA hybridization. Double-stranded DNA may be separated by heating into single strands, eager to reunite upon cooling (Fig. 1–11). If small sequences of DNA, radioactively tagged, are mixed in before cooling, they will bind to complementary areas of the longer DNA molecules, labeling that area as their home (locus). Since it is possible to create sequences of nucleotides in any order and the order of amino acids in some proteins is known, a DNA probe specific for that protein can be constructed and used to search a DNA molecule for its locus. Using DNA hybridization, bacterial amplification techniques, and restriction endonucleases in conjunction with classic genetic methods, the location of many of the genes on a chromosome can be determined. Further, if the locus of a particular gene is known and a DNA probe fails to bind to it, it may be inferred that base sequences have been altered or are absent (i.e., that a mutation exists) (Kazazian, 1985).

Using DNA probes for specific genes or for base sequences known to be near a gene, it is possible to diagnose genetic disease on the molecular level, even before birth. By collecting fetal cells shed into the amniotic fluid using amniocentesis or by collecting fetal placental cells with a procedure known as chorion villus sampling, one can diagnose with accuracy a variety of hemoglobinopathies, including sickle cell anemia and beta-thalassemia, and Duchenne muscular dystrophy. The development of genetic diseases as diverse as cystic fibrosis, Huntington chorea, Alzheimer disease, and retinoblastoma can be predicted in childhood from DNA analysis (Garver, 1987). Finally, if someday a gene's "unhealthy" DNA could be replaced with new DNA, it might be possible to treat genetic disease.

While great strides have been made in the understanding of genes and gene products, the issue of how

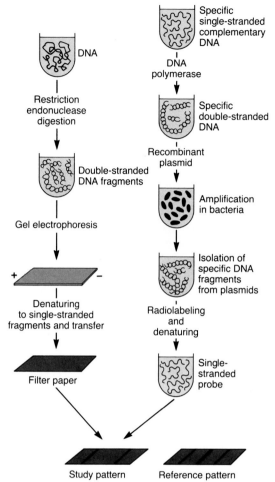

Figure 1–11. DNA hybridization as a gene probe. (Modified after Kazazian, H. H. 1985. The nature of mutation. Hosp. Pract. 2:55.)

interfere with differential growth. The saddle nose deformity seen in fetal hydantoin syndrome may be the result of underdevelopment of the nasal septum associated with this known teratogen. An example of failed induction is seen in the cerebral and craniofacial malformations that comprise the holoprosencephaly series (see Chapter 3). A critical tissue area called the prechordal mesoderm is responsible for inducing sagittal division of the anterior portion of the brain and for the formation of the nasofrontal process. Failure of this induction results in a single cerebral ventricle and underdevelopment of the midface.

During fetal and postnatal life, there is a continuation of differential growth and development. This includes the precocious growth of the nervous system, which results in enlargement of the calvaria in the fetus and infant out of proportion to enlargement of the face and the remainder of the body. The concepts of this chapter furnish the basis for understanding normal postnatal growth and possible abnormalities of the craniofacial complex.

SELECTED REFERENCES

Ayala, F. 1978. The mechanisms of evolution. Scientific American 239:56.
  A well-illustrated article that explains the concepts of molecular biology as related to evolution. This entire issue is devoted to evolution.
Burdi, A. 1976. Biological forces which shape the human midface before birth. In McNamara, J. (ed.): Craniofacial growth series, Monograph No. 6. Ann Arbor, MI, Center for Human Growth and Development, the University of Michigan.
  A comprehensive article that relates molecular biology to embryonic and fetal growth.
Enlow, D. 1975. Handbook of Facial Growth. Philadelphia, W. B. Saunders Co.
  This book is written primarily in atlas style and illustrates craniofacial growth from embryonic to adult life.
Isaacson, G. 1986. Atlas of Fetal Sectional Anatomy. New York, Springer-Verlag.
  An excellent atlas of fetal sectional anatomy that correlates gross, MRI, and ultrasound findings.
May, M. 1986. The Facial Nerve. New York, Thieme, Inc.
  An outstanding review of the anatomy, physiology, and disease states of the facial nerve.
Moore, K. L. 1983. Before We Are Born: Basic Embryology and Birth Defects, 2nd ed. Philadelphia, W. B. Saunders Co.
  A clinically oriented embryology text that is well-illustrated.
Stewart, R. 1976. Genetic factors in craniofacial morphogenesis. In Stewart, R., and Prescott, G. (eds.): Oral Facial Genetics. St. Louis, The C. V. Mosby Co.
  This is a comprehensive text with extensive references that describes the genetic aspects of craniofacial abnormalities and gives other extensive descriptions of oral abnormalities.

REFERENCES

Avery, T, 1974. Developmental Anatomy, 7th ed. Philadelphia, W. B. Saunders Co.
Ayala, F. 1978. The mechanisms of evolution. Scientific American 239:56.
Bergsma, D. 1979. Birth Defects Compendium, 2nd ed. New York, Alan R. Liss, Inc., p. 433.
Burdi, A. R. 1976. Biological forces which shape the human midface

DNA controls growth and development remains largely unexplored. We know why eyes are blue, but not how eyes come to be.

Recently, several genes have been discovered that seem to control morphogenesis, or at least their absence predicts its failure. In the fruit fly, for instance, a specific DNA sequence controlling the development of the insect's hind parts has been identified. Still, the regulation of embryogenesis is poorly defined on the molecular level. We know that gravity affects the development of the early frog embryo and determines which half of the structure will be the head and which the tail. Further, physical contact between developing structures in the embryo seems to be necessary for the induction of those body parts, implying that there must be surface "sensors" or transmitted chemical substances that allow cell-to-cell communication. These factors influence the rate of growth of particular groups of cells, allowing the proportional growth of structures and the proper migration of tissues. This process is seen in the medial "migration" (actually differential growth) of the lateral shelves during palatal formation.

These phenomena introduce another level at which developmental deviations can occur. Teratogens can before birth. *In* McNamara, J. (ed.): Craniofacial growth series. Monograph No. 6, Ann Arbor, MI, Center for Human Growth and Development, the University of Michigan.

Burdi, A. R. 1977. Early development of the human basicranium: Morphogenic basicranium: Morphogenic controls, growth patterns and relations. *In* Bosma, J. F. (ed.): NIH symposium on development of the basicranium. U.S. Government Printing Office, pp. 81–92. (Available from Superintendent of Documents as No. 017–047–00011–61).

Darnell, J., Lodish, H., and Baltimore, D. 1986. Molecular Cell Biology. New York, Scientific American Books, pp. 985–1033.

DeMyer, W. 1975. Median facial malformations and their implications for brain malformations. *In* Bergsma, V. (ed.): Morphogenesis and Malformation of Face and Brain. New York, Alan Rhise, Inc., pp. 155–181.

Enlow, D. 1975. Handbook of Facial Growth. Philadelphia, W. B. Saunders Co.

Garver, K. L. 1987. From the editor. Genet. Pract. 4(2):1.

Gasser, R. 1961. The development of the facial nerve in man. Ann. Otol. Rhinol. Laryngol. 76:37.

Johnston, M. 1975. The neural crest in abnormalities of the face and brain in birth defects. Original Article Series II, no. 7, pp. 1–18.

Kazazian, H. H. 1985. The nature of mutation. Hosp. Pract. 2:55.

Kier, S. 1971. Fetal skull. *In* Newton, T., and Potts, D., (eds.): Radiology of the Skull and Brain, Vol. 1, Chap. 7. St. Louis, The C. V. Mosby Co.

Krogman, W. 1974. Craniofacial Growth and Development: An Appraisal. Yearb. Phys. Anthropol. 18:31.

Latham, R. 1976. An appraisal of the early maxillary growth mechanism. *In* McNamara, J. (ed.): Craniofacial growth series, Monograph No. 6, Ann Arbor, MI, Center for Human Growth and Development, the University of Michigan.

Maue-Dickson, W., and Trefler, M. 1977. Image quality in computerized and conventional tomography in the assessment of craniofacial anomalies. SPIE 127:353.

Moore, K. 1977. The Developing Human, 2nd ed. Philadelphia, W. B. Saunders Co.

Prewitt, J. 1976. Prospective medical advances in computerized tomography. *In* Bosma, J. (ed.): Development of the Basicranium. DHEW Publication No. (NIH) 789.

Roberts, J. A. 1973. An Introduction to Medical Genetics. London, Oxford University Press.

Stark, R. 1977. Embryology of cleft palate. *In* Converse, J. (ed.): Reconstructive Plastic Surgery. Philadelphia, W. B. Saunders Co., pp. 1941–1949.

Stewart, R. 1976. Genetic factors in craniofacial morphogenesis. *In* Stewart, R., and Prescott, G. (eds.): Oral Facial Genetics, St. Louis, The C. V. Mosby Co., pp. 46–66.

Vogel, F., and Motulsky, A. G. 1986. Human Genetics: Problems and Approaches, 2nd ed. New York, Springer-Verlag, pp. 87–127.

Watson, J. D., Hopkins, N. H., Roberts, J. W., et al. 1987. Molecular Biology of the Gene, 4th ed. Menlo Park, CA, The Benjamin/Cummings Publishing Co., pp. 65–94 and 606–618.

White, R. L. 1985. Diagnosis when the gene locus is unknown. Hosp. Pract. 5:103.

Williams, P., and Wendell-Smith, C. 1969. Basic Human Embryology, 2nd ed. Philadelphia, J. B. Lippincott Co.

Chapter 2

POSTNATAL CRANIOFACIAL GROWTH AND DEVELOPMENT

Sylvan E. Stool, M.D.   William A. Marasovich, D.D.S., M.D.

Growth implies an increase in dimension and mass, whereas development implies a progression to more adult characteristics. In this chapter, we shall start by describing the appearance of the soft tissues of the human head and then examine the underlying skeletal components in order to relate the development of these components to some of the basic principles and concepts of cartilage and bone growth. The infant face rarely projects an image of the adult configuration. Conversely, attempting to identify an adult by examination of his or her "baby pictures" is usually impossible. The face of the infant or child is not a miniature of an adult face but has definite proportions that are different from those of the adult. The changes that take place during maturation are part of a differential growth process. In general, newborns, regardless of their ethnic backgrounds, resemble each other more than each one does his or her parents. The different proportions of infant and adult faces have been studied extensively by artists and anthropologists and are appreciated almost instinctively by the layperson (Hogarth, 1965; Ligett, 1974). These changes in the facial configuration and proportions are illustrated in Figure 2–1.

The infant has a very prominent forehead because of the early development of the cerebral hemispheres in relation to the face. About 90 per cent of the child's facial height is achieved by 5 years of age, whereas 90 per cent of the facial width is attained by 2 years. Thus, the young child's head appears round.

The *face* of the infant is diminutive compared with the calvaria. As seen in Figure 2–1, the proportion of facial mass to cranial mass, as viewed laterally, is 1 to 3. Subsequent growth in childhood alters this proportion so that the ratio becomes about 1 to 2½, whereas in the adolescent and the adult, the proportion becomes 1 to 2. However, if this proportion does not change as described, the adult is frequently referred to as having a "baby face." In addition, because the soft tissues of the face include fat, the external appearance does not necessarily reflect the underlying musculoskeletal structure of the face. Thus, the underlying proportions may change but the general outline of the adult face may still appear childlike. The infant face

has a "flat" configuration, which changes during adolescence when sharper angles develop as a result of orbital, mandibular, and nasal growth. The maxilla and mandible will grow to accommodate the primary dentition (20 teeth), followed by the permanent dentition (32 teeth) (see Fig. 2–7). The *chin* of the infant is almost nonexistent but is usually a prominent adult structure as a result of mandibular growth and development. The cheekbones are notable in the adult because of loss of baby fat and rotation of the skeletal components. The *ears* of the infant appear to be very low-set because the head in general is more ovoid than elongated; the ears appear to "rise" with growth because of the increase in the vertical dimension of the lower facial height. The configuration of the ear remains the same throughout life, although its mass increases.

The most prominent facial features, the relationship of which has become characteristic of human faces, are the nose and the eyes. The *nose* of the infant has a distinctive pug appearance. It is diminutive and remains so throughout most of childhood. During adolescence and later, especially in the male, there is an increase in length, breadth, and protrusion of the nose, which is related to the increase in airway requirements at this age and which is accompanied by a similar increase in the size of the internal airway. The growth of the face can more easily be explained if a subordinate position is given to the craniofacial skeleton, while a leading role is designated to the soft tissues and the functional components that play a part in the activities of the face. In these, the maintenance of the airway is predominant (Moss and Salentijn, 1969). Humans are the only animals with a truly external nose, and this particularly human trait is subject to many variations, depending in part on ethnic background.

The *eyes* of the infant appear to be wide-set and have a very prominent inner canthal fold, giving an appearance of hypertelorism because of the lack of vertical dimension of the face. If the infant's face is bisected horizontally, the eyes are located in the inferior half of the face. During childhood, the eyes appear to move upward, but in actuality the lower half

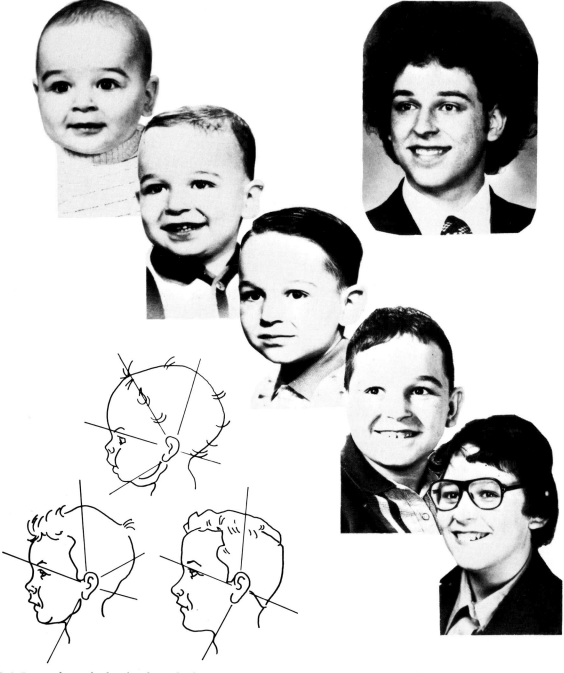

Figure 2–1. Postnatal growth of a white boy. The diagonal from above downward shows the boy at ages 6 months, 2 years, 4 years, 8 years, and 12 years: the photograph in the upper right corner is the same child at 18 years. Drawings in the lower left show the changes in proportion of face mass to cranial mass. In the infant, it is 1 to 3; during childhood, it gradually changes to 1 face mass to 2½ cranial mass. From adolescence through adult life, it is 1 face mass to 2 cranial mass.

of the face grows more than the upper half, so the maxilla and mandible become more prominent. In the older child, the eyes are placed midway in the face. In adolescence, with further growth and development of the lower half of the face relative to the upper half, the eyes finally appear to be just above the dividing line. This adult configuration is the result of differential growth of facial components. The same principle may be used to explain why in adults the eyes are less prominent than they appear to be in children: with growth of the supraorbital rim during adolescence, less of the eye is exposed.

Even though growth is often measured through its performance early in life, there is no reason to assume that it terminates at any specific period. A study conducted by Behrents (1985) as an extension of the Bolton-Brush growth studies revealed continuing growth of the craniofacial complex throughout all age levels, similar in direction to adolescent alterations but of lesser magnitude and rate.

GROWTH CONCEPTS

"Parallel evaluation of the cranium and of other parts of the skeleton is at the present time the basis for the clinical distinction of generalized skeletal disorders from cranial abnormalities" (Pierce et al., 1977). Therefore, in order to understand the normal morphologic changes that occur with growth, as well as craniofacial abnormalities, it is important to describe some basic concepts of skeletal growth: *bone formation, remodeling,* and *displacement.* The information presented in the following section may be studied more fully in Williams and colleagues (1969), Sokoloff and Bland (1975), Rubin (1964), and Enlow (1982).

Bone Formation

Humans possess an endoskeleton that is fabricated from specialized connective tissue—cartilage and bone. Cartilage is a special, tough, pliable tissue that has the capacity to form in regions that experience direct pressure; it does not always calcify and does not necessarily have a surface membrane. Its most important feature in the craniofacial complex is its ability to function as a precursor or model for bone. The characteristics of bone are hardness and rigidity and the possession of a surface membrane, or periosteum. It is a complex substance that is viewed by the chemist as a compound of protein, polysaccharide, mineral, and cellular constituents. To the histologist, it is a tissue composed of osteogenic cells and intracellular matrix. To the gross anatomist, it is an organ with vascular and nerve supplies.

The cells of cartilage and bone are derived from fetal mesenchymal tissue, which has a fairly uniform and undifferentiated appearance. These cells differentiate into chondroblasts and osteoblasts. Osteoblasts secrete a matrix that mineralizes and surrounds and encases them; they mature into osteocytes. Multinucleated giant cells called osteoclasts, which are known to destroy mineralized bone, also develop. They do not act on uncalcified bone—a fact of some importance in certain dysplasias—but they play an important role in the process of destruction and deposition that results in bone formation. A more detailed description of these cells and factors affecting their function has been described by Canalis (1983) and Centrella and Canalis (1985).

Bone always forms in preexisting connective tissue. When this tissue is cartilage, the process is called endochondral ossification; when it is noncartilaginous, it is called intramembranous ossification. The sequence of events is illustrated in Figure 2–2. Regulation of bone formation is further discussed by Raisz and Kream (1983).

Membranous bone in the skull forms as a layer of mesenchyme with foci of condensation. These areas of condensation begin to ossify, and the process extends until the areas meet to form suture lines. Craniosynostosis will result if premature closure of sutures in the cranium occurs. This condition is described thoroughly by Cohen (1986).

Endochondral ossification is a more complex process that is easier to visualize in the tubular bones. The mesenchyme condenses and then undergoes chondrification. This forms a precise model for future bone surrounded by a limiting membrane. Formation of a periosteal collar is followed by development of a primitive marrow cavity and an ossification center, which forms at the end of the bone. It is possible to identify four distinct segments in the tubular bone. The epiphysis is covered by an articular cartilage in tubular bones and includes the ossification center. The physis, or growth plate, is a very narrow but highly active region that consists of four zones all related to chondrogenesis. The metaphysis is a zone where the transformation, or change of growing cartilage into bone, takes place. Growth in length is achieved primarily through the activities of cells in the metaphysis. This is also an important region in the remodeling process. Eventually, when growth ceases, the physis will undergo ossification and disappear. The diaphysis is the shaft of the bone.

Remodeling and Displacement

In the craniofacial complex, growth and development depend on two separate but interrelated processes; displacement, which involves motion of segments of bone, and remodeling, which involves a change in the configuration of the bone while displacement is occurring. Bone grows by a continuous process of deposition and resorption. This is not a uniform process throughout the entire bone but is a differential growth process. If this were not so, the adult skeleton would be the same as the fetal configuration. The mechanism by which these two different but complementary functions are achieved is influenced by a

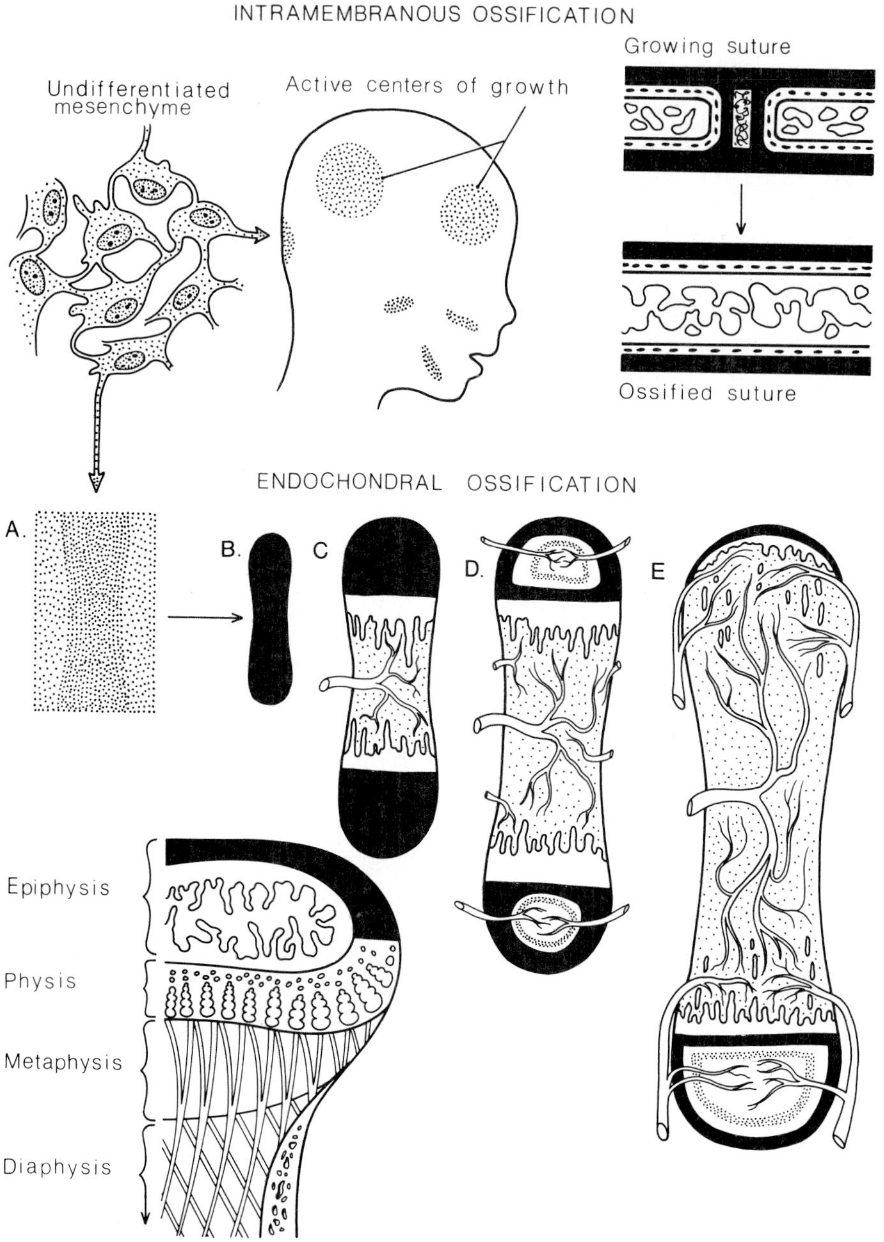

INTRAMEMBRANOUS OSSIFICATION

ENDOCHONDRAL OSSIFICATION

Figure 2–2. This figure illustrates the mechanism of formation of the two types of bone found in the skull. Undifferentiated mesenchyme is the precursor of both. *Intramembranous ossification:* Mesenchyme condenses to form centers of growth, which enlarge until they meet to form a suture. Growth proceeds at these sutures and remains active until the stimulus is removed and the suture ossifies. *Endochondral ossification:* *A,* Endochondral bone formation also begins with condensation. *B,* Cartilage *anlage* is formed. *C,* Vascular mesenchyme forms a primary marrow, and a periosteal collar forms. *D,* Ossification centers develop at the extremities, resulting in the four segments illustrated in the lower left. *E,* Eventually the bone is completely ossified, and the segmental differences disappear. The segments of a typical long bone are shown in the lower left. Epiphysis—a secondary ossification center, covered with cartilage. Physis—the cartilage growth plate. Metaphysis—the segment in which cartilage is transformed to bone by endochondral bone formation. Diaphysis—the shaft separating the growing ends. (Redrawn in part from Williams et al., 1969, and Rubin, 1964.)

number of factors, such as stress on the surface and various nutritional, hormonal, and genetic influences. The biodynamics have been studied for years and are still undergoing conceptual changes (Bassett, 1972).

In the simplest terms, bone grows because of osteoblastic activity and is resorbed by osteoclastic activity; anything that interferes with this process will result in an abnormal configuration. In the tubular bones, this concept is fairly easy to visualize. In order for a

bone to increase in length and retain its normal shape, it is necessary to add and subtract bone. This is illustrated in Figure 2–3.

The craniofacial region is a much more complex area, and perhaps the process of bone growth in this region can best be visualized by describing the technique by which an artist working with clay might construct a bowl, using coils. A basic hollow form is constructed, to which clay is added superficially. The

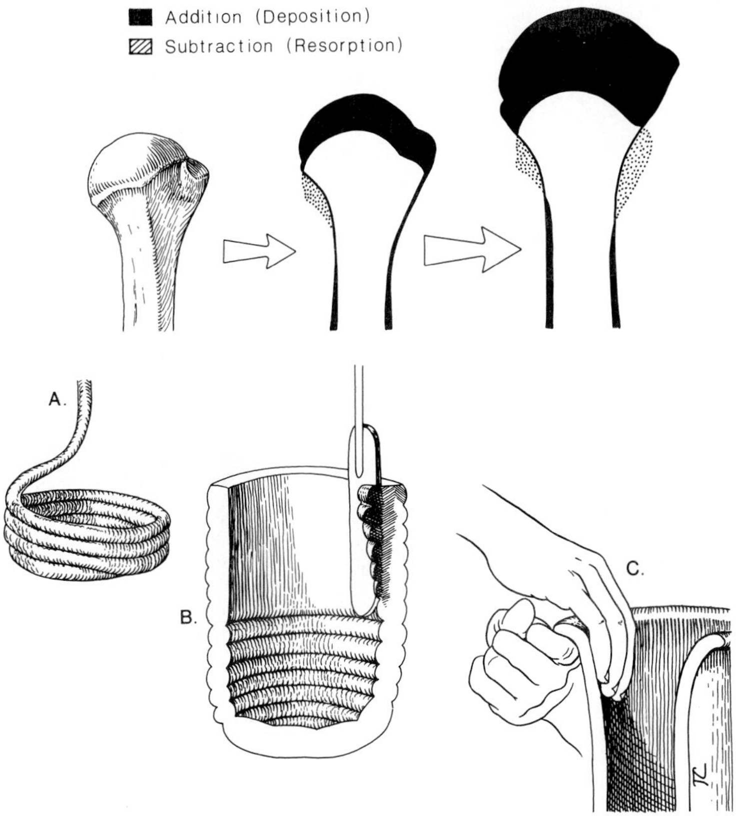

Addition (Deposition)
Subtraction (Resorption)

Figure 2–3. The concept of remodeling is illustrated. In order to prevent distortion of growing bone, there is osteoclastic cut-back at the metaphysis. An example is this tubular bone, in which there is addition—deposition—at the epiphysis and subtraction—resorption—at the metaphysis.

The concepts involved in skeletal growth and development are illustrated using the analogy of the ancient coil technique of clay construction. *A,* The initial step is formation by deposition (addition); during this process, there is concomitant removal, resorption (subtraction) resulting in differential growth. *B,* The final configuration is achieved by these two processes as well as an additional one, displacement *(C).*

edges may be smoothed in order to achieve a pleasing configuration. In order to keep the wall thickness uniform, it may be necessary to remove (subtract) some clay from the inner surface of the bowl (resorption). If a change in the configuration is desirable, it can be accomplished by applying pressure on the inner surface (displacement) and modeling the outer surface. Although this simple explanation is of some help in understanding the mechanics of bone formation, it does not explain why these events occur in the human.

For the clinician, it is important to realize that bone formation begins in the fetus and undergoes constant changes throughout life. This twofold process is important not only in the formation of craniofacial structures but also in the growth of other bones. In a series of investigations utilizing both cross-sectional and longitudinal material, Israel (1967, 1968, 1973, 1977) came to the conclusion that with aging the cranial skeleton and vertebrae basically gained in all dimensions studied.

The effects of abnormal bone formation can well be illustrated in human skull growth (Fig. 2–4). In achondroplasia, all bone forming from cartilage (having a cartilaginous precursor) is abnormal, including the chondrocranium. This results in a shortened skull base, a flattened palate, a sunken bridge to the nose, and a general reduction in the development and size of the facial region (Sullivan, 1986) (Fig. 2–4B). The growth

of the calvaria, which does not rely on ossification of cartilage for growth, is unhindered.

A certain group of disorders are affected by alterations in membranous bone formation. For instance, a craniometaphyseal abnormality involves alterations of the remodeling process, which are best understood by examination of the extremities. Some systemic diseases, such as hemolytic and iron deficiency anemias, may first be recognized in the cranium. Obviously, complete diagnosis of some cranial abnormalities necessitates evaluation of the remainder of the skeleton.

Postnatal Skeletal Growth

The external features and some of the basic concepts of bone growth of the craniofacial complex have been discussed. We will now examine the changes that occur in the skeleton. Skeletal growth is more readily assessed and easier to document than soft tissue growth, as it is subject to radiographic examination and physical measurements (Dorst, 1971). These methods yield good estimates of skeletal proportions. Because of the availability of these tools, skeletal growth parameters have come to be widely used as indices for general growth evaluation. "Skeletal age" is one of the "biologic ages" used to ascertain the normality of growth and development. Usually, this is evaluated

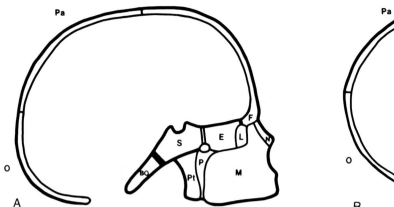
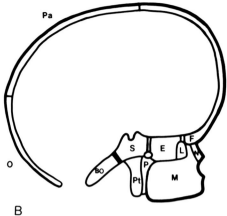

Figure 2–4. A, Normal skull. The bones of the calvaria, cranial base, and upper face. Position of the sphenooccipital synchondrosis shown in black. M, maxilla; N, nasal bone; F, frontal bone; L, lacrimal bone; E, ethmoid; P, vertical plate of the palatine bone; S, body of the sphenoid; Pt, pterygoid plate; O, occipital; BO, basioccipital; Pa, parietal. (*Note:* Any relative forward growth of the anterior cranial base will *carry* the "upper facial region" with it into a more anterior position.) *B*, Achondroplastic skull. Note the shortened skull base, sunken bridge of the nose, and general reduction in the development and the size of the facial region.

not only with cephalometric radiography but also by examination of the extremities, most commonly the wrist.

The skull is a complex structure formed from many component bones that articulate along an intricate network of sutures. The final location of each bone is determined by a composite of many different localized growth processes as well as regional changes. Figure 2–5A presents frontal views of the skulls of a newborn, a child, and an adult; Figure 2–5B shows three-quarter views. Figure 2–5C shows these same skulls with the infant and the child enlarged to the same size as the adult so that the vertical dimensions are equal. This provides a graphic means of illustrating changes in proportion.

Growth and development of the craniofacial complex will be discussed as involving the cranium, the mandible, and the nasomaxillary complex. The bones that compose the cranium must be considered in two parts—the calvaria (roof) and the basicranium (floor)—because distinctly different circumstances and modes of growth are involved for each.

Cranium

CALVARIA. The calvaria is constructed from the frontal, parietal, and portions of the temporal, occipital, and sphenoid bones. At birth, the bones are separated by six fontanelles that are bridged by fibrous tissue. The anterior fontanelle is the last to close (at about 18 months). As can be seen in Figure 2–5C, the skull of an infant is almost round. Sullivan (1986) makes the following comparison: The curvature of the surface of a large sphere is less than that of a small sphere. The adult calvaria is larger than the infant's and shows a corresponding reduction in curvature.

At birth, the brain weighs about half as much as the adult brain, and by ages 5 to 8 years it attains 90 per cent of its adult weight. In conjunction with the expansion of the underlying hemispheres, the bones

of the skull base are *carried* outward; they do not grow in an ectocranial dimension by their own depository and resorptive activity. As the bones are all displaced circumferentially, tension fields are established in the sutural membranes; this is believed to trigger (directly or indirectly) the progressive deposition of new bone by the sutures (Enlow, 1981). This enlarges the perimeter of each bone.

BASICRANIUM. The basicranium is a particularly fascinating region that has been the subject of much investigation (Bosma, 1976). Phylogenetically, it is the oldest skeletal component; anatomically, it has been considered the cornerstone of craniofacial growth. The basicranium is formed from the basal part of the occipital, the sphenoid, the petrous part of the temporal, and the ethmoid bones. It is primarily composed of bones formed by the ossification of cartilage precursors. Synchondroses, in addition to sutures, are present in the cranial base. They represent regional adaptation to the pressure-located areas of the growing cranium. In the case of the sphenooccipital synchondrosis, ossification takes place on both the sphenoidal and the occipital faces of the cartilage. (This is in contrast to ossification in the epiphyseal cartilage of a long bone, which occurs on only one surface.)

Investigators have not agreed as to the exact role of cartilage in craniofacial development (Babula et al., 1970; Koski, 1981). The sphenooccipital synchondrosis has been presumed to represent the primary growth site of the basicranium. This assumption has been the subject of much controversy, and whether the synchondrosis acts as a primary growth center or not, it must not be regarded as the only mechanism participating in cranial base growth.

It is difficult to visualize the basicranium from the anterior view. Figure 2–6, which is a tangential view of the inferior aspect of the skull, reveals that the nasomaxillary complex covers the anterior portion, beneath the anterior cranial fossa. The posterior portion of the cranial base provides the roof of the

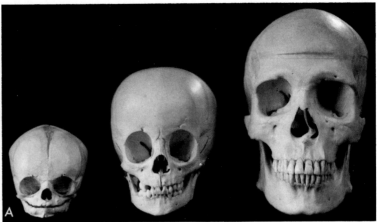

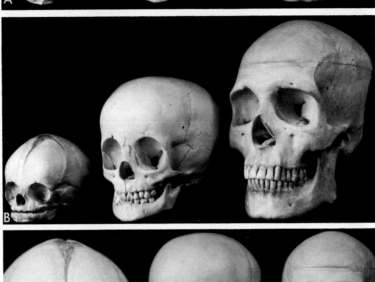

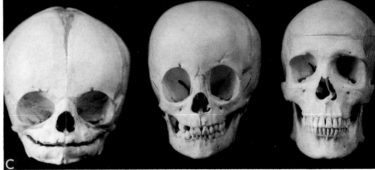

Figure 2–5. Skulls of a newborn, a child, and an adult illustrate skeletal changes during growth and development. A, Frontal view. B, Three-quarter view. C, The newborn and the child skulls have been enlarged to the same size as the adult skull to demonstrate the changes in proportion with growth.

nasopharynx. In Figure 2–6, the shape of this region has been traced on three skulls from different age groups. In the infant (I), this line is relatively flat, but with growth and development it assumes a more curved appearance in the child (C). This is due not only to increased depth, which results from remodeling of the palate, but also to the flexure of the basicranium. These changes provide an enlarged nasal airway to meet the requirements of gas exchange and speech resonance in the adult.

For the otolaryngologist, this region is important for several reasons. Many bone dysplasias affecting the skeleton may also affect the cranial base. As major nerves and vessels passing through foramina in the basicranium become involved, classic symptomatology results. One such example is osteopetrosis and facial palsy which is thoroughly discussed by Hamersma and

May (1986). Also, the size of the nasopharyngeal airway is in part determined by the configuration of the basicranium, and this has an effect on respiration and middle ear function because of the dynamics of airflow. Finally, the ear may also be affected as the osseous eustachian tube passes through the cranial base, and the muscles that control the cartilaginous portion of the tube originate from it.

Mandible

The human mandible is a membrane bone that forms in close association with Meckel's cartilage, the first branchial arch cartilage. At birth, the bone is in two parts joined in the midline by the symphysis menti, which closes by the end of the first year of life. The mandible is unusual in having a secondary growth

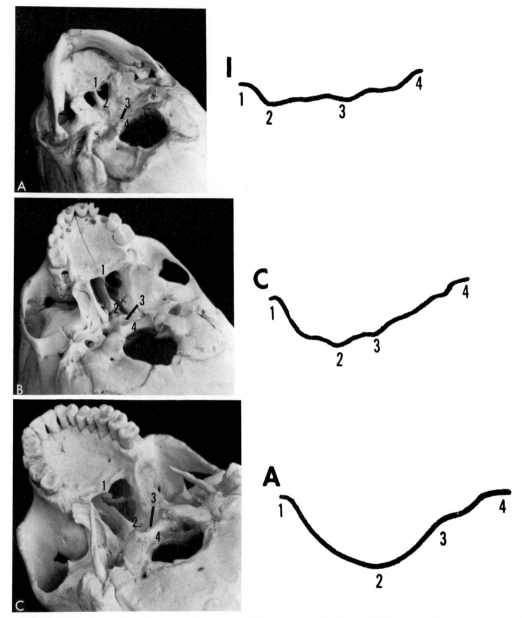

Figure 2–6. Tangential views of the inferior aspect of the skulls of *(A)* an infant (I); *(B)* a child (C); and *(C)* an adult (A). All illustrate the change in configuration of the nasopharynx. The anatomic landmarks indicated are *1*, posterior nasal spine; *2*, junction of vomer with the base of the skull; *3*, sphenooccipital synchondrosis; and *4*, edge of the foramen magnum. The change in size and configuration of the posterior choanae and the nasal airway with age can be appreciated.

cartilage under the surface of the articular condyle (Sullivan, 1986).

In studying craniofacial growth, it is often helpful to recognize that remodeling or displacement of a bone or region of bones will have an effect on growth and development of a neighboring bone or region. In other words, a counterpart exists. The two principal parts of the mandible (ramus and corpus) are often considered separately, as each relates to different regions in the face and the cranium. (The corpus counterpart is the anterior cranial base; the ramus counterpart is the middle cranial base.) The corpus is progressively enlarged to match the erupting primary and secondary dentitions and also the hyoid muscles and other soft

tissues attached to it. The ramus enlarges to accommodate the masticatory muscles, airway, oral and nasal mucosae, tongue, salivary glands, tonsils, and pharyngeal muscles. The vertical lengthening of the ramus must match the extent of vertical nasal enlargement. Any uncompensated mismatch between the nasal-ramus relationship may lead to an open bite (Enlow, 1986). Mandibular growth is multidirectional but primarily downward and forward.

The condyle grows in whatever direction and to whatever extent it must to provide a functional occlusal position for the dental arch. Although controversy still exists, many investigators currently hold that the condylar cartilage may not perform an actual primary role

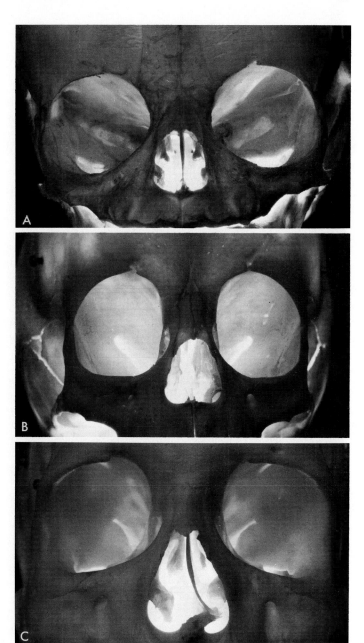

Figure 2–7. Skulls of *(A)* a newborn, *(B)* a child, and *(C)* an adult that have been transilluminated to emphasize the change in the relationship of the floor of the orbit to the floor of the nose. In the newborn and the child, there is little separation; however, in the adult the distance increases because of downward growth and displacement of the floor of the nose and upward growth of the floor of the orbit.

in mandibular growth and development, but rather that it is an important adaptive site of growth (Enlow, 1982). In a study regarding shape change in the mandible during adolescence, Dibbets and colleagues (1987) found further support for the theories that postulate local control factors for mandibular growth. They noted that the growth process of the mandible does not always proceed at a uniform rate for corpus and ramus, concluding that the growing mandible may favor either at any specific time.

Nasomaxillary Complex

The nasomaxillary complex consists of the nasal, lacrimal, maxillary, zygomatic, palatine, and pterygoid bones and the vomer. It can be seen (see Fig. 2–4A)

that this regional complex is closely related to the anterior segment of the cranium formed by the frontal, ethmoid, and sphenoid bones. Any relative forward growth of the anterior cranial base will *carry* the "upper facial region" with it into a more anterior position. Development of the nasomaxillary complex has been the subject of extensive investigation (McNamara, 1976). Although long ago it was observed that growth of these structures occurs downward and forward, the mechanism of such growth has been the subject of debate. The problem has been that it is difficult to design studies in which the variables are effectively controlled (Enlow, 1973). In addition, this is a complex anatomic region that is difficult to visualize from one perspective. Growth in this region occurs in both the horizontal and the vertical planes, and different segments grow at varying rates. This can be appreciated by examining Figure 2–7, which shows the change in configuration and relationship of the orbits and the nasal apertures with age. Figure 2–7A is a photograph of a newborn; Figure 2–7B, a child; and Figure 2–7C, an adult skull; all have been transilluminated so that the changes in density of the bone and the outline of the nasal apertures are more apparent.

The remodeling changes in the orbit are very complex, as many bones are involved, each of which undergoes different amounts of growth and displacement. One of the most marked changes is the difference in the relationship of the floor of the nose to the floor of the orbit. In the newborn, they are almost level, and in the child there is some separation. However, in the adult, there is a marked change due to the downward displacement of the entire maxilla. This change is more complex, as the floor of the orbit it displaced superiorly and the floor of the nose is displaced inferiorly. The change in the bony septum with age is rather dramatic. In the newborn the septum appears straight, and in the adult skull shown, there is marked septal deviation, a common finding. It is interesting that the breadth of the nasal bridge does not increase noticeably from early childhood to adulthood, although the shape of the nasal aperture changes from almost circular to pear shaped—a characteristic that shows marked racial variation.

The biomechanical force for displacement of the nasomaxillary complex is the subject of much controversy. According to Scott (1953), it is due to the expansion of the nasal septum, whereas Latham (1970) believes that it is due to traction on the septopremaxillary ligaments. Early principles noted by van der

Klaauw (1948–1952) were strengthened and advanced by Moss (1962, 1976) as the "functional matrix" theory, which proposes that the genetic determinants of skeletal growth do not reside within the actual bony part itself. That is, the pacemakers of the displacement and the bony remodeling processes occur in the surrounding soft tissue parts. It is important to understand that the functional matrix concept describes essentially what happens during displacement and remodeling but is not intended to explain how this growth happens or what the regulating processes actually are at the tissue and cellular levels.

Another factor that influences the nasomaxillary complex is dentition. There is little evidence in the newborn's jaw of the dental structures that will develop. However, inspection of Figure 2–8, which shows the maxilla and mandible of a child, reveals a palisade of multitiered primary and permanent teeth in many stages of development (Enlow, 1975). The growth and development of teeth and related dental architecture have been studied extensively, and methods of evaluation and modalities of treatment of these structures are discussed in Chapters 50 and 51.

The development of the craniofacial skeleton has been investigated widely by means of standardized cephalometric radiographs. Currently, work is being completed at Children's Hospital of Pittsburgh employing this technique to explore relationships between upper airway obstruction and craniofacial growth. Cephalometric studies have also been undertaken to examine sexual dimorphism in the craniofacial complex. Ingerslev and Solow (1975) found that the cranium was, on the average, smaller in the female than in the male group except as regards the nasal bone, the foramen magnum, and the inner orbital distance. The female group showed a more prominent frontal bone and a less prominent nasal bone than the male group. Bibby (1979) noted that the patterns of craniofacial morphology in males and females appear to be identical except in posterior facial height. In addition, the male skulls were 8.5 per cent larger than the female skulls.

Many factors have been shown to affect craniofacial growth and development (van Limborgh, 1972; Harris et al., 1973; Susanne, 1980; Sinclair, 1985; Schumaker, 1985). A detailed description of each will not be given, but rather Figure 2–9A and B may be studied to obtain an overall view of both the general growth factors and the local factors postulated to influence craniofacial growth. In strong contrast to the many factors known to influence general growth, little information is available concerning the local control mechanisms that guide the growth of the bones and the development of the craniofacial skeleton. Whereas much is known of what happens, little is known about how it happens.

FUNCTIONS OF THE HUMAN CRANIOFACIAL COMPLEX

In these first two chapters, we have discussed prenatal and postnatal development and have alluded to

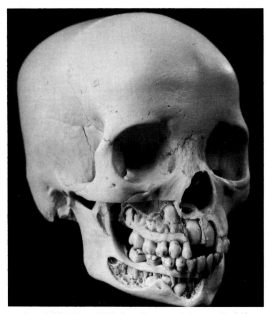

Figure 2–8. Skull of a child that demonstrates a mixed dentition. The multitiered battery of teeth is partially responsible for the increase in the vertical and horizontal dimensions of the jaws with increasing age.

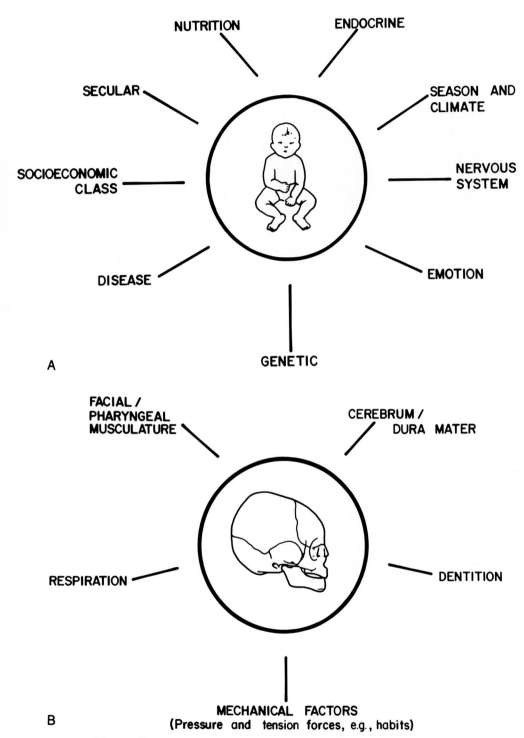

Figure 2–9. *A,* General factors affecting growth and development. *B,* Local factors postulated to affect craniofacial growth.

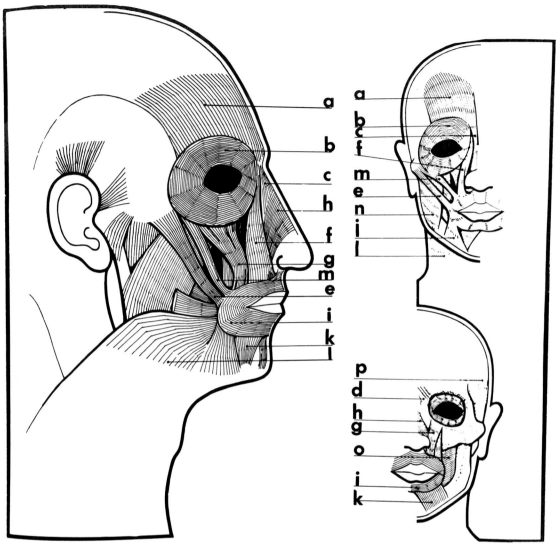

Figure 2–10. The distribution of the facial muscles and the complexity of this musculature are illustrated in this figure. The muscles originate in laminal form and segment into specific muscles, as described by Gasser (1967), a, frontalis; b, orbicularis oculi; c, procerus; d, corrugator; e, zygomaticus major; f, levator labii superioris et alae nasi; g, levator labii; h, compressor naris; i, orbicularis oris; j, depressor anguli oris; k, depressor labii inferioris; l, platysma; m, zygomaticus minor; n, masseter nonexpressive; o, buccinator nonexpressive; p, temporal nonexpressive.

some of the many functions of the craniofacial complex: respiration, olfaction, speech, digestion, hearing, balance, vision, and neural integration. The tissue components of this complex can be classified as skeletal tissue, soft tissue, and functional spaces (nasopharyngeal and oropharyngeal). Space permits only a brief discussion of these functions, but since the musculature is intimately related to skeletal development, it will be discussed in more detail.

EYE. One of the most salient elements of human evolution has been the development of vision as a dominant sense. It was this sense that enabled primitive humans to survive as a species and to develop our present state of technology. The development of binocular vision enabled humans to evolve a system of eye-hand coordination that their increased cerebral function can utilize.

EAR. The ear has the dual functions of hearing and balance. The balance mechanism is of earlier phylogenetic development and is represented by paired organs that are connected to the brain. Hearing is a person's most important contact with his or her environment, for without adequate hearing, speech and communication will not develop.

NOSE. The sense of smell, which is of such importance in the lower animals, is one of the less important basic functions in humans. However, the conditioning of inhaled air and the provision of a nasal airway are two important functions of the nose in respiration.

MOUTH. As the initial portion of the digestive tract, the mouth has a vital function, and, although it may be temporarily bypassed by artificial means, the ultimate growth and development of the organism will be affected if the anatomy of this area is altered.

Speech, which utilizes both the air and food passages, is a relatively recent phylogenetic function.

However, for the human, speech is one of the major achievements and represents the most important means of communication and expression. The neuromuscular functions of the craniofacial complex are concerned with both the aesthetic and the expressive functions of the face. The human face covers a highly complicated skeletal framework with extremely flexible and expressive soft tissue. It is capable of an amazing number of motions and has the ability to convey emotion. Since the face is not covered, even slight facial deformities may be difficult to conceal and can seriously affect the appearance, and thus the interpersonal relationships, of a child. This was expressed beautifully by Charles Bell in 1821.

> The human countenance performs many functions—in it we have combined the organs of mastication, of breathing, of natural voice and speech, and of expression. These motions are performed directly by the will; here also are seen signs of emotions, over which we have but a very limited or imperfect control; the face serves for the lowest animal enjoyment, and partakes of the highest and most refined emotions.

The distribution of the facial musculature is illustrated in Figure 2–10, which demonstrates the relationship of the various facial muscle masses. Facial movements that occur during fetal life were described by Hooker (1939) and have been discussed in detail by Humphrey (1970).

At birth, the infant's musculature is primarily involved with the functions of suckling and swallowing. The airway is maintained, and there are primitive facial reflexes that provide some expression. Experiments have shown that there are responses to taste such as sweet and sour (Steiner, 1973). Early postnatal facial expressions are largely imitations, but most of the facial muscles are used for mandibular stabilization and airway functions. During subsequent postnatal growth and development, there will be tremendous changes in the facial neuromusculature. According to Enlow (1975), more attention has been given to the study of the growth of the craniofacial skeleton than to the neuromusculature. One of the reasons for this is that it is much more difficult to study the neuromusculature of the face than it is to study bone structures of the face; consequently, we know less about the facial and jaw muscles and are less certain of what we do know than we are about the knowledge of bones and teeth.

During the early periods of embryonic growth, an intimate functional relationship exists between the muscles and the bones to which they are attached. Obviously, when the bones grow, the muscles also must change their size and shape. As a consequence, the muscles occupy different positions, and there is constant adjustment in the attachments of muscles to the skeleton. For instance, changes in the vertical dimensions of the skull will result in a reorientation of the angles at the musculoosseous junctions.

The influence of the facial musculature on skeletal growth will depend on the region involved. Since the most powerful of the facial muscles are involved with mastication, the influence of musculature on the dentition and especially on the mandible will be considerable. Muscles of the airway and food passages compete for influence with the tongue, one of the most powerful muscles of the head.

As a final comment on postnatal craniofacial growth and development, just as the embryo begins as an undifferentiated cell mass, the newborn appears as an undifferentiated craniofacial complex. Because of differential growth, highly developed individual characteristics will appear as the newborn matures. In the skeleton, osteoblastic and osteoclastic activity lead to bone deposition, resorption, and displacement. The stimuli for alterations in skeletal development are both genetic and environmental, and it is a balance of these two factors that is responsible for the ultimate craniofacial configuration. The functions of the craniofacial complex, the most characteristic of which in humans are binocular vision (so important in eye-hand coordination), speech, and an infinite variety of facial expressions, have evolved over millions of years. It is understandable that we should desire to know more about this very important area of development, but it is also obvious why study of the craniofacial complex involves deep concentration and unusual effort to yield results.

SELECTED REFERENCES

Dorst, J. P. 1971. Changes of the skull during childhood. *In* Newton, T. H., and Potts, D. G. (eds.): Radiology of the Skull and Brain, Vol. 1. St. Louis, The C. V. Mosby Co.
This is a concise description of skeletal growth during childhood; it also discusses some cranial abnormalities.
Enlow, D. H. 1982. Handbook of Craniofacial Growth. 2nd ed. Philadelphia, W. B. Saunders Co.
This well-organized text illustrates the various growth concepts and also includes an extensive bibliography.
Rubin, P. 1964. Dynamic Classification of Bone Dysplasias. Chicago, Yearbook Medical Publishers, Inc.
This book describes some of the anomalies of the craniofacial complex and also discusses the growth mechanisms by which they occur.
Sullivan, P. G. 1986. Skull, jaw, and teeth growth patterns. *In* Falkner, F., and Tanner, J. M. (eds.): Human Growth, Vol. 2, Postnatal Growth. New York, Plenum Press, pp. 243–268.
This well-written chapter discusses in detail the differential growth of the skull and jaw.

REFERENCES

Babula, W. J., Smiley, G. R., and Dixon, A. D. 1970. The role of the cartilaginous nasal septum. Am. J. Orthod. 58:250.
Bassett, A. H. 1972. The biophysical approach to craniofacial morphogenesis. Acta Morphol. Neerl. Scand. 10:71.
Behrents, R. G. 1985. Growth in the aging craniofacial skeleton. Craniofacial Growth Series, Monograph No. 17. Ann Arbor, MI, Center for Human Growth and Development. University of Michigan.
Bell, C. 1833. The nervous system of the human body. Papers delivered to the Royal Society on the Subject of the Nerves. Stereotyped by Duff Green, for the Register and Library of Medical and Chirurgical Science.
Bibby, R. E. 1979. A cephalometric study of sexual dimorphism. Am. J. Orthod. 76:256.

Bosma, J. (ed.). 1976. Symposium on the Development of the Basicranium. Bethesda, MD, U.S. Dept. of Health, Education and Welfare. DHEW Pub. No. (NIH) 76–989.

Canalis, E. 1983. The hormonal and local regulation of bone formation. Endocr. Rev. 4:62.

Centrella, M., and Canalis, E. 1985. Local regulators of skeletal growth: A perspective. Endocr. Rev. 6:544.

Cohen, M. M. 1986. Craniosynostosis: Diagnosis, Evaluation, and Management. New York, Raven Press.

Dibbets, J. M., deBruin, R., and Van der Weele, L. 1987. Shape change in the mandible during adolescence. In Carlson, D. S., and Ribbens, K. A.: Craniofacial Growth During Adolescence. Craniofacial Growth Series, Monograph No. 20. pp. 69–85. Ann Arbor, MI, Center for Human Growth and Development. University of Michigan.

Dorst, J. P. 1971. Changes of the skull during childhood. In Newton, T. H., and Potts, D. G. (eds.): Radiology of the Skull and Brain, Vol. 1. St. Louis, The C. V. Mosby Co.

Enlow, D. H. 1973. Growth and the problem of the local antral mechanism. Am. J. Anat. 178:2.

Enlow, D. H. 1975. Handbook of Craniofacial Growth. Philadelphia, W. B. Saunders Co.

Enlow, D. H. 1981. Postnatal facial growth. In Forrester, D. J., Wagner, M. L., and Fleming, J. (eds.): Pediatric Dental Medicine. Philadelphia, Lea & Febiger, pp. 40–54.

Enlow, D. H. 1986. Normal Craniofacial Growth. In Cohen, M. M. (ed.): Craniosynostosis: Diagnosis, Evaluation, and Management. New York, Raven Press, pp. 131–156.

Gasser, R. F. 1967. The development of the facial muscles in man. Am. J. Anat. 120:357.

Hamersma, H., and May, M. 1986. Osteopetrosis and facial palsy. In May, M. (ed.): The Facial Nerve. New York, Thieme Inc., pp. 469–483.

Harris, J. E., Kowalski, C. J., and Watnick, S. S. 1973. Genetic factors in the shape of the craniofacial complex. Angle Orthod. 43:107.

Hogarth, B. 1965. Drawing the Human Head, 9th ed. New York, Watson-Guptill Publications.

Hooker, D. 1939. Fetal behavior. Association for Research in Nervous and Mental Disease XIX. Interrelationship of Mind and Body, pp. 237–243, Baltimore, Williams & Wilkins Co.

Humphrey, T. 1970. Reflex activity in the oral and facial area of the human fetus. In Bosma, J. (ed.): Second Symposium on Oral Sensation and Perception. Springfield, IL, Charles C Thomas Pub.

Ingerslev, C. H., and Solow, B. 1975. Sex differences in craniofacial morphology. Acta Odont. Scand. 33:85.

Israel, H. 1967. Loss of bone and remodeling—redistribution in the craniofacial skeleton with age. Fed. Proc. 26:1723.

Israel, H. 1968. Continuing growth in the human cranial skeleton. Arch. Oral Biol. 13:133.

Israel, H. 1973. Age factor and the pattern of change in craniofacial structures. Am. J. Phys. Anthropol. 39:111.

Israel, H. 1977. The dichotomous pattern of craniofacial expansion during aging. Am. J. Phys. Anthropol. 47:47.

Koski, K. 1981. Mechanisms of craniofacial skeletal growth. In Barrer, H. G. (ed.): Orthodontics: The State of the Art. Philadelphia, University of Pennsylvania Press, pp. 209–222.

Latham, R. A. 1970. Maxillary development and growth: The septomaxillary ligament. J. Anat. 107:471.

Ligett, J. 1974. The Human Face. London, Constable & Co., Ltd.

McNamara, J. 1976. Factors Affecting the Growth of the Midface. Craniofacial Growth Series, Monograph No. 6. Ann Arbor, MI, Center for Human Growth and Development. University of Michigan.

Moss, M. L. 1962. The functional matrix. In Kraus, B. S., and Riedel, R. A. (eds.): Vistas in Orthodontics. Philadelphia, Lea & Febiger, pp. 85–98.

Moss, M. L. 1968. The primacy of functional matrices in one facial growth. Dent. Pract. Dent. Rec. 19:65.

Moss, M. L. 1976. The role of the nasal septal cartilage in midfacial growth. In McNamara, J. A. (ed.): Factors Affecting the Growth of the Midface. Craniofacial Growth Series, Monograph No. 6., pp. 169–204. Ann Arbor, MI, Center for Human Growth and Development. University of Michigan.

Moss, M. L., and Salentijn, L. 1969. The primary role of functional matrices in facial growth. Am. J. Orthod. 55:566.

Pierce, R., et al. 1977. The Cranium of the Newborn Infant. Bethesda, MD, U.S. Dept. of Health, Education and Welfare, DHEW Pub. No. (NIH) 76–788.

Raisz, L., and Kream, B. 1983. Regulation of Bone Formation. N. Engl. J. Med. 309:83.

Rubin P. 1964. The Dynamic Classification of Bone Dysplasias. Chicago, Yearbook Medical Publishers, Inc.

Schumaker, G. H. 1985. Factors influencing craniofacial growth. In Dixon, A. D., and Sarnat, B. G. (eds.): Normal and Abnormal Bone Growth: Basic and Clinical Research. New York, Alan R. Liss, Inc., pp. 3–22.

Scott, J. A. 1953. The cartilage of the nasal septum. Br. Dent. J. 95:37.

Sinclair, D. 1985. Human Growth after Birth. 4th ed. Oxford, Oxford University Press, pp. 148–169.

Sokoloff, L., and Bland, J. 1975. The Musculoskeletal System. Baltimore, Williams & Wilkins Co.

Steiner, J. 1973. The gustofacial response: Observations on normal and anencephalic infants. In Bosma, J. (ed.): Oral Sensation and Perception. Bethesda, MD, U.S. Dept. of Health, Education, and Welfare, DHEW Pub. No. (NIH) 73–546.

Sullivan, P. G. 1986. Skull, jaw, and teeth growth patterns. In Falkner, F., and Tanner, J.M. (eds.): Human Growth, Vol. 2, Postnatal Growth. New York, Plenum Press, pp. 243–268.

Susanne, C. 1980. Developmental genetics of man. In Johnston, F. E., Roche, A. F., and Susanne, C. (eds.): Human Physical Growth and Maturation: Methodologies and Factors. New York, Plenum Press, pp. 221–242.

van der Klaauw, C. J. 1948–1952. Size and position of the functional components of the skull. Arch. Neerl. Zool. 9:1.

van Limborgh, J. 1972. The role of genetic and local environmental factors in the control of postnatal craniofacial morphogenesis. Acta Morphol. Neerl. Scand. 10:37.

Williams, P. L., et al. 1969. Basic Human Embryology. 2nd ed. Philadelphia, J. B. Lippincott Co.

Chapter 3

CRANIOFACIAL ANOMALIES AND SYNDROMES

M. Michael Cohen, Jr., D.M.D., Ph.D.   **Sylvan E. Stool, M.D.**

William A. Marasovich, D.D.S., M.D.

The first two chapters of this text have discussed normal prenatal and postnatal growth and development and have mentioned how alterations in these processes may result in abnormalities. In this chapter, we will discuss some of the current concepts regarding genesis of the abnormalities that are seen by the physician who is interested in ear, nose, and throat disorders in children. This vast and complex field encompasses the concepts of a number of disciplines, such as embryology, chemistry, molecular biology, and genetics, and information is increasing at such a rapid rate that it is not possible for any text to remain current. However, several general principles have now been well-established that will enable the physician to develop an orderly approach to the evaluation of the abnormal child. Even though there are great variations among individuals with abnormal characteristics, those individuals with syndrome complexes by definition will resemble each other more than each will resemble the normal members of his or her family.

Progress in describing errors of morphogenesis has been hindered by difficulties with nomenclature. To clarify various concepts, an international working group (Spranger et al., 1982) recommended the definitions in Table 3–1 to describe individual alterations of form or structure. In studying patterns of morphologic defects, the terms in Table 3–2 have been suggested to describe the types of relationships between abnormalities observed in an individual. Each reflects a different level of knowledge on the causation and genesis of the pattern.

EPIDEMIOLOGY OF DEVELOPMENTAL DEFECTS

Many epidemiologic studies of congenital malformations have been undertaken, based on either retrospective (birth records, death certificates, or questionnaires) or prospective data. Persaud (1985) notes that because of varying terminology and differences in diagnostic criteria, it is seldom possible to compare the results of these studies. Moreover, because of

these discrepancies in definition and terminology, the frequency of occurrence reported may vary considerably (Kennedy, 1974; Leck, 1977; Rumeau-Rouquette et al., 1980). Similarly, confounding variables become apparent when studying the prevalence of malformations in different ethnic groups. Young (1987) notes that when comparing ethnic differences in prevalence within a large community, allowance should be made for differences in antenatal care, diet, maternal age and parity, social class, and occupation.

In most retrospective studies, the population sample is uncontrolled. Hospital records are often inadequate or incomplete, leading to those cases being rejected. Thus, the resultant sample to be analyzed becomes biased. Persaud (1985) notes that, for these reasons, the overall frequency of congenital malformations reported might be of limited value unless carefully planned prospective studies are undertaken.

Kennedy (1974) presented one of the most comprehensive reviews of the world literature on the fre-

TABLE 3–1. Definitions to Describe Individual Alterations of Form or Structure

MALFORMATION

A malformation is a morphologic defect of an organ, a part of an organ, or a larger region of the body resulting from an intrinsically abnormal developmental process.

Examples

Cleft lip and palate, septal defects of the heart, polydactyly.

DISRUPTION

A disruption is a morphologic defect of an organ, a part of an organ, or a larger region of the body resulting from the extrinsic breakdown of, or an interference with, an originally normal developmental process.

Example

Phocomelia seen in thalidomide embryopathy.

DEFORMATION

A deformation is an abnormal form, shape, or position of a part of the body caused by mechanical forces.

Examples

Congenital torticollis, clubfoot associated with oligohydramnios, plagiocephaly.

TABLE 3–2. Suggested Terms to Describe the Types of Relationships between Abnormalities Observed in an Individual

SEQUENCE*

A sequence is a pattern of *multiple* anomalies derived from a single known or presumed prior anomaly or mechanical factor.

Examples

Robin sequence, which causes failure of tongue descent, thought to be the result of a hypoplastic mandible or one that is small by intrauterine constraint; arthrogryposis caused by intrauterine limitation of fetal movement; and the Potter sequence, resulting from oligohydramnios.

SYNDROME

A syndrome is a pattern of *multiple* anomalies thought to be pathogenetically related and not known to represent a single sequence.

Example

Down syndrome.

ASSOCIATION

An association is a nonrandom occurrence in two or more individuals of multiple anomalies not known to be a sequence or a syndrome.

Examples

CHARGE association, VATER association.

*The term *sequence* conveys the same basic concept for which *anomalad* or *complex* had been used in the past.

quency and geographic distribution of congenital malformations. Reporting more than 20 million births (including the records of 238 studies), the overall percentage of congenital malformations was found to range from 1.08 (data obtained from hospital records, birth certificates, and retrospective questionnaires) to 4.50 (intensive examination of the children).

Polani (1973) estimated that at least 6 per cent of all newborns show genetic (2 per cent) or developmental (4 per cent) defects. Major malformations are present in at least 2 per cent of all live-born infants, and such malformations account for approximately 20 per cent of all neonatal deaths. Not unexpectedly, the high frequency of developmental defects among neonatal deaths is a consistent observation in other related studies (Buckfield, 1973; Harris et al., 1975; Norman, 1984).

Myrianthopoulos (1985) refined an earlier analysis of the Collaborative Perinatal Study data (Myrianthopoulos and Chung, 1974) and reported that significantly more children had malformations from ages 1 to 7 years than through the first year of life. Tuchmann-Duplessis (1975) reported that in western countries the prevalence of obvious malformations at birth was estimated at 2 to 3 per cent and 4 to 6 per cent after a follow-up period of two years because of cardiovascular, renal, and central nervous system anomalies that only later became evident.

In examining sex differences in the prevalence of malformations, this same study (Myrianthopoulos, 1985) reported that males are more often malformed and have significantly more single and multiple, as well as major and minor, malformations than do fe-

males. Among malformations with a frequency of five or more per 10,000 births, 12 major and 8 minor malformations are significantly more frequent in males than in females, whereas only three major and no minor malformations are significantly more frequent in females than in males. Regarding racial differences in malformations, Myrianthopoulos (1985) found a higher prevalence of malformations in blacks than in whites. This difference was entirely due to a higher frequency among blacks of a few minor malformations, specifically polydactyly, branchial arch anomalies, and pigmentation defects. There is no difference between blacks and whites in the prevalence of major malformations, and whites have a significantly higher prevalence of multiple malformations than do blacks.

Congenital anomalies were the fifth leading cause of years of potential life lost (YPLL) before age 65 in both 1985 and 1984. The leading cause of premature mortality was congenital anomalies of the cardiovascular system, such as transposition of the great vessels, followed by the nervous and respiratory systems, respectively. It has been noted that YPLL statistics do understate the full public health impact of congenital anomalies, as anomalies in infants who die shortly after birth may not be diagnosed. Therefore, the infants' deaths are not attributed to congenital anomalies. Perhaps more important, YPLL statistics are based only on live-born infants. This leads to underestimation because a substantial number of babies with anomalies are stillborn, and even a greater number of malformed fetuses are aborted spontaneously (MMWR, 1987). Boué and colleagues (1975) found that more than 60 per cent of 1498 abortuses (younger than 12 weeks of age) were associated with chromosomal anomalies.

SYNDROMES

The word "syndrome" is of Greek derivation and means "running together." Minimally, a syndrome is viewed as several abnormalities in the same individual. One of the misconceptions about this term relates to the logic that many use when they see a unique patient. They do not acknowledge that a single patient can represent a syndrome. This is the same as saying that if you were the first person to see an aardvark, the animal could not exist until a herd of aardvarks was found. The conclusion is obvious; a syndrome can exist with a single patient (Fig. 3–1 A and B).

Syndrome Delineation

Because craniofacial anomalies are associated with a great many syndromes, the physician who treats children may see a wide variety of anomalies, many of which are not readily recognized as being associated with any one syndrome. The process of syndrome delineation can be divided into stages (Cohen, 1977, 1982) (Table 3–3). In a large study of newborn infants with multiple anomalies of all kinds (syndromes), only

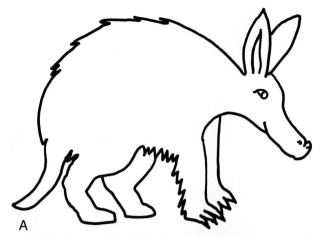

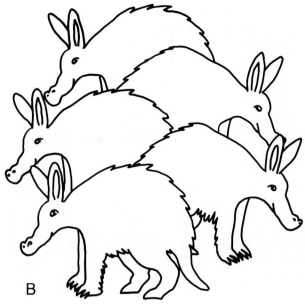

Figure 3–1. *A* and *B*, The aardvark is an unusual-appearing animal. If you subscribe to the school that says it takes more than one case to make a syndrome, then the presence of a single animal cannot be explained. Obviously, you can have a syndrome with a single patient.

40 per cent had known, recognized syndromes (Marden et al., 1964). The other 60 per cent had provisionally unique-pattern syndromes that needed to be further delineated. A major task in medicine is to delineate the unknown-genesis syndromes as rapidly as possible because such delineation fosters good patient care. As an unknown-genesis syndrome becomes delineated, its phenotypic spectrum, its natural history, and its risk of recurrence become known, allowing for better patient care and family counseling. The process of syndrome delineation also aids in the study of pathogenesis by sorting anomalies into meaningful biologic categories (Cohen, 1982).

In an *unknown-genesis syndrome* (Type A) the cause is simply not known. In a *provisionally unique-pattern syndrome* (Type A-1), two or more abnormalities are observed in the same patient in such a way that the clinician does not recognize the overall pattern of defects from his or her own experience, or from searching the literature, or from consultation with the most learned colleagues in the field. The patient shown in Figure 3–2 has a provisionally unique-pattern syndrome. This baby has craniosynostosis involving the sagittal suture, as well as prominent veins, strabismus, micrognathia, an umbilical hernia, complete anterior

TABLE 3–3. Syndrome Delineation

TYPE

A	Unknown-genesis syndrome
	A-1 Provisionally unique-pattern syndrome
	A-2 Recurrent-pattern syndrome
B	Known-genesis syndrome
	B-1 Pedigree syndrome
	B-2 Chromosomal syndrome
	B-3 Biochemical-defect syndrome
	B-4 Environmentally induced syndrome

Data from Cohen, M. M., Jr. 1982. The Child with Multiple Birth Defects. New York, Raven Press.

dislocation of the tibia, and deformed feet. It is more likely that these abnormalities have a common cause (even though we do not yet know what that is) than that they are caused by different factors acting independently. The probability that such abnormalities occur in the same patient by chance becomes less likely the more abnormalities the patient has and the rarer these abnormalities are individually in the general population. Obviously, if a second example comes to light, the condition is no longer unique. A provisionally unique-pattern syndrome is a one-of-a-kind syndrome to a particular observer at a particular point in time (Cohen, 1977).

The next stage in syndrome delineation is the *recurrent-pattern syndrome* (Type A-2). A recurrent-pattern syndrome can be defined as a similar or identical set of abnormalities in two or more unrelated patients. A recurrent-pattern syndrome is illustrated in Figure 3–3. These two patients from different families share a wide bifrontal diameter, ocular hypertelorism, large ears, micrognathia, finger contractures at the proximal interphalangeal joints, deeply set fingernails, umbilical hernias, excessive growth, and a variety of other abnormalities. The presence of the same abnormalities in two or more patients suggests (but does not prove) that the pathogenesis in both cases is the same. At the recurrent-pattern stage of syndrome delineation, the etiology is still unknown. In general, the validity of a recurrent-pattern syndrome increases the more abnormalities there are in the condition and the more patients who are known to have the syndrome (Cohen, 1977).

A *known-genesis syndrome* (Type B) can be defined as two or more abnormalities causally related on the basis of (1) occurrence in the same family or, less conclusively, the same mode of inheritance in different families; (2) a chromosomal defect; (3) a specific defect in an enzyme or structural protein; or (4) a teratogen or environmental factor (Cohen, 1977). These four

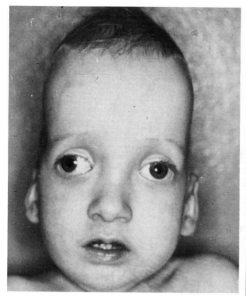

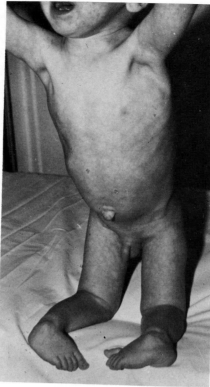

Figure 3–2. Provisionally unique-pattern syndrome. Craniosynostosis involving the sagittal suture, prominent veins, strabismus, micrognathia, and other extracephalic abnormalities. (From Cohen, M. M., Jr. 1977. Genetic perspectives on craniosynostosis and syndromes with craniosynostosis. J. Neurosurg. 47:886.)

types of known-genesis syndromes have been respectively termed pedigree, chromosomal, biochemical-defect, and environmentally induced syndromes.

A *pedigree syndrome* (Type B-1) is of known genesis on the basis of pedigree evidence alone. The basic defect itself remains undefined, although the condition is known to represent a monogenic disorder. A good example is the Treacher Collins syndrome (Fig. 3–4).

A *chromosomal syndrome* (Type B-2) is cytogenetically defined and may be typified by the trisomy 13 syndrome (Fig. 3–5). This condition is characterized by holoprosencephaly, microphthalmia, posterior scalp defects, forehead hemangiomas, orofacial clefting, polydactyly, hyperconvex fingernails, cardiac defects, and many other abnormalities (Cohen, 1982).

In a *biochemical-defect syndrome* (Type B-3), specific enzymatic defects are known in recessive syndromes. The term is also meant to include specific defects in structural proteins when these become known in some of the dominant disorders. The Lesch-Nyhan syndrome (Fig. 3–6), characterized by

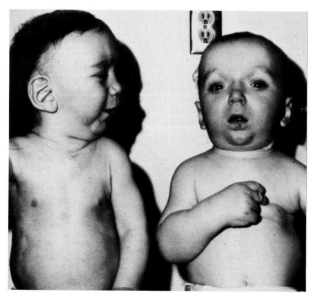

Figure 3–3. Recurrent-pattern syndrome in two patients. Note wide bifrontal diameter, ocular hypertelorism, large ears, long philtrum, and micrognathia. (From Weaver, D. D., et al. 1974. A new overgrowth syndrome with accelerated skeletal maturation, unusual facies, and camptodactyly. J. Pediatr. 84:547.)

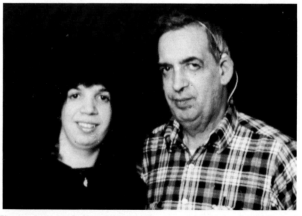

Figure 3–4. A father and daughter with Treacher Collins syndrome. This is a pedigree autosomal dominant syndrome with high penetrance and marked variability in expressivity. Note the downward slanting palpebral fissures, micrognathia, and the father's use of a hearing aid. Audiometric tests show a nonprogressive conductive hearing loss.

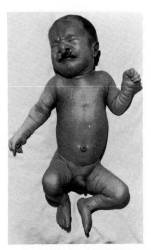

Figure 3–5. Trisomy 13 syndrome. (With permission from Smith, D. W., Patau, K., Therman, E., et al. 1963. The D-1 trisomy syndrome. J. Pediatr. 62:326–341.)

hypoxanthine-guanine-phosphoribosyl-transferase deficiency, is an X-linked recessive biochemical-defect syndrome (Cohen, 1982).

An *environmentally induced syndrome* (Type B-4) is defined in terms of the causative teratogen or environmental factor. Infants born to mothers who are chronic alcoholics during their pregnancies have an increased risk of having growth deficiency of prenatal onset persisting into postnatal life, microcephaly, mental deficiency, narrow palpebral fissures, mild maxillary hypoplasia, short nose (Fig. 3–7), cardiac malformations, and other anomalies (Cohen, 1982).

Comments

The process of syndrome delineation is summarized in Figure 3–8. Generally, a syndrome can be placed

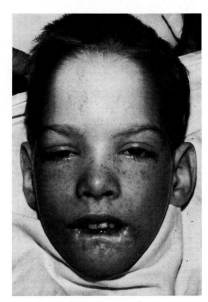

Figure 3–6. Biochemical-defect syndrome of the enzymatic type. Lesch-Nyhan syndrome with enzymatic defect in purine metabolism that leads to self-mutilation of lips. (From Cohen, M. M., Jr. 1982. The Child with Multiple Birth Defects. New York, Raven Press.)

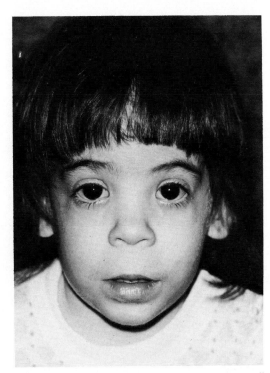

Figure 3–7. Known-genesis syndrome of the environmentally induced type. Fetal alcohol syndrome. Note microcephaly, narrow palpebral fissures, mild maxillary hypoplasia, and short nose. (From Clarren, S. K., and Smith, D. W. 1978. The fetal alcohol syndrome. N. Engl. J. Med. 289:1063. Reprinted, by permission of The New England Journal of Medicine.)

into one of the categories discussed previously. Occasionally, a syndrome may be delineated in a one-step delineation, thus bypassing several of the stages mentioned earlier. For example, if a new chromosomal abnormality is discovered during the laboratory investigation of a patient clinically defined as having a provisionally unique-pattern syndrome, the patient represents a known-genesis syndrome of the chromosomal type in a one-step delineation. However, the variability of the clinical expression must await the discovery of more patients with that syndrome. In other instances, such as a large dominant pedigree with many affected individuals, a known-genesis syndrome of the pedigree type and much of its phenotypic variability can be determined in one step (Cohen, 1982, 1986).

Figure 3–8 makes reference to an association. An association is defined as a nonrandom occurrence in two or more individuals of multiple anomalies not known to be a sequence or syndrome. An example is the CHARGE association (Dobrowski et al., 1985; Goldson et al., 1986).

Significance

The significance of syndrome delineation cannot be overestimated. If the phenotypic spectrum is known, the clinician can search for suspected defects that may not be apparent immediately but that may produce clinical problems at a later date, such as a hemivertebra in the Goldenhar syndrome (Cohen and Rollnick, 1989) (Fig. 3–9). If a certain complication may occur in a

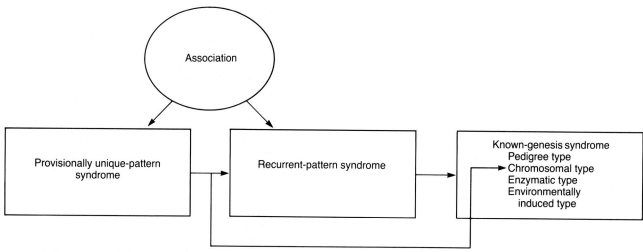

Figure 3–8. Diagram of the process of syndrome delineation. See text. (With permission from Cohen, M. M., Jr. 1982. The Child with Multiple Birth Defects. New York, Raven Press, p. 46.)

given syndrome, such as a Wilms tumor in the Beckwith-Wiedemann syndrome, the clinician is forewarned to monitor the patient with intravenous pyelograms. Finally, if the recurrence risk is known, the parents can be counseled properly about future pregnancies. This is especially important if the risk is high and the disorder is severely handicapping or disfiguring, has mental deficiency as one component, or entails a dramatically shortened life span. For example, cleft palate or the Robin sequence is a common feature of the Stickler syndrome, an autosomal dominant disorder with a 50 per cent recurrence risk when one parent is affected. In this condition, retinal detachment occurs in 20 per cent of reported cases, and blindness occurs in 15 per cent. Genetic counseling is of great importance because the risk of developing serious ocular problems is high. This relatively common condition also illustrates the importance of syndrome delineation because the entity was unrecognized before 1965, although surely it existed before that time (Fig. 3–10).

The Robin sequence consists of micrognathia, cleft

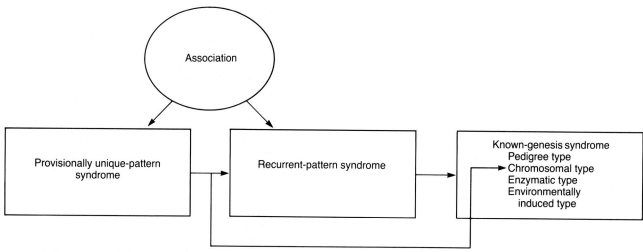

Figure 3–9. An infant with oculoauriculovertebral dysplasia (Goldenhar syndrome). There are multiple obvious facial defects. This cluster should alert the clinician that there are cryptic anomalies of the vertebrae that may later become symptomatic.

palate, and glossoptosis. The terminology has undergone a number of changes. First, the condition was considered a syndrome, then an anomalad; currently, it is considered a sequence. It is an important group of anomalies for the pediatric otolaryngologist, as affected patients often have difficulty with the airway. It is obvious that this group of findings is related to a number of conditions (Table 3–4). The different etiologies and pathogenetic mechanisms are summarized in Figure 3–11.

Thus, syndrome delineation fosters good patient care; the overall treatment program gains rationality. In contrast, with a provisionally unique-pattern syndrome, the treatment program and overall manage-

TABLE 3–4. Conditions Associated with the Robin Sequence

MONOGENIC SYNDROMES
Beckwith-Wiedemann syndrome
Camptomelic syndrome
Cerebrocostomandibular syndrome
Diastrophic dysplasia
Donlan syndrome
Myotonic dystrophy
Persistent left superior vena cava syndrome
Radiohumeral synostosis syndrome
Spondyloepiphyseal dysplasia congenita
Stickler syndrome

CHROMOSOMAL SYNDROMES
dup (11q) syndrome

TERATOGENICALLY INDUCED SYNDROMES
Fetal alcohol syndrome
Fetal hydantoin syndrome
Fetal trimethadione syndrome

UNKNOWN-GENESIS SYNDROMES
Digitopalatal syndrome
Femoral dysgenesis–unusual facies syndrome
Martsolf syndrome
Robin-amelia syndrome

Modified and updated from Cohen, M. M., Jr. 1976. The Robin anomalad—its nonspecificity and associated syndromes. J. Oral Surg. 34:587–593.

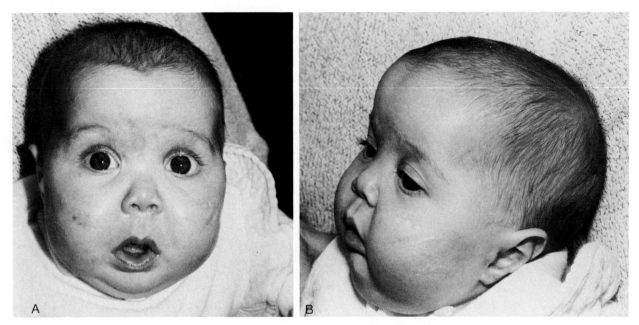

Figure 3–10. Identical twins with Stickler syndrome. In addition to the Robin sequence, there are cranial nerve abnormalities.

ment frequently leave something to be desired (Cohen, 1982, 1986).

Biologic Types of Syndromes and Syndrome Models

Syndromes can be analyzed at different levels of organization. In the broadest possible context, there are perhaps four general classes of syndromes: dysmetabolic syndromes, dyshistogenetic syndromes, malformation syndromes, and deformation syndromes. They represent disturbances in metabolism, tissues, organs, and regions, respectively. The four types of syndromes and their relationships are illustrated by the inverted triangle shown in Figure 3–12. It will be

observed that the syndromes are stratified. For example, a malformation syndrome has dyshistogenetic and dysmetabolic levels underlying it. However, the syndrome expresses itself at the organ formation level (Cohen, 1982).

The four different syndrome models and their characteristics are summarized in Table 3–5 and will be discussed in detail in the following section. The term syndrome model is used to convey the notion that not necessarily every finding in a given syndrome can be accounted for. In fact, the power of any model is that it is an abstract conception, and, as such, it can ignore some of the realities in the same manner as the law of gravity ignores friction. "Science," says the noted philosopher Morris Cohen, "must abstract some phenomena and neglect others because not all things that

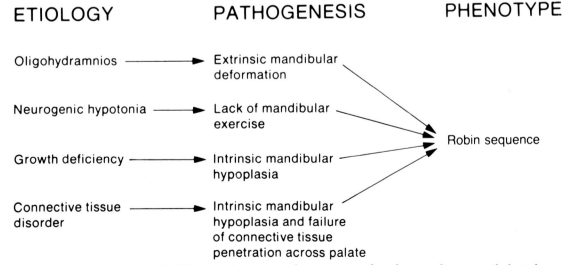

Figure 3–11. Several possible etiologies with different pathogenetic mechanisms can produce the anomalies seen with the Robin sequence. (With permission from Cohen, M. M., Jr. 1979. Syndromology's message for craniofacial biology. J. Maxillofacial Surg. 7:89–109.)

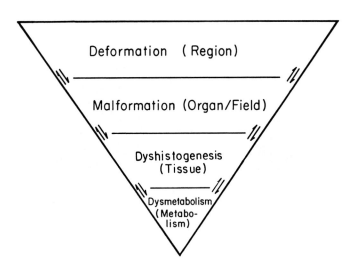

Figure 3–12. Stratification of syndromes into dysmetabolic, dys-histogenetic, malformation, and deformation syndromes that represent expression at the metabolic, tissue, organ, and regional levels, respectively. (From Cohen, M. M., Jr. 1982. The Child with Multiple Birth Defects. New York, Raven Press.)

TABLE 3–5. Syndrome Prototypes

TYPE	LEVEL OF DISTURBANCE	FEATURES	EXAMPLES
Dysmetabolic syndrome	Metabolism	Frequently normal at birth with generalized progressive disturbances after birth Clinical features relatively uniform compared with other types of syndromes Not associated with congenital malformations Biochemically defined or potentially so Commonly recessive mode of inheritance	Hurler syndrome, Lesch-Nyhan syndrome, Tay-Sachs disease

Dyshistogenetic syndrome	Tissues	Simple dyshistogenetic syndrome
		  Characterized by involvement of only one germ layer
		  Inheritance may be dominant or recessive
			Marfan syndrome, achondroplasia

		Hamartoneoplastic syndrome
		  Characterized by hamartomas, hyperplasia, and a propensity for neoplasia
		  May involve one, two, or all three germ layers
		  Inheritance is commonly dominant
			Gardner syndrome, Peutz-Jeghers syndrome

Malformation syndrome	Organs/fields	Several noncontiguous malformations in the same patient Characterized by embryonic pleiotropy in which the several malformation sequences are developmentally unrelated at the embryonic level Lack of biochemical definition; highest state of definition is a known-genesis syndrome of the chromosomal or pedigree type	Trisomy 13 syndrome, Meckel syndrome, Rubinstein-Taybi syndrome
Deformation syndrome	Regions	Characterized by alterations in the shape or structure of previously normal parts Most important cause is lack of fetal movement whether the cause be a mechanical, functional, or malformational disturbance Commonly affects musculoskeletal system	Potter sequence based on a nonmalformational cause such as amniotic rupture; Rosenmann-Arad syndrome*

*Most multiple deformations are based on malformational or deformational sequences.
With permission from Cohen, M. M., Jr. 1982. The Child with Multiple Birth Defects. New York, Raven Press.

exist together are relevant together." Thus, the models provide us with a framework for analyzing various types of syndromes by giving us convenient points from which to move in our thinking. Some syndromes closely fit the proposed models; others have features that overlap one model and another (Cohen, 1982).

Dysmetabolic Syndromes

Dysmetabolic syndromes are characterized by inborn errors of metabolism. Metabolism is carried out as a stepwise series of reactions, each step being catalyzed by a specific enzyme. The pathway may be blocked at any step, either completely or partially, by impaired activity of the required enzyme resulting from a mutation in the gene that codes for the normal enzyme. Enzymatic blocks have various consequences: (1) A precursor substance may accumulate just proximal to the block and may itself be harmful; (2) a usually minor pathway may become active, resulting in overproduction of toxic metabolites; (3) the deficient product itself may be a substrate for a subsequent reaction, which cannot proceed because of insufficient quantities of substrate; and (4) a feedback inhibition type of control mechanism may be impaired because of an enzymatic block (Cohen, 1982, 1986).

The clinical manifestations of dysmetabolic syndromes depend upon the particular metabolic pathway involved, the availability of alternative pathways, the solubility of metabolites, the particular organ systems involved, and a variety of other factors. A typical example of a dysmetabolic syndrome is the Hurler syndrome—an autosomal recessive disorder characterized by alpha-L-iduronidase deficiency, which inhibits degradation of alpha-L-iduronide–containing mucopolysaccharides. Accumulation of undegraded or partially degraded acid mucopolysaccharides interferes with the normal function of affected cells and leads to the characteristic clinical symptoms, which are progressive: a coarse facial appearance, thick lips, and a large tongue are evident by 2 years of age. Other progressive features include growth deficiency, mental retardation, cloudy corneas, hepatosplenomegaly, cardiomegaly, and excessive urinary excretion of dermatan sulfate and heparan sulfate. Another example of a dysmetabolic syndrome is the Lesch-Nyhan syndrome, discussed earlier under known-genesis syndromes of the biochemical-defect type. In this X-linked recessive disorder, the enzyme hypoxanthine-guanine-phosphoribosyl-transferase, which plays a role in regulating purine synthesis, is missing. Features include uric aciduria, mental retardation, and self-mutilation of the lips and fingers (Fig. 3–6).

Dysmetabolic syndromes have enzymatic defects and are primarily recessively inherited. Some dominantly inherited dysmetabolic syndromes may be caused by basic defects in structural proteins in some instances and by regulator mutations that result in excessive or reduced enzyme reduction rates in other instances (Cohen, 1982, 1986).

In low molecular weight dysmetabolic syndromes, a patient is usually normal at birth, since intrauterine compensation has taken place by placental or maternal metabolism. In high molecular weight dysmetabolic syndromes, abnormalities may be present during fetal life or at birth. Generalized progressive disturbances may appear after birth in some instances, or considerably later in other instances, or only under special circumstances in still other instances (Cohen, 1982, 1986).

Pure dysmetabolic syndromes are not associated with congenital malformations such as cleft lip, ventricular septal defect, and syndactyly. There are a few exceptions to this general rule of thumb. First, it is possible for a malformation to occur coincidentally in a dysmetabolic syndrome. However, the frequency would not be expected to be any more common than the frequency of isolated malformations in the general population. Second, it has been observed that albinism (a dysmetabolic disorder in which melanin is not produced) is associated with a defect in decussation of the optic nerve fibers. Finally, pseudovaginal perineoscrotal hypospadias accompanies the 5-alpha-reductase deficiency (Cohen, 1982, 1986).

Dyshistogenesis and Dyshistogenetic Syndromes

The term dyshistogenesis is used here to signify a developmental disturbance of tissue structure. There are two classes of dyshistogenetic syndromes: simple dyshistogenetic syndromes and hamartoneoplastic syndromes (Cohen, 1982, 1986).

In simple dyshistogenetic syndromes, only one germ layer is involved, and either dominant or recessive inheritance may be encountered. The Marfan syndrome is a good example. Its features include tall stature with a disproportionately long lower segment, long fingers and toes, detachment of the lens from the zonular fibers in the eye, and aortic aneurysms. All these features trace their origin to a basic defect in connective tissue (derived from the mesodermal germ layer), even though the exact nature of the defect is unknown. The Marfan syndrome is inherited as an autosomal dominant trait (Cohen, 1982, 1986).

Craniometaphyseal dysplasia is another example of an autosomal dominant syndrome. It is characterized by bone growth without remodeling. The facial features become more distorted with age (Fig. 3–13). This condition is further discussed in Chapter 25.

In hamartoneoplastic syndromes, one, two, or all three germ layers are involved. The major distinguishing features consist of hamartomas and a marked propensity for neoplasia. Autosomal dominant inheritance is characteristically observed, although a few such conditions occur only sporadically (Cohen, 1982).

Hamartomas are tumorlike, nonneoplastic admixtures of tissues indigenous to the part with an excess of one or more of these. Hamartomas are either present at birth or appear later during postnatal maturation of the tissue. Hemangiomas are excellent examples of hamartomas. They may occur singly or multiply, and,

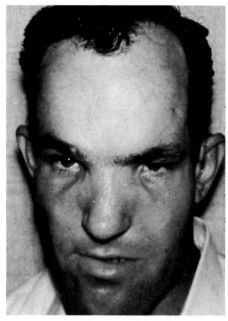 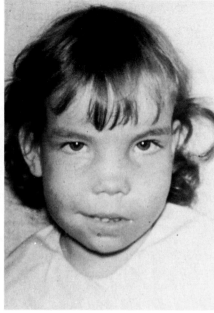

Figure 3–13. A father and a daughter with craniometaphyseal dysplasia. The nose is broad. The father is prognathic and has a profound hearing loss.

in contrast to malformations such as cleft lip, hamartomas are located variably throughout the body, with the consequences of the abnormality depending upon the location. For example, a large hemangioma of the face has an obvious psychologic impact, while the same lesion on a limb may result in hemihypertrophy. If such a lesion occurs in the gastrointestinal tract, bleeding may occur that results in anemia (Cohen, 1982).

The impact of a hamartoma on the patient depends upon (1) the type, (2) the location, (3) the size, and (4) the number of lesions. On this basis, hamartomas may be classified as major or minor. A small hemangioma and an intradermal nevus are examples of minor hamartomas. Minor hamartomas differ from minor malformations in being much more common in the general population; for example, the average white person has 20 melanotic nevi. Hemangiomas are common and frequently occur internally (e.g., hemangiomas of the liver) as well as on the skin (Cohen, 1982).

Both hamartomas and neoplasms are nonspecific. Each may occur as an isolated abnormality or may be a component part of various syndromes. For instance, a hemangioma may occur alone or together with multiple enchondromas in the Maffucci syndrome. An olipoma may occur alone or as part of tuberous sclerosis, and a Wilms tumor may occur alone, with hemihypertrophy, or as part of trisomy 18 syndrome (Cohen, 1982).

Hamartomatous tissue varies in its predisposition to neoplasia. The lesions of neurofibromatosis are prone to neurofibrosarcomatous degeneration. On the other hand, malignant transformation of angiomyolipomas of the kidney in tuberous sclerosis is uncommon, and neoplasia in the angiomatous lesions of the Klippel-Trénaunay-Weber syndrome is virtually unknown (Cohen, 1982).

Hamartoneoplastic syndromes can be divided into unilaminar, bilaminar, or trilaminar types, depending on which germ layers are involved. A good example of a hamartoneoplastic syndrome is the dominantly inherited Gardner syndrome, characterized by osteomas, odontomas, colonic polyposis, fibromas, and, sometimes, lipomas and leiomyomas.

Malformations and Malformation Syndromes

A *malformation* may be defined as a primary structural defect resulting from a localized error of morphogenesis (Anonymous, 1975). Malformations are defects of organ structure that arise during the formation or developmental placement of an organ. Approximately 3 per cent of all newborns have significant malformations, and approximately 1 per cent have multiple malformations or malformation syndromes.

There are three general classes of malformations—incomplete morphogenesis, redundant morphogenesis, and aberrant morphogenesis. The most common class is incomplete morphogenesis, which has a number of different subtypes (Cohen, 1982).

In *incomplete morphogenesis*, embryogenesis proceeds normally until the time of developmental arrest. Of the many different types of incomplete morphogenesis, only three will be considered here. In *aplasia*, there is total failure of development. If, for instance, the optic vesicle fails to contact the surface ectoderm, the lens fails to form. In *hypoplasia*, there is partial failure of development. Micrognathia is an example of such underdevelopment. *Failure of fusion* is a third type of incomplete morphogenesis. For example, if the palatine processes fail to contact each other during embryogenesis, a cleft palate results (Cohen, 1982).

Redundant morphogenesis is much less common. In this class of malformations, the redundant organ passes through the same stage of morphogenesis at the same time as does its normal counterpart. A good example of redundant morphogenesis is an ear tag in the presence of a perfectly normal ear. Such a tag may be interpreted as having developed from a supernumerary auricular hillock (Cohen, 1982).

Aberrant morphogenesis is rare and has no counterpart in normal morphogenesis. A good example is a mediastinal thyroid gland. During normal morphogenesis, the thyroid gland is never found in the mediastinum (Cohen, 1982).

Malformations may be relatively simple or complex. The later the defect is initiated during development, the simpler the malformation. Examples of simple malformations include microphthalmia, cleft lip, and choanal atresia. Malformation sequences are initiated earlier during organogenesis and have more far-reaching consequences. A *malformation sequence* may be defined as a malformation together with its subsequently derived structural changes. The primary defect sets off a morphologic chain of secondary and tertiary events, resulting in what appear to be multiple malformations. However, all such malformations are developmentally interrelated. Holoprosencephaly and facial dysmorphism represent an example of a

malformation sequence (Fig. 3–14). In holoprosencephaly, the embryonic forebrain fails to cleave sagittally into cerebral hemispheres, transversely into telencephalon and diencephalon, and horizontally into olfactory and optic bulbs. Holoprosencephaly varies in its degree of severity. At the mild end of the spectrum is simple absence of the olfactory tracts and bulbs. Holoprosencephaly is associated with facial dysmorphism, which also varies from mild to severe (Fig. 3–14). A single eye or closely set eyes, proboscis formation, a single-nostril nose, a flattened nose, and a median cleft lip may be observed variably or in combination. All the malformations encountered trace their origins developmentally to a single primary defect in morphogenesis (Cohen, 1982; Cohen et al., 1971) (Fig. 3–15, *top*).

Malformations may be minimally or maximally expressed. For example, bifid uvula is a minimal expression of cleft palate. Malformation sequences may also be minimally or maximally expressed.

Major malformations are of surgical, medical, or cosmetic importance and may lead to secondary func-

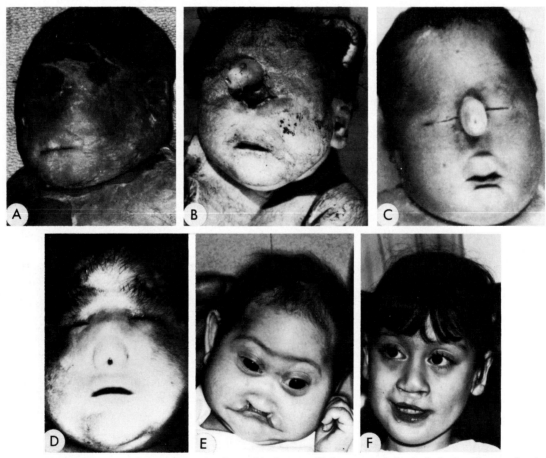

Figure 3–14. Spectrum of dysmorphic facies associated with variable degrees of holoprosencephaly. *A*, Cyclopia without proboscis formation; note single central eye. *B*, Cyclopia with proboscis. *C*, Ethmocephaly. Ocular hypotelorism with proboscis formation. *D*, Cebocephaly; ocular hypotelorism with single-nostril nose. *E*, Premaxillary agenesis, flat nose, and ocular hypotelorism. *F*, Ocular hypotelorism and surgically repaired cleft lip. (*A* and *F* from Cohen, M. M., Jr. 1976. Etiologic heterogeneity in holoprosencephaly and facial dysmorphia and comments on the facial bones and cranial base. *In* Bosma, J. F. [ed.]: Development of the Basicranium. Bethesda, MD, U.S. Dept. of Health, Education, and Welfare. [NIH] 76–989, p. 384. *B*, *C*, and *D* from Cohen, M. M., Jr., et al.: Holoprosencephaly and facial dysmorphia: Nosology, etiology, and pathogenesis. *In* Bergsma, D. [ed.]: Part XI. Orofacial Structures. Baltimore: Williams & Wilkins for the National Foundation–March of Dimes, BD:OAS VII[7]:125–135, 1971, with permission. *E* from DeMyer, W. E., and Zeman, W.: Alobar holoprosencephaly [arhinencephaly] with median cleft lip and palate. Confinia Neurologia 23:1, 1963, with permission.)

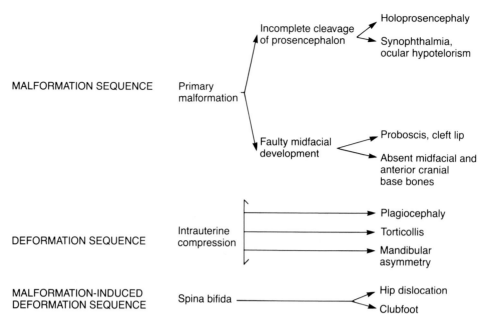

Figure 3–15. Malformation sequence with holoprosencephaly as an example (top). Deformation sequence with intrauterine compression as an example (middle). Malformation-induced deformation sequence with spina bifida as an example (bottom). (Modified from Cohen, M. M., Jr. 1982. The Child with Multiple Birth Defects. New York, Raven Press.)

tional disturbances. Examples of major malformations include cleft lip, congenital heart defects, and omphaloceles. *Minor malformations* are generally not of surgical or medical significance, although in some instances, they may be of cosmetic concern, such as webbed neck, ptosis of the eyelids, or prominent epicanthic folds. Rarely, they may cause complications such as an infected branchial arch fistula (Marden et al., 1964). Some minor anomalies are pictured in Figure 3–16. A representative but by no means exhaustive list of minor malformations of the head and neck is presented in Table 3–6.

The occurrence of single minor malformations is common in the general population, being found in 15 per cent of all newborns. The occurrence of two is less common, and the presence of three or more minor anomalies is distinctly unusual, occurring in approximately 1 per cent of all newborns. Of great interest is the occurrence of a major malformation in 90 per cent of all newborns with three or more minor malformations (Marden et al., 1964). The implication is clear that any newborn with three or more minor malformations should be carefully evaluated for possible hidden major malformations such as cardiac, renal, or vertebral defects.

Minor malformations occur with high frequency in many malformation syndromes. For example, in the Down syndrome, 79 per cent of all malformations

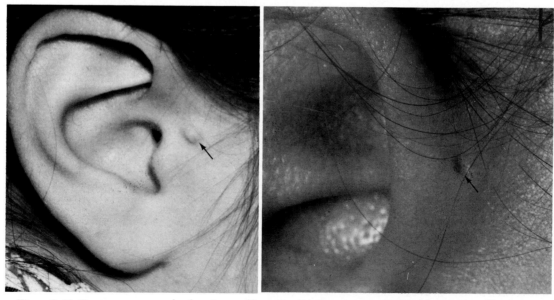

Figure 3–16. Ear tag as an example of a minor malformation *(A)*. Ear pit as an example of a minor malformation *(B)*.

TABLE 3–6. Minor Malformations

HEAD
Aberrant scalp hair patterning
Flat occiput
Bony occipital spur
Third fontanelle

EYES
Epicanthic folds
Epicanthus inversus
Upward-slanting palpebral fissures
Downward-slanting palpebral fissures
Short palpebral fissures
Dystopia canthorum
Minor hypertelorism
Minor hypotelorism
Minor ptosis
Coloboma (eyelid, iris)

EARS
Primitive shape
Lack of helical fold
Asymmetric size
Posterior rotation
Small ears
Protuberant ears
Absent tragus
Double lobule
Auricular tag
Auricular pit
Narrow external auditory meatus

NOSE
Small nares
Notched alae

ORAL REGIONS
Borderline small mandible
Incomplete form of cleft lip
Bifid uvula
Aberrant frenulum
Enamel hypoplasia
Malformed teeth
Malocclusion

NECK
Mild webbed neck
Branchial cleft fistula

Adapted from Cohen, M. M., Jr. 1982. The Child with Multiple Birth Defects. New York, Raven Press. Modified from Marden, P. M., et al. 1964. J. Pediatr. 64:358.

TABLE 3–7. Significance of Minor Anomalies

FACT	IMPLICATION
In newborns with three or more minor anomalies, 90 per cent have a major anomaly	Search for major occult anomalies
Minor anomalies are present in many multiple congenital anomaly syndromes	Aid in diagnosis
42 per cent of idiopathic mental retardation patients have three or more anomalies, of which 80 per cent are minor anomalies	Aid in prognosis

With permission from Cohen, M. M., Jr. 1982. The Child with Multiple Birth Defects. New York, Raven Press, p. 15.

detectable by clinical examination are minor malformations; in trisomy 18 syndrome, 38 per cent of the malformations are minor; in trisomy 13, 50 per cent of the malformations are minor; and in the Turner syndrome, 73 per cent of detectable malformations are minor. Thus, minor malformations serve as diagnostic aids for many malformation syndromes.

Finally, 42 per cent of patients with idiopathic mental retardation have three or more malformations, of which 80 per cent are minor (Smith and Bostian, 1964). Thus, minor malformations may be considered aids in the prediction of mental deficiency associated with other abnormalities.

The significance of minor malformations is summarized in Table 3–7. Of all minor anomalies, 71 per cent occur in the head and neck region and the hand—easily accessible areas for the pediatric otolaryngologist to evaluate (Fig. 3–17).

All malformations, whether major or minor, and all malformation sequences are nonspecific. Each may occur as an isolated abnormality; each may also occur as a component part of various syndromes. Cleft palate, for example, may occur alone or as part of the autosomal dominant Stickler syndrome, characterized by high myopia, retinal detachment, and various abnormalities of bones and joints. A minor malformation

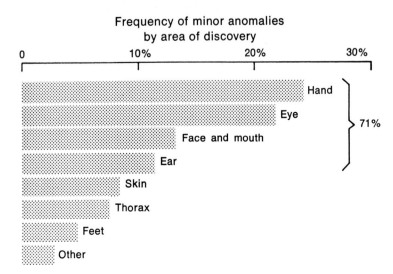

Figure 3–17. Frequency of minor anomalies by region. Of all minor anomalies, 71 per cent occur in the head and neck region and the hand. (Modified from Smith, D. W., and Bostian, K. E. 1964. Congenital anomalies associated with idiopathic mental retardation. J. Pediatr. 65:189.)

such as epicanthic folds may occur alone or as part of the Down syndrome. Holoprosencephaly and facial dysmorphism may occur alone or as part of the trisomy 13 syndrome (Cohen, 1982).

Because malformations occur with various frequencies in different syndromes, they are facultative rather than obligatory; that is, they may or may not be present in a given example of a condition in which they are known to be features. For example, two common features of the Beckwith-Wiedemann syndrome are macroglossia and omphalocele, yet cases are known in which both malformations are absent. Pathognomonic abnormalities for various syndromes, are rare.

Since malformations are both nonspecific and facultative for various disorders, syndrome diagnosis is made from the overall pattern of abnormalities. It cannot be stressed strongly enough that diagnosis is never made on the basis of specific abnormalities but on the basis of the overall pattern. The more abnormalities there are in a given syndrome, the easier the condition is to diagnose because even if some of the features are not expressed, the overall pattern is still discernible. Conversely, the fewer abnormalities there are in a given syndrome, the more difficult the condition is to diagnose if some of the features are not expressed. In general, diagnosis of any syndrome with some of its features not expressed is more of a problem in a sporadic case than in a familial instance. For example, if an 8-year-old child has ocular hypertelorism and bifid ribs but no other abnormalities, the diagnosis of the basal cell nevus syndrome is extremely probable if the child comes from a family in which one or more members are known to have the syndrome. It is highly likely that such a child will go on to develop other features of the syndrome, such as jaw cysts, bridging of the sella turcica, and basal cell carcinomas. On the other hand, the diagnosis is extremely uncertain if a child with the same anomalies comes from a perfectly normal family (Cohen, 1982, 1986).

A *malformation syndrome* may be defined as two or more malformations or malformation sequences in the same individual. A true malformation syndrome is characterized by *embryonic pleiotropy* in which a pattern of developmentally unrelated malformations or malformation sequences occurs. The difference between a malformation syndrome and a malformation sequence is diagrammed in Figure 3–18. We have already discussed holoprosencephaly and facial dysmorphism as an isolated malformation sequence. In the trisomy 13 syndrome—a true malformation syndrome—holoprosencephaly and facial dysmorphism occur together with congenital heart defects, polydactyly, and other anomalies (Fig. 3–5). These malformations are unrelated at the embryonic level, although at a more basic level, they have a common cause—an extra chromosome no. 13.

Deformations and Deformation Syndromes

A *deformation* is an alteration in the shape or structure of a previously normal part (Anonymous,

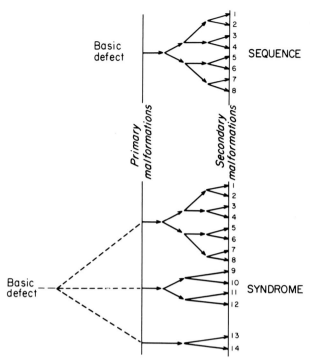

Figure 3–18. Diagram comparing malformation sequence (top) with true malformation syndrome (bottom). Isolated holoprosencephaly is an example of a malformation sequence. When holoprosencephaly occurs with polydactyly, congenital heart defects, and other anomalies as in trisomy 13 syndrome, the condition is a malformation syndrome. (From Cohen, M. M., Jr. 1982. The Child with Multiple Birth Defects. New York, Raven Press.)

1975). Deformations arise most frequently during fetal life. Since the most common cause is intrauterine molding, the musculoskeletal system is usually affected. The most important factor contributing to deformations is lack of fetal movement, whatever the cause. Important deformations include clubfoot, congenital hip dislocation, congenital postural scoliosis, plagiocephaly in the absence of craniosynostosis, and some cases of sternomastoid torticollis. An example of a mandibular deformation is illustrated in Figure 3–19. Approximately 2 per cent of all newborns have deformations (Dunn, 1976).

A sequence of events leading to deformation is diagrammed in Figure 3–20. First pregnancies tend to be associated with unstretched uterine and abdominal muscles. This can result in uteroplacental insufficiency, which, in turn, can lead to decreased amnionic fluid (oligohydramnios). Breech presentation is common since the uterus is too compressed to allow the fetus to rotate into the cephalic position. Uterine restraints on fetal movement allow the mild but persistent extrinsic forces to deform the fetus (Dunn, 1976).

The characteristic features of deformations and malformations are contrasted in Table 3–8. Malformations tend to arise during the organogenetic period of embryonic life. Deformations, on the other hand, tend to arise during the fetal period, after organogenesis is already completed. Thus, deformations affect intact regions. A clubfoot is not an organ defect but a regional

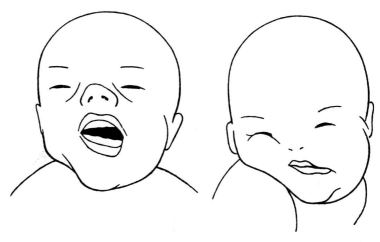

Figure 3–19. Mandibular deformation resulting from sharply lateroflexed position of the head *in utero* with the shoulder pressed against the mandible for a long period of time. (Courtesy of Mead Johnson and Company.)

defect, since the limbs have already formed. Furthermore, deformations tend not to have structural defects, in contrast to malformations, which do. With clubfoot, for example, five digits and the proper number of phalanges and metatarsals are present. This is not true of malformations such as ectrodactyly (missing digits) or polydactyly (extra digits). Some degree of perinatal mortality accompanies every statistical survey of malformations because of the high incidence of central nervous system and cardiovascular anomalies. In contrast, the perinatal mortality tends to be extremely low in surveys of deformations. Finally, spontaneous correction in some instances or, more commonly, correction by posturing is possible for many deformations. Tibial torsion present in newborns, for example, undergoes spontaneous correction in most cases. Postural correction is feasible in many cases of scoliosis, congenital hip dislocation, and clubfoot. In contrast, spontaneous correction of malformations is rare (except for septal defects of the heart), and correction by posturing is not possible.

Since the deformations discussed thus far have a common mechanical origin, more than one deformation might be expected to occur in some patients. In a study of approximately 4500 newborns, Dunn (1976) indicated that one third of all patients with deformations had multiple deformations or deformation sequences. A *deformation* sequence may be defined as two or more deformations in the same patient that have a common cause. For example, plagiocephaly, torticollis, and mandibular asymmetry in the same patient all may be caused by intrauterine compression. A deformation sequence is contrasted with a malformation sequence in Figure 3–15 (*top, middle*).

Comments on Syndrome Models

To reiterate, syndrome models provide us with a framework for analyzing various syndromes by giving us convenient points from which to move in our thinking. As we indicated earlier, some syndromes closely fit the models proposed, and others have overlapping features that express themselves at more than one level. Figure 3–21 shows the four types of syndromes and how they are stratified. The representative syndromes at the margins of the inverted triangle all express themselves at two different levels. As we have already noted, bilateral renal agenesis results in oligohydramnios, producing the Potter syndrome. Here, we have a malformation-induced deformation syndrome. The basal cell nevus syndrome has dyshistogenetic features such as basal cell carcinomas and medulloblastoma. True malformations, such as ocular hypertelorism, bifid ribs, and cervical spina bifida

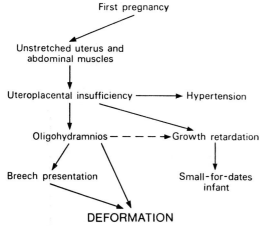

Figure 3–20. Diagram illustrating sequence of events leading to deformation. (From Dunn, P. M. 1976. Congenital postural deformities. Br. Med. Bull. 32:71.)

TABLE 3–8. Comparison of Malformations and Deformations

	MALFORMATION	DEFORMATION
Time of occurrence	Embryonic period	Fetal period
Level of disturbance	Organ	Region
Structural changes	Present	Absent
Perinatal mortality	Present	Absent
Spontaneous correction	Absent	Present
Correction by posture	Absent	Present

With permission from Cohen, M. M., Jr. 1982. The Child with Multiple Birth Defects. New York, Raven Press, p. 21.

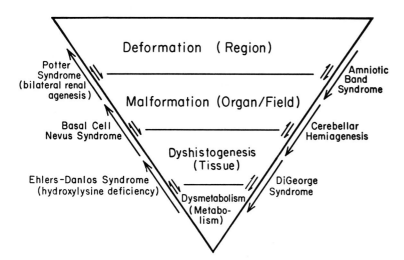

Figure 3–21. Examples of compound syndromes that express themselves at more than one level.

occulta, are also present. In one form of the Ehlers-Danlos syndrome, hydroxylysine deficiency results in dyshistogenetic skin changes (Cohen, 1982).

SYNDROME DESIGNATION

From the preceding text, it can be concluded that the designation of syndromes is rather arbitrary. A number of methods are used (Cohen, 1976, 1982).

BASIC DEFECT. Describing the basic defect is the ideal approach to syndrome designation; however, it may be cumbersome. For example, Lesch-Nyhan syndrome is caused by hypoxanthine-guanine-phosphoribosyl-transferase deficiency. The eponym is easier to use.

EPONYMS. An example is Down syndrome, which can also be designated by the chromosomal abnormality. This is a common syndrome (Fig. 3–22). The more rarely occurring Apert syndrome is another example of syndrome designation by an eponym (Fig. 3–23).

CHARACTERISTIC FEATURES. Syndromes have been designated by their characteristic features or anatomic findings. An example is whistling face syndrome. The child in Figure 3–24 has microstomia, an "H" groove on the chin, a flat midface, a long philtrum, and a small nose. In addition, she has a rare associated malformation, choanal atresia. The mother also exhibits a puckered mouth despite her attempt at smiling.

ACRONYMS. An example is the leopard syndrome, which stands for lentigines, electrocardiographic condition abnormalities, ocular hypertelorism, pulmonic stenosis, atrial septal defect, retardation of growth, and sensorineural deafness.

NUMERIC NOMENCLATURE. Generally, numeric nomenclature has found its most important use in those areas in which knowledge at the biochemical level has rapidly demonstrated etiologic heterogeneity. Examples are the designation of the various mucopolysaccharidoses.

GEOGRAPHIC NOMENCLATURE. The least common method of designating various syndromes is to identify the geographic location of the initial patient. The Brazilian-type achondrogenesis is an example.

COMPOUND DESIGNATIONS. Finally, compound designations of various types may be used. An example is Hurler syndrome, which may be designated as an alpha-L-iduronidase deficiency or as Hurler syndrome (MPS-I-H).

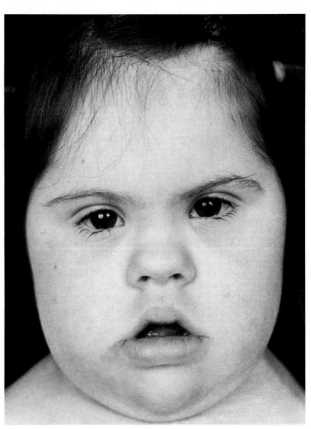

Figure 3–22. A child with Down syndrome. Note the upward slanting palpebral fissures and brachycephalic skull with flattening of the occiput. Development of the midface is poor, with relative prognathism and ocular hypotelorism and hypoplasia of the nasal bones.

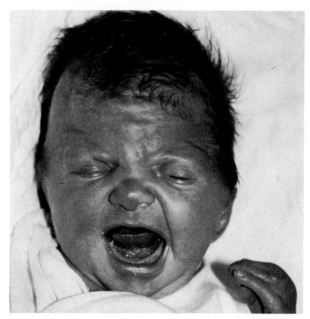

Figure 3–23. An infant with Apert syndrome. The midface is usually underdeveloped, thus making the mandible appear more prominent. The skull is malformed as the frontal and occipital bones are flattened. Irregular early obliteration of the cranial sutures is common, especially the coronal.

AN APPROACH TO SYNDROME DIAGNOSIS AND PATIENT MANAGEMENT

Establishing an accurate diagnosis is a challenge that often faces physicians caring for newborn infants with malformations. As previously stated, because a great many syndromes have craniofacial anomalies as a component, the clinician who is interested in ear, nose, and throat disorders may become involved in the evaluation of the child. Because many syndromes have been described, it is difficult to remember those seen very infrequently. An organized approach to syndrome evaluation and diagnosis is important.

Initially, a thorough history must be obtained (Fig. 3–25). This should include family history at least over three generations, the presence or absence of parental consanguinity, maternal and paternal ages at the time of conception, possible maternal exposure to environmental teratogens (e.g., occupational), parental ethnic origins, and prior miscarriages, stillbirths, neonatal deaths, or birth defects.

Physical examination should include documentation of major and minor anomalies as well as general growth parameters. The examiner should also consider the possibility of internal malformations when obvious external malformations exist. Otoscopic and audiometric evaluation may be of special value because of the cryptic nature of this system and the fact that, when identified early, hearing loss may be amenable to therapy. It is important to be aware of certain specific association patterns such as ear malformations with renal abnormalities, asymmetric crying facies with

cardiovascular anomalies, hypotelorism with midline brain malformations, cleft palate with atrial septal defect, and anal atresia with tracheoesophageal fistula, among many (Chudley, 1985). Clinical photographs should be obtained, as these will be invaluable additions to the record and can be used for future reference, especially in circumstances of stillbirths.

Even the most experienced dysmorphologist sees a limited number of patients of any given genetic disorder, since these are individually rare, and wide variation in phenotypic expression usually exists. A logical approach to any patient who exhibits anomalies is to narrow the possibilities systematically by first using the least expensive and least invasive techniques. It is essential to go beyond individual limited experience and utilize the collective observations of others by consulting texts devoted exclusively to the subject of syndromology (Gorlin et al., 1990; Nyhan and Sakati, 1976; Goodman and Gorlin, 1983; Borgaonkar, 1984; McKusick, 1986; Shepard, 1986; Jones, 1988).

Since the syndromes of known genesis and many of the recurrent-pattern syndromes can be found in syndromology textbooks, they can be properly identified, and a rational workup of such patients may be planned from the description of the syndrome. This cannot be done for provisionally unique-pattern syndromes or for some of the less well-known recurrent-pattern syndromes. With the aid of the child's history and physical examination, the clinician should strive to classify unknown-genesis syndromes as dysmetabolic, dyshis-

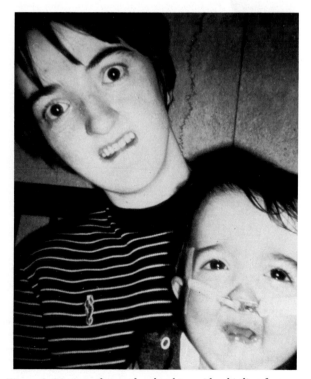

Figure 3–24. A mother and a daughter with whistling face syndrome. The child has microstomia, an "H" groove on the chin, a flat midface, a long philtrum, and a small nose. The mother also exhibits a puckered mouth despite her attempt at smiling.

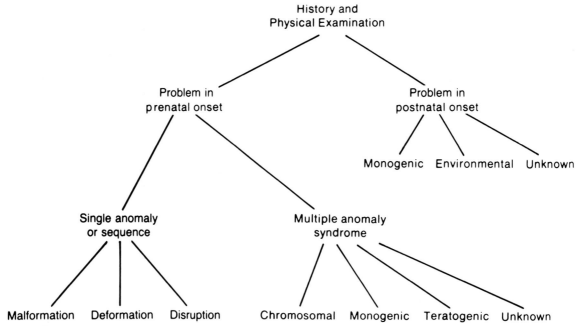

Figure 3–25. The approach to the diagnosis of patients with structural defects. (With permission from Cohen, M. M., Jr. 1982. The Child with Multiple Birth Defects. New York, Raven Press.)

togenetic, malformational, or deformational. Such classification allows the physician to evaluate the patient rationally. One of the first steps in evaluating an unusual-appearing child is to decide whether the manifestations had their origin prenatally or postnatally (Fig. 3–26). If the patient has no malformations of the embryonic type, was normal at birth, and shows progressive deterioration with time, the patient has a dysmetabolic syndrome. It is unlikely, although not impossible, that the unknown metabolic defect will be discovered in the patient in question. Nevertheless, consultation in an academic medical center should be sought in selected cases, since it is sometimes possible to define a new dysmetabolic disorder. Even if the patient represents a sporadic instance in the family, the highest recurrence risk for future affected offspring

is 25 per cent, since all known dysmetabolic syndromes are recessive.

If the unknown-genesis syndrome is dyshistogenetic, is it simple or hamartoneoplastic? If the syndrome is the latter type, the patient should be monitored frequently for the possibility of neoplasms.

If the unknown-genesis syndrome is malformational, it is not rational to perform amino acid screening and similar tests, since pure malformation syndromes are not known to be dysmetabolic. Certainly, a chromosomal study is indicated.

Many patients with multiple malformations may have growth deficiency of prenatal onset, in which the infant is small for gestational age. If this type of growth deficiency is regarded as a malformation, that is, as hypoplasia of the whole individual, it is not surprising

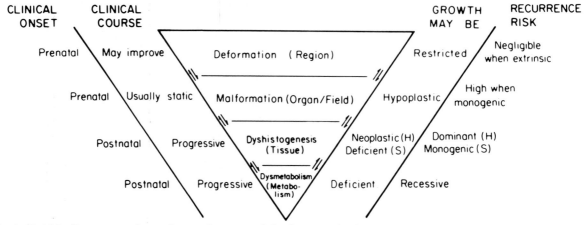

Figure 3–26. This diagram may be used to predict some of the features of unknown-genesis syndromes. H, Hamartoplastic type of dyshistogenetic syndrome; S, simple type of dyshistogenetic syndrome. (With permission from Cohen, M. M., Jr. 1982. The Child with Multiple Birth Defects. New York, Raven Press.)

that other malformations, especially those of incomplete morphogenesis, frequently accompany the growth deficiency. Organ formation and developmental placement are susceptible to malformation if hypoplasia occurs during the period of rapid differentiation and growth. Endocrine studies and various other tests for humorally mediated growth deficiency are contraindicated in pure malformation syndromes. Such growth deficiency usually persists into postnatal life, and there is no known treatment.

In the patient with multiple malformations of unknown genesis, it is important to sort out malformation sequences from true malformation syndromes whenever this is possible. Malformation sequences tend to have a multifactorial recurrence risk, whereas true malformation syndromes are more likely to be monogenic or chromosomal.

The finding of multiple deformations of unknown genesis defines a deformation syndrome. When growth deficiency accompanies multiple deformations, it is usually caused by intrauterine compression or uteroplacental insufficiency. Endocrine studies and various tests for humorally mediated growth deficiency are contraindicated. Catch-up growth is expected following birth, once the fetus is no longer compressed within the uterus.

There are, of course, many syndromes of unknown genesis that may express their phenotypes at more than one level. When malformations and deformations occur together in the same syndrome of unknown genesis, the clinician should strive to explain the deformations in terms of the malformations when this is possible. Some unknown-genesis syndromes with phenotypic expression at more than one level are occasionally refractory to the type of analysis proposed here.

As an aid to the physician's understanding of congenital anomalies and syndromes, each section of this text has a review of the embryology and development of the organ system discussed, as well as a detailed review of the congenital anomalies usually associated with that particular region. It is possible, in many instances, that if the most obvious abnormality is recognized and reviewed, insight may be gained into the biologic type and possible associated manifestations of the specific abnormality.

SELECTED REFERENCES

Borgaonkar, D. S. 1984. Chromosomal Variation in Man: A Catalog of Chromosomal Variants and Anomalies, 4th ed. New York, Alan R. Liss, Inc.
    A bibliographic listing of chromosomal abnormalities.
Cohen, M. M., Jr. 1982. The Child with Multiple Birth Defects. New York, Raven Press.
    A comprehensive guide to syndrome delineation.
Goodman, R. M., and Gorlin, R. J. 1983. The Malformed Infant and Child: An Illustrated Guide. New York, Oxford University Press.
    A well-organized illustrated guide describing the more frequently encountered syndromes.
Gorlin, R. J., Cohen, M. M., Jr., and Levin, L. S., 1990. Syndromes of the Head and Neck, 3rd ed. New York, Oxford Univ. Press (in press).
    An encyclopedic text that catalogs well over 1000 syndromes that have various head and neck components.
Jones, K. L. 1988. Smith's Recognizable Patterns of Human Malformations, 4th ed. Philadelphia, W. B. Saunders Co.
    The previous editions of this monograph were the most widely used pediatric references for identifying malformation syndromes.
McKusick, V. A. 1986. Mendelian Inheritance in Man: Catalogs of Autosomal Dominant, Autosomal Recessive, and X-linked Phenotypes, 7th ed. Baltimore, The Johns Hopkins University Press.
    One of the world's foremost experts provides a catalog of genetic diseases.
Nyhan, W. L., and Sakati, N. O. 1976. Genetic and Malformation Syndromes in Clinical Medicine. Chicago, YearBook Medical Publishers, Inc.
    A practical illustration of malformations.
Shepard, T. H. 1986. Catalog of Teratogenic Agents, 5th ed. Baltimore, The Johns Hopkins University Press.
    A comprehensive listing of the agents identified as teratogens.

REFERENCES

Anonymous. 1975. Classification and nomenclature of morphological defects. Lancet 1:513.
Borgaonkar, D. S. 1984. Chromosomal Variation in Man: A Catalog of Chromosomal Variants and Anomalies, 4th. ed. New York, Alan R. Liss, Inc.
Boué, J., Boué, A., and Lazar, P. 1975. Retrospective and prospective epidemiological studies of 1500 karyotyped spontaneous abortions. Teratology 12:11.
Buckfield, P. 1973. Major congenital faults in newborn infants: A pilot study in New Zealand. N.Z. Med. J. 78:195.
Chudley, A. E. 1985. Genetic contribution to human malformations. In Persaud, T. V. N., Chudley, A. E., and Skalko, R. G. (eds.): Basic Concepts in Teratology. New York, Alan R. Liss, Inc., pp. 31–68.
Clarren, S. K., and Smith, D. W. 1978. The fetal alcohol syndrome. N. Engl. J. Med. 289:1063.
Cohen M. M., Jr. 1976. Syndrome designations. J. Med. Genet. 13:266.
Cohen, M. M., Jr. 1977. On the nature of syndrome delineation. Acta Genet. Med. Gemellol. (Rome) 26:103.
Cohen, M. M., Jr. 1982. The Child with Multiple Birth Defects. New York, Raven Press.
Cohen, M. M., Jr. 1986. Children, birth defects, and multiple defects: Part 1. Ann. R. Coll. Phys. Surg. Can. 19:375.
Cohen, M. M., Jr. 1986. Children, birth defects, and multiple defects: Part 2. Ann. R. Coll. Phys. Surg. Can. 19:465.
Cohen, M. M., Jr., and Rollnick, B. R. 1989. Oculoauriculovertebral spectrum: An updated critique. Cleft Palate J. (in press).
Cohen, M. M., Jr., Jirasek, J. E., Guzman, R. T., et al. 1971. Holoprosencephaly and facial dysmorphia: Nosology, etiology, and pathogenesis. Birth Defects 7(7):125.
Conen, P. E., Phillips, K. G., and Manntuer, L. S. 1962. Multiple developmental anomalies and trisomy of a 13–15 group chromosome ("D" syndrome). Can. Med. Assoc. J. 87:709.
DeMyer, W. E., and Zeman, W. 1963. Alobar holoprosencephaly (arhinencephaly) with medial cleft lip and palate. Confin. Neurol. 23:1.
Dobrowski, J. M., Grundfast, K. M., Rosenbaum, K. N., et al. 1985. Otorhinologic manifestations of CHARGE association. Otolaryngol. Head Neck Surg. 93:798.
Dunn, P. M. 1976. Congenital postural deformities. Br. Med. Bull. 32:71.
Goldson, E., Smith, A. C., and Stewart, J. M. 1986. The CHARGE Association: How well can they do? Am. J. Dis. Child. 140:918.
Goodman, R. M., and Gorlin, R. J. 1983. The Malformed Infant and Child: An Illustrated Guide. New York, Oxford University Press.

Gorlin, R. J., Pindborg, J. J., and Cohen, M. M., Jr. 1976. Syndromes of the Head and Neck, 2nd ed. New York, McGraw-Hill.

Harris, L. E., Stayura, L. A., Ramirez-Talavera, P. F., et al. 1975. Congenital and acquired abnormalities observed in live-born and stillborn neonates. Mayo Clin. Proc. 50:85.

Jones, K. L. 1988. Smith's Recognizable Patterns of Human Malformations, 4th ed. Philadelphia, W. B. Saunders Co.

Kennedy, W. P. 1974. Epidemiologic aspects of the problem of congenital malformation. Birth Defects Orig. Article Ser. 3, 2:1–18.

Leck, I. 1977. Correlation of malformation frequency with environmental genetic attributes in man. In Wilson, J. G., and Clarke, F. F. (eds.): Handbook of Teratology. New York, Plenum Press, pp. 243–324.

Marden, P. M., Smith, D. W., and McDonald, M. J. 1964. Congenital anomalies in the newborn infant, including minor variations. J. Pediatr. 64:358.

McKusick, V. A. 1986. Mendelian Inheritance in Man: Catalogs of Autosomal Dominant, Autosomal Recessive, and X-Linked Phenotypes, 7th ed. Baltimore, The Johns Hopkins University Press.

MMWR June 19, 1987, Vol. 36, no. 23.

Myrianthopoulos, N. C. 1985. Malformations in Children from One to Seven Years: A Report from the Collaborative Perinatal Project. New York, Alan R. Liss, Inc.

Myrianthopoulos, N. C., and Chung, C. S. 1974. Congenital Malformations in Singletons: Epidemiologic Survey. Birth Defects Orig. Article Ser. 10, 11:1–58.

Norman, M. G. 1984. Pediatric Pathology. Ann. R. Coll. Phys. Surg. Can. 17:23–27.

Nyhan, W. L., and Sakati, N. O. 1976. Genetic and Malformation Syndromes in Clinical Medicine. Chicago, YearBook Medical Publishers, Inc.

Persaud, T. V. N. 1985. Genetic contributions to human malformations. In Persaud, T. V. N., Chudley, A. E., and Skalko, R. G. (eds.): Basic Concepts in Teratology. New York, Alan R. Liss, Inc., pp. 13–22.

Polani, P. E. 1973. The Incidence of developmental and other genetic abnormalities. Guy's Hosp. Rep. 122:53.

Rumeau-Rouquette, C., Goujard, J., and Kaminski, M. 1980. Problems in conducting prospective surveys. Acta Morphologica Acad. Sci. Hung. 28:167.

Shepard, T. H. 1986. Catalog of Teratogenic Agents, 5th ed. Baltimore, The Johns Hopkins University Press.

Smith, D. W., and Bostian, K. E. 1964. Congenital anomalies associated with idiopathic mental retardation. J. Pediatr. 65:189.

Spranger, J., Benirschke, K., Hall, J. G., et al. 1982. Errors of morphogenesis: Concepts and terms. J. Pediatr. 100:160.

Tuchmann-Duplessis, H. 1975. Drug Effect on the Fetus. Sydney, ADIS Press.

Weaver, D. D., Graham, C. B., Thomas, I. T., et al. 1974. A new overgrowth syndrome with accelerated skeletal maturation, unusual facies, and camptodactyly. J. Pediatr. 84:547.

Young, I. D. 1987. Malformations in different groups. Arch. Dis. Child. 62:109.

Chapter 4

MALFORMATIONS AND SYNDROMES

William S. Crysdale, M.D.

Congenital abnormalities stem from errors in morphogenesis and genetic factors. An anomaly is an isolated local structural defect, or malformation, that results in a structural change, such as an isolated cleft of the bony or secondary palate. A syndrome comprises several defects in a recognizable pattern and is not a consequence of a single local error of morphogenesis (for example, Crouzon syndrome). Thus, each craniofacial syndrome has certain clinical features (albeit of varied frequency and degree), and the condition has a recognized natural history and an established mode of inheritance, or risk of occurrence. Syndrome labels are confusing because they are described by different types of terms: eponyms, anatomic terms, enzyme deficiencies, or chromosome abnormalities, for instance. As medical knowledge expands, the descriptions of syndromes may become obsolete, may change, or may be eliminated. In the meantime, we use various catalogues to describe the incidence and association of congenital defects in anomalies and syndromes (Jones, 1988; Gorlin et al., 1976; Konigsmark and Gorlin, 1976). This chapter discusses the aspects of interest to the otolaryngologist of the normal growth and development and the pathogenesis of congenital anomalies that have been described in the preceding chapters.

THE TEAM APPROACH

Children with craniofacial abnormalities are best managed by a team of specialists (Munro, 1975). The head of the team should accept the responsibility for coordinating the patient's needs from birth to adulthood. Good communication within the team is essential and can be achieved only by group review of the patients and delineation of their needs in open discussion. Team review of patients is time-consuming and hence relatively inefficient, but the byproducts of good intrateam communication and the increased appreciation of other team members' problems, concerns, and special skills are worth the effort. At The Hospital for Sick Children, Toronto, we have two such teams: the maxillofacial team, for treating children with isolated oral clefts, and the craniofacial team, for treating children with other (usually more severe) craniofacial anomalies.

The maxillofacial team, traditionally headed by a plastic surgeon, routinely includes a dentist, orthodontist, otolaryngologist, pediatrician, social worker, and speech pathologist (Fig. 4–1). They meet once a week to review current cases, usually five or six patients. Other specialists are consulted as the need arises. All patients with isolated orofacial clefts are reviewed by the team at 5 and 15 years of age; most children are also reviewed between 2 and 3 years of age by a "miniteam" composed of a dentist, an otolaryngologist, and a speech pathologist. Usually, most patients have been assessed individually by an otolaryngologist during the first year of life.

The craniofacial team, headed by a craniofacial surgeon, has members from 15 other disciplines—anesthesiology, audiology, dentistry, facial anthropology, genetics, medical art, neuroophthalmology, neuroradiology, neurosurgery, orthodontics, otolaryngology, psychiatry, psychology, social work, and speech pathology. During the past 14 years, this team has evaluated over 600 children and adults.

In our center, the otolaryngologist on the teams is involved in the assessment and management of disorders of the upper airway, such as hearing loss, airway obstruction, speech disorders, infections, and disorders of olfaction.

HEARING LOSS

The importance of early detection and expeditious management of significant hearing loss cannot be overemphasized. Even mild hearing losses, if not detected early, can significantly retard the acquisition of language skills (Holm and Kumze, 1969). Untreated hearing losses of moderate or greater degree have a measurable—even devastating—effect on speech and intellectual development.

All infants with craniofacial anomalies have a high risk of having a hearing loss and require diligent otologic and audiologic follow-up until their audiologic status has been established (Downs and Silver, 1972). Unfortunately, detection of hearing loss is delayed in a large percentage of children with craniofacial anomalies but without any obvious structural aural defects. This occurs because many people, lay persons and

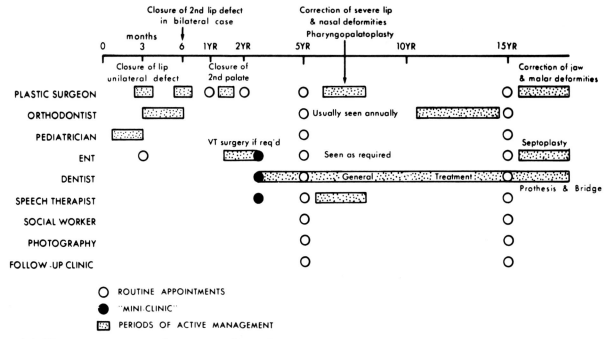

Figure 4–1. Diagrammatic summary of routine specialist involvement in the maxillofacial clinic through which children with cleft lip and palate deformities are followed.

medical personnel alike, hold the erroneous belief that because of their odd appearance, such children are mentally retarded (Crysdale, 1978). Thus, the delayed acquisition of communication skills is attributed to mental deficiency and not to a possible hearing loss (Fig. 4–2).

Hearing loss in children with craniofacial anomalies may be congenital or acquired. The loss is congenital when there is present at birth significant malformation of the structures of the external, middle, or inner ear. Acquired hearing loss is a consequence of any postnatal process, perhaps a consequence of the malformation that interferes with auditory function.

Assessment of hearing is found in Chapter 9.

Congenital Hearing Loss

Congenital hearing loss, usually conductive, is an intrinsic component of many craniofacial syndromes. Deafness associated with an aural anomaly may be due to a primary defect of the temporal bone or secondary defects in bone contiguous to the temporal bone (Caldarelli, 1977). In most craniofacial anomalies, sensorineural hearing loss is thought to be coincidental only.

Atresia of the external auditory meatus, with various degrees of obliteration of the middle ear cleft, is usually associated with microtia. The latter anomaly is frequently seen in Treacher Collins syndrome (mandibulofacial dysostosis) and hemifacial microsomia (Fig. 4–3). Bilateral atresia of the external auditory meatus with microtia was seen in one patient who had Crouzon disease. Microtia, being visible, is "helpful" to the

patient, as it usually stimulates the physician to determine the patient's level of auditory function. In patients who have a craniofacial syndrome with bilateral microtia and atresia, the middle ear cleft is almost invariably obliterated, and reconstructive middle ear surgery is not possible. However, these patients manage quite well when provided with an appropriate hearing aid, as their intelligence has been found to be normal except when the condition is part of Apert syndrome (acrocephalosyndactyly). We do not recommend reconstructive middle ear surgery for patients with unilateral microtia and atresia, but CROS (Contralateral Routing of Signal) hearing aids may be helpful in auditory rehabilitation.

If a child's ears have a normal appearance, a congenital conductive hearing loss—an invisible deformity—may not be detected until it has adversely affected the development of speech and language. In the absence of microtia, a conductive hearing loss may be a consequence of ossicular deformity or ankylosis or fixation of the stapes. In many of these patients, the tympanic membrane is small and oblique and has abnormal landmarks, an otoscopic finding that should make the physician suspect the presence of a hearing loss. Middle ear surgery may improve hearing in these children.

Studies of a temporal bone from a patient with Apert syndrome showed the stapedial vestibular joint region to be abnormal, with incomplete development of the annular ligament and fixation of the stapes by undifferentiated cartilage in two areas (Lindsay et al., 1975). In another patient with this syndrome, the stapes was found to be fixed when it was inspected at tympa-

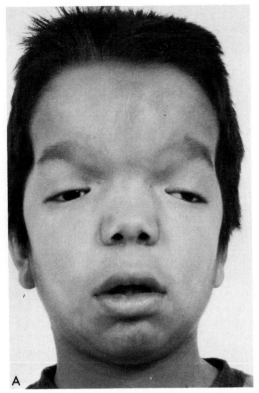

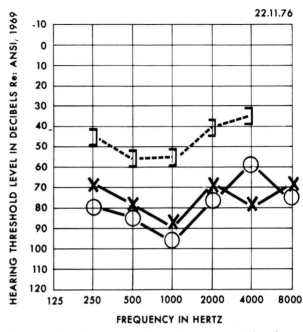

Figure 4–2. *A,* Poor language development in this North American Indian boy with isolated primary hypertelorism was attributed to mental retardation. *B,* The mixed congenital hearing loss was finally detected at 10 years of age. Psychologic reassessment now suggests above-normal intelligence. (With permission from Crysdale, W. S. [1978]. Abnormal facial appearance and delayed diagnosis of congenital hearing loss. J. Otolaryngol. 7:349–352.)

Figure 4–3. Left hemifacial microsomia in an 11-year-old boy. Bony ankylosis of the left temporomandibular joint severely limits the jaw movement. Left-sided microtia with 60-dB conductive hearing loss is present. Airway control prior to mandibular surgery was established by inserting a rigid bronchoscope through the opening to the left of the upper incisors after unsuccessful attempts at nasal intubation.

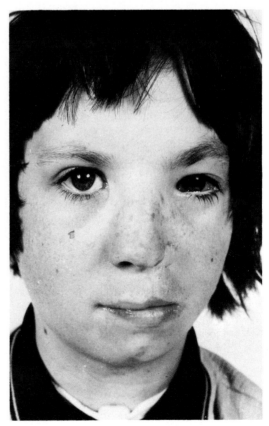

notomy; a gush of perilymphatic fluid occurred from the oval window when the stapes was removed (Bergstrom et al., 1972).

Some patients with hypertelorism have a congenital sensorineural hearing loss; this combination may represent a variant of Waardenburg syndrome.

Congenital anomalies of the ear are discussed in Chapter 18.

Acquired Hearing Loss

Acquired hearing loss is usually conductive and is most often the consequence of eustachian tube dysfunction. The degree of middle ear pathology is in proportion to the duration and severity of this eustachian tube dysfunction. Thus, one may observe patients with middle ear effusions or various degrees of middle ear atelectasis or even attic cholesteatoma. Perforations of the pars tensa and extensive tympanosclerosis may be a consequence of middle ear infection or therapeutic procedures such as tympanostomy tube insertion.

Eustachian tube insufficiency is most frequently seen in patients with a cleft secondary palate. It is present also in patients with a craniosynostosis in whom the nasopharynx is distorted, obstructed, or both as a result of aberrant growth of the midface and skull base. It has been suggested that in patients with Apert syndrome, the ciliated epithelium in the eustachian tube is abnormal, retarding clearance of middle ear secretions (Selder, 1973).

Successful management of middle ear effusions in patients with palatal clefts usually requires the insertion of tympanostomy tubes, as middle ear effusions in these patients rarely respond to conservative measures. At our center, palatal clefts are repaired at 18 months of age, and the decision to insert tympanostomy tubes is usually deferred for a further three months; then, if the middle ear effusion has not resolved, the tubes are inserted (Crysdale, 1976). Care should be taken when performing myringotomy on patients with craniosynostosis; we found unilateral dehiscence of the jugular bulb in three of our patients (Witzel et al., unpublished observations).

Other pathology related to eustachian tube dysfunction, such as atelectasis of the middle ear and attic cholesteatoma, is observed in older patients; the management of these problems is discussed in another chapter. In our experience, tympanoplastic procedures in children with a history suggestive of eustachian tube dysfunction are unsuccessful in the majority of cases and should be deferred until late adolescence. Extensive tympanosclerosis may cause significant conductive hearing loss. If the condition is bilateral, amplification may be required, as surgery is rarely beneficial.

AIRWAY OBSTRUCTION

The otolaryngologist is responsible for managing problems that may compromise the airway from the anterior nares to the segmental bronchi. In children with craniofacial abnormalities, the causes of obstruction may be legion, and the effects of the obstruction may be dependent on the age of the child. Neonates may experience life-threatening nasal or oropharyngeal obstruction; older children may have obstructive apneic episodes during sleep or troublesome nasal obstruction from day to day; and some children undergoing maxillofacial or craniofacial surgery may also experience difficulty in airway maintenance.

Airway obstruction is further discussed in Chapter 71.

Neonatal Nasal Airway Obstruction

Neonates are obligate nose-breathers for the first two to three months of life (Stool and Houlihan, 1977) and therefore experience respiratory distress, even asphyxia, if nasal airway obstruction is unrelieved. Newborn infants whose nasal passages are blocked exhibit "paradoxic cyanosis": They become cyanotic when quiet with their mouths closed but lose their cyanosis when crying and, hence, using the oral airway. Characteristically, paradoxic cyanosis occurs in infants with bilateral choanal atresia and in neonates with midfacial hypoplasia (such as those with Crouzon or Apert syndrome). It has also been observed in patients with frontal nasal dysplasia, who have a defect of the cribriform plate and a nasal encephalocele. Neonatal nasal airway obstruction can usually be relieved by taping an oral airway in place. Conscientious nursing care is necessary for these children. When the infant learns to use his or her oral airway (by 2 to 3 months of age), the danger of asphyxia is past.

Neonatal Oropharyngeal Obstruction

Neonatal respiratory distress may be a consequence of glossoptosis, which will occur when the relationship of mandible to hyoid is altered (as in infants with retrognathia or micrognathia) so that the tongue falls back and obstructs the oropharynx (Farnsworth and Pacik, 1971) (Fig. 4–4). This obstructing posture of the tongue seems to occur more readily, hence causing more problems clinically, when associated with cleft palate. Cor pulmonale has been detected as early as 5 weeks of age in an infant with Pierre Robin syndrome who was experiencing airway distress (Cogswell and Easton, 1974); certainly, asphyxia will occur in severe cases.

The author's experience is that this type of airway obstruction can usually be relieved by nursing the infant carefully in the prone position for the first few months of life. Creating a tongue-lip adhesion and suturing the tongue in front of this (Hawkins and Simpson, 1974) is rarely helpful; nasopharyngeal intubation (Stern et al., 1972) or tracheotomy is the treatment of choice in refractory cases. Before tracheotomy, the airway obstruction is relieved by inserting a rigid

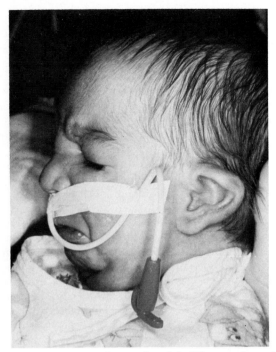

Figure 4–4. This boy was born with a cleft of the secondary palate and experienced increasing respiratory distress secondary to glossoptosis (Pierre Robin syndrome). Tracheotomy at 5 weeks of age eliminated the respiratory obstruction and was maintained for five months.

bronchoscope—a challenging task for a pediatric endoscopist to accomplish in a hypoxic but struggling retrognathic infant. The rigid bronchoscope (3 or 3.5 mm in diameter) must be inserted without the aid of a laryngoscope and in the absence of anesthesia; it is passed through the glottis from the lateral retromolar position, and the tracheotomy proceeds in an orderly fashion with the bronchoscope in place. By 6 months of age, mandibular growth has usually been sufficient to decrease glossoptosis to an insignificant level, and decannulation is possible. If the palate is cleft in these infants, some physicians prefer to maintain the tracheotomy until this defect has been repaired.

Obstructive Apneic Episodes

Obstructive apneic episodes during sleep, in some cases associated with the development of cor pulmonale, have been documented in children with normal craniofacial configurations but in whom adenoidal hypertrophy is causing chronic nasopharyngeal obstruction (Mangat et al., 1977). Children with craniofacial anomalies that affect the configuration of the upper airway may also experience similar obstruction during sleep.

Children with craniofacial anomalies in which there is severe posterior displacement of the midfacial structures (as in Apert and Crouzon syndromes) have very narrow nasopharyngeal airways and will suffer apneic episodes during sleep. In fact, the development of cor pulmonale in a 3-year-old child with Crouzon disease and clinical improvement after adenotonsillectomy have been reported (Don and Siggers, 1971). The author has observed substantial reduction in obstructive apneic episodes during sleep, with near disappearance of the associated stridor, after adenotonsillectomy in several such children younger than 3 years of age. Relief of this early airway obstruction in patients with craniosynostosis permitted the craniofacial surgeon to defer surgery to a more appropriate age.

Retrognathia is frequently a significant factor with respect to obstructive sleep apnea syndrome. Noisy, stridorous breathing during sleep, with occasional obstructive apneic episodes, increased in severity over several months in a 5-year-old child with retrognathia. This nighttime airway obstruction was almost eliminated by removing the palatine tonsils, which were large and pedunculated. Presumably, tonsillar hypertrophy in this child with glossoptosis caused significant oropharyngeal obstruction when the pharyngeal musculature was relaxed, as is normal during deep rapid eye movement (REM) sleep. A 15-year-old boy with a similar clinical picture was not cured by tonsillectomy; however, obstructive apneic episodes were eliminated by performing sliding mandibular osteotomies and placing him in a Class III occlusion. This latter procedure "pulled" the hyoid and associated tongue and pharyngeal musculature forward. Severe retrognathia or micrognathia with associated hypoplasia of the hypopharynx is common in patients with Treacher Collins syndrome, and these patients in particular are at high risk for developing obstructive sleep apnea (Johnston et al., 1981).

Life-threatening obstructive apneic episodes will occur if palatopharyngoplasty is performed in a child who has glossoptosis. Cor pulmonale developed in two of three children with Pierre Robin syndrome who had undergone palatopharyngoplasty to overcome velopharyngeal incompetence (VPI), and one of these children died of respiratory obstruction at 8 years of age (Jackson et al., 1976). A 3-year-old patient who had Treacher Collins syndrome experienced moderately severe obstructive apneic episodes during sleep after successful palatopharyngoplasty. To have some periods of uninterrupted sleep, she formed the habit of sleeping prone in the knee-chest position. Eventually, the child became hypersomniac, and tracheotomy was necessary four months after the successful palatopharyngoplasty to eliminate the obstructive episodes. The girl now sleeps well with a tracheotomy tube in place at night but wears a small Silastic stent during the daytime that plugs the tracheocutaneous fistula and permits speech. Children with a history that suggests airway obstruction and who have retrognathia or micrognathia are poor candidates for pharyngeal flap surgery, as they may experience significant upper airway obstruction during sleep postoperatively. Thus, surgeons correcting VPI with pharyngeal surgery must evaluate their patients for and question parents about clinical suggestions of obstructive apnea syndrome. One of our surgeons (as a result of an unhappy clinical circumstance) routinely has all his patients who are scheduled for pharyngoplasty undergo a preoperative sleep study.

Less troublesome nighttime obstruction may develop in adolescents in whom palatopharyngoplasty has been "too successful." These patients with repaired palatal clefts and persistent VPI have normal mandibular configurations. Following palatopharyngoplasty, they develop almost total nasal obstruction and speech that is noticeably hyponasal. Characteristically, they sleep poorly, with frequent nightmares. One girl reported waking frequently and "gasping for air." Dilatation of the small lateral ports with Tucker bougies gave only transient relief, and surgical revision of the pharyngeal flap was necessary.

Flexible nasopharyngoscopy is most helpful in evaluating these patients. With the endoscope in place, children are asked to breathe in with both the nose and the mouth temporarily occluded. One can then frequently determine the level and the cause of the obstruction to be removed—palatine tonsils, base of the tongue, or redundant supraglottic structures or pharyngeal folds. Despite such evaluation or if such an evaluation is not possible because of lack of patient cooperation, one frequently is left with proceeding empirically through an escalating series of operative procedures (each of which is followed by a sleep study to determine effectiveness)—tonsillectomy, laser resection of the midportion of the base of the tongue, uvulopalatopharyngoplasty, laser resection of redundant supraglottic structures or pharyngeal folds, creation of a Class III malocclusion, and, finally, permanent tracheotomy. It has been suggested (Lauritzen et al., 1986) that all patients with severe craniofacial anomalies and significant breathing problems, regardless of their planned subsequent treatment, have a tracheotomy as an initial measure because asphyxiation may occur.

Chronic Nasal Obstruction

Individuals with craniofacial anomalies commonly are open-mouthed. However, mouth-breathing is not always indicative of nasal airway obstruction; it may be a consequence of malocclusion or retrognathia. If it is due to nasal obstruction, the latter may be secondary to causes (allergic rhinitis, adenoidal hypertrophy) unrelated to the anomaly. However, in most of these patients, nasal obstruction is consequent upon distortion of the midfacial anatomy. Differentiation of mouth-open posture and true nasal airway obstruction and various causes thereof is greatly facilitated by using rhinometry; the author now has experience with the use of active posterior rhinometry in over 1000 patients (Parker et al., 1989).

As clefts of the primary and secondary palate are a common anomaly, nasal obstruction is most frequently observed in that group of patients. Reduction in the caliber of the nasal airway may be a consequence of

several factors unique to these children: distortion of nasal soft tissue, nasal mucosa edema, and deviation of the nasal septum. In children who have a unilateral cleft of the primary palate, slumping and collapse of the ipsilateral lower lateral cartilage may cause obstruction. Significant nasal mucosa edema may be a consequence of an ipsilateral oronasal fistula, heterotopic dental eruption in the floor of the nose, or sinusitis. If the cleft is unilateral, the nasal septum is deviated: The anterior aspect of the nasal septum is visible in the contralateral nostril; posteriorly, however, the septum angulates sharply to the cleft side, to articulate with the tilted, malpositioned vertical plate of the vomer bone (Fig. 4–5).

In the absence of anterior nasal obstruction due to alar collapse, successful septoplasty with improvement of the airway will be achieved by removing the septal obstruction and reducing mucosa edema. The former is accomplished by relatively conservative excision of the caudal aspect of the quadrilateral cartilage, maintaining dorsal and caudal struts, combined with radical removal of the nasal crest of the maxilla and the thickened, tilted vomer bone. Management of mucosa edema with turbinate hypertrophy is difficult. Elimination of sinusitis and closure of the oronasal fistula is helpful, as may be out-fracturing of the ipsilateral turbinate; turbinate bulk can be reduced by cauterization, cryosurgery, or laser application. We reserve aggressive management of nasal obstruction until early adolescence, when the patients are embarking upon more active orthodontic management, as persistent mouth-breathing then will have a deleterious effect on the teeth.

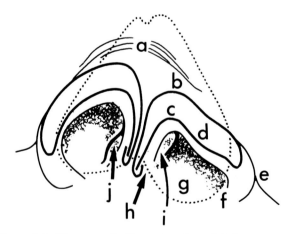

Figure 4–5. Diagrammatic illustration of nasal deformity in the patient with unilateral cleft of primary palate. (a) Nasal tip deviated to normal side. (b) Ipsilateral upper lateral cartilage flatter. (c) Dome of lower lateral cartilage lower, retroposed, and less well-developed. The angle between medial and lateral crurae is less acute. (d) Lateral crus of lower lateral cartilage flatter, and alar base (f) displaced downward in association with flat, underdeveloped maxilla (e). (g) Nasal floor wider. (h) Columella and cartilaginous septum deviated to normal side. (i) Posterior cartilaginous deviation usually will cause ipsilateral nasal obstruction, while anteriorly, the caudal strut of the quadrilateral cartilage is visible in the normal side (j).

Airway Obstruction and Craniofacial Surgery

During surgical correction of craniofacial anomalies under general anesthesia, the airway is protected and controlled by the use of an endotracheal tube (nasal or oral) or tracheotomy tube. In many cases, this operative protection must be maintained postoperatively to prevent aspiration of blood from the oropharynx or if airway obstruction by swollen soft tissues is anticipated. Ninety-eight of 542 patients (18 per cent) who underwent craniofacial surgery between 1972 and 1984 inclusively required a tracheotomy for airway management (Crysdale et al., 1987).

Elective tracheotomy is now required less often in this group of patients than was the case even ten years ago. Anesthetists are more facile with flexible endoscopes and now are able to intubate patients who previously were impossible or extremely difficult to intubate. The increasing use of miniplates across osteotomy sites to stabilize the facial skeleton has frequently eliminated the need for intermaxillary fixation—one of the indications for tracheotomy. Appropriate communication is necessary between the craniofacial surgeon, the otolaryngologist, the anesthetist, and, perhaps, even the intensivist as the patient's preoperative, intraoperative, and postoperative airway management is considered. Generally speaking, elective tracheotomy should be considered in the following situations. First, tracheotomy is recommended if endotracheal intubation for the intended surgical procedure is impossible or is anticipated to be very difficult or traumatic. In this type of patient, tracheotomy becomes mandatory if postsurgery or extubation distress is anticipated, as airway control at that point may be difficult or impossible. Next, tracheotomy may be indicated to facilitate surgery and postoperative care, especially if extensive midfacial procedures are performed (e.g., Le Fort III). A less common indication is poor patient cooperation in a situation in which endotracheal intubation is normally utilized (e.g., mandibular osteotomy). Most children undergoing mandibular osteotomy will be managed postoperatively with nasoendotracheal tubes, whereas those who have already undergone palatopharyngoplasty may require tracheotomy prior to the osteotomy. However, it is possible to nasally intubate a teenager with a preexisting palatopharyngoplasty flap if the lateral ports are relatively commodious. In children who have severe retrognathia or ankylosis of the temporomandibular joint (Fig. 4–3) and who require tracheotomy, blind nasal intubation may be possible (Sklar and King, 1976), or, alternatively, a rigid bronchoscope can usually be inserted without using a laryngoscope. If severe retrognathia is accompanied by cervical spondylosis, tracheotomy can be performed without airway control but under light anesthesia induced intravenously and supplemented with local infiltration of an anesthetic agent.

Discussion between the anesthetist and the otolaryngologist is essential, to plan preoperative, operative, and postoperative airway management. From 1972 to 1984, 97 of 541 patients underwent elective tracheotomy before a craniofacial operation. One additional patient required an emergency tracheotomy when airway obstruction developed at the time of induction. A total of 12 significant complications occurred in this group of 98 patients—one patient suffered permanent neurologic damage as a result of tracheotomy tube obstruction during the postoperative period. To reduce morbidity rates, all tracheotomies should be done with the airway controlled by a bronchoscope or endotracheal tube.

Intraoperative aspiration of blood is minimized by the routine use of cuffed tracheotomy tubes. In children younger than 6 years of age, the author uses a cuffed armored endotracheal tube, which is sutured in place; 24 hours after surgery, this tube is replaced by a metal, noncuffed tracheotomy tube. Decannulation usually occurs within one week. Children in whom a tracheotomy has been created because intubation would be difficult or impossible and who will require further surgery within six months should be fitted after decannulation with a solid Silastic plug, to maintain the tracheocutaneous fistula. Twenty-two of the 98 children in our series had their tracheocutaneous fistula maintained for these reasons.

After mandibular osteotomy, nasotracheal intubation is maintained until soft tissue swelling subsides. Most children have been extubated uneventfully within five days postoperatively. Between 1972 and 1984, 42 complications were recorded in 278 patients who were nasally intubated for more than six hours postoperatively after craniofacial surgery (usually mandibular osteotomy). Thirty-three patients experienced postextubation airway distress, and recontrol of the airway was required in 11 of these patients: oral endotracheal tube (3), nasal endotracheal tube (5), and urgent tracheotomy (3). Two of the three patients who underwent an urgent tracheotomy developed subglottic stenosis that responded to endoscopy, and decannulation was achieved within six months. Also during this 13-year period, persistent laryngeal granulomas developed in three adolescent girls who had been nasoendotracheally intubated for six days after mandibular osteotomies (Fig. 4–6A). Their symptoms were surprisingly minor—mildly husky speech, transient aphonia, and slight dyspnea with exercise. The granulomata were readily removed by microlaryngoscopy (Fig. 4–6B).

SPEECH DISORDERS

Hypernasality

Hypernasality is most often observed in children who have velopharyngeal incompetence (VPI) after cleft palate repair. It may also be apparent (and it is important that the otolaryngologist stress this to other team members) as "deaf speech" in a child who does not have VPI but who has a craniofacial anomaly and a hearing loss exceeding 30 dB (Yules, 1970). In most

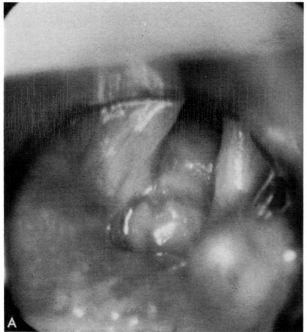

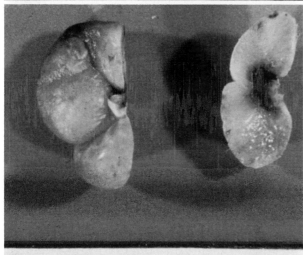

Figure 4–6. *A*, Larynx at time of microlaryngoscopy in 16-year-old girl who had nasoendotracheal intubation for seven days following bilateral mandibular osteotomies four months previously. A mature epithelialized polyp is attached by a narrow stalk to the arytenoid process of the left vocal cord. *B*, Surgical specimen.

youngsters, hypernasal speech can be reduced to an acceptable degree with speech therapy. Persistent VPI has been eliminated in some children by injecting Teflon beneath the mucous membrane of the nasopharynx (Smith and McCabe, 1977), but palatopharyngoplasty is the treatment of choice in most centers. This procedure is usually done when the child is 5 years of age when speech therapy has been unsuccessful. Cineradiography and nasopharyngoscopy with a flexible tube are helpful adjuncts in determining the degree of VPI.

Hyponasality

Hyponasality indicates lack of nasal resonance and is invariably due to nasal airway obstruction. It occurs in patients with severe posterior displacement of the midface, persistent congenital choanal atresia, or iatrogenic velopharyngeal atresia consequent on too successful palatopharyngoplasty. Ironically, in these last patients, their original speech disorder was hypernasality. Removal of nasal airway obstruction diminishes and may eliminate hyponasality.

Nasality is further discussed in Chapter 94.

Hoarseness

Nodules of the vocal cords are present in approximately 20 per cent of children who have VPI; they are thought to be a result of increased laryngeal activity to compensate for loss of vocal power. The nodules and the hoarseness disappear after elimination of the VPI and the evolution of normal speech patterns. Hoarseness—even transient aphonia in some cases—develops after nasotracheal intubation in a minority of patients.

INFECTIONS OF THE UPPER RESPIRATORY TRACT

Purulent otitis media seems to occur more often in children who have craniofacial anomalies. Persistent, painless otorrhea without pyrexia or other evidence of coalescent mastoiditis probably indicates dysfunction of the eustachian tube. The condition may be unresponsive even to rigorous conservative measures, including daily aural toilet under microscopy, instillation of topical medications, and the parenteral administration of aminoglycoside antibiotics. Frequently, at this juncture the therapy is abandoned; then, two to three months later, the ear is found to be dry. In such cases, presumably, cessation of the otorrhea marks the resumption of some degree of eustachian tube function.

In patients with unremitting, recurrent, acute otitis media, adenoidectomy may be advised, even in children who have a repaired cleft of the secondary palate. Velopharyngeal insufficiency will occur postoperatively, and the parents must be advised that palatopharyngoplasty will be required later to eliminate the hypernasality that will be present after adenoidectomy. Adenoidectomy is also indicated before palatopharyngoplasty if there is excessive adenoid tissue obstructing the nasal airway.

Sinusitis is more common than usual in cleft palate patients (Jaffe and DeBlanc, 1971). In our five-year study, unilateral maxillary sinusitis developed in a few adolescents after nasal intubation for four or five days following mandibular osteotomy. Presumably, the nasoendotracheal tube obstructed the ostium of the sinus, preventing normal drainage and providing ideal conditions for opportunistic infection.

Purulent, foul-smelling rhinorrhea indicates the presence of infected foreign material in the nasal airway or paranasal sinuses. The foreign material may be autogenous. Infected bone sequestra and teeth, driven into the sinus during Le Fort osteotomy, have been removed from antra via an anterior approach through the canine fossa; preoperative tomography and intraoperative use of an image intensifier were most helpful to localize and remove these foreign bodies. Foreign material may also be exogenous in origin. It may be food that has been forced into the anterior aspect of the nasal cavity through an oronasal fistula or into the posterior choana past an incompetent palate. In one of our patients, a foul-smelling gauze pack was removed from the back of the nose six months after palatopharyngoplasty.

Tonsillitis does not seem to occur with increased frequency in this group of patients. Tonsillectomy can be done safely if recurrent infections are a problem; in many cleft palate patients, articulation is markedly improved afterwards.

DISORDERS OF OLFACTION

We have not attempted evaluation of the sense of smell in patients with craniofacial anomalies, but some adolescents have commented spontaneously after major corrective surgery that their sense of smell has improved. Presumably, partial or total anosmia is not uncommon in patients with congenital obstruction of the nasal airway.

REFERENCES

Bergstrom, L., Neblett, L. M., and Hemenway, W. G. 1972. Otologic manifestations of acrocephalosyndactyly. Arch. Otolaryngol. 96:117.

Caldarelli, D. E. 1977. Congenital middle ear anomalies associated with craniofacial and skeletal syndromes. In Jaffe, B. F. (ed.): Hearing Loss in Children. A Comprehensive Text. Baltimore, University Park Press, pp. 310–340.

Cogswell, J. J., and Easton, D. M. 1974. Cor pulmonale in the Pierre Robin syndrome. Arch. Dis. Child. 49:905.

Crysdale, W. S. 1978. Abnormal facial appearance and delayed diagnosis of congenital hearing loss. J. Otolaryngol. 7:349.

Crysdale, W. S. 1976. Rational management of middle ear effusions in the cleft palate patient. J. Otolaryngol. 5:463.

Crysdale, W. S., Kohli-Dang, N., Mullins, G. C., et al. 1987. Airway management and craniofacial surgery: Experience in 542 patients. J. Otolaryngol. 16:207.

Don, N., and Siggers, D. C. 1971. Cor pulmonale in Crouzon's disease. Arch. Dis. Child 46:394.

Downs, M. P., and Silver, H. K. 1972. The A.B.C.D.'s to H.E.A.R.; Early identification in nursery, office and clinic of the infant who is deaf. Clin. Pediatr. 11:563.

Farnsworth, P. B., and Pacik, P. T. 1971. Glossoptotic hypoxia and micrognathia—the Pierre Robin syndrome reviewed. Early recognition and prompt surgical treatment is important for survival. Clin. Pediatr. 10:600.

Gorlin, R. J., Pindborg, J. J., and Cohen, M. M., Jr. (eds.) 1976. Syndromes of the Head and Neck, 2nd ed. New York, McGraw-Hill.

Hawkins, D. B., and Simpson, J. V. 1974. Micrognathia and glossoptosis in the newborn. Clin. Pediatr. 13:1066.

Holme, V. A., and Kumze, L. H. 1969. Effect of chronic otitis media on language and speech development. Pediatrics 43:833.

Jackson, P., Whitaker, L. A., and Randall, P. 1976. Airway hazards associated with pharyngeal flaps in patients who have the Pierre Robin syndrome. Plast. Reconstr. Surg. 58:184.

Jaffe, B. F., and DeBlanc, C. B. 1971. Sinusitis in children with cleft lip and palate. Arch. Otolaryngol. 93:479.

Johnston, C., Taussig, L. M., Koopmann, C., et al. 1981. Obstructive sleep apnea in Treacher Collins syndrome. Cleft Palate J. 18:39.

Jones, K. L. 1988. Smith's Recognizable Patterns of Malformation, 4th ed. Philadelphia, W. B. Saunders Co.

Konigsmark, B. W., and Gorlin, R. J. 1976. Genetic and Metabolic Deafness. Philadelphia, W. B. Saunders Co.

Lauritzen, C., Lilja, J., and Jarlstredt, J. 1986. Airway obstruction and sleep apnea in children with craniofacial anomalies. Plast. Reconstr. Surg. 77:1.

Lindsay, J. R., Black, F. O., and Donelly, W. H., Jr. 1975. Acrocephalosyndactyly (Apert's syndrome): Temporal bone findings. Ann. Otol. Rhinol. Laryngol. 84:174.

Mangat, D., Orr, W. C., and Smith, R. O. 1977. Sleep apnea, hypersomnolence, and upper airway obstruction secondary to adenotonsillar enlargement. Arch. Otolaryngol. 103:383.

Munro, I. R. 1975. Orbito-cranio-facial surgery: The team approach. Plast. Reconstr. Surg. 55:170.

Parker, L. P., Crysdale, W. S., Cole, P., et al. 1989. Rhinomanometry in children. Int. J. Pediatr. Otorhinolaryngol. (in press).

Robson, M. C., Stankiewicz, J. A., and Mendelsohn, J. S. 1977. Cor pulmonale secondary to cleft palate repair. Case report. Plast. Reconstr. Surg. 59:754.

Selder, A. 1973. Hearing disorders in children with otocraniofacial syndromes. In Proceedings of the Conference: Orofacial Anomalies. Clinical and Research Implications, April 15–17, 1972. Phoenix, Ariz., American Speech and Hearing Assoc., ASHA Report #8, 95–110.

Sklar, G. S., and King, B. D. 1976. Endotracheal intubation and Treacher Collins syndrome. Anesthesiology 44:247.

Smith, J. K., and McCabe, B. F. 1977. Teflon injection in the nasopharynx to improve velopharyngeal closure. Ann. Otol. Rhinol. Laryngol. 86:559.

Stern, L. M., Fonkalsrud, E. W., Hassakis, P., et al. 1972. Management of Pierre Robin syndrome in infancy by prolonged nasoesophageal intubation. Am. J. Dis. Child. 124:78.

Stool, S. E., and Houlihan, R. 1977. Otolaryngologic management of craniofacial anomalies. Otolaryngol. Clin. North Am. 10:41.

Witzel, M. A., Crysdale, W. S., and Munro, I. R. Speech and hearing problems in 38 patients with Apert's, Crouzon's and Pfeiffer's syndrome. Unpublished observations, the Hospital for Sick Children, Toronto.

Yules, R. B. 1970. Hearing in cleft palate patients. Arch. Otolaryngol. 91:319.

Chapter 5

PRINCIPLES AND METHODS OF MANAGEMENT

Linton A. Whitaker, M.D.   Dennis J. Hurwitz, M.D.

The surgery of craniofacial malformations is an evolving discipline that includes a variety of dental, medical, surgical, and other specialized procedures. Each anomaly must be thoroughly analyzed through meticulous physical examination, advanced imaging techniques, and, at times, extensive surgical exposure. Soft tissue–bone relationships must be appreciated, and the effect of repositioning one on the other needs to be anticipated. Osseous correction involves the isolation of bone segments by osteotomies; alteration of the position of bone in space and fixation by wires or small metal plates; or manipulation of undesirable contours by shaving, burring, or staggering incomplete osteotomies. Soft tissue realignment, coordinated with underlying osseous procedures, is the movement of skin, fat, muscle, and mucous membranes from a nearby or distant location to achieve a desirable correction of the deformity. The surgical exposure of the craniofacial skeleton and the raising of soft tissue flaps should not injure nearby vital structures. A conscientious effort is made to avoid direct cerebral and ocular injuries, fistulas, infections, and inadequate correction of the deformity.

As this surgery is performed primarily in children, the dynamics of growth must be understood and anticipated in the timing and execution of the operations. Successful rehabilitation of the patient is more likely to occur when treatment is performed by an experienced craniofacial team in centers where this surgery is frequently done. Most of the surgical groups have been developed from existing cleft palate teams by adding neurosurgical and ophthalmologic personnel and utilizing more sophisticated imaging techniques and operative methods.

Modern craniofacial surgery began in the 1960's with the pioneering work of plastic surgeon Paul Tessier and has been greatly expanded in North America by other plastic surgeons who have studied with him in Paris, France. His innovative and thoughtful work continues to the present time.

HISTORICAL PERSPECTIVES

From the Trojan War chronicle of Homer to the syndrome report of Crouzon in 1912, the study of congenital craniofacial deformities was largely descriptive.* Limited strip craniectomies were advocated in 1921 (Mehner, 1921); more extensive craniectomies were reported in 1927 (Faber and Towne, 1927). In 1950, the orbital cranial deformity was camouflaged by a variety of extraorbital procedures (Webster and Deming, 1950; Lewin, 1952). Longacre (1968) popularized serial split-rib onlay bone grafts to the hypoplastic midface skeleton of patients with Crouzon syndrome.

In 1949 Gillies performed the first elective craniofacial osteotomy for Crouzon syndrome along the Le Fort III fracture lines (Gillies and Harrison, 1950). Severe midfacial relapse in their patient some years later prompted more limited secondary contour corrections and halted their investigation of this procedure. Between 1949 and 1965, there were scattered attempts at craniofacial reconstruction. Joined by neurosurgeon Rougiere, Tessier approached patients with craniofacial dysostosis with an intracranial exposure through a coronal scalp incision. Tessier modified Gillies' craniofacial dysjunction osteotomies and supported his orbitofacial advancements with bone graft stops.

Since this pioneering work in the mid-1960's, a dozen craniofacial teams have developed worldwide. Careful reviews of extensive and lengthy clinical experiences are becoming available. Computed radiographic and magnetic imaging is being applied to the head and neck. There are innovative ways to harvest and shape bone grafts. Surgical exposure, soft tissue flaps, and osteotomies are being refined. The timing of surgery and psychologic effects are being analyzed.

SPECTRUM OF CORRECTABLE ANOMALIES

Craniofacial surgery, by definition of those working in the field, means surgery concentrated about the orbits and has indeed been called orbitocranial surgery (Whitaker et al., 1976). To qualify as a craniofacial

---

*In the *Iliad*, Thersites is an ugly man whose head comes to a point. This led to the French term *tête à la Thersite* for acrocephaly.

operation, at least one orbit must be entirely stripped of soft tissue except for the attachments at the nasolacrimal apparatus and the point of entry of the optic nerve. The most common structural deformities that can be corrected by a craniofacial technique are acrocephalosyndactyly and craniofacial dysostosis (Apert and Crouzon syndromes), orbital hypertelorism, mandibulofacial dysostosis, hemifacial microsomia, and certain instances of craniofacial trauma and tumors of the midface and orbit. Although these deformities primarily involve the middle and upper thirds of the face, the lower third is often an integral part of the abnormality, as when dealing with deformities of the external ears. Maldevelopment of portions of these interrelated areas often results in distorted growth of adjacent structures, producing a complex deformity of bony and soft tissue (Goodman and Gorlin, 1977).

Mandibulofacial dysostosis, or Treacher Collins syndrome, generally represents the simplest form of deformity correctable by craniofacial surgical techniques. It is characterized by zygomatic hypoplasia of a subtle to extreme degree, often with absent areas of bone in the zygomas, antimongoloid slant of the eyes, nasal deformity, and low-set ears; sometimes with other ear abnormalities; and frequently with mandibular and palatal abnormalities. The basis for correction of the deformity is addition of bone in areas of bony deficiency, with simultaneous correction of the antimongoloid slant of the eyes and correction of the ears. Mandibular osteotomies may also be necessary for correction of such deformities. Hemifacial microsomia is structurally similar to a unilateral form of mandibulofacial dysostosis, manifesting zygomatic and mandibular hypoplasia and ear abnormalities that may be particularly prominent (Franceschetti, 1968).

Craniofacial dysostosis, or Crouzon syndrome, can be identical in appearance to acrocephalosyndactyly and usually involves craniostenosis with forehead and skull abnormalities, as well as orbits that are too shallow for the ocular globes, producing exorbitism. Minimal grades of orbital hypertelorism may be associated with the exorbitism in the craniofacial dysostoses, and typically midface hypoplasia with retromaxillism is present. Correction of these deformities involves a more complicated procedure that includes advancing the areas of bony deficiency and holding the advanced bone in place with bone grafts (Block, 1957; Dingman, 1956; Lewin, 1952; Tessier, 1971c and d).

Orbital hypertelorism and similar craniofacial defects represent perhaps the most complicated of the deformities correctable by craniofacial techniques. The orbits in these patients are too far apart, not having achieved adequate rotation toward the midline *in utero*. The inadequate rotation can be a result of several intrauterine events, including encephaloceles at the frontonasal area, paramedian facial clefts, craniosynostosis, or other as yet unknown reasons (Currarino and Silverman, 1960; Gonzales-Ulloa, 1964; Tessier, 1971a, 1972, 1976; Trautman et al., 1962).

In certain instances the residua of craniofacial trauma, particularly of secondary reconstructions with displacement of the orbit or structures about the upper face, can be corrected using craniofacial techniques (Whitaker and Schaffer, 1977; Jones et al., 1977).

PLANNING RECONSTRUCTION

The major craniofacial abnormalities can be considered as a group for the purposes of operative planning. Because the abnormalities are predominantly structural, with few functional and physiologic problems, the goal of surgical correction is normal facial structure and function. Standards of normality that have been widely described in the plastic surgery, physical anthropology, and dental literature are used for evaluating craniofacial procedures and problems. Such norms are the basis for determining what is abnormal and for defining the goal of the surgery (Broadbent and Mathews, 1957; Cameron, 1931; Duke-Elder and Wybar, 1961; Gonzales-Ulloa, 1962, 1964; Whitaker et al., 1975).

Physical examination of the craniofacial structure as a whole must be performed, utilizing concepts of symmetry and facial form. Operations on soft tissue, the nose, and the ears are based on the principles of symmetry in facial form. The hairline in the frontal region should be more or less horizontal, and the eyebrows should be in the same plane. The medial and lateral canthi normally are on the same horizontal line, approximately parallel to the eyebrows. Slight variations from this can exist, but in general there should be a straight line from the lateral canthi through the medial canthi. The upper edge of the ear is normally at approximately the lower edge of the eyebrow on each side.

Bony shifts represent the foundation of craniofacial surgery, and measurements between bones are the basis for such shifts. The interpupillary distance is measured between the midpoints of the pupils. Although the measurement is often inaccurate because of strabismus, it is a useful preliminary guide; the normal range is 58 to 71 mm in the adult. The medial intercanthal distance is obtained by using calipers to measure between the medialmost extents of the palpebral fissures; this distance is the final determinant of the success of the correction. However, the measurement that is used as the basis for planning orbital shifts is the bony interorbital distance. It is determined by using standard 2-m films (to reduce magnification errors) and making measurements directly on radiographs. Cephalograms also may be utilized for this. The normal medial intercanthal distance is 5 to 8 mm more than the bony interorbital distance.

Orbital volume and globe-orbit relationships can be measured in a variety of ways. An indirect clinical indicator of orbital volume is the hand-held Luedde exophthalmometer. It measures the distance from the lateral orbital margin to the apex of the cornea. This distance normally is from 12 to 16 mm. The difference between the measured and expected values is the distance that an orbit of insufficient volume at the level of the lateral orbital rim must be advanced to produce an orbit of normal depth and volume. However, if the remaining orbital walls relate abnormally to the lateral orbital wall, special compensation in the operative planning is made. Computed tomography (CT) scans and three-dimensional reformations can be used to more directly measure the globe and orbital relationships, as well as the orbital volume.

By measuring the medial intercanthal distance and obtaining a direct exophthalmometer reading on the patient, determinations can be made as to how far medially or forward to shift the orbits. In addition, measuring levels of the orbital rims, pupils, and canthi aids in determining how far superiorly or inferiorly to move an orbit. By such determinations, precise planning can be made for movement of orbits in any direction.

Bitemporal distance may be considered also, because if it is too wide, it must be narrowed, and if too narrow, expanded. The same is true for the zygomas. Prominence of the zygomatic bones is essential to normal facial appearance, and because they are often hypoplastic in the syndromes referred for corrective surgery and may be completely absent, they must be considered in reconstruction of the face. The zygomatic arches are the key to reconstruction of defects in mandibulofacial dysostosis. They average 1.5 cm at the widest, and 0.5 cm anterior-to-posterior in the adult. The distance from the external auditory canal to the zygomaticomaxillary sutures averages 6 cm in the adult. The exact length can be determined in each individual by direct measurement from the tragus to the lateral side of the nose. Bone grafts to correct defects must approximate these dimensions.

Photographs are essential in planning the craniofacial operative procedures, as they give a fixed point of reference for soft tissue and bony shifts. Life-sized black and white photographs in full face and profile views are utilized, with plans for orbital and jaw shifts as well as ear and nose changes based on such photographs. They are used in conjunction with direct patient measurements, radiographic measurements, and dental study models in planning the corrective surgery.

Dental study models determine the jaw shifts that are necessary to correct the malocclusion that usually occurs in these syndromes. The lips must be taken into consideration with such jaw shifts, and changes in the form of the lips must be made if necessary to accommodate shifts of either the mandible or maxilla.

Standard 2-m radiographs in the posteroanterior and lateral views or cephalometrograms are essential for measurements of the bony distances of the face. They are particularly necessary in determining the cribriform plate level, which is important in deciding whether or not to operate intracranially to correct hypertelorism. Standardized radiographs are essential for long-term follow-up and for determining whether growth or relapse has occurred.

Tomograms may be useful in defining abnormalities within the orbits or in the cranial base: computed tomography is a precise tool for determining structures within the orbit and cranium. Recently three-dimensional surface imaging from CT scans has become a routine part of the diagnostic evaluation. Special computed programs and sophisticated editing of high-quality, abutting CT slices reconstruct images to resemble anatomic dry skulls. Cryptic anatomic deformity is visualized, greatly assisting in planning osteotomies (Fig. 5–1A and B). The visual composite offered by the three-dimensional image is of inestimable advantage to grasp the artistic implication of the deformity in this treatment. CT-based surgical simulation with model reconstruction is now cumbersome and time consuming. However, further advances in technology should make this approach feasible, thereby minimizing surgical error and predicting the amount of soft tissue change that will accompany a given bony improvement.

Multispecialty evaluation of the patient's condition and potential for rehabilitation is essential in craniofacial surgery (Munro, 1975); thus, the team concept is extremely important. In particular, neurosurgeons must work in conjunction with plastic surgeons in all operative procedures performed on patients with intracranial problems. Airway problems are handled by the otolaryngology service: Elective tracheostomies are performed infrequently. Abnormal laryngeal position or anatomy, especially as encountered in Treacher Collins syndrome, might require a preoperative tracheostomy, particularly when the child is younger than 3 years of age or lower facial or neck surgery is contemplated. All patients having surgery to correct orbit deformities are seen by ophthalmologists (strabismus following craniofacial surgery is frequent, although most of the time it is self-limiting). Input from the anesthesiology group is essential because of the frequent difficulties that occur with airway maintenance and the prolonged time that the patient is anesthetized. In the authors' institution the anthesiologists regularly evaluate the patients prior to their admission to the hospital. The need for specialized radiographs means that an unusual amount of input is necessary from the radiology department. Dental help, particularly from orthodontics and pedodontics, is necessary both for planning and in providing methods of fixation following surgical reconstructive procedures about the jaws. Physical anthropology has been useful in helping to determine the normal values for facial measurements and the proper goals for surgical procedures. The nursing services and intensive care units are alerted to provide the special care required by these patients, who have massive facial swelling and often large bandages following surgery.

SURGICAL METHODS

PRELIMINARY SURGICAL PREPARATION. Preparations for a major, prolonged operative procedure must be made (Davies and Munro, 1975; Munro, 1975). All patients in whom the oral or nasal cavities or any of

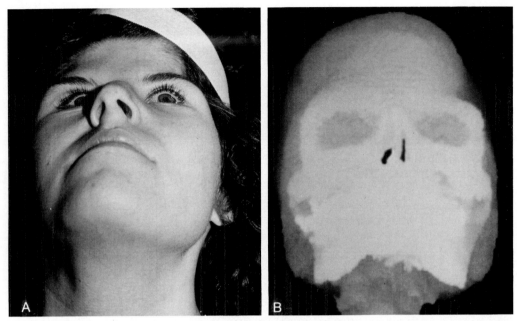

Figure 5–1. A, This teenage female patient had bicoronal synostosis that failed to respond to extended strip craniectomy in infancy. B, CT scan. In addition to deep supraorbital and temporal depressions, which are more extensive on the left side than on the right side, she has marked asymmetry of the orbits. The right orbit is much wider than the left, with the lateral orbital rim being 50 per cent wider on the right than on the left. The nasal bone deviation to the right is well visualized.

the sinuses is entered receive preoperative antibiotics in the highest appropriate dose for their body weight and age. The antibiotic is started 12 hours before surgery and is given at 4-hour intervals during the operative procedure.

Because of the prolonged nature of the procedure and because frequently a large volume of blood is lost, the following must be prepared by the anesthesia group:

1. Standard intravenous lines
2. Central venous pressure line
3. Arterial lines
4. Indwelling urinary catheter
5. Rectal thermometer probe
6. Electrocardiograph leads connected to a visual display screen
7. Endotracheal anesthesia tube
8. Preparation for hypotensive anesthesia
9. Cerebrospinal fluid drainage catheter which is optional and may be left open to drip during intracranial operations
10. Oxygen pulse oximeter

THE EXPOSURE. The unique feature of and, in fact, the foundation of craniofacial surgery is the coronal incision. This incision is carried from the superior tragal notch on one side to the superior tragal notch on the opposite side, going directly across the vertex of the skull. The scalp flap and forehead tissue are then turned down and a subperiosteal dissection of the entire upper facial skeleton is carried out (Fig. 5–2). Unusually good visualization of the upper face and midface is thus provided, and the orbits and nasal bones can be exposed in case plating or wiring of bony fragments is necessary about the infraorbital rim. A conjunctival incision is done to allow visualization of

the area from the nasolacrimal apparatus medially to the juncture of the inferior and lateral orbital walls. Only when a considerable amount of bone grafting has to be done on the anterior zygoma is an external eyelid incision used. If scars are present, particularly after trauma, they may be used for access. External nasal incisions are sometimes made in instances of hypertelorism; other than in these two exceptions, all incisions are kept in the hairline and in the conjunctival area so that visible scars are kept to a minimum.

The lower face, below the level of the zygomas, is approached by means of buccal sulcus incisions, in combination with conjunctival or eyelid incisions (Fig. 5–3). By means of the buccal sulcus incision, the entire maxilla and lower portion of the zygoma including the zygomatic arch can be cleared. Such incisions are used for midface osteotomies such as in a Le Fort I, II, or III osteotomy. When possible, entry into the oral cavity is avoided because of concern about contaminating the wound, although infections have been rather rare.

By means of these combined approaches, all soft tissue is stripped from the face from the level of the forehead to the level of the maxilla, leaving the orbital contents attached only at the optic foramen and the nasolacrimal apparatus. The soft tissue orbits are, therefore, circumferentially mobilized, and the nose is detached of all soft tissue in most instances to a level below the nasal bones (Tessier, 1971d).

EXTRACRANIAL CORRECTIONS. In its simplest form, craniofacial surgery involves adding bone to areas of deficiency. This occurs primarily in instances of mandibulofacial dysostosis, hemifacial microsomia, and posttraumatic problems, as well as in a host of other, rare problems.

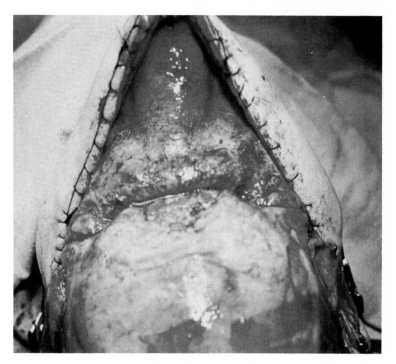

Figure 5–2. Coronal incision showing subperiosteal dissection to base of nose and exposing upper portions of both orbits.

The most common donor sites for bone grafts have been the ribs, calvaria, and ilium. Up to four ribs can be taken without concern by skipping one rib in the middle and taking two on either side of the strut. In general, a 4- to 5-cm inframammary incision is made and the ribs are dissected out subperiosteally in 8- to 15-cm segments, depending on the size of the patient. Rib regrowth can then be expected and the same ribs reharvested at a later date (Longacre and deStefano, 1957; Pagnell, 1960).

As an alternative, especially when cancellous bone is specifically desired or when larger amounts of bone are needed, iliac bone can be used, but there is the disadvantage of greater and more prolonged donor site discomfort. The scarring is also generally more obvious. The thickness of the ilium allows for more freedom to sculpt the grafts to fit the facial contours and optimize bony contact between recipient bed and graft. Cancellous bone is also useful in areas of marginal vascularity where a more certain take of the bone graft is desirable, so that in certain instances the disadvantages are outweighed by better results.

The bone grafts are tailored to the appropriate size and shape and wired into place. In mandibulofacial dysostosis, two or three layers of split ribs are usually needed across the body of the zygoma and one or two

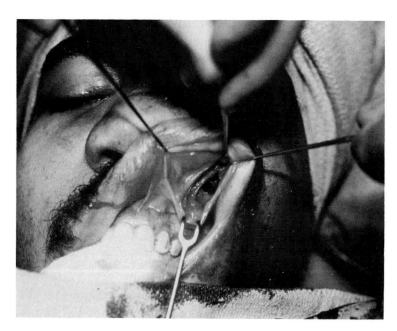

Figure 5–3. Buccal sulcus incision for exposure of lower face.

layers are needed along the lateral orbit of each side of the face. In hemifacial microsomia, the reconstruction is similar but usually unilateral (Converse et al., 1973a and b, 1974a and b; Longacre et al., 1963; Obwegeser, 1974) (Figs. 5–4 and 5–5).

With care, large segments of split- or full-thickness bone grafts can be harvested from the temporoparietal bones. The donor sites of full-thickness calvarial grafts can be reconstructed with split-thickness portions of the graft or by curing methyl methacrylate at room temperature. The membranous cranial bone grafts resorb less than bone grafts from other donor sites but are difficult to shape and contour because of variable thickness and brittleness. In highly selected situations, such as if there is zygomaticomaxillary bone and soft tissue deficiency, vascularized parietal bone grafts transferred to the face on a pedicle of the superficial temporal artery may result in permanent improvement (Cutting et al., 1984) (Fig. 5–6A and B). Free autogenous bone grafts, with the occasional use of the pedicled bone graft, are preferred to obtain bony stability and augmentation. A variety of implantable materials, including laminated carbonized Teflon (Proplast), ceramics, irradiated bone, and cartilage, have become available. These materials tend to be used for secondary augmentation of bone.

Osteotomies with *en bloc* movements of segments of bone are sometimes done extracranially. In particular, subcranial Le Fort III osteotomies or movements of segments of hypoplastic zygomas are instances in which this technique is used. The segments of bone to be moved are cut loose using power tools and osteotomes and moved into position. Bone grafts are placed behind them to fill the gap and to hold the segment in its new position. Wires are used to fix the bones in place when necessary, although interlocking segments of bone held by tension are preferred if possible (Murray and Swanson, 1968). Small bone plates, with self-tapping screws, are increasingly being used to stabilize maxillary and mandibular osteotomies.

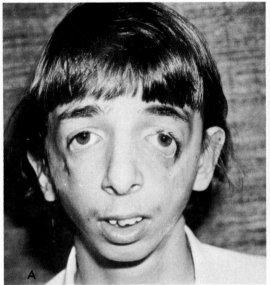
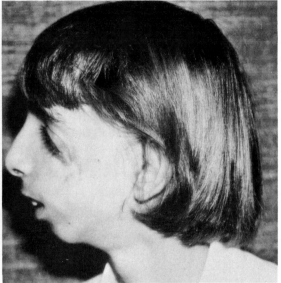
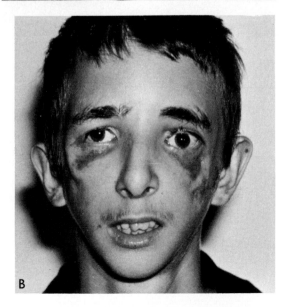

Figure 5–4. *A,* Preoperative full face and profile views of patient with Treacher Collins syndrome, showing pseudocolobomas, extreme zygomatic hypoplasia, and hypoplasia of the chin. *B,* Postoperative view showing correction of colobomas, zygomatic hypoplasia, and chin deficiency. The zygomatic hypoplasia was corrected with onlay grafts and the chin deformity with a combination of sliding genioplasty and onlay grafts.

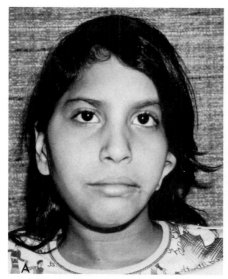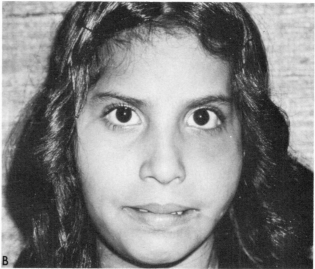

Figure 5–5. *A*, Preoperative view of patient with left hemifacial microsomia. *B*, Postoperative view of same patient, following onlay grafts to zygoma, dermal graft, and lateral canthopexy on the left. (Reproduced by permission from Whitaker, L. A. 1978. Evaluation and treatment of upper facial asymmetry. *In* Whitaker, L. A., and Randall, P. (eds.): Symposium on Reconstruction of Jaw Deformity. St. Louis, 1978, The C. V. Mosby Co.)

Postoperative intermaxillary fixation has been eliminated or reduced to only several weeks.

Following corrections, the wounds are generally closed with single layer sutures.

LIMITED INTRACRANIAL APPROACHES WITH EN BLOC MOVEMENTS. These approaches involve limited intracranial dissection, typically with burr holes to protect the frontal or temporal lobes of the brain. This is most applicable in an extended Le Fort III osteotomy, in procedures to move the lateral wall of the orbit, or in certain instances of Le Fort II osteotomies. The burr holes are made in the frontal and temporal regions in the Le Fort III procedure so that the extended Le

Fort III can be carried up to the supraorbital area with the frontal lobes protected by the burr holes, using packing to move the frontal lobe of the brain and to move the temporal lobe backward (Fig. 5–7*A* through *D*).

In all instances in which the jaws are moved, some form of fixation is necessary. Generally, this means intermaxillary fixation, often with cast-capped splints or with orthodontic bands. This must be carefully planned with the orthodontists preoperatively (Freihofer, 1973; Hogemann and Willmar, 1974; Jabaley and Edgerton, 1969; Longacre, 1968; Obwegeser, 1969; Tessier, 1971*b*, *c*, and *e*).

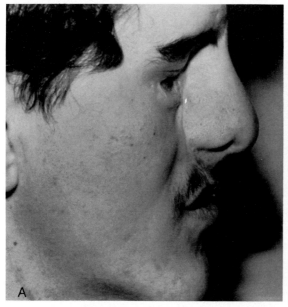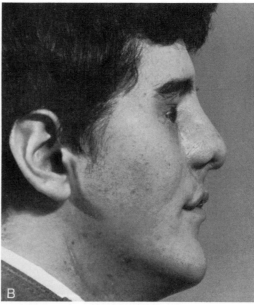

Figure 5–6. *A*, This young man, with bilateral oblique facial cleft, has severe maxillomalar retrusion despite a prior Le Fort I advancement osteotomy and recession of the mandible. In addition, he has congenital anophthalmic orbit on the right. *B*, The postoperative view shows the result after a superficial temporal artery full-thickness parietal bone graft, which has maintained its projection owing to its enhanced vascularity.

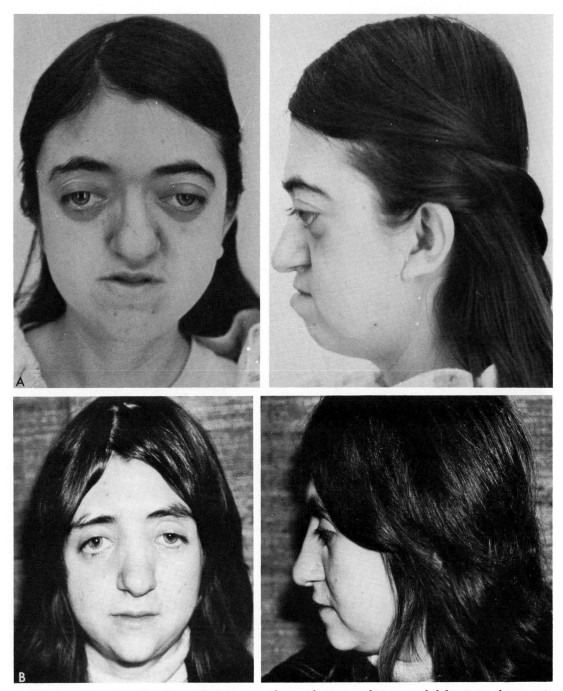

Figure 5–7. A, Preoperative views of patient with Crouzon syndrome, showing exorbitism, nasal deformity, and zygomaticomaxillary hypoplasia. B, Postoperative views showing deformities corrected following Le Fort III midface advancement.

Illustration continued on following page

INTRACRANIAL PROCEDURES. Full-scale intracranial approaches are required in the most complex craniofacial procedures. These involve complete shifts of one or both orbits or of any of the bones about the skull. The orbits may be cut loose posteriorly near the apex and shifted in any direction desired to correct the structural deformities (Fig. 5–8). It is only by means of such an intracranial approach that techniques can be used to protect the frontal lobe of the brain.

The neurosurgeon does a unilateral or bilateral cra-

niotomy after stripping of the soft tissue has been completed. The frontal lobes of the brain and, if necessary, the temporal lobes are retracted after the craniotomy is done, and the osteotomies of the orbits are next accomplished. Protecting both the brain and the orbital contents and using power instruments, the orbits are cut loose and moved in the direction desired. In the correction of orbital hypertelorism, a segment of bone is removed from the region of the glabella and the nose; both orbits are cut loose and are moved

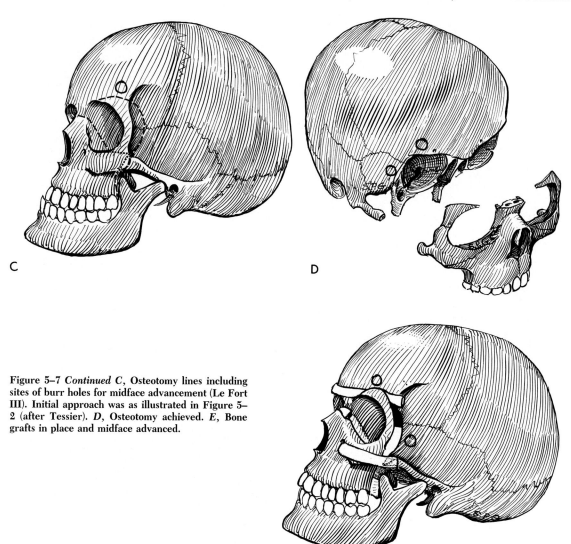

Figure 5–7 *Continued C*, Osteotomy lines including sites of burr holes for midface advancement (Le Fort III). Initial approach was as illustrated in Figure 5–2 (after Tessier). *D*, Osteotomy achieved. *E*, Bone grafts in place and midface advanced.

medially. For downward displacement of an orbit, it is cut and moved into the position desired. Inferior orbital movement can be accomplished if an orbit is, as occasionally occurs with craniostenosis, positioned too high. Orbits may be advanced by cutting them near the apex, moving them into a forward position, and holding them there with bone grafts. This is particularly applicable in the correction of exorbitism (Converse et al., 1970, 1975; Converse and Wood-Smith, 1971; Edgerton et al., 1970; Longacre, 1968; Tessier, 1972, 1974).

After orbital movements, gaps should be filled with bone grafts—typically split rib—and the segments wired in place. Interlocking bone segments, if possible, are preferred.

Shifts of areas of skull to correct deformities of any area but particularly about the frontal or temporal region may be made by cutting the bones loose, repositioning them, and molding or shaping them as necessary by burring, cutting, or refashioning with bone grafts (Munro, 1976).

PREVENTIVE SURGERY. Surgery on children younger than 1 year old is an exciting clinical area in the correction of craniofacial deformities. It is particularly applicable in structural deformities of the upper face and utilizes the developing brain and globes as molding influences on reconstructed structures. The brain nearly triples in volume during the first year of life, and the ocular globes follow a similar pattern of growth. After 3 months of age, it is technically simpler to do the soft tissue dissection required in a craniofacial exposure, and the bones are much more pliable and easily cut. At the same time, the neurosurgeon does a craniectomy for craniostenosis; in children with deformities about the upper face, the orbits can be partially advanced into new positions, or less severe cases of hypertelorism can be corrected. Following that correction, and after placement of structures into more normal relation with one another, growth progresses normally under the influence of the developing brain and ocular globes (Fig. 5–9). In addition to the technical and psychologic advantages of early correction, distant bone graft donor sites are not necessary, because bone obtained from a craniectomy can be used

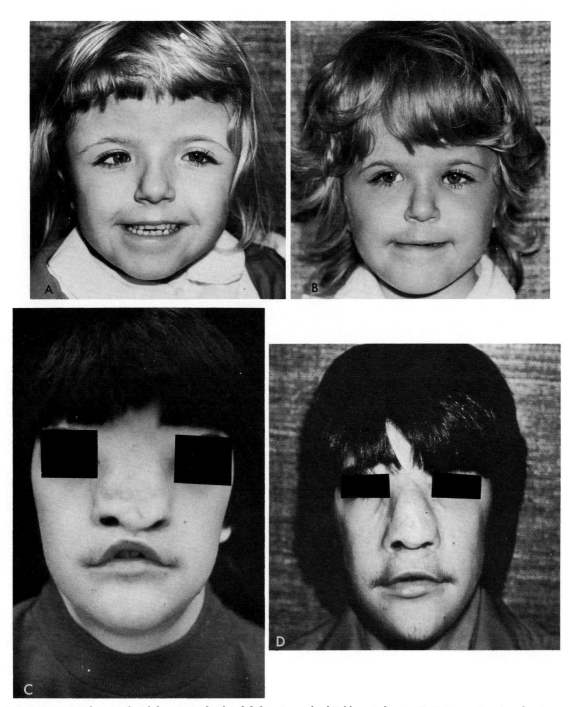

Figure 5–8. *A*, Patient with craniofacial dysostosis, forehead deformity, and orbital hypertelorism. *B*, Postoperative view showing correction of orbital hypertelorism and reshaping of forehead intracranially. *C*, Preoperative view of patient with orbital hypertelorism, nasal deformity, and extremely short upper lip. *D*, Postoperative view showing correction of orbital hypertelorism, correction of nasal deformity, and lengthening of lip.

Illustration continued on following page

for grafting (Edgerton et al., 1974*a* and *b*; Freihofer, 1974; Ingraham et al., 1948; Longacre et al., 1961; Whitaker and Randall, 1974; Whitaker et al., 1976*b*, 1977).

RESULTS

ANCILLARY PROCEDURES. By means of alterations in the major bony and soft tissues of the face, the basic architecture of the face is changed. Additional procedures are usually required to attain the best corrections of facial deformities: medial canthopexies with orbital hypertelorism; lateral canthopexies with hypertelorism, mandibulofacial dysostosis, and craniofacial dysostosis; and corrections of nasolacrimal apparatus problems. Various forms of osteoplasty may be necessary. Nasolacrimal apparatus drainage problems are frequent in orbital hypertelorism, in which an inadequate drain-

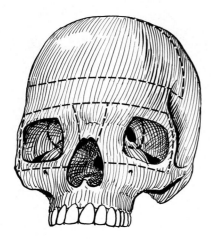

E

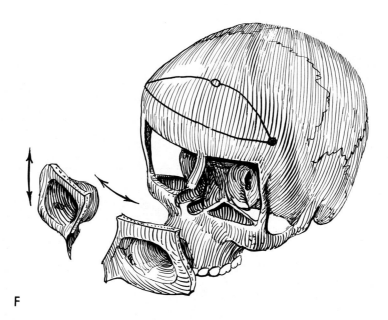

F

Figure 5–8 *Continued E*, Basic osteotomy sites for orbital shifts used with variations in the two patients. Full craniotomy was necessary for brain protection. *F*, Orbits mobilized. *G*, Orbits in place with bone grafts. (*A* and *B* with permission from Whitaker, L. A., et al. 1980. Improvements in craniofacial reconstruction: Methods evolved in 235 consecutive patients. Plast. Reconstr. Surg. 65:561.)

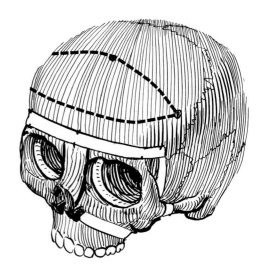

G

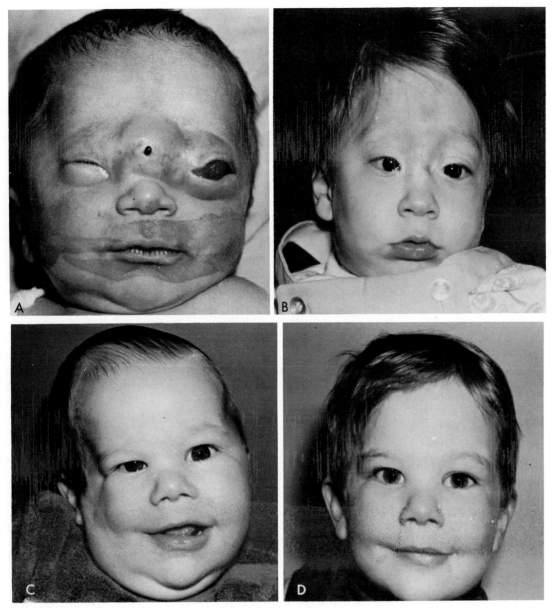

Figure 5–9. *A,* Preoperative view of patient with encephalocele and orbital hypertelorism. *B,* Postoperative view of same patient. *C,* Preoperative view of patient with isolated craniostenosis. *D,* Postoperative view of same patient. (*A* and *B* with permission from Whitaker, L. A., et al. 1980. Improvements in craniofacial reconstruction: Methods evolved in 235 consecutive patients. Plast. Reconstr. Surg. 65:561. *C* and *D* with permission from Whitaker, L. A., et al. 1977. Early surgery for isolated craniofacial dysostosis. Plast. Reconstr. Surg. 60:575.)

age system often exists. Often canthoplasties are advisable in addition to canthopexies in instances of webbing at the medial canthi following correction of orbital hypertelorism. Eyebrows may have to be repositioned. Nasal soft tissue changes may be necessary, particularly in patients with clefts going through the nose and the interorbital area. These are done in tandem with bony changes about the orbit. Plastic procedures on the lip and the ear and changes in the lower jaw may be essential to completing the reconstruction. Mandibular and maxillary osteotomies may be required, particularly in patients with mandibulofacial dysostosis and in those with hemifacial microsomia or other types of facial asymmetry.

Improvement in the stability of medial orbital trans-

position and simultaneous correction of anterior openbite with expansion of the maxillary arch can be achieved by a total facial bipartition procedure introduced by Van der Muelen (1983) and promoted by Caronni (1986). In this operation, the two halves of the maxilla are split at the level of the midpalate; as the orbits are drawn together, the hemimaxillas are distracted.

PROBLEMS AND COMPLICATIONS. The involved and major nature of this surgery makes it hazardous: The mortality rate worldwide has been approximately 1.5 per cent. Death is generally related to intracranial problems associated with the length of the surgery, brain damage during surgery, or intracranial infections. Blindness has been reported, but is rare, and has generally occurred as a result of shifts of the orbits for orbital hypertelorism.

Infection has been the most frequent serious problem occurring in this surgery, with an approximate 7 per cent infection rate documented in one large series (Whitaker et al., 1976a). There is a slightly higher incidence of infection associated with intracranial procedures in which the oral cavity is entered, but in general the infection rate has been rather uniform for intra- and extracranial procedures. By means of the routines outlined earlier, the infection rate has been diminished considerably in the authors' patients. Generally temporary, although sometimes permanent, damage to the cranial nerves has been reported, particularly to the sixth nerve and to a frontal branch of the seventh nerve. Areas of hypesthesia with fifth nerve deficit are frequent following the surgery but are usually transient.

Canthal drift following medial repositioning or upward or downward repositioning of the lateral canthus is a significant problem that has not been satisfactorily solved. Telecanthus following reconstruction for orbital hypertelorism is minimized by preliminary dissection of the medial canthal ligaments. External compression plates have not been satisfactory and may cause skin necrosis. Direct deep suturing of the skin of the nose and medial canthal region to the repositioned orbital and nasal bones has minimized lateral drift of the medial canthal region. Nevertheless, local soft tissue revisionary surgery for the canthi is often necessary.

Growth patterns following surgery in craniofacial dysostosis are unpredictable. Extensive early frontoorbital reconstruction of the Apert deformity is usually followed by some recurrence of the original turribrachycephaly. Moreover, in older patients, the bony deformity is so extensive and the soft tissues so poorly malleable to the reconstructed skeleton that the results are frequently less than satisfactory.

Strabismus is another problem that occurs in the orbital region, following stripping of the orbits. In most instances, this is self-correcting, but a small number of patients will require strabismus surgery. Velopharyngeal incompetence following midface advancement has been reported but is seemingly rare.

Structural losses, or bony resorption, are difficult to measure accurately. There is undoubtedly a small amount of this in every case, but the precise amount is difficult to determine. It is believed that *en bloc* movements have less tendency to resorb or relapse, whereas onlay grafts result in unpredictable amounts of resorption.

Although the facial structures may be repositioned to reflect normal or nearly normal relations to each other, the most difficult structural problem remaining is still the soft tissue deformity in overall facial form and function. With the less severe deformities, a normal facial appearance can often be achieved, but with increasingly severe deformities the residua of correction, especially the soft tissue problems, continue to be difficult to deal with.

Growth has seemed to progress normally in faces following upper face surgery. Midface surgery at an early age is not followed by normal growth (Kaban et al., 1986; Kreiborg and Aduss, 1986). Therefore, major procedures should probably be delayed except for the most severely deformed and psychosocially handicapped individuals.

It is to be remembered that the recovery period is long, and that postoperatively the face is bandaged and the patients frequently are intubated with an endotracheal tube, so communication is difficult. This situation is extremely well tolerated, particularly in younger children. The facial bandages are removed 2 to 3 days postoperatively, but postoperative swelling is present for weeks, and patients are advised to wait at least 6 weeks before attempting to return to normal activities. One year is necessary for all changes to "settle in" and for the final result to be observed (Converse et al., 1974b, 1975; Salyer et al., 1975; Whitaker et al., 1976b).

TIMING OF SURGERY

The planning of the surgical rehabilitation of a patient with a major craniofacial deformity ideally begins at birth. The decision as to timing of surgery is a judgment balancing the indications for surgery and the knowledge that a repositioned, but nongrowing maxilla will ultimately thwart facial balance. The release of coronal synostosis with frontoorbital advancement is performed at about 6 months of age, when cranial bones have become firm enough for stability and the brain growth potential is considerable. The treatment of asymmetric deformities has been more successful than that of the symmetric ones (Whitaker and Bartlett, 1987). The early frontoorbital advancement performed in infancy should have the temporal and lateral orbital structures reconstructed with cranial bone so that healthy, normal-thickness bone can be advanced at the time of midfacial surgery some years later. Craniectomized cranium is replaced by thin and brittle bone that is difficult to recontour. In general, the rare infant with Crouzon or Apert syndrome with compromised airway, increasing visual loss, or feeding problems should be treated with local procedures such as tracheostomy, eyelid tarsorrhaphies, and gastrostomy. Life-threatening hemorrhage and poor stability have inhibited the performance of frontofacial advancements in early infancy by most surgeons. However, Mühlbauer and associates (1987) have shown excellent early results with the temporary use of miniplates for holding monoblock advancements in infant surgery for craniofacial dysostosis. Marchac and Renier (1987) advocated early craniofacial approach for the most severe deformities. Severe midfacial retrusion, particularly with complicating nasopharyngeal obstruction, dislocation of the globe from the orbit, recurrent corneal ulcerations, and possible irreversible psychologic problems, may prompt a Le Fort III facial advancement by the age of 3 years. Unless there are significant functional or psychosocial indications, midface advancement by Le Fort I, II, or III, if not performed by preschool age, should be postponed until facial growth is complete.

It appears that the stability of the correction of orbital hypertelorism is good and that inhibition of growth, even with complete nasal septal resection, is minimal, so the operation can be performed anytime after the age of 2 years (Lejoyeux et al., 1986). Mulliken and Kaban (1986) agreed that growth is minimally affected but were disappointed with the early relapse that occurred after more extensive orbital translocations and with the excessive resorption of the nasal bridge bone graft. Malar and maxillary reconstructions in patients with Treacher Collins syndrome have shown an unusual degree of resorption. Temporal fascia grafts appear to have a role in these problematic situations, but it is not clear at this time whether early use of these grafts will be followed by normal growth. The timing of treatment of hemifacial microsomia is directly related to the severity of the deformity. The more severe deformity should be corrected in early childhood (Mulliken and Kaban, 1986; Munro, 1986), with the expectation that more reconstructive surgery will be necessary later.

Careful monitoring of the psychosocial adjustment of the affected patient throughout childhood is important. Pertschuk and Whitaker (1986) have observed that "left uncorrected, craniofacial malformations are associated in adolescence and childhood with measurable disturbances in mood, self-concept, and socialization. Individuals are typically able to perform well enough to avoid psychiatric intervention; however, relative to the general population, these patients are at a distinct psychosocial disadvantage." Improvement in appearance through corrective surgery in young children appears to enhance psychosocial development, but there is often no change in self-concept and adaptability after surgery in adults.

REFERENCES

Block, F. C. 1957. Developmental anomalies of the skull affecting the eye. Arch. Ophthalmol. 57:593.

Broadbent, T. R., and Mathews, V. L. 1957. Artistic relationships in surface anatomy of the face: Application to reconstructive surgery. Plast. Reconstr. Surg. 20:1.

Cameron, J. 1931. Interorbital width, new cranial dimension. Am. J. Phys. Anthropol. 15:509.

Caronni, E. P. 1986. Facial bypartition in hypertelorism. Cleft Palate J. (Suppl.) 23:19.

Converse, J. M., Coccaro, P. J., Becker, M., and Wood-Smith, D. 1973a. On hemifacial microsomia. Plast. Reconstr. Surg. 51:268.

Converse, J. M., Horowitz, S. L., Coccaro, P. J., and Wood-Smith, D. 1973b. Corrective treatment of skeletal asymmetry in hemifacial microsomia. Plast. Reconstr. Surg. 52:221.

Converse, J. M., McCarthy, J. G., and Wood-Smith, D. 1975. Orbital hypertelorism: Pathogenesis, associated faciocerebral anomalies and surgical correction. Plast. Reconstr. Surg. 56:389.

Converse, J. M., Ransohoff, J., Mathews, E. S., Smith, B., and Molenaar, A. 1970. Ocular hypertelorism and pseudohypertelorism. Plast. Reconstr. Surg. 45:1.

Converse, J. M., and Wood-Smith, D. 1971. An atlas and classification of midfacial and craniofacial osteotomies. Transactions of

the Fifth International Congress of Plastic and Reconstructive Surgery. Melbourne, Butterworth's, p. 931.

Converse, J. M., Wood-Smith, D., and McCarthy, J. G. 1975. Report on a series of 50 craniofacial operations. Plast. Reconstr. Surg. 55:283.

Converse, J. M., Wood-Smith, D., McCarthy, J. G., and Coccaro, P. J. 1974a. Craniofacial surgery. Clin. Plast. Surg. 1(3):499.

Converse, J. M., Wood-Smith, D., McCarthy, J. G., Coccaro, P. J., and Becker, M. H. 1974b. Bilateral facial microsomia. Plast. Reconstr. Surg. 54:413.

Currarino, G., and Silverman, F. N. 1960. Orbital hypertelorism, arhinencephaly and trigonocephaly. Radiology 74:206.

Cutting, C. B., McCarthy, J. G., and Berenstein, A. 1984. The blood supply of the upper craniofacial skeleton. The search for composite calvarial bone grafts. Plast. Reconstr. Surg. 74:603.

Davies, D. W., and Munro, I. R. 1975. The anesthetic management and intra-operative care of patients undergoing major facial osteotomies. Plast. Reconstr. Surg. 55:50.

Dingman, R. D. 1956. A syndrome of craniofacial dysostosis. Report of 2 cases. Plast. Reconstr. Surg. 18:113.

Duke-Elder, S., and Wybar, K. C. 1961. The Anatomy of the Visual System (Vol. 2, System of Ophthalmology Series). St. Louis, C. V. Mosby Co.

Edgerton, M. T., Jane, J. A., and Berry, F. 1974a. Craniofacial osteotomies and reconstructions in infants and young children. Plast. Reconstr. Surg. 54:13.

Edgerton, M. T., Jane, A., Berry, F. A., and Fuher, J. C. 1974b. Feasibility of craniofacial osteotomies in infants and young children. Scand. J. Plast. Reconstr. Surg. 8:164.

Edgerton, M. T., Udvarhely, G. B., and Knox, D. L., 1970. The surgical correction of ocular hypertelorism. Ann. Surg. 172:3.

Faber, H. K., and Towne, E. B. 1927. Early craniectomy as a preventive measure in oxycephaly and allied conditions, with special reference to the prevention of blindness. Am. J. Med. Sci. 173:701.

Franceschetti, A. 1968. Craniofacial dysostoses. In Symposium on Surgical and Medical Management of Congenital Anomalies of the Eye. New Orleans Academy of Ophthalmology, 16th Symposium. St. Louis, C. V. Mosby Co., p. 77.

Freihofer, H. P. 1973. Results after midface osteotomies. J. Maxillofac. Surg. 1:30.

Freihofer, H. P. 1974. Kieferorthopadische operationen im jugendalter—ja oder nein? Vortrag Dtsch Ges Kiefer-u Gesichtschir (Hamburg).

Gillies, H. D., and Harrison, S. H. 1950. Operative correction by osteotomy of recessed malar maxillary compound in a case of oxycephaly. Br. J. Plast. Surg. 3:123.

Gonzales-Ulloa, M. 1962. Quantitative principles in cosmetic surgery of the face (profileplasty). Plast. Reconstr. Surg. 29:186.

Gonzales-Ulloa, M. 1964. Quantum method for the appreciation of the morphology of the face. Plast. Reconstr. Surg. 34:241.

Goodman, R. M., and Gorlin, R. J. 1977. Atlas of the Face in Genetic Disorders, 2nd ed. St. Louis, C. V. Mosby Co.

Hogemann, K. E., and Willmar, K. 1974. On LeFort III osteotomy for Crouzon's disease in children. Scand. J. Plast. Reconstr. Surg. 8:169.

Ingraham, F. D., Alexander, E., Jr., and Matson, D. D. 1948. Clinical studies in craniosynostosis; analysis of 50 cases and description of a method of surgical treatment. Surgery 24:518.

Jabaley, M. E., and Edgerton, M. T. 1969. Surgical correction of congenital midface retrusion in the presence of mandibular protrusion. Plast. Reconstr. Surg. 44:1.

Jones, W. D., III, Whitaker, L. A., and Murtagh, F. 1977. Applications of reconstructive craniofacial techniques to acute upper facial trauma. J. Trauma 17:339.

Kaban, L. B., Conover, M., Mullikan, J. B. 1986. Midface position after LeFort III advancement. A long term study. Cleft Palate J. (Suppl.) 23:75.

Kreiborg, S., and Aduss, H. 1986. Pre- and postsurgical facial growth in patients with Crouzon's and Apert's syndrome. Cleft Palate J. 23:78.

Lejoyeux, E., Tulasne, J. F., and Tessier, P. L. 1986. Maxillary growth following total septal resection in correction of orbital hypertelorism. Cleft Palate J. (Suppl.) 23:27.

Lewin, M. L. 1952. Facial deformity in acrocephaly and its surgical correction. Arch. Ophthalmol. 47:321.

Longacre, J. J. 1968. The early reconstruction of congenital hypoplasia of the facial skeleton and skull: Surgical management of facial deformation secondary to craniosynostosis. *In* Longacre, J. J. (ed.): Craniofacial Anomalies: Pathogenesis and Repair. Philadelphia, J. B. Lippincott Co., p. 151.

Longacre, J. J., and deStefano, G. A. 1957. Reconstruction of extensive defects of the skull with split rib grafts. Plast. Reconstr. Surg. 19:186.

Longacre, J. J., DeStefano, A., and Holmstrand, K. E. 1961. The early versus the late reconstruction of congenital hypoplasia of the facial skeleton and skull. Plast. Reconstr. Surg. 27:489.

Longacre, J. J., Stevens, G. A., and Holmstrand, K. E. 1963. The surgical management of first and second branchial arch syndrome. Plast. Reconstr. Surg. 31:507.

Marchac, D., and Renier, D. 1987. Treatment of craniosynostosis in infancy. Clin. Plast. Surg. 14:61.

Mehner, A. 1921. Beitrage zu den Augenveranderungen bei der Schadeldeformitat des sog. Turmschadels mit besonderer Berucksichtigung des Rontgenbildes. Klin. Monatsbl. Augenheilkd. 61:204.

Mühlbauer, W., Anderl, H., Ramatschi, P., et al. 1987. Radical treatment of craniofacial anomalies in infancy and the use of miniplates in craniofacial surgery. Clin. Plast. Surg. 14:101.

Mulliken, J. B., and Kaban, L. B. 1986. Analysis and treatment of hemifacial microsomia in childhood. Clin. Plast. Surg. 14:91.

Munro, I. R. 1975. Orbito-cranio-facial surgery: The team approach. Plast. Reconstr. Surg. 55:170.

Munro, I. R. 1976. Cranial vault reshaping. Presented at the Second International Conference on the Diagnosis and Treatment of Craniofacial Anomalies, New York, May 1976.

Munro, I. R. 1986. Treatment of craniofacial microsomia. Clin. Plast. Surg. 14:77.

Murray, J. E., and Swanson, L. T. 1968. Midface osteotomy and advancement for craniostenosis. Plast. Reconstr. Surg. 41:299.

Obwegeser, H. 1969. Surgical correction of small or retrodisplaced maxillae. Plast. Reconstr. Surg. 43:351.

Obwegeser, H. L. 1974. Correction of skeletal anomalies of otomandibular dysostosis. J. Maxillofac. Surg. 2:73.

Pagnell, A. 1960. The use and behavior of bone grafts to the deformed facial skeleton. *In* Transactions of the Second International Congress of Plastic Surgery. Edinburgh, E and S Livingstone, Ltd.

Pertschuk, M. J., and Whitaker, L. A. 1986. Psychosocial considerations in craniofacial deformity. Clin. Plast. Surg. 14:163.

Salyer, K. E., Munro, I. R., Whitaker, L. A., et al. 1975. Difficulties and problems to be solved in the approach to craniofacial malformations. Birth Defects 11:315.

Tessier, P. 1971a. Orbitocranial surgery. Transactions of the Fifth International Congress of Plastic and Reconstructive Surgery. Melbourne, Butterworth's, p. 903.

Tessier, P. 1971b. Relationship of craniostenoses to craniofacial dysostoses, and to faciostenoses. Plast. Reconstr. Surg. 48:224.

Tessier, P. 1971c. The definitive plastic surgical treatment of the severe facial deformities of craniofacial dysostosis. Plast. Reconstr. Surg. 48:419.

Tessier, P. 1971d. The scope and principles—dangers and limitations—and the need for special training—in orbitocranial surgery. Transactions of the Fifth International Congress of Plastic and Reconstructive Surgery. Melbourne, Butterworth's, p. 903.

Tessier, P. 1971e. Total osteotomy of the middle third of the face for faciostenosis or for sequelae of Le Fort III fractures. Plast. Reconstr. Surg. 48:533.

Tessier, P. 1972. Orbital hypertelorism. 1. Successive surgical attempts, material and methods, causes and mechanisms. Scand. J. Plast. Reconstr. Surg. 6:135.

Tessier, P. 1974. Experiences in the treatment of orbital hypertelorism. Plast. Reconstr. Surg. 53:1.

Tessier, P. 1976. Anatomical classification of facial, craniofacial and laterofacial clefts. J. Maxillofac. Surg. 4:69.

Trautman, R. C., Converse, J. M., and Smith, B. 1962. Plastic and Reconstructive Surgery of the Eye and Adnexa. Washington, Butterworth's.

Van der Meulen, J. C. 1983. Surgery related to the correction of hypertelorism. Plast. Reconstr. Surg. 71:1.

Webster, J. P., and Deming, E. G. 1950. Surgical treatment of bifid nose. Plast. Reconstr. Surg. 6:1.

Whitaker, L. A., and Bartlett, S. P. 1987. The craniofacial dysostoses: Guidelines for management of the symmetric and asymmetric deformities. Clin. Plast. Surg. 14:73.

Whitaker, L. A., and Randall, P. 1974. The developing field of craniofacial surgery. Pediatrics 54:571.

Whitaker, L. A., LaRossa, D., and Randall, P. 1975. Structural goals in craniofacial surgery. Cleft Palate J. 12:23.

Whitaker, L. A., Munro, I. R., Jackson, I. T., and Salyer, K. E. 1976a. Problems in craniofacial surgery. J. Maxillofac. Surg. 4:131.

Whitaker, L. A., and Schaffer, D. 1977. Severe traumatic oculo-orbital displacement: Diagnosis and treatment. Plast. Reconstr. Surg. 59:352.

Whitaker, L. A., Schut, L., and Randall, P. 1976b. Craniofacial surgery: Present and future. Ann. Surg. 184:558.

Whitaker, L. A., Schut, L., and Kerr, L. P. 1977. Early surgery for isolated craniofacial dysostosis. Plast. Reconstr. Surg. 60:575.

Zins, J. E., and Whitaker, L. A. 1979. Membranous vs. endochondral bone autografts: Implications for craniofacial reconstruction. Surg. Forum 30:521.

Section II

THE EAR AND RELATED STRUCTURES

Chapter 6

EMBRYOLOGY AND DEVELOPMENTAL ANATOMY OF THE EAR

Margaret A. Kenna, M.D.

To understand ear disease, both congenital and acquired, knowledge of the embryology and anatomy of the ear is essential. Anatomically, the ear is divided into the external ear, the middle ear, and the inner ear. The middle ear and the inner ear develop in the lateroinferior portion of the skull called the temporal bone. A basic understanding of the developmental anatomy of the branchial arch system is necessary to comprehend the embryology of the ear. There is some disagreement among authors about the exact timing of different developmental events; the timing of such events given here is an attempt to represent the most current consensus.

EXTERNAL EAR

The external ear is divided into the pinna, or auricle, and the external auditory canal. During the fourth week of gestation, the pinna develops around the first branchial groove from first (mandibular) and second (hyoid) branchial arch mesoderm. During the fifth and sixth weeks, these arches give rise to six outgrowths, the hillocks of His, that condense and fuse by the third month to form the pinna. The exact adult structures that form from these hillocks are controversial. One view asserts that the tragus is derived from the first arch, and the rest of the pinna, with the exception of the concha, is derived from the second arch. A second, more widely accepted theory is that the first hillock gives rise to the tragus, the second forms the crus of the helix, the third forms the majority of the helix, the fourth becomes the antihelix, the fifth produces the antitragus, and the sixth gives rise to the lower helix and lobule. The first three hillocks derive from the mandibular arch, and the second three from the hyoid arch (Pearson, 1988). The concha is formed from ectoderm from the first branchial groove. Initially, the developing pinna is located caudal to the mandibular area, but by the 20th fetal week, as the mandible grows and develops, the pinna attains the adult configuration and location (Fig. 6–1A and B). In the child aged 4 to 5 years, the pinna is almost adult-sized; in the 9-year-old child, the pinna has attained complete

adult size. In the newborn, the cartilage of the pinna is soft and pliable, with relatively more chondrocytes and an immature matrix. In the child aged 9 years, the cartilage is firmer and histologically mature (Wong, 1983).

The postnatal anatomy of the pinna is shown in Figure 6–1C through E. Anteriorly the skin is firmly adherent to the elastic cartilage of the pinna, with an absence of subcutaneous tissue, while posteriorly the skin is separated from the cartilage by a distinct subcutaneous layer. The lobule is devoid of cartilage and contains only fibrous tissue and fat. Three extrinsic muscles (the anterior, superior, and posterior auricular muscles) attach the pinna to the scalp and the skull. These muscles, when well developed, can move the auricle as a whole. In humans, there are several intrinsic auricular muscles that are indistinguishable grossly and are functionally insignificant.

The external auditory canal (EAC) develops from the first branchial groove between the mandibular and hyoid arches. At 4 to 5 weeks of gestation, the ectoderm of the first groove comes into contact with the endoderm of the first pharyngeal pouch. Then, mesoderm grows between the ectoderm and the endoderm, and the contact is disrupted. At eight weeks, the cavum conchae (first branchial groove) deepens, forming a funnel-shaped tube, the "primary meatus," that becomes surrounded by cartilage and eventually becomes the outer one third of the EAC. During the ninth week, the groove deepens, grows toward the middle ear, and comes into contact with the epithelium of the first pharyngeal pouch. A solid epidermal plug extends inward from the primary meatus to the primitive tympanic cavity, forming the meatal plate. Then, mesenchyme forms between epithelial cells of the tympanic cavity and the meatal plate and becomes the fibrous layer of the substantia propria of the tympanic membrane (Fig. 6–2). During the 21st fetal week, the cord of epithelial cells begins to resorb, forming a canal. By the 28th week, the deepest cells of the ectodermal plug remain, forming the superficial layer of the tympanic membrane. The medial two thirds of the external auditory canal is derived from the new ectodermal tube and becomes the bony portion of the canal (Pearson, 1988; Schuknecht and Gulya, 1986).

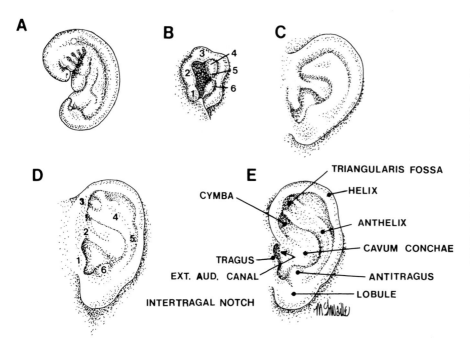

Figure 6–1. Auricular development and anatomy. *A*, Fetus (5 mm): Branchial arch development is evident. *B*, First and second branchial arches in 11-mm fetus: Six hillocks are present; hillocks 1, 2, and 3 are from the first (mandibular) arch; hillocks 4, 5, and 6 are from the second (hyoid) arch. *C*, Newborn auricle: adult configuration but smaller. *D*, Auricle, fully developed, showing hillocks' relationship to anatomy. *E*, Auricle fully developed, showing anatomic parts. (Adapted from Anson, B., and Donaldson, J. 1973. *Surgical Anatomy of the Temporal Bone and Ear*, 2nd ed. Philadelphia, W. B. Saunders Co., p. 31.)

At birth, the external auditory canal is not ossified, except for the tympanic ring, and is not of adult size. Completion of ossification occurs by the second year of life, and adult size is reached by age 9 years. After ossification, the lateral one third of the ear canal is cartilaginous, and the medial two thirds is bony. The skin of the cartilaginous portion contains hair follicles and sebaceous and ceruminous glands.

The intrinsic and the extrinsic auricular muscles are innervated by the facial nerve. The nerve supply to the medial portion of the EAC is from the auriculotemporal (mandibular branch of trigeminal) nerve. The nerve supply to the posterior ear canal and the area around the tympanic membrane proceeds from Arnold's nerve, the only cutaneous branch of the vagus. Arterial supply to both the pinna and the EAC is from the superficial temporal and the posterior auricular arteries (Donaldson and Miller, 1980).

Tympanic Membrane

The tympanic membrane (TM) develops from structures associated with both the external ear and the middle ear. At 4 to 5 weeks of gestation, the primitive TM is represented by the area of contact between the ectodermal meatal cord forming the external auditory meatus (first branchial groove) and the lateral end of the endodermal tubotympanic recess (first pharyngeal pouch). At 8 weeks, mesodermal tissue grows between the first pharyngeal pouch and the first branchial groove. The mesoderm thins out in the area of the meatal plate and becomes the fibrous layer of the TM. The fibrous layer consists of outer radial fibers and inner circular fibers. As previously noted, at 21 weeks the epidermal plug hollows out, becoming the EAC. The most medial portion of this plug becomes the superficial portion of the tympanic membrane. The completed TM has three layers: (1) an outer epithelial layer, from ectoderm of the first branchial groove; (2) a middle fibrous layer, from the mesoderm in between the first groove and the first pouch; and (3) an inner mucosal layer, derived from endoderm of the tympanic cavity.

The TM inserts into the tympanic ring. The ring is formed during the ninth week, from four ossification

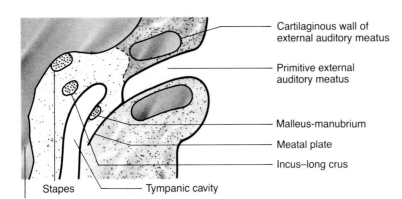

Figure 6–2. Development of meatus and meatal plate in relation to tympanic cavity at 9 weeks' gestation. (Redrawn from English, G. M. [ed.]. 1988. *Otolaryngology*, Vol. I, Diseases of the Ear and Hearing. Revised edition. Philadelphia, J. B. Lippincott Co., p. 12.)

centers, in membranous bone. These centers fuse and grow rapidly; the development of the tympanic ring is nearly complete by 16 weeks. The ring is deficient at the superior cranial aspect, the notch of Rivinus. Laterally, innervation to the tympanic membrane is the same as that to the EAC. Medially, innervation is supplied by the tympanic branch of the ninth nerve. Laterally, the blood supply is from the deep auricular branch of the internal maxillary artery, whereas medially it is supplied by the stylomastoid branch of the posterior auricular artery and the anterior tympanic branch of the internal maxillary artery.

At birth, the TM is almost adult-sized and is nearly horizontal; however, it becomes more vertical with development of the EAC (Anson and Davies, 1980). The mature eardrum consists of two parts, the pars tensa and the pars flaccida. The pars flaccida is located superiorly, over the notch of Rivinus and the epitympanum, and is composed of only a lateral squamous and a medial mucosal layer. The pars tensa, constituting most of the tympanic membrane, overlies the middle ear and is composed of all three layers (squamous, fibrous, and mucosal) (Fig. 6–3).

MIDDLE EAR

The middle ear consists of the TM, the tympanic cavity, three ossicles, two muscles, tendons, and the eustachian tube. Connection to the mastoid bone is via the aditus ad antrum from the middle ear. The eustachian tube connects the middle ear to the nasopharynx.

During the third week of gestation, expansion of the first (and, in some sources, the second) pharyngeal pouch, lined with endoderm, forms the tubotympanic recess. During weeks 4 to 6, there is progressive expansion; at week 7, constriction of the midportion of the recess by the second branchial arch leads to the formation of the eustachian tube (medially) and the tympanic cavity (laterally). At about week 18, the epitympanum, which leads into the antrum and the mastoid, forms from an extension of the tympanic cavity.

During the development of the tympanic cavity, differentiation of mesenchymal tissue above, medial to, and posterior to the tympanic cavity produces the ossicles, muscles, and tendons of the middle ear. Eventually, these structures will extend into the cavity and will be covered by the epithelial lining of the cavity (Pearson, 1988).

The roof of the tympanic cavity, the tegmen tympani, is formed laterally by an extension of the otic capsule and medially by fibrous tissue. This roof becomes ossified at the beginning of the 23rd week of gestation. The anterior epitympanic wall and part of the lateral tympanic cavity are formed from the tympanic process of the squamous portion of the temporal bone (Anson and Davies, 1980). One view holds that the main part of the floor of the middle ear is formed from an offshoot of the petrous pyramid; another view theorizes that the floor of the middle ear arises from a separate bone formed between the pyramid and the tympanic ring.

During development, the tympanic cavity is filled with mucoid tissue. Beginning during the third month, this tissue becomes looser and vacuolated, allowing expansion of the tympanic cavity. During this expansion, the ossicles, muscles, and tendons become wrapped with tympanic cavity epithelium (Fig. 6–4).

During the third to seventh months, the mucoid tissue is absorbed. Four pouches, or sacs, are formed, with mucosal folds between them. These four sacs become distinct anatomic areas. The saccus anticus becomes the anterior pouch of Tröltsch. The saccus medius develops into the epitympanum and petrous area. The saccus superior becomes the posterior pouch of Tröltsch, the inferior incudal space, and part of the

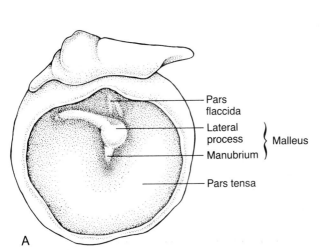

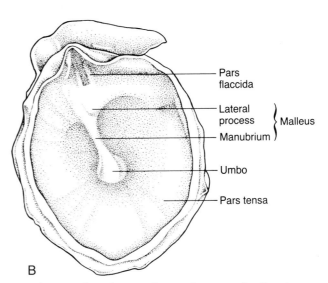

Figure 6–3. Tympanic membrane development. *A*, Newborn: Tympanic membrane is almost horizontal. Lateral process of malleus is most prominent. Pars flaccida is thicker and more vascular. *B*, Adult: Tympanic membrane is more vertical. Lateral process of malleus is less prominent. Manubrium of malleus is more vertical. Pars flaccida appears less vascular.

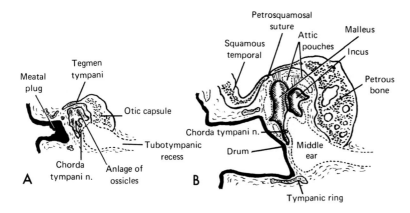

Figure 6–4. A and B, Expansion of middle ear. (From Anson, B. J., and Davies, J. 1980. Embryology of the ear. In Paparella, M. M., and Shumrick, D. A. [eds.]: Otolaryngology, Vol. I. 2nd ed. Philadelphia, W. B. Saunders Co., p. 11.)

mastoid. The saccus posterior becomes the round window, the oval window, and the sinus tympani.

By the 30th week, expansion of the tympanic cavity is complete, followed four weeks later by that of the epitympanum. (Pneumatization starts at approximately the 30th week and is nearly complete at birth.)

There are two middle ear muscles. The tensor tympani and its tendon are derived from mesoderm of the first branchial arch; innervation is by the mandibular branch of the trigeminal nerve. This muscle is contained in a bony semicanal above the eustachian tube and attaches via the tendon to the manubrium of the malleus. The stapedius muscle is derived from mesoderm of the second arch and is innervated by the seventh cranial nerve. This muscle originates from the pyramidal eminence and inserts via its tendon onto the neck of the stapes.

Middle Ear Ossicles

There are three middle ear ossicles: the malleus, the incus, and the stapes. They are formed from the mesenchyme of the mandibular and the hyoid arches and from the otic capsule (stapes only). Specifically, the head of the malleus, and the short crus and body of the incus, arise from the mandibular arch. The manubrium of the malleus, the long process of the incus, and the head, neck, crura, and tympanic surface of the footplate of the stapes arise from the hyoid arch. The medial surface of the stapedial footplate and the annular stapedial ligament arise from the otic capsule.

At 4½ weeks, the mesenchyme of the second arch forms the blastema, which is then divided by the seventh nerve into the stapes, interhyale and laterohyale. The stapes ring forms around the stapedial artery during weeks 5 to 6, and otic capsule mesenchyme appears, forming the medial footplate and the annular ligament. At 8½ weeks, the incudostapedial joint forms. During the tenth week, the shape of the stapes changes from that of a ring to that of a stirrup. The interhyale forms stapedius muscle and tendon, and the laterohyale becomes the posterior wall of the middle ear. The laterohyale also joins with the otic capsule to partially form the anterior wall of the facial canal and the bone of the stapedial pyramid.

All three ossicles begin to develop during the fourth to sixth fetal weeks. During the next 3 to 4 weeks, the mesenchyme develops into cartilaginous models of the ossicles. The models for the incus and the malleus grow to adult size by 15 weeks; the model for the stapes reaches full size by 18 weeks. The incus and the malleus, which start as a single mass, separate, and the malleoincudal joint is formed at 8 to 9 weeks. Ossification of the malleus and the incus begins at 15 weeks and appears first at the long process of the incus. Remodeling of the bone of the incus and the malleus continues throughout postfetal life. Ossification of the stapes begins at week 18. There is no remodeling of the fetal bone of the stapes during postfetal life. At birth, all the ossicles are of adult size and shape. When the mesenchyme resorbs and the ossicles are free, the endodermal epithelium of the tympanic cavity connects the ossicles to the cavity wall in a mesenterylike manner. The supporting ossicular ligaments develop in these epithelial connections (Anson and Davies, 1980; Schuknecht and Gulya, 1986; Pearson, 1988) (Fig. 6–5).

Tympanic Antrum, Mastoid Air Cells, and Related Spaces

The antrum is usually the largest and, in poorly pneumatized mastoids, often the only identifiable air cell in the mastoid air cell system. The antrum appears as a lateral extension of the epitympanum at 21 to 22 weeks. The lumen of the antrum is well developed by the 34th week, and its pneumatization is complete during the first year of life.

In the adult, nearly all parts of the temporal bone are extensively pneumatized, including the zygoma, squama, petrous apex, and jugular wall areas. Air cell formation is usually completed during postfetal life but may continue into old age. Pneumatization of the petrous pyramid, which is highly variable, begins at approximately the 28th fetal week, whereas pneumatization of the mastoid air cells starts at the 33rd week. The mastoid itself is formed when the bone of the

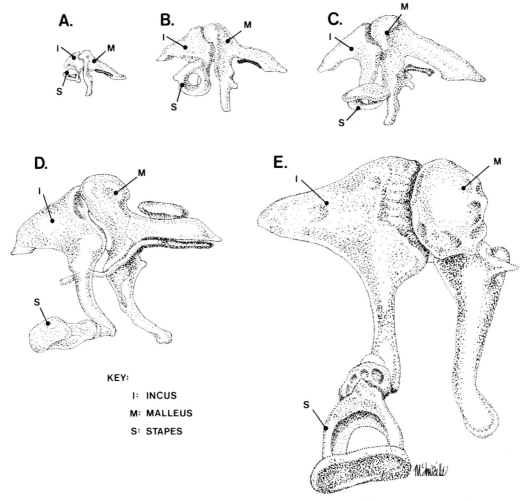

Figure 6–5. Ossicular development. *A*, Fetus, 2 months: cartilaginous ossicles recognizable, *B*, Fetus, 3 months. *C*, Fetus, 4 months: attaining adult configuration but cartilaginous. *D*, Fetus, 6 months: adult configuration and size; ossification begins. *E*, Adult ossicles. (Adapted from Anson, B. J., and Davies, J. 1980. Developmental anatomy of the ear. *In* Paparella, M., and Shumrick, D. [eds.]: Otolaryngology, Vol I. 2nd ed. Philadelphia, W. B. Saunders Co., p 8.)

antrum and the tympanic plate expand, with air cells formed by the extension of epithelium from the antrum into the developing mastoid bone area. In the infant, the antrum is nearly adult-sized, and the bulge of the lateral semicircular canal can be seen in its floor. The pattern of mastoid pneumatization is generally symmetric; however, it is highly variable among individuals. The mastoid process appears at the age of 1 year. The various forms of otitis media are often found to be associated with poorly pneumatized mastoids; however, the cause-and-effect relationship between these two findings is very controversial. Currently, it is thought that mastoid air cell development can be hindered by early and repeated middle ear disease (Tos et al., 1984; Palva and Palva, 1966). Heredity also may play a role in mastoid size.

Temporal Bone

There are four parts to the adult temporal bone: petrous, squamous, tympanic and mastoid; however, only the petrous, squamous, and tympanic parts have formed at birth. The squamous and the tympanic portions form by membranous bone development. The squamous portion begins to develop at approximately week 8, and the tympanic during weeks 9 to 10. The petrous portion is formed from cartilage (endochondral bone) of the periotic capsule, with ossification starting in the sixth month. All portions of the temporal bone, except the petrous, continue to develop in postfetal life. The mastoid bone develops primarily after birth, with a mastoid process evident by the age of 1 year and well developed by age 3 years. Mastoid development is mainly lateral and posterior to the antrum. After birth, the styloid process is formed from ossification of the mesoderm in the upper part of the second arch.

At birth, the middle ear cavity is approximately adult-sized, as are the oval and the round windows and the TM. The malleus, the incus, and the stapes reach adult size by the sixth month of gestation. At birth, the eustachian tube is about 1.7 cm long, about half as long as in the adult. It is fairly horizontal, with the pharyngeal opening being at the level of the hard palate. With growth, the tube angles downward, with the opening at the level of the inferior nasal turbinate by the age of 6 years.

During the newborn period and during infancy, the lateral surface of the temporal bone differs from that in the adult. There is no bony ear canal, except superiorly, and no mastoid process. The facial nerve is very superficial as it emerges from the stylomastoid foramen behind the tympanic membrane and can be injured by obstetric forceps or the usual posterior auricular incision used in mastoid surgery (Shambaugh and Glasscock, 1980.)

The lateral surface anatomy of the temporal bone is important surgically. In postnatal life, the spine of Henle marks the posterosuperior aspect of the external ear canal, and the antrum is usually found medial to the spine. In the infant, the bone over the antrum is cribriform, allowing infection to extend subperiosteally, with posterior auricular edema, erythema, and abscess formation. The temporal line, the inferior margin of the temporal muscle, marks the approximate level of the middle fossa. There are two suture lines in the bony external canal, the tympanomastoid, posteriorly, and the tympanosquamous, superiorly. The surgeon uses these suture lines as landmarks when making incisions in the EAC. The mandibular fossa, involved in articulation of the condyle of the mandible, is a concavity on the inferior surface of the squamous part of the temporal bone (Fig. 6–6).

Facial Nerve

The facial nerve (seventh cranial nerve) is the nerve of the second branchial arch. At the end of the third gestational week, a collection of cells, the acousticofacial ganglion (also called crest or primordium), can be identified as an aggregation of neural crest cells dorsolateral to the rhombencephalon and rostral to the otic placode. By the end of the fourth week, the facial and the acoustic portions of the primordium have become more distinct. The facial division extends ventrally to a thickened area of surface ectoderm, the epibranchial placode, located on the upper surface of the second branchial arch. During the fifth week, the neuroblasts of the geniculate ganglion appear in the facial portion of the primordium, in the area where the placode and the neural crest cells are contiguous. Then, the distal portion of the primordium divides equally, with one portion going caudally into the second arch mesenchyme and eventually becoming the main facial nerve trunk. The other division extends rostrally into the first arch and becomes the chorda tympani nerve (at 5 weeks). The terminal branches of the chorda tympani end in the same region that the lingual nerve (termination of a branch of the mandibular nerve) ends in; there the two nerves unite (Gasser, 1967; Schuknecht and Gulya, 1986; Pearson, 1988).

The facial motor nucleus develops separately from the acousticofacial primordium and is derived from

neuroblasts in the upper portion of the rhombencephalon. The motor nuclei of the sixth and seventh cranial nerves develop in close proximity in the pons, which explains the involvement of both sixth and seventh nerves in the congenital Möbius syndrome as well as the findings in other neoplastic, inflammatory, and vascular disorders.

The sensory nervus intermedius develops from the geniculate ganglion at 7 weeks of gestation, and extends to the brain stem between the motor root of the seventh nerve and the eighth nerve. The greater superficial petrosal nerve, the second branch of the seventh nerve to develop, comes from the most ventral part of the geniculate ganglion, at about 5 weeks. The branch to the stapedius muscle develops at about 8 weeks, and geniculate ganglion development is completed by week 15. This separate development of the sensory and motor parts of the seventh nerve allows patients with congenital facial paralysis to have intact sensation and taste.

The seventh nerve is located in the facial canal that develops as a sulcus on the lateral aspect of the otic capsule by the eighth fetal week. The future canal is still cartilaginous and contains the stapedius muscle, the facial nerve, and blood vessels. Closure of the canal is nearly complete by the seventh month.

At birth, facial nerve development is complete. The fully developed facial nerve originates from the facial nucleus, leaving the brain stem at the inferior border of the pons between the olive and the inferior cerebellar peduncle. It enters the internal acoustic meatus (internal auditory canal) accompanied by the nervus intermedius and travels in a bony canal, the fallopian canal, laterally to the geniculate ganglion. The greater and the lesser superficial petrosal nerves diverge at this point, and the remainder of the facial nerve turns posteriorly and traverses the middle ear, still in the bony canal. The facial nerve lies just above the oval window niche and, at the pyramidal eminence, turns again to take a vertical, or mastoid, course. There, the nerve is located just lateral and inferior to the lateral semicircular canal and, finally, exits from the stylomastoid foramen at the anterior end of the digastric groove. The chorda tympani nerve leaves the facial nerve in the vertical mastoid portion, passing in its own canal to the posterior iter. There it passes lateral to the long process of the incus and medial to the malleus handle to the anterior iter, entering the anterior petrotympanic fissure (canal of Huguier) to leave the middle ear (May, 1985). In as many as 55 per cent of cases, the bony facial canal is found to be dehiscent in part of its course, most commonly in the horizontal portion (Baxter, 1971; Gasser, 1967).

There are several important spaces and landmarks in the completed, adult form of the middle ear. The canal of Huguier, already mentioned, is located in the anterior middle ear and contains the chorda tympani nerve. The *ponticulus* is the bony ridge between the oval window and the sinus tympani; the *subiculum* is the bony ridge between the round window niche and the sinus tympani. The *sinus tympani* is bounded

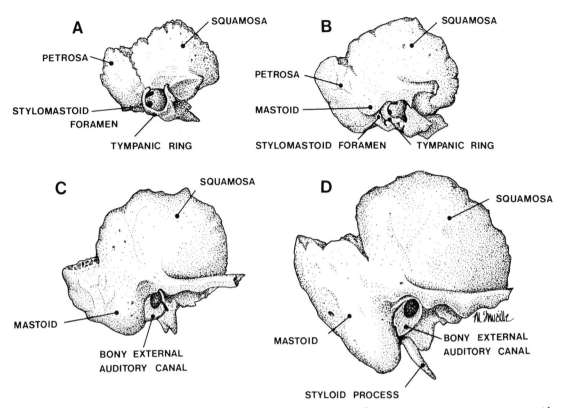

Figure 6–6. Lateral temporal bone development. *A*, Newborn: Petrous, squamous, and tympanic portions are present; mastoid portion is not developed. Stylomastoid foramen (exit of facial nerve) is just behind tympanic ring. *B*, Infant, 1.5 years old: Mastoid development is under way. Stylomastoid foramen can still be exposed and is not covered by mastoid process. Tympanic ring is ossifying. *C*, Child, 5 years: Mastoid process is well developed and covers stylomastoid foramen. Tympanic ring has completely ossified, and entire bony external auditory canal is osseous. *D*, Adult: normal anatomy.

medially by the bony labyrinth, laterally by the pyramidal eminence, superiorly by the lateral semicircular canal and ponticulus, inferiorly by the subiculum and the jugular wall, and posteriorly by the posterior semicircular canal. The *facial recess* is bounded medially by the facial nerve, laterally by the bony tympanic annulus and chorda tympani, and superiorly by the short process of the incus. When middle ear cholesteatoma is present, both the facial recess and the sinus tympani can be involved; cholesteatoma can be very difficult to detect and remove from these areas. On the anterior medial wall of the middle ear is located the cochleariform process, the curved end of the tensor tympani semicanal. In revision mastoid surgery, this may be one of the few safe remaining landmarks (Shambaugh and Glasscock, 1980).

INNER EAR

The inner ear is located in the petrous portion of the temporal bone and consists of a membranous labyrinth inside a bony labyrinth. At birth, it is adult in size and configuration except for changes in the periosteal layer of the bony labyrinth and continued postfetal growth of the endolymphatic sac and duct.

Membranous Labyrinth

The adult membranous labyrinth consists of the utricle, saccule, semicircular ducts, endolymphatic sac and duct, and the cochlear duct. It is housed in the bony labyrinth, contains endolymph, and is bathed by perilymph.

The membranous labyrinth develops from surface ectoderm at the end of the third week of gestation. An area of plaquelike thickening appears on the lateral aspect of the neural fold dorsal to the first branchial groove and in close relation to the hindbrain (rhombencephalon). During the fourth week, the placode invaginates to become the auditory pit, then the auditory vesicle (otocyst). During this process, it becomes surrounded by mesenchyme that will become the cartilaginous capsule of the otocyst (otic capsule) (Li and McPhee, 1979). The auditory vesicle becomes divided into two pouches by three folds: The ventral (cochlear, pars inferior) pouch will form the saccule and the cochlear duct, and the dorsal component (vestibular, pars superior) will give rise to the utricle, the semicircular ducts, and the endolymphatic duct. As differentiation of the membranous labyrinth progresses, the adult configuration is recognizable by 2½ months of fetal life, and the membranous labyrinth without the end organ is complete by 6 months of fetal life (Fig. 6–7). However, the endolymphatic sac and

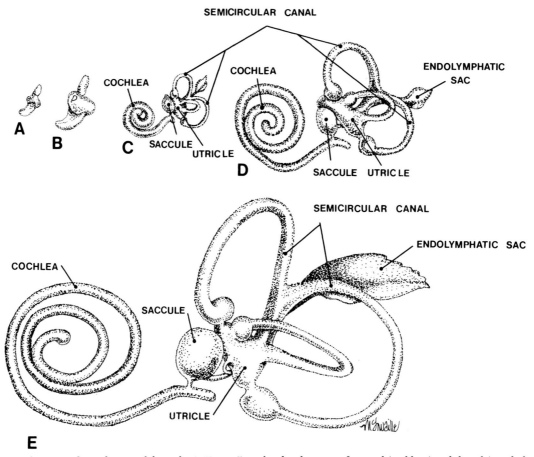

Figure 6–7. Development of membranous labyrinth. *A*, Fetus, 5 weeks: development of ventral (cochlear) and dorsal (vestibular) pouches. *B*, Fetus, 6 weeks: rapid growth. *C*, Fetus, 2.5 months: Adult structures easily recognizable. Cochlea has attained its 2.5 turns; semicircular canals, utricle, saccule, and endolymphatic sac and duct are well developed. *D*, Fetus, 6 months: Membranous labyrinth development is complete, except endolymphatic sac and duct continue to grow postfetally. *E*, Adult: fully developed labyrinth. (Adapted from Anson, B. J., and Davies, J. 1980. *In* Paparella, M.M., and Shumrick, D.A. [eds.]: Otolaryngology, Vol. I. 2nd ed. Philadelphia, W. B. Saunders Co., p. 14. After Bast, T. H., and Anson, B. J. 1949. The Temporal Bone and Ear. Springfield, IL: Charles C Thomas.)

duct continue to grow after birth, in conjunction with the rest of the temporal bone and with the enlargement of the posterior cranial fossa.

Utricle and Saccule

The utricle and the saccule are otolithic organs. The utricle is sensitive to linear acceleration, but the function of the saccule in humans is unclear. The utricle is derived from the dorsal (vestibular) pouch of the auditory vesicle, while the saccule comes from the ventral (cochlear) pouch. The utricle, saccule, and endolymphatic duct begin to develop at about week 6 of gestation and, by week 8, have an adult configuration. The ductus reuniens, which connects the saccule to the cochlear duct, forms at about 7 weeks. A Y-shaped duct connects the utricle to the saccule and is composed of the utriculoendolymphatic duct and the sacculoendolymphatic duct.

Neuroepithelial cells develop in the maculae of the saccule and the utricle and the crests of the semicircular canals. By week 11 of gestation, development of this neuroepithelium and the supporting cells is complete. These areas of neuroepithelium secrete a gelat-

inous substance that becomes the otolithic membranes of the cupulae of the crests. This gelatinous substance contains rhombic crystals of calcium carbonate, called otoconia. The macula of the saccule lies in the vertical plane on the medial wall, whereas the macula of the utricle lies on the anterolateral wall, perpendicular to the utricular macula. The primary receptor cells in the maculae are Type I and Type II hair cells. Cilia from these sensory cells extend upward into the otolithic membrane, which contains the otoconia. The hair cells are supported by columnar supporting cells.

The utricle and the saccule both are contained in the vestibule of the inner ear. The utricle is ovoid and flattened, with a rounded end that occupies the elliptical recess of the posterosuperior vestibule. The semicircular canals open into its posterior wall, and the utriculosaccular duct opens into it anteriorly. The saccule, smaller and rounded, is located in the anteroinferior portion of the vestibule, near the oval window footplate, and connects to the cochlea via the ductus reuniens. The utricle connects posteriorly with the semicircular canals and anteriorly with the saccular and endolymphatic ducts (Donaldson and Miller, 1980).

Endolymphatic Duct and Sac

The endolymphatic duct and sac develop from the dorsal component of the otocyst at about 6 weeks of gestation, and growth continues in postfetal life. The fully developed duct lies mainly in the vestibular aqueduct, is surrounded by perilymph and periotic tissue, and is connected to the utriculosaccular duct. At its distal end lies the endolymphatic sac, in a fossa on the posterior portion of the petrous temporal bone. The duct's two main functions are endolymph absorption and pressure equalization between the cerebrospinal fluid and the endolymphatic systems.

Semicircular Ducts

During week 6 of gestation, the semicircular ducts (canals) begin to develop from the dorsal component of the auditory vesicle. The superior duct develops first, followed by the posterior and then the lateral. During week 7, a ridgelike structure, the crista ampullaris, composed of neuroepithelial cells, develops at the dilated, or ampulla, end of each semicircular duct. The ampullated ends of each duct open into the utricle, while the nonampullated ends of the posterior and the superior ducts fuse to form the common crus, which opens into the middle part of the utricle. The nonampullated end of the lateral duct opens separately into the utricle. By week 11, the neuroepithelium and supporting cells of the cristae are complete. The superior semicircular duct reaches maximum growth by week 19, followed by the posterior canal. The lateral canal reaches maximum growth by the 22nd week. Like the macula, the crista contains Type I and Type II hair cells with cilia that extend upward into the cupula. The cupula is a gelatinous mass of mucopolysaccharides within a keratin framework and forms a flap, or partition, across the ampulla.

Cochlear Duct and Organ of Corti

During the sixth week of gestation, the cochlear duct develops from the ventral (saccular) pouch of the auditory vesicle. At week 7, one turn of the cochlea is formed, and by week 8 the entire 2½ to 2¾ turns have been completed. The narrow tube connecting the cochlear duct to the saccule is called the ductus reuniens.

The organ of Corti arises in the wall of the cochlear duct. The epithelium in the area of the future organ of Corti differentiates into two ridges of tall columnar cells that extend the entire length of the cochlear duct. The cells of these ridges secrete a gelatinous substance that becomes the tectorial membrane.

The larger, inner ridge becomes the spiral limbus, and the outer, smaller ridge the organ of Corti. At the 22nd week, this outer ridge develops inner and outer hair cells, pillar cells, and Hensen cells. Differentiation of the inner and outer ridges begins at the basal turn of the cochlear duct and spreads to the apex. At week 8, the stria vascularis begins to develop in the external wall of the cochlear duct; it is well developed by week 20. The organ of Corti completes its development during the fifth month of gestation, with the tunnel of Corti and the canal of Nuel being formed at the 26th week.

The organ of Corti itself contains the sensory receptors for hearing and has two types of cells: sensory cells and supporting cells. The afferent fibers of the auditory (eighth) nerve and the efferent fibers of the olivocochlear bundle enter the organ of Corti from beneath the basilar membrane and innervate the sensory cells. The sensory cells are of two types, the inner and the outer hair cells, so named by the cells' relative proximity to the tunnel of Corti (located medially in the spiral cochlea). Each cell has stereocilia extending from its surface, and each cell surface contains a small cuticle-free region (the stereocilia extend from the region where the thick cuticle is located in the upper surface of the hair cell) that indicates where a kinocilium was located during embryonic life. The supporting cells are known as Deiter, Hensen, Claudius, and Boettcher cells, the inner border cells, the inner phalangeal cells, the inner and outer pillar cells, and the outer sulcus cells (Fig. 6–8).

In the adult, the cochlear duct extends from the cochlear recess of the vestibule and ends in a blind pouch, the cupular cecum, at the apex. At its basal end, the small ductus reuniens communicates with the saccule.

In the completed state, the cochlear duct is triangular and divides the bony cochlear canal into three separate compartments: the scala media (cochlear duct); the scala vestibuli, adjoining Reissner membrane; and the scala tympani, adjacent to the basilar membrane. The scala media contains endolymph, and both the scala tympani and the scala vestibuli contain perilymph. The "floor" of the cochlear duct is the basilar membrane, and the "roof" is Reissner membrane, which extends from the vestibular crest of the spiral ligament to the spiral limbus and divides the scala media from the scala vestibuli. Reissner membrane has two layers: a single layer of connective cells that faces the scala vestibuli and a single layer of epithelial cells that faces the scala media. These two layers of cells are joined by tight junctions, which prevent the free mixing of perilymph and endolymph, although selective transport does occur (Johnson, 1971). The basilar membrane is suspended between the spiral limbus and the spiral ligament. The organ of Corti overlies the basilar membrane.

Auditory Nerve

It is currently thought that the cells that form the eighth nerve ganglion are derived from the auditory vesicle (otocyst). During the fourth week of gestation, these cells migrate between the epithelium and basement membrane of the otic vesicle and form the auditory ganglion. The eighth nerve ganglion then divides into a superior part (pars superior) and an inferior part (pars inferior). The pars superior gives

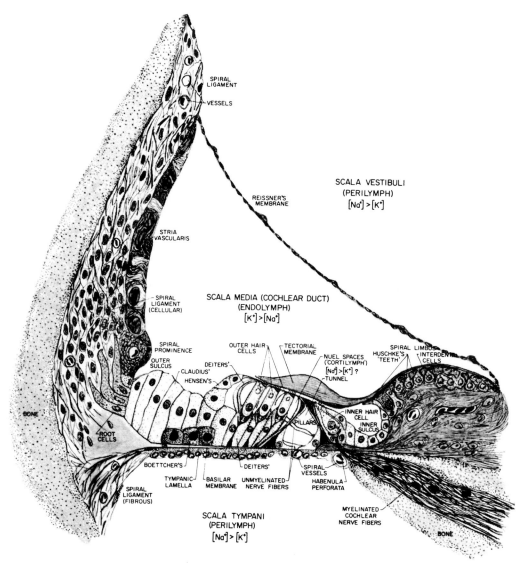

Figure 6–8. Diagram of transverse midmodiolar view of cochlear duct. (With permission from Hawkins, J. E. 1966. Hearing: anatomy and acoustics. *In* Best, C. H., and Taylor, W. B. [eds.]: Physiological Basis of Medical Practice, 8th ed. Chapter 17. © 1966, The Williams & Wilkins Co., Baltimore.)

rise to the superior (utricular) branch of the vestibular nerve, which supplies the utricular macula and the ampullar crests (cristae) of the lateral and the superior semicircular ducts. The pars inferior becomes the inferior portion of the vestibular nerve supplying the saccular macula and the crista of the posterior semicircular duct, and the cochlear nerve supplying the organ of Corti. The nerve cells in the cochlear and vestibular nerve ganglia are unusual in that they remain bipolar throughout life, the central processes terminating in the brain stem, and the peripheral processes terminating in the sensory areas of the developing inner ear (Pearson, 1988; Schuknecht and Gulya, 1986).

Bony Labyrinth, or Auditory Capsule

The bony labyrinth encloses the membranous labyrinth and consists of the cochlea, three semicircular canals, vestibule, and perilymphatic spaces. Its devel-

opment occurs in three stages. The first stage involves condensation of mesenchyme around the developing membranous labyrinth during the fourth to sixth weeks of gestation. Areas marking the location of the internal auditory canal, the entrance of the eighth nerve, and the developing endolymphatic duct can be seen. Precartilage formation begins and continues during weeks 6 and 7, when true cartilage formation begins. In the areas where the membranous semicircular duct is expanding, dedifferentiation of cartilage and precartilage allows for growth, while redifferentiation into cartilage is found in the "trailing edge" areas of membranous labyrinth growth (i.e., where expansion has stopped). The process continues until the membranous labyrinth attains adult size in midterm. Perichondrium of the otic capsule appears at week 12.

The second stage in otic capsule development involves the formation of perilymphatic spaces. The vestibule, enclosing the utricle, saccule, and part of the cochlear duct, begins to develop at week 8. Then follows development of the scala tympani during weeks 8 to 9. The scala tympani begins under the round window, and the scala vestibuli starts slightly later as an outpouching of the vestibule, near the oval window. The growth and development of the scalae closely follows that of the cochlear duct, and the scalae attain adult size by 16 weeks. The perilymphatic spaces around the semicircular ducts begin to develop after the scalae, with the one around the lateral semicircular duct being the most greatly developed.

There are four projections from the perilymphatic space: the perilymphatic (periotic) duct, the fossula post fenestram, the fissula ante fenestram, and an unnamed projection around the endolymphatic duct. The fissula traverses the bony partition between the inner and the middle ear anterior to the oval window and is thought to provide an overflow channel for perilymph. The perilymphatic duct runs in a canal through the petrous bone and connects the scala tympani with the subarachnoid space. The fossula post fenestram is located posterior to the oval window and is found in only about two thirds of embryos.

The third stage of otic capsule development involves ossification. This begins at about the 15th fetal week, from 14 centers, and forms the petrous part of the temporal bone. Calcification in the 14 centers precedes ossification. By the 23rd week, all the centers have fused to form a complete bony capsule. Ossification of the inner ear does not occur until each portion has attained adult size. In the adult, the bony capsule has three layers: (1) an outer layer of perichondrial (periosteal) bone, (2) a middle layer of intrachondral and endochondral bone, and (3) an inner layer of internal perichondrial bone. In the adult, the middle and inner layers can still be identified. In the region of the fissula ante fenestram, the middle layer is considered a favored site for development of otosclerosis.

SUMMARY

The embryology and developmental anatomy of the ear are quite complex, but an understanding of them can help explain many congenital anomalies of the ear. Depending on the time during gestation that the abnormalities occurred, anomalies of the outer ear (pinna, EAC) and the middle ear may or may not be related to anomalies of the inner ear. Sophisticated evaluation of audiologic function (brain stem evoked responses) as well as radiographic evaluation of the middle and inner ear (by computed tomography and magnetic resonance imaging) make comprehensive investigation of these structures possible in young children and infants.

REFERENCES

Anson, B. J., and Davies, J. 1980. Embryology of the ear. *In* Paparella, M. M., and Shumrick, D. A. (eds.): Otolaryngology, 2nd ed. Philadelphia, W. B. Saunders Co., pp. 3–25.

Baxter, A. 1971. Dehiscence of the fallopian canal. An anatomical study. J. Laryngol. Otol. 85:587.

Donaldson, J. A., and Miller, J. M. 1980. Anatomy of the ear. *In* Paparella, M. M., and Shumrick, D. A. (eds.): Otolaryngology, 2nd ed. Philadelphia, W. B. Saunders Co., pp. 26–62.

Gasser, R. F. 1967. The development of the facial nerve in man. Ann. Otol. Rhinol. Laryngol. 76:37.

Gerhardt, J. J., and Otto, H. D. 1981. The infratemporal course of the facial nerve and its influence on the development of the ossicular chain. Acta Otolaryngol. 91:567.

Johnson, L. G. 1971. Reissner's membrane in the human cochlea. Ann. Otol. Rhinol. Laryngol. 80:425.

Li, C. W., and McPhee, J. 1979. Influences on the coiling of the cochlea. Ann. Otol. Rhinol. Laryngol. 88:280.

May, M. 1985. Anatomy of the facial nerve for the clinician. *In* May, M. (ed.): The Facial Nerve. New York, Thieme Medical Pubs., pp. 21–62.

Palva, T., and Palva, A. 1966. Size of the human mastoid air cell system. Acta Otolaryngol. 62:237.

Pearson, A. A. 1988. Developmental anatomy of the ear. *In* English, G. M. (ed.): Otolarynology, revised ed. 5 vols. (Loose Leaf Reference Services). New York, Harper Medical, pp. 1–68.

Schuknecht, H. F., and Gulya, A. J. 1986. Phylogeny and embryology. *In* Schuknecht, H. F., and Gulya, A. J. (eds.): Anatomy of the Temporal Bone with Surgical Implications. Philadelphia, Lea & Febiger, pp. 235–273.

Shambaugh, G. E., and Glasscock, M. E. 1980. Surgical anatomy of the temporal bone. *In* Shambaugh, G. E., and Glasscock, M. E. (eds.): Surgery of the Ear, 3rd ed. Philadelphia, W. B. Saunders Co., pp. 31–52.

Tos, M., Stangerup, S. E., and Hvid, G. 1984. Mastoid pneumatization. Evidence of the environmental theory. Arch. Otolaryngol. 110:502.

Wong, M. L. 1983. Embryology and developmental anatomy of the ear. *In* Bluestone, C. D., and Stool, S. E. (eds.): Pediatric Otolaryngology. Philadelphia, W. B. Saunders Co., pp. 85–111.

Chapter 7

PHYSIOLOGY OF THE EAR

John D. Durrant, Ph.D.

AUDITORY RESPONSE AREA

Sound is created by a vibratory source (e.g., the vibrating prongs of a tuning fork) that causes molecules of the substance of the surrounding medium (e.g., air) to be displaced. As the source vibrates, it alternately compresses and rarefies the particles of the surrounding medium, creating local alterations of the static pressure. These changes are minute. For instance, at sound pressures in air capable of causing pain to the ear, the static or steady-state pressure equivalent equals only 10^{-1} atmosphere, whereas the minimum sound pressure detectable by the normal human ear is one-ten-millionth of this value, or 10^{-8} atm. This illustrates both the exquisite sensitivity of the auditory system and its impressive dynamic range.

The quantification of sound actually requires two measures. The first alluded to is amplitude or magnitude. Sound is, of course, a form of energy, which means that it has the ability to do work. The most fundamental measure of sound is acoustic intensity—a powerlike quantity measured in units such as watts per square meter. However, it is more practical to measure sound pressure, which is quantified in pascals (1 Pa = 1 newton/m²). For instance, the minimally detectable sound is on the order of 20 μPa (2×10^{-5} Pa). Sound pressure is proportional to the square root of acoustic intensity and is the vibratory "force" created by a given acoustic intensity or "power" acting on the medium. It is the intensity of sound that primarily determines the sense of loudness.

The other of the two measures in question is frequency, which is the primary determinant of the sense of pitch. Because sound is vibratory, the number of vibrations, or cycles, per second is also an important specification. The unit of measure cycles per second has been given the name hertz (Hz). It is important to realize that simple sounds, such as that produced by the tuning fork, reflect oscillations at a single frequency; however, sounds in nature are much more complex. Nevertheless, these sounds can be analyzed and represented in terms of their frequency components and the magnitude of each. This is called spectrum analysis. Not only do sounds such as speech have complicated spectra, but also their spectra change rapidly over time. Clearly, the auditory system must be able to perform some form of spectrum analysis; in addition, it must be able to carry out such analyses at rather high rates. Not only does sound spectrum determine the loudness and the pitch of a given sound, but also its nuances give rise to the perceived sound qualities, such as timbre, volume, and density. It is the ability of the auditory system to analyze even complex sounds that permits one to distinguish between, for instance, a clarinet and a trumpet, even when both are playing the same note or pitch.

A further appreciation of the abilities of the auditory system can be gained by examining the auditory response area, as shown in Figure 7–1A. This is a two-dimensional space, mapped with axes of frequency and sound pressure level. The units of measure of the former are hertz. The units of measure of sound pressure level (SPL) are decibels (dB). Decibels are logarithmic numbers and are favored over units of sound pressure for their compression of the tremendous range of numbers covered by the dynamic range of hearing. Again, this range is defined by the smallest sound intensity or pressure detectable versus that which causes a sense of feeling or even pain. This range in acoustic intensity is $10^{14}:1$ and in sound pressure is $10^7:1$ (because sound pressure is proportional to the square root of acoustic intensity). The decibel is equal to 10 times the log of the intensity ratio or 20 times the log of the pressure ratio, so this dynamic range is 140 dB. Because the decibel is based on a ratio, it is a dimensionless number. Therefore, for representing sound pressures (or acoustic intensities) in an absolute sense, a reference quantity is required. It should not be surprising from the earlier discussion that the generally accepted reference for sound pressure level measurements is 20 μPa.

As noted earlier, the lower limit of the dynamic range of hearing reflects the exquisite sensitivity of the auditory system. Indeed, it has been speculated that further improvement in hearing sensitivity is limited by the "floor" set by thermal noise (i.e., that created by the random bombardment of particles of the medium). However, for humans, this noise floor appears to be more than 20 dB below the limits of hearing for even the most sensitive normal-hearing individuals (Green, 1976). Further improvements in hearing sensitivity actually would be of little practical value owing to masking by biologic noise (i.e., noise in the "system"), and, as discussed below, sensitivity is not everything.

The upper limit is no less remarkable but for much different reasons. It is an expression of the limit of physiologically appropriate stimulation of the auditory system. Sounds on the order of 140-dB SPL are, of course, quite loud. They also stimulate the tactile sense and pain. However, well below this limit there are warning signs that the ear's limit of tolerance for sound is beng reached; for example, prolonged exposures to sounds as low as 85-dB SPL (A-scale weighted) can cause permanent damage to the hearing organ. Indeed, it is this level (previously 90 dBA) that the National Institute of Occupational Safety and Health has stipulated as the maximum limit of noise permissible for a worker to be exposed to for 8 hours/day on a daily basis without wearing hearing protection (Sutter, 1986). Exposure to higher levels of sound is safe only for shorter and shorter lengths of time. Even brief exposures to intense sounds (e.g., explosive noises) can cause permanent damage, called acoustic trauma.

The limits of hearing along the frequency dimension are expressed by the minimal audibility curve (Fig. 7-1A). This curve is obtained by measuring the SPL required for a group of otologically normal young subjects to just detect the presence of sound as a function of frequency (Robinson and Dadson, 1956). Although the auditory system is quite sensitive over a limited range of frequencies, sensitivity becomes poorer and poorer at extreme high and low frequencies (Fig. 7-1A). What is "high" and "low" is species dependent. For humans, the usable frequency range is fairly well centered on the spectrum of speech, although the entire hearing frequency range is not required for reproduction of intelligible speech. For instance, the telephone is engineered to reproduce only the range of about 300 to 3000 Hz. The low- and high-frequency limits of hearing are not clearly demarked and are somewhat matters of definition. The range of 20 to 20,000 Hz is generally accepted as the nominal useful range of hearing for humans, although auditory responses to sound are demonstrable significantly below (Yeowart and Evans, 1974) and above this range (Corso, 1965). Still, beyond these limits, rather high SPLs of sound are required to reach threshold and may cause distortion (Wever and Bray, 1937) or may be devoid of a clear sense of pitch (Corso and Levine, 1965).

In the final analysis, it is not enough for the auditory system to have extraordinary sensitivity, a tremendous dynamic range, and an extensive frequency range unless relatively small changes in intensity and frequency can be detected or small intensity and frequency differences can be discriminated. The ability to distinguish between sounds with complex but similar spectra, such as the spoken words "bad" and "pad," is a testimonial to the impressive discriminatory ability of the human auditory system. Psychophysical measures of discrimination ability, called difference limens

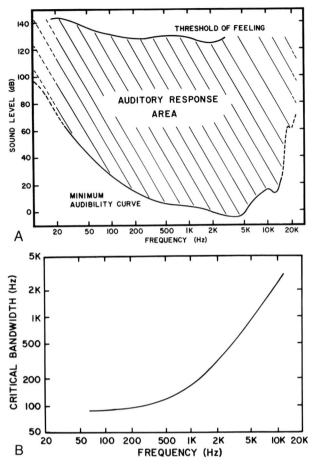

Figure 7–1. A, The auditory response area. The minimal audibility curve is based on data of Robinson and Dadson (1956). The extreme low- and high-frequency portions of the curve (broken lines) have been extended based on data of Yeowart and Evans (1974) and Corso (1965), respectively. The representation of the threshold-of-feeling curve is based on data of Wegel (1932). B, The critical bandwidth as a function of frequency at the center of the band. (After Zwicker, E., et al. 1957. Critical bandwidth in loudness summation. J. Acoust. Soc. Am. 29:548–557.)

(or differential thresholds), provide an indication of the basic differential sensitivity of the auditory system. The difference limen (DL) for intensity is about 1 dB (Jestead et al., 1977), which amounts to a 12 per cent change in intensity or about 0.7 per cent of the dynamic range. The difference limen for frequency is approximately 0.2 per cent (Wier et al., 1977), meaning that with careful listening one should be able to distinguish between a tone of 1000 Hz and one of 1002 Hz. However, these specifications of differential sensitivity, particularly the difference limen for frequency, are valid only for the central region of the auditory response area. Decreased discriminatory ability is observed as the extremes of the frequency range, the limits of hearing sensitivity, or both are approached (Licklider, 1951).

The difference limen for frequency also does not realistically characterize the limits of the frequency-resolution capability of the auditory system for sounds more complex than single-frequency or "pure" tones or for simultaneously occurring sounds in general. For instance, were the 1000- and 1002-Hz tones in the preceding example presented together, two tones would not be perceived. Rather, a tone of one pitch (based on the average of the two frequencies) would be heard, but its loudness would wax and wane, or "beat," at the difference frequency of 2 Hz (Wever, 1929).

There are other perceptual attributes that reflect this inability of the auditory system to resolve fine differences in the spectral components of sound, including the manner in which loudness grows as a function of the range of frequencies covered by a sound (i.e., its bandwidth) and how different sounds interfere with or mask one another (Plomp, 1971). A measure of this resolution limit is the critical bandwidth (Zwicker et al., 1957; Scharf, 1970), which also varies across frequency (Fig. 7–1*B*). Within a critical bandwidth, the loudness of a sound, for example, will depend primarily on the total energy of the sound, whereas the loudness of sounds whose spectra spread beyond a critical bandwidth will depend, as well, on how many critical bands are spanned. Thus, beyond one critical band, loudness itself summates. For instance, speech presented at the same intensity as a single pure tone will sound louder than the tone. Although the critical band is a much more pessimistic specification of the auditory system's spectral resolving power, its capabilities continue to be impressive for several reasons: First, the frequency range of hearing spans over 25 critical bands. Second, the critical bands are not fixed intervals but rather are sliding intervals, along the frequency axis. Last, again, the system is capable of carrying out its spectrum analyses at quite rapid rates and in "real" time, providing the free-running speech communication ability that human beings enjoy.

Many of the auditory functions previously described are determined by events in the auditory periphery, that is, the processes of transferring the energy of sound to the organ of hearing and its subsequent transduction to electrochemical events that will lead to neural impulses transmissible by the acoustic nerve to the brain. It is in the periphery that some, if not all, of the limits previously described are established. It is also the peripheral system that is, at least in part, accessible to noninvasive medical examination and is most accessible to both therapeutic and surgical treatment. Therefore, the peripheral auditory system and its workings will be described most extensively.

ROUTING OF SOUND ENERGY TO THE COCHLEA

The human ear is divided into three parts—the external, middle, and internal portions. The outer and middle ear collect sound energy and funnel it to the inner ear. These physical functions cannot be fully appreciated without considering the basic acoustic and mechanical principles involved. When examining the anatomy of the ear of various submammalian species

(e.g., frogs, lizards, and birds), the outer ear at first seems expendable, and, indeed, the middle ear makes the more substantial contribution to auditory capabilities. The function of the middle ear can be appreciated by considering the problem of transmitting sound energy from one medium to another. For example, when sound waves in air encounter water, under the most ideal circumstances (i.e., plane wave propagation with a zero angle of incidence), only 0.1 per cent of the energy will be transmitted; 99.9 per cent will be reflected! This represents a 30-dB (i.e., 10 log [1000/1]) loss of sound energy from air to water. Given that the organ of Corti is housed in the fluid-filled cochlea, it is clear that optimal hearing sensitivity will not be possible via direct transmission of sound from air to cochlea.

It is well known from physics that sound (or, more generally, vibratory) energy transfer from one medium or one vibratory system to another is optimal only when the media or systems are matched in terms of their impedances. Impedance is a form of opposition to vibratory motion that arises from the combined mass (or density), elasticity, and friction of each medium or system. Mathematically, impedance is a complex number, meaning that it has both magnitude and phase; however, for our purposes here, it is not necessary to delve into such details. To reiterate the simple but important rule, optimal power transfer is possible only when the impedances of the media or systems involved are matched. This is true in electric, mechanical, and acoustic systems; thus, the output impedance of a high-fidelity amplifier must be matched to the input impedance of the loudspeaker to achieve the greatest frequency response and efficiency of power transfer. In vacuum tube amplifiers, for instance, the amplifier's output impedance is much higher than the input impedances of typical loudspeakers, so a transformer is used to match their impedances (whereas in transistor amplifiers such transformers are not needed owing to their naturally low-impedance characteristics). So too does the middle ear mechanism serve as a transformer to match the impedance of air to that of the cochlear input—the oval window.

The classic description of the elements of the middle ear is illustrated in Figure 7–2. In that figure, the middle ear system is modeled as a network of plates or pistons and levers. The analysis of this system has been described extensively by various writers (Dallos, 1973; Durrant and Lovrinic, 1984; Zwislocki, 1975) and is presented only conceptually here. The most obvious transformation, and indeed the largest component (numerically) of the transformation, is the large areal ratio of the tympanic membrane and the stapes footplate. Like the diaphragm of a loudspeaker, not all of the surface of the eardrum is free to vibrate, but even allowing for this factor, the ratio is relatively large (approximately 13:1). Thus, the force of a sound wave acting over the eardrum piston is funneled to the much smaller footplate area, yielding sound pressure amplification (because pressure equals force divided by area). There is an additional force amplifica-

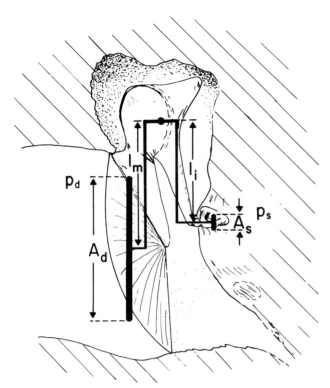

Figure 7–2. Components of the middle ear transformer, viewed as a system of two pistons connected by a folded lever. A, Area; p, sound pressure; l, length. Subscripts: d, eardrum; m, manubrium of the malleus; i, long crus of the incus; s, stapes footplate. (Inspired by drawing of Zwislocki, 1965.)

tion through the leverage of the ossicular chain system amounting to about 1.3:1. The total pressure amplification can be expressed as $13 \times 1.3 = 17$, which can be represented in decibels, equaling about 25 dB.

At first glance, this number seems to offer the sort of match that was needed, if the air-to-water analogy were valid. However, the input impedance of the cochlea does not appear to be as great as that of water (Zwislocki, 1975), thus limiting the validity of this analogy. Additionally, pressure amplification is not the only consideration. For instance, tremendous pressure might be generated by a given system. Yet, if no motion results, work (in the physical sense) has not been accomplished, and no power transfer will occur. Therefore, a more comprehensive analysis requires consideration of both sound pressure and velocity transformation, which in turn is reflected in the impedance transformation through the system. Results of such analyses have suggested the human middle ear system to be only about 60 per cent efficient and to be "worth" only about 13 dB. Of course, such estimates are only as good as the measures available and the assumption of validity of the piston model.

The classic piston model has been of great heuristic value, it is an easy-to-understand model, and it serves to illustrate the concepts of pressure amplification and impedance transformation. However, there is experimental evidence that this model's validity is limited. Holograms of the tympanic membrane in motion suggest that the curvature of the eardrum is the major

component of the transformer, rather than the eardrum-footplate areal ratio per se (Tonndorf and Khanna, 1970). The idea of transformation via the curvature of the eardrum was suggested first by Helmholtz over 100 years ago and can be appreciated from the analogy of a cable suspended between two poles (Wever and Lawrence, 1954). To pull the cable sufficiently taut to eliminate sag requires a great amount of force at the ends. Conversely, an upward push on the sagging part of the cable can create substantial force at the ends (assuming the cable to be sufficiently stiff to convey the applied and subsequently transformed force to the ends). Similarly, force acting on the eardrum might be transformed along the manubrium.

Another aspect of the mechanics of the middle ear that has been investigated is the proper model for the impedance of the stapes footplate, namely as a source impedance looking into the cochlea (Killion and Dallos, 1979). Results of the analysis of this problem suggest the possibility that the middle ear transformer could be more efficient than previously thought and that the total pressure amplification gain of the combined outer (see later) and middle ear might be realized, thereby yielding a substantially more favorable estimate of the "worth" of the middle ear. Indeed, the fenestration operation (predecessor of stapes mobilization surgery), in which the eardrum is essentially connected directly to a surgically formed window in the osseous labyrinth, yielded improvements in hearing at times approaching 25 dB (Davis and Walsh, 1950).

There is yet another value of the middle ear that is not as easily quantified but is easy to appreciate. Were it not for the middle ear transformer the round window would not be "protected." Sound waves then would reach both windows and could cause phase cancellation within the cochlea. However, only partial phase cancellation would occur at most frequencies, owing to the different planes of the windows.

Perhaps the most perplexing aspect of the workings of the middle ear transformer for the clinician is the dilemma of how hearing losses due to middle ear diseases, malformations, or other pathologic conditions can exceed even the most liberal estimate of its worth (e.g., sometimes exceeding 50 dB). The answer is that pathologic changes can actually cause the system to work even less efficiently than with no middle ear transformer at all! For example, atretic ears demonstrate air conduction hearing losses on the order of 50 dB. Additionally, when unilaterally deaf subjects are tested under earphones, transcranial conduction is observed to occur at 40 to 70 dB. These values largely reflect the air-to-skull impedance mismatch, although there is some acoustic leakage under the earphone cushion. It is not difficult to imagine that as outer or middle ear pathologic changes worsen, a specific pathway into the inner ear is lost. The physical problem then is no longer the one confronting nature in the evolution of the hearing mechanism, that of the air-to-cochlea impedance mismatch, but that of the air-to-skull mismatch.

Actually, even the most pessimistic estimates of the worth of the middle ear by physical systems standards make it appear quite efficient overall. Yet, this efficiency is realized at a price; the frequency response of the system is not without bounds, as noted earlier. In other words the middle ear filters sound. It efficiently transfers sound energy over the midfrequency range but becomes increasingly inefficient at the extremes of the hearing range, as was demonstrated by the minimal audibility curve (see Fig. 7–1). This point is further demonstrated by the graphs in Figure 7–3, in which the sound pressure transformation between (in effect) the cochlea and the eardrum yields a derived sensitivity curve remarkably similar to the minimal audibility curve. In short, the overall shape of the minimal audibility curve, and therefore the frequency limits of hearing, are ostensibly determined by the transfer characteristics of the middle ear system (Dallos, 1973; Durrant and Lovrinic, 1984). That is not to say that, for example, the cochlea of the bat would work in the elephant, or vice versa. Certainly, the inner and middle ear have evolved symbiotically, and it is the structures and mechanics of the organ of Corti that determine the overall sensitivity of the ear. Rather, the point is that the mechanical efficiency and response-versus-frequency characteristics reflected by the minimal audibility curve are largely determined by the middle ear.

The middle ear impedance and response characteristics are not entirely static but are subject to slight changes, even in the normal ear. First, there is the effect of changes in air pressure, which can push or pull on the eardrum and effectively alter the stiffness of the middle ear system. (This is done purposefully in tympanometry; see Chapters 9 and 21.) Of course, these pressure changes are generally relieved by opening the eustachian tube during swallowing and other maneuvers. Second, and more interesting from a physiologic acoustics point of view, are those changes caused by activation of the acoustic reflex (alternatively referred to as the middle ear muscle reflex or stapedius reflex, the latter term reflecting the prevalence of contribution of the stapedius muscle to sound activation of the reflex). This reflex can be monitored by observing the change in the input impedance (primarily stiffness or, its reciprocal, compliance) during intense sound stimulation. Clinically, this is accomplished with an emittance test instrument, the electroacoustic bridge, as used in tympanometry. Of particular interest is the possible role of the reflex.

Perhaps the most commonly assumed role of the reflex is that of protecting the ear from overstimulation. Given that the activation of the reflex does reduce the transmission of sound through the middle ear, some protection is likely to be afforded by this mechanism. However, this protection is also limited to the low frequencies, at which the increased stiffening of the ossicular chain is most effective (Møller, 1965, 1972). The reflex also seems too sluggish to protect the ear from impulsive sounds (Solomon and Starr, 1963), and it probably adapts too much to offer protection against

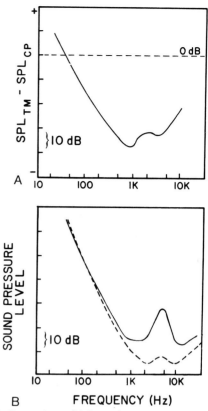

Figure 7–3. Comparison of *(A)* sound pressure gradient across the cochlear partition and *(B)* behavioral thresholds (minimal audibility curve) in the cat. The dashed line is the minimal audibility curve. The solid line is also the minimal audibility curve, but it has been corrected for the effects of resonance in the ear canal. In *A* the middle ear cavity or bulla was open, contributing to a slightly different slope of the low-frequency portion of these curves. SPL, Sound pressure level; TM, tympanic membrane; CP, cochlear partition. (Based on *(A)* data of Nedzelnitsky [1974] and *(B)* Dallos' adaptation [1973] of data from Miller et al. [1963].)

relatively constant noises (Tonndorf, 1976). Furthermore, it is not clear why such a protective mechanism would evolve, as noise pollution is a relatively modern phenomenon and is clearly synthetic.

Certainly, the acoustic reflex does provide the central auditory system with one means of controlling sound input at the periphery, albeit limited. However, the contribution of the musculature does not rest entirely on activation of the reflex arc because the normal tonus of the muscles affects the response characteristics of the middle ear mechanism (Simmons, 1964). They help to damp resonances and antiresonances of the system. The reflex is also activated just before and during vocalization, thus somewhat attenuating one's own voice (Borg and Zakrisson, 1975).

The outer ear also plays a role in matching the mechanics of the ear to the air medium outside. In various subhuman species, the pinnas are large and mobile and serve additionally to enhance the animal's ability to locate sounds. Even in humans, the role of the outer ear is not trivial. The combined acoustics of the head (acting as a baffle) and the ear canal (acting like a pipe with one end closed) contribute as much as 20-dB sound pressure amplification at the eardrum in the 2000- to 5000-HZ region (Shaw, 1974). Comparison of the graphs in panels A and B of Figure 7–3 shows (in this case in the cat) how there would be a progressive decrease in sensitivity above about 1000 Hz were sound energy fed directly to the tympanic membrane. The ear canal demonstrates a resonance point of approximately 3400 Hz (Wiener and Ross, 1946), the fundamental mode of this "pipe." Thus, it is the ear canal resonance, together with the head-baffle effect, that tends to reverse the upward swing in the sensitivity curve to provide additional sensitivity in the 2000- to 5000-Hz region (see Fig. 7–1A). This certainly must benefit the reception of consonant sounds, which have relatively less energy than vowels, and the fundamental pitch of the voice. It is unfortunate that this additional amplification may (at least in part) predispose the 4000-Hz region of hearing to damage from noise exposure, regardless of the spectrum of the noise (Tonndorf, 1976). Last, the human auricle, although not mobile and relatively small, does appear to be important for front-to-back and vertical sound localization. This contribution to audition is attributable to the acoustic baffle represented by the appendage per se, plus the convolution of its structure, which may cause discriminable spectral changes according to the elevation of the sound source (Butler and Helwig, 1983; Searle et al., 1975; Shaw, 1974). (This point will be elaborated later.) So, the human auricle is by no means vestigial, and the contributions of the outer ear are significant indeed.

STIMULATING HAIR CELLS

As described previously, the purpose of the outer and middle ear is to efficiently transfer sound energy from air to the inner ear. The role of the cochlea and many of the structures of the hearing organ is to couple the vibratory energy delivered to the oval window by the stapes footplate to the hair cells. To appreciate the mechanical mechanisms and events involved, it is worthwhile to first consider just what it takes to stimulate hair cells and, as a class of mechanoreceptors, how they work fundamentally.

For many years understanding of the workings of the cochlear hair cell was limited to a combination of theory, observations of the extracellularly recorded "gross" electric potentials of the cochlea, and extra- and intracellular recordings from hair cells of the lateral line organs found, for example, on the skin of fishes and frogs (Flock, 1965). Observations on the latter were supplemented by observations on vestibular hair cells (Duvall et al., 1966). The hair cells of these two systems have both stereocilia and a single kinocilium. As illustrated by Figure 7–4, the kinocilium provides a clear morphologic indicator of the preferred direction of deflection of the sensory hairs. Bending of the hairs in the direction of the kinocilium (from the group of stereocilia) causes maximal depolarization of the hair cell, which in turn leads to increased spike action

potentials in the neuron to which it is connected. In addition, it is significant that the deflection of the hairs in the opposite direction causes hyperpolarization and inhibits discharges of the primary neuron. Displacement of the hairs from side to side is essentially ineffective.

The reflection of signs of both excitation and inhibition in the pattern of discharges in the associated nerve fiber is an important aspect of neural encoding in vestibular and auditory systems. The vast majority of neurons exhibit some amount of spontaneous activity, often 20 or more spikes per second. In the auditory system, this spontaneous activity is random. The important point is that, even in the absence of sound stimulation, most primary auditory neurons are active (Kiang, 1965; Evans and Palmer, 1980). Thus, the excitation of auditory neurons is less a matter of turning them on and off than it is of altering the probability of discharge. The occurrence of spontaneous activity is important because it ultimately says something about the basic physiology of the hair cell and reflects the underlying mechanisms responsible for the keen mechanical sensitivity of the hair cell receptors. Indeed, higher spontaneous-rate neurons tend to exhibit the greater sensitivity (Evans and Palmer, 1980).

The model of hair cell transduction that has guided research in this area for years is that of Davis (1965). Davis postulated that the bending of the sensory hairs depolarizes (and alternately hyperpolarizes) the hair cell membrane by altering the membrane resistance. The hair cell membrane appears to be "leaky" so that there is a small but constant amount of ionic current flow across the cell membrane. This leakage current is presumably the "stimulus" for the spontaneous background activity in the associated nerve fiber. Deflection of the hairs in the excitatory direction then increases the current flow and causes increased release of transmitter substance at the base of the hair cell (Flock et al., 1973). This is illustrated conceptually in Figure 7–5. Only over the past decade or so has the actual membrane biophysics involved begun to be understood (Hudspeth, 1985). Suffice it to say, these details largely represent elaborations of the Davis model, the major tenet of which has (reasonably) withstood the test of time (Tonndorf, 1975).

A pivotal component of the Davis model, which dealt specifically with the cochlear hair cell, was the suggested role of the endolymphatic potential (EP)— the resting potential measured within the scala media, which is generated by the stria vascularis (Tasaki and Spyropoulos, 1959). The EP is viewed as providing an extra "force" for driving current through the hair cell (Davis, 1965). Visualizing the EP as a battery in the stria vascularis and the resting membrane potential of the hair cell as a battery, one can consider these batteries as effectively wired in series; this doubles the transmembrane potential relative to the membrane potential of the hair cell alone.

That the EP is found in an extracellular space filled with a high concentration of potassium represents an intriguing physiologic phenomenon and gives rise to a

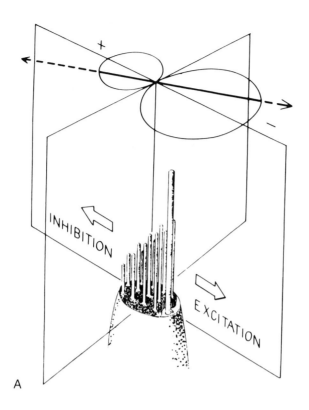

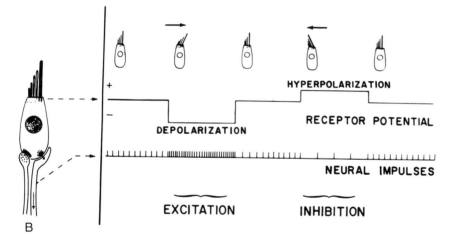

Figure 7–4. *A,* Diagram illustrating the directional sensitivity of the hair cell. *B,* Relationship of discharge rate of action potentials in the afferent neuron connected to the hair cell in response to different directions of shearing of the hairs. (Adapted from Flock, Å. 1965. Transducing mechanisms in lateral line canal organ receptors. Cold Spring Harbor Symp. Quant. Biol. 30:133–146.)

Figure 7–5. Schematic representation of excitatory current flow through the hair cell *(left)* and mechanism of chemical transmission between the hair cell and the afferent nerve ending *(right).* (Adapted with permission from Flock, Å., et al. 1973. The physiology of individual hair cells and their synapses. *In* Møller, A. R. [ed.]: Basic Mechanisms in Hearing. New York, Academic Press, pp. 273–306.)

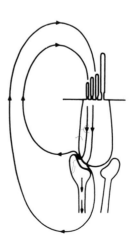
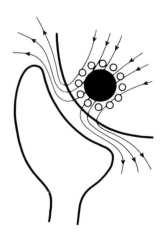

long-standing argument: is the EP a by-product of the biochemical mechanisms needed to create the high potassium (and low sodium) concentration or vice versa? A somewhat separate issue is whether the endolymph itself might enhance the sensitivity of the hair cells, if the hairs, in fact, are bathed in endolymph—yet another point of debate. These mysteries have yet to be fully unraveled. Revelations of actin filaments in stereocilia (Tilney et al., 1980), other microstructural details (Lim, 1986), and the possible effector role of outer (versus the pure receptor role of inner) hair cells (Brownell et al., 1985) create even more questions as to the significance of endolymph and the EP. Whatever its direct purpose, or *raison d'être*, the presence of a normal EP appears to be requisite for a completely normally functioning hearing organ. Indeed, it appears to influence the sensitivity of the cochlear hair cell system, at least as reflected by changes in the cochlear potentials (Honrubia and Ward, 1969), discussed later.

Stimulating the Cochlear Hair Cell

Although cochlear hair cells have no kinocilia, there are anatomic signs and electrophysiologic evidence that they too exhibit directional sensitivity. The pattern of the stereocilia on the outer hair cells seems to point to the direction of maximally excitatory displacements because the base of the W pattern is, and the locations of the tallest stereocilia are, oriented radially away from the modiolus. Thus, they appear to be stimulated optimally by radial deflections of the hairs (Fig. 7–6). Although the stereocilia of inner hair cells form only slight crescent patterns, these crescents also "bulge" in the radial direction.

The problem of stimulating cochlear hair cells is how to cause bending of the hairs via an up-and-down motion of the hearing organ. A workable solution to this puzzle is suggested by Figure 7–6 and relies heavily on the structural relation between the tectorial membrane and the body of the hearing organ (Ryan and Dallos, 1984). The former pivots effectively at the lip of the internal sulcus, whereas the organ of Corti, supported by the basilar membrane, effectively pivots at or near its attachment to the osseous spiral lamina. Because the two pivot points are displaced from one another, up-and-down motion of the organ creates a radial shear between them. A simple demonstration of this can be made using an unsharpened pencil. The pencil is held on end between the two hands with the arms fully extended. The right hand is placed with the palm turned up, and the left with palm down, thus orienting the pencil vertically. The left hand represents the tectorial membrane, the pencil represents a stereocilium, and the right hand represents the basilar membrane and supporting cells of the organ of Corti. The left and right shoulders represent the respective pivot points and, of course, are displaced from each other. Keeping the arms perfectly straight while moving the hands together up and down, it can be seen that an alternating shearing force is created between

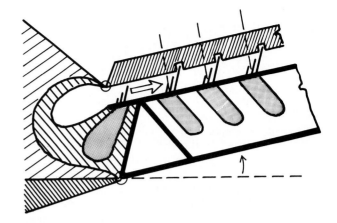

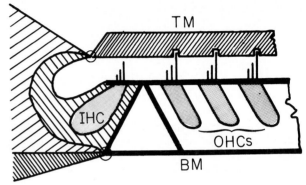

Figure 7–6. Schematic representation of the organ of Corti illustrating how shearing displacements of the stereocilia can result from displacement of the basilar membrane. BM, Basilar membrane; TM, tectorial membrane; IHC, inner hair cell; OHCs, outer hair cells. (Adapted with permission from Ryan, A., and Dallos, P. 1984. Physiology of the cochlea. *In* Northern, J. L. [ed.]: Hearing Disorders, 2nd ed. Boston, Little, Brown and Co., pp. 253–266.)

the two hands, causing the stereocilium to be "rocked" toward and away from the body (i.e., "radially").

The stereocilia have been shown to be stiff normally (Flock and Cheng, 1977), and, as illustrated in Figure 7–6, the tallest of the hairs of the outer hair cells clearly impale the underbelly of the tectorial membrane (Hunter-Duvar, 1978). So, it is fairly clear that the shearing displacements created by the up-and-down motion of the basilar membrane will lead to deflection of the hairs. Indeed, these structural factors might figure significantly in the entire scheme of the mechanical characteristics of the cochlear partition (see later). The mode of displacement of the stereocilia of the inner hair cells, on the other hand, is less obvious and more controversial, beginning with the controversy of whether the hairs of inner hair cells are as tightly coupled to the tectorial membrane at those of the outer hair cells. The consensus is that hairs of inner hair cells, at most, just touch the tectorial membrane. However, even if these stereocilia are freestanding, it is probable that they still would be displaced by the virtual flow of fluid created in the channel between the tectorial membrane and the surface of the organ, which in turn would be alternately compressed by the transformation of up-and-down to shearing motion (Ryan and Dallos, 1984). Therefore, the hairs of outer hair cells would be most directly stimulated by basilar membrane displacements, whereas the velocity of the basilar membrane would be critical for bending the hairs of the inner hair cells. Electrophysiologic evidence strongly supports the notion of the outer hair cells' being displacement sensitive (Dallos et al., 1972), whereas both velocity and displacement responses have been observed for inner hair cells (Zwislocki and Sokolich, 1973). In any event, the hairs of the inner hair cells do not appear to be tightly coupled to the tectorial membrane. For instance, microscopy has failed to provide convincing evidence of any pockets for the stereocilia of the inner hair cells on the underbelly of the tectorial membrane, which are so clearly organized into the distinctive pattern of the stereocilia of the outer hair cells.

MOTION OF THE BASILAR MEMBRANE

As intimated in the foregoing, the essential mechanical event for stimulating auditory hair cells is the back-and-forth shearing displacement of the stereocilia, which in turn requires the up-and-down motion of the organ of Corti and, therefore, motion of the basilar membrane. Actually, the entire cochlear partition (i.e., Reissner membrane, organ of Corti, basilar membrane, and fluid contained by the cochlear duct) moves together, namely in response to fluid displacement caused by motion of the stapes. The basis of this motion is illustrated in Figure 7–7; it was revealed by the classic experiments of von Békèsy (1960) and verified more recently by researchers using highly sophisticated measurement techniques (Rhode, 1986). It is noteworthy that stapes displacement does not lead to bulk fluid displacement via the helicotrema, except perhaps for very-low-frequency vibrations or static displacements of the stapes (Dallos, 1970). In other words, throughout most of the audible frequency range, it is as if the helicotrema did not exist. Rather, an inward displacement of the stapes displaces perilymph in the scala vestibuli, which pushes down on the cochlear partition, displacing fluid in the scala tympani, which then pushes out on the round window membrane. The opposite series of events occurs in response to a pull on the stapes. In this manner, the round window membrane vibrates sympathetically with vibration of the stapes (von Békèsy, 1960).

In Figure 7–7A the cochlea is uncoiled for illustrative purposes, and the cochlear partition is represented as a single membrane, the mechanics of which is determined extensively by the properties of the basilar membrane. A displacement of the cochlear partition (or basilar membrane) caused by a push on the stapes does not lead to uniform displacement along the entire

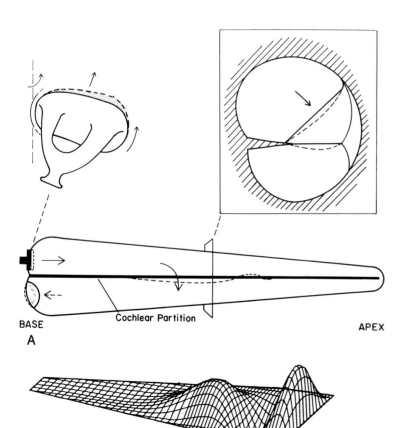

BASE

Cochlear Partition

APEX

A

B

Figure 7–7. **A, Illustration of the manner in which displacement of the stapes leads to displacement of the cochlear partition (the basilar membrane, in particular). Cross-sectional (longitudinal) view of the uncoiled cochlea. Inset drawings indicate in more detail the actual modes of displacement of the stapes and, subsequently, the cochlear partition. Note: The stapes appears to move about an axis defined by the ligament along the posterior aspect of the footplate, although a certain amount of its motion is also piston-like (i.e., in and out). (After von Békèsy, G. 1960. Experiments in Hearing, translated and edited by E. G. Wever. New York, McGraw-Hill Book Co.) B, Three-dimensional view of displacement of the basilar membrane at one instant. (From Holmes, M. H. 1980. An analysis of a low-frequency model of the cochlea. J. Acoust. Soc. Am. 68:482–488.)**

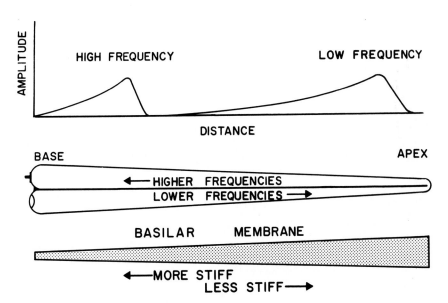

Figure 7–8. Peak displacement of the traveling wave at different frequencies of the sound stimulus and its dependence on the stiffness gradient of the basilar membrane, which in turn increases in width toward the apex. (Based on drawings and data of von Békèsy, G. 1960. Experiments in Hearing, translated and edited by E. G. Wever. New York, McGraw-Hill Book Co.; also data of Rhode, W. S. 1973. An investigation of postmortem cochlear mechanics using the Mossbauer effect. *In* Møller, A. R. [ed.]: Basic Mechanisms in Hearing. New York, Academic Press, pp. 39–63.)

length of the partition. The displacement is regional owing to the peculiar wave motion that is excited along the basilar membrane in response to the application of vibratory energy (see preceding discussion). Von Békèsy (1960) described this motion as traveling waves. These waves build up from the basalward aspect of the basilar membrane and crest as they progress apicalward, namely at or near a place that is uniquely related to the frequency of vibration applied at the stapes (Fig. 7–8). It is at this place that eventually (i.e., over several cycles of vibration) the overall maximum displacement will occur and after which vibration of the partition decays quickly, because the basilar membrane is critically damped. In this way, frequency is transformed into a place code.

Whether the central auditory system actually makes use of the frequency-to-place transformation is discussed later. The more basic issue is the fundamental importance of the underlying hydromechanical events and what mechanical properties of the cochlea make them possible. The first issue is somewhat speculative, that is, would the cochlea work the way it does were the place encoding of frequency per se not necessary? One should consider, however, the most obvious alternative—a simple vibrating membrane. It is not a trivial matter to get a membrane, diaphragm, or plate to vibrate uniformly across its surface over a wide range of frequencies. There is also the matter of mechanical impedance, which also will vary across frequency. What one has in the cochlea, then, is a clever mechanical system for handling a broad frequency range efficiently, much as horns are used to match loudspeakers. How traveling waves occur is a matter too involved to deal with here, but the primary mechanical feature that governs their behavior over frequency is well known and simple to describe. As shown by Figure 7–8, the gradient of stiffness along the basilar membrane primarily determines the frequency-to-place transformation. Toward the base, the basilar membrane becomes more stiff, whereas it is

less stiff near the apex. This change in stiffness, in turn, is due to the change in width of the membrane—narrower toward the base and wider toward the apex (Fig. 7–8). The gradient of stiffness along the entire length of the basilar membrane amounts to a 100:1 change from base to apex.

Of course, there are many other aspects of the structure of the cochlea and the organ of Corti that contribute to the detailed mechanical events of the cochlea, and these may include such microstructural features as the change in the number and lengths of the stereocilia, angle of orientation of the **W** pattern, and the tectorial membrane–stereocilia interface from base to apex (Lim, 1986). For purposes here, knowledge of the details is perhaps less important than an appreciation of the extent to which the mechanical events of the cochlea are translated into a code useful to the central auditory system.

NEURAL ENCODING OF THE SOUND STIMULUS AND BASIC AUDITORY INFORMATION PROCESSING

Frequency

The links between the hair cell receptors and the central auditory system are, naturally, the primary auditory neurons that richly innervate the organ of Corti. The response of an individual neuron can be examined using microelectrodes. Much as one can determine the minimal audibility curve, the response area of an individual primary auditory neuron can be ascertained (Kiang, 1965). As illustrated in Figure 7–9, the SPL at which a criterion increase in spike discharge rate (above the spontaneous rate) is measured against the frequency of stimulation. This minimal audibility curve for neurons is called a tuning function; as seen in Figure 7–9A, it has a sharp minimum or

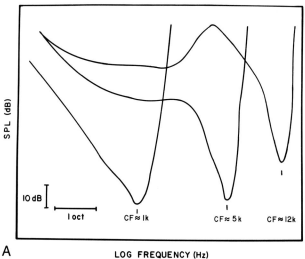

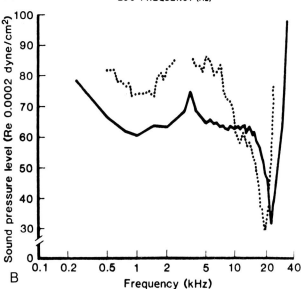

Figure 7–9. A, Tuning functions illustrating the frequency response of primary auditory neurons (in this case, from cat). (Based on data of Kiang and Moxon [1974] as presented by Zwicker [1974].) **B,** Comparison of tuning functions for the response of the basilar membrane versus that of a first-order neuron. The solid line is a plot of the SPL required for 3×10^{-8} cm basilar membrane displacement at the point of observation in the base of the cat cochlea. The dotted line is a single-unit tuning function (obtained in a different animal and in another laboratory by M. C. Liberman); the data shown are from a unit whose characteristic frequency is near that at which the minimum of the mechanical tuning function occurs. (With permission from Khana, S. M., and Leonard, D. G. 1982. Basilar membrane tuning in the cat cochlea. Science 215:305–306. Copyright 1982 by the AAAS.)

peak of sensitivity at one frequency—the characteristic frequency (CF). The value of the CF depends on the place of origin of the neuron along the basilar membrane. In other words, nerve fibers originating from more basalward regions will have higher CFs, and those from more apical regions will have lower CFs. It is evident from the tuning function that, although the primary auditory neurons are quite selective in their sensitivity, they are not discretely sensitive to a single frequency. In addition, the roll-off in sensitivity

is much steeper for frequencies above the CF and much less steep for lower frequencies, particularly after the SPL has been increased to approximately 40 dB above that at which CF occurs. The question that baffled researchers for many years is whether the observed pattern of the tuning function and the degree of frequency selectivity represented by the "tip" region of the tuning function around CF are completely attributable to the cochlear hydromechanical events described earlier or whether additional filtering is needed between the receptor and nerve cells. The answer, as illustrated in Figure 7–9B, is now known to be the former; the peripheral mechanical events provide all the selectivity necessary to account for the neural tuning curves (Khanna and Leonard, 1982; Russell and Sellick, 1977). Because tuning curves derived from psychoacoustic measures (Zwicker, 1974) show little increase in selectivity over the tuning functions of primary auditory fibers, it would appear that the cochlear mechanics accounts largely for the frequency discrimination ability of the auditory system. However, as further discussed later, some central processing is required for pitch perception, particularly for complex sounds such as those created by musical instruments. This is because, for such complex sounds, there inevitably are considerably complex patterns of motion of the basilar membrane arising from overlapping traveling waves excited by the spectral components of the given sound (Keidel, 1980). If place is the primary cue for frequency encoding, it should be possible to reconstruct the pattern of motion of the basilar membrane from activity recorded from neurons throughout the acoustic nerve (Fig. 7–10A). Through tedious and meticulous electrophysiologic experiments, such demonstrations can be made (Pfeiffer and Kim, 1975), as shown by Figure 7–10B.

Because the auditory neurons leave the hearing organ in an orderly fashion, the frequency-to-place code is also expected to be reflected in the organization of the central nuclei to which the primary fibers radiate. This organizational scheme, known as tonotopic organization, also has been demonstrated for all major nuclei of the central pathways and the primary auditory cortex (Brugge and Geisler, 1978; Merzenich et al., 1975; Walzl, 1947). As illustrated in Figure 7–11, this is accomplished by the observation of a systematic progression in CFs of neurons encountered as a recording microelectrode is advanced along an appropriate axis. It is as if the cochlea were mapped along this axis. Because there are multiple nuclei (e.g., dorsal and ventral cochlear nuclei) or major subdivisions of nuclei (e.g., posterior and anterior ventral cochlear nuclei), there are actually multiple maps at most, if not all, levels of the ascending auditory pathway.

The pervasiveness of tonotopic organization in the auditory system bespeaks the importance of the place code in the encoding and processing of frequency information. Yet, it is most certainly not the only cue. The auditory neurons show considerable ability to encode temporal features of the stimulus. It is true that individual neurons are not capable of following

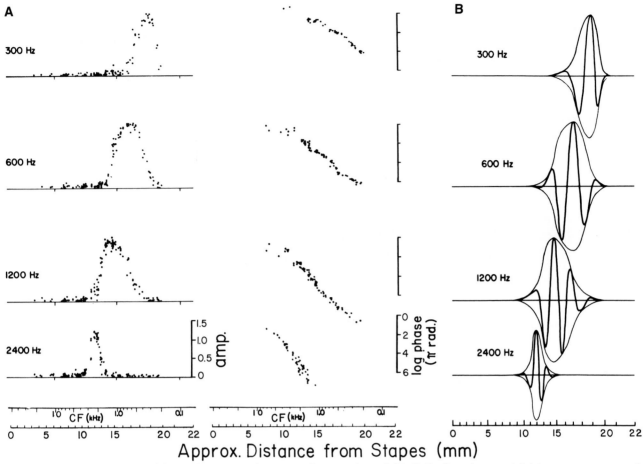

Figure 7–10. *A*, Amplitudes and phases of responses of an array of neurons (recorded individually and sequentially) in response to tones of the frequencies indicated, presented at 20-dB SPL. *B*, Traveling wave patterns derived from data in *A*. (Adapted from Pfeiffer, R. R., and Kim, D. O. 1975. Cochlear nerve fiber responses: Distribution along the cochlear partition J. Acoust. Soc. Am. 58:867–869.)

Figure 7–11. Diagrammatic illustration of concept of tonotopic organization. A tonal map of the cochlea is projected onto this hypothetic auditory nucleus by virtue of the orderly connection between it and the hair cells along the basilar membrane (inset). Thus, an electrode traversing the path indicated by the arrow records activity from neurons with characteristic frequencies (CF) that systematically vary from low to high. (With permission from Durrant, J. D., and Lovrinic, J. H. 1984. Bases of Hearing Science, 2nd ed. © 1984, the Williams & Wilkins Co., Baltimore)

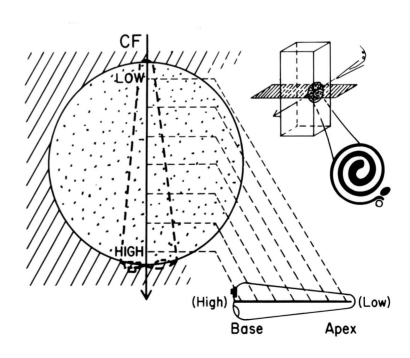

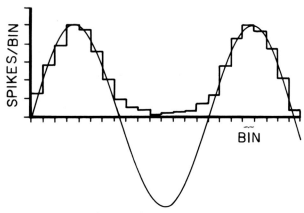

Figure 7–12. Periodicity in the pattern of neural discharges reflected by a histogram of the spikes occurring in each time bin over the period observed. (Based on Brugge et al. 1969. J. Neurophysiol. 32:386.)

each cycle of the stimulus in a one-to-one fashion, except for relatively low frequencies. Even the notion of volleying, once believed to be the mechanism for overcoming this limitation (Wever, 1949), is oversimplified. A more statistical concept (as was invoked in describing the spontaneous activity of auditory neurons) is necessary to describe the temporal pattern of discharges, as illustrated in Figure 7–12. Here it is shown that, although individual discharges are not locked to a particular phase of the time history or waveform of the stimulus, their probability of occurrence at any time does reflect the stimulus waveform (Brugge et al., 1969; Rose et al., 1967). In this way, auditory neurons appear to be able to represent the periodicity of the stimulus to frequencies at least up to 5000 Hz. Not only is this information available to be extracted by the central system to provide a sense of fundamental pitch for complex sounds, but also it is available for other temporal discriminations. For now, it is sufficient to acknowledge that the auditory system is indeed capable of impressive high-frequency, and therefore "high-speed," temporal encoding, as expected of any system capable of encoding and processing of such complex stimuli as speech.

Intensity

The intensity of the sound is important too and must be encoded for neural transmission in and processing by the central auditory system. At the first level of encoding, the auditory system works like most sensory systems, and, as illustrated in Figure 7–13A, intensity is translated into rate of spike discharge (Kiang, 1968). Therefore, the more intense the stimulus, the more vigorous the rate of discharge of the auditory neuron. However, there are limits. First, the stimulus must be sufficiently strong to cause a significant increase in discharges above the background (spontaneous) rate, although for relatively low-frequency stimuli it may be sufficient that there be only a significant increase in the degree of synchronization of the discharges with the phase of the stimulus (Rose et al., 1967) (i.e., with

no net increase in discharge rate). Here, again, the temporal pattern of discharges may be important. The other limit is that the discharge rate ultimately saturates. At CF, this typically occurs at only 20 to 30 dB, and off CF perhaps to levels as high as 40 dB above the intensity that just causes a significant increase in discharges over the spontaneous rate (Sachs and Abbas, 1974). At higher intensities, the discharge rate saturates. This limit raises an interesting question. If the dynamic range of the individual neuron is a mere 20 to 40 dB, how is it that the dynamic range of the auditory system is 140 dB? Would not this saturation degrade intensity discrimination and hopelessly muddle the discharge pattern created by complex stimuli such as speech, even at conversational levels?

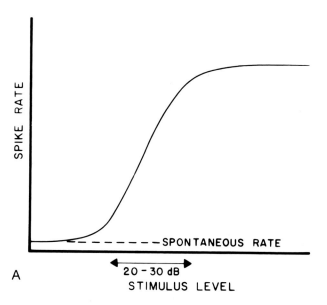

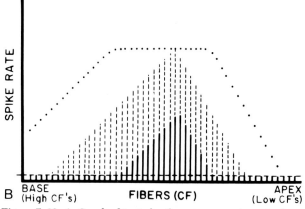

Figure 7–13. *A,* Graph of typical spike rate–versus–intensity function for a first-order neuron monitored at the characteristic frequency. (Based on data from the cat from Kiang [1968].) *B,* Hypothetic histogram-type plot of the spike rate of an array of fibers. The activity of these fibers is shown at only a few levels. The dotted line demarks the upper limits of the histogram at saturating levels of the stimulus for fibers with characteristic frequencies that approximate the frequency that gives rise to the peak of the traveling wave in the cochlea. (Modified after Whitfield, I. C. 1956. Electrophysiology of the central auditory pathway. Br. Med. Bull. 12:105–109.)

The dynamic range puzzle has yet to be fully solved, but a workable (although not infallible) solution has been put forth and some relevant observations have been made. First, it is significant that the primary neurons are tuned to a certain frequency but, as noted earlier, are still responsive to other frequencies. This occurs because the traveling wave represents a pattern of displacement, not a discrete bump, despite the keen sensitivity and selectivity represented by the tip of the tuning function. Thus, as the intensity of the sound increases, there is a spread of excitation (Fig. 7–13B). Looking across the many neurons, then, the central auditory system sees continued growth in the total density of neural discharges, even after neurons tuned to the stimulus have saturated (Whitefield, 1967a, b). However, listening off frequency does not appear necessary to maintain intensity discrimination ability because essentially the same difference limens are obtained in the presence of stop-band noise (Viemeister, 1983), that is, a masker with energy above and below (but not within) the desired frequency range. The density-of-discharge code also does not address necessarily, and indeed may complicate, the problem of preservation of the spectral features of speech and other complex stimuli. Thus, the extraction of the features of such sounds may require further processing centrally. The central system perhaps can set some rules for weighting activity from different neurons (e.g., based on synchrony of discharges), which can preserve spectral features in the neural code (Sachs and Young, 1979; Young and Sachs, 1979). It has been observed that there are central neurons, at least at the cortex in primates, that show sharp tuning characteristics for intensity, much as most neurons show selectivity for frequency (Pfingst and O'Connor, 1981).

OTHER ASPECTS OF CENTRAL AUDITORY PROCESSING

With the entry of the acoustic nerve into the brain stem, there immediately begins, in effect, a multiplication of the auditory neurons. Thus, as noted earlier, multiple tonotopic maps of the cochlea can be found throughout the auditory system. This may seem redundant, but there also appears to be increased specialization of the response patterns of auditory neurons at the level of the cochlear nuclei and higher centers. Whereas discharge patterns are much the same from one primary neuron to the next, no less than five different patterns of discharge have been identified within the cochlear nucleus complex (Kiang, 1975). As suggested by Figure 7–14, these different patterns may be linked to the different morphologic cell types, although the association of discharge pattern with cell morphology may not be exactly as shown nor as simple. Still, the observed variations in discharge patterns represent one mechanism of feature detection by central auditory neurons; for instance, the pattern of discharge of some neurons is somewhat selectively sensitive to stimulus onset alone (e.g., cell 4 in Fig.

7–14B) or onset and offset (e.g., cell 5 in Fig. 7–14B). More centrally, neurons may be found to be more sensitive to frequency modulation than to the mere onset of the stimulus and thus appear to be dedicated more to the detection of particular features of the stimulus (Keidel, 1974; Suga, 1971). Additionally, the circuitry of the central system is elaborated, as manifested by the multiplicity of ordering of neurons in the ascending pathways, branching of ascending fibers, and the formation of feedback loops. Of course, there is a substantial descending or efferent auditory pathway (Harrison and Howe, 1974a), although it is only the lower part of the system, the olivocochlear system, that is still well known (Galambos, 1958; Klinke and Gallay, 1974). Therefore, the central system does have some ability to vary the input sensitivity, namely at the periphery, which is further facilitated via the middle ear muscle reflex system. There also is suspicion that the efferent system could even influence frequency discrimination ability via changes in peripheral frequency tuning. This suspicion has been heightened by the observations of actin in the stereocilia of hair cells and the demonstration of motile responses of isolated hair cells to electric current (as discussed previously), but clear experimental evidence of such facilitation is still forthcoming.

A truly impressive aspect of central auditory processing is binaural sound localization. Although the primary ascending auditory pathway is a crossed pathway, the ipsilateral ascending pathway is quite robust (Harrison and Howe, 1974b). With decussation of fibers at several levels of the central system, it is clear that there must be substantial interaction of information from the two ears. More centrally, nerve cell specialization or "wiring" is encountered, which facilitates the comparator functions that underlie binaural processing (Cassedy and Neff, 1975; Erulkar, 1972; Irving and Harrison, 1967; Masterson et al., 1982; Moushigian et al., 1971; Rose et al., 1966). Thus, there are neurons at the levels of the superior olive and the inferior colliculus that receive inputs from both ears and may, for example, be excited by binaural stimuli while being inhibited by monaural stimuli. Rather than belaboring these features, the basic abilities of the binaural system and the fundamental cues for binaural sound localization (Mills, 1972; Neff, 1968) will be discussed briefly.

The basic cues for binaural sound localization are most easily appreciated from observations of the phenomenon of binaural lateralization, although the two phenomena are not identical (Plenge, 1974). Lateralization is generally demonstrated via presentation of sound to the two ears by earphones. Earphones create the impression that the sounds presented are located somewhere between the two ears within the head (whereas the sound image is generally externalized with loud speaker presentation). The task for the subject is the same as that which the physician asks of patients during the Weber test—to determine from which side of the head the sound seems to come. As shown in Figure 7–15, signals presented in phase and

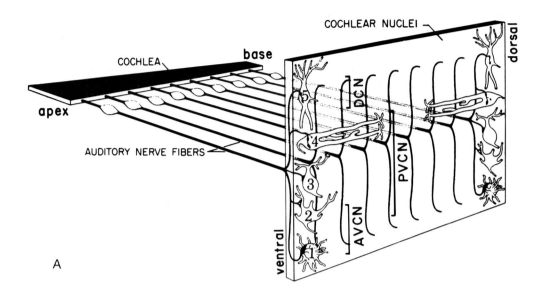

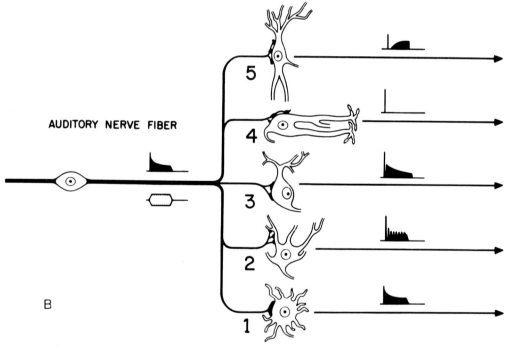

Figure 7–14. *A*, Highly schematic representation of connections between the peripheral auditory system and the cochlear nuclei. AVCN, Anterior, and PVCN, posterior ventral cochlear nuclei; DCN, dorsal cochlear nucleus. Some of the complexity of the morphology of the second-order neurons is indicated (five different types shown). *B*, Possible relation between cell types and discharge patterns as reflected in poststimulus time histograms. Response types are as follows: 1, primarylike; 2, "chopper"; 3, primarylike with notch; 4, "on"; and 5, "pauser." (Adapted with permission from Kiang, N. Y.-S. 1975. Stimulus representation in the discharge patterns of auditory neurons. *In* Eagles, E. L. [ed.]: The Nervous System, Vol. 3: Human Communication and Its Disorders. New York, Raven Press.)

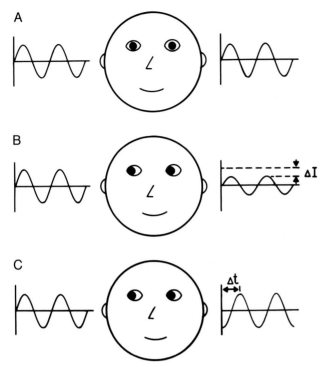

Figure 7–15. Illustration of the binaural lateralization of the sound image obtained when the same frequency tone is presented via earphones *(A)* at the same intensity and time/phase, *(B)* at different intensities (ΔI), and *(C)* at different times/phases (Δt) to the two ears. (With permission from Durrant, J. D., and Lovrinic, J. H. 1984. Bases of Hearing, 2nd ed. © 1984, the Williams & Wilkins Co., Baltimore.)

at identical intensities to the two ears will be perceived as coming from the center of the head owing to binaural fusion. With either a larger amplitude or leading phase (or earlier arrival) of the sound to one ear, the sound image is lateralized toward that ear. The binaural system is quite sensitive to interaural time and intensity disparities. In listening to sounds from the environment, such disparities are created by the separation of the two ears, as illustrated by Figure 7–16, but the time and intensity cues subserve binaural localization for different frequency ranges (Mills, 1972). This is attributable to the acoustics involved. At lower frequencies, the diameter of the head is shorter than the wavelengths of the sound waves, so diffraction occurs (Kinsler and Frey, 1962) (Fig. 7–16A). This means that the sound waves tend to scatter around the head, the result being that the intensity of the sound at the two ears is not appreciably different, regardless of which way the head is turned with respect to the sound source. Still, it takes longer for the sound to reach the ear farthest from the sound source, so a temporal disparity is created. As frequency increases, the auditory system has less ability to accurately represent the temporal structure of the sound, but at these frequencies, diffraction no longer occurs (Fig. 7–16A and B). The head tends to shadow the ear farthest from the sound source, so an intensity disparity is thus created. At the two ears, additionally, the head (and at high frequencies even the auricle) acts as an acoustic baffle

and enhances the sound pressure in the vicinity of the "near" ear (Shaw, 1974).

This is not to say that sound localization is entirely dependent on binaural processing. Monaural localization is possible but is much less precise. Monaural localization is, in part, an adaptation of intensity discrimination and takes advantage of the head shadow effect. Monaural localization may also take advantage of mechanisms underlying the auditory system's ability to localize sounds at different elevations, even in the midsagittal plane. Here the auricle again makes a special contribution (Butler and Helwig, 1983), its convolutions apparently creating subtle changes in the high-frequency sound spectrum as the sound source is raised or lowered or as the head is tilted. In general, the importance of the mobility of the head must not be underestimated in sound localization (e.g., the head may be turned to nullify binaural differences and "zero" in on a source).

The emphasis here on binaural sound localization is not meant to imply that binaural processing is singularly dedicated to this function. Binaural processing also facilitates the detection and discrimination of sounds in a background of noise (McFadden, 1968), as well as selective attention (Cherry, 1959). The most common complaints of unilaterally hearing-impaired people and hearing-impaired individuals wearing only one hearing aid pertain to their difficulties in understanding speech in noisy places, at meetings, or in other situations in which there are "competing messages."

CORTICAL PROCESSING

Much, if not all, of the processing previously discussed can and is likely to be accomplished at the brain stem level of the central auditory system. Indeed, several of the basic auditory abilities appear to be attributable to subcortical processing. For example, it has been shown that auditory decorticate animals are capable of detecting the presence of sound and

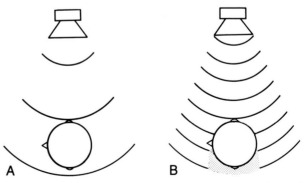

Figure 7–16. Simplified representation of the acoustic effects of the head on sound waves. *A,* Wavelengths greater than the head diameter, wherein diffraction occurs. *B,* Sound waves with shorter wavelengths, wherein the head casts a "shadow." (With permission from Durrant, J. D., and Lovrinic, J. H. 1984. Bases of Hearing, 2nd ed. © 1984, the Williams & Wilkins Co., Baltimore.)

changes in intensity, frequency, and location of sound (Canford, 1979; Cassedy and Neff, 1975; Heffner, 1978; Massopust et al., 1971; Neff, 1959). So impressive are the capabilities of the brain stem auditory processing that one may wonder just what auditory abilities, if any, are attributable to cortical processing. Of course, there is no doubt of the necessity of cortical processing for cognition and deciphering speech information, which in turn doubtlessly requires more than the primary auditory cortex. Additionally, auditory decorticate animals have been found to be incapable of distinguishing between tonal patterns (in which the same tones are included in the different patterns presented), discriminating changes in sound duration, and, in general, discriminating between stimulus conditions that involve ro net change in neural activity (Neff, 1959). Although such animals show amazing abilities to compensate, they appear not to truly localize sound in space. This requires an internal map of auditory space (Knudsen and Konishi, 1978), which is apparently relegated to the cortex (Benson et al., 1981).

The neuroanatomic and neurophysiologic bases for cortical auditory processing are many, but the gross manifestations are tonotopic organization over the surface of the primary auditory cortex (Merzenich et al., 1975; Romani et al., 1982; Woolsey, 1971) and perhaps columnar organization throughout different layers (Abeles and Goldstein, 1970; Galaburda and Sanides, 1980; Imig et al., 1982; Kelly and Wong, 1981). The former is perhaps a mere by-product of the orderly arrangement of neurons in the ascending pathway. Still, this system should serve to presort information according to frequency. Columnar organization, which is known better in other sensory systems, is perhaps the basis for the more advanced processing for which the cortex is responsible. At the cortex, one also expects even further specialization in the response of the neurons, and it is through the layers of the cortex that the morphologic variants in the cells and the intracellular circuits are found that would be expected, intuitively, to be required for this advanced processing.

AUDITORY ELECTROPHYSIOLOGY AND CLINICAL APPLICATIONS

Throughout this overview of the auditory system, great reliance has been placed on information obtained from single-unit recordings in infrahuman species, that is, bioelectrical recordings made utilizing microelectrodes (e.g., micropipette) capable of picking up activity from just outside or even inside single cells. However, there are also a number of gross or compound potentials that can be recorded in the auditory system; one of these, the endolymphatic potential, was already mentioned. These potentials represent the activity of many cells (receptor, neural, or other); they have provided valuable electrophysiologic indexes for use in basic research in auditory function; and most have

proved subsequently to be recordable in humans and to have clinical utility, as discussed in part in Chapter 9.

Electrocochleography

The stimulus-related electric potentials of the organ of Corti and the acoustic nerve compose an electric response, the recorded waveform of which has been called the electrocochleogram. First, there are two cochlear potentials that arise from hair cell receptor potentials: cochlear microphonics (CM) and summating potentials (SP) (Dallos, 1973), as shown in Figure 7–17. An electrode placed within the cochlea or even externally (e.g., on the round window membrane or the promontory, eardrum, or more remote sites with signal processing) will pick up these potentials simultaneously. The CM has a waveform that mimics that of the sound stimulus. Therefore, if the stimulus is a tone burst, the CM will appear as a sinusoidal pulse. However, the CM waveform will often appear to be offset; that is, in the case of the sinusoidal pulse, the zero axis will be displaced above or below the baseline of the recording (Fig. 7–17). If the CM is "stripped" away via low-pass filtering or averaging with phase cancellation, this offset (a direct current pulse) can be isolated. This is the summating potential. The CM and SP are products of mechanoelectric transduction processes of the hair cells (Dallos, 1973). However, as extracellular manifestations of the unit receptor potentials, they reflect much more because they are distributed through the elaborate electroanatomic structure of the cochlea (Durrant, 1979). Even with fairly selective intracochlear recording techniques, the yield represents the responses of many cells. If there is damage to the cells in the vicinity of the recording electrode or electrodes, the recorded activity may be dominated or contaminated with potentials conducted from other regions of the cochlea. The SP also may have a small component that arises from the dendrites of the primary auditory neurons, reflecting generator potentials (Dallos, 1981). Additionally, at a given site of recording, the activity "seen" by the electrodes will depend on the location of the site relative to the pattern of the traveling wave created by the stimulus. In general, the genesis of these grossly recorded potentials is somewhat complex, yet they do provide useful indexes of the hydromechanical events of the cochlea and the integrity of the hair cells.

The other component of the electrocochleogram is the whole-nerve action potential (AP). This is the compound action potential of the acoustic nerve in response to the onset, and to a lesser degree cessation, of a sound stimulus (Fig. 7–18). Of course, primary auditory neurons discharge repeatedly in the presence of sound, but it is at the onset of sound that they respond most vigorously (see Fig. 7–14) and at which the discharges from different neurons are synchronized best. (Note: The magnitude of compound action potentials is proportional to the number of neurons activated

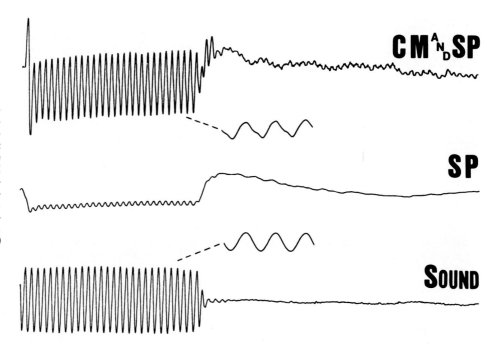

Figure 7–17. Tracings from recordings of the cochlear microphonic (CM) and summating potential (SP) along with the output of the monitoring microphone (Sound). Insets show details of CM and sound tracings via an expanded time base. (With permission from Durrant, J. D. 1981. Auditory physiology and an auditory physiologist's view of tinnitus. J. Laryngol. Otol. Suppl. 4:21–28.)

[Katz, 1966].) The AP, then, provides an indication that not only have the hair cells been stimulated, but also the activity of the hair cells has led successfully to the excitation of the auditory neurons. By its nature, the AP does not provide highly specific information about the response of the system; it is clearly dominated by transient events. Because of the importance of synchronization, the AP tends to be dominated by more basalward fiber populations (Kiang, 1975). This is where the traveling wave velocity is high; thus traveling wave propagation delays, and therefore phase dispersions, are minimal. However, through the use of tone bursts and masking tricks to limit the effective spectrum of the stimulus, it also is possible to obtain some frequency-specific information from the AP (Dallos and Cheatham, 1976). Like the cochlear potentials, the AP also can be recorded from inside or outside the cochlea, even from sites as remote as the ear lobe or the mastoid process.

Recording the AP and other components of the electrocochleogram at extracochlear sites that are accessible clinically requires appropriate recording meth-

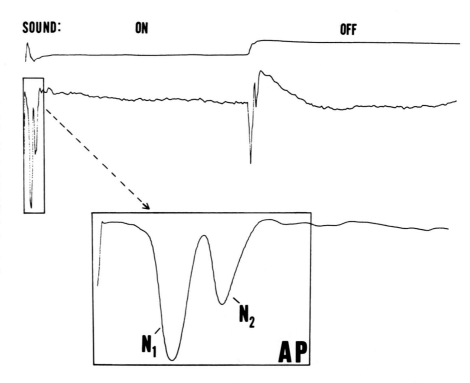

Figure 7–18. Recording of the whole-nerve action potential (AP). Inset, Time base expanded to illustrate major component waves of the AP (N_1 and N_2). The top tracing is actually the SP−, used here to indicate exactly when the stimulus has been turned on and off at the level of the hair cell transducer (thus eliminating inherent time delays due to propagation of sound down the ear canal and of the traveling wave in the cochlea). (With permission from Durrant, J. D. 1981. Auditory physiology and an auditory physiologist's view of tinnitus. J. Laryngol. Otol. Suppl. 4:21–28.)

ods and signal processing using computer-based signal averaging. For greatest sensitivity the transtympanic method (Aran et al., 1972) is superior. A needle electrode is pushed through the eardrum with its tip resting on the promontory. Of course, this method requires local or, in children and some others, general anesthesia. On the other hand, with an acceptable loss of sensitivity for most purposes, it is possible to obtain usable electrocochleograms from the surface of the tympanic membrane (Cullen et al., 1972) or the surface of the skin of the external auditory meatus (Coates, 1974; Ferraro et al., 1986). The farther away from the eardrum, naturally, the poorer is the sensitivity of the recording. Nevertheless, the AP is still reasonably prominent (at least in normal-hearing subjects or those with only mild hearing losses) in surface recordings from the ear lobe or mastoid and represents the initial segment of the so-called auditory brain stem response (see below). Even the CM can be detected at such remote sites, although extreme precautions are necessary to eliminate stimulus artifact (Sohmer and Pratt, 1976). Which of the various methods is the method of choice depends on the purpose for the recording (i.e., what information is being sought) and cost-benefit considerations (i.e., the need to know) versus potential risks involved should sedation or anesthesia be required.

Brain Stem and Cortical Evoked Potentials

The excitation of the whole-nerve AP by an abrupt sound stimulus actually initiates a series of electric waves reflecting a relatively long-lasting response of the nervous system (Picton et al, 1974). Within the first few milliseconds or so after stimulus onset, the action potentials of the primary auditory neurons are triggered and propagate through the nerve trunk to the cochlear nuclei. Because the nerve trunk is insulated well (electrically) within the internal auditory meatus, the electric manifestations of this initial bioelectric activity, as seen from surface electrodes, are two waves—one essentially from the distal end and the other from the proximal end of the nerve (Møller and Janetta, 1982). Then the second and higher order neurons are excited. Subsequent events are less clearly defined and more controversial as to which specific structures are most responsible for which "bumps" in the waveform of the potential, but at least three, perhaps four or five, are presumed to arise sequentially from generators in the brain stem auditory pathways (Buchwald and Huang, 1975; Møller et al., 1981). Therefore, whereas the time difference between the occurrence of the first and third waves reflects peripheral propagation of action potentials, the interval, for example, between the third and fifth waves appears to reflect transmission primarily through the pontine level pathways.

The components of the electrocochleogram and the previously mentioned brain stem potentials constitute the class of auditory evoked potentials known as short-latency potentials, or the fast components. As discussed in Chapter 9, the whole-nerve AP and brain stem potentials collectively constitute the so-called auditory brain stem response (ABR), which occurs approximately within the first 10 msec of stimulus onset (depending on the intensity and the spectrum of the stimulus and maturational and other factors). As more time is permitted between stimuli, still other potentials emerge. The time window of approximately 10 to 50 msec contains the so-called middle latency response (MLR) (Fig. 7–19). The components of the MLR arise from higher auditory brain stem centers, primary auditory cortex, or both (Picton et al., 1974). Last, there are the long-latency potentials that are cortical potentials (Reneau and Hnatiow, 1975). The P_1-N_2 components demark what has traditionally been called the auditory evoked potential (AEP), but the long-latency responses include still other components, such as the P_{300}, contingent negative variation, and sustained potentials. The long-latency potentials presumably reflect activity of much more than the primary auditory cortex and appear to reflect integrative and cognitive processing (Polich and Starr, 1983). All these potentials can be recorded from common electrodes placed on the surface of the scalp (e.g., one electrode on the mastoid and the other at the vertex). However, the analysis filter and time windows are varied to emphasize one class of potentials over the other, and the shortest-latency potentials are the smallest and require the most stimulus repetitions to acquire enough signal averaging to extract them from the overwhelming background noise. Thus, specific sets of recording variables are generally adopted for the desired class of potentials, and the same stimulus paradigm will not be optimal necessarily for all classes of potentials. Here, too, the potentials recorded and the techniques used are matters of what information is desired and the need to know. Additionally, because the long-latency potentials are quite sensitive to the level of arousal, and even the state of attention (Schwent et al., 1976), the clinical application of these potentials tends to be more restricted than that of the short-latency potentials, which in turn are relatively unaffected by the level of arousal (from comatose to awake and alert) or by most sedatives or anesthetics.

Clinical Utility

The long-latency, or cortical, AEPs have been known for over three decades and have commanded attention from otologists, neurologists, audiologists, psychologists, and psychiatrists. The breadth of clinical investigations and applications reflects this wide range, but by far the greatest interest in evoked potentials for otologic, neurotologic, and audiologic clinical applications has been displayed for the ABR. Within a decade of the first description of the ABR in the literature, ABR evaluations became a routine offering of audiology clinics, otology and neurology practices,

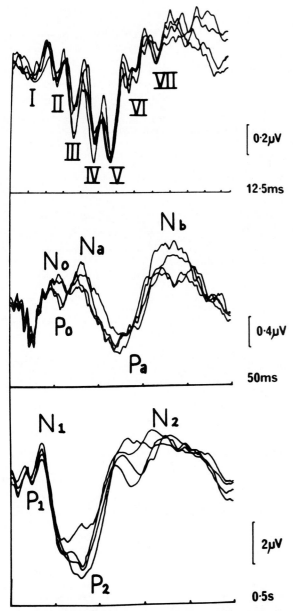

Figure 7–19. Components of the auditory evoked response recorded with scalp electrodes from a human subject and elicited by an acoustic click (presented 60 dB above the subject's behaviorally determined threshold). Tracings obtained in four different trials are overlaid to demonstrate repeatability of the responses; each tracing is the result of about 1000 repetitions of the click. Top, Fast or brain stem components. Middle, Middle latency components. Bottom, Late or cortical components. Major wavelets are labeled according to convention. Note: Vertex positive voltages are plotted in the downward direction, for consistency between tracings here and in Figure 7–18; this is the opposite of the most popular convention but is merely a matter of how the electrodes are connected to the recording amplifier. (Adapted with permission from Picton, T. W., et al. 1974. Human auditory evoked potentials. I: Evaluation of components. Electroencephalogr. Clin. Neurophysiol. 36:179–190.)

and electroencephalography laboratories. These evaluations have proved valuable in several areas:

1. Determination of the intergrity of the auditory nerve and brain stem to detect and distinguish between cochlear and retrocochlear lesions (i.e., so-called site-of-lesion testing).

2. Screening for possible hearing defects in newborns and other difficult-to-test patients.

3. Estimation of hearing thresholds in uncooperative patients.

4. Surgical monitoring and screening of brain stem function in comatose patients (e.g., as a component of evaluations of brain death).

However, it is important to note that, although the ABR is a sensitive indicator of auditory nerve and brain stem pathologic change (Starr and Achor, 1975; Selters and Brackmann, 1977; Glattke, 1983) and although it can be used to estimate hearing sensitivity (McGee and Clemis, 1980), as discussed in Chapter 9, ABR evaluations are not tests of hearing per se and are not equivalent to audiometry. The stimuli used are brief transients, such as clicks and tone pips (typically 3-msec duration or less) unlike the relatively long-duration tone bursts used in audiometry. More important, a normal ABR does not guarantee hearing, and not all normal-hearing subjects have normal ABRs. The ABR certainly reflects some aspects of auditory processing but is not necessarily dependent on the same neural events that are essential for perception and the auditory capabilities discussed earlier. Indeed, as a compound neural potential, it merely reflects the most robust, and at the same time the most redundant, feature of auditory neuronal response—stimulus onset.

During the early development of the ABR evaluation as a clinical tool, clinical electrocochleography also was developing and vying for acceptance as a routine test procedure. Although interest in electrocochleography has faded in the United States, there remains some interest in noninvasive electrocochleographic methods for supplementing the ABR evaluation. First, it can be useful for improving the identification of the auditory nerve component (i.e., the first wave of the ABR) (Durrant, 1986). Second, the SP is known to be especially sensitive to cochlear hydrops, or Ménière disease (Coats, 1981). On the far side of the ABR time interval, the middle-latency responses also have generated interest and may be used singly or in conjunction with ABR evaluations. These potentials may provide the basis for a more comprehensive analysis of auditory function for two reasons. First, at least some components of the MLR appear to arise from the primary auditory cortex. Second, MLRs exhibit reasonably good responsivity to low-frequency stimuli (Mendel and Wolf, 1983), in contrast to the ABRs elicited by low-frequency stimuli, which are much less robust.

In summary, it is now technically feasible to record electric potentials from essentially any level of the auditory system, using noninvasive techniques. When appropriately applied and integrated with other diagnostic tests, evoked potential evaluations can be of great clinical value.

Acknowledgment: The author wishes to express his appreciation to his friend and associate, Professor Jean H. Lovrinic, Temple University, for her helpful comments and criticisms.

SELECTED REFERENCES

Durrant, J. D., and Lovrinic, J. H. 1984. Bases of Hearing Science, 2nd ed. Baltimore, Williams & Wilkins Co.
> *Comprehensive introductory text providing not only depth of coverage of physiologic acoustics and psychoacoustics but also underlying fundamentals from physics and acoustics.*

Haggard, M. P., and Evans, E. F. (eds.). 1987. Hearing. Br. Med. Bull. 43:775.
> *Collection of brief but detailed and up-to-date reviews of topics in hearing, nearly half of which deal with physiologic acoustics.*

Møller, A. R. 1983. Auditory Physiology. New York, Academic Press.
> *In-depth treatise on the physiology of hearing.*

REFERENCES

Abeles, M., and Goldstein, M. H., Jr. 1970. Functional architecture in cat primary auditory cortex: Columnar organization and organization according to depth. J. Neurophysiol. 33:172.

Aran, J. M., Portmann, M., Portmann, C., et al. 1972. Electrocochleography in adults and children. Electrophysiological study of the peripheral receptor. Audiology 11:77.

Benson, D. A., Hienz, R. D., and Goldstein, M. H. 1981. Single-unit activity in the auditory cortex of monkeys actively localizing sound sources: Spatial tuning and behavioral dependency. Brain Res. 219:249.

Borg, E., and Zakrisson, J. E. 1975. The activity of the stapedius muscle in man during vocalization. Acta Otolaryngol. 79:325.

Brownell, W. E., Bader, C. R., Bertrand, D., et al. 1985. Evoked mechanical responses of isolated cochlear outer hair cells. Science 227:194.

Brugge, J. F., and Geisler, C. D. 1978. Auditory mechanisms of the lower brainstem. Annu. Rev. Neurosci. 1:363.

Brugge, J. F., Anderson, D. J., Hind, J. E., et al. 1969. Time structure of discharges in single auditory nerve fibers of the squirrel monkey in response to complex periodic sounds. J. Neurophysiol. 32:386.

Buchwald, J. S., and Huang, C. M. Far-field acoustic response: Origins in the cat. Science 189:382.

Butler, R. A., and Helwig, C. C. 1983. The spatial attributes of stimulus frequency in the median sagittal plane and their role in sound localization. Am. J. Otolaryngol. 4:165.

Canford, J. L. 1979. Auditory cortex lesions and interaural intensity and phase-angle discrimination in cats. J. Neurophysiol. 42:1518.

Casseday, J. H., and Neff, W. D. 1975. Auditory localization: Role of auditory pathways in brain stem of the cat. J. Neurophysiol. 38:842.

Cherry, C. 1959. Two ears—but one world. In Rosenblith, W. A. (ed.): Sensory Communication. Cambridge, MA, MIT Press, pp. 99–117.

Coats, A. C. 1974. On electrocochleographic electrode design. J. Acoust. Soc. Am. 56:708.

Coats, A. C. 1981. The summating potential and Meniere's disease. Arch. Otolaryngol. 107:199.

Corso, J. F. 1965. Cited in Corso, J. F. 1967. The Experimental Psychology of Sensory Behavior. New York, Holt, Reinhart and Winston, p. 280.

Corso, J. F., and Levine, M. 1965. Pitch discrimination at high frequencies by air- and bone-conduction. Am. J. Psychol. 78:557.

Cullen, J. K., Jr., Ellis, M. S., Berlin, C. I., et al. 1972. Human acoustic nerve action potential recordings from the tympanic membrane without anesthesia. Acta Otolaryngol. 74:15.

Dallos, P. 1970. Low-frequency auditory characteristics: Species dependence. J. Acoust. Soc. Am. 48:489.

Dallos, P. 1973. The Auditory Periphery: Biophysics and Physiology. New York, Academic Press.

Dallos, P. 1981. Cochlear physiology. Annu. Rev. Psychol. 32:153.

Dallos, P., and Cheatham, M. A. 1976. Compound action potential (AP) tuning curves. J. Acoust. Soc. Am. 59:591.

Dallos, P., Billone, M. C., Durrant, J. D., et al. 1972. Cochlear inner and outer hair cells: Functional differences. Science 177:356.

Davis, H. 1965. A model for transducer action in the cochlea. Cold Spring Harbor Symp. Quant. Biol. 30:181.

Davis, H., and Walsh, T. E. 1950. The limits of improvement of hearing following the fenestration operation. Laryngoscope 60:273.

Durrant, J. D. 1979. Comments on the effects of overstimulation on microphonic sensitivity. J. Acoust. Soc. Am. 66:597.

Durrant, J. D. 1981. Auditory physiology and an auditory physiologist's view of tinnitus. J. Laryngol. Otol. (Suppl.) 4:21.

Durrant, J. D. 1986. Combined EcochG-ABR versus conventional ABR recordings. Semin. Hearing 7:289.

Durrant, J. D., and Lovrinic, J. H. 1984. Bases of Hearing Science, 2nd ed. Baltimore, Williams & Wilkins Co.

Duvall, A. J., Flock, A., and Wersall, J. 1966. The ultrastructure of the sensory hairs and associated organelles of the cochlear inner hair cell with reference to directional sensitivity. J. Cell Biol. 29:497.

Erulkar, S. D. 1972. Comparative aspects of spatial localization of sound. Physiol. Rev. 52:238.

Evans, E. F., and Palmer, A. R. 1980. Relationship between the dynamic range of cochlear nerve fibers and their spontaneous activity. Exp. Brain Res. 40:115.

Ferraro, J. A., Murphy, G. B., and Ruth, R. A. 1986. A comparative study of primary electrodes used in extratympanic electrocochleography. Semin. Hearing 7:279.

Flock, Å. 1965. Transducing mechanisms in the lateral line canal organ receptors. Cold Spring Harbor Symp. Quant. Biol. 30:133.

Flock, Å., and Cheung, H. C. 1977. Actin filaments in sensory hairs of inner ear receptor cells. J. Cell Biol. 75:339.

Flock, Å., Jorgensen, M., and Russell, I. 1973. The physiology of individual hair cells and their synapses. In Møller, A. R. (ed.): Basic Mechanisms in Hearing. New York, Academic Press, pp. 273–302.

Galaburda, A., and Sanides, F. 1980. Cytoarchitectonic organization of the human auditory cortex. J. Comp. Neurol. 190:597.

Galambos, R. 1958. Neural mechanisms in audition. Laryngoscope 68:388.

Glattke, T. J. 1983. Short-Latency Auditory Evoked Potentials. Baltimore, University Park Press.

Green, D. M. 1976. An Introduction to Hearing. Hillsdale, NJ, Lawrence Erlbaum Associates.

Harrison, J. M., and Howe, M. E. 1974a. Anatomy of the descending auditory system (mammalian). In Keidel, W. D., and Neff, W. D. (eds.): Handbook of Sensory Physiology, Vol. V/1, Anatomy, Physiology (Ear). Berlin, Springer-Verlag, pp. 363–388.

Harrison, J. M., and Howe, M. E. 1974b. Anatomy of the afferent auditory nervous system of mammals. In Keidel, W. D., and Neff, W. D. (eds.): Handbook of Sensory Physiology, Vol. V/1, Anatomy, Physiology (Ear). Berlin, Springer-Verlag, pp. 183–336.

Heffner, H. 1978. Effect of auditory cortex ablation on localization and discrimination of brief sounds. J. Neurophysiol. 41:963.

Holmes, M. H. 1980. An analysis of a low-frequency model of the cochlea. J. Acoust. Soc. Am. 68:482.

Honrubia, V., and Ward, P. H. 1969. Dependence of the cochlear microphonics and the summating potential on the endocochlear potential. J. Acoust. Soc. Am. 46:388.

Hudspeth, A. J. 1985. The cellular basis of hearing: The biophysics of hair cells. Science 230:745.

Hunter-Duvar, I. M. 1978. Electron microscopic assessment of the cochlea. Acta Otolaryngol. (Suppl.) 351:2.

Imig, T. J., Reale, R. A., and Brugge, J. F. 1982. The auditory cortex: Patterns of corticocortical projections related to physiological maps in the cat. In Woolsey, C. N. (ed.): Cortical Sensory Organization, Vol. 3—Multiple Auditory Areas. Clifton, NJ, Humana Press, pp. 1–41.

Irving, R., and Harrison, J. M. 1967. The superior olivary complex and audition: A comparative study. J. Comp. Neurol. 130:77.

Jesteadt, W., Wier, C. C., and Green, D. M. 1977. Intensity discrimination as a function of frequency and sensation level. J. Acoust. Soc. Am. 61:169.

Katz, B. 1966. Nerve, Muscle, and Synapse. New York, McGraw-Hill Book Co.

Keidel, W. D. 1974. Information processing in higher parts of the auditory pathway. In Zwicker, E., and Terhardt, E. (eds.): Facts and Models in Hearing. New York, Springer-Verlag, pp. 216–226.

Keidel, W. D. 1980. Neurophysiological requirements for implanted cochlear prostheses. Audiology 19:105.

Kelly, J. P., and Wong, D. 1981. Laminar connections of the cat's auditory cortex. Brain Res. 212:1.

Khanna, S. M., and Leonard, D. G. B. 1982. Basilar membrane tuning in the cat cochlea. Science 215:305.

Kiang, N. Y.-S. 1965. Discharge Patterns of Single Fibers in the Cat's Auditory Nerve. Cambridge, MA, MIT Press.

Kiang, N. Y.-S. 1968. A survey of recent developments in the study of auditory physiology. Ann. Otol. 77:656.

Kiang, N. Y.-S. 1975. Stimulus representation in the discharge patterns of auditory neurons. In Eagles, E. L. (ed.): The Nervous System, Vol. 3: Human Communication and Its Disorders. New York, Raven Press, pp. 81–96.

Kiang, N. Y.-S., and Moxon, E. C. 1974. Tails of tuning curves of auditory-nerve fibers. J. Acoust. Soc. Am. 55:620.

Killion, M. C., and Dallos, P. 1979. Impedance matching by the combined effects of the outer and middle ear. J. Acoust. Soc. Am. 66:599.

Kinsler, L. E., and Frey, A. R. 1962. Fundamentals of Acoustics. New York, John Wiley & Sons.

Klinke, R., and Galley, N. 1974. Efferent innervation of vestibular and auditory receptors. Physiol. Rev. 54:316.

Knudsen, E. I., and Konishi, M. 1978. A neural map of auditory space in the owl. Science 200:795.

Licklider, J. C. R. 1951. Basic correlates of the auditory stimulus. In Stevens, S. S. (ed.): Handbook of Experimental Psychology. New York, John Wiley & Sons, pp. 985–1039.

Lim, D. J. 1986. Cochlear micromechanics in understanding otoacoustic emission. Scand. Audiol. (Suppl.) 25:17.

Massopust, L. C., Wolin, L., and Frost, V. 1971. Frequency discrimination thresholds following auditory cortex ablations in the monkey. J. Aud. Res. 11:227.

Masterson, R. B., Glendenning, K. K., and Nudo, R. J. 1982. Anatomical pathways subserving the contralateral representation of a sound source. In Gatehouse, R. W. (ed.): Localization of Sound: Theory and Applications. Groton, CT, Amphora Press, pp. 113–125.

McFadden, D. 1968. Masking-level differences determined with and without interaural disparities in masker intensity. J. Acoust. Soc. Am. 44:212.

McGee, T. J., and Clemis, J. B. 1980. The approximation of audiometric thresholds by auditory brain stem responses. Otolaryngol. Head Neck Surg. 88:295.

Mendel, M. I., and Wolf, K. E. 1983. Clinical applications of the middle latency responses. Audiology 8:141.

Merzenich, M. M., Knight, P. L., and Roth, G. L. 1975. Representation of cochlea within primary auditory cortex in the cat. J. Neurophysiol. 38:231.

Miller, J. D., Watson, C. S., and Covell, W. P. 1963. Deafening effects of noise on the cat. Acta Otolaryngol. (Suppl.) 176:1.

Mills, A. W. 1972. Auditory localization. In Tobias, J. V. (eds.): Foundations of Modern Auditory Theory, Vol. 1. New York, Academic Press, pp. 303–348.

Møller, A. R. 1965. An experimental study of the acoustic impedance of the middle ear and its transmission properties. Acta Otolaryngol. 60:129.

Møller, A. R. 1972. The middle ear. In Tobias, J. J. (eds.): Foundations of Modern Auditory Theory, Vol. 2. New York, Academic Press, pp. 135–194.

Møller, A. R., and Jannetta, P. J. 1982. Comparison between intracranially recorded potentials from the human auditory nerve and scalp recorded auditory brainstem responses (ABR). Scand. Audiol. 11:33.

Møller, A. R., Jannetta, P. J., Bennett, M., and Møller, M. B. 1981. Intracranially recorded responses from the human auditory nerve: New insights into the origin of brainstem evoked potentials (BSEP). EEG Clin. Neurophysiol. 52:18.

Moushegian, G., Stillman, R. D., and Rupert, A. L. 1971. Characteristic delays in superior olive and inferior colliculus. In Sachs, M. B. (ed.): Physiology of the Auditory System: A Workshop. Baltimore, National Educational Consultants, Inc., pp. 245–254.

Nedzelnitsky, V. 1974. Measurement of sound pressure in the cochleae of anesthetized cats. In Zwicker, E., and Terhardt, E. (eds.): Facts and Models in Hearing. New York, Springer-Verlag, pp. 45–53.

Neff, W. D. 1959. Neural mechanisms of auditory discrimination. In Rosenblight, W. A. (ed.): Sensory Communications. Cambridge, MA, MIT Press, pp. 259–278.

Neff, W. D. 1968. Localization and lateralization of sound in space. In DeReuck, A. J. S., and Knight, J. (eds.): Hearing Mechanisms in Vertebrates. Boston, Little, Brown and Co., pp. 207–231.

Pfeiffer, R. R., and Kim, D. O. 1975. Cochlear nerve fiber responses: Distribution along the cochlear partition. J. Acoust. Soc. Am. 58:867.

Pfingst, B. E., and O'Connor, T. A. 1981. Characteristics of neurons in auditory cortex of monkeys performing a simple auditory task. J. Neurophysiol. 45:16.

Picton, T. W., Hillyard, S. A., Krausz, H. I., et al. 1974. Human auditory evoked potentials. I: Evaluation of components. EEG Clin. Neurophysiol. 36:179.

Plenge, G. 1974. On the differences between localization and lateralization. J. Acoust. Soc. Am. 56:944.

Plomp, R. 1971. Old and new data on tone perception. In Neff, W. D. (ed.): Contributions to Sensory Physiology, Vol. 5. New York, Academic Press, pp. 179–216.

Polich, J. M., and Starr, A. 1983. Middle-, late-, and long-latency auditory evoked potentials. In Moore, E. J. (ed.): Bases of Auditory Brain-Stem Evoked Responses. New York, Grune & Stratton, pp. 345–361.

Reneau, J. P., and Hnatiow, G. Z. 1975. Evoked Response Audiometry: A Topical and Historical Review. Baltimore, University Park Press.

Rhode, W. S. 1973. An investigation of post-mortem cochlear mechanics using the Mossbauer effect. In Møller, A. R. (ed.): Basic Mechanisms in Hearing. New York, Academic Press, pp. 39–63.

Rhode, W. S. 1986. Basilar membrane motion: Results of Mossbauer measurements. Scand. Audiol. (Suppl.) 25:7.

Robinson, D. W., and Dadson, R. S. 1956. A re-determination of the equal loudness relations for pure tones. Br. J. Appl. Phys. 7:166.

Romani, G. L., Williamson, S. J., and Kauffman, L. 1982. Tonotopic organization of the human auditory cortex. Science 216:1339.

Rose, J. E., Brugge, J. F., Anderson, D. J., et al. 1967. Phase-locked response to low-frequency tones in single auditory nerve fibers of the squirrel monkey. J. Neurophysiol. 30:769.

Rose, J. E., Gross, N. B., Geisler, C. D., et al. 1966. Some neural mechanisms in the inferior colliculus of the cat which may be relevant to localization of a sound source. J. Neurophysiol. 29:288.

Russell, I. J., and Sellick, P. M. 1977. Tuning properties of cochlear hair cells. Nature 267:858.

Ryan, A., and Dallos, P. 1984. Physiology of the cochlea. In Northern, J. L. (ed.): Hearing Disorders, 2nd ed. Boston, Little, Brown and Co., pp. 253–266.

Sachs, M. B., and Abbas, P. J. 1974. Rate versus level functions for auditory-nerve fibers in cats: Tone-burst stimuli. J. Acoust. Soc. Am. 56:1835.

Sachs, M. B., and Young, E. D. 1979. Encoding of steady-state vowels in the auditory nerve: Representation in terms of discharge rate. J. Acoust. Soc. Am. 66:470.

Scharf, B. 1970. Critical bands. In Tobias, J. V. (ed.): Foundations of Modern Auditory Theory, Vol. 1. New York, Academic Press, pp. 159–202.

Schwent, V. L., Hillyard, S. A., and Galambos, R. 1976. Selective attention and the auditory vertex potential. I. Effects of stimulus delivery rate. EEG Clin. Neurophysiol. 40:604.

Searle, C. L., Braida, L. D., Cuddy, D. R., et al. 1975. Binaural pinna disparity: Another auditory localization cue. J. Acoust. Soc. Am. 57:448.

Selters, W. A., and Brackmann, D. E. 1977. Acoustic tumor detection with brain stem electric response audiometry. Arch. Otolaryngol. 103:181.

Shaw, E. A. G. 1974. The external ear. In Keidel, W. D., and Neff, W. D. (eds.): Handbook of Sensory Physiology, Vol. V/1, Anatomy, Physiology (Ear). Berlin, Springer-Verlag, pp. 455–490.

Simmons, F. B. 1964. Perceptual theories of middle ear muscle function. Ann. Otol. Rhinol. Laryngol. 73:724.

Sohmer, H., and Pratt, H. 1976. Recording of the cochlear microphonic potential with surface electrodes. EEG Clin. Neurophysiol. 40:253.

Solomon, G., and Starr, A. 1963. Electromyography of middle ear muscles in man during motor activities. Acta Neurol. Scand. 39:161.

Starr, A., and Achor, L. J. 1975. Auditory brain stem responses in neurological disease. Arch. Neurol. 32:761.

Suga, N. 1971. Feature detection in the cochlear nucleus, inferior colliculus, and auditory cortex. *In* Sachs, M. B. (ed.): Physiology of the Auditory System: A Workshop. Baltimore, National Educational Consultants, Inc., pp. 197–206.

Sutter, A. H. 1986. Hearing conservation. *In* Berger, E. H., Ward, W. D., Morrill, S. C., and Royster, L. H. (eds.): Noise and Hearing Conservation Manual. Akron, OH, American Industrial Hygiene Association, pp. 1–18.

Tasaki, I., and Spyropoulos, C. S. 1959. Stria vascularis as a source of endocochlear potential. J. Neurophysiol. 22:149.

Tilney, L. G., Derosier, D. J., and Mulroy, M. J. 1980. The organization of actin filaments in the stereocilia of cochlear hair cells. J. Cell Biol. 86:244.

Tonndorf, J. 1975. Davis—1961 revisited: Signal transmission in the cochlear hair cell–nerve junction. Arch. Otolaryngol. 101:528.

Tonndorf, J. 1976. Relationship between the transmission characteristics of the conductive system and noise-induced hearing loss. *In* Henderson, D., Hamernik, R. P., Dosanjh, D. S., et al. (eds.): Effects of Noise on Hearing. New York, Raven Press, pp. 159–177.

Tonndorf, J., and Khanna, S. M. 1970. The role of the tympanic membrane in middle ear transmission. Ann. Otolaryngol. 79:743.

Viemeister, N. F. 1983. Auditory intensity discrimination at high frequencies in the presence of noise. Science 221:1206.

von Békèsy, G. 1960. Experiments in Hearing (translated and edited by E. G. Wever). New York, McGraw-Hill Book Co.

Walzl, E. M. 1947. Representation of the cochlea in the cerebral cortex. Laryngoscope 57:778.

Wegel, R. L. 1932. Physical data and physiology of excitation of the auditory nerve. Ann. Otol. Rhinol. Laryngol. 41:740.

Wever, E. G. 1929. Beats and related phenomena resulting from the simultaneous sounding of two tones. Phychol. Rev. 36:402.

Wever, E. G. 1949. Theory of Hearing. New York, Dover Publications, Inc.

Wever, E. G., and Bray, C. M. 1937. The perception of low tones and the resonance volley theory. J. Psychol. 3:101.

Wever, E. G., and Lawrence, M. 1954. Physiological Acoustics. Princeton, Princeton University Press.

Whitfield, I. C. 1967*a*. Coding in the auditory nervous system. Nature 213:756.

Whitfield, I. C. 1967*b*. The Auditory Pathway. Baltimore, Williams & Wilkins Co.

Wiener, F. M., and Ross, D. A. 1946. The pressure distribution in the auditory canal in a progressive sound field. J. Acoust. Soc. Am. 18:401.

Wier, C. C., Jesteadt, W., and Green, D. M. 1977. Frequency discrimination as a function of frequency and sensation level. J. Acoust. Soc. Am. 61:178.

Woolsey, C. N. 1971. Tonotopic organization of the auditory cortex. *In* Sachs, M. B. (ed.): Physiology of the Auditory System: A Workshop. Baltimore, National Educational Consultants, Inc., pp. 271–282.

Yeowart, N. S., and Evans, M. J. 1974. Thresholds of audibility for very low-frequency pure tones. J. Acoust. Soc. Am. 55:814.

Young, E. D., and Sachs, M. B. 1979. Representation of steady-state vowels in the temporal aspects of the discharge patterns of populations of auditory-nerve fibers. J. Acoust. Soc. Am. 66:1381.

Zwicker, E. 1974. On a psychoacoustical equivalent of tuning curves. *In* Zwicker, E., and Terhardt, E. (eds.): Facts and Models in Hearing. New York, Springer-Verlag, pp. 132–141.

Zwicker, E., Flottrop, G., and Stevens, S. S. 1957. Critical bandwidth in loudness summation. J. Acoust. Soc. Am. 29:548.

Zwislocki, J. 1965. Analysis of some auditory characteristics. *In* Luce, R., Bush, R., and Galanter, E. (eds.): Handbook of Mathematical Psychology, Vol. 3. New York, John Wiley & Sons, pp. 1–97.

Zwislocki, J. 1975. The role of the external and middle ear in sound transmission. *In* Eagles, E. L. (ed.): The Nervous System, Vol. 3: Human Communication and Its Disorders. New York, Raven Press, pp. 45–55.

Zwislocki, J. J., and Sokolich, W. G. 1973. Velocity and displacement in auditory-nerve fibers. Science 182:64.

Chapter 8

METHODS OF EXAMINATION: CLINICAL EXAMINATION

Charles D. Bluestone, M.D.   Jerome O. Klein, M.D.

Of the various methods currently used in the diagnosis of ear disease in children, the medical history and a physical examination that includes pneumatic otoscopy are usually sufficient to establish a clinical diagnosis when inflammation is present. Although less common than the inflammatory diseases, congenital, traumatic, and neoplastic problems are also of importance.

SIGNS AND SYMPTOMS

There are eight prominent signs and symptoms primarily associated with diseases of the ear and temporal bone. *Otalgia* is most commonly associated with inflammation of the external and middle ear but may also be of nonaural origin, as from the temporomandibular joint, the teeth, or the pharynx. In young infants, pulling at the ear or general irritability, especially when it is associated with fever, may be the only sign of ear pain (Chap. 12). Purulent *otorrhea* is a sign of otitis externa, otitis media with perforation of the tympanic membrane, or both. Bloody discharge may be associated with acute or chronic inflammation, trauma, or neoplasm. A clear drainage may be indicative of a perforation of the drum with a serous middle ear effusion or cerebrospinal fluid otorrhea draining through a defect in the external auditory canal or through the tympanic membrane from the middle ear (Chap. 13). *Hearing loss* is a symptom that may be the result of disease of either the external or the middle ear (conductive hearing loss) or the result of a pathologic condition in the inner ear, retrocochlea, or the central auditory pathways (sensorineural hearing loss) (Chap. 14). *Swelling* about the ear is most commonly the result of inflammation (e.g., external otitis, perichondritis, or mastoiditis), trauma (e.g., hematoma), or, on rare occasions, neoplasm. *Vertigo* is not a common complaint in children but is present more often than was formerly thought. The most common cause is eustachian tube–middle ear–mastoid disease, but vertigo may be due also to labyrinthitis; perilymphatic fistula between the inner and middle ear resulting from a congenital defect, trauma, or choleste-

atoma; vestibular neuronitis; benign paroxysmal positional vertigo; Ménière disease; or disease of the central nervous system. Older children may describe a feeling of spinning or turning, whereas younger children may not be able to verbalize concerning the symptom but manifest the dysequilibrium by falling, stumbling, or "clumsiness." Unidirectional horizontal jerk *nystagmus*, usually associated with vertigo, is vestibular in origin (Chap. 15). *Tinnitus* is another symptom that children infrequently describe but that is commonly present, especially in patients with eustachian tube–middle ear disease or conductive or sensorineural hearing loss (Chap. 16). *Facial paralysis* is an infrequent but frightening condition both for the child and for his or her parents. When it is due to disease within the temporal bone in children, it most commonly occurs as a complication of acute or chronic otitis media; however, facial paralysis also may be idiopathic (Bell palsy) or the result of temporal bone fracture or neoplasm, or, on rare occasions, oticus due to *Herpes zoster* (Chap. 17). Other signs and symptoms of conditions that may be associated with ear disease may also be present, such as symptoms of upper respiratory allergy associated with otitis media (Chap. 21).

PHYSICAL EXAMINATION

Aside from the history, the most useful method for diagnosing ear disease is a physical examination that includes pneumatic otoscopy. Adequate examination of the entire child, with special attention to the head and neck, can lead to the identification of a condition that may predispose to or be associated with ear disease. The appearance of the child's face and the character of his or her speech may be important clues to the possibility of an abnormal middle ear. Many of the craniofacial anomalies, such as mandibulofacial dysostosis (Treacher Collins syndrome) and trisomy 21 (Down syndrome), are associated with an increased incidence of ear disease (Chap. 4). Mouth breathing and hyponasality may indicate intranasal or postnasal obstruction, while hypernasality is a sign of velopha-

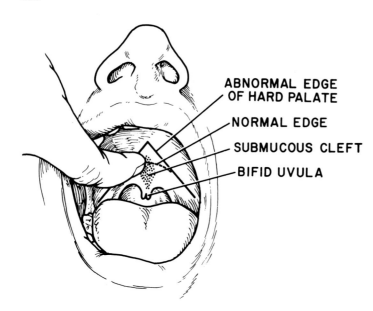

ABNORMAL EDGE
OF HARD PALATE

NORMAL EDGE

SUBMUCOUS CLEFT

BIFID UVULA

Figure 8–1. Bifid uvula, widening and attenuation of the median raphe of the soft palate, and V-shaped midline notch, rather than a smooth curve, are diagnostic of a submucous cleft palate.

ryngeal incompetence. Examination of the oropharyngeal cavity may uncover an overt cleft palate or a submucous cleft (Fig. 8–1), both of which predispose the infant to otitis media with effusion (Stool and Randall, 1967; Paradise et al., 1969). Although a bifid uvula has been associated with an increased incidence of middle ear disease (Taylor, 1972), more recent studies fail to corroborate this finding (Schwartz et al., 1985; Fischler et al., 1987). An examination of the child's head and neck may also reveal posterior nasal or pharyngeal inflammation and discharge. Other pathologic conditions of the nose, such as polyposis, severe deviation of the nasal septum, or a nasopharyngeal tumor, may also be associated with otitis media (Chaps. 4, 21, 31, 95).

Examination of the ear itself is the most critical part of the clinician's assessment of the patient, but it must be performed systematically. The auricle, periauricular area, and external auditory meatus should be examined first; all too frequently these areas are overlooked in the physician's haste to make a diagnosis by otoscopic examination, but the presence or absence of signs of infection in these areas may aid later in the differential diagnosis or evaluation of complications of ear disease. For instance, eczematoid external otitis may result from acute otitis media with discharge, or inflammation of the postauricular area may be indicative of a periosteitis or subperiosteal abscess that has extended from the mastoid air cells. Palpation of these areas will determine if tenderness is present; exquisite pain on palpation of the tragus would indicate the presence of acute diffuse external otitis (Chap. 20).

After the examination of the external ear and canal, the clinician may proceed to the most important part of the physical assessment, the otoscopic examination.

OTOSCOPIC EXAMINATION

Positioning the Patient for Examination

The position of the patient for otoscopy depends on the patient's age, his or her ability to cooperate, the

clinical setting, and the preference of the examiner. Otoscopic evaluation of an infant is best performed on an examining table. The presence of a parent or assistant is necessary to restrain the baby, as undue movement usually prevents an adequate evaluation (Fig. 8–2). Some clinicians prefer to place the infant prone on the table, whereas others prefer the patient to be supine. Use of the examining table is also desirable for older infants who are uncooperative or when a tympanocentesis or myringotomy is performed without general anesthesia. Figure 8–3 shows that infants and young children who are only apprehensive and not struggling actively can be evaluated adequately while sitting on the parent's lap. When necessary, the child may be restrained firmly on an adult's lap if the parent holds the child's wrists over the abdomen with one hand and holds the patient's head against the adult's chest with the other hand. If necessary, the child's legs can be held between the adult's thighs. Some infants can be examined by placing the child's head on the parent's knee (Fig. 8–4). Cooperative children sitting in a chair or on the edge of an examination table can usually be evaluated successfully. The examiner should hold the otoscope with the hand or finger placed firmly against the child's head or face, so that the otoscope will move with the head rather than cause trauma (pain) to the ear canal if the child moves suddenly (Fig. 8–5). Pulling up and out on the pinna will usually straighten the ear canal enough to allow exposure of the tympanic membrane. In the young infant, the tragus must be moved forward and out of the way.

Removal of Cerumen

Before adequate visualization of the external canal and tympanic membrane can be obtained, all obstructing cerumen must be removed from the canal. Many children with acute otitis media have moderate to large accumulations of cerumen in the ear canal. For optimal visualization of the tympanic membrane, mechanical

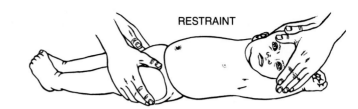

RESTRAINT

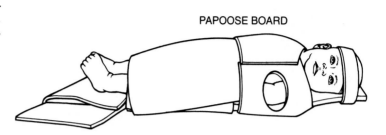

PAPOOSE BOARD

Figure 8–2. Methods of restraining an infant for examination and for procedures such as tympanocentesis or myringotomy. (From Bluestone, C. D., and Klein, J. O. 1988. Otitis Media in Infants and Children. Philadelphia, W. B. Saunders Co., p. 71.)

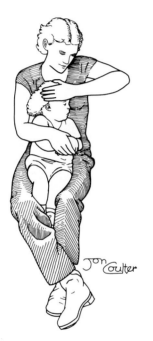

Figure 8–3. Method of restraining child for examination of the ear.

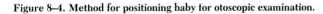

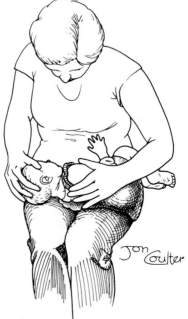

Figure 8–4. Method for positioning baby for otoscopic examination.

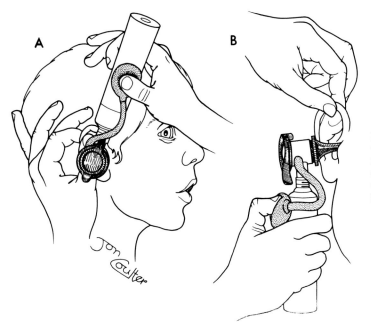

Figure 8–5. Methods of positioning otoscope to enhance visualization and to minimize the chance that head movement will result in trauma to the ear canal. Both of the otoscopist's hands can be used *(A)*, or, when the child is cooperative, a finger touching the child's cheek is sufficient *(B)*.

removal was necessary in approximately one third of 279 patients observed by Schwartz and colleagues (1983); necessity for cerumen removal was inversely proportional to age, with more than half of cerumen removal procedures performed in infants younger than 1 year of age. Removal of cerumen can usually be accomplished by use of an otoscope with a surgical head and a wire loop or a blunt cerumen curette (Fig. 8–6) or by irrigating the ear canal *gently* with warm water delivered through a dental irrigator (Water Pik) (Fig. 8–7).

Instillation of hydrogen peroxide (3 percent solution) in the ear canal for 2 to 3 minutes softens cerumen and may facilitate removal with subsequent irrigation.

Reported use of some commercial preparations (e.g., triethanolamine polypeptide oleate-condensate [Cerumenex]) may cause dermatitis of the external canal. These materials may be of value, if used infrequently and under the physician's supervision.

Otoscope

For proper assessment of the tympanic membrane and its mobility, a pneumatic otoscope in which the diagnostic head has an adequate seal should be used.

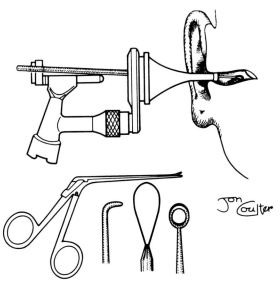

Figure 8–6. Method for removing cerumen from the external ear canal employing the surgical head attached to the otoscope and instruments that can be used.

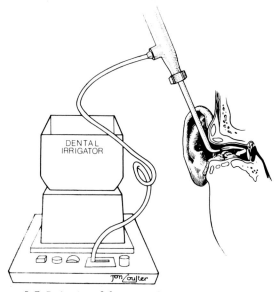

Figure 8–7. Irrigation of the external canal with a dental irrigator to remove cerumen.

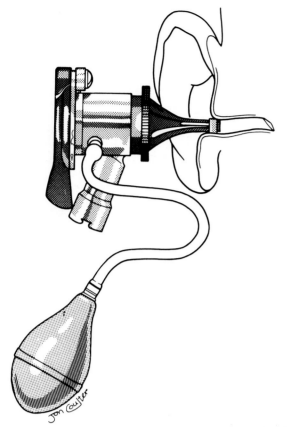

Figure 8–8. Pneumatic otoscope with rubber tip on the end of the ear speculum to give a better seal in the external auditory canal. (From Bluestone, C. D., and Klein, J. O. 1988. Otitis Media in Infants and Children. Philadelphia, W. B. Saunders Co., p. 73.)

The quality of the otoscopic examination is limited by deficiencies in the designs of commercially available otoscopes. The speculum employed should have the largest lumen that comfortably can fit in the child's cartilaginous external auditory meatus. If the speculum is too small, adequate visualization may be impaired and the speculum may touch the bony canal, which can be painful. In most models, an airtight seal is usually not possible because of a leak of air within the otoscope head or between the stiff ear speculum and the external auditory canal, although leaks at the latter location can be stopped by cutting a small section of rubber tubing and slipping it over the tip of the ear speculum (Fig. 8–8).

Many otolaryngologists prefer to use a Bruening or Siegle otoscope with the magnifying lens. Both of these instruments allow for excellent assessment of drum mobility because they have an almost airtight seal. A head mirror and lamp or a headlight (Fig. 8–9) is necessary to provide light for the examination.

Examination of Tympanic Membrane

Inspection of the tympanic membrane should include evaluation of its position, color, degree of translucency, and mobility. Assessment of the light reflex is of limited value because it does not indicate the

status of the middle ear in the evaluation of tympanic membrane–middle ear disorders.

POSITION OF THE TYMPANIC MEMBRANE. The positions of the tympanic membrane when the middle ear is aerated and when effusion is present are illustrated in Figure 8–10.

The *normal eardrum* should be in the neutral position, with the short process of the malleus visible but not prominent through the membrane.

Mild retraction of the tympanic membrane usually indicates the presence of negative middle ear pressure, an effusion, or both. The short process of the malleus and posterior mallear fold are prominent, and the manubrium of the malleus appears to be foreshortened.

Severe retraction of the tympanic membrane is characterized by a prominent posterior mallear fold and short process of the malleus and a severely foreshortened manubrium. The tympanic membrane may be severely retracted, presumably owing to high negative pressure in association with a middle ear effusion.

Fullness of the tympanic membrane is apparent initially in the posterosuperior portion of the pars tensa and pars flaccida, because these two areas are the most highly compliant parts of the tympanic membrane (Khanna and Tonndorf, 1972). The short process of the malleus is commonly obscured. The fullness is caused by increased air pressure, effusion, or both within the middle ear. When bulging of the entire tympanic membrane occurs, the malleus is usually obscured, which occurs when the middle ear–mastoid system is filled with an effusion.

APPEARANCE OF THE TYMPANIC MEMBRANE. The normal tympanic membrane has a ground-glass appearance; a blue or yellow color usually indicates a middle ear effusion seen through a translucent tympanic membrane. A red tympanic membrane alone may not be indicative of a pathologic condition, because the blood vessels of the drum head may be

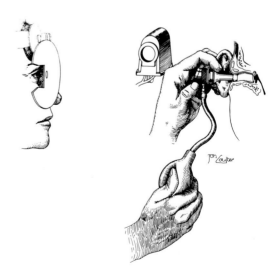

Figure 8–9. Observation of eardrum mobility with the Bruening otoscope with magnifying lens. The light source is from a lamp reflected off of a head mirror.

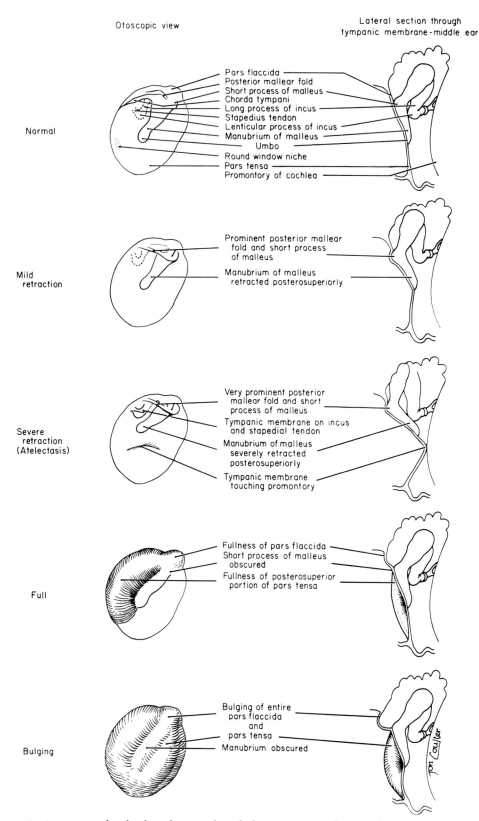

Figure 8–10. Otoscopic view compared with a lateral section through the tympanic membrane and middle ear to demonstrate the various positions of the drum with their respective anatomic landmarks (see text).

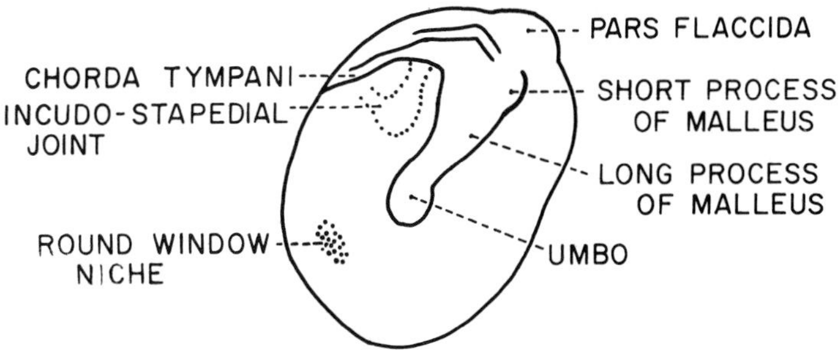

CHORDA TYMPANI --
INCUDO-STAPEDIAL
JOINT

PARS FLACCIDA

SHORT PROCESS
OF MALLEUS

LONG PROCESS
OF MALLEUS

ROUND WINDOW
NICHE

UMBO

Figure 8–11. Diagrammatic view of the tympanic membrane depicting important landmarks that usually can be visualized with the otoscope.

engorged as the result of the patient's crying, sneezing, or nose blowing. It is critical to distinguish between translucency and opacification of the eardrum to identify a middle ear effusion. The normal tympanic membrane should be translucent, and the observer should be able to look through the drum and visualize the middle ear landmarks (the incudostapedial joint promontory, the round window niche, and, frequently, the chorda tympani nerve) (Fig. 8–11). If a middle ear effusion is present medial to a translucent drum, an air-fluid level or bubbles of air admixed with the liquid may be visible (Fig. 8–12). An air-fluid level or bubbles can be differentiated from scarring of the tympanic membrane by altering the position of the head while observing the drum with the otoscope (if fluid is present, the air-fluid level will shift in relation to gravity) or by seeing movement of the fluid during pneumatic otoscopy. The line frequently seen when a severely retracted membrane touches the cochlear

promontory will disappear (the drum will pull away from the promontory) if sufficient negative pressure can be applied with the pneumatic otoscope. Inability to visualize the middle ear structures indicates opacification of the drum, which is usually the result of thickening of the tympanic membrane, the presence of an effusion, or both.

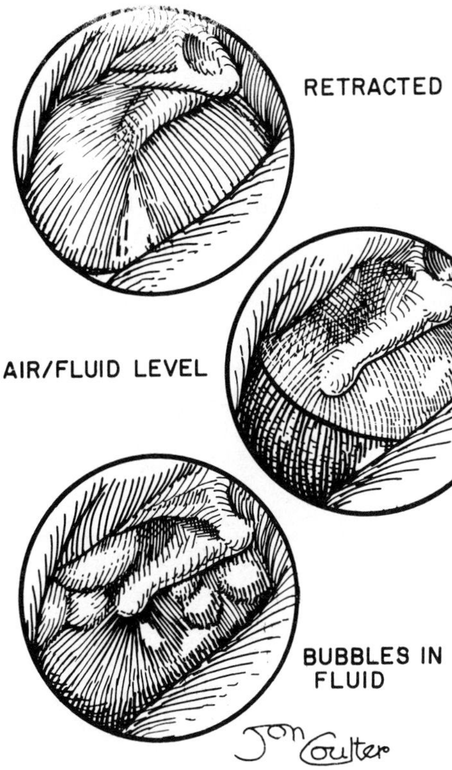

A bright light is necessary for accurate otoscopy. Barriga and colleagues (1986) surveyed otoscopes in physicians' offices and hospital clinics and found that many were inadequately maintained. A light output of 100 foot-candles or more was optimal for clinical otoscopy. Replacement of the bulb rather than replacement of the battery was more likely to restore adequate light to the units with poor performance (Barriga et al., 1986). Otoscope batteries should be replaced frequently so that the ability of the examiner to "look through" the tympanic membrane will not be impaired (Barriga et al., 1986). The electric otoscope is better than the battery type.

MOBILITY OF THE TYMPANIC MEMBRANE. Abnormalities of the tympanic membrane and the middle ear are reflected in the pattern of tympanic membrane mobility when first positive and then negative pressure is applied to the external auditory canal with the pneumatic otoscope (Bluestone and Shurin, 1974). As shown in Figure 8–13, this is achieved by first applying slight pressure on the rubber bulb (positive pressure) and then, after momentarily breaking the seal, releasing the bulb (negative pressure). The presence of effusion, high negative pressure, or both within the middle ear can markedly dampen the movements of the eardrum. When the middle ear pressure is ambient, the normal tympanic membrane moves inward with slight positive pressure in the ear canal and outward toward the examiner with slight negative pressure. The motion observed is proportionate to the applied pressure and is best visualized in the posterosuperior quadrant of the tympanic membrane (Fig. 8–14). If a two-layered membrane or atrophic scar (due to a healed perforation) is present, mobility of the tympanic membrane can also be assessed more readily by observing the movement of the flaccid area.

Figure 8–15, Frame 1, shows the normal tympanic membrane when the middle ear contains only air at ambient pressure. A hypermobile eardrum (Frame 2) is seen most frequently in children whose membranes are atrophic or flaccid. The mobility of the tympanic membrane is greater than normal (the drum is said to

RETRACTED

AIR/FLUID LEVEL

BUBBLES IN
FLUID

Figure 8–12. Three examples of otoscopic findings (right ear).

TO OBTAIN POSITIVE PRESSURE:

1. Insert speculum with
   no pressure on bulb

2. Depress bulb

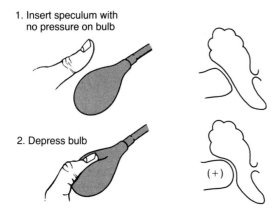

(+)

TO OBTAIN NEGATIVE PRESSURE:

1. Insert speculum with
   bulb depressed

2. Release
   bulb

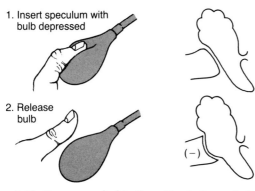

(−)

Figure 8–13. Pressure applied to the rubber bulb attached to the pneumatic otoscope will deflect the normal tympanic membrane inward with applied positive pressure and outward with applied negative pressure if the middle ear pressure is ambient. The movement of the eardrum is proportionate to the degree of pressure exerted on the bulb until the tympanic membrane has reached its limit of compliance. (From Bluestone, C. D., and Klein, J. O. 1988. Otitis Media in Infants and Children. Philadelphia, W. B. Saunders Co., p. 75.)

be highly compliant) if the drum moves when even slight positive or negative external canal pressure is applied; if the drum moves equally well to both applied positive and negative pressures, the middle ear pressure is approximately ambient. However, if the tympanic membrane is hypermobile to applied negative pressure but is immobile when positive pressure is applied, the tympanic membrane is flaccid and negative pressure is present within the middle ear. A middle ear effusion is rarely present when the tympanic membrane is hypermobile, even though high negative middle ear pressure is present. A thickened tympanic membrane (caused by inflammation, scarring, or both) or a partly effusion-filled middle ear (in which the middle ear air pressure is ambient) shows decreased mobility to applied pressures, both positive and negative (Frame 3).

Normal middle ear pressure is reflected by the neutral position of the tympanic membrane as well as by its response to both positive and negative pressures

in each of the previous examples (Frames 1 through 3). In other cases, the eardrum may be retracted—usually because negative middle ear pressure is present (Frames 4 through 6). The compliant membrane is maximally retracted by even moderate negative middle ear pressure and hence cannot visibly be deflected inward further with applied positive pressure in the ear canal. However, negative pressure produced by releasing the rubber bulb of the otoscope will cause a return of the eardrum toward the neutral position if a negative pressure equivalent to that in the middle ear can be created by releasing the rubber bulb (Frame 4), a condition that occurs when air, with or without an effusion, is present in the middle ear. When the middle ear pressure is even lower, there may be only slight outward mobility of the tympanic membrane (Frame 5) because of the limited negative pressure that can be exerted through the otoscopes currently available. If the eardrum is severely retracted with extremely high negative middle ear pressure, if middle ear effusion is present, or if both occur, the examiner is not able to produce significant outward movement (Frame 6).

The tympanic membrane that exhibits fullness (Frame 7) will move to applied positive pressure but not to applied negative pressure if the pressure within the middle ear is positive and air, with or without an effusion, is present. In such an instance, the tympanic membrane is stretched laterally to the point of maximum compliance and will not visibly move outward any farther to the applied negative pressure but will move inward to applied positive pressure as long as some air is present within the middle ear—mastoid air cell system. When this system is filled with an effusion and little or no air is present, the mobility of the bulging tympanic membrane (Frame 8) is severely decreased or absent to both applied positive and negative pressure. Gates (1986), using these principles, compared the sensitivity, specificity, and predictive value of pneumatic otoscopy and tympanometry in the detection of middle ear effusion. As the skill of the

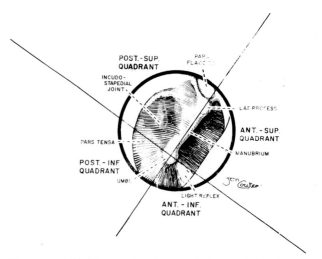

Figure 8–14. The four quadrants of a right tympanic membrane.

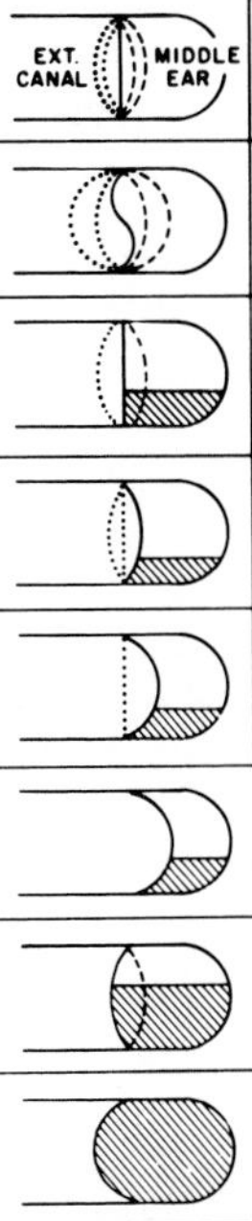

PNEUMATIC OTOSCOPY						MIDDLE EAR	
EARDRUM POSITION*	EARDRUM MOVEMENT† POSITIVE ▽ PRESSURE		NEGATIVE PRESSURE			CONTENTS	PRESSURE
	LOW	HIGH	LOW	HIGH			
I. NEUTRAL	1+	2+	1+	2+		AIR	AMBIENT
2. NEUTRAL	2+	3+	2+	3+		AIR	AMBIENT
3. NEUTRAL	0	1+	0	1+		AIR OR AIR AND EFFUSION	AMBIENT
4. RETRACTED	0	0	1+	2+		AIR OR AIR AND EFFUSION	LOW NEGATIVE
5. RETRACTED	0	0	0	1+		AIR OR EFFUSION AND AIR	HIGH NEGATIVE
6. RETRACTED	0	0	0	0		AIR OR EFFUSION OR BOTH	VERY HIGH NEGATIVE OR INDETERMINATE
7. FULL	0	1+	0	0		AIR AND EFFUSION	POSITIVE OR INDETERMINATE
8. BULGING	0	0	0	0		EFFUSION	POSITIVE OR INDETERMINATE

* POSITION OF EARDRUM
— AT REST; --- POSITIVE PRESSURE APPLIED (BULB COMPRESSED);
··· NEGATIVE PRESSURE APPLIED (RELEASE BULB)

† DEGREE OF TYMPANIC MEMBRANE MOVEMENT AS VISUALIZED THROUGH
THE OTOSCOPE; 0 = NONE, 1+ = SLIGHT, 2+ = MODERATE, 3+ = EXCESSIVE

▽ COMPRESSION OF BULB EXERTS POSITIVE PRESSURE; RELEASE OF A
COMPRESSED BULB INDUCES NEGATIVE PRESSURE

Figure 8–15. Pneumatic otoscopic findings related to middle ear contents and pressure (see text). (From Bluestone, C. D., and Klein, J. O. 1988. Otitis Media in Infants and Children. Philadelphia, W. B. Saunders Co., p. 76.)

otoscopist increases, the reliance on tympanometry in the diagnosis of effusion should decrease.

Figure 8–16 shows examples of common conditions of the middle ear as assessed with the otoscope, in which position, color, degree of translucency, and mobility of the tympanic membrane are diagnostic aids.

Otoscopy in the Newborn Infant

The tympanic membrane of the neonate is in a position different from that of the older infant and child; if this is not kept in mind, the examiner may perceive the eardrum to be smaller and retracted because in the neonate the tympanic membrane appears to be as wide as it is in older children but not as high (Fig. 8–17). Figure 8–18 shows that this perception is due to the more horizontal position of the neonatal eardrum, which frequently makes it difficult for the examiner to distinguish the pars flaccida of the tympanic membrane from the skin of the wall of the deep superior external canal.

In the first two days of life, the ear canal is filled with vernix caseosa, but this material is readily removed with a small curette or suction tube. Low-birth-weight (< 1200 gm) infants have external canals that may be so narrow as not to permit entry of the 2-mm diameter speculum. The canal walls of the young infant are pliable and tend to expand and collapse with insufflation during pneumatic otoscopy. Because of the pliability of the canal walls, it may be necessary to advance the speculum farther into the canal than would be the case for the older child. The tympanic membrane often appears thickened and opaque during the first few days. In many infants, the membrane is in an extreme oblique position, with the superior aspect proximal to the observer (Fig. 8–17). The tympanic membrane and the superior canal wall may appear to lie almost in the same plane, so that it is often difficult to distinguish the point where the canal ends and the pars flaccida begins. The inferior canal wall bulges loosely over the inferior position of the tympanic membrane and moves with positive pressure, simulating the movement of the tympanic membrane. The examiner must distinguish the movement of the canal walls and the movement of the membrane. The following should be considered to distinguish the movement of these structures: Vessels are seen within the tympanic membrane but not in the skin of the ear canal; the tympanic membrane moves during crying or respiration; and, inferiorly, the wall of the external canal

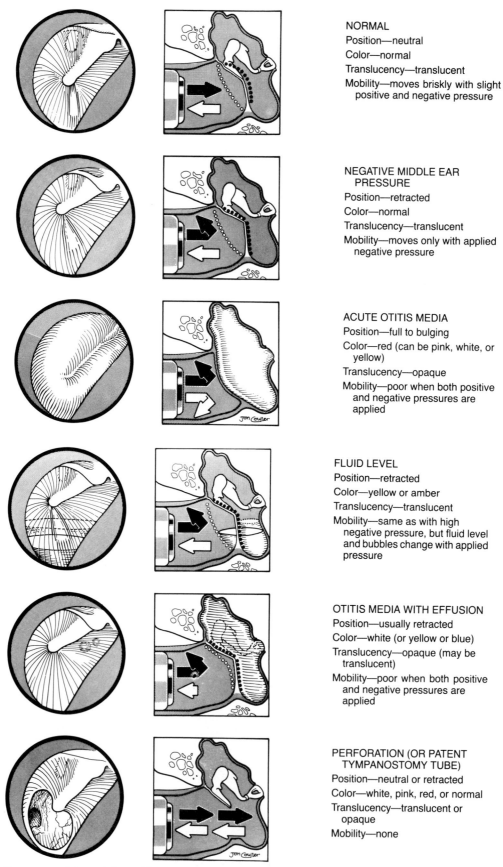

NORMAL
Position—neutral
Color—normal
Translucency—translucent
Mobility—moves briskly with slight positive and negative pressure

NEGATIVE MIDDLE EAR PRESSURE
Position—retracted
Color—normal
Translucency—translucent
Mobility—moves only with applied negative pressure

ACUTE OTITIS MEDIA
Position—full to bulging
Color—red (can be pink, white, or yellow)
Translucency—opaque
Mobility—poor when both positive and negative pressures are applied

FLUID LEVEL
Position—retracted
Color—yellow or amber
Translucency—translucent
Mobility—same as with high negative pressure, but fluid level and bubbles change with applied pressure

OTITIS MEDIA WITH EFFUSION
Position—usually retracted
Color—white (or yellow or blue)
Translucency—opaque (may be translucent)
Mobility—poor when both positive and negative pressures are applied

PERFORATION (OR PATENT TYMPANOSTOMY TUBE)
Position—neutral or retracted
Color—white, pink, red, or normal
Translucency—translucent or opaque
Mobility—none

Figure 8–16. Common conditions of the middle ear as assessed with the otoscope. (From Bluestone, C. D., and Klein, J. O. 1988. Otitis Media in Infants and Children. Philadelphia, W. B. Saunders Co., p. 78.)

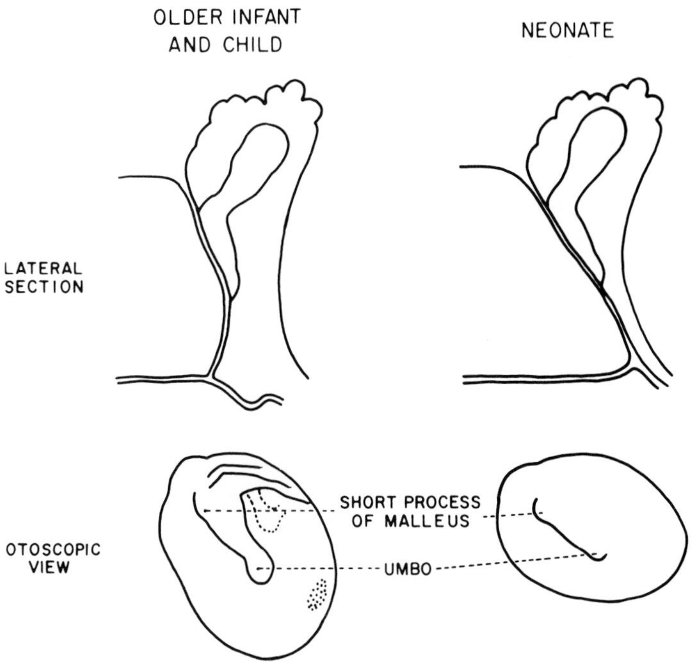

OLDER INFANT
AND CHILD

NEONATE

LATERAL
SECTION

OTOSCOPIC
VIEW

SHORT PROCESS
OF MALLEUS

UMBO

Figure 8–17. Comparison of the tympanic membrane of an older infant or a child with that of a neonate. The lateral section shows the greater angulation of the neonate's external canal with regard to the tympanic membrane. The appearance of the eardrums and canals on otoscopy is depicted in the lower drawings; the neonate appears to have a smaller tympanic membrane because of angulation of the eardrum.

and the tympanic membrane lie at an acute angle. By 1 month of age, the tympanic membrane has assumed an oblique position, one with which the examiner is familiar in the older child. However, during the first few weeks of life, examination of the ear requires patience and careful appraisal of the structures of the external canal and the tympanic membrane.

Accuracy, Validation Techniques, and Interexaminer Reliability of Otoscopy

Otoscopy is subjective and thus usually is an imprecise method of assessing the condition of the tympanic membrane and the middle ear. Many clinicians still

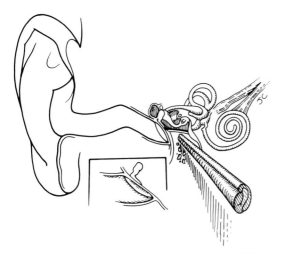

Figure 8–18. Position of tympanic membrane in the child is more vertical than it is in the neonate. (From Bluestone, C. D., and Klein, J. O. 1988. Otitis Media in Infants and Children. Philadelphia, W. B. Saunders Co., p. 79.)

do not use a pneumatic otoscope, and few have been trained adequately to make a correct diagnosis. The primary reason for this lack of proper education is the method of teaching employed. Because otoscopy involves a monocular assessment of the tympanic membrane, the teacher cannot verify that the student actually visualized the anatomic features that led to the diagnosis. An otoscope with a second viewing port is available (Fig. 8–19). Teacher and student can make observations together, and student errors can be corrected immediately. One of the most effective means of education currently available is the correlation of the otoscopic findings with those obtained by an otomicroscope that has an observer tube for the student. In this manner, the instructor can point out the critical landmarks and can demonstrate tympanic mobility using the Bruening otoscope.

Assessment techniques can also be improved by correlating otoscopy findings with a tympanogram taken immediately after the otoscopic examination (Bluestone and Cantekin, 1979; Cantekin et al., 1980). Lack of agreement between the otoscopic findings and tympanometry usually results in a second otoscopic examination, because tympanometry is generally accurate in distinguishing between normal and abnormal tympanic membranes and middle ears (specifically, in the identification of middle ear effusions). The presence or absence of negative pressure within the middle ear as measured by pneumatic otoscopy can be verified only by similar results on the tympanogram. Validation of the presence or absence of effusion as observed by otoscopy is best achieved by performing a tympanocentesis or myringotomy immediately after the examination. When surgical opening of the tympanic membrane is indicated, preliminary otoscopy by several examiners is an effective way of teaching many students to evaluate the state of the middle ear.

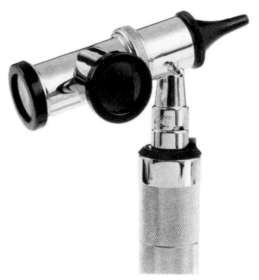

Figure 8–19. Teaching otoscope with sidearm viewer. (From Welch-Allyn and Co., New York.)

In most studies of otitis media, the disease has been identified by otoscopy; however, in many such studies no information has been offered to enable the reader to evaluate the ability of the otoscopist to make the diagnosis correctly. In an attempt to classify tympanometric patterns, Paradise and colleagues (1976) validated the diagnosis of the otoscopist by performing a myringotomy shortly after the otoscopic examination. This method of validation of otoscopic findings was also used in studies of infants with cleft palates in which two otoscopists were involved (Paradise et al., 1969; Paradise and Bluestone, 1974). However, most other studies of otitis media have not reported validation of the diagnostic criteria, and, when attempts have been made to determine interexaminer reliability in these studies, the results have been so poor as to infer that the data reported are not accurate. Jordan (1972) reported the consistency of descriptions of middle-ear appearance by otologists. In assessing normality or abnormality of the tympanic membrane, the examiners agreed in only 60 per cent of the observations in ten children.

In the design of a study in which otoscopic examination is used in the identification of otitis media with effusion and related conditions, the diagnostic abilities of all otoscopists included in the study must be validated, and interexaminer reliability must be established. If the primary ear disease being studied is otitis media with effusion, each otoscopist should have a high degree of accuracy in identifying otitis media with effusion. This can be achieved by performing otoscopy on a group of children immediately prior to tympanocentesis or myringotomy (Cantekin et al., 1980). The sensitivity (the total number of otoscopic diagnoses of otitis media with effusion absent in ears without otitis media with effusion divided by the total myringotomy findings when otitis media with effusion is present) and specificity (total number of otoscopic diagnoses of otitis media with effusion absent in ears without otitis

media with effusion divided by the total myringotomy findings when otitis media with effusion is absent) should be as high as possible. Interexaminer reliability can be tested by having all the otoscopists involved in the study independently make an otoscopic diagnosis prior to the tympanocentesis or myringotomy.

In more recent studies, such as the one by Mandel and coworkers (1987), the diagnosis of middle ear effusion is based on a decision-tree algorithm (Cantekin, 1983) that combines the findings of a validated otoscopist, as described previously, with the results of tympanometry and middle ear muscle reflex testing (Chap. 9).

OTOMICROSCOPY

Many otolaryngologists use the otomicroscope to improve the accuracy of diagnosis of otitis media and related conditions. For the assessment of tympanic membrane mobility, the microscope, when used with the Bruening otoscope and nonmagnifying lens (Fig. 8–20), is superior to conventional otoscopes; this is because the microscope provides binocular vision (and therefore depth perception), a better light source, and greater magnification. Under most conditions, otomicroscopic examination is impractical and generally not necessary. However, when a diagnosis by otoscopy is

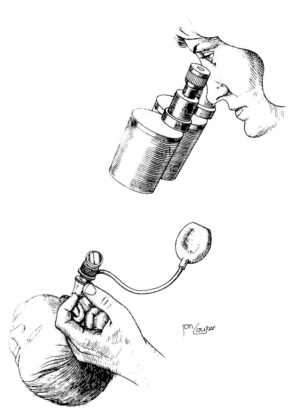

Figure 8–20. Precise assessment of tympanic membrane mobility employing the otomicroscope and a Bruening otoscope with a nonmagnifying lens.

in doubt, the otomicroscope is an invaluable diagnostic aid and frequently is essential in arriving at the correct diagnosis (e.g., in differentiating a deep retraction pocket in the posterosuperior quadrant of the tympanic membrane from a cholesteatoma). In addition to the advantages offered by the otomicroscope for certain diagnostic problems, it is superior to the conventional otoscopes for minor surgical procedures, such as tympanocentesis, because it allows for a more precise visualization of the field.

Even though several studies reported in the past have used the otomicroscopic examination as a validator for the presence or absence of middle ear disease (otitis media with effusion), no study has reported on the sensitivity and specificity of the microscopic examination for detecting middle ear effusion. It is purported to be superior to the standard otoscopic examination, but its superiority to tympanometry with otoscopy has not yet been shown. However, as a teaching device, the otomicroscope with an observer tube attachment is preferable to the currently available otoscope.

Whenever the otoscopic examination is unsatisfactory owing to inability to adequately visualize the tympanic membrane (e.g., narrow external canal, uncooperative child), an examination under general anesthesia employing the otomicroscope may be indicated in selected infants and children, such as when a suppurative complication is present.

HEARING TESTS

Tuning Fork Tests

Prior to the widespread availability of audiometric evaluation of hearing, tuning forks were an essential part of the physical examination of patients who had a suspected hearing loss. In the modern era, many otolaryngologists have not included tuning fork tests as part of their routine examination of the ear and hearing. Sheehy and coworkers (1971) advocate their continued use to validate the audiometric assessment, and Yung and Morris (1981) believe tuning forks are of value in screening for hearing loss. Their usefulness in children has been questioned, and they are considered by many to be unreliable in this age group. Capper and colleagues (1987) compared the Rinne and Weber test responses to audiometric findings in 125 children and reported that about one third of tuning fork responses were incorrect, especially in children younger than 6 years of age. Tuning fork tests can be helpful in older children and teen-agers in assessing hearing when audiometry is unavailable or unreliable or when serial evaluation of hearing is desired after an initial audiogram is obtained. Examples of the latter indication would be following the course of otitis media or during the immediate postoperative period following middle ear surgery.

The Weber test is performed by placing a tuning fork (usually 512 Hz) at the vertex or against the teeth and asking the child if the sound lateralizes to one ear or not. The Rinne test is performed by asking the child to compare the loudness level of the tuning fork applied to the mastoid bone and opposite the external auditory canal. (An extensive description of these and other tuning fork tests is provided in Shambaugh and Glasscock [1980].)

Other Subjective Tests of Hearing

Although not ideal, testing a child's ability to hear conversational and whispered speech can be helpful as an alternative to frequent periodic audiometric tests. An example of the usefulness of such testing is when the clinician wants to serially assess the hearing of a child who has a middle-ear effusion and a previously documented conductive hearing loss, as an aid in management decisions (e.g., watchful waiting versus surgical intervention), since the hearing loss may fluctuate.

When performing the testing, the clinician should present words that are familiar to the child, first at a conversational level and then in a whisper. The clinician should be behind the child on the side being tested, to prevent lip reading, while masking the opposite ear; gently rubbing a small sheet of paper over the non–test ear is usually sufficient for masking. A child who fails to repeat words spoken at a conversational level will have about a 60-dB loss or greater, whereas if conversational speech is heard and whispered speech is not, the loss can be judged to be between 30 and 60 dB. These tests should not replace behavioral or nonbehavioral audiometric tests, because their reliability is questionable, especially in young children; but these tests can be a cost-effective way of periodically assessing hearing after audiograms have been obtained.

When the findings of audiometry reveal that the child has no hearing in one ear, (i.e., anacousis), the use of a Bárány noisemaker (Fig. 8–21) as a masking

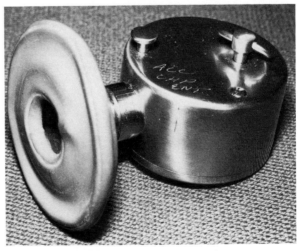

Figure 8–21. A Bárány noisemaker.

device may be helpful to further verify the loss. When the noisemaker is inserted into the hearing ear, the patient with an anacoustic ear will not be able to repeat words that are presented in a loud voice (e.g., shouted words).

REFERENCES

Barriga, R., Schwartz, R. H., and Hayden, G. F. 1986. Adequate illumination for otoscopy: Variations due to power source, bulb, and head and speculum design. Am. J. Dis. Child. 140:1237.

Bluestone, C. D., and Cantekin, E. I. 1979. Design factors in the characterization and identification of otitis media and certain related conditions. Ann. Otol. Rhinol. Laryngol. 88:13.

Bluestone, C. D., and Shurin, P. 1974. Middle-ear disease in children: Pathogenesis, diagnosis and management. Pediatr. Clin. North Am. 21:370.

Cantekin, E. I. 1983. Algorithm for diagnosis of otitis media with effusion. Ann. Otol. Rhinol. Laryngol. 92:6.

Cantekin, E. I., Bluestone, C. D., Fria, T. J., et al. 1980. Identification of otitis media with effusion. Ann. Otol. Rhinol. Laryngol. 89:190.

Capper J. W. R., Slack, R. W. T., and Maw, A. R. 1987. Tuning fork tests in children. J. Laryngol. Otol. 101:780.

Elner, A., Ingelstedt, S., and Ivarsson, A. 1971. The elastic properties of the tympanic membrane system. Acta Otolaryngol. 72:397.

Fischler, R. S., Todd, N. W., and Feldman, C. 1987. Lack of association of cleft uvula with otitis media in Apache Indian children. Am. J. Dis. Child. 141:866.

Gates, G. A. 1986. Differential otomanometry. Am. J. Otolaryngol. 7:147.

Jordan, R. E. 1972. Epidemiology of otitis media. In Glorig, A., and Gerwin, K. S. (eds.): Otitis Media. Proceedings of the National Conference, Gallier Hearing and Speech Center, Dallas, TX. Springfield, IL, Charles C Thomas.

Khanna, S. M., and Tonndorf, J. 1972. Tympanic membrane vibrations in cats studied by time-averaged holography. J. Acoust. Soc. Am. 51:1904.

Mandel, E. M., Rockette, H. E., Bluestone, C. D., et al. 1987. Efficacy of amoxicillin with and without decongestant-antihistamine for otitis media with effusion in children. N Engl. J. Med. 316:432.

Paradise, J. L., and Bluestone, C. D. 1974. Early treatment of universal otitis media of infants with cleft palate. Pediatrics 53:48.

Paradise, J. L., Bluestone, C. D., and Felder, H. 1969. The universality of otitis media in fifty infants with cleft palate. Pediatrics 44:3542.

Paradise, J. L., Smith, C. G., and Bluestone, C. D. 1976. Tympanometric detection of middle-ear effusion in infants and young children. Pediatrics, 58:198.

Schwartz, R. H., Hayden, G. F., Rodriguez, W. J., et al. 1985. The bifid uvula: Is it a marker for an otitis-prone child? Laryngoscope 95:1100.

Schwartz, R. H., Rodriguez, W. J., McAveney, W., et al. 1983. Cerumen removal: How necessary is it to diagnose acute otitis media? Am. J. Dis. Child. 137:1064.

Shambaugh, G. E., and Glasscock, M. E. 1980. Surgery of the Ear, 3rd ed. Philadelphia, W. B. Saunders Co.

Sheehy, J. L., Gardner, G., and Hambley, W. M. 1971. Tuning fork tests in modern otology. Arch. Otolaryngol. 94:132.

Stool, S. E., and Randall, P. 1967. Unexpected ear disease in infants with cleft palate. Cleft Palate J. 4:99.

Taylor, G. D. 1972. The bifid uvula. Laryngoscope 82:771.

Yung, M. W., and Morris, T. M. D. 1981. Tuning fork tests in the diagnosis of serous otitis media. Br. Med. J. 283:1576.

Chapter 9

THE ASSESSMENT OF HEARING AND MIDDLE-EAR FUNCTION IN CHILDREN

Robert J. Nozza, Ph.D.   Thomas J. Fria, Ph.D.

From the time of birth, a child exists in a world of sensory experiences. The reception and perception of these experiences provide the framework for communication and other interactive links to the environment. Consequently, a decrement in sensory experience endangers the normal development of cognitive skills vital to the child's successful interaction with his or her environment. If a child has an undetected or unremediated sensory impairment in the months crucial to learning, a developmental lag results. This lag may prove irreversible, and the child may never realize his or her potential capabilities.

The long-term effects of hearing loss cannot be dismissed as trivial even when the impairment appears to be mild or transient. As a result, we are obligated to identify children with impaired hearing, to assess the nature and the extent of the impairment, and to manage the child's present and future environmental interactions in the context of the impairment. This chapter will focus on the procedures used to assess hearing in children. The philosophies and the techniques for the habilitation or rehabilitation of children with impaired hearing are presented in Chapters 96 and 97. (Physiology is in Chap. 7.)

To understand the auditory system and its function, one must understand the anatomy, physiology, and psychology of hearing. The development of this complex process is largely unknown, and our ability to assess it during development has limitations. However, it is during development that disordered hearing has its greatest impact, so assessment of hearing in infants and children is one of the greatest challenges facing audiologists today. It is impossible to cover in a comprehensive way material on assessment of hearing and middle-ear function in children in one chapter. Several of the topics that are subheadings in this chapter have entire textbooks devoted to them. Therefore, this chapter cannot be the only resource in pediatric audiology used by the medical professional or student. It is at best a guide to some of the many possible avenues and approaches to the evaluation of the ear with respect to its primary purpose, sensing and interpreting meaningful acoustic information in the environment.

The methods for assessing hearing in children are either behavioral or physiologic. Behavioral methods of assessment include behavioral observation audiometry (BOA), conditioned orientation reflex (COR) audiometry, visual reinforcement audiometry (VRA), "play" audiometry, tangible reinforcement operant conditioning audiometry (TROCA), and conventional audiometry.

Electroacoustic immittance measurements and measures of auditory evoked potentials are the two most commonly used physiologic techniques. Such methods provide information regarding the integrity of the auditory system but do not assess directly the perceptual event we call hearing.

Regardless of the assessment technique employed, the examiner must interpret the behavioral or physiologic responses obtained and judge whether a given child's hearing is normal or impaired. However, the reliability and validity of this judgment does depend on the particular assessment technique employed and the skill and experience of the observer. For this reason, a judgment of impaired or unimpaired hearing, based on a single evaluation or a single technique, should be regarded with caution, and often a combination of several techniques and multiple evaluations over time are necessary to arrive at a valid assessment of hearing in the very young.

In addition, the age of the child will significantly influence the precision with which assessment information may be obtained. The nature of the auditory response is inherently gross and nonvolitional in the neonate and becomes more refined and voluntary as the child develops. However, the common belief that some children are too young to be properly evaluated is not true. Reasonably precise estimates of hearing are obtainable in most cases. The methods used and their limitations are described in detail in the following sections.

BEHAVIORAL METHODS OF ASSESSMENT

Early in life, there is a change with age in the ability to respond to sound, so the discussion that follows will be organized around appropriate tests for various age groups. The test methods described were designed, or evolved, to capitalize on response capabilities and proclivities at different stages of development. The age and the developmental level of a child dictate which behavioral assessment method has the greatest probability of yielding meaningful information.

Behavioral Observation Audiometry

Behavioral observation audiometry (BOA) is a term used to describe procedures typically used for assessing auditory function in infants younger than approximately 5 months of age. BOA is any procedure in which the examiner presents a stimulus sound and observes the associated behavioral response of the child. True BOA procedures do not incorporate conditioning procedures. Rather, the procedure relies on the observer's understanding of naturally occurring responses to auditory stimulation early in life and the conditions under which they will most probably occur. Involuntary responses that often occur following sound stimulation in the young infant include eye blinks, eye widening, startle or Moro reflex, leg kicks, crying, and quieting. The more complex the spectrum of the sound (e.g., speech or noise as opposed to a tone) and the greater the intensity, the more likely the infant is to respond (Eisenberg, 1976; Hoversten and Moncur, 1969). Also, an infant in a quiet or lightly sleeping state is more inclined to provide an involuntary response to sound than an alert and active one, a crying and fussing one, or even one in a deep sleep. BOA is a viable screening procedure in the physician's office, or it can be used as a more diagnostic assessment tool in major audiology centers devoted to pediatric testing.

In the office setting, the baby typically is seated on the mother's lap, and the physician or examiner presents the stimulus to either side of the baby and observes the associated behavioral response. Simple noisemakers, such as rattles, squeak toys, Oriental bells, and crinkled onion-skin paper are common stimulus devices in the office setting. These devices produce sounds composed of a broad range of frequencies of indeterminate relative intensities, and consequently their use provides only a gross qualitative estimate of the normality of hearing. The chance for false-positive judgments of impairment is usually small, since the child who fails to respond is at high risk for significant hearing impairment. Such a child must be referred for more extensive testing at a center devoted to pediatric hearing assessment. However, false-negative judgments of impairment could be more serious, since a child with a significant high-frequency hearing loss may respond to a broad-frequency noisemaker in an apparently normal fashion. Concomitant persistence of parental or grandparental concern about the hearing of such children should alert the physician to the need for referral for more extensive tests. A comprehensive discussion of the use of noisemakers is presented by

Northern and Downs (1984), and the reader intending to use these devices will profit from their suggestions.

In audiology centers concerned with assessing hearing in children, BOA is conducted in a manner different from the way it is performed in the office setting. The test environment is carefully controlled, and only calibrated stimuli are used. To avoid the unwanted influence of background sounds, the child is tested in a sound-treated test booth designed to attenuate ambient noise. To permit stimulation from either side, the child is situated (usually on the mother's lap) between two loudspeakers. Stimuli are presented through the loudspeakers from an adjoining control room with calibrated pure tone and speech audiometric equipment. The examiner is usually an experienced audiologist who observes the child through a window between the control room and the test booth. In some centers, two examiners conduct the test: One presents the stimuli from the control room, and the other, located in the test booth, observes the child's responses.

BOA in an audiology center is aimed at determining minimum response levels (MRLs) for various stimuli, that is, the minimum intensity necessary to elicit a response during at least 50 per cent of the trials at that intensity. Tones, noise, and speech signals are commonly employed. When tones through loudspeakers are used, the tones are "warbled," which means they are electronically modulated in frequency to avoid standing waves in the test booth that would make stimulus intensity calibration impossible. Warbled tones with center frequencies of 500, 1000, 2000, and 4000 Hertz (Hz) are commonly used. Narrow bands of noise, with energy concentrated around the same frequencies, are used in some centers as alternatives to warbled tone signals. Speech stimuli are also used and usually consist of the examiner's live voice, a recording of the parent's voice, or other recorded speech materials.

The ability to elicit a response varies widely as a function of the stimulus used in a BOA procedure. Hoversten and Moncur (1969) and Thompson and Thompson (1972) observed large differences in responses to speech stimuli as opposed to noise or tones. Speech was a more powerful stimulus for young and older infants. The Auditory Behavioral Index for Infants, suggested by Northern and Downs (1974), is shown in Table 9–1 and serves as an example of BOA response norms that can be used to interpret the responses of a given child. Table 9–1 shows the nature of the responses that can be expected for a child of a given age and the average stimulus levels necessary to produce the response for noisemakers, warbled pure tones, and speech signals. Noisemaker data are included in this table. However, specific noisemakers were selected by the authors, and an analysis of the frequency and intensity characteristics of the sounds produced by the selected devices was conducted.

As the data in Table 9–1 illustrate, the stimulus level necessary to produce a response decreases as the age of the child increases. This is apparent for all three

TABLE 9–1. Auditory Behavioral Index for Infants

AGE	NOISEMAKERS (APPROX. SPL)	WARBLED PURE TONES (RE: AUDIOMETRIC ZERO)	SPEECH (RE: AUDIOMETRIC ZERO)	EXPECTED RESPONSE	STARTLE TO SPEECH (RE: AUDIOMETRIC ZERO)
0–6 wk	50–70 dB	78 dB	40–60 dB	Eye-widening, eye-blink, stirring or arousal from sleep, startle	65 dB
6 wk–4 mo	50–60 dB	70 dB	47 dB	Eye-widening, eye-shift, eye-blink, quieting, beginning rudimentary head turn by 4 mo	65 dB
4–7 mo	40–50 dB	51 dB	21 dB	Head-turn on lateral plane toward sound; listening attitude	65 dB
7–9 mo	30–40 dB	45 dB	15 dB	Direct localization of sounds to side, indirectly below ear level	65 dB
9–13 mo	25–35 dB	38 dB	8 dB	Direct localization of sounds to side, directly below ear level, indirectly above ear level	65 dB
13–16 mo	25–30 dB	32 dB	5 dB	Direct localization of sound on side, above and below	65 dB
16–21 mo	25 dB	25 dB	5 dB	Direct localization of sound on side, above and below	65 dB
21–24 mo	25 dB	26 dB	3 dB	Direct localization of sound on side, above and below	65 dB

From Northern, J. L., and Downs, M. P. 1984. Hearing in Children, 3rd ed. © 1984, The Williams & Wilkins Co., Baltimore. Modified from McConnell, F., and Ward, P. H. 1967. Deafness in Childhood. Nashville, Vanderbilt University Press.

stimulus types shown. It is interesting also to note that only speech MRLs approximate normal adult threshold levels and only for the child 12 months or older. Consequently, the responses obtained with BOA are interpreted as either age-appropriate or age-inappropriate, with impairment inferred in the latter case, particularly for children younger than 12 months of age.

Murphy (1961) and Thompson and Weber (1974) also published norms that can be used to interpret BOA results. Murphy (1961) found that, in normal infants, less stimulus intensity was required to elicit a response than that suggested by Northern and Downs (1984). Thompson and Weber (1974) found, using BOA, that there was great variability (over 50 dB) in the MRLs of a group of normal infants. These discrepancies have motivated many centers to generate their own norms for BOA. Moreover, it has been demonstrated that knowledge of the loudness, the spectrum, and the time of onset of a stimulus in the BOA procedure can influence an observer's decision regarding the presence or absence of a response (Moncur, 1968; Weber, 1969). This bias is increased in the office setting, where additional cues are available to the infant and there is less control over the stimulus. Wilson and Thompson (1984) suggest that the response variability and observer bias inherent in BOA preclude its use as an assessment tool and that it should serve only as an initial screening procedure to determine levels for further testing.

BOA, then, is a term used to describe a technique whereby a child's behavioral response to a variety of stimulus sounds is observed. The procedure is most commonly used to evaluate neonates and infants younger than 6 months of age. The nature of the stimulus, the child's prestimulus activity, response habituation, and the unpredictable bias of the observer are factors that can weaken the reliability of the procedure as an assessment tool. BOA should be considered as a subjective screening procedure that serves best to detect significant auditory impairment.

Visual Reinforcement Audiometry

Visual reinforcement audiometry (VRA) also involves the presentation of a stimulus sound and the observation of the child's associated behavioral response. The response, a head turn toward the source of the sound, is rewarded with a visual stimulus such as a blinking light, an illuminated picture or toy, or an animated toy that is located above the loudspeaker. The visual stimulus serves to strengthen the child's response to the sound, to decrease the effects of response habituation, and to increase the examiner's control of the child's responses. As such, the visual stimulus is referred to as the visual reinforcer.

Suzuki and Ogiba (1960, 1961) suggested a technique to condition the "orientation" or localization reflex in young infants, and many clinics refer to the test as conditioning orientation reflex (COR) audiometry. However, as Wilson (1978) points out, the technique can be used for children who do not exhibit an unconditional orientation reflex, and consequently the general term visual reinforcement audiometry (VRA) is probably more appropriate. VRA is most successful for assessing infants from 6 to 24 months of age.

In the early VRA approaches, a simple visual reinforcer, such as a blinking light or an illuminated toy, was used to reward localization responses. However,

Moore and colleagues (1975; 1977) showed that a complex visual reinforcer (an animated toy) elicited a greater number of responses in normal 6- to 18-month-old infants than did a simple blinking light reward.

Wilson and Thompson (1984) cited the work of Wilson and coworkers (1976) and Thompson and Weber (1974) to demonstrate that VRA with an animated toy reward yielded MRLs that were significantly lower than those obtained with conventional BOA. In addition, the range of stimulus intensities required to elicit a response was significantly less with the VRA procedure, and the MRLs were not far removed from normal adult thresholds.

Consequently, VRA is a particularly viable procedure for assessing auditory responses in infants as young as 5 months. This assessment tool is reliable, reduces variability among infants, and reflects MRLs in normal infants that approximate adult values.

Tangible Reinforcement Operant Conditioning Audiometry

Tangible reinforcement operant conditioning audiometry (TROCA) uses tangible reinforcement, such as candy, sugar-coated cereal, or other edibles, to reward the child for pressing a bar when the stimulus is heard. A special apparatus is used that dispenses the reward when the bar is pressed. TROCA is described by Lloyd and coworkers (1968) as a technique applicable for use with severely retarded children. Subsequent studies (Fulton et al, 1975; Wilson, 1978) have reported the utility of TROCA in obtaining auditory MRLs in infants. Fulton and colleagues (1975) used earphones in their study and obtained thresholds at the standard audiometric test frequencies, but they were able to do so only in infants 12 months of age or older. These same investigators found that an average of 11.4 test sessions was required for earphone testing.

In 1977, Wilson and Decker (Wilson, 1978) used both TROCA and VROCA (the same technique using visual reinforcement instead of a tangible reward) to assess 7- to 20-month-old infants with warbled tone stimuli presented through loudspeakers. These investigators found that an average of four test sessions was required to establish MRLs. Of the infants younger than 12 months of age, 64 per cent were successfully tested, while 84 per cent of the 13- to 20-month-old children were successfully evaluated.

Owing to the special equipment required and the inordinate amount of time necessary for accurate results, TROCA has not been used widely in clinical settings as a primary assessment procedure. Yet, the technique is quite promising as a tool for the assessment of difficult-to-test children such as the severely mentally retarded.

Play Audiometry

The behavioral assessment techniques discussed thus far are applied best to children younger than 3 years of age. At 2 years of age, a child can yield voluntary responses to sound that are premature prototypes of the adult response. Conventional audiometric techniques can be used, but they must be modified to be more interesting for the young child. This is accomplished by structuring the test situation in such a manner that the child can appropriately respond to stimuli by participating in a form of "play" activity. For this reason, the technique is often called "play" audiometry. It can be used for assessing hearing levels for both speech and pure tone stimuli.

Play audiometry requires a considerable amount of flexibility and creativity on the part of the examiner. A play activity must be used that (1) interests the child and (2) permits the child to respond appropriately while "playing." A common approach is to use a series of colored disks of different sizes that are stacked on a peg. The child is instructed to hold a disk up to his or her ear, and when the "bell" comes on to stack the disk on the peg. With a short practice session, the child can be taught to respond appropriately as stimulus frequency and intensity are varied. This technique is ideal for the 2- to 5-year-old child but can also be helpful for evaluating chronologically older children who are mentally retarded or emotionally disturbed (Barr, 1955; Darley, 1961). Of course, there is nothing sacred about the colored disk on a peg, and a variety of other activities can be and have been used successfully. However, the general principle underlying the technique is the same.

Conventional Audiometry

The use of conventional audiometric techniques is traditionally reserved for the child aged 5 years or older. Yet there are a surprising number of 3½ and 4 year olds who can be tested with conventional means. Simply, the child is instructed to listen quietly for the test sound and indicate when it is heard by raising a hand. The intensity is varied from trial to trial, depending on the response of the child during the previous trial. The lowest intensity at which at least 50 per cent of the presentations are correctly detected is taken as the threshold estimate. Thresholds can be obtained with conventional audiometry in children aged 5 years or older.

Bone Conduction Testing and Masking

Bone conduction testing and the use of masking are no less valuable in the identification, differential diagnosis, and management of hearing impairment in children than they are in adults. Responses to bone-conducted stimuli can be obtained in children, using most of the techniques previously described. Head-turn responses can even be elicited using bone-conducted stimuli and VRA. Calibration standards for bone-conducted signals on the heads of infants and children have not been established, but, in infants, the presence of an air-bone gap can be determined grossly using the bone-conduction oscillator. As with the fitting of earphones, infants sometimes object to wearing the bone-conduction oscillator, but it is always worth a try when there is a question about conductive versus sensorineural hearing loss.

Masking to eliminate the participation of the nontest ear in either air-conduction or bone-conduction testing is often necessary. A discussion of masking and masking techniques requires greater attention than can be devoted in this chapter, but the concept should not be ignored. The interested reader can consult Goldstein and Newman (1985) for a review of masking considerations. Because infants are typically not tested while wearing earphones or with a bone vibrator, asymmetries in hearing that require masking are often not identified. However, with training, many infants can perform the VRA task reliably with earphones and masking noise (Nozza and Wilson, 1984; Nozza, 1987). Children capable of performing play audiometry or TROCA should be able to perform with earphones and maskers without difficulty. It is important that the professionals who interpret hearing test results be aware of the possible cross-over of stimuli to the nontest ear and the need for masking to produce a valid result. Likewise, in situations in which masking cannot be accomplished because of a fatigued or uncooperative child, the professional who interprets the results should use caution in drawing conclusions about the nature and the extent of hearing loss.

Speech Audiometry

Speech can be used as a stimulus in any of the procedures previously described. Speech awareness threshold (SAT), the lowest level at which a listener can reliably respond to the presence of speech, provides only limited information with respect to the nature and the degree of impairment. More meaningful information is obtained when the ability of the patient to recognize words can be assessed.

SPEECH-RECOGNITION THRESHOLD (SRT). The SRT is a threshold for recognition of words that are entirely familiar to the listener. For older children and adults, spondee words (two-syllable words with equal stress on each syllable, such as baseball and airplane) are typically used. For younger children, the test is usually altered to accommodate the language level of the child being tested. Rather than asking the young child to repeat the words, a different response mode must be used. Young children are frequently reluctant to say words back to the audiologist or may have poor articulation, confounding the assessment of auditory skills with limitations in production. Alternative approaches include asking the child to point to pictures of familiar objects displayed on a table or to respond by pointing to a selection of objects or to body parts. For older children, simple verbal repetition is appropriate as a response.

The SRT is most often administered by the audiologist using live-voice presentation. However, commercial tapes are available, with calibrated lists of spondee words that can be used for greater reliability and validity in testing. Individual ear SRTs provide a check on the threshold estimates made using more frequency-specific stimuli, such as pure tones, warbled tones, and narrow-band noises. The SRT typically is within 8 dB of the pure-tone average (PTA: average of thresholds at 500, 1000, and 2000 Hz; see later) when it has been obtained reliably, and can provide a check on the reliability of the pure-tone thresholds. However, a word of caution about the relationship between the PTA and the SRT is necessary. The correspondence between the two measures is quite good only when several criteria are met. First, the person being tested must respond in a reliable and consistent way. Second, the words used to estimate the SRT must be from a large set of possible words rather than a small set. The fewer words used, the greater the chance that guessing will influence performance and improve the score. Third, and most important, the configuration and the type of hearing loss can influence the degree to which the SRT and the PTA correspond. The most common cause of discrepancy between the PTA and the SRT occurs in cases of sharply sloping high-frequency sensorineural hearing loss. In such a case, the PTA might be quite high because of elevated thresholds at 1000 or 2000 Hz. The SRT, on the other hand, may appear quite good because of the information available to the listener in the low frequencies of the speech sound. Again, a small closed set of words from which to choose and a reasonably careful listener can provide an SRT that is considerably better (lower) than the PTA. Conversely, the SRT can be considerably poorer than the PTA in cases of sensorineural hearing loss in which there is severe distortion. The listener may detect the words but may be unable to recognize what is being said. These possibilities should be considered carefully before a child is labeled unreliable or inconsistent based on lack of agreement between the PTA and the SRT. (See also below for testing of functional hearing loss). Such possibilities also serve to alert us to the limitations of speech recognition testing alone as a means to identify and describe a hearing loss.

WORD INTELLIGIBILITY TESTING. Word intelligibility testing, or speech discrimination testing as it is sometimes called, serves a different purpose from that of the SRT. Monosyllabic words are presented to the child at a level that is well above the SRT or the PTA, for example, 30 or 40 dB sensation level (SL; refers to an individual's behavioral hearing threshold for a particular stimulus). The word lists are commonly "phonetically balanced" so that an appropriate sampling of all phonemes in the language is represented. Lack of ability to recognize words, even when presented at levels well above threshold, provides important diagnostic information as well as information necessary in making a prognosis for rehabilitation. Performance versus intensity on word intelligibility tests, for example, can be useful in locating the site of the lesion producing the hearing loss as well as providing important information with respect to fitting and use of amplification.

Word intelligibility test scores are usually the percentage of words correctly understood at a given decibel level. Most lists used in intelligibility testing have 50 words, so each word represents two points. Sometimes half-lists can be used with good reliability, but then each word has a value of four points. Scoring is usually done simply as correct or incorrect. Efforts to develop tests that use finer analyses of errors, such as phoneme omissions and replacements, have not been used widely in the clinical setting with children.

It is important to always be aware of the circumstances under which the word intelligibility test score was obtained. In isolation, the percentage of words correctly identified is virtually meaningless. Performance on the test depends very heavily on the intensity level at which the words are presented, the configuration of the hearing loss, the difficulty of the test words, the receptive vocabulary of the child being tested, and, perhaps, whether the words are presented "live-voice" or using a professional recording. The audiologist reports on the audiogram, in addition to the score, the level of presentation, the test and the list used, and the manner of presentation so that other professionals can interpret the result properly.

In many clinics, word intelligibility tests are presented routinely at 30 or 40 dB SL (SRT). Ordinarily, this level is adequate for the child to achieve maximum performance. However, in cases of sensorineural hearing loss with recruitment, a 40 dB SL may be too great and may make it difficult for the child to achieve maximum performance. Again, the configuration of the loss influences the relationship between the SL of the words and the word intelligibility score. The child with a high-frequency hearing loss, for example, may have a low SRT. However, presentation of words at 30 or 40 dB SL may not be sufficient to permit maximum performance. A presentation level at which speech sounds comfortably loud is often used and often is a good way to achieve a maximum score with a single test. As a rule, a low discrimination score for a child with hearing loss should indicate to the audiologist that testing at other intensity levels should be done regardless of how the intensity level for the initial test was chosen. In no case should word intelligibility test scores be reported or interpreted without the presentation level, manner of presentation, and word list taken into account.

In some cases, hearing-aid evaluations in particular, word intelligibility lists may be presented in a sound field at intensity levels that more closely represent the levels of conversational speech, for example, 50 to 60 dB hearing level (HL; refers to normal hearing for a group of young adults). Performance can then be compared to intelligibility scores obtained monaurally under earphones at higher intensity levels relative to threshold. This information is useful in predicting potential performance with amplification. Thus, testing with hearing aids at conversational levels provides the audiologist with an index (albeit limited) of the benefit gained with specific amplifying devices. In addition, assessment can be done with noise or competing messages in the background to help define the ability of the child to use the hearing aid in less favorable listening conditions.

Children older than about 7 years of age can typically perform the word intelligibility test designed for adults (e.g., CID W-22 word list; Hirsh et al., 1952). There also have been a number of tests developed for word intelligibility testing in younger children. Haskins (1949), recognizing the need for a test better suited to the level of a child, developed a list of words considered to be within the vocabulary of kindergarten children. The PBK series (Haskins, 1949) is commonly used today for children aged 4 to 7 years, vocabulary level permitting. Tests for even younger children have also been developed. The same problem that faces the audiologist in obtaining an SRT from a young child exists with respect to testing word intelligibility. That is, a response mode other than verbal repetition is required. This is particularly important when testing hearing impaired children who may have poor articulation.

Ross and Lerman (1970), addressing the need for a word intelligibility test suitable for hearing-impaired children, developed a test that utilizes a picture-pointing response. It is called the Word Intelligibility by Picture Identification Test, or the WIPI. The norms for this test were derived from a group of hearing-impaired youngsters, so it has greatest validity with that population. However, the WIPI works well with many young children in audiology clinics.

Elliott and Katz (1980) developed a word intelligibility test that is suitable for children with a receptive language level of as young as 3 years. Like the WIPI, it incorporates a picture-pointing response; thus, very young children can respond. The test, which was developed at Northwestern University and is called NU-CHIPS, has good normative data and is fairly easy to administer.

Finally, Susan Jerger and others (1980; 1981) have developed the Pediatric Speech Intelligibility (PSI) Test. This test was designed to provide not only a useful word intelligibility test for young children but also a means of assessing central auditory processing. In this test, sentences or words in isolation are used. In addition, words and sentences can be presented in the presence of a competing message, either diotically or dichotically, to better assess central auditory function. The test also uses a picture-pointing task and has applications for children as young as 2 years of age.

Each of the aforementioned word intelligibility tests for children is available in tape-recorded lists. The audiologist is sometimes more successful, in the tests that permit it, when presenting word lists using monitored live-voice presentation. However, differences in voice characteristics from one tester to another, careless monitoring of vocal output, or both tend to weaken the reliability and validity of speech test results. With small children, the need for flexibility is great. Therefore, sometimes the objectivity and control provided by professionally recorded materials must be sacrificed, and methods more likely to produce results used. The professional who must interpret speech results should be aware of the limitations inherent in live-voice, half-list tests and the increase in test-retest variability when testing is done by more than one audiologist.

It should also be noted that each test has its own characteristics with respect to performance as a function of age. Audiologists should be able to interpret word intelligibility test scores appropriately if they are aware of the age-appropriate norms for the test used. A low score by a young child may be age-appropriate if the test is designed for an older child. Therefore, the consumer of audiologic information should be aware of all the limitations of looking at a test score in isolation.

The Audiogram and Hearing Loss

The audiogram is a graphic representation of a child's hearing thresholds for air- and bone-conducted pure-tone stimuli at octave frequencies from 250 to 8000 Hz.* The octave stimulus frequencies are represented on the audiogram abscissa, and stimulus intensities, in decibels referenced to hearing level (dBHL, ANSI, 1969), are shown on the ordinate. At each stimulus frequency, coded symbols are used to denote the threshold. An example of the audiogram form and coded symbols suggested by the American Speech and Hearing Association (ASHA, 1974) is shown in Figures 9–1a and b, respectively.

A child's air-conduction thresholds at the tested stimulus frequencies are connected with a solid line, and in some centers bone-conduction thresholds are linked with a dashed line. Ordinarily, the thresholds for both ears are plotted on the same graph, but some clinicians prefer to use a separate graph for each ear. For clarity, when a single graph is used, the right ear threshold symbols are circles written in red, and those of the left ear are Xs in blue.

The audiogram most often represents the threshold obtained with either play or conventional audiometry through earphones. Thresholds obtained with warbled pure tones or narrow-band noise through loudspeakers can be plotted using a "W" to denote thresholds for the former and "NBN" for the latter.

The audiogram indicates whether hearing is normal or impaired and, if hearing is impaired, the nature and degree of the hearing loss. Several guidelines can be used to retrieve this information from the audiogram. The decision as to whether certain results indicate normal or impaired hearing has been the subject of considerable disagreement among various clinicians and investigators, particularly in the context of hearing loss in children. It has been suggested that impairment begins when the PTA exceeds 25 dB HL (ANSI, 1969), but this is based on adult data. Northern and Downs (1984) suggest that significant impairment begins when

*Owing to equipment limitations, bone-conduction thresholds are not tested for an 8000-Hz stimulus.

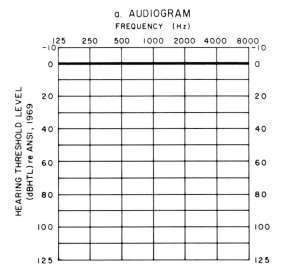

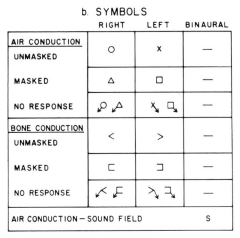

Figure 9–1. The audiogram (a) and the symbols (b) used to denote hearing thresholds suggested by the American Speech and Hearing Association (1974).

the average threshold exceeds 15 dB HL, and such children may benefit from trial amplification with a hearing aid. As a compromise, one may consider 20 dB HL as the limit of normal hearing, with impairment beginning when air-conducted sound thresholds exceed this level. As we shall see, however, this compromise may overlook significant conductive hearing loss.

Consequently, when the air and bone conduction thresholds of a given child are equal (or within 10 dB of each other) and 20 dB HL or better, hearing is within normal limits. When the audiogram reflects impaired hearing, the relative threshold of air and bone conduction will indicate the nature of the hearing loss—conductive, sensorineural, or mixed.

The audiogram of a child with a conductive hearing loss shows normal bone conduction thresholds and elevated air conduction thresholds (Fig. 9–2A). The exception to this general guideline would be a case in which air conduction thresholds were within the 20 dB normal limit but the bone conduction thresholds were at least 15 dB better. In other words, the bone

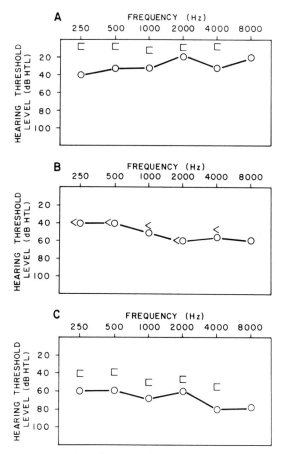

Figure 9–2. Sample audiograms showing three different types of hearing loss in the right ear: *A*, conductive hearing loss; *B*, sensorineural hearing loss; and *C*, mixed hearing loss.

conduction scores could be −5 or 0 dB HL, and the air conduction scores would be 15 or 20 dB HL. This, too, would be considered a conductive impairment owing to the significant air-bone "gap" of 15 dB or more.

The nature of the hearing loss is sensorineural when the audiogram shows both air and bone conduction thresholds to be elevated but within 10 dB of each other (Fig. 9–2*B*). When both air and bone conduction thresholds are elevated but are separated by more than 10 dB, the hearing loss is mixed in nature, as shown in Figure 9–2*C*.

Aside from indicating the nature of the hearing impairment, if any, the audiogram also suggests the degree of impairment based on the average decibel threshold elevation for air conduction scores at 500, 1000, and 2000 Hz. A preferable way of denoting the degree of hearing loss in a child is to rate the loss as mild, moderate, moderately severe, severe, or profound. The average hearing thresholds (ANSI, 1969) associated with these ratings are 21 to 40 dB (mild), 41 to 55 dB (moderate), 56 to 70 dB (moderately severe), 71 to 90 dB (severe), and 91 dB or greater (profound).

Hence, the audiogram can describe the nature and the degree of hearing impairment. This information, along with much more, is helpful in estimating the

handicap a child might realize. In this context, a description of the loss as either unilateral or bilateral is relevant. A bilateral impairment has more serious implications than a unilateral loss. However, Bess and Tharpe (1984) and Matkin (1986) have independently concluded that children with unilateral hearing loss are educationally handicapped. Limited ability to hear optimally in the poor signal-to-noise ratios common in classrooms seems to be a major factor. Schwartz and Bess (Chapter 96) present an interesting discussion of the impact of unilateral versus bilateral impairment.

The effects of bilateral hearing impairment on a child's function will depend, in part, on the degree of impairment, whether the impairment is conductive or sensorineural, and, if sensorineural, whether the loss is congenital or acquired. Downs (1974) outlined the interplay of these factors, and her suggestions are shown in Table 9–2. The more severe the hearing loss, and the earlier the onset with respect to language acquisition, the more factors other than the hearing loss influence the child's outcome. Brookhouser and Moeller (1986) have suggested that factors such as parental involvement, intelligence, medical status, and multiple handicaps are at least as important to the ability of the severely hearing-impaired child to achieve academically and to learn language and speech as the degree and the configuration of the hearing loss.

Behavioral Assessment Techniques—Summary

The material presented thus far has shown that a variety of age-dependent behavioral techniques are available for the audiologic assessment of neonates, infants, and young children. Ordinarily, the techniques for neonates and infants up to about 5 or 6 months of age provide only qualitative information about the auditory function of the child in question (hearing is either normal or impaired). At about 6 months of age, quantitative threshold information is obtainable with some behavioral techniques, particularly those involving conditioning procedures. By 3 years of age, most children can be assessed with "play" audiometric techniques. From this age, a pure-tone audiogram, which can indicate the nature and degree of impairment, is obtainable.

The various assessment techniques rely on a continuum of auditory responsivity from gross auditory reflexes to refined voluntary responses. Certain techniques are better suited for evaluating behavior at opposite ends of this continuum, whereas other techniques (e.g., VRA and TROCA) can assess responsivity throughout the continuum. By knowing where on the continuum the child falls, the appropriate test can be employed, and the judgment as to whether the hearing is normal or impaired can be made on the basis of the appropriateness of the child's responses.

PHYSIOLOGIC ASSESSMENT TECHNIQUES

Obtaining a reliable test of hearing in the pediatric patient can be difficult when using behavioral test

TABLE 9–2. Probable Handicapped Conditions Associated with Hearing Loss

CONDUCTIVE HEARING LOSS

Condition	Degree of Loss at Present	Probable Effect on Function
Evidence of past ear disease 1. Perforation 2. Scarring	5–20 dB	1. Subtle auditory dysfunction 2. Infantile speech 3. Articulation problems 4. Language retardation
Serous otitis	10–30 dB	1. Inattention 2. Speech and language retardation if persistent
Chronic otitis	15–55 dB	1. Inattention 2. Speech and language retardation if persistent
Middle-ear anomaly	30–65 dB	1. Marked articulation problems 2. Serious language retardation

SENSORINEURAL HEARING LOSS

Condition	Degree of Loss	Probable Effect on Function	
Congenital loss	25–40 dB	Mild speech and language retardation	
	40–65 dB	Moderate to severe speech and language retardation	
	70–85 dB	Severe speech and language retardation	If habilitation is not started very early
	85 dB +	No speech or language	
Acquired loss	25–100 dB	If acquired after 2 years of age, speech and language need not be retarded if rehabilitation begins promptly. Speech deterioration occurs if loss is profound.	

From Downs, 1974, personal communication.

methods. Therefore, tests that do not require a behavioral response are quite helpful to the pediatric audiologist and otolaryngologist. The two physiologic assessment techniques most often used are acoustic immittance measures (admittance or impedance) and auditory evoked potentials. Both tests are often considered "objective" tests because rather than requiring a voluntary response from the patient, they take advantage of naturally occurring physiologic responses. However, the information obtained by such tests must still be interpreted by a human observer and is still susceptible to artifact and error. Therefore, the objectivity of such tests should be treated with a healthy skepticism.

Acoustic Immittance Measurements

Immittance is a term used to describe the transfer of acoustic energy, whether measured in terms of acoustic admittance (flow of energy) or acoustic impedance (opposition to flow of energy). Admittance and impedance are reciprocals and so provide similar information in a different way. Clinical immittance measures, which are measures of either acoustic admittance or acoustic impedance at the tympanic membrane, provide information from which inferences about the integrity of the entire middle-ear system can be made. Immittance measures commonly used are tympanometry, static acoustic immittance, and immittance changes that result from the stapedial reflex. They can be used with adults as well as children but are particularly valuable in children because they require little cooperation and no voluntary response from the patient. Also, among children, there is a high prevalence of middle-ear disease, especially otitis media with effusion, which can be identified and monitored with reliability and ease using immittance measures.

To fully understand and interpret acoustic immittance test results, one should first have an understanding of the basic underlying physical principles. Only a brief introduction to some of the many and complex factors involved in acoustic immittance is presented here. The interested reader should consult Margolis (1981), Northern and Grimes (1978), Van Camp and colleagues (1986), Van Camp and Creten (1976), and Wiley and Block (1985) for more comprehensive information on the development of acoustic immittance instruments and the principles of acoustic immittance testing.

Impedance Versus Admittance

IMPEDANCE. The opposition to the flow of acoustic energy that is attributable to mass and stiffness is called *reactance*. In reactance, energy is stored. That portion of reactance that is due to stiffness is called negative, or compliant, reactance, and that part attributable to mass is called positive, or mass, reactance. *Resistance* is the portion of the impedance attributable to friction in the system, in which case, energy is dissipated. If a system has stiffness and mass, the overall reactance will be the sum of the two reactances contributed. Because one component is negative (compliant) and the other is positive (mass), the absolute magnitude of the reactance will be *less* than either one alone. The reactance and the resistance together determine the total impedance. However, because the reactance and the resistance are out of phase with each other, the combining of components requires the use of complex (i.e., real and imaginary) numbers, which, for simplicity, are not discussed in this chapter. Mass reactance is proportional to frequency, and compliant reactance is inversely proportional to frequency; thus, their relative effects depend on the frequency of the driving force. Compliant reactance increases as frequency decreases. Mass reactance increases with increases in frequency. If a system has greater compliant reactance than mass reactance, it is called a stiffness-controlled system. If a system has greater mass reactance, it is called a mass-controlled system.

ADMITTANCE. The reciprocal of impedance is admittance. The terms used to describe the components of admittance are susceptance (the reciprocal of reactance) and conductance (the reciprocal of resistance). The reciprocal of negative (compliant) reactance is positive susceptance or compliance. The reciprocal of positive (mass) reactance is negative susceptance.

Middle-Ear Immittance

The middle-ear system has all three elements of the mechanical systems previously described. There is stiffness provided by the tympanic membrane, ossicular chain, and the volume of air in the middle ear. Mass is provided primarily by the ossicles. The resistance (or conductance) component comes primarily from the cochlea.

The basis for acoustic immittance testing in the auditory system is the ability to determine the input acoustic immittance of the middle-ear system at the tympanic membrane. This is done by introducing a controlled force (sound pressure in the form of a probe tone) into the ear canal and measuring the resulting sound pressure level (SPL). The degree to which the middle ear permits the flow of acoustic energy determines how much acoustic energy will be reflected from the tympanic membrane and, as a result, how much can be measured in the ear canal. The SPL of the signal in the ear canal is proportional to the immittance in the system (Wiley and Block, 1985). The greater the flow of acoustic energy through the middle ear (greater admittance, less impedance), the lower the overall SPL in the ear canal. The poorer the flow of acoustic energy through the middle ear (less admit-

tance, greater impedance), the greater the SPL in the ear canal.

Probe-Tone Effects

The normally functioning middle-ear system is a stiffness-controlled system when immittance is measured using a low-frequency probe tone (e.g., 220 Hz). For all practical purposes, the measure is one of compliant reactance (or compliance). For this reason, acoustic immittance measures using a low-frequency probe tone are often called measures of middle-ear compliance. The measure may be reported in terms of a volume of air (ml or cc) with equivalent compliance.

Some instruments incorporate a higher-frequency probe tone in addition to one around 220 Hz. A probe tone of about 660 Hz is closer to the resonant frequency of the middle ear and is less dominated by the stiffness in the system. A change in the stiffness of the middle ear resulting from a pathologic condition will cause a greater proportional change in immittance with a high-frequency probe tone than with a low-frequency probe tone, making abnormalities easier to detect with the higher-frequency probe. This is true for pathologic conditions that increase stiffness (e.g., otosclerosis) as well as those that decrease stiffness (e.g., disarticulation of the ossicles) (Fig. 9–3). In addition, the high-frequency probe tone is a more sensitive indicator of

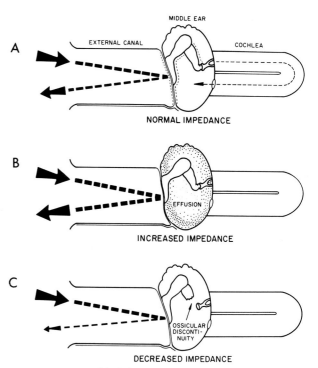

Figure 9–3. A simplified diagram demonstrating that middle-ear conditions influence impedance and, consequently, the transmission/reflection of an input sound. In the normal ear (*A*), more input sound energy is transmitted than is reflected. The increased impedance caused by a middle-ear effusion (*B*) results in a decrease in transmitted energy and an increase in the amount reflected. An ossicular discontinuity (*C*) results in decreased impedance and an increase in transmitted energy with a much smaller proportion of reflected energy (even less than observed in the normal ear).

changes in mass, such as those that accompany cholesteatoma and adhesions.

Instrumentation

Instruments measure or report immittance values in different ways. Some use impedance values (Z) and some admittance values (Y). Some also have circuitry that permits the separation of admittance into its susceptance (B) and conductance (G) components. Combined with low- and high-frequency probe tones, the capability to evaluate in detail the immittance characteristics of the middle-ear system is greatly enhanced when there is separation of the B and G components. As shown later, some characteristics of the abnormal middle-ear system can be obscured when one assumes that there is only a stiffness-controlled system and uses only a low-frequency probe tone.

In clinical immittance measuring systems, the probe signal is introduced into the ear canal via a probe assembly and tip made to fit snugly into the ear canal. The assembly includes a driver, or transducer, to deliver the probe signal to the ear and a microphone used in the measurement of ear-canal SPL. The other important component of the delivery system is a pump that allows the tester to vary the pressure in the ear canal. Figure 9–4 is a simplified diagram of an electroacoustic impedance bridge. When the probe assembly is fit hermetically into the ear canal with the soft tip, acoustic immittance of the ear canal and middle-ear system can be measured with different amounts of air pressure in the ear canal. That is, the air pressure in the ear canal can be increased or decreased with the pump, and changes in the SPL of the probe signal in the ear canal can be used to derive measures of immittance. The changes in immittance as a function of changing air pressure in the ear canal are plotted graphically as a tympanogram.

The different types of immittance instruments previously described are found in many clinics and practitioners' offices. First, a review of the information provided by the impedance bridge using a 220-Hz probe tone will be described. Much of the early clinical study in immittance testing was based on the system with low-frequency probe tone and relative, or arbitrary, measures of "compliance." Following that, a description of the admittance meter will be provided to illustrate the use of both low- and high-frequency probe-tone immittance, with separation of the susceptance (B) and conductance (G) components.

Tympanometry with Impedance Instrument

The interaction of the impedance bridge and the ear in generating a tympanogram can be understood with the assistance of Figure 9–5. With 200 mm H_2O pressure in the ear canal, the tympanic membrane is effectively clamped, and compliance is minimal (Fig. 9–5). In our example, impedance changes are recorded in arbitrary units. Some impedance instruments record impedance changes using absolute physical units (ml or cc) by using a slightly different electronic design than that described earlier. The impedance bridge is arbitrarily set to a value corresponding to minimal compliance, and the plotter begins recording at the intersection of +200 mm H_2O and minimal compliance. As pressure is decreased, the tympanogram begins to rise, indicating increased compliance. As pressure is decreased further, the tympanogram will continue to rise until, at a certain air pressure value, it reverses direction and begins to fall (Fig. 9–5). This reversal indicates that compliance is now decreasing.

Consequently, tympanic membrane compliance is maximal at the point where the tympanogram reverses direction. This reversal point is often called the "peak" of the tympanogram (Fig. 9–5C).

The tympanogram can be interpreted on the basis of three features: (1) the height of the peak, (2) the horizontal position of the peak in relation to atmospheric pressure, and (3) the rate of change in the curve height at the peak—the peak gradient (Brooks, 1969).

The height of the tympanogram peak reflects the degree of tympanic membrane compliance and the relative mobility of at least a portion of the membrane. The peak is normally located between half and full

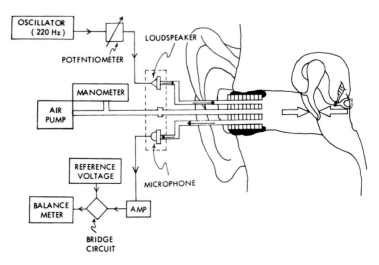

Figure 9–4. A component diagram of the electroacoustic impedance bridge.

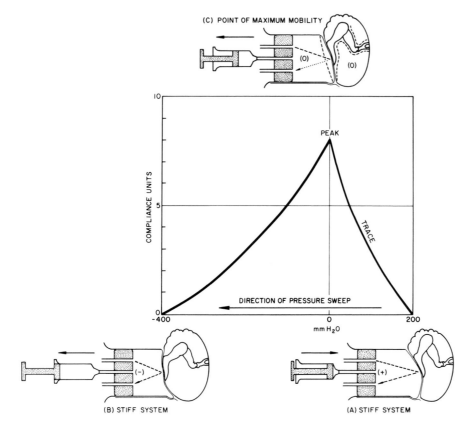

Figure 9–5. The interaction of the impedance bridge and the ear in the generation of a tympanogram (see text).

vertical scale on the tympanogram recorded using arbitrary units. A peak height of less than half scale is generally associated with middle-ear conditions that reduce compliance or mobility. A peak height exceeding full vertical scale deflection is generally associated with conditions that increase compliance or mobility. For instruments reporting in equivalent volume units (ml or cc), normative values are similar to those reported later for admittance instruments using a low-frequency probe tone.

The horizontal location of the tympanogram peak in relation to atmospheric pressure gives an indirect approximation of the air pressure in the middle-ear space. This is based on the principle that tympanic membrane compliance is maximal when the air pressure on both sides of the membrane is the same (Terkildsen and Thomsen, 1959). A number of investigators (Flisberg et al., 1963; Ingelstedt et al., 1967; Peterson and Liden, 1970; Elner et al., 1971; Renvall et al., 1975) have demonstrated that the tympanometrically determined and actual middle-ear pressures can differ and that the air pressure suggested by the tympanogram is influenced by tympanic membrane mobility and the volume of the middle-ear space. Although the tympanometrically determined pressure may not be precisely that of the middle-ear space, the horizontal position of the peak gives a general indication of pressure conditions in the middle ear, and it is consequently helpful in interpreting the tympanogram.

Figure 9–6 demonstrates how shifts in the horizontal position of the tympanogram peak reflect pressure conditions in the middle ear. Positive and negative pressures produce corresponding shifts in the horizontal peak position, and in fact the absence of a peak can reflect extreme negative pressure in the middle-ear space.

The normal range of tympanometric peak pressure has been the subject of some debate, and several values have been reported (Brooks, 1969; Jerger, 1970; Holmquist and Miller, 1972; Renvall et al., 1973; Paradise et al., 1976). In young children, there is support (Paradise et al., 1976; Schwartz et al., 1978) for a range of -150 to 50 mm H_2O pressure, inclusive, as normal. Deviations from this range can be rated as either abnormally negative or positive peak pressure. In children, it should be realized that middle-ear pressure tends to fluctuate from day to day (Cooper et al., 1974; Lewis et al., 1975; Schwartz et al., 1978), and a determination of abnormal pressure should be made on the basis of the persistence of the condition with time.

It follows that the height and horizontal position of the tympanogram peak, respectively, indicate tympanic membrane mobility and air pressure in the middle-ear space. The gradient of the peak is also worthy of consideration. Recall that this feature represents the rate of change in curve height in the region of the peak. Typically, the gradient is rated as either "sharp" or "gradual." A gradual peak gradient implies a slower rate of change in curve height, which in turn implies a subtle degree of tympanic membrane "sluggishness" or a general dampening of the system's responsiveness to changes in external conditions. Gradient of the curve is a particularly pertinent feature in

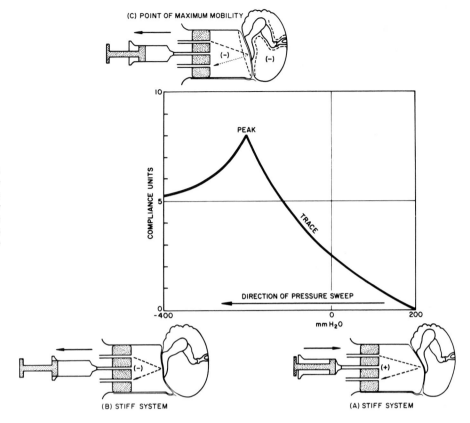

Figure 9–6. The manner in which the tympanogram can reflect negative air pressure in the middle ear. Compliance is low when positive pressure (A) or negative pressure (B) is applied. The air pressure at the peak of the trace is an approximation of middle-ear pressure (C).

the tympanograms of children, since it has been found to be related to the presence of otitis media with effusion (Paradise et al., 1976; Fiellau-Nikolajsen, 1983).

Figure 9–7 illustrates some commonly encountered types of tympanograms, with their associated middle-ear pressures, tympanic membrane compliances, and presumptive conditions of the middle ear. This figure demonstrates how, in a very general way, the status of the middle ear can be inferred from the tympanogram. To make such an inference, one must consider pressure and mobility of the tympanic membrane and, in certain instances, peak gradient of the tympanogram curve.

Figure 9–7 is intended to present general principles for the interpretation of tympanograms on the basis of pressure mobility and peak gradient. The reader must realize that the implied one-to-one relationship between tympanogram shape and specific middle-ear conditions is an oversimplification. The conditions are "presumed" to be associated with given tympanograms, or, in other words, they are the "probable" associated conditions. There will be exceptions to the apparently simple relationships shown in Figure 9–7, and tympanograms must be interpreted in the context of other clinical information. For example, otoscopic examination and acoustic middle-ear muscle reflex tests are important to the interpretation of tympanometric findings.

Several authors (Jerger, 1970; Liden et al., 1970; Paradise et al., 1976; Feldman, 1978) have suggested grouping various tympanograms into specific categories

or types to facilitate their interpretation. The tympanogram categorizations of Jerger (1970) and Paradise and colleagues (1976) are of particular interest; the former has received widespread clinical use, and the latter is relevant to the pediatric population.

Jerger's (1970) classification has been used widely in the clinical setting, but it is based on only two of the three tympanogram features—peak height and horizontal position. The tympanogram types suggested by Jerger (1970) tend to oversimplify interpretation and are not validated, but since they are used in many centers, they will be given brief mention here (Fig. 9–8).

In Jerger's tympanogram types A, A_S, and A_D the peaks are all placed horizontally to approximate atmospheric pressure ($\pm$ 100 mm H_2O), but the peak heights differ. The Type A tympanogram has a peak height between half and full scale on the ordinate, and it is associated with a normal middle-ear system. Type A_S has a shallow peak, less than half scale on the ordinate, and is associated with conditions such as ossicular fixation and a thickened tympanic membrane in which the middle-ear system demonstrates decreased mobility. The Type A_D tympanogram has a peak that exceeds full scale on the ordinate and is associated with a highly compliant system such as that found in ossicular disruption.

Jerger (1970) also described Type B and C tympanograms. Type B is the tympanogram with no peak and is associated with otitis media with effusion, tympanic membrane perforation, or impacted cerumen. Type C tympanograms show a horizontal peak position

TYMPANOGRAM	PRESSURE	MOBILITY	PRESUMED TYMPANIC MEM-BRANE/MIDDLE EAR CONDITION
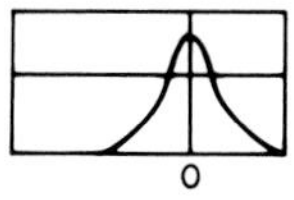	NORMAL	NORMAL	NORMAL
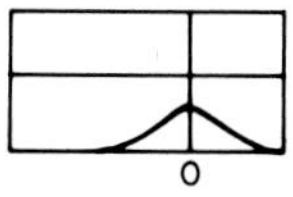	NORMAL	LOW	MIDDLE EAR EFFUSION, &/OR THICKENED TYMPANIC MEM-BRANE, &/OR OSSICULAR FIX-ATION
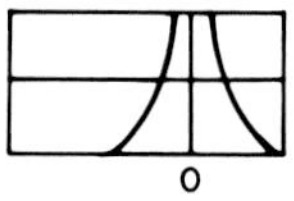	NORMAL	HIGH	FLACCID TYMPANIC MEM-BRANE OR OSSICULAR DISCON-TINUITY
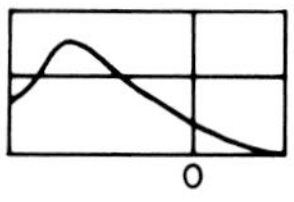	NEGATIVE	NORMAL	HIGH NEGATIVE PRESSURE WITH OR WITHOUT MIDDLE EAR EFFUSION
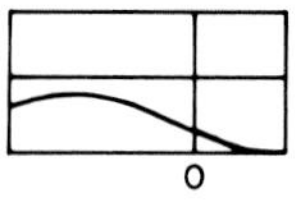	NEGATIVE	LOW	MIDDLE EAR EFFUSION, &/OR THICKENED TYMPANIC MEM-BRANE, &/OR OSSICULAR FIX-ATION
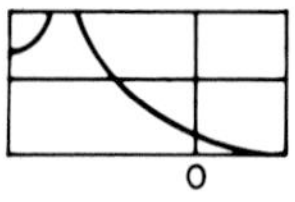	NEGATIVE	HIGH	FLACCID TYMPANIC MEMBRANE & HIGH NEGATIVE PRESSURE (OR OSSICULAR DISCONTINUITY & HIGH NEGATIVE PRESSURE)
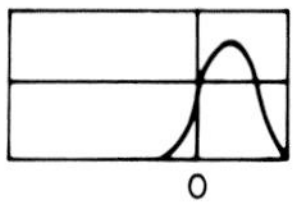	POSITIVE	NORMAL	HIGH POSITIVE PRESSURE WITH OR WITHOUT MIDDLE EAR EFFUSION

Figure 9–7. Tympanogram types and property variants related to clinical findings.

at a pressure more negative than -100 mm H_2O and are generally associated with eustachian tube dysfunction.

It is of particular interest in children to identify those tympanogram types that are associated with the presence of otitis media with effusion. Several investigators (Jerger et al., 1974b; Paradise et al., 1976; Orchik et al., 1978) have confirmed the association of the so-called Type B tympanogram with effusion, but with one exception (Paradise et al., 1976), these authors concluded that other tympanogram types are poor predictors of the presence of otitis media.

Paradise and coworkers (1976) found that the probability of otitis media with effusion being present was, in tympanograms of other than Type B (which they called Type EFF), related to the gradient of the tympanogram peak and to a lesser extent to the height of the peak. These authors divided tympanogram shapes into seven types on the basis of the horizontal position, height, and gradient of the peak. These types represented regions on the tympanogram as shown in Figure 9–9. The regions included normal (NL), high negative pressure (HN), high positive pressure (HP), transitional (TR), and effusion (EFF). The percentages shown in Figure 9–9 denote the probability that ears with that tympanogram type contained effusions. The authors studied 141 children between the ages of 7 months and 6 years; the data are based on these

examinations. The figure also shows a percentage dichotomy for the HN and TR regions. Tympanograms falling in these regions were found to reflect a higher probability of effusion if the peak gradient was gradual (g) rather than sharp (s).

Paradise and associates (1976) consequently found that tympanogram shapes or variants could be grouped into seven types—NL, HN-s, HN-g, HP, TR-s, TR-g, and EEF—and that these types were useful in detecting effusion in the children they studied.

Tympanometry with Admittance Instrument

When total admittance (Y) is measured using a low-frequency probe tone, tympanometric shape is very similar to that obtained using an impedance bridge as previously described. Admittance is measured in absolute units (millimhos or mmhos) or equivalent volume (ml or cc) rather than arbitrary units, so information regarding actual transfer of acoustic energy can be derived directly from the tympanogram.

Variations in tympanogram shape can occur when admittance is separated into the susceptance (B) and conductance (G) components and when a higher-frequency probe tone is used. A scheme for categorizing middle-ear status using Y, B, and G tympanograms was proposed by Vanhuyse and associates (1975) and has been discussed by Margolis and Shanks (1985) and

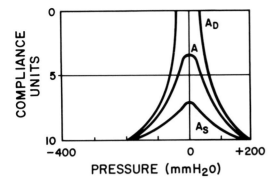

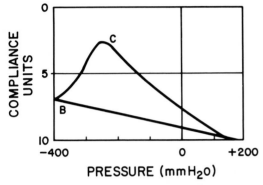

Figure 9–8. Tympanogram classification according to Jerger (1970): A, A_D, A_S (top graph) and B and C (bottom graph).

Van Camp and coworkers (1986). A detailed review of the categorization scheme is beyond the scope of this chapter, but some general relationships between the different tympanograms will be presented.

In most normal ears, the Y, B, and G tympanograms maintain the shape of the normal tympanograms illustrated in the previous section. However, the use of the high-frequency probe tone will sometimes cause

notching (Fig. 9–10) in the B, and perhaps the Y, tympanograms in a normal ear.

In cases of middle-ear effusion, the tympanometric shapes are generally flat or rounded. Gradient (shape) has been quantified in a variety of ways using admittance measures and low-frequency probe tones (de Jonge, 1986; Koebsell and Margolis, 1986). Margolis and Heller (1987) found that gradient was the single most useful tympanometric variable in identifying young children for medical referral. The Y and B tympanograms with a 220-Hz probe tone often will be quite similar because the admittance is predominated by the compliance in a stiffening pathologic condition such as otitis media with effusion. The flat tympanogram can be recorded in cases of probe-tip occlusion due to wax or canal wall or due to an opening in the tympanic membrane from a perforation or tympanostomy tube. An estimate of ear canal volume provides a good indication of the problem in either of those cases. In small children, a measure of greater than 1.5 cc at 220 Hz is suggestive of an opening in the tympanic membrane.

In other stiffening pathologic conditions, such as otosclerosis or other forms of ossicular fixation, the tympanograms have peaks of reduced amplitude. Sometimes, such a tympanometric configuration is difficult to discern from a normal tympanogram, but it is in such a case that the higher frequency probe tone can be of value. In a normal middle-ear system, the peak susceptance (B) and peak conductance (G) should have similar values when the high-frequency probe is used. However, in cases of fixation, the patterns will be separated, with the susceptance being much greater than the conductance.

In ears with ossicular discontinuity or other conditions that increase the admittance of the system,

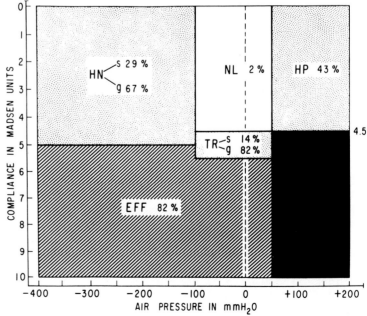

Figure 9–9. Tympanogram classification suggested by Paradise and colleagues (1976). Percentages denote the associated incidence of effusion.

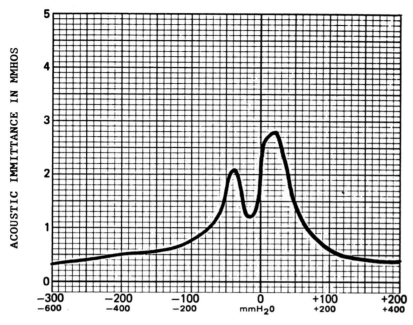

Figure 9–10. Hand-drawn example of a "notched" tympanogram. Abscissa (mm H₂O) reflects two possible ranges, selectable at the time of the test. Ordinate is in acoustic mmho (see text).

sometimes a broad, shallow notching can occur in the B tympanogram, whereas the Y and G tympanograms appear normal. This occurs with both low- and high-frequency probe tones, although there are some normal ears that produce a similar configuration with the high-frequency tone. Tympanic membrane abnormalities can cause similar tympanograms. Also, ears with abnormally high admittance characteristics may produce notching in all three tympanograms (Y, B, and G) when the high-frequency probe tone is used. This rarely occurs in normal ears and does not occur using the low-frequency probe tone.

There are some things to be aware of when performing tympanometry and interpreting tympanometric information. First is the understanding that the immittance of the system is measured at the plane of the tympanic membrane. If there are abnormalities of the tympanic membrane that cause it to have very high admittance, such as scarring, the lower admittance of the rest of the system will be obscured in the measurement. The high admittance of the tympanic membrane will be recorded, and the remainder of the system will not reveal its ability to transfer acoustic energy.

Also, differences in instrumentation can cause differences in tympanometric configuration. The rate and the direction of air pressure change, for example, can cause differences in peak pressure and amplitude from one instrument to the next.

TYMPANOMETRY WITH INFANTS. Tympanometry with infants younger than 6 months of age is controversial. Paradise and colleagues (1976) found that impedance testing using a 220-Hz probe tone was not sensitive in identifying ears filled with fluid in young infants. Apparently, compliance of the ear canal wall interferes with the recording of impedance at the tympanic membrane. More recently, Marchant and colleagues

(1986) reported success in identifying otitis media with effusion in young infants, using a 660-Hz probe tone and the susceptance (B) tympanogram. Static admittance greater than 0 mmho correctly indicated effusion (as determined by myringotomy) in a high percentage of ears of young infants. Northern (1988) has also suggested that tympanometry provides useful diagnostic information in infants. However, Margolis and Shanks (1985), in reviewing data from infant studies, have concluded that the utility of tympanometry in young infants has not yet been determined adequately and that additional research is required.

Tympanometry, then, is a graphic representation of tympanic membrane immittance when air pressure is varied in the ear canal. The tympanogram provides an estimate of middle-ear pressure and tympanic membrane mobility. The tympanogram peak height, horizontal position, and gradient can be used to infer the status of the middle ear. However, tympanometry is only one of three acoustic impedance measurements, and clinical judgments should not be made without consideration of static immittance measurements and the results of the acoustic middle-ear muscle reflex test. In addition, the results of the entire battery of acoustic immittance tests must be viewed in the context of other clinical findings.

Static Immittance Measurements

IMPEDANCE BRIDGE: 220-Hz PROBE TONE. Static immittance measurements compare tympanic membrane immittance under two air pressure conditions: (1) with 200 mm H₂O pressure in the ear canal and (2) with a pressure in the canal that corresponds to the tympanometric peak pressure. Using the 220-Hz probe tone, the static immittance is virtually equivalent to compliant reactance and is often reported in terms of the volume of air (in ml or cc) with equivalent compliance. The compliance under the first condition is subtracted from that under the second condition, and the result is an estimate of the compliance of the middle-ear system. The reason for the subtraction is to eliminate the contribution of the volume of air in the ear canal (i.e., between the probe tip and the tympanic membrane) from the total estimate of compliance. This yields the compliance of the middle-ear system alone. Determining static impedance in kOhms requires some computation and is not readily estimated from the tympanogram itself.

Extremely stiff middle-ear systems generally yield very low static compliance values, and extremely compliant systems yield very high values. However, between these extremes, the static compliance values of normal and abnormal systems tend to overlap. The extent of this overlap has essentially precluded using static compliance measurements as clinically important indicators of pathologic conditions.

When the tympanogram shows negative middle-ear pressure and reduced mobility with little or no evidence of a peak, the static compliance value with 200 mm H_2O in the ear canal can be important. In these situations, a low compliance value (less than 0.4 cc) can suggest the presence of excessive cerumen or that the probe tip is resting against the canal wall. A high compliance value (greater than 1.5 cc) is suggestive of an opening in the tympanic membrane; this could be due to a perforation or the presence of a patent tympanostomy tube. Lower compliance values are found in infants and small children, for whom 1.0 or 1.5 cc may be the upper limit.

Consequently, the static compliance value with 200 mm H_2O in the ear canal can be used to confirm the reliability of the tympanogram and to detect a tympanic membrane perforation or patent tympanostomy tube. The application of this compliance value has been termed the physical volume test (PVT) by Northern and Grimes (1978) and is reported as such by some clinicians.

ADMITTANCE—220-Hz PROBE TONE. Static compliance using an admittance meter is done in essentially the same way as with the impedance bridge. However, there is an advantage in using the admittance meter, because the static admittance may be provided in units of equivalent volume (ml or cc) or in absolute units (mmho), which can be extracted directly from the tympanogram. The admittance at either very high or very low ear canal air pressure, whichever gives the lower admittance value, should be subtracted from the admittance at the tympanogram peak. The static admittance is the difference, then, between the maximum (ear canal and middle ear) and the minimum (ear canal alone) admittance values recorded on the tympanogram.

Van Camp and associates (1986) have suggested norms for static acoustic admittance. First, they suggest that values be obtained using only the low-frequency probe tone, because it is more difficult to estimate ear canal volume when the tympanogram is notched, an occurrence more common with the high-frequency probe tone, and because of error associated with measuring ear canal volume using the high-frequency probe. They report that the range of static admittance values (in acoustic mmho) for adults is 0.50 to 1.75 for pump speeds less than 50 daPa/second and 0.57 to 2.0 for a pump speed of 200 daPa/second. Children between 3 and 5 years of age have lower static admittance values and were reported separately by Van Camp and colleagues (1986). In this younger group, the range was 0.35 to 0.90 for the slower pump speeds and 0.4 to 1.03 for the faster pump speed.

Acoustic Middle-Ear Muscle Reflex

Acoustic impedance instrumentation can be used also to detect the contraction of the middle-ear muscles, the stapedius and tensor tympani, to intense sound stimulation. This contraction is called the acoustic middle-ear muscle reflex or simply the acoustic reflex.

The anatomy of the acoustic reflex arc is described in Chapter 7. The afferent portion of the arc, up to and including the superior olivary complex, is shared with the hearing mechanism. The efferent fibers of the acoustic reflex arc arise from brain stem neuronal connections between the olivary complex and the facial nerve nucleus for the stapedius muscle and the trigeminal nerve nucleus for the tensor tympani muscle (Jepsen, 1963).

The acoustic immittance instrument indicates the status of the acoustic reflex in two ways: first, the reflex results in a stiffening of the ossicular chain and a concomitant change in immittance; second, because the reflex is bilateral to a unilateral stimulus (the muscles of both sides contract when one ear is stimulated), an earphone can be placed on one ear to deliver an intense stimulus, and the probe tip of the immittance instrument inserted in the opposite ear can detect the change in immittance caused by the reflex.

When the immittance instrument is used to detect an acoustic reflex elicited by stimulating the opposite ear, the response is commonly called the contralateral, or crossed, acoustic reflex. Many acoustic immittance instruments marketed today have probe tips designed both to stimulate and to detect the acoustic reflex in the same ear; the reflex is elicited and its effect on immittance is detected in the same ear. Under these conditions, the response is called the ipsilateral, or uncrossed, acoustic reflex.

For clinical purposes, three acoustic reflex parameters are commonly considered. These include the reflex threshold intensity, its response amplitude decay in time, and the differential response to different types of sound stimuli. These features enable the examiner to make qualitative judgments about hearing, such as the type of impairment and the probable site of a lesion, as well as quantitative judgments, such as an estimation of the degree of hearing loss and hearing aid effectiveness.

The threshold of the acoustic reflex is operationally

defined as the minimal stimulus intensity required to produce an observable change in monitored immittance. This minimal intensity, or acoustic reflex threshold, is typically specified as a certain number of decibels (dB) referenced to either "sensation level" or "hearing level." Sensation level (SL) refers to the individual's behavioral hearing threshold for a given stimulus, and hearing level (HL) refers to normal hearing for a group of young adults (i.e., 0 dB on the audiogram). For example, a reflex threshold of 85 dB HL for a 1000-Hz pure tone can also be expressed as 85 dB SL if the individual's hearing threshold for that stimulus is 0 dB HL. If the individual's hearing threshold for the same 1000-Hz pure tone is 30 dB HL, then the reflex threshold of 85 dB HL can also be expressed as 55 dB SL. These relationships between sensation level and hearing level are important to an understanding of the acoustic reflex parameters.

In adults with normal hearing, the contralateral acoustic reflex threshold for pure tones of different frequencies is approximately 85 dB poorer than behavioral hearing thresholds (i.e., 85 dB SL). The range of effective stimulus intensities is 70 to 95 dB SL (Metz, 1952; Jepsen, 1963; Alberti and Kristensen, 1970; Jerger, 1970). Approximately 20 dB less intensity is required to elicit a reflex with a broad-band noise stimulus (Metz, 1952; Jepsen, 1963; Skinner et al., 1978). Ipsilateral reflex thresholds are approximately 10 dB better than contralateral thresholds (Møller, 1962; Fria et al., 1975).

Age is an important factor relating to the presence of the acoustic reflex and its threshold. Only a small percentage of neonates exhibit an acoustic reflex when an impedance bridge with a 220-Hz probe-tone frequency is used to detect the response (Kieth, 1971; McCandless and Allred, 1978). McCandless and Allred (1978) found that significantly more neonates (89 per cent) yielded acoustic reflexes if a bridge with a 660-Hz probe-tone frequency was employed. In one population of 1600 ears of school-age children (Liden and Renvall, 1978), 13 per cent had absent acoustic reflexes.

When the acoustic reflex is present in infants and young children, its threshold is slightly higher than that found in adults (Jepsen, 1963; Robertson et al., 1968). Average thresholds in neonates and infants approximate 95 dB HL (Kieth, 1971; McCandless and Allred, 1978). In school-age children the threshold is on the average 92 dB HL (Liden and Renvall, 1978). The adult with normal hearing, on the other hand, has an average threshold of about 85 dB HL (Metz, 1952; Jepsen, 1963; Jerger, 1970).

Various types of hearing impairment can influence the acoustic reflex. As Jerger and colleagues (1978) point out, the influence on the acoustic reflex of sensorineural impairment of cochlear origin is complex, but generally less difference exists between hearing and reflex thresholds (Metz, 1952). The reflex can occur at about the same absolute level as found in normal ears, but because of the elevated hearing threshold, ears with a sensorineural impairment ap-

parently require less stimulus intensity above the hearing threshold to elicit the responses. Jerger and associates (1972) reported that the likelihood of eliciting the acoustic reflex was significantly reduced when the degree of sensorineural hearing loss exceeded 80 dB HL.

The influence of middle-ear impairment and attendant conductive hearing loss on the reflex is not as straightforward, as a result of the mode of reflex stimulation. Recall that ipsilateral acoustic reflex tests stimulate and detect the response in the same ear through the immittance instrument probe-tip assembly. In an impaired middle ear, the impedance is already abnormally altered, and further changes in impedance due to middle-ear muscle contraction may not be observable; to be detectable, these changes may require elevated stimulus intensity levels.

It follows that ipsilateral acoustic reflex testing in an impaired middle ear will most probably yield no response; if the response is present, the threshold of the response will tend to be elevated.

The influence of middle-ear impairment on the contralateral acoustic reflex may be somewhat harder to understand. The contralateral reflex will probably be absent if the middle ear having the probe-tip assembly is impaired or if the impaired middle ear having the stimulus earphone has a moderate to moderately severe conductive hearing loss (Jerger et al., 1974c). The reason for the first situation was given in the previous paragraph. In the second situation, the conductive hearing loss necessitates reflex stimulus levels that may be beyond the instrument's output capabilities. For these reasons, the contralateral acoustic reflex is generally absent in cases of bilateral middle-ear impairment. When the impairment is unilateral, the contralateral reflex will also be absent for both ears, if the impaired ear has a moderate to moderately severe conductive hearing loss.

Lesions beyond the cochlea (at the eighth cranial nerve or brain stem level) can result in either an absent or an elevated reflex or a reflex response amplitude that rapidly decays in time to a continuous stimulus (Anderson et al., 1970; Greisen and Rasmussen, 1970; Jerger et al., 1974a; Bosatra et al., 1975; Sheehy and Inzer, 1976; Jerger and Jerger, 1977). Anderson and colleagues (1970) first demonstrated that, for tones of 500 and 1000 Hz, the acoustic reflex in eighth cranial nerve tumor cases tends to have a response amplitude that decays to half strength or less in less than 5 seconds of continuous pure-tone stimulation.

Jerger and associates (1974a) and Sheehy and Inzer (1976) reported reflex findings in a larger series of such tumor cases and substantiated the clinical significance of reflex decay. However, these investigators found the reflex to be absent in most of the cases reviewed. In these studies, an abnormal reflex (absent or decaying) correctly identified 80 to 86 per cent of such retrocochlear impairments. Greisen and Rasmussen (1970) and Jerger and Jerger (1977) have demonstrated how the comparison of ipsilateral and contralateral reflexes can be used to identify eighth nerve and brain stem level impairments.

It should be apparent that the presence or absence of the acoustic reflex, its threshold, and degree of response amplitude decay can suggest a variety of underlying pathologic conditions. Consequently, the acoustic reflex alone cannot pinpoint a specific pathologic condition. Reflex findings must be viewed in the context of the tympanometric and behavioral audiometric results in order to infer the nature of hearing impairment and the possible location of the underlying lesion.

An absent acoustic reflex or a significantly elevated acoustic reflex threshold is highly suggestive of an impairment at some level of the auditory system. If the tympanogram is also abnormal, the level of impairment is likely to be the middle ear. An absent or elevated reflex with a normal tympanogram usually suggests a sensorineural impairment of either cochlear or retrocochlear origin, depending on the degree of associated sensorineural hearing loss. The probability of retrocochlear involvement is increased when the reflex is absent or elevated, and the tympanometrically normal ear has a sensorineural hearing loss of less than 80 dB HL. When the associated sensorineural hearing loss is 80 dB HL or more, an absent or elevated reflex can suggest either severe cochlear damage or a retrocochlear lesion. If the reflex occurs at essentially normal levels (70 to 100 dB HL) and does not decay in a tympanometrically normal ear with less than 80 dB HL sensorineural hearing loss, a probable location of the lesion is the cochlea.

Certain children are unable or unwilling to yield reliable behavioral hearing test results. In these cases, the reflex and tympanogram can provide evidence that corroborates impressions of the child's suspected impairment. If both the reflex and the tympanogram are normal, the likelihood of a sensorineural hearing loss exceeding 80 dB HL is low. Although some small proportion of otherwise normal children will not have a recordable acoustic reflex, a child with absent reflexes and a normal tympanogram in both ears may have a severe sensorineural hearing loss. Consequently, when less than reliable behavioral hearing tests suggest an impairment, measurements of the reflex and recording a tympanogram can add credence to associated clinical impressions.

Niemeyer and Sesterhenn (1974) first suggested that the difference between acoustic reflex thresholds for pure tones and broad-band noise could be used to estimate the degree of hearing loss. Recall that ordinarily the reflex threshold for broad-band noise is approximately 20 dB better than that for pure tones. Niemeyer and Sesterhenn (1974) observed that this difference was reduced in ears with sensorineural hearing losses and that the reduction was systematically related to the degree of the sensorineural loss. Consequently, these authors concluded that the degree of loss could be predicted from the tone-noise difference in reflex thresholds.

The use of the acoustic reflex as a predictor of degree of hearing loss has been further investigated by several authors (Jerger et al., 1974d; Johnsen et al., 1976; Schwartz and Sanders, 1976; Kieth, 1976; Margolis and Fox, 1977; Van Wagoner and Goodwine, 1977; Jerger et al., 1978). Generally, these investigations have shown that the tone-noise reflex threshold difference is best used to differentiate normal from impaired hearing but cannot accurately estimate the degree of associated hearing loss. An estimation of the degree of hearing loss is most effectively provided on the basis of the acoustic reflex threshold for broadband noise, which tends to increase along with increased sensorineural impairment (Johnsen et al., 1976; Jerger et al., 1978).

A number of investigators (McCandless and Miller, 1972; Tonnison, 1975; Denenberg and Altshuler, 1976; Rappaport and Tait, 1976; Snow and McCandless, 1976; Rainville, 1977) have evaluated the utility of the acoustic reflex in choosing an appropriate hearing aid. In this context, the reflex is most useful in pediatric and geriatric populations when behavioral indices of hearing ability are unavailable.

In these cases, the acoustic reflex can provide information about the most effective hearing aid volume setting to avoid exceeding an individual's loudness discomfort level with a particular hearing aid. A more extensive discussion of this acoustic reflex application is given in Chapter 96. Because of the many variables involved and the lack of definitive experimental evidence, the use of the acoustic reflex in fitting hearing aids in children should be approached with caution.

The qualitative and quantitative uses of acoustic reflex data should be apparent at this point. The reflex, when interpreted in the context of tympanometry and behavioral hearing test results, can suggest the nature of impairment and the location of an underlying lesion. The response also shows promise as a tool for estimating or predicting the degree of hearing loss and for determining the suitability of a particular hearing aid for a given child.

Emphasis has been placed here on interpreting the three acoustic immittance measurements—tympanometry, static compliance, and the acoustic reflex—as a whole. This approach provides the best opportunity for accurate diagnostic assessment. However, there have been numerous attempts to separate certain immittance measurements as screening tools, particularly for the detection of middle-ear disease in children.

Several published investigations have evaluated the screening effectiveness of tympanometry and the acoustic reflex (Brooks, 1973; Renvall et al., 1973; Ferrer, 1974; Harker and Van Wagoner, 1974; Lewis et al., 1974; McCandless and Thomas, 1974; Orchik and Herdman, 1974; Cooper et al., 1974; Brooks, 1976; McCurdy et al., 1976; Roberts, 1976; Brooks, 1977). Brooks (1978) supported the utility of the acoustic reflex alone as a screening tool for detection of middle-ear disease in children. These investigators commonly agree that immittance measurements are easy to perform, noninvasive, reliable, and highly sensitive to the presence of middle-ear disease. These factors would favor the use of tympanometry and the acoustic reflex as screening measurements for the detection of disease. However, definitive data supporting the validity of using immittance measurements for screening are still lacking. Although the measurements are sensitive to disease when it is present, they are considerably less accurate in sorting out children without disease, and the percentage of false-positive errors obtained is uncomfortably high (Paradise and Smith, 1978; Fria et al., unpublished). The resulting over-referral rate argues against the cost-effectiveness of mass screening for middle-ear disease with acoustic immittance measurements. An excellent review of the state of the art and suggested guidelines for immittance screening for middle-ear disease in children was presented at a symposium on this topic, the proceedings of which were published by Harford and colleagues in 1978. Arguments for and against immittance screening in children were presented at a workshop in Washington, D.C. (Bluestone et al., 1986). The recommendation of the workshop participants was that a national task force be formed to study issues related to screening children for middle-ear disease. Until such a task force reports its findings, it was suggested that screening programs designed to reach children at risk for developing complications and sequelae of otitis media continue.

Auditory Evoked Potentials

Many chapters and even texts have been devoted to auditory evoked potentials. Those by Gardi and Mendel (1977), Glattke (1978), McCandless (1978), Mendel (1977a, 1977b), Skinner (1978), Moore (1983), Jacobson (1985), Jacobson and Hyde (1985), and Davis and Owen (1985) are quite thorough in their treatment of the topic. The monograph entitled "Principles of Electric Response Audiometry" by Davis (1976) is an additional excellent reference. The present chapter will not attempt to cover the entire area in as much depth but instead will offer a brief description of component auditory evoked potentials and how they are measured. A more extensive discussion will be given for those responses that are particularly valuable for evaluating hearing in children. Finally, a pragmatic approach will be taken that identifies the children to whom the procedure is most applicable.

There are several component auditory evoked potentials, and each component response occurs in a different time frame following stimulus onset. These components and their related time frames include (1) the "cochlear" components—0 to 4 msec, (2) the "fast" components—4 to 12 msec, (3) the "middle" components—12 to 50 msec, (4) the "slow" components—50 to 300 msec; and (5) the "late" components—300 to 800 msec.

Each of these components reflects electrical activity from different anatomic levels in the auditory system; the earlier components are from peripheral and brain stem levels, and the latter components are from midbrain and cortical levels.

Figure 9–11 shows a diagram of the equipment used for evoked potential tests. Three miniature electrodes are used to record these responses. An "active" electrode is placed either in close proximity or in a favorable orientation to the neural generators responsible for the response component of interest. The "reference" electrode is placed on a site that is presumably "quiet" with respect to the component being measured. The third, or "ground," electrode is placed on an indifferent site—usually the forehead or contralateral neck or mastoid process. The actual placement of active, reference, and ground electrodes will vary with the component of interest.

The activity from the recording electrodes is then amplified, filtered, and analyzed by the ABR system. In essence, a computer serves to "average out" background EEG and myogenic activity, thereby enhancing the response associated with multiple stimulus presentations. The computer analysis is "triggered" at the onset of each stimulus and continues to include the time frame corresponding to the response component being measured.

Excessive muscle activity, as well as electrical artifacts from the surrounding environment, or line current inadequacies, can obliterate an otherwise observable electric response. Consequently, the child must be relaxed or preferably asleep. In addition, the test environment must be conducive to accurate recordings; the environment must be void of nearby sources of electrical artifacts, such as transformers or fluorescent light ballasts, and adequate line current grounding is essential.

In general, auditory electric responses provide perhaps the best data for physiologic assessment of the auditory system's responsivity in children. However, all response components are not equally useful: The validity of the slow (50 to 300 msec) and late (300 to 800 msec) components for evaluating infants and children is still open to question (Mendel, 1977b), although these components can provide useful clinical information in an older child who is awake, cooperative, and alert (however, such a child is not often referred for such testing). Usually the child who is a candidate for auditory evoked potentials testing is either unable or unwilling to cooperate for conventional hearing tests.

With regard to the slow component, the inherent degree of intersubject and intrasubject variability, and of the variability due to the age and attentive state of the child can lead to significant clinical error (Barnet and Goodwin, 1965; Rapin and Bergman, 1969; Goodhill et al., 1970). In addition, if drugs are used to induce sleep in the child, the reliability of the slow components is adversely influenced (Davis, 1973; Skinner and Shimota, 1975). According to Davis (1976), the middle components show promise as tools for evaluating infants and children, but the clinical acceptance of these components has not been widespread. Mendel (1977b) has discussed the use of the middle-

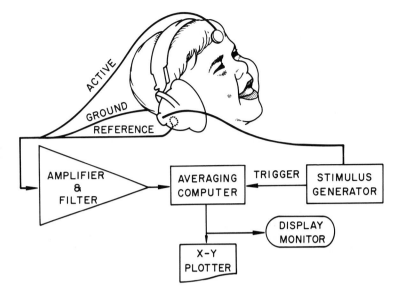

Figure 9–11. Recording electrode placement and equipment diagram for auditory brain stem response tests.

latency responses in infants and children. Kraus and colleagues (1985) found that there were significant age effects in the middle-latency response and that hearing sensitivity could be estimated in cases in which there was an observable response. However, absent responses do not necessarily mean hearing loss, limiting the utility of the middle components with respect to auditory assessment.

The cochlear (0 to 4 msec) and fast (4 to 12 msec) components are rapidly gaining acceptance as clinical tools for assessing children. The common names for these components are electrocochleography (ECochG) and the auditory brain stem response (ABR), respectively.

Electrocochleography (ECochG)

These first components reflect cochlear and eighth cranial nerve activity; the latter is also known as the whole-nerve action potential or simply the eighth nerve action potential. The eighth nerve action potential is the response of interest in the procedure.

ECochG requires that the active electrode be placed in close proximity to the neural generator of the response (the eighth cranial nerve). For this reason, the most effective active electrode placement is through the tympanic membrane and onto the promontory in the middle ear (Aran, 1976; Eggermont et al., 1974). Because this electrode placement requires a surgical procedure and a general anesthetic in children, other less invasive electrode placements have been tried. The ear canal appears to be a reasonable compromise location for the active electrode in ECochG (Yoshie et al., 1967; Coats and Dickey, 1970; Salomon and Elberling, 1971; Cullen et al., 1972; Elberling, 1974). The compromise involved, however, is that the response is an order of magnitude smaller at this location, and consequently response sensitivity and reliability are open to question. However, Ruth

and Lambert (1987) have recently reported on tympanic-membrane placement of electrode with success.

ECochG with a promontory electrode has been demonstrated to be useful in establishing the validity of the behavioral audiogram (Eggermont et al., 1974) and in the detection of eighth cranial nerve impairments (Brackmann and Selters, 1976; Odenthal and Eggermont, 1976).

The major limitation of ECochG as a tool for evaluating infants and children is the required surgical procedure for placing the active electrode and the related use of general anesthesia. The availability of the ABR, which is noninvasive and requires at most a sedative to induce sleep, has prompted many clinicians to choose the ABR in lieu of ECochG for evaluating infants and children. In addition, the ABR reflects activity not only of eighth cranial nerve fibers but also of central auditory centers. The reader interested in the principles and clinical application of ECochG is referred to Eggermont and associates (1974), Ruben and colleagues (1976), and Durrant (1986).

The Auditory Brain Stem Response (ABR)

The evoked potentials recorded in the first 10 msec have been referred to as brain stem evoked response (BSER), brain stem auditory evoked response (BAER), or auditory brain stem response (ABR). ABR will be used in this chapter. The ABR consists of five to seven vertex-positive* waves, labeled I to VII, occurring in the first 10 msec following stimulus onset (Fig. 9–12). The response was first reported by Sohmer and Feinmesser (1967), but the landmark papers in this area were published by Jewett and his colleagues (Jewett,

---

*"Vertex-positive" refers to the condition in which the active electrode, on the vertex of the skull, is connected to the positive input of the preamplifier. The waves can also be referred to as "vertex-negative" if the active electrode is connected to the negative input of the preamplifier. The former situation, however, is becoming an accepted convention.

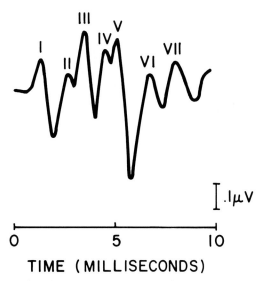

Figure 9–12. The auditory brain stem response (ABR) for a young adult with normal hearing. Component waves are labeled I through VII.

1970; Jewett et al., 1970; Jewett and Williston, 1971; Jewett and Romano, 1972).

The neural generators of the ABR have been difficult to determine precisely. Møller and Jannetta (1985) have discussed the complexity of establishing a relationship between ABR waves and specific regions of the ascending pathways using a far-field recording method. Relating findings in animals to those in humans is also not appropriate. Nevertheless, numerous carefully conducted studies have led Møller and Jannetta to conclude the following regarding the relationship between neural generators and ABR waves. Wave I is associated with activity from the distal portion of the eighth nerve; Wave II originates from the proximal portion of the eighth nerve; Wave III is associated primarily with activity in neurons of the cochlear nucleus; and Wave IV has its origin primarily from neurons of the superior olivary complex, although there are probably contributions from neurons at the level of the cochlear nucleus and the lateral lemniscus as well. In general, Wave V receives contributions from both the lateral lemniscus and the inferior colliculus. Waves VI and VII are dominated by activity from the inferior colliculus. Møller and Jannetta caution that there are multiple generators for each of the ABR waves beyond Wave III and that each generator beyond the cochlear nucleus contributes to more than one of the ABR waves.

The electrode configuration for the ABR includes the active electrode on the vertex of the skull or the midforehead at the hairline and the reference and ground electrodes respectively on the ipsilateral and contralateral mastoid processes or earlobes. The ABR is a far-field recording of minute electric discharges from multiple neurons. Therefore, the stimulus must be one that can cause simultaneous discharges of large numbers of the neurons involved. Stimuli with very rapid onset, such as clicks or tone bursts, must be

used. It is unfortunate that the rapid onset required to create a measurable ABR also creates a spread of energy in the frequency domain, reducing the frequency-specificity of the response. The responses to 1000 to 2000 clicks, filtered clicks, or brief, pure-tone bursts are typically averaged for each stimulus intensity employed. The stimuli are presented at a rapid rate (10 to 30 per second). The length of time required for a test depends on such factors as the number of stimuli and intensity levels tested per ear, the rate of presentation, and the number of stimuli "averaged" per test. Total test duration is usually one hour or more.

The deleterious effects of excessive muscle activity were mentioned earlier, and this factor is particularly pertinent to obtaining accurate ABR recordings. For this reason, a child must be completely relaxed, preferably asleep, for the procedure. Natural sleep can often be facilitated by feeding babies up to about 6 months of age immediately prior to the test. Often, children 7 years or older can lie quietly for the procedure. The ABR is not affected by sedation or general anesthesia. Infants and children between about 6 months and 6 or 7 years of age routinely are sedated to avoid problems related to muscle activity during testing. Also, ABR testing can be done in the operating room when a child is anesthetized for another procedure.

Investigations subsequent to the early descriptions of the ABR have shown the response to be consistent between and within subjects and to be unchanged in awake and sleeping subjects. Of the five to seven waves constituting the ABR, Waves I, III, and V can be obtained consistently, whereas Waves II and IV appear inconsistently between and within subjects. The latency (the time of occurrence following stimulus onset) of the various waves increases, and wave amplitudes decrease with reductions in stimulus intensity; at stimulus intensities close to behavioral hearing threshold, only Wave V can be discerned (Fig. 9–13). These and other ABR properties have emerged from the extensive research efforts of a number of investigators, which have been adequately reviewed in two texts (Moore, 1983; Jacobson, 1985).

There are developmental changes in the response morphology, wave amplitudes, and wave latencies of the ABR. Very early in life, only Waves I, III, and V are evident, with Wave I having a much greater amplitude than that of V. Over time, the relationship changes, with Wave V becoming much more prominent than the other waves in the normal adult ABR. For the most part, changes in latency provide the most consistent index of development of the ABR. All ABR waves decrease in latency during early life. However, the rate of maturation of the various waves varies. Wave I has the shortest developmental time course, reaching adult latency value by about 2 to 3 months. Wave V has the longest course, reaching adult latency value sometime in the second year of life (Hecox, 1975; Salamy and McKean, 1976; Teas et al., 1982; Hecox and Burkard, 1982; Cox, 1985). Wave III matures at a point in time between the ages at which Wave I and

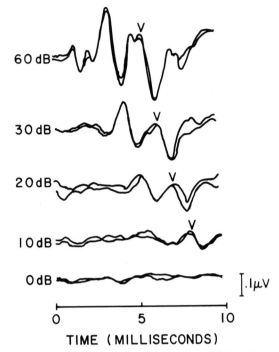

Figure 9–13. The auditory brain stem response (ABR) to decreasing stimulus intensity. Each trace represents the averaged response to 1500 stimuli of the same intensity, and for the four lower traces stimulus intensity has been reduced by 10 dB. Note the reduction in amplitude and the increase in response time (latency) of Wave V with decreased stimulus intensity.

Wave V mature. Interwave latencies (I–III; III–V; and I–V) show developmental change as well.

It is not clear what accounts for the developmental change in ABR wave latency, but some mechanisms have been suggested. They include maturation of the cochlea, increasing myelination of the central fibers, changes in transmission characteristics of the middle ear, increased synchrony, and greater synaptic efficiency (Hecox, 1975; Hecox and Burkard, 1982).

The ABR is commonly used in two ways in the pediatric setting. First, it is used as an audiometric test, providing information regarding the ability of the peripheral auditory system to transmit information to the auditory nerve and beyond. Second, the test can be used in the differential diagnosis or monitoring of central nervous system pathologic conditions (Jacobson, 1985).

For the audiometric approach, a search is conducted for the minimum stimulus intensity yielding an observable ABR. ABR thresholds using click stimuli are correlated best with behavioral hearing thresholds in the higher frequencies (1000 to 4000 Hz). The conventional ABR is unable to assess adequately responsivity to lower stimulus frequencies (Davis, 1976). Efforts have been made to obtain more frequency-specific information using the ABR. Stapells and colleagues (1985) reviewed the various ways of altering the stimulus ensemble and the recording parameters to yield more frequency-specific information than is provided by using the predominantly high-frequency click stim-

ulus. Filtering clicks and rapidly gating tones to make tone bursts have been mentioned. Many investigators have used a variety of masking techniques, including high-pass filtered noise masking, notched-noise masking, and pure-tone masking. All these methods have limitations in their ability to limit the response to the frequency desired or in their ability to generate a clear ABR. While progress has been made in recent years, there is still no reliable and valid method for predicting the audiogram from low to high frequencies using the ABR.

While one must be cognizant of the frequency-specificity limitations of the ABR used for audiometric purposes, it is also important to realize that the technique does not assess the perceptual event called "hearing." The ABR reflects auditory neuronal electric responses that are adequately correlated to behavioral hearing thresholds, but a normal ABR only suggests that the auditory system, up to the midbrain level, is responsive to the stimulus employed, and it does not guarantee normal "hearing." Conversely, failure to elicit the ABR indicates an impairment of the system's synchronous response, but it does not prove that a child is totally "deaf" or that he or she has profoundly impaired "hearing." Consequently, ABR interpretation for audiometric purposes must be qualified by other clinical assessment data, either available at the time or resulting from follow-up evaluations.

As an otoneurologic technique, the ABR may be used to infer the level of the auditory system—middle ear, cochlea, eighth cranial nerve, or brain stem—at which an impairment exists. The latency of the ABR waves is the primary consideration in these applications. For middle-ear and cochlear impairments, wave latency as a function of stimulus intensity is important. Wave latencies at a fixed stimulus intensity provide the basis for detecting eighth cranial nerve and brain stem impairments.

In cases of middle-ear impairment, the entire series of ABR waves is delayed in time by an amount commensurate with the degree of conductive hearing loss (Hecox and Galambos, 1974; Yamada et al., 1975; Fria and Sabo, 1980; Finitzo-Hieber and Friel-Patti, 1985). Typically, Wave V latency as a function of decreasing stimulus intensity is used to detect such impairment, but other evidence (Mendelson et al., 1979) suggests that Wave I latency provides a better index of middle-ear impairment.

The ABR in cases of cochlear impairment generally yields a steeper latency-intensity function. In other words, wave latencies are essentially normal at a high stimulus intensity but become excessively prolonged as stimulus intensity is decreased (Picton et al., 1977). Consequently, the characteristic ABR finding in cochlear impairment includes a normal I-to-V interwave latency in addition to the steep latency-intensity function. However, the problem is complicated by the fact that the slope or configuration of the hearing loss may influence results.

The ABR has also proved to be effective in detecting eighth cranial nerve impairment (Selters and Brackmann, 1977; Terkildsen et al., 1977; Coats and Martin, 1977; Clemis and McGee, 1979; Thomsen et al., 1978) and brain stem impairment (Starr and Achor, 1975; Stockard and Rossiter, 1977; Stockard et al., 1977). In general, such impairments show an increased latency difference between Waves I and V.

The ABR, then, is a series of positive waves occurring in the first 10 msec following stimulus onset that apparently reflect activity in successively higher levels of the auditory tract, up to and perhaps including lower midbrain centers. Within limits, the response can be used audiometrically to estimate hearing acuity, and it also has utility for inferring at which level of the auditory system impairment might exist. The consistent nature of the ABR in newborns as well as in older children, and in sleeping as well as in awake subjects, makes the test a particularly useful tool for evaluating hearing in pediatric populations. However, it is important to remember that the ABR is evidence of synchronous neural firing and that, in some cases of central nervous system dysfunction, behavioral response to sound can be normal but no ABR can be recorded.

The ABR and other electric responses are extremely complex and difficult to interpret. A number of factors, including instrumentation design and settings, environment, and patient characteristics, may influence the quality of the recording. Testing and interpretation of electrophysiologic activity must be done by people adequately trained; otherwise there is the risk that unreliable and perhaps erroneous conclusions will affect patient care.

Referral Criteria

REFERRAL CRITERIA FOR THE ABR. As was stated earlier, the ABR has great advantages for evaluating the auditory system of the young or uncooperative patient. It is a very stable phenomenon that is essentially free from the effects of state. The ABR can be measured in a patient who is awake, under sedation, or under anesthesia. Disadvantages include the fact that measurement of the ABR is not a test of hearing but of electric responses in the pathways of the eighth nerve and brain stem that occur as a result of auditory stimulation. It lacks frequency specificity as well.

Nevertheless, the ABR test has become an irreplaceable component of the audiologic test battery. The ABR test is not an assessment technique that should be applied to every patient in need of audiologic services. However, there are situations for which the ABR can provide information essential to identification, diagnosis, or management that could not be acquired in any other way. There are other situations in which the ABR supplements or corroborates other clinical or audiologic evidence.

Infants who should be referred for ABR testing include newborns meeting the high-risk criteria of the Joint Committee on Infant Hearing (see later), postmeningitic infants; infants with recurrent acute otitis media, persistent otitis media with effusion, or both;

children with significant mental retardation, emotional disturbance, or both for whom ear-specific behavioral hearing testing is not possible; children with suspected eighth nerve or brain stem disorders; children with sudden onset, fluctuating, progressive, or unilateral sensorineural hearing loss; other difficult-to-test patients; patients (especially infants) for whom ear-specific auditory responses are needed; and those for whom confirmation of suspected auditory or central nervous system dysfunction is required.

THE ABR AND NEWBORN HEARING SCREENING. The ABR has also proved useful in screening the hearing of neonates. Many programs use the ABR to screen the hearing of infants who meet the high-risk criteria published in 1982 by the Joint Committee on Infant Hearing. These criteria are neonatal asphyxia, bacterial meningitis, congenital infection, defects of the head or neck, elevated bilirubin, family history of hearing loss, and low birth weight (less than 1500 gm). Sabo and colleagues (1986) reported on a screening program that has successfully tested nearly 2000 infants, meeting similar high-risk criteria, with the ABR over a six-year period. Sensitivity and specificity values are quite high using the combined high-risk register, and, in all, about 15 per cent of the neonates meeting high-risk criteria were referred for follow-up. About 3.5 per cent of the screened group were identified as hearing impaired. Others have reported studies of the cost-effectiveness of the ABR relative to the Crib-o-gram (Simmons et al., 1979) or the high-risk register alone. Shimizu and associates (1986) and Prager and colleagues (1987) have reported that ABR testing compares quite favorably with the other methods with respect to cost per child identified as hearing impaired.

AUTONOMIC RESPONSES. Over the years, the autonomic nervous system has been utilized for assessment of hearing in difficult-to-test populations. In routine clinical practice, such measures, which include changes in respiration, heart rate, and electrodermal activity in the skin, have not gained great acceptance. The interested reader can consult Hogan (1975) for a review of the autonomic correlates of audition.

TESTS FOR FUNCTIONAL (NONORGANIC) HEARING LOSS. One of the problems that audiologists face in assessing hearing behaviorally is the identification of the child with functional, or nonorganic, hearing loss. Because much of our routine clinical assessment requires a voluntary behavioral response, we must take precautions that a child is not exaggerating hearing loss. Children might wish to exhibit a hearing loss because of the secondary gains that accrue from added attention or because it can help explain other undesirable behaviors, such as poor performance in school or personality problems (Martin, 1985). The consequences of falsely labeling a child as hearing impaired can come in the form of parental distress, inappropriate management of the child, or reinforcement of the child's psychologic difficulties, depending on the origin of the functional hearing loss.

Northern and Downs (1984) point out that the child who exaggerates or invents hearing loss is most probably doing so for reasons that are important to him or her. The audiologist or other professional encountering a suspected nonorganic hearing loss should consider whether the child has a psychologic or emotional need that is being met by the consequences of a hearing loss. Therefore, it is necessary in such patients that the audiologist first assess as accurately as possible the true status of the auditory system. Second, assistance in determining what needs of the child are being met by feigning hearing loss should be offered to the family.

In many cases, the child with functional hearing loss is suspected from the beginning. Observations of the child outside of the test room may reveal exaggerated efforts to hear. However, observation may belie any hearing loss at all. The child's behavior may be very different once he or she is involved with the structured task of the hearing test. A competent pediatric audiologist will notice exaggerated efforts to hear the sound, inconsistencies on repeated attempts to obtain threshold for a given stimulus, widely different thresholds depending on method used, and lack of correspondence between SRT and PTA (although the caution previously offered regarding the effect of hearing loss configuration on this relationship should be heeded when functional hearing loss is considered). Current test methods now allow us virtually to rule out hearing loss in normal hearing individuals by so-called objective test measures. Immittance testing, especially the acoustic reflex test, and ABR testing can usually provide enough hard evidence to establish whether hearing is really impaired to the degree exhibited. These tests can be used to corroborate results and impressions from informal observation and behavioral testing.

There are behavioral assessment techniques used with adults to obtain estimates of thresholds in patients who seem to be exaggerating. The use of such complicated tests in children is not common because of the lack of sophistication on the part of subjects to perform the tasks or to provide convincing performances in traditional testing. The Stenger test, beneficial in identifying functional hearing loss in patients with unilateral or asymmetric hearing loss, can be used with older children.

With small children, there are often large discrepancies in the results of routine tests, so identification of nonorganicity is not difficult. Sometimes, young children can be instructed to say "yes" when they hear a tone and to say "no" when they do not. A youngster too immature to appreciate the stimulus-response contingency will respond "no" to the sounds that are heard but that are below the selected minimum response level. Infants and children with unusual configurations of hearing loss can respond in atypical ways on standard tests. The trained pediatric audiologist must use experience and creativity, along with a test battery, to establish accurate and reliable estimates of hearing.

THE ROLE OF THE AUDIOLOGIST

This chapter has described the various techniques available for assessing hearing in infants. The reader should now have a basic understanding of the techniques for such assessment and an awareness of sources where more extensive treatment of a particular technique can be found. Throughout this chapter, it has been emphasized that no one method of assessment is definitive and that accurate assessment involves the consideration of information provided by several tests of hearing used in combination. Although certain techniques can be used in isolation as screening tools in certain situations (e.g., BOA in the office situation), comprehensive assessment is based on the results of a combination of these tests.

The audiologist plays a multifaceted role in the assessment process. He or she must devise and implement an assessment strategy composed of procedures that are applicable to the child in question and must interpret the results in the context of the impairment suspected. The audiologist must also convey assessment results to the referral source and must provide suggestions that are meaningful for the management of the child. In concert with the referral source, the audiologist can also play an important role in interpreting the results to concerned family members and in counseling the family with regard to the impact an impairment may have on the child's future interaction with the environment from a social and educational point of view.

The audiologist can serve as a valuable resource for the implementation of habilitative or rehabilitative plans for a hearing-impaired child. In addition, the audiologist is usually aware of the public and special school programs in the community that will play an active role in the child's education. The audiologist maintains contact with such programs, so the long-term follow-up of a particular child is maintained.

In conclusion, the audiologist should be an active team member in the general pediatric assessment of any child, regardless of age. At his or her disposal are the knowledge, experience, and techniques required to make a meaningful assessment of hearing in infants and children. Owing to the importance of adequate hearing in infancy and childhood, we as health care professional are obligated to give the assessment of hearing the high priority it deserves.

SELECTED REFERENCES

Pediatric Audiology

Jerger, J. 1984. Pediatric Audiology. Current Trends. San Diego, College Hill Press.
  Contributed chapters from experts in pediatric audiology. Major topics include behavioral assessment, immittance, evoked potentials, hearing aid selection, and aural rehabilitation.
Bess, F. H. (ed.). 1988. Hearing Impairment in Children. Parkton, MD, York Press.
  Proceedings of the Third International Symposium on Childhood Deafness, held in Nashville, Tennessee, in July 1986. Contributed chapters cover three major areas: etiology/audiology disorders; identification and assessment; and management. Excellent, up-to-date reviews make it an important reference to have.

Immittance Testing

Margolis, R. H., and Shanks, J. E. 1985. Tympanometry. *In* Katz, J. (ed.): Handbook of Clinical Audiology, 3rd ed. Baltimore, Williams & Wilkins.

This short chapter provides a good explanation of the fundamentals of tympanometry. It includes the latest methods of interpreting tympanograms.

Wilber, L. A., and Feldman, A. S. 1976. Acoustic Impendance and Admittance—The Measure of Middle Ear Function. Baltimore, Williams & Wilkins.

Complete text on fundamentals of immittance testing. Has chapters on clinical application, including acoustic and nonacoustic stapedial reflex tests and detailed information on the physics of the middle-ear system.

Audiology Brain Stem Response (ABR)

Fria, T. J. 1980. The auditory brain stem response. Background and clinical applications. Monographs in Contemporary Audiology. Minneapolis, MN, Maico Hearing Instruments. 2(2):1–44.

Complete but not lengthy explanation of the fundamentals of the ABR. Good basic publication for reference.

Jacobsen, J. T. 1985. The Auditory Brain Stem Response. San Diego, College Hill Press.

Contributed chapters from many authors. Topics range from basic technical issues of the ABR, to neuroanatomy, to the clinical application of the ABR. It has an entire section devoted to pediatric assessment as well.

Moore, E. J. 1983. Brain Stem Evoked Responses. New York, Grune & Stratton.

Multiple contributing authors. This book has more detail on the fundamentals and less detail on the clinical applications than the Jacobsen book (just noted). There is also some discussion of other potentials.

REFERENCES

Alberti, P. W., and Kristensen, R. 1970. The clinical application of impedance audiometry. Laryngoscope 80:735.

American National Standard Institute, 1969. Standard specifications for Audiometers. ANSI–S3.6–1969 (R 1973). American National Standards Institute, Inc., New York.

Anderson, H., Barr, B., and Wedenberg, E. 1970. Early diagnosis of VIIIth nerve tumors by acoustic reflex tests. Acta Otolaryngol. 263:232.

Aran, J. M. 1976. The electro-cochleogram: Recent results in children and in some pathological cases. Arch. Klin. Ohren. Nasen. Kehlkopf. 198:128.

ASHA, 1974. Committee on Audiometric Evaluation, Guidelines for audiometric symbols. ASHA 16:260.

Barnet, A. B., and Goodwin, R. S. 1965. Averaged evoked electro-encephalographic responses to clicks in the human newborn. EEG Clin. Neurophysiol. 18:441.

Barr, B. 1955. Pure-tone audiometry for pre-school children. Acta Otolaryngol. Suppl. 121.

Bess, F. H., and Tharpe, A. M. 1984. Unilateral hearing impairment in children. Pediatrics 74:206.

Bluestone, C. D., Fria, T. J., Arjona, S. K., et al. 1986. Controversies in screening for middle ear disease and hearing loss in children. Pediatrics 77:57.

Bosatra, A., Russolo, M., and Poli, P. 1975. Modifications of the stapedius muscle reflex under spontaneous and experimental brain stem impairment. Acta Otolaryngol. 80:61.

Brackman, D. E., and Selters, W. A. 1976. Electrocochleography in Meniere's disease and acoustic neuromas. *In* Ruben, R. J., Elberling, C., and Salomon, G. (eds.): Electrocochleography. Baltimore, University Park Press, pp. 315–330.

Brookhouser, P. E., and Moeller, M. P. 1986. Choosing the appropriate habilitative track for the newly identified hearing-impaired child. Ann. Otol. Rhinol. Laryngol. 95:51.

Brooks, D. N. 1969. The use of the electroacoustic impedance bridge in the assessment of middle ear function. Int. Audiol. 8:563.

Brooks, D. N. 1973. Hearing screening: A comparative study of an impedance method and pure tone screening. Scand. Audiol. 2:67.

Brooks, D. N. 1976. School screening for middle ear effusions. Ann. Otol. Rhinol. Laryngol. 25(85):223.

Brooks, D. N. 1977. Mass screening with acoustic impedance. Proceedings of the Third International Symposium on Impedance Audiometry. New York, American Electromedics, May.

Brooks, D. N. 1978. Impedance screening for school children—State of the art. *In* Harford, E. R., Bess, F. H., Bluestone, C. D., et al. (eds.): Impedance Screening for Middle Ear Disease in Children. New York, Grune & Stratton, pp. 173–180.

Clemis, J. D., and McGee, T. 1979. Brain stem electric response audiometry in the differential diagnosis of acoustic tumors. Laryngoscope 89(1):31.

Coats, A. C., and Dickey, J. R. 1970. Non-surgical recording of human auditory nerve action potentials from the tympanic membrane. Ann. Otol. Rhinol. Laryngol. 29:844.

Coats, A. C., and Martin, J. L. 1977. Nerve action potentials and brain stem evoked responses: Effects of audiogram shape and lesion location. Arch. Otolaryngol. 103:605.

Cooper, J. C., Gates, G., Owen, J., et al. 1974. An abbreviated impedance bridge technique for school screening. J. Speech Hear. Disord. 40:260.

Cox, L. C. 1985. Infant assessment: Developmental and age-related considerations. *In* Jacobson, J. T. (ed.): The Auditory Brainstem Response. San Diego, College Hill Press, pp. 297–316.

Cullen, J. K., Ellis, M. S., Berlin, C. I., et al. 1972. Human acoustic nerve action potential recordings from the tympanic membrane without anesthesia. Acta Otolaryngol. 74:15.

Darley, F. L. 1961. Identification audiometry. J. Speech Hear. Disord. Suppl. 9.

Davis, H. 1973. Sedation of young children for evoked response audiometry (ERA). Summary of a symposium. Audiology 12:55.

Davis, H. 1976. Principles of electric response audiometry. Ann. Otol. Rhinol. Laryngol. (Suppl.) 85:1.

Davis, H., and Owen, J. H. 1985. Auditory evoked potentials. *In* Owen, J. H., and Davis, H. (eds.): Evoked Potential Testing: Clinical Applications. New York, Grune & Stratton.

Denenberg, L. J., and Altshuler, M. W. 1976. The clinical relationship between acoustic reflexes and loudness perception. J. Am. Audiol. Soc. 2(3):79.

Downs, M. P. 1974. Personal communication.

Durrant, J. D. 1986. Observations on combined noninvasive electrocochleography and auditory brainstem response recording. Semin. Hear. 7:289.

Eggermont, J. J., Odenthal, D. W., Schmidt, P. H., et al. 1974. Electrocochleography. Basic principles and clinical application. Acta Otolaryngol. Suppl. 316.

Eisenberg, R. B. 1976. Auditory Competence in Early Life. Baltimore, University Park Press.

Elberling, C. 1974. Action potentials along the cochlear partition recorded from the ear canal in man. Scand. Audiol. 3:13.

Elliott, L. L., and Katz, D. R. 1980. Development of a new children's test of speech discrimination. Auditec of St. Louis, St. Louis, Mo.

Elner, A., Ingelstedt, S., and Ivarsson, A. 1971. Indirect determination of middle ear pressure. Acta Otolaryngol. 72:255.

Feldman, A. S. 1978. Acoustic impedance-admittance battery. *In* Katz, J. (ed.): Handbook of Clinical Audiology, 2nd ed. Baltimore, Williams & Wilkins.

Ferrer, H. 1974. Use of impedance audiometry in school screening. Public Health 88:153.

Fiellau-Nikolajsen, M. 1983. Tympanometry and secretory otitis media. Acta Otolaryngol. 394:1.

Finitzo-Hieber, T., and Friel-Patti, S. 1985. Conductive hearing loss and the ABR. *In* Jacobson, J. T. (ed.): The Auditory Brainstem Response. San Diego, College Hill Press, pp. 113–132.

Fria, T. J. 1980. The auditory brain stem response. Background and clinical applications. Monographs in Contemporary Audiology. Maico Hearing Instruments. Minneapolis, Minn., 2(2):1–44.

Fria, T. J. 1985a. Identification of congenital hearing loss with the auditory brainstem response. *In*: Jacobson, J. T. (ed.): The Auditory Brainstem Response. San Diego, College Hill Press, pp. 317–334.

Fria, T. J. 1985b. Threshold estimation with early latency auditory potentials. In Katz, J. (ed.): Handbook of Clinical Audiology, 3rd ed. Baltimore, Williams & Wilkins, pp. 549–564.

Fria, T. J., and Sabo, D. L. 1980. Auditory brainstem responses in children with otitis media with effusion. Ann. Otol. Rhinol. Laryngol. 68:200.

Fria, T. J., Leblanc, J., Kristensen, R., et al. 1975. Ipsilateral acoustic reflex stimulation in normal and sensorineural impaired ears: A preliminary report. Can. J. Otolaryngol. 4:695.

Fria, T. J., Sabo, D., and Beery, Q. C. 1979. The acoustic reflex in the identification of otitis media with effusion, unpublished.

Fulton, R. T., Gorzycki, P. A., and Hull, W. L. 1975. Hearing assessment with young children. J. Speech Hear. Disord. 40:397.

Gardi, J. N., and Mendel, M. 1977. Evoked brainstem potentials. In Gerber, S. E. (ed.): Audiometry in Infancy. New York, Grune & Stratton, pp. 205–246.

Glattke, T. J. 1978. Electrocochleography. In Katz, J. (ed.): Handbook of Clinical Audiology, Baltimore, Williams & Wilkins, pp. 328–343.

Goldstein, B. A., and Newman, C. W. 1985. Clinical masking: A decision-making process. In Katz, J. (ed.): Handbook of Clinical Audiology, 3rd ed. Baltimore, Williams & Wilkins, pp. 170–201.

Goodhill, V., Lowell, E. L., and Lowell, M. O. 1970. Computerized objective auditory testing in infancy. Final report of project DHEW H-181.

Greisen O., and Rasmussen, P. 1970. Stapedius muscle reflexes and otoneurological examinations in brain stem tumors. Acta Otolaryngol. 70:366.

Harford, E. R., Bess, F. H., Bluestone, C. D., et al. 1978. Impedance Screening for Middle Ear Disease in Children. New York, Grune & Stratton.

Harker, L. A., and Van Wagoner, R. 1974. Application of impedance audiometry as a screening instrument. Acta Otolaryngol. 77:198.

Haskins, H. 1949. A phonetically balanced test of speech discrimination for children. Master's thesis, Northwestern University.

Hecox, K. 1975. Electrophysiological correlates of human auditory development. In Cohen, L. B., and Salapatek, P. L. (eds.): Infant Perception from Sensation to Cognition, Vol. 2. Perception of Space, Speech and Sound. New York, Academic Press.

Hecox, K. E. 1985. Neurologic application of the auditory brainstem response to the pediatric age group. In Jacobson, J. T. (ed.): The Auditory Brain Stem Response. San Diego, College Hill Press, pp. 287–295.

Hecox, K., and Burkard, R. 1982. Developmental dependencies of the human brainstem auditory evoked response. Ann. N.Y. Acad. Sci. 388:538.

Hecox, K., and Galambos, R. 1974. Brainstem auditory evoked responses in human infants and adults. Arch. Otolaryngol. 99:30.

Hirsh, I. J., Davis H., Silverman, S. R., et al. 1952. Development of materials for speech audiometry. J. Speech Hear. Disord. 17:321.

Hogan, D. D. 1975. Autonomic correlates of audition. In Fulton, R. T., and Lloyd, L. L. (eds.) Auditory Assessment of the Difficult-to-test. Baltimore, Williams & Wilkins.

Holmquist, J., and Miller, J. 1972. Eustachian tube evaluation using the impedance bridge. Mayo Foundation Impedance Symposium. Mayo Clinic, Rochester, MN, 297–307, June.

Hoversten, G. H., and Moncur, J. P. 1969. Stimuli and intensity factors in testing infants. J. Speech Hear. Res. 12:687.

Ingelstedt, S., Ivarsson, A., and Jonsson, B. 1967. Mechanics of the human middle ear. Acta Otolaryngol. Suppl. 228.

Jacobson, J. T. (ed.): 1985. The Auditory Brainstem Response. San Diego, College Hill Press.

Jacobson, J. T., and Hyde, M. L. 1985. An introduction to auditory evoked potentials. In Katz, J. (ed.): Handbook of Clinical Audiology, 3rd ed. Baltimore, Williams & Wilkins, pp. 496–533.

Jepsen, O. 1963. Middle ear muscle reflexes in man. In Jerger, J. (ed.): Modern Developments in Audiology. New York, Academic Press, pp. 193–239.

Jerger, J. 1970. Clinical experience with impedance audiometry. Arch Otolaryngol. 92:311.

Jerger, J. 1984. Pediatric Audiology: Current Trends. San Diego, College Hill Press.

Jerger, J., Jerger, S., and Mauldin, L. 1972. Studies in impedance audiometry. I. Normal and sensorineural ears. Arch. Otolaryngol. 96:513.

Jerger, J., Harford, E., Clemis, J., et al. 1974a. The acoustic reflex in eighth nerve disorders. Arch. Otolaryngol. 99:409.

Jerger, J., Anthony, L., Jerger, S., et al. 1974c. Studies in impedance audiometry. III. Middle ear disorders. Arch. Otolaryngol. 99:165.

Jerger, J., Burney, P., Mauldin, L., et al. 1974d. Predicting hearing loss from the acoustic reflex. J. Speech Hear. Disord. 18:11.

Jerger, J., Hayes, D., Anthony, L., et al. 1978. Factors influencing prediction of hearing level from the acoustic reflex. Monographs in Contemporary Audiology. 1:1–20. Minneapolis, Maico Hearing Instruments, Inc.

Jerger, S., and Jerger, J. 1977. Diagnostic value of crossed vs. uncrossed acoustic reflexes: Eighth nerve and brainstem disorders. Arch. Otolaryngol. 103:445.

Jerger, S., Jerger, J., and Lewis, S. 1981. Pediatric speech intelligibility test. II. Effect of receptive language age and chronological age. Int. J. Pediatr. Otorhinolaryngol. 3:101.

Jerger, S., Lewis, S., Hawkins, J., et al. 1980. Pediatric speech intelligibility test. I. Generation of test materials. International J. Pediatric Otorhinolaryngol. 2:217.

Jerger, S., Jerger, J., and Mauldin, L. 1974b. Studies in impedance audiometry. II. Children less than six years old. Arch. Otolaryngol. 99:1.

Jewett, D. L. 1970. Volume-conducted potentials in response to auditory stimuli as detected by averaging in the cat. EEG Clin. Neurophysiol. 28:609.

Jewett, D. L., and Romano, M. N. 1972. Neonatal development of auditory system potentials averaged from the scalp of the rat and cat. Brain Res. 36:101.

Jewett, D. L., and Williston, J. S. 1971. Auditory evoked far fields averaged from the scalp of humans. Brain 94:681.

Jewett, D. L., Romano, M. N., and Williston, J. S. 1970. Human auditory evoked potentials: Possible brainstem components detected on the scalp. Science 167:1517.

Johnsen, N. J., Osterhammel, D., Terkildsen, K., et al. 1976. The white noise middle ear muscle reflex thresholds in patients with sensorineural hearing impairment. Scand. Audiol. 5:313.

de Jonge, R. 1986. Normal tympanometric gradient: A comparison of three methods. Audiology 25:299.

Kieth, R. W. 1971. Impedance audiometry with neonates. Presented at the Annual Convention of the American Speech and Hearing Association. November.

Kieth, R. W. 1976. An evaluation of predicting hearing loss from the acoustic reflex. Presented at the Annual Convention of the American Speech and Hearing Association. Houston, Texas, November.

Koebsell, K. A., and Margolis, R. H. 1986. Tympanometric gradient measured from normal preschool children. Audiology 25:149.

Kraus, N., Smith, D. I., Reed, N. L., et al. 1985. Auditory middle latency responses in children: Effects of age and diagnostic category. Electroencephalogr. Clin. Neurophysiol. 62:343.

Lewis, A. N., Barry, M., and Stuart, J. 1974. Screening procedures for the identification of hearing and ear disorders in Australian aboriginal children. J. Laryngol. Otol. 88:335.

Lewis, N., Dugdale, A., Canty, A., et al. 1975. Open-ended tympanometric screening: A new concept. Arch. Otolaryngol. 101:722.

Liden, G., and Renvall, U. 1978. Impedance audiometry for screening middle ear disease in school children. In Harford, E. R., Bess, F. H., Bluestone, C. D., et al. (eds.): Impedance Screening for Middle Ear Disease in Children. New York, Grune & Stratton, pp. 197–206.

Liden, G., Peterson, J., and Bjorkman, G. 1970. Tympanometry. Arch. Otolaryngol. 92:248.

Lloyd, L. L., Spradlin, J. E., and Reed, M. J. 1968. An operant audiometric procedure for difficult-to-test patients. J. Speech Hear. Disord. 33:236.

Marchant, C. D., McMillan, P. M., Shurin, P. A., et al. 1986. Objective diagnosis of otitis media in early infancy by tympanometry and ipsilateral acoustic reflex thresholds. J. Pediatr. 109:590.

Margolis, R. H. 1981. Fundamentals of acoustic immittance. In Popelka, G. R. (ed.): Hearing Assessment with the Acoustic Reflex. New York, Grune & Stratton, pp. 117–143.

Margolis, R. H., and Fox, C. M. 1977. A comparison of three methods for predicting hearing loss from acoustic reflex thresholds. J. Speech Hear. Res. 20:241.

Margolis, R. H., and Heller, J. W. 1987. Screening tympanometry: Criteria for medical referral. Audiology 26:197.

Margolis, R. H., and Shanks, J. E. 1985. Tympanometry. In Katz, J. (ed.): Handbook of Clinical Audiology, 3rd ed. Baltimore, Williams & Wilkins.

Martin, F. N. 1985. The pseudohypacusic. In Katz, J. (ed.): Handbook of Clinical Audiology, 3rd ed. Baltimore, Williams & Wilkins.

Matkin, N. D. 1986. Diagnostic case study in pediatric audiology. Presented at the annual convention of American Speech-Language-Hearing Association, Detroit, MI, November 21–24.

McCandless, G. A. 1978. Neuroelectric measures of auditory function. In Rose, D. E. (ed.): Audiological Assessment, 2nd ed. Englewood Cliffs, Prentice Hall, pp. 420–443.

McCandless, G. A., and Allred, P. L. 1978. Tympanometry and emergence of the acoustic reflex infants. In Harford, E. R., Bess, F. H., Bluestone, C. D., et al. (eds.): Impedance Screening for Middle Ear Disease in Children. New York, Grune & Stratton, pp. 57–68.

McCandless, G. A., and Miller, D. 1972. Loudness discomfort and hearing aids. Natl. Hear. Aid. J. 7:28.

McCandless, G. A., and Thomas, G. K. 1974. Impedance audiometry as a screening procedure for middle ear disease. Trans. Am. Acad. Ophthalmol. Otolaryngol. 78:98.

Mendel, M. 1977a. Evoked cochlear potentials. In Gerber, S. E. (ed.): Audiometry in Infancy. New York, Grune & Stratton, pp. 183–204.

Mendel, M. 1977b. Electroencephalic tests of hearing. In Gerber, S. E. (ed.): Audiometry in Infancy. New York, Grune & Stratton, pp. 151–182.

Mendelson, T., Salamy, A., Lenoir, M., et al. 1979. Brainstem evoked potential findings in children with otitis media. Arch. Otolaryngol. 105:17.

Metz, O. 1952. Threshold of reflex contractions of muscles of the middle ear and recruitment of loudness. Arch. Otolaryngol. 55:536.

Møller, A. R. 1962. The sensitivity of contraction of the tympanic muscles in man. Ann. Otol. Rhinol. Laryngol. 71:86.

Møller, A. R., and Jannetta, P. J. 1985. Neural generators of the auditory brainstem response. In Jacobson, J. T. (ed.): The Auditory Brainstem Response. San Diego, College Hill Press, pp. 13–32.

Moncur, J. P. 1968. Judge reliability in infant testing. J. Speech Hear. Res. 11:348.

Moore, E. J. 1983. Brain Stem Evoked Responses. New York, Grune & Stratton.

Moore, J. M., Thompson, G., and Thompson, M. 1975. Auditory localization of infants as a function of reinforcement conditions. J. Speech Hear. Dis. 40:29.

Moore, J. M., Wilson, W. R., and Thompson, G. 1977. Visual reinforcement of head-turn responses in infants under 12 months of age. J. Speech Hear. Dis. 42:328.

Murphy, K. P. 1961. Development of hearing in babies. Hearing Instruments, November 9–11.

Niemeyer, W., and Sesterhann, G. 1974. Calculating the hearing threshold from the stapedius reflex threshold for different sound stimuli. Audiology 13:421.

Northern, J. L., and Downs, M. P. 1984. Hearing in Children, 3rd ed. Baltimore, Williams & Wilkins.

Northern, J. L., and Grimes, A. M. 1978. Introduction to acoustic impedance. In Katz, J. (ed.): Handbook of Clinical Audiology. Baltimore, Williams & Wilkins, pp. 344–355.

Nozza, R. J. 1987. The binaural masking level difference in infants and adults: Developmental change in binaural hearing. Infant Behavior and Development 10:105.

Nozza, R. J., and Wilson, W. R. 1984. Masked and unmasked pure-tone thresholds of infants and adults: Development of auditory frequency selectivity and sensitivity. J. Speech Hear. Res. 27:613.

Odenthal, D. W., and Eggermont, J. J. 1976. Electrocochleography study in Meniere's disease and pontine angle neuronoma. In Ruben, R. J., Elberling, C., and Salomon, G. (eds.) Electrocochleography. Baltimore, University Park Press, pp. 331–352.

Orchik, D. J., and Herdman, S. 1974. Impedance audiometry as a screening device with school age children. J. Aud. Res. 14:283.

Orchik, D. J., Dunn, J. W., and McNutt, L. 1978. Tympanometry as a predictor of middle ear effusion. Arch. Otolaryngol. 104:4.

Paradise, J. L., and Smith, C. G. 1978. Impedance screening for preschool children—State of the art. In Harford, E. R., Bess, F. H., Bluestone, C. D., et al. (eds.): Impedance Screening for Middle Ear Disease in Children. New York, Grune & Stratton, pp. 113–124.

Paradise, J. L., Smith, C. G., and Bluestone, C. D. 1976. Tympanometric detection of middle ear effusion in infants and young children. Pediatrics 58:198.

Peterson, J., and Liden, G. 1970. Tympanometry in human temporal bones. Acta Otolaryngol. 92:258.

Picton, T. W., Woods, D. L., Baribeau-Braun, J., et al. 1977. Evoked potential audiometry. J. Otolaryngol. 6(2):90.

Prager, D. A., Stone, D. A., and Rose, D. N. 1987. Hearing loss screening in the neonatal intensive care unit: Auditory brain stem response versus Crib-O-Gram; a cost-effectiveness analysis. Ear Hear. 8:213.

Rainville, M. 1977. Hearing aid fitting using stapedial reflex measurement. Proceedings of Third International Symposium on Impedance Audiometry, Acton, Maine, American Electromedics Corp., 49–50.

Rapin, I., and Bergman, M. 1969. Auditory evoked responses in uncertain diagnosis. Arch. Otolaryngol. 90:307.

Rappaport, B. E., and Tait, C. A. 1976. Acoustic reflex threshold measurement in hearing aid selection. Arch. Otolaryngol. 102:129.

Renvall, U., Liden, G., and Bjorkman, G. 1975. Experimental tympanometry in human temporal bones. Scand. Audiol. 4:135.

Renvall, U., Liden, G., Jungert, S., et al. 1973. Impedance audiometry as a screening method in school children. Scand. Audiol. 2:133.

Roberts, M. E. 1976. Comparative study of pure tone, impedance, and otoscopic hearing screening methods. Arch. Otolaryngol. 102:690.

Robertson, E. O., Peterson, J. L., and Lamb, L. E. 1968. Relative impedance measurements in young children. Arch. Otolaryngol. 88:162.

Ross, M., and Lerman, J. 1970. A picture identification task for hearing-impaired children. J. Speech Hear. Res. 13:44.

Ruben, R. J., Elberling, C., and Salomon, G. 1976. Electrocochleography. Baltimore, University Park Press.

Ruth, R. A., and Lambert, P. A. 1987. Electrocochleography: Tympanic membrane versus promontory electrode. Presented at the 10th Biennial International Symposium of the International ERA study group. Charlottesville, VA, August 23–27.

Sabo, D. L., Nozza, R. J., Delano, S. E., et al. 1986. ABR screening in the NICU: Alternative design. Presented at the annual convention of American Speech-Language-Hearing Association, Detroit, MI, November 21–24.

Salamy, A., and McKean, C. M. 1976. Postnatal development of human brainstem potentials during the first year of life. EEG Clin. Neurophysiol. 40:418.

Salomon, G., and Elberling, G. 1971. Cochlear nerve potentials recorded from the ear canal in man. Acta Otolaryngol. 71:319.

Schwartz, D. M., and Sanders, J. 1976. Critical bandwidth and sensitivity prediction in the acoustic stapedial reflex. J. Speech Hear. Disord. 41:244.

Schwartz, D. M., Schwartz, R. H., Rosenblatt, M., et al. 1978. Variability in tympanometric pattern in children below five years of age. In Harford, E. R., Bess, F. H., Bluestone, C. D., et al. (eds.): Impedance Screening for Middle Ear Disease in Children. New York, Grune & Stratton, pp. 145–152.

Selters, W. E., and Brackmann, D. E. 1977. Acoustic tumor detection with brainstem electric response audiometry. Arch. Otolaryngol. 103:181.

Sheehy, J. L., and Inzer, B. E. 1976. Acoustic reflex test in neuro-otologic diagnosis. Arch. Otolaryngol. 102:647.

Shimizu, H., Walters, R. J., Kennedy, D. W., et al. 1986. A comparative study of neonatal hearing screening procedures. Paper presented at the annual convention of the American Speech-Language-Hearing Association, Detroit, MI, November 21–24.

Simmons, F. B., McFarland, W. H., and Jones, F. R. 1979. An automated hearing screening technique for newborns. Acta Otolaryngol. 87:1.

Skinner, B. K., Norris, T. W., and Jirsa, R. E. 1978. Contralateral-ipsilateral acoustic reflex thresholds in preschool children. *In* Harford, E. R., Bess, F. H., and Bluestone, C. D., et al. (eds.): Impedance Screening for Middle Ear Disease in Children. New York, Grune & Stratton, pp. 161–170.

Skinner, P. H. 1978. Electroencephalic response audiometry. *In* Katz, J. (ed.): Handbook of Clinical Audiology. Baltimore, Williams & Wilkins, pp. 311–327.

Skinner, P. H., and Shimota, J. 1975. A comparison of the effects of sedatives on the auditory evoked cortical response. J. Am. Audiol. Soc. 1:71.

Snow, T., and McCandless, G. 1976. The use of impedance measures in hearing aid selection. Natl. Hear. Aid J. 7:32.

Sohmer, H., and Feinmesser, M. 1967. Cochlear action potentials recorded from the external ear in man. Ann. Otol. Rhinol. Laryngol. 76:427.

Stapells, D. R., Picton, T. W., Perez-Abalo, M., et al. 1985. Frequency specificity in evoked potential audiometry. *In* Jacobson, J. T. (ed.): The Auditory Brainstem Response. San Diego, College Hill Press, pp. 147–177.

Starr, A., and Achor, L. J. 1975. Auditory brainstem responses in neurological disease. Arch. Neurol. 32:761.

Stockard, J. J., and Rossiter, U. S. 1977. Clinical and pathologic correlates of brainstem auditory response abnormalities. Neurology, 27(4):316.

Stockard, J. J., Stockard, J. E., and Sharbrough, F. W. 1977. Detection and localization of occult lesions with brainstem auditory responses. Mayo Clin. Proc. 52:761.

Suzuki, T., and Ogiba, Y. 1960. A technique of pure tone audiometry for children under three years of age: Conditioned orientation reflex (COR) audiometry. Rev. Laryngol. 81:33.

Suzuki, T., and Ogiba, Y. 1961. Conditioned orientation reflex audiometry. Arch. Otolaryngol. 74:192.

Teas, D. C., Klein, A. J., and Kramer, S. J. 1982. An analysis of auditory brainstem responses in infants. Hear. Res. 7:19.

Terkildsen, K., and Thomsen, K. A. 1959. The influence of pressure variations on the impedance of the human ear drum. J. Laryngol. Otol. 73:409.

Terkildsen, K., Huis in't Veld, F., and Osterhammel, P. 1977. Auditory brainstem responses in the diagnosis of cerebellopontine angle tumors. Scand. Audiol. 3:123.

Thompson, G., and Weber, B. A. 1974. Responses of infants and young children to behavioral observation audiometry (BOA). J. Speech Hear. Disord. 39:140.

Thompson, M., and Thompson, G. 1972. Responses of infants and young children as a function of auditory stimuli and test methods. J. Speech Hear. Res. 15:699.

Thomsen, J., Terkildsen, K., and Osterhammel, P. 1978. Auditory brain stem responses in patients with acoustic neuromas. Scand. Audiol. 7:179.

Tonnison, W. 1975. Measuring in-the-ear gain of hearing aids by the acoustic-reflex method. J. Speech Hear. Res. 18:5.

Van Camp, K. J., and Creten, W. L. 1976. Principles of acoustic impedance and admittance. *In* Feldman, A. S., and Wilber, L. A. (eds.): Acoustic Impedance and Admittance. The Measurement of Middle Ear Function. Baltimore, Williams & Wilkins, pp. 300–334.

Van Camp, K. J., Margolis, R. J., Wilson, R. H., et al. 1986. Principles of Tympanometry: ASHA Monographs, No. 24.

Vanhuyse, J. J., Creten, W. L., and Van Camp, K. J. 1975. On the W-notching of tympanogram. Scand. Audiol. 4:45.

Van Wagoner, R. S., and Goodwine, S. 1977. Clinical impressions of acoustic reflex measures in an adult population. Arch. Otolaryngol. 103:582.

Weber, B. 1969. Validation of observer judgments in behavioral observation audiometry. J. Speech Hear. Disord. 34:350.

Wilber, L. A., and Feldman, A. S. 1976. Acoustic Impedance and Admittance—The Measure of Middle Ear Function. Baltimore, Williams & Wilkins.

Wiley, T. L., and Block, M. G. 1985. Overview and basic principles of acoustic immittance measurements. *In* Katz, J. (ed.): Handbook of Clinical Audiology, 3rd ed. Baltimore, Williams & Wilkins.

Wilson, W. R. 1978. Behavioral assessment of auditory function in infants. *In* Minifie, F. D., and Lloyd, L. L. (eds.): Communicative and Cognitive Abilities—Early Behavioral Assessment, Baltimore, University Park Press.

Wilson, W. R., and Thompson, G. 1984. Behavioral audiometry. *In* Jerger, J. (ed.): Pediatric Audiology: Current Trends. San Diego, College Hill Press.

Wilson, W. R., Moore, J. M., and Thompson, G. 1976. Sound field auditory thresholds of infants utilizing visual reinforcement audiometry (VRA). Presented at the annual convention of the American Speech and Hearing Association, Houston, Texas, November.

Yamada, O., Yagi, T., Yamane, H., et al. 1975. Clinical evaluation of the auditory evoked brainstem response. Auris Nasus Larynx 2:92.

Yoshie, N., Ohasi, T., and Suzuki, T. 1967. Non-surgical recording of auditory nerve action potentials in man. Laryngoscope 77:76.

Chapter 10

METHODS OF EXAMINATION: RADIOLOGIC ASPECTS

Hugh D. Curtin, M.D.

Imaging has evolved rapidly in the past decade, and the advances have had a profound effect on imaging of the ear. The progress has been so rapid that most textbook descriptions of imaging are outdated by the time of or shortly after publication. The descriptions found in this chapter are unlikely to be exceptions, so consultation with a knowledgeable radiologist is really the only way one can remain up to date in regard to optimal methods of imaging for the problem of a specific patient. First, the imaging modalities most commonly used will be described, and then specific points about several common clinical situations will be discussed.

IMAGING MODALITIES

Plain Film Radiography

Plain films remain a cost effective, low-radiation-exposure examination. They are useful as surveys of larger regions such as the mastoids (Etter, 1965; Bergeron et al., 1984). Their value relies on large differences in radiographic density between bone, soft tissue, and air (Figs. 10–1 and 10–2). The mastoids are normally filled with air, which is easily defined when contrasted against the surrounding bony structures. The pathologic condition is identified as soft tissue or fluid replacing the air density.

The bony skeleton is well evaluated by plain film because of the difference in density between bone and adjacent air or soft tissues. The major problem in conventional radiography is superimposition of one structure on another. However, if an area can be projected away from other overlying bony structures, plain films give excellent bony detail. For instance, the internal auditory canal can be measured if superimposed on the orbit (transorbital view) (Fig. 10–2) or away from the skull base (Stenvers view).

Tomography

Pluridirectional tomography (plain film) has been all but replaced by computed tomography (CT). Tomog-raphy gives images of the bone with high spatial resolution (ability to precisely define small structures). The spatial resolution is actually slightly better than with CT. However, soft tissue definition is poor. Any angle or obliquity of an image can be produced (Figs. 10–3 and 10–4).

The high resolution, the ability to do oblique images, and excellent bone images allow good characterization of congenital labyrinthine anomalies. The extremely high density of metal allows good images of metal prostheses. CT has problems with imaging metals and actually gives a distorted image (Fig. 10–5).

The examination has a fairly high radiation exposure because of the multiple slices and usually requires sedation or even anesthesia in young patients.

Computed Tomography

Computed tomography (CT) has lead the revolution in imaging and has moved radiology into the computer age (Valvassori et al, 1982; Bergeron et al., 1984). The x-ray beams are seen by detectors rather than captured on a film. Computers calculate how much x-ray density comes from each small region (pixel) within a slice. The resultant picture rivals tomography in spatial resolution and far surpasses tomography in the ability to differentiate one tissue density from another. Brain is easily separated from cerebrospinal fluid, and muscles are clearly defined when contrasted against various fat planes.

Radiation exposure is low, especially when one considers that the tissues outside the slice of interest receive very little dosage. There are no "ghost" shadows on CT, so the air-bone and air–soft tissue interfaces are clearer than in conventional tomography.

The technical advancement that allowed CT to surpass tomography of the temporal bone is the so-called "bone algorithm." The image generated during the scanning process shows soft tissues well. However, the data can be remanipulated by the computer to accentuate margins between tissues with high density differences. This is called a "bone algorithm" because of the excellent depiction of bone and soft tissue margins. The program does equally well with air–soft tissue and

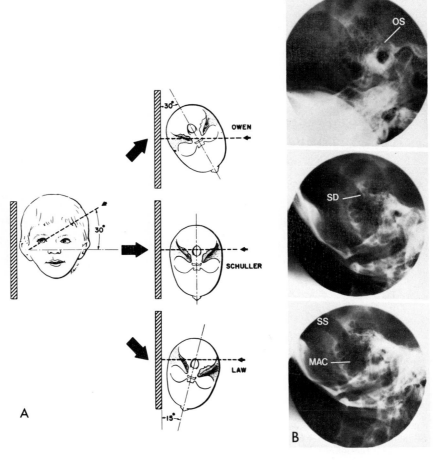

Figure 10–1. Lateral-type projections. *A*, Diagram illustrating, on the left, the primary caudal angulation of 30 degrees used to project the mastoid closest to the cassette away from the image of the contralateral mastoid. (In the Law projection, this angle is reduced to 15 degrees.) On the right, the secondary angulations for three commonly used projections are shown as being achieved by rotation of the patient's head. Sophisticated skull units achieve the same projections by a second angulation of the x-ray tube without moving the patient. *B*, The resultant radiographs. In this patient, the ossicles and sinodural angle are best demonstrated in Owen projection.

air-bone interfaces. Thus, minute structures, such as the facial nerve canal and the ossicles, are now easily seen on CT (see Figs. 10–8*A* and *B* and 10–10*A*).

The soft tissue algorithm is the usual image that has been available since the advent of CT (see Fig. 10–8*B*). The bone window (see Fig. 10–10*A*) is the routine soft tissue algorithm seen at a wider window. More density levels are seen at once. The bone algorithm is actually a computer program that sharpens bone margins, giving a far clearer image than a bone window (Figs. 10–8*A* and 10–24).

Currently, CT is used when plain films will not suffice. Indeed, in many situations, CT is done before plain films are taken. For instance, in the middle ear and mastoid, a few well-chosen slices on CT can give more definite information than plain films, with very little radiation in general and essentially no exposure to such radiation-sensitive structures as the thyroid or the lens of the eye.

The disadvantages of CT include the necessity to sedate many young patients, even for short examinations. Axial CT images are routinely used. Other orientations easily obtained by tomography are much more difficult to achieve with CT. Metal, such as is found in dental fillings, can provide streaklike artifacts that obscure an area of interest. The temporal bone is dense enough to cause streak artifacts; these are a problem because they obscure important areas in the posterior fossa.

More advanced data manipulation has helped solve the problem created by the difficulty in obtaining multiple projections. The slices are taken serially and are contiguous. The computer can stack the slices and figure out an approximation of other views (Fig. 10–6). This is called re-formatting and gives a reasonable coronal, sagittal, or oblique slice, with no additional scan time or radiation. The resolution is not as good as that of the direct coronal view (taken with the patient's head tilted back), which may still be necessary if a small, thin structure must be vizualized.

Magnetic Resonance Imaging

Magnetic resonance imaging (MRI) relies on the behavior of certain nuclei when subjected to a magnetic field (Brant-Zawadzki and Norman, 1987). These nuclei behave as though they were spinning. Because the nucleus is charged, the motion creates a minute magnetic field that interacts with any other magnetic field either related to neighboring spinning charges or to an externally applied field. Magnetic resonance imaging takes advantage of the fact that these atoms can be stimulated using very specific radio frequencies. As the stimulated nuclei relax, the radio signals of the same specific frequency are limited by the nuclei and can be detected. This characteristic radio frequency is directly related to the strength of the magnetic field.

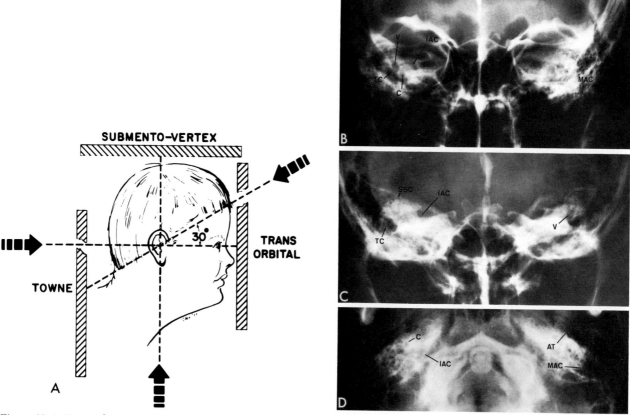

Figure 10–2. Towne, base, and posteroanterior projections. A, Diagram indicating the cassette position, incident beam, centering, and positioning for Towne, base (submentovertex), and posteroanterior (transorbital) projections of the temporal bones. B, Transorbital projection radiograph. The internal auditory canals, vestibules, and lateral and superior semicircular canals are usually well displayed. C, Towne projection radiograph. D, Submentovertex projection radiograph. TC, Tympanic cavity.

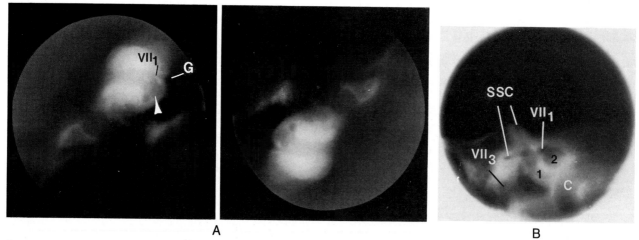

Figure 10–3. A, Pöschl projection. Tomographic slice through the cochlea. The slice is taken perpendicular to the long axis of the petrous bone. This gives a perfect cross-section through the cochlea. VII₁, Labyrinthine segment of the facial nerve canal; G, geniculate. Arrowhead indicates separation between second and apical turns of the cochlea (demonstration of this bony partition excludes a Mondini malformation). B, Pluridirectional tomography, Stenvers view. Slice parallel to the long axis of the petrous bone (45-degree angle from frontal projection). 1, Basilar turn of the cochlea; 2, apical turns of the cochlea; VII₁, labyrinthine segment of the facial nerve canal; VII₃, mastoid segment of the facial nerve canal; SSC, superior semicircular canal and horizontal semicircular canal; C, carotid canal.

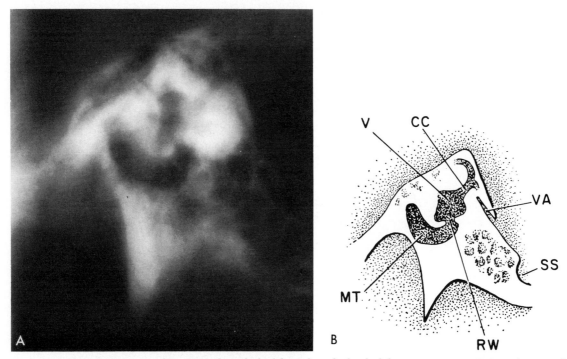

Figure 10–4. *A*, Lateral (sagittal) tomographic section through the labyrinth at the level of the crus commune. *B*, Line drawing of *A*. VA, Vestibular aqueduct; V, vestibule; CC, crus commune; MT, mesotympanum; RW, round window; SS, sigmoid sinus.

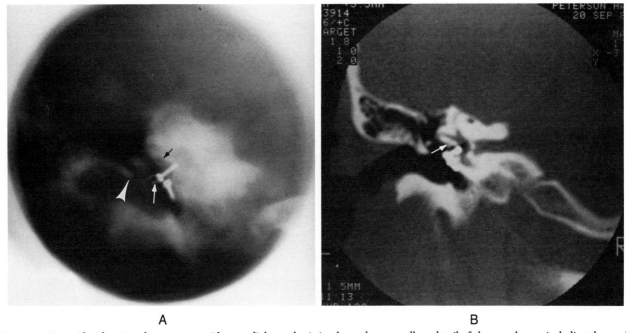

Figure 10–5. *A*, Pluridirectional tomogram, with stapedial prosthesis in place, shows excellent detail of the prostheses, including the small wires used to attach the prosthesis to an ossicle. The second prosthesis is seen adjacent to the promontory. The resolution is higher than on CT (see *B*). Attachment wire indicated by white arrow. Facial nerve canal shown by black arrow. Arrowhead marks scutum. Note how the actual bony cortex of the facial nerve canal can be defined. *B*, CT of the same patient. The demonstration of the two prostheses is much less precise because of the high density of the metal. The position of the prostheses is much more precisely defined on the tomogram. Note also the less sharp image of the facial nerve canal (white arrow) compared with that on the tomogram.

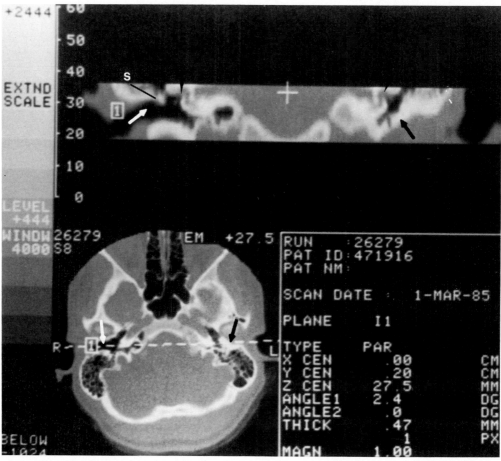

Figure 10–6. Coronal re-format. External auditory canal atresia. Axial slices were initially done, and coronal re-format was performed by the computer. The external auditory canal is seen on the normal side (white arrow) in both the axial and the coronal re-formatted images. Note the atretic plate (black arrow) on the abnormal side again in both axial and re-formatted images. Oval window indicated by arrowheads. S, Scutum.

Thus, an image can be produced by varying the magnetic field. An imaginary grid is laid across an area of interest. Each point on this grid is subjected to a slightly different magnetic field and, therefore, has a slightly different characteristic frequency. The signal coming from each point can be identified. These slight variations in local magnetic field are accomplished by a complex system of magnets or coils. There is an overall baseline magnetic field that remains constant, and there are gradient magnets or coils that essentially give a stronger magnetic field at one side of the body than at the other. The last components are the radio-frequency coils (functioning like antennas), which emit the radio-frequency pulse, listen for the returning signal, or both.

An extensive description of MRI is beyond the scope of this book, but several terms and ideas are very useful and recur frequently in the discussions of MRI.

1. Almost all imaging is currently done by stimulating hydrogen nuclei.

2. On most systems, signal is indicated by whiteness or brightness.

3. T_1 relaxation is a measure of how fast the stimulated nuclei return to their baseline magnetic field level. This type of imaging provides good anatomic information. Fat is very bright, whereas muscle tends to be dark. Cerebrospinal fluid is dark (Fig. 10–7A).

4. T_2 relaxation measures how fast the stimulated nuclei lose phase coherence after the stimulating signal is turned off. This is a more complicated principle but nonetheless can be measured. Images may not be quite as pleasing but often give more specific information about various tissues. Cerebrospinal fluid becomes bright (Fig. 10–7B). Brain becomes darker, fat darkens, and muscle remains dark. Even though the image is not as sharp, a lesion might be better defined because the T_2 characteristics may differ more from surrounding structures than the T_1 characteristics.

5. Cortical bone, air, and rapidly flowing blood are black (signal void) (Fig. 10–7B).

There are many more extensive sources available. (Interested readers are referred to the work by Brant-Zawadzki and Norman [1987]).

The advantages of MRI over CT are several. There is no ionizing radiation. The radio frequencies used are not considered harmful. Even strong magnetic fields are considered safe as long as patients do not have certain ferromagnetic metals in or near their

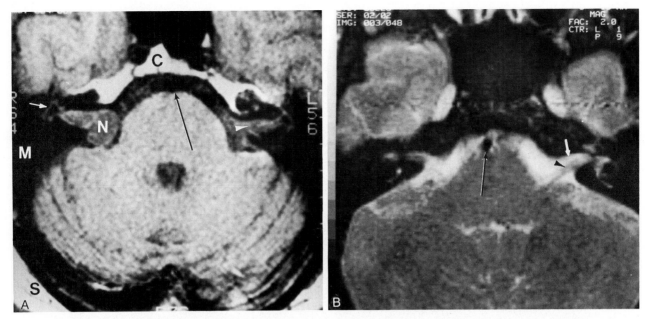

Figure 10–7. *A*, T$_1$-weighted image (short TR, short TE). Acoustic neuroma. Cerebrospinal fluid is dark (long arrow) and can be seen entering the left internal auditory canal (arrowhead). The acoustic neuroma (N) fills the abnormal internal auditory canal and bulges into the cerebellopontine angle cistern. In the mastoid (M), neither bone nor air gives enough signal to be seen, so they cannot be differentiated. The fat in the subcutaneous area (S) as well as in the clivus (C) gives a very bright signal. The tumor produces an intermediate signal, and the facial nerve canal (short white arrow) has enough tissue to give an intermediate signal as well. *B*, Normal internal auditory canal T$_2$-weighted image. T$_2$-weighted image shows bright cerebrospinal fluid contrasted against the nerves extending into the internal auditory canal. Cerebrospinal fluid in the internal auditory canal is indicated by the white arrow. Cranial nerves in the internal auditory canal are shown by the arrowhead. Note the signal void in the basilar artery (black arrow).

bodies. Currently, intravenous contrast enhancement is not used routinely. However, work is being done in developing paramagnetic contrast materials such as gadolinium, which can be made to give a very bright signal.

The blood vessels are often well seen on MRI. Rapidly flowing blood often gives no signal (Fig. 10–7*B*). The stimulated protons in blood have moved on by the time one listens for the returning signal. Therefore, blood vessels (especially arteries) are seen as black holes within the surrounding tissue.

MRI artifacts differ from those produced with CT. The posterior fossa is better seen on MRI than CT. Local artifacts are seen around metal and dental amalgams, but the streak artifacts that degrade the entire image are not present.

Any orientation can be obtained. Sagittal, coronal, and oblique views are as easily obtained as axial views.

Using various "pulse sequences" of radio stimulation, one can vary the signal of different tissues to obtain better tissue specificity.

Negative aspects of MRI that may be less relevant in the future are (1) the long imaging time often requiring sedation or anesthesia in the young; (2) its inability to distinguish air from cortical bone (this limits, for example, the usefulness of MRI in the middle ear and mastoid); and (3) the fact that the minimum slice thickness currently available is slightly higher than that with CT.

Angiography

Angiography defines the blood vessels and is helpful in establishing the blood supply of a tumor or the course of an artery. The anatomic definition of the

Figure 10–8. Patient with mastoiditis, epidural abscess, and jugular vein occlusion. *A*, Axial CT with *bone algorithm* shows opacification of the attic and the antrum, with minimal demineralization of bone (arrowhead) next to the sinodural angle. Note the air within the attic (short arrow) on the opposite side. 1, Internal auditory canal; 2, vestibular aqueduct; 3, horizontal semicircular canal; 4, posterior semicircular canal; 5, malleus; 6, incus; 7, facial nerve canal. *B*, *Soft tissue algorithm* shows lucency (black arrow) with some small enhancement medially that may represent on this image a small amount of residual flow or could be enhancement of the dura. *C*, Lower slice shows decreased density or attenuation in the vascular portion of the jugular foramen (arrow) compared with the normal side (arrowhead) or with the carotid arteries (C). This raises the possibility of a jugular vein thrombosis. *D*, Magnetic resonance scan with intermediate weighting. The bright signal in the mastoid (arrow) indicates retained secretions or fluid. Compare with the opposite side. Note that there is some signal from the vestibule (V) and cochlea (C), and part of the horizontal semicircular canal (3) can be seen. *E*, On a lower slice, T$_1$-weighted image, there is a stronger signal in the sigmoid sinus (S) and the jugular vein (J) than is usually seen with rapidly flowing blood. (*Caution*: It must be noted that the jugular vein can have various appearances.) *F*, Sagittal T$_1$-weighted image shows a definite difference in signal between the jugular vein (J) and the carotid artery (C). Note the curve of the jugular (arrow) passing toward the sigmoid sinus. Again, this suggests jugular vein thrombosis.

See illustration on following page

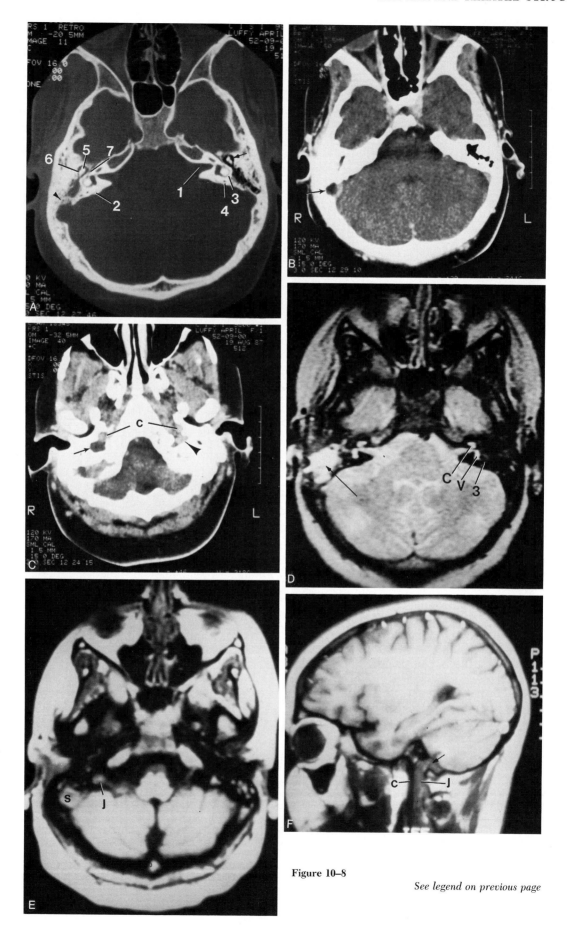

Figure 10–8

See legend on previous page

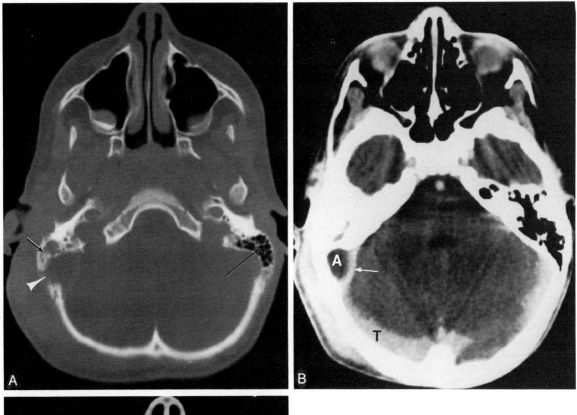

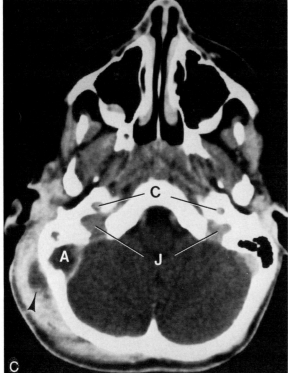

Figure 10–9. Patient with acute mastoiditis and epidural and superficial abscesses. *A, Bone algorithm* showing definite demineralization of the septations in the mastoid (shorter arrow) and around the sigmoid sinus (arrowhead). Note the black density of air within the normal side (longer arrow). *B,* Soft tissue algorithm shows decreased attenuation (A) at the abscess collection. Again, the enhancement medial to the collection (arrow) could represent residual blood flow or enhancing dura. Note that this enhancement is of the same density as that of the transverse sinus (T). *C,* Slightly lower slice shows the abscess (A) in the region of the sigmoid sinus but also in the superficial soft tissue (arrowhead). Note that in this patient, in contrast to the previous patient, the jugular bulb on the involved side is approximately the same as that on the normal side as well as approximately the same as the carotid arteries. This suggests that there is no jugular vein thrombosis. J, Jugular bulbs; C, carotid arteries.

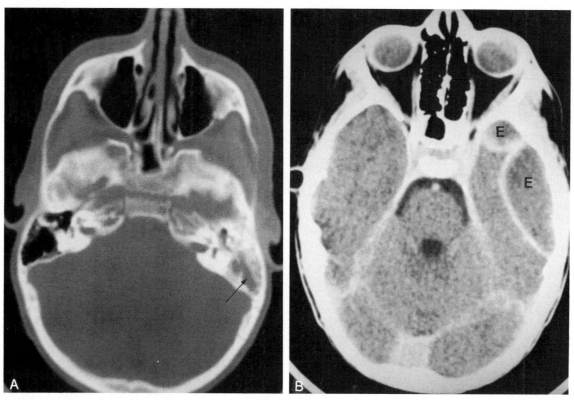

Figure 10–10. *A*, Axial *bone window* (not algorithm) shows fluid in the mastoid (arrow) and in the attic (arrowhead). Compare with the opposite side. The bone is less distinct than would be expected in a bone algorithm. *B*, Slightly higher slice shows several loculations of epidural abscess (E). Note how they taper toward the calvarium.

margins of a lesion are currently better defined with either CT or MRI. Recently, progress has been made in the embolization procedures that can be used to diminish the blood supply of a tumor preoperatively or actually to treat some arteriovenous abnormalities.

CLINICAL SITUATIONS

Certain clinical situations have been chosen to illustrate points about the various radiologic modalities as they pertain to the temporal bone.

Infections

Plain films are used as a survey. The development of the mastoid can be appreciated, as can clarity or opacity of the air cells. However, a few slices with CT can define very small amounts of fluid and can give excellent definition of the bony septation within the mastoid (Fig. 10–8). Small erosions are easier to appreciate on CT than on plain films or pluridirectional tomography (Fig. 10–9). Thus, when a concomitant cholesteatoma is suspected, CT is ideal.

Magnetic resonance imaging does not give the resolution needed for subtle evaluation of the temporal bone. However, MRI does detect fluid, as there is signal where there should be none (Fig. 10–8). Obstruction or fluid filling air cells gives a bright signal.

If the middle ear and mastoid are being evaluated, intravenous administration of contrast material may not be necessary. However, if there is suspicion of any intracranial complication, intravenous contrast material is administered to increase the sensitivity of the examination in detecting such pathologic conditions as epidural abscess and brain abscess (Fig. 10–10). The epidural abscess tapers toward the bone at either end of the collection. The dura enhances. A common location of an otogenic epidural abscess is directly lateral to the sigmoid sinus (Figs. 10–8 and 10–9). The sinus is actually within the dura and can be elevated and compressed. The blood flow may be "squeezed" into the medial portion of the sigmoid sinus, which remains patent. Further or continued involvement can lead to actual occlusion. When occlusion occurs, the clot can propagate along the jugular vein (Fig. 10–8).

Determination of patency of the sigmoid sinus and the jugular vein can be difficult. On CT, the appearance of an obstructed sigmoid can be very close to that of an epidural abscess (Figs. 10–8 and 10–9). Both show a lucency between the bone and the enhancing dural margin. Some help comes from the appearance of the jugular vein. If the vein is clotted, there is usually a lower attenuation in the vascular compartment of the jugular foramen when intravenous contrast material is used. In questionable cases, a bolus of contrast material can be injected to optimize the "opacification" of vessels.

Dynamic scanning is a combination of bolus injection

with multiple slices taken rapidly at the same level. The changes in density reflect the blood opacification and can determine a normal arterial or venous pattern.

Magnetic resonance imaging may also be useful in the analysis of blood vessel patency (Figs. 10–8 and 10–9). Usually, a vessel will look "black" if flow is sufficiently high. However, the jugular vein may have a variable appearance because of tortuosity and variable rates of flow. Limited flip angle imaging or gradient echo (a more recently developed pulse sequence) makes vessels appear bright. More experience is needed to assess reliability in this determination.

Cholesteatoma and Chronic Inflammatory Disease

In patients with cholesteatoma, CT is the examination of choice. Contrast enhancement is not needed unless there is concern regarding a concurrent intracranial pathologic condition. CT has problems differentiating actual cholesteatoma from fluid or granulation tissue. The radiologist can identify bone erosion (Figs. 10–11 through 10–13). The horizontal semicircular canal is carefully inspected along the lateral curve. The tegmen tympani, lateral wall of the attic, and facial nerve canal all are evaluated. Coronal imaging is very helpful in evaluating the facial nerve canal, tegmen, and lateral wall of the attic as well as the lateral aspect of the horizontal semicircular canal. Detection of erosion of the ossicles is less reliable. Large erosions can be seen, but small erosions are difficult to exclude. Erosion of bone is presumptive evidence of cholesteatoma.

Rarely, an encephalocele occurring as a postoperative complication can clinically mimic recurrent cholesteatoma. The tegmen is again a key landmark (Fig. 10–14).

Atticoantral disease or blockage has an appearance like cholesteatoma but with no bone erosion. Below the level of the head of the malleus and the body of the incus, the middle ear is clear (Fig. 10–15).

Automastoidectomy occurs when a cholesteatoma breaks into the external auditory canal and evacuates. The bone erosion is characteristic of cholesteatoma, but the eroded area is filled with air rather than soft tissue.

Dystrophic calcification, often referred to as tympanosclerosis, is considered a sequela of chronic inflammation and can sometimes be visualized on CT. Calcification can be seen in the tympanic membrane or in the middle ear interfering with ossicular formation (Fig. 10–16).

Tumors

CT is excellent in the determination of tumor extent. Tumor destroys bone. Below the temporal bone, tumor obliterates soft tissue and fat planes and so is detectable (Fig. 10–17). Intracranial extension of the tumor has a higher CT density than that of the cerebrospinal fluid space and often can be differentiated from brain.

Magnetic resonance imaging has some advantages, although spatial resolution is lower. Because pulse sequences can be varied to optimize the contrast (different appearance) between tissue, tumor margin

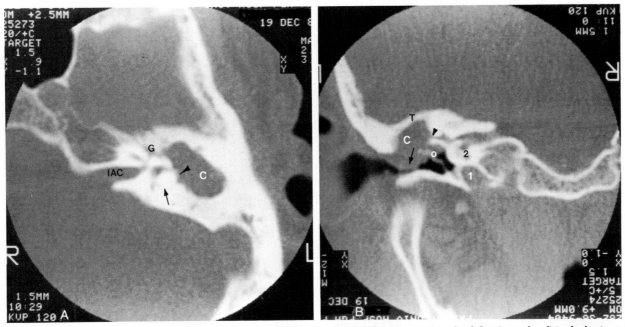

Figure 10–11. Axial slice of cholesteatoma. A, Cholesteatoma (C) fills the attic and the antrum. Note the defect (arrowhead) in the horizontal semicircular canal. IAC, Internal auditory canal; G, geniculate ganglion. Posterior limb of the horizontal semicircular canal is indicated by the arrow. B, Coronal image of cholesteatoma. There is absence of the scutum as the cholesteatoma (C) grows down into the external auditory canal (arrow). Again, there is erosion of the horizontal semicircular canal (arrowhead). The ossicle (O) is displaced. 1, Carotid artery; 2, cochlea; T, tegmen.

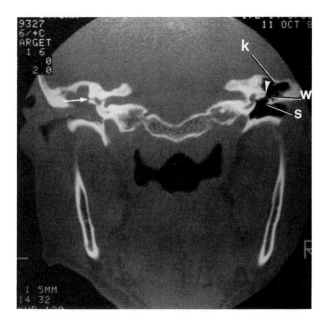

Figure 10–12. Coronal CT scan in a patient with cholesteatoma. Note complete erosion of the scutum and ossicles and erosion into the horizontal semicircular canal (arrow). Note the normal anatomy on the opposite side. s, Scutum; w, lateral wall of the attic; k, Koerner septum. Intact horizontal semicircular canal is shown by the arrowhead.

can be most easily seen. For instance, below the temporal bone, CT may have trouble separating tumor and muscle. Magnetic resonance imaging usually can show the muscle-tumor interface, using T_1 and T_2.

The appearance of cerebrospinal fluid can be varied. On T_1, cerebrospinal fluid is dark; on T_2, it is bright. This aids in detecting tumor–cerebrospinal fluid interfaces. The classic example is detection of small acoustic neuromas, in which MRI is considered the examination of choice. Tumors can be seen on either T_1 or T_2 images contrasted against cerebrospinal fluid. Gadolinium is a paramagnetic contrast agent that makes demonstration of acoustic neuromas easier. The tumor

"lights up" on the relatively brief T_1-weighted image, thus hopefully allowing quicker and more cost effective examinations. Acoustic neuromas are rare but do occur occasionally in children.

Magnetic resonance imaging is considered better than CT in defining the relation of tumor to brain. Again, this is due to increased soft tissue discrimination. The ability to do coronal and sagittal imaging is also helpful.

Initially, the temporal bone was considered a poor subject for tumor evaluation because neither the cortical bone nor the air gave signal and thus everything looked "black." However, as tumor replaces either

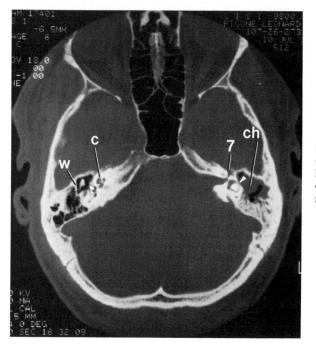

Figure 10–13. Cholesteatoma (ch) partially filling the attic and eroding the anterolateral margin of the horizontal semicircular canal (arrowhead). Note the metallic density of a stapes prosthesis in the opposite oval window. w, Lateral wall of the attic normal side; c, cochlea; 7, geniculate ganglion.

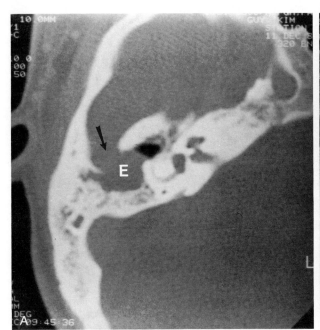

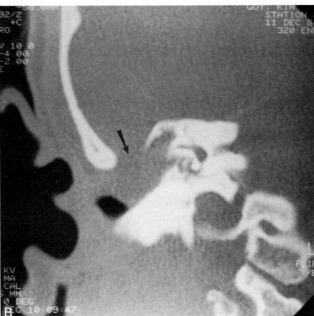

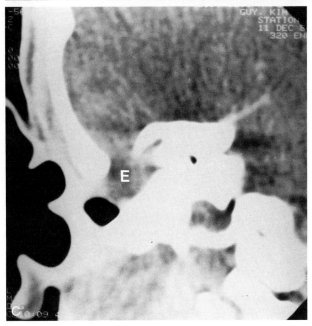

Figure 10–14. Postmastoidectomy encephalocele. *A*, Axial scan shows an appearance much like that of a recurrent cholesteatoma. However, there is a large defect (arrow) in the tegmen of the mastoid. The tissue within the mastoid represents a herniation of brain (encephalocele [E]). *B*, Coronal image better demonstrates the defect in the tegmen (arrow). *C*, Soft tissue image shows the density of the encephalocele (E) to be approximately that of the brain.

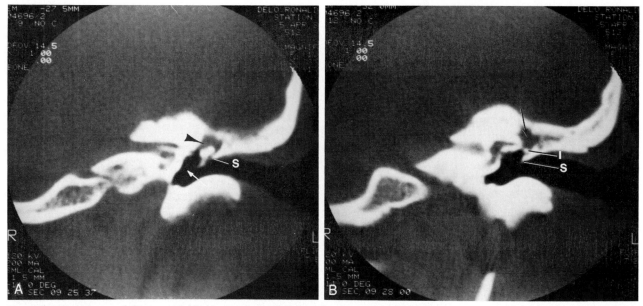

Figure 10–15. Atticoantral disease with blockage at the level of the isthmus. *A*, The lower middle ear (arrow) is normal. However, the attic (arrowhead) is filled with fluid, which does not extend below the scutum (s). *B*, Slightly posterior slice shows the uneroded scutum (s) and the short process of the incus (i), with opacification of the upper attic and antrum (arrow).

cortical bone or air, one finds signal (brightness) where there should be none. Thus, one does indeed see the image of the actual tumor rather than the hole that the tumor makes. There is often a significant amount of fat in the apex of the petrous bone. Fat is very bright on T_1-weighted images. As tumor replaces this fat, the brightness is replaced by the lower signal of the tumor.

Another advantage of MRI is its potential ability to differentiate tumor and fluid trapped in the mastoid. The signal of the tumor is usually less than that of the retained fluid, allowing definition of the tumor margin.

Congenital Anomalies

Currently, the initial radiographic procedure for congenital anomalies is CT (Figs. 10–18 through 10–25). The anomalies are separated into those of the inner ear and those of the middle or external ear. To exclude an anomaly, the radiologist checks certain landmarks.

The cochlea should be normal in size and should have the normal number of turns (Figs. 10–18 through 10–20). The most important structure is the bony separation between the second and the apical turns

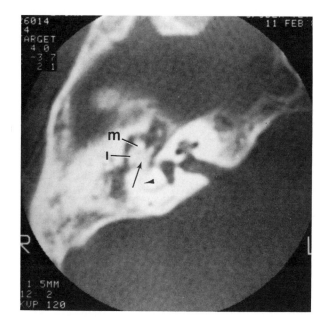

Figure 10–16. Tympanosclerosis and a chronic middle-ear inflammatory problem. Dense calcification (arrow) is shown between the horizontal semicircular canal and the incus. There is opacification of the attic and the antrum as well. The horizontal semicircular canal is indicated by the arrowhead. i, Incus; m, malleus.

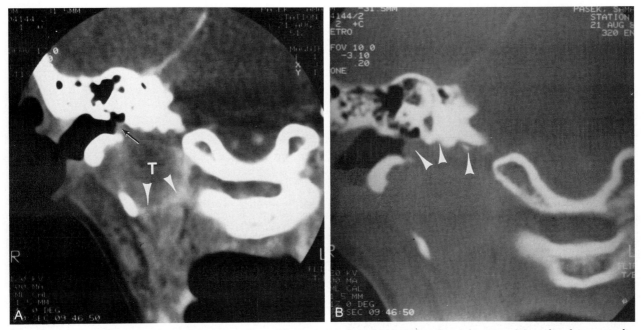

Figure 10–17. Rhabdomyosarcoma eroding up into the middle ear. *A*, Soft tissue algorithm shows the tumor (T) eroding bone extending into the middle ear (arrow). Note that the lower margin of the tumor (arrowheads) can be defined, as it is contrasted against the normal fat planes beneath the skull base. *B*, Bone algorithm shows the erosion of the bone (arrowheads), but the lower margin of the lesion is less well defined.

(Figs. 10–3A and 10–24A). This is usually identifiable on CT and essentially excludes the Mondini anomaly. The semicircular canals should form a ring rather than a sac (Fig. 10–21). Most frequently affected is the horizontal or lateral semicircular canal. The vestibular and cochlear aqueducts can be readily seen on CT (Fig. 10–22).

External auditory canal atresia can be staged using CT (Figs. 10–23 and 10–24). Coronal views can be very helpful but often are not necessary if the axial images are done so that sagittal and coronal re-formatted sections can be made (see Fig. 10–5). The width of the atretic plate and the patency of the middle ear can be evaluated (Fig. 10–25). The degree of ossicular fusion can be approximated. Minor anomalies of the ossicular chain cannot be completely excluded.

The facial nerve can migrate anteriorly either in relation to an underdeveloped cochlea (Fig. 10–26) or

Text continued on page 172

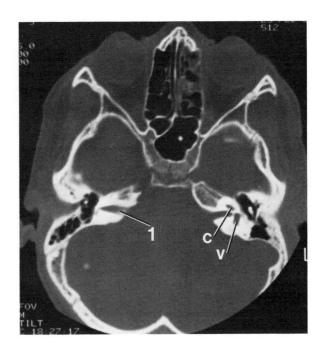

Figure 10–18. Michel deformity. Level of the internal auditory canal (1). No cochlea or vestibule is seen on the right side. V, Vestibule on the normal side; C, cochlea. (Reprinted with permission from Curtin, H. D.: Congenital Malformations of the Ear. *In* Valvassori, G. E., and Mafee, M. F. [eds.]: Diagnostic Imaging in Otolaryngology—I. The Ear. Otolaryngologic Clinics of North America. Philadelphia, W. B. Saunders Co., 1988.)

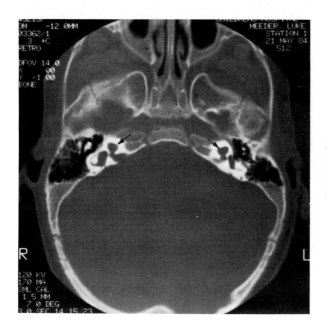

Figure 10–19. Mondini malformation. Note the cystic dilatation of the cochlea (arrows) bilaterally. (Reprinted with permission from Curtin, H. D.: Congenital Malformations of the Ear. *In* Valvassori, G. E., and Mafee, M. F. [eds.]: Diagnostic Imaging in Otolaryngology—I. The Ear. Otolaryngologic Clinics of North America. Philadelphia, W. B. Saunders Co., 1988.)

Figure 10–20. Severe deformity of the cochlea and the vestibule. The internal auditory canal appears to communicate widely (arrow) with the vestibule and the cochlea, which are represented by a single large, dilated sac (arrowhead). The ossicular chain is relatively normal.

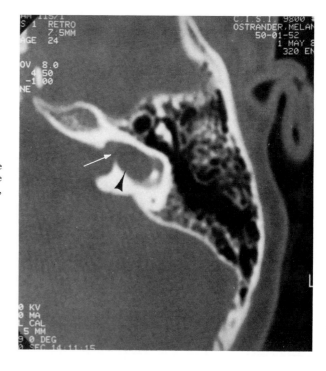

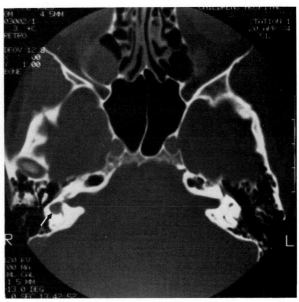

Figure 10–21. Horizontal semicircular canal (arrow) is represented by a cystic dilated remnant. (Reprinted with permission from Curtin, H. D.: Congenital Malformations of the Ear. *In* Valvassori, G. E., and Mafee, M. F. [eds.]: Diagnostic Imaging in Otolaryngology—I. The Ear. Otolaryngologic Clinics of North America. Philadelphia, W. B. Saunders Co., 1988.)

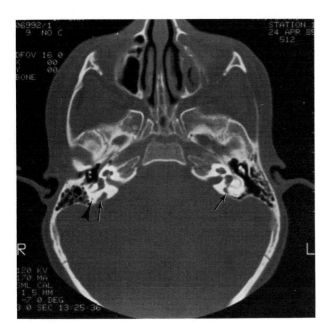

Figure 10–22. Dilatation of the vestibular aqueduct. The vestibular aqueducts (arrows) are larger than usual. Normal maximums are approximately the same as that of the posterior semicircular canal (arrowhead).

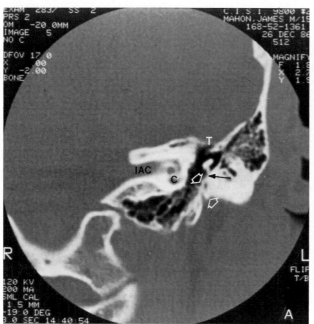

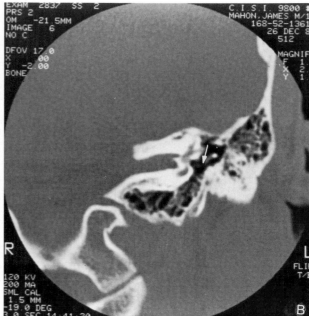

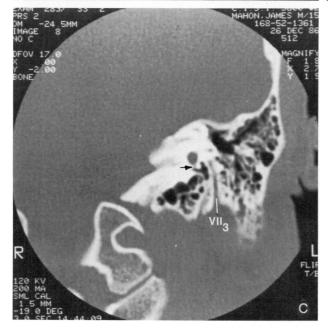

Figure 10–23. *A,* Coronal external auditory canal atresia. There is fusion of the ossicle to the atretic plate (black arrow). The thickness of the atretic plate (between open arrows) is easily demonstrated. *C,* Cochlea; *IAC,* internal auditory canal; *T,* tegmen. *B,* The incus and the stapes (arrow) are relatively normal, but, again, note the absence of the external auditory canal. *C,* Coronal image, level of the round window (arrow), shows the facial nerve canal (VII$_3$) in its mastoid segment. Normally, this should be seen on a more posterior cut. (*A, B,* and *C,* Reprinted with permission from Curtin H. D.: Congenital Malformations of the Ear. *In* Valvassori, G. E., and Mafee, M. F. [eds.]: Diagnostic Imaging in Otolaryngology—I. The Ear. Otolaryngologic Clinics of North America. Philadelphia, W. B. Saunders Co., 1988.)

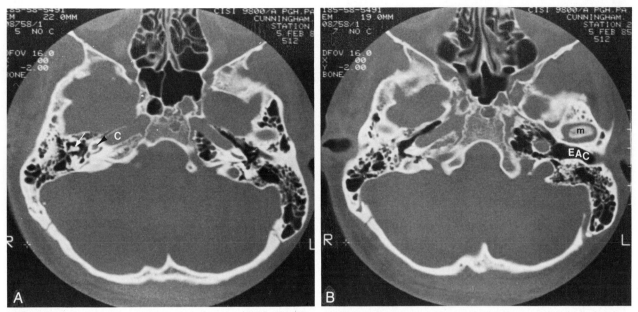

Figure 10–24. *A*, External auditory canal atresia with fusion of the ossicular chain. Note the fusion of malleus and incus (arrow). The cochlea is normal. The bony separation between the second and apical turns (arrowhead) is the finding that essentially excludes a Mondini malformation of the cochlea. C, Carotid canal. *B*, External auditory canal atresia, lower slice than that shown in *A*. The normal external auditory canal (EAC) contrasted with that on the opposite side. M, Mandibular condyle. (*A* and *B*, Reprinted with permission from Curtin, H. D.: Congenital Malformations of the Ear. *In* Valvassori, G. E., and Mafee, M. F. [eds.]: Diagnostic Imaging in Otolaryngology—I. The Ear. Otolaryngologic Clinics of North America. Philadelphia, W. B. Saunders Co., 1988.)

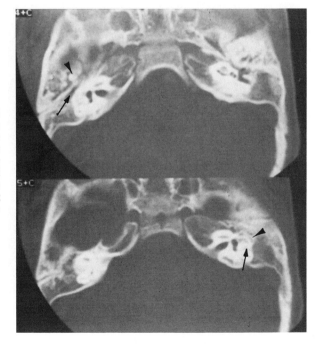

Figure 10–25. External auditory canal atresia, with very underdeveloped middle ear. Upper image shows very narrow middle ear (arrow), with some minimal ossicular differentiation (arrowhead). On the lower image (actually more superior in the patient), bone (arrowhead) is immediately contiguous with the horizontal semicircular canal (arrowhead). The very narrow middle ear may be filled with fluid or with tissue. (Reprinted with permission from Curtin, H. D.: Congenital Malformations of the Ear. *In* Valvassori, G. E., and Mafee, M. F. [eds.]: Diagnostic Imaging in Otolaryngology—I. The Ear. Otolaryngologic Clinics of North America. Philadelphia, W. B. Saunders Co., 1988.)

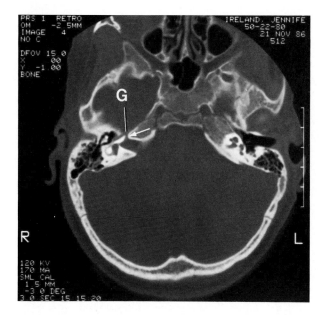

Figure 10–26. Anterior migration of the facial nerve canal. Bone algorithm. Facial nerve canal has migrated anteriorly and medially along the petrous apex. An inferior slice showed a very small cochlear remnant. G, Geniculate ganglion. Arrow indicates labyrinthine segment of the facial nerve canal. (Reprinted with permission from Curtin, H. D.: Congenital Malformations of the Ear. *In* Valvassori, G. E., and Mafee, M. F. [eds.]: Diagnostic Imaging in Otolaryngology—I. The Ear. Otolaryngologic Clinics of North America. Philadelphia, W. B. Saunders Co., 1988.)

more commonly in conjunction with an atretic external ear canal (Fig. 10–23). These abnormal positions can be a problem at surgery and are readily detected on CT. The tympanic segment of the facial nerve can "drop" down to the level of the stapes or rarely can cross the promontory (Fig. 10–27).

Perhaps the most important anomaly in the ear is the aberrant carotid artery (Fig. 10–28). This is readily detected on CT, as the lateral bony wall of the carotid canal is absent and the vessel can be followed into the middle ear. The foramen spinosum is usually absent

because the middle meningeal artery derives supply via a persistent stapedial artery that passes from the aberrant segment of the carotid artery through the middle ear (and stapes) before reaching the middle cranial fossa close to the geniculate ganglion. Dehiscent jugular bulbs are also visible, but they are less potentially catastrophic.

Although CT is the initial procedure in most evaluations of the temporal bone, tomography can be done to take advantage of the variety of projections easily available. For instance, slices taken either along the

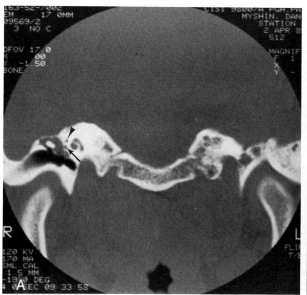
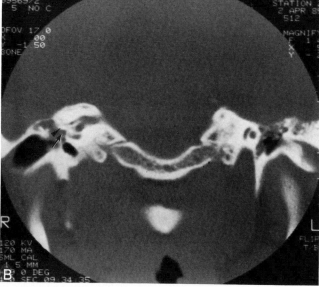

Figure 10–27. Coronal image. Inferior migration of the tympanic segment of the facial nerve canal. *A,* The tympanic segment of the facial nerve canal (arrow) is much more inferior than usual. Normally, it is more lateral to the labyrinthine segment (arrowhead). There is also opacification of the attic. *B,* More posterior slice through the region of the oval window shows an indistinct density representing the facial nerve canal (arrow). It is inferiorly displaced and very close to the oval window. No lucency is seen immediately beneath the horizontal canal in the normal location of the facial nerve (arrowhead). (*A* and *B,* Reprinted with permission from Curtin, H. D.: Congenital Malformations of the Ear. *In* Valvassori, G. E., and Mafee, M. F. [eds.]: Diagnostic Imaging in Otolaryngology–I. The Ear. Otolaryngologic Clinics of North America. Philadelphia, W. B. Saunders Co., 1988.)

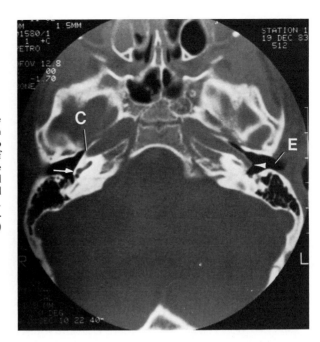

Figure 10–28. Aberrant carotid artery. Carotid artery extends more laterally than usual, extending out over the promontory, where it can be seen through the external auditory canal. Compare its position to that on the normal, opposite side. Arrowhead indicates lateral extent of the aberrant carotid. E, External auditory canal. Arrow indicates the promontory. Note the intact bony wall of the carotid canal on the normal side (C). (Reprinted with permission from Curtin, H. D.: Congenital Malformations of the Ear. *In* Valvassori, G. E., and Mafee, M. F. [eds.]: Diagnostic Imaging in Otolaryngology—I. The Ear. Otolaryngologic Clinics of North America. Philadelphia, W. B. Saunders Co., 1988.)

axis of the petrous bone (Stenvers view) or perpendicular to it (Pöschl view) can be very helpful in evaluating congenital abnormalities of the cochlea if the individual turns are not definitely identified on CT (Fig. 10–3A). Sagittal views are helpful for evaluating the ossicles.

Trauma

Trauma to the ear is also evaluated by CT (Figs. 10–29 and 10–30). Fractures are more easily seen because of fluid in air cells adjacent to fracture lines (Fig. 10–29). Fractures through the septations of the mastoid are easily appreciated. Ossicular disruption can be defined (Fig. 10–30). One must keep in mind that neither CT nor tomography can completely exclude a fracture, especially a "hairline" undisplaced fracture. The fractures most easily missed are those that are parallel to, or in the plane of, a CT slice rather than perpendicular to the slice. For instance, a vertical (superioinferior) fracture in the squamous temporal bone would be in the plane of a coronal slice and could

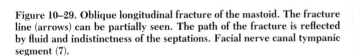

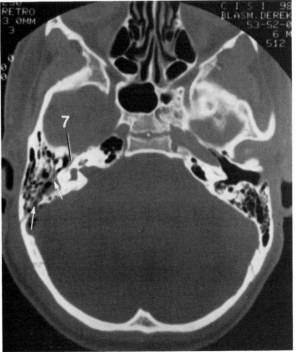

Figure 10–29. Oblique longitudinal fracture of the mastoid. The fracture line (arrows) can be partially seen. The path of the fracture is reflected by fluid and indistinctness of the septations. Facial nerve canal tympanic segment (7).

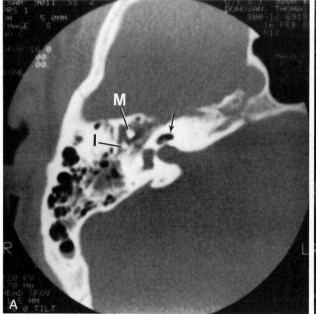

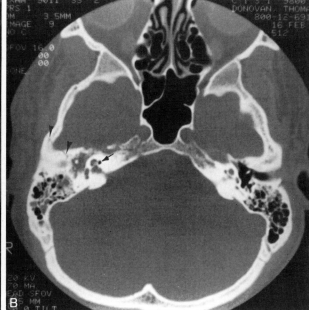

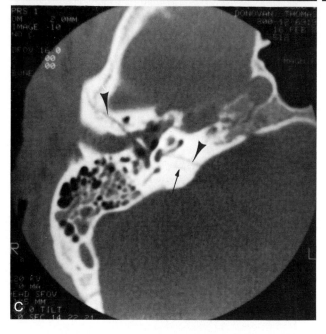

Figure 10–30. Longitudinal fracture, with ossicular dislocation and with violation of the labyrinth. *A,* Separation of the malleus (**M**) and the incus (**I**). Note the air within the cochlea, which is much blacker than normal (arrow). *B,* Fracture line (arrowheads). Air in the cochlea is indicated by the arrow. *C,* Inferior slice. Fracture lines (arrowheads). The fracture line through the petrous portion, more medially, should not be confused with the cochlear aqueduct (arrow), which can be seen indistinctly slightly posteriorly.

be missed. Such a fracture would "cross" an axial slice and so should be apparent.

Computed tomography also gives excellent visualization of the more vital intracranial structures in a traumatized patient. Hematomas (acute) are white on an unenhanced scan (Fig. 10–31).

Miscellaneous

Various bony dysplasias can be diagnosed and staged using CT, especially with bone algorithms. Fibrous dysplasia's characteristic density is slightly darker (less dense) than that of normal cortical bone. Areas of soft tissue can be seen within, depending on the degree of mineralization (Fig. 10–32).

Similarly, CT can demonstrate the demineralized bone of otosclerosis contrasted against the denser otic capsule (Fig. 10–33). Cochlear otosclerosis has a very characteristic appearance, with a lucency abutting the cochlear lumen. Although early changes can be missed, narrowing of the oval window and demineralization of the fissula ante fenestram can often be detected.

SUMMARY

Plain films remain as survey views. Computed tomography has almost completely replaced pluridirec-

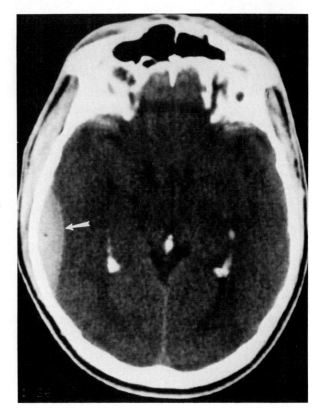

Figure 10–31. Epidural hematoma (arrow) showing the hyperdensity on the uncontrasted scan and the usual tapering toward the calvarium.

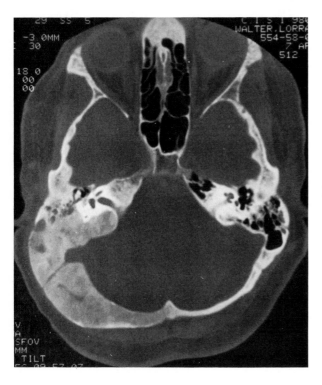

Figure 10–32. Fibrous dysplasia showing thickening of the occipital and temporal bones, with intermediate mineralization.

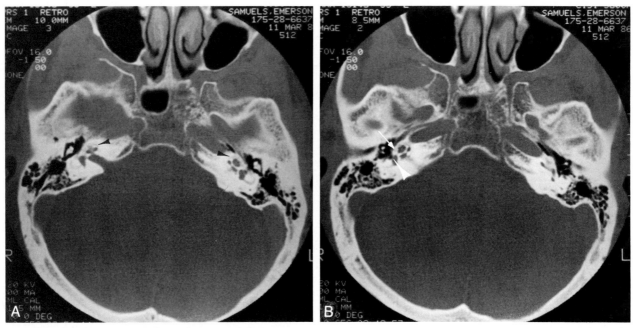

Figure 10–33. *A*, Cochlear otosclerosis showing indistinctness of the otic capsule close to the cochlea (arrowheads). *B*, Slightly inferior slice shows slight thickening of the bone, which is undermineralized (arrow), in the region of the fissula ante fenestram just anterior to the footplate of the stapes. Footplate of the stapes (arrowhead).

tional tomography. Magnetic resonance imaging is advancing rapidly and, as the technology improves, may replace CT in many cases, if for no other reason than the fact that ionizing radiation is not used.

SELECTED REFERENCES

Bergeron, R. T., Osborn, A. G., and Som, P. M. 1984. Head and Neck Imaging Excluding the Brain. St. Louis, MO, The C.V. Mosby Co.
A complete text dealing with all aspects of head and neck radiology.
Brant-Zawadzki, M., and Norman, D. 1987. Magnetic Resonance Imaging of the Central Nervous System. New York, Raven Press.
A good general descriptive text on magnetic resonance. Some sections specifically discuss head and neck problems.
Mancuso, A. A., and Hanafee, W. N. 1985. Computed Tomography and Magnetic Resonance Imaging of the Head and Neck, 2nd ed. Baltimore, Williams & Wilkins.
An excellent text examining computed tomography and magnetic resonance. Excellent anatomic and pathologic illustrations.
Swartz, J. D. 1986. Imaging of the Temporal Bone. New York, Thieme Medical Pub., Inc.
A book dealing with evaluation of the temporal bone.

Valvassori, G. E., and Mafee, M. F. May 1988. Otolaryngologic Clinics of North America. Diagnostic Imaging in Otolaryngology I: The Ear. Philadelphia, W. B. Saunders Co.
A recent publication exploring multiple aspects of radiologic imaging in various regions of the head and neck.
Valvassori, G. E., Potter, G. D., Hanafee, W. N., et al. 1982. Radiology of the Ear, Nose, and Throat. Philadelphia, W. B. Saunders Co.
An excellent text. Very good sections on normal anatomy as seen on plain films and tomography.
Vignaud, J., Jardin, C., and Rosen, L. 1986. The Ear, Diagnostic Imaging. New York, Masson Publishing USA, Inc.
Complete text dealing with the temporal bone. This update of a French text now includes CT and some magnetic resonance.

REFERENCES

Etter, L. E. 1965. Roentgenography and Roentgenology of the Middle Ear and Mastoid Process. Springfield, IL, Charles C Thomas.
Valvassori, G. E., and Mafee, M. F. August 1988. Otolaryngologic Clinics of North America. Diagnostic Imaging in Otolaryngology II: Sinuses and Neck. Philadelphia, W. B. Saunders Co.

Chapter 11

THE NEUROVESTIBULAR TESTING OF INFANTS AND CHILDREN

Lydia Eviatar, M.D.   Abraham Eviatar, M.D.

Vestibular dysfunction in children may present in a variety of ways, from the subtle lag in acquisition of head and postural control seen in infants with delayed maturation of vestibular function (e.g., premature babies) to the acute episodes of vertigo and loss of postural control encountered in diseases of the labyrinth. Because of the close interaction of the vestibular system with the visual, auditory, proprioceptive, cerebellar, and motor pathways in the maintenance of postural control and equilibrium in space, it is often difficult to single out which of the systems is directly responsible for a noted deficit. It is by a process of elimination that a correct diagnosis can be established. This implies that neurologic testing of sensory channels such as vision, hearing, and proprioception as well as of cerebellar motor pathways will be required. Both the neurologic examination and vestibular testing are adapted to the patient's age and the level of maturation of the central nervous system.

BASIS OF THE EXAMINATION

A good history of the presenting signs and symptoms from the parents of the patient and a detailed description of associated symptoms and signs are essential. It is important to review motor developmental milestones, history of drug intake (especially ototoxic drugs), and prior illnesses that may have affected the eighth nerve (Table 11–1).

The method of examining children presented in this chapter has been tested in more than 500 children, and normative data were obtained and published (Eviatar and Eviatar, 1979). The method evolved from information from embryologists, anatomists, neurophysiologists, and clinical investigators.

EMBRYONIC DEVELOPMENT OF THE NEUROVESTIBULAR SYSTEM

A review of the basic information on the development of the labyrinth and its gradual contribution to various postural and oculomotor reflexes is pertinent

TABLE 11–1. Review of History of Neurovestibular Examination

I. Pregnancy
  1. Intrauterine infections: *Toxoplasmosis, rubella, cytomegalic inclusion disease, herpes* (TORCH); AIDS
  2. Rh incompatibility
  3. Ingestion of ototoxic drugs
  4. Toxemia of pregnancy or gestational diabetes
II. Neonatal period
  1. Neonatal asphyxia
  2. Neonatal jaundice
  3. Respiratory distress syndrome
  4. Central nervous system infection, sepsis, ingestion of ototoxic drugs, AIDS, or ARC
  5. Craniofacial anomalies
III. Developmental milestones
  1. Sitting, standing, walking, speech
IV. History of otitis, mastoiditis, central nervous system infections, ingestion of ototoxic drugs, vertigo, head trauma
V. Hereditary diseases affecting hearing or balance: Degenerative or metabolic neurocutaneous syndrome (e.g., neurofibromatosis)
VI. Tumors: cerebellopontine angle tumors, brain stem gliomas, cerebellar tumors, supratentorial tumors
VII. Vascular malformations
VIII. Collagen disorders: Systemic lupus erythematosus

to a discussion of neurovestibular examination. From studies in embryos, it is known that brain stem reflexes controlling eyeball movements begin to operate at about the 15th week of gestation and become well established by the 24th week (Gesell and Amatruda, 1945; Hooker, 1952; Bergstrom, 1969).

Organized regional reflex responses to movements of the head and neck also emerge at about the 28th week (Gesell and Amatruda, 1945). The vestibular receptors in the inner ear become fully active by the 32nd week of gestation, at which time a well-developed Moro reflex can be elicited. This reflex persists until the child is between 3 and 5 months old (Schulte et al., 1969). Centripetal activity from the maturing ampullary cristae is detectable as a feeble Moro reflex as early as the eighth to ninth week of fetal life (Gesell and Amatruda, 1945; Humphrey, 1969; Cratty, 1970). Myelination of the vestibular nerve fibers and of the intersegmental tract systems of the cervical spinal cord begins around 16 weeks of gestation and is virtually completed at birth, whereas the pyramidal tract is fully myelinated only by 2 years of age.

DEVELOPMENT OF THE VESTIBULAR SYSTEM AND ITS FUNCTIONS

The vestibular part of the inner ear consists of the three semicircular canals, the utricle, and the saccule. They are concerned with orientation in three-dimensional space, equilibrium, and modification of muscle tone (see Chap. 6).

The vestibular receptors of the semicircular canals are the cristae ampullares. The receptors of the utricle and saccule are the maculae. Angular acceleration causes movement of endolymphatic fluid of the semicircular canals and deflection of hair cells in the sensory epithelium of the cristae. This aspect of labyrinthine function is referred to as kinetic equilibrium. The utricular macula responds to changes in gravitational forces and to linear acceleration and conveys information concerning the position of the head in space (static equilibrium) (Carpenter, 1974).

It is as yet unclear what the exact role of the saccular macula is. The maculae and cristae are innervated by peripheral nerve endings originating in the bipolar cells of the vestibular ganglia. The central processes of the bipolar cells are primary vestibular fibers forming a vestibular nerve root, which enters the cerebellopontine angle, where the root fibers pass dorsally between the inferior cerebellar peduncle and the spinal trigeminal tract. While entering the vestibular nuclear complex, which lies on the floor of the fourth ventricle, the fibers bifurcate into short ascending and long descending fibers. A small number of fibers will pass directly to the ipsilateral cerebellar cortex of the nodulus, uvula, and flocculus as mossy fibers. The peripheral processes of the ganglion cells, which innervate the cristae in the semicircular canals, project primarily to the superior vestibular nucleus and rostral parts of the medial vestibular nucleus (Stein and Carpenter, 1967). Cells of the inferior vestibular ganglion, which innervate the saccular maculae, give rise to central fibers that descend and terminate mainly in the dorsolateral portions of the inferior vestibular nucleus. Secondary vestibular fibers arise from the vestibular nuclei and project to the cerebellum, to the nuclei of the oculomotor nerves, and to all spinal levels. From the vestibular nuclei arise ascending fibers, crossed and uncrossed, which run in the medial longitudinal fasciculus (MLF) and project to the nuclei of the extraocular muscles (abducens, trochlear, and oculomotor). These secondary vestibular fibers in the MLF play an important role in conjugate eye movements. Selective stimulation of the nerve endings from the ampulla of each semicircular canal produces specific deviation of both eyes, which is considered to be a primary vestibular response. Lesions of the MLF rostral to the abducens nuclei produce a disturbance

of conjugate horizontal eye movements known as anterior internuclear ophthalmoplegia. Lesions or sectioning of the MLF rostral to the abducens nuclei abolish oculomotor responses, but nystagmus still results from labyrinthine stimulation, suggesting that impulses essential for nystagmus probably pass via the reticular formation. At the brain stem level, the descending secondary vestibular fibers in the MLF fibers are the medial vestibulospinal (crossed) and lateral vestibulospinal (uncrossed) tracts. Almost all the fibers reaching the spinal level are ipsilateral. Most fibers end at the cervical level, although some descend to the thoracic level. They terminate in the medial part of the anterior horn. The medial vestibulospinal tract plays an important role in the interaction of neck and vestibuloocular reflexes. The lateral vestibulospinal tract extends to the level of the sacral cord. In animal experiments, excitation by electric stimulation of the vestibulospinal fibers or the lateral nucleus produces excitation of extensor motor neurons and inhibition of flexor motor neurons (Baloh and Honrubia, 1979). Their influence is exerted primarily on axial and proximal extensor muscles by assisting local myotactic reflexes and producing enough extra force to support the body against gravity and to maintain an upright posture. A small number of primary vestibular fibers end in the reticular formation. The main influence on the reticulospinal outflow is mediated by way of secondary vestibular neurons. Muscular tone is highly dependent on myotactic reflexes (deep tendon reflexes), which in turn are under the influence of the combined excitatory and inhibitory influence of multiple supraspinal neural centers.

After transection of the midbrain, the inhibitory influence of the cortex on the basal ganglia is removed, and the animal exhibits decerebrate rigidity manifested by increased tone in the extensor antigravity muscles. A significant decrease in tone will result if a bilateral labyrinthectomy is performed. Unilateral destruction of the labyrinth or of the lateral vestibular nucleus will result in an ipsilateral decrease in tone. Changes of position of the head in a decerebrate animal produce remarkable changes in posture and tone called tonic neck reflexes. Similar postural changes resulting from changes of position of the head will be seen in newborns until 4 months of age and are broadly designated as tonic neck reflexes.

An understanding of the anatomy and function of vestibular pathways is necessary to recognize the various symptoms and signs of labyrinthine dysfunction. Vestibular irritation or disease causes the individual to experience vertigo, which is the illusion that he or his surroundings are moving. It may cause postural deviation, unsteadiness in the upright position, oculomotor deviation, or nystagmus. The presence of nystagmus is a good objective sign that the vestibular system is malfunctioning.

Nystagmus consists of rhythmic, involuntary oscillations of the eyes, characterized by alternating slow and rapid ocular excursions. Although the slow excursion represents the primary response to stimulation and the rapid phase is the reflex realignment, it is customary to name the nystagmus after the direction of the rapid phase.

The majority of laboratory tests for vestibular dysfunction rely on the evaluation of nystagmus evoked by stimulation of nerve endings in the semicircular canals by rotation or caloric irrigation. The vestibular impulses will then be transmitted to the vestibular nuclei and from there through the ascending secondary vestibular nerve fibers to the nuclei of the extraocular muscles in the brain stem.

The evaluation of postural responses of the head and extremities as a result of changes of position in space and changes in the center of gravity will test the integrity of the descending secondary vestibular fibers, the medial and lateral vestibulospinal tracts.

The central connections of the vestibular pathways are extensive and not well known. In addition to their close connections with the cerebellum and the reticular activating system of the brain stem, they also connect with the thalamus, specifically the ventroposterolateral nucleus (VPL), which projects to the precentral and postcentral gyrus. The cortical representation of the vestibular system is in the posterosuperior aspect of the temporal lobe, dorsal to Heschl gyrus and at the intraparietal sulcus. Electric stimulation of these areas can produce an illusion of rotation (de Morsier, 1938; Penfield and Kristiansen, 1951; Penfield and Jasper, 1954). Excitatory foci in these areas can produce focal seizures, with vertigo as the presenting symptom.

METHODS OF EXAMINATION

The neurovestibular examination consists of the following procedures.

1. A neurodevelopmental evaluation adapted to the patient's age and level of central nervous system maturity.

2. A comprehensive ear, nose, and throat examination to rule out the presence of infection, trauma, tumor, congenital anomalies, or fistula. The examiner should look for anomalies of the external ear and preauricular pits and branchial cleft fistulae. The use of the pneumatic otoscope in the diagnosis of middle-ear disease and perilymphatic fistula (Hennebert sign) is helpful. In the presence of an intact tympanic membrane, negative pressure can be applied with a pneumatic otoscope and will presumably cause utriculofugal flow in the horizontal canal of the affected ear. A positive response is a slow ocular deviation (toward or away from the affected ear) followed by a few (three to four) nystagmic beats, even when pressure is sustained.

3. A hearing test adapted to the patient's age and level of responsiveness should be performed. Infants can be tested by observing their behavioral responses to an infant auditory screener or with the help of a Crib-o-gram. Orienting responses to sound in a free field will appear by 4 or 5 months of age. Play audiometry can be initiated after age 2 years. When

responses to free-field screening are questionable, brain stem and cortical evoked responses will provide additional information.

4. On radiographic examination, a transorbital view of the skull will demonstrate the inner ears and the internal auditory canals. Such an examination is helpful in screening for congenital anomalies, tumors in the acoustic meatus, and sometimes cerebellopontine angle tumors. If a lesion is suspected, computerized axial tomography (with or without contrast) will help establish the diagnosis. Magnetic resonance imaging (MRI) is also very helpful in delineating pathologic conditions around the cerebellopontine angle.

5. To help rule out some of the major blood dyscrasias and metabolic dysfunctions that may cause dizziness, one should perform laboratory tests, including a complete blood count with sickle cell preparation and baseline metabolic studies, such as fasting blood sugar and a two-hour postprandial blood sugar, determinations of blood urea nitrogen, calcium, electrolytes, and triiodothyronine (T_3) and thyroxine (T_4) levels.

Neurologic Examination

Tables 11–2 and 11–3 present the basic procedures used in neurologic examinations of children of all ages. In infants younger than 2 years of age, information is obtained through observation, play, and evaluation of

TABLE 11–2. Neurologic Examination of Children from Birth to 4 Years Old

CRANIAL NERVES (NO. TO BE TESTED)	FUNCTION (TEST)
III, IV, VI	Following objects 2–4 weeks—wandering gaze 4–6 weeks—from midline to 90° to either side From 6 weeks—sideways for 180° up and down Nystagmus: Is it positional or spontaneous?
II	Funduscopy, visual fields
V	Corneal reflex and mastication
VII	Facial expression
VIII	Hearing test appropriate to patient's age Vestibular: doll's-eye phenomenon (newborn), rotatory nystagmus, verticular acceleration
IX, X	Palatal motions, gag reflex
XII	Tongue movements (rooting in the infant) Muscle tone, muscle power, deep tendon reflexes Posture: Head and body control (supine, prone, sitting, and standing) Developmental reflexes: Primitive reflexes (birth to 4 months), righting reflexes (6 months on) Fine motor coordination: Finger-light pursuit, building with blocks, copying figures

TABLE 11–3. Neurologic Examination of Children 4 Years Old to Adult

I. Traditional examination in Table 11–2
II. Additional coordination and balance tests
1. Finger-nose
2. Heel-shin
3. Tandem gait (blindfolded)
4. Romberg
5. Reinforced Romberg
6. Stepping test
7. Past-pointing test
8. Diadochokinesia
9. Kinesthesia
10. Expanded sensory examination
11. Equilibrium reactions
12. Electronystagmography

postural responses. Since many of the classic neurologic tests cannot be performed on children this young, additional tests of fine motor and gross motor coordination are not added until the child is older than 2 years. By age 4, the general neurologic examination is comparable to the one performed in adults.

Assessment of postural responses in infants includes the evaluation of head control when in the prone position, when pulled from the supine position, while sitting, and while standing. Neck and trunk postures in response to various changes in position are noted. Tonic neck reflexes are normally present in the infant up to 4 months of age and gradually disappear thereafter (Paine and Oppe, 1966); in premature infants, they may last longer. In the infant, muscle tone and power can be assessed mostly through play. The presence of hypotonia or tremor may suggest cerebellar disease. Rigidity, posturing, or choreiform movements may suggest disease of the basal ganglia. The various preparatory stages of locomotion and finally gait are evaluated according to the norms expected for each age. All 12 cranial nerves can be evaluated even in the young child, as can fundi and visual fields (Paine and Oppe, 1966). Particularly important to evaluate are extraocular motions. Newborn infants may focus for a few seconds on the examiner's face but will not follow objects. After 14 days of age, the infant may follow objects or faces from the midline to 90 degrees laterally. By 6 weeks of age, the infant will follow objects throughout the horizontal and vertical fields of vision. Thus, ocular alignment can be evaluated as well as the presence of nystagmus and its characteristics.

Congenital nystagmus is usually pendular on straight gaze and may convert to oscillatory when gaze is directed to the fast component. It is almost always dependent on fixation, disappearing or decreasing with fixation or during convergence. Occasionally, a reverse nystagmus, in the opposite direction, may be recorded when the infant's eyes are closed. The optokinetic response may also be inverted. A latent congenital nystagmus may appear only during monocular vision (when one eye is covered) and is commonly associated with congenital ocular defects such as concomitant squint and alternating hyperphoria (Baloh and Hon-

rubia, 1979). Other types of nystagmus may be diagnosed later in life. A comprehensive discussion of the various types of nystagmus can be found elsewhere (Cogan, 1972).

Coordination tests used in evaluating infants are different from those used in older children: In the young infant, the finger-nose test is substituted by finger-light pursuit and the finger-apposition or alternate-motion tests by clapping hands, building with blocks, picking up raisins, and scribbling.

Proprioception is difficult to evaluate in infants and may be inferred from tests that involve foot and hand placing, supporting, and stepping as well as from manipulation of objects. The sensory examination of young infants is also rather crude.

By age 4 years, a complete, detailed neurologic evaluation can be performed (Table 11–3), including more specific vestibular tests such as the sharpened Romberg test described by Fregly (1974). The patient is tested with feet aligned in the tandem heel-to-toe position, with eyes closed and arms folded. A normal person can maintain this position for about 30 seconds. With unilateral or bilateral vestibular impairment, the patient can rarely sustain this position and may fall, mostly toward the affected side. Unilateral labyrinthine dysfunction or labyrinthectomy will cause transient hypotonia and loss of righting reflexes on the side of the lesion. With time, other supraspinal reflexes will compensate for the loss of tonic labyrinthine signals. However, difficulties in maintaining balance may persist in the blindfolded individual. With bilateral loss of labyrinthine function, righting reflexes are deficient, and the blindfolded patient is unable to maintain the upright position or ambulate in the dark.

Stepping tests may also be helpful in the diagnosis of labyrinthine dysfunction. A variation of the Fukuda test (1959) is used in our laboratory. The patient is asked to mark time in place at the intersection of two perpendicular lines for 60 seconds with arms extended and eyes closed. A deviation over 45 degrees may signify vestibular disease, just as may falling or the past-pointing test. This test is usually performed with the patient seated, arms extended, his index finger touching that of the examiner. With eyes closed, the patient is asked to raise his extended arm and index finger and attempt to return it to the original position, touching the examiner's finger. In the presence of vestibular dysfunction, there is consistent pointing past the examiner's finger toward the side of the lesion.

A detailed sensory examination, including stereognosis, proprioception, two-point discrimination, and determination of position and vibration sense, is performed on children older than 4 years.

DEVELOPMENTAL REFLEXES

We divide children into four groups according to their ages and levels of maturation of the central nervous system.

Group I: Birth to 4 Months

In this group, tonic neck reflexes predominate. They are demonstrated by passive or active motions of the head relative to fixed positions of the body, which elicit movement of the endolymphatic fluid in the semicircular canals and stimulate the sensory nerve endings in the cristae ampullares. At the same time, proprioceptive stimuli arise from the cervical vertebrae and muscles. Appropriate tonic neck responses will depend on the integrity of the vestibular and proprioceptive afferents and of the efferent motor pathways. Although one cannot separate proprioceptive from labyrinthine stimuli, a well-coordinated reflex indicates a normal overall integrated response.

NECK RIGHTING. Active or passive rotation of the head from the midline to one side in an infant lying supine produces a rotation of the whole body in the direction of the head turn (Fig. 11–1).

ASYMMETRIC TONIC NECK REFLEX. Asymmetric tonic neck reflex (ATN) (Fig. 11–2) is obtained with the baby lying supine with the head in the midline position. Active or passive rotation of the head to one side while the infant's chest is restrained will produce flexion of the extremities on the side of the occiput and extension of the extremities on the side of the face.

SYMMETRIC TONIC NECK REFLEX. Symmetric tonic neck reflex (STN) (Fig. 11–3) has two stages. In the first stage, the baby is held in the horizontal prone position, with the baby's chest on the examiner's arm or with the baby's chest on the examiner's lap. Dorsi-

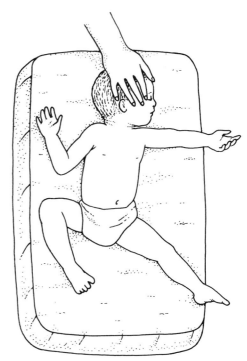

Figure 11–2. Asymmetric tonic neck reflex.

flexion of the head will produce extension of the upper extremities and flexion of the lower extremities (Fig. 11–3A). In the second stage, abrupt ventroflexion of the head will produce flexion of the upper extremities and extension of the lower extremities (Fig. 11–3B).

MORO REFLEX. For testing the Moro reflex (Fig. 11–4), the baby lies in the supine position with the head ventroflexed and supported by the examiner's hand. An abrupt backward deflexion of the head about 30 degrees in relation to the trunk will produce an exten-

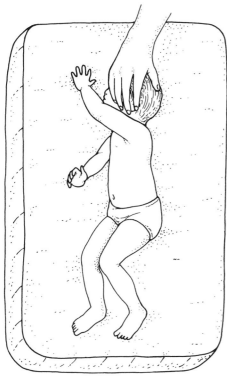

Figure 11–1. Neck righting.

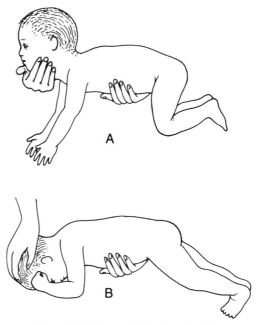

Figure 11–3. Symmetric tonic neck reflex.

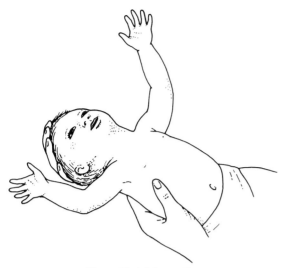

Figure 11–4. Moro reflex.

sion and abduction of the arms, followed by an embrace.

Absent tonic neck reflexes, including an absent Moro reflex, may occur in the severely asphyxiated hypotonic child with severe central nervous system depression and in those with severe myopathic disorders. Complete absence of labyrinthine function may also produce hypotonia, poor head control, and depressed tonic neck reflexes.

Specific vestibular reflexes are the response to vertical acceleration (introduced by the authors) and the doll's-eye phenomenon.

VERTICAL ACCELERATION. With the vertical acceleration test (Fig. 11–5), the baby is held in the supine position on the examiner's extended forearms. The head and trunk must be aligned and parallel to the

ground. A rapid downward acceleration is the stimulus produced to the baby's horizontal body by the examiner, who bends rapidly on his or her knees to a crouched position. A normal response consists of abduction and extension of the arms, with fanning of the hands. The response is similar to the Moro reflex. The difference is the absent dorsiflexion of the head, which eliminates proprioceptive input from the cervical vertebrae. Since the stimulus is vertical acceleration, it most probably stimulates the maculae of the utricle as opposed to the cristae of the semicircular canals that are stimulated with the Moro reflex.

DOLL'S-EYE PHENOMENON. In testing for the doll's-eye phenomenon (Fig. 11–6), the baby is held vertically under the armpits, with the head bent forward 30 degrees over the chest, and is rotated for 360 degrees around an axis passing through the examiner's head. Ten rotations in one direction are sufficient and provide a strong vestibular stimulus. The normal response is deviation of the eyes and head opposite the direction of rotation. The doll's-eye phenomenon usually persists for the first 2 weeks of life in full-term neonates and up to 6 weeks in the full-term baby small for gestational age. Premature babies may have persistent doll's-eye responses until 3 months of age. Gradually, as vestibular responses mature, nystagmus is superimposed, with a quick component in the direction of rotation. This response can be recorded with electronystagmography. In most cases, it is sufficient to observe the response visually during and following rotation.

Group 2: 4 to 6 Months

Babies in this age group vary in terms of their development achievements. Many normal infants will

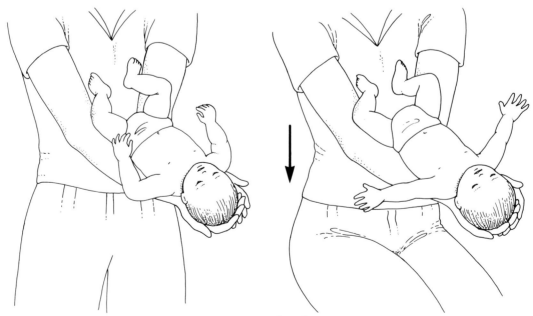

Figure 11–5. Vertical acceleration.

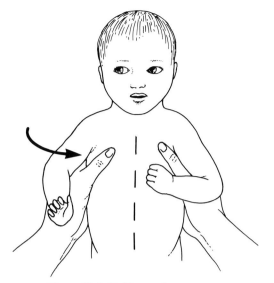

Figure 11–6. Doll's-eye phenomenon.

still have residual primitive tonic neck reflexes, while in others, righting responses will appear. Both conditions are normal.

Group 3: 6 to 18 Months

This is a period of rapid motor and sensory development. Myelination of the pyramidal tract proceeds, as do dendritic arborization of the cerebral cortex and cerebellar cortical differentiation. Integration of visual, labyrinthine, and proprioceptive stimuli occurs, re-

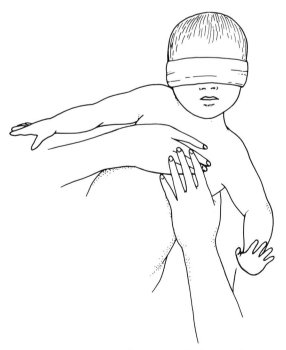

Figure 11–7. Head righting in vertical suspension.

sulting in more elaborate motor responses to changes in head position, called righting reflexes. Righting reflexes are elicited by an abrupt tilt of the patient and change in the patient's center of gravity. The acceleration imposed on the labyrinth elicits stimuli that bring on righting of the head and protective reactions of the extremities in the direction of tilt. Since optical and vestibular righting responses are identical, the individual must be tested blindfolded in order to eliminate visual cues.

The most important reflexes are the head-righting responses. They can be obtained by picking up the infant from the prone or supine position and bringing him or her to the upright position or by tilting the seated infant sideways, frontward, or backward (Fig. 11–7). Every abrupt change of the head position in space will elicit vestibular head-righting responses whereby the mouth and eyes of the infant will become parallel to the ground. At the same time, propping reactions of the extremities may be noted, especially in the sitting position. The presence of this reflex will enable the child to maintain his or her equilibrium in sitting (Fig. 11–8).

PARACHUTE REFLEX. This reflex is also called a sentinel reaction because it is a basic protective body mechanism that remains present throughout life. During the testing procedure, the baby is held under his or her armpits with the back toward the examiner, and vertical downward acceleration toward the examining table is applied. The normal response consists of extension and abduction of the arms, with extension of fingers as well as righting of the head.

HOPPING REACTION. The hopping reaction (Fig. 11–9) appears in the normal full-term infant by 8 to 10 months of age. The baby is tested in the standing position, with the examiner holding him or her around the chest and gently tilting him or her sideways, frontward, or backward. A normal response consists of the initiation of a few steps in the direction of tilt, accompanied by righting of the head. Acquisition of this reflex is preparatory for independent walking.

EQUILIBRIUM RESPONSES: AGE 4 YEARS TO ADULT

Although equilibrium reactions may be present before age 4, it is difficult to test them in the very young child, who may be too frightened to cooperate and relax when major changes in his or her center of equilibrium are made. Essentially, the equilibrium responses are more sophisticated and highly integrated righting reactions involving the whole body. They can be tested in the sitting position or the kneeling position, with the examiner pulling the child by his or her arm sideways (Fig. 11–10). The normal response consists of righting of the head and extension with abduction of the extremities on the side opposite the direction of tilt. Postural reactions can also be elicited by tilting the patient, either prone (Fig. 11–11) or supine (Fig. 11–12), on a tilting board. The angle of tilt of the

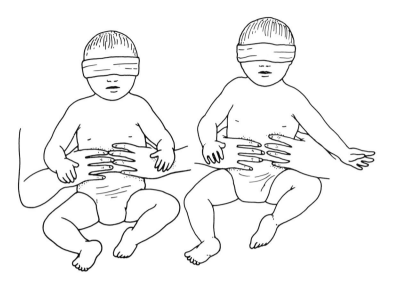

Figure 11–8. Head righting in sitting position (buttress response).

board is about 45 degrees sideways, and the examiner looks for righting responses of the head and extension with abduction reactions of the extremities.

ELECTRONYSTAGMOGRAPHY

Electronystagmography is a method of recording nystagmic eye movements elicited by positional testing or during labyrinthine stimulation by rotation and caloric irrigation (Table 11–4). The test is performed in a partially darkened room with the patient blind-folded in order to eliminate fixation of gaze or optokinetic nystagmus. It is beyond the scope of this chapter to discuss in detail the rationale of this method and the equipment that can be used. Several good monographs on the subject are available (Barber and Stockwell, 1976; Yongkees and Philipson, 1964). For routine clinical testing, a one-channel AC dinograph recorder is sufficient. In patients with spontaneous nystagmus, MLF lesions, or nuclear lesions, a more sophisticated monocular horizontal and vertical simultaneous recording on a four-channel DC dinograph is more suitable. Microelectrodes are applied bitemporally for recording

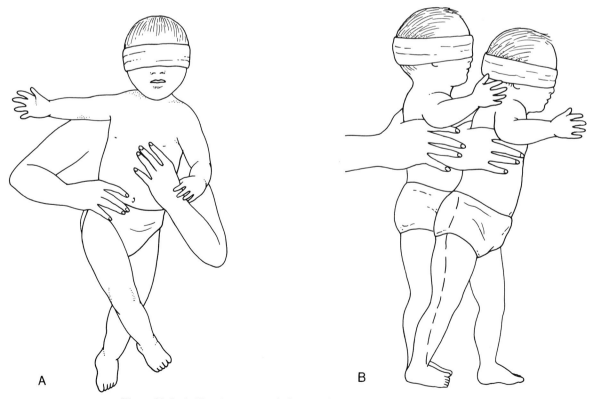

Figure 11–9. A, Hopping reaction (sideways). B, Hopping reaction (forward).

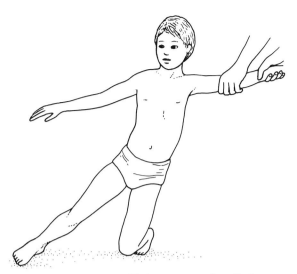

Figure 11–10. Equilibrium response (kneeling).

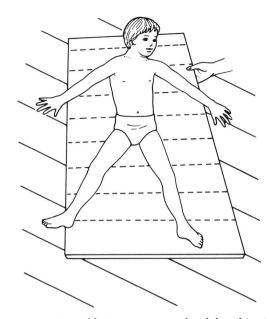

Figure 11–12. Equilibrium response on the tilt board (supine).

of eye movements, and a neutral electrode is applied on the nasion. A position test is first performed with the infant in supine, right lateral, and left lateral positions. In the older child, a position test is also done in the sitting position.

The perotatory stimulation is provided by a commercially available torsion swing (TS) with the application of manual force. In children with monocular nystagmus or strabismus, monocular recording is recommended. Recording of both horizontal and vertical eye movements in these patients adds important information regarding the direction of motion of each individual eye and contributes to the diagnostic capability of the test. The TS provides a sinusoidal acceleration of progressively decreasing intensity from a 90-degree angle to the right and left of the patient until a spontaneous stop. Two perotatory stimulations are usually recorded with a five-minute interval between the two stimulations.

The stimulus provided by the torsion swing elicits good oculomotor responses and provides the type of

stimulation that closely mimics the physiologic conditions encountered in daily situations. The young infant is seated in his or her parent's lap on the torsion swing. The parent's right hand maintains the baby's head flexed 30 degrees over the body in order to align the lateral semicircular canals parallel to the ground. The parent's left hand props the baby's trunk in the vertical position, close to the parent's chest, so the axis of rotation is through the baby's head. The torsion swing is a nonthreatening experience for children, who like to be rocked back and forth and, in most cases, cooperate well throughout the test. Recording the eye movements is done during stimulation with the torsion swing. In the majority of cases, the response ceases with cessation of perotatory stimulation.

In the very young infant, a sinusoidal curve may be the only response obtained, recording the conjugate eye movements in the direction opposite the direction of rotation (doll's-eye phenomenon), over which slowly will be superimposed a few nystagmoid beats, changing direction with the direction of rotation. As the response fully matures, a good alternating nystagmus is obtained. The response thus recorded is the result of a summation of responses elicited from both labyrinths. About 50 per cent of full-term appropriate-for-gestational-age (FTAGA) infants develop nystagmus during

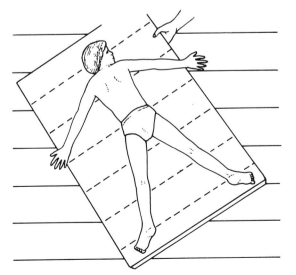

Figure 11–11. Equilibrium response on the tilt board (prone).

TABLE 11–4. Electronystagmography

I. Positional test: prone, supine, right lateral, left lateral
   1. Sitting—head right
               head left
               ventroflexed 30°
               dorsiflexed 30°
II. Perotatory (torsion swing)
III. Ice-cold caloric irrigation (10 sec)
IV. Bithermal caloric irrigation (only children older than 4 years)
V. Pendulum tracking from 6 months
VI. Optokinetic stimulation from 6 months

perotatory stimulation within the first 10 to 20 days of postnatal life. The majority of full-term small-for-gestational-age (FTSGA) infants (95 per cent) have nystagmus in response to perotatory stimulation within the first 20 to 30 days of life. However, premature infants have a significant delay (up to 90 days) in the appearance of perotatory evoked nystagmus (Eviatar et al., 1974). These maturational factors, which correlate with gestational age and weight at birth, are taken into account when evaluating the perotatory response in such infants as those treated with aminoglycosides. Indeed, one of the effects produced by aminoglycoside treatment may be a delay in acquiring perotatory responses (Eviatar and Eviatar, 1980).

In normal infants and children, values for the speed of the slow component, amplitude, and number of beats per torsion swing excursion are identical for the right- and left-beating nystagmus. The total number of beats of nystagmus to right or left is also identical. Directional preponderance is considered when the total number of beats in one direction exceeds by 25 per cent the number of beats in the other direction. A directional preponderance may be found in the presence of a strong positional nystagmus and may be secondary to it. When present, it suggests vestibular dysfunction.

There is no significant increase over time in the mean values of amplitude or the number of beats per torsion swing excursion of the perotatory nystagmus. The speed of the slow component of perotatory nystagmus increases from the time of its appearance until age 4 years, from a mean of 35.0 degrees per second to an average of 40.0 degrees per second. Sleep and drowsiness can inhibit responses significantly (Eviatar et al., 1979).

Ice-Cold Caloric (ICC) Irrigation

Additional testing with ICC irrigation of each ear canal may be performed in order to evaluate the response from each labyrinth individually.

The test is performed with the blindfolded baby in the supine position, restrained on a papoose board, with the head ventroflexed 30 degrees. A 10-second irrigation with ice-cold water is the stimulus used (temperature of the water at the spout is about 5°C). Recording of the oculomotor response starts at the onset of irrigation. The direction of nystagmus will be opposite the ear stimulated. As soon as a good response appears, the baby is turned to the prone position, and the direction of nystagmus is reversed if the labyrinth is intact. As soon as this new response begins to fade, the baby is turned back to the supine position. The direction of nystagmus reverts to the initial direction, away from the ear stimulated. If the child is sleepy or very irritable during the test, the response may be inhibited or incomplete (e.g., a response only in the supine and prone positions). The test is performed in three positions (supine, prone, and back to supine) with each irrigation in order to eliminate false re-

sponses, such as intensification of a latent nystagmus or a response from the other labyrinth (Eviatar and Eviatar, 1974). Ten minutes should elapse before stimulating the other ear canal with ice-cold water.

The ICC stimulation is a crude method in that it tests for a response to a vigorous, nonphysiologic stimulus. Thus, it is performed only in cases where serious doubts exist regarding the function of the vestibular apparatus, such as when there is significant delay in the development of head and postural control, when there are abnormal responses to torsion swing, when there is a history of ingestion of ototoxic drugs, or in the congenitally deaf child in whom abnormal vestibular function is suspected. Twenty-five per cent of the full-term infants tested in our laboratory had a positive response to the caloric test within the first 10 to 20 days of life, and the majority of infants responded within the first month. About 40 per cent of the small-for-gestational-age babies responded by 1 month of age, while the majority responded by 6 to 8 weeks of age. Many premature babies did not respond until 3 months of age (Eviatar et al., 1974). Therefore, it is important not to confuse the absence of positive response due to delayed maturation with the lack of response due to acquired or congenital vestibular damage. When a positive response is present, the quality of the response becomes an indicator of the maturity and integrity of vestibular responses.

There is a maturational pattern in the development of the caloric evoked nystagmus response: Increases in the number of beats per 10 seconds, in the amplitude, and in the speed of the slow component are apparent in the first three months of life for all gestational groups. The intensity of nystagmus is directly proportional to gestational age and weight at birth (Eviatar et al., 1979). Full-term babies, appropriate- or large-for-gestational-age, acquire a mature pattern of nystagmus within three to six months of birth. However, premature and small-for-gestational-age babies show progressive maturation of caloric responses throughout the first year of life. The frequency and the speed of the slow component are the most reliable variables in the qualitative evaluation of induced caloric nystagmus. These variables are directly proportional to gestational age and weight at birth in the first six months of life.

While the intensity of evoked nystagmus increases with age, the latency of the response decreases in direct relation to the length of gestation and the weight at birth. Latency provides a good estimate of the maturity of vestibular responses. Because of the method used, the total duration of evoked nystagmus is poorly correlated with the degree of maturation. However, since normative values are available, estimates of dysfunction can be made by evaluating the total duration of the response (Eviatar and Eviatar, 1979).

Optokinetic Stimulation

Optokinetic nystagmus can be evaluated in most children within three to six months of birth. As the children grow older and pay more attention to the content of images seen, better responses are obtained by projecting a rotating filmstrip on a screen. The nystagmus can be recorded in response to two speeds of rotation: 3 degrees and 16 degrees per second, respectively. The frequency, amplitude, and speed of the slow component can be analyzed in response to the two rotation speeds. Abnormalities of tracing may be related to ocular problems, damage to optic tracts, optic radiation, or frontal or cerebellar lesions. The information obtained is helpful in the evaluation of the overall quality of neurovestibular function.

Bithermal Caloric Irrigation

Bithermal irrigation of the external auditory meatus for 30 seconds with 30°C and 44°C water is used in children aged 4 years and older. A 10-minute interval is allowed between two consecutive irrigations. The intensity of nystagmus, represented by the speed of the slow component at the culmination of nystagmus, is used for calculation. Calculation of labyrinthine preponderance (Jongkee's formula) is as follows.

$$\frac{(R30 \text{ degrees} + R44 \text{ degrees}) - (L30 \text{ degrees} + L44 \text{ degrees}) \times 100}{R30 \text{ degrees} + R44 \text{ degrees} + L30 \text{ degrees} + L44 \text{ degrees}}$$

A difference between the two labyrinths of more than 22 per cent suggests labyrinthine preponderance.

Calculation of directional preponderance is done using the following formula.

$$\frac{(R30 \text{ degrees} + L44 \text{ degrees}) - (R44 \text{ degrees} + L30 \text{ degrees}) \times 100}{R30 \text{ degrees} + L44 \text{ degrees} + R44 \text{ degrees} + R30 \text{ degrees}}$$

A difference of more than 18 per cent suggests directional preponderance.

This procedure lasts about 45 minutes and requires the child's cooperation and patience. Therefore, it cannot be used in children younger than 4 years of age. The significance of directional and labyrinthine preponderance in children has been discussed elsewhere (Eviatar and Wassertheil, 1971; Eviatar and Eviatar, 1977).

SELECTED REFERENCES

Abel, L. A., Troost, B. T., and Dell'Osso, L. 1983. The effects of age on normal saccadic characteristics and their variability. Vision Res. 23:33.
    Maturational aspects of saccadic eye movements are emphasized.
Cyr, D. G., Brookhaven, P. E., Valente, M., et al. 1985. Vestibular evaluation of infants and preschool children. Otolaryngol. Head Neck Surg. 93:4, 463.
    The article describes a technique of testing the vestibular system in young children by using the closed loop irrigation system devised by Gram. The authors also elaborate on simple methods of calibration of eye movements in infants 6 months and older.
Ornitz, E. M., Brow, M. B., Mason, A., et al. 1974. The effects of visual input on post-rotatory nystagmus in normal children. Acta Otolaryngol. 77:418.

Ornitz, E. M., Atwell, C. W., Walter, D. O., et al. 1979. The maturation of vestibular nystagmus in infancy and childhood. Acta Otolaryngol. 88:244.
    Ornitz and coworkers describe the maturation of vestibular responses to rotatory stimulation, emphasizing the differences between the nystagmus elicited during rotation and the postrotatory nystagmus. They also emphasize the inhibitory effect of visual input on rotatory nystagmus of normal children.
Supance, J. S., and Bluestone, C. D. 1983. Perilymph fistulas in infants and children. Otolaryngol. Head Neck Surg. 19:663.
    The importance of considering perilymph fistula in the differential diagnosis of sudden hearing loss and vertigo is addressed.

REFERENCES

Baloh, R. W., and Honrubia, V. 1979. Clincal neurophysiology of the vestibular system. *In* Pulm, F., and McDowell, F. (eds.): Contemporary Neurology Series, Vol. 18. Philadelphia, F. A. Davis Co., pp. 115–118.
Barber, H. O., and Stockwell, C. W. 1976. Manual of Electronystagmography. St. Louis, The C. V. Mosby Co.
Bergstrom, L. 1969. Electrical parameters of the brain during ontogeny. *In* Robinson, R. J., et al. (eds.): Brain and Early Behavior Development in the Fetus and Infant. CASDS Study Group on Brain Mechanisms of Early Behavior Development. New York, Academic Press, pp. 15–37.
Carpenter, B. 1974. Core Text of Neuroanatomy. Baltimore, Williams & Wilkins.
Cogan, D. G. 1972. Neurology of the Ocular Muscles. Springfield, IL, Charles C Thomas.
Cratty, B. T. 1970. Perceptual and Motor Development in Infants and Children. London, Macmillan.
de Morsier, J. 1938. Contribution à l'étude des centres vestibulaires corticaux et des hallucinations illiputienes. Encephal 33:57.
Eviatar, A. 1970. The torsion swing as a vestibular test. Arch. Otolaryngol. 92:437.
Eviatar, A., and Eviatar, L. 1974. A critical look at the cold calorics. Arch. Otolaryngol. 99:361.
Eviatar, L., and Eviatar, A. 1977. Vertigo in children: Differential diagnosis and treatment. Pediatrics 59:833.
Eviatar, L., and Eviatar, A. 1979. The normal nystagmic response of infants to caloric and perotatory stimulation. Laryngoscope 89:1036.
Eviatar, A., and Eviatar, L. 1980. Vestibular Effect of Aminoglycosides in Humans. Chicago International Symposium on Aminoglycosides. Boston, Little, Brown and Co.
Eviatar, A., and Wassertheil, S. 1971. The clinical significance of directional preponderance concluded by electronystagmography. J. Laryngol. Otol. 85:355.
Eviatar, L., Eviatar, A., and Naray, I. 1974. Maturation of neurovestibular responses in infants. Dev. Med. Child. Neurol. 16:435.
Eviatar, L., Miranda, S., Eviatar, A., et al. 1970. Development of nystagmus in response to vestibular stimulation in infants. Ann. Neurol. 5:508.
Fregly, A. R. 1974. Vestibular ataxia and its measurement in man. *In* Kornhuber, H. H. (ed.): Handbook of Sensory Physiology, Vol. 6, Part 2. New York, Springer-Verlag.
Fukuda, T. 1959. The stepping test: Two phases of the labyrinthine reflex. Acta Otolaryngol. 50:95.
Gesell, A., and Amatruda, C. S. 1945. The Embryology of Behavior: The Beginning of the Human Mind. New York, Harper.
Hamilton, W. T., and Mossman, H. W. 1972. Human Embryology: Prenatal Development of Form and Function, 4th ed. Cambridge, Hoffer.
Hooker, D. 1952. The Prenatal Origin of Behavior. Lawrence, KS, University of Kansas Press.
Humphrey, T. 1969. Postnatal repetition of human prenatal activity sequences with some suggestions of their neuroanatomical lesions. *In* Robinson, R. J., et al. (eds.): Brain and Early Behavior Development in the Fetus and Infant. CASDS Study Group on Brain Mechanisms of Early Behavioral Development. New York, Academic Press, pp. 43–84.

Paine, R. S., and Oppe, T. E. 1966. Neurological examination of children. Clin. Dev. Med. 20/21, 98–142.

Penfield, W., and Jasper, H. 1954. Epilepsy and the Functional Anatomy of the Human Brain. Boston, Little, Brown and Co.

Penfield, W., and Kristiansen, D. 1951. Epileptic Seizure Patterns: A study of the Localizing Value of Initial Phenomena in Focal Cortical Seizures. Springfield, IL, Charles C Thomas.

Schulte, F. T., Linke, I., Michaelis, E., et al. 1969. Excitation, inhibition, and impulse conduction in spinal motoneurones of preterm, term and small for date newborn infants. In Robinson, R. J., et al. (eds.): Brain and Early Behavior Development in the Fetus and Infant. CASDS Study Group on Brain Mechanisms of Early Behavioral Development. New York, Academic Press.

Stein, B. M., and Carpenter, M. D. 1967. Central projections of portions of the vestibular ganglia innervating specific parts of the labyrinth in the Rhesus monkey. Am. J. Anat. 120:281.

Yongkees, L. B. W., and Philipson, A. T. 1964. Electronystagmography. Acta Otolaryngol. Suppl. 189.

Chapter 12

OTALGIA

Werner D. Chasin, M.D.

This chapter discusses otologic and nonotologic causes of ear pain. Referred pain and the multiple sensory innervation of the ear lead to problems in localizing pain; indeed, disorders of various parts of the head and neck may result in pain being perceived in or about the ear (Table 12–1). The skin, perichondrium, and periosteum of the external ear, the tympanic membrane, the lining of the middle ear, and the mastoid periosteum all possess rich sensory innervation (Warwick and Williams, 1973h).

The nerves that contribute to this complex innervation originate from several segments of the brain and spinal cord and include the trigeminal, facial, glossopharyngeal, vagus, and spinal accessory nerves and the cervical plexus (C_2–C_3). Tremble (1965) has described the specific portions of the ear that are innervated by the various nerves and has related these to the evaluation of otalgia.

The manner in which children react to otalgia is a function of their ages, level of maturation, and personalities (Hayden and Schwartz, 1985). Infants may not be able to localize the pain and may simply cry and be irritable, although some will manipulate the ear. An infant with ear pain due to a middle-ear infection is likely to act as if he or she is ill and has a fever. If the otalgia is referred, as during teething, the manifestations may be similar, but the fever is absent. As the child becomes more verbal, he or she is apt to tell the parent that that there is pain in the ear, or the child may continue to "act out" the pain by crying and scratching the ear. Children, like adults, have varying pain thresholds and may fail to give indication of a localized discomfort even when suffering from acute otitis media. They may simply act listless, reject food, vomit, and develop some fever. However, by the time they reach school age, most children can describe their ear pain clearly to their parents. A symptom that is most useful in helping to differentiate otalgia due to middle-ear inflammation from otalgia that is referred is the feeling of fullness, blockage, or pressure in the ear. However, this symptom, when present, can be elicited only from older children. The author continues to remain surprised that many children, even those as old as 6 or 7 years, will not admit to a feeling of blockage in an infected ear or in one harboring an obvious effusion, even when they are questioned directly.

EVALUATION OF THE CHILD WITH OTALGIA

History

When evaluating a child with ear pain, the physician should first obtain an accurate history. In addition, the physician (1) should have an understanding of the principle of referred pain, (2) should possess a knowledge of the multiple sensory innervation of the ear, and (3) should ask appropriate questions to differentiate intrisic from referred otalgia. (For example. when the pain is aggravated by chewing of food or gum, this would lead one to evaluate carefully the temporomandibular joints and the teeth.)

Examination of the Ears

The examination of the ears must be thorough. Both the cranial and the lateral surfaces of the auricle, as well as the postauricular areas, should be inspected for traumatic or inflammatory lesions. Special attention must be paid to the sites of possible sinus tracts in front of the root of the helix and in the cranial surface of the superior half of the auricle. The external auditory canal should be inspected for anomalies, such as a duplicated external auditory canal.

Next, the tympanic membrane should be inspected for disorders intrinsic to the drumhead as well as for signs of those middle-ear disorders that it may reflect. The author has found the Hallpike-Blackmore monocular ear microscope with a pneumatic attachment and 6× magnification to be the most useful otoscope for routine clinical use in examining the ears of infants and children. This instrument has excellent coaxial illumination and specula that are atraumatic and that afford a perfect pneumatic seal. The otologic examination may need to be supplemented by a tympanometric evaluation to detect possible negative intratympanic pressure, which can be a subtle cause of intrinsic otalgia (Chap. 8).

Evaluation for Referred Otalgia

In children, the cause of otalgia most commonly can be found within the temporal bone. Nevertheless, like adults, they may also have ear pain that originates from disorders outside the ear—referred otalgia. To successfully discover the cause of such ear pain, the physician must, in a systematic manner, evaluate the territory of each of the nerves that may mediate referred otalgia (White and Sweet, 1969). However, considerable controversy exists about the proportional territories within the ear of the various nerves that innervate this structure. Recent evidence points to the trigeminal nerve as the most probable somatic sensory nerve of the tympanic membrane (Saunders and Weider, 1985).

The clinical evaluation may need to be supplemented by such radiologic studies as roentgenograms of the mastoids, paranasal sinuses, bony and soft tissue structures of the neck, and a barium-enhanced evaluation of the esophagus. Computed tomography (CT) is useful in disclosing the presence of lesions deep in the neck, in the infratemporal fossa and parapharyngeal space, and in the skull that may cause otalgia (Chap. 10). Magnetic resonance imaging (MRI) holds the advantage of not using radiation, but it does not display osseous structures to good advantage. Therefore, the author prefers CT enhanced with intravascular contrast material for diagnostic studies to uncover the causes of otalgia, both intrinsic and referred (Chap. 10).

In the vast majority of patients with otalgia, the cause of the pain can be discovered. Seldom indeed should one make the diagnosis of "otalgia of undetermined etiology."

OTALGIA DUE TO INTRINSIC EAR DISEASE

External Ear

When ear pain is due to a disorder of the external ear, this should be obvious on clinical examination. The pain is localized to the ear, with little radiation elsewhere, and an abnormality is seen in either the auricle, the external auditory canal, or both. Some common causes of such pain in children are listed in Table 12–1 and include external otitis (dermatitis—bacterial, fungal, or allergic), foreign bodies, perichondritis of the auricle, infected preauricular cyst, insects and magots, herpes zoster, myringitis bullosa, fractures of the tympanic ring, and tumors of the external auditory canal. The management of these disorders is fairly direct and is described in Chapter 20.

The pain-sensitive structures of the external ear include the skin of the auricle and the external auditory canal, the perichondrium of the auricle, and the outer portion of the external auditory canal.

TABLE 12–1. Causes of Otalgia in Children

INTRINSIC

I. *External Ear*	
A. External otitis	E. Insects
B. Foreign body	F. Myringitis
C. Perichondritis	G. Trauma
D. Preauricular cyst or sinus	H. Tumor

II. *Middle Ear, Eustachian Tube, and Mastoid*	
A. Barotrauma	G. Masked mastoiditis
B. Middle-ear effusion	H. Intracranial complication
C. Negative intratympanic pressure	I. Tumor
D. Acute otitis media	J. Histiocytosis X
E. Mastoiditis	K. Wegener granuloma
F. Aditus block	

EXTRINSIC

I. *Trigeminal Nerve*	IV. *Vagus Nerve*
A. Dental	A. Laryngopharynx
B. Jaw	B. Esophagus
C. Temporomandibular joint	C. Thyroid
D. Oral cavity	V. *Cervical Nerves*
II. *Facial Nerve*	A. Lymph nodes
A. Bell palsy	B. Cysts
B. Tumors	C. Cervical spine
C. Herpes zoster	D. Neuralgia
III. *Glossopharyngeal Nerve*	IV. *Miscellaneous*
A. Tonsil	A. Migraine
B. Oropharynx	B. Aural neuralgia
C. Nasopharynx	C. Salivary gland
	D. Paranasal sinuses
	E. Central nervous system

Middle Ear

The pain-sensitive structures of the middle ear and mastoid include the tympanic membrane, periosteum of the mastoid cortex, and the mucoperiosteum of the middle ear and mastoid. The osseous structures of the middle ear and the other parts of the temporal bone do not appear to be supplied with pain receptors. The factors that stimulate these receptors are (1) stretching, (2) pressure, (3) toxic products of infection, and (4) direct nerve invasion by tumors.

When a disease process involves the middle ear and mastoid system, there exists potentially a large constellation of symptoms in addition to the pain itself. This constellation is broader in the older child who can express them adequately. The infant expresses middle-ear otalgia by crying, irritability, and sometimes scratching the ear, sticking the finger into it, or pulling it. He or she may have associated systemic signs and symptoms such as fever, vomiting, and a toxic manifestation. As the child becomes older and more verbal, the physician may be able to elicit the description of such additional symptoms as blockage or fullness in the ear (or ears), "popping," "bells ringing," diminished hearing, and noise intolerance. In general, the more symptoms and signs that exist and that are referable directly to the ear, the more likely it is that the otlagia is due to intrinsic disease of the ear than that it is referred. For example, in an older child with otalgia as the only ear symptom, the pain will, after suitable evaluation, probably turn out to be referred. On the other hand, if the primary complaint of otalgia is accompanied by symptoms of ear blockage, popping, and hearing loss, it becomes much more likely that the otalgia is a symptom of intrinsic ear disease.

The causes and characteristics of otalgia due to intrinsic disease of the middle ear, mastoid, and deeper portions of the temporal bone include acute otitis media, an incompetent eustachian tube, chronic middle-ear effusions, negative middle-ear pressure, mastoiditis, aditus block syndrome, masked mastoiditis, tympanomastoiditis, tumors of the ear, histiocytosis, and Wegener granulomatosis; each of these will be discussed further.

Acute otitis media is, of course, the most common cause of otalgia due to intrinsic ear disease in the pediatric age group (Chap. 21).

Acute environmental pressure changes in the presence of an *incompetent eustachian tube* may cause otalgia. This is seen in children, usually with a history suggestive of eustachian tubal incompetence, when they develop otalgia during flights, automobile rides up or down significant land elevations, or when diving into the water. The otologic findings may be negative or may show an acute hemorrhagic otitis with a red or blue tympanic membrane, with or without evidence of a middle-ear effusion or hemorrhage as detected by pneumatic otoscopy. If hemorrhagic otitis is present and if the child is old enough to be tested with tuning forks or audiometry a conductive hearing loss will be found. The pain is most probably due to the sudden intratympanic and intramastoid pressure changes, with resultant pressure or tension on the mucosa.

Children with *chronic middle-ear effusions* are subject to episodes of otalgia. These may be due either to pressure changes, as in barotrauma, or to bacterial infection of the middle-ear effusion. These two different causes of otalgia in middle-ear effusions may be difficult to differentiate. Generally, pain due to superinfection is more persistent and may be accompanied with the other symptoms of acute otitis media (e.g., fever, toxicity, and vomiting), and with a well-developed superinfection, the tympanic membrane is apt to be full or even bulging with vesicular surface changes. In cases of middle-ear effusion without infection, the drumhead is retracted, and no inflammatory changes are noticeable.

In some children, the cause of otalgia is intrinsic in the ear, but the result of the otoscopic examination is quite negative. The pain may be due to simple *negative pressure* without a middle-ear effusion and can be diagnosed with the aid of the acoustic impedance bridge.

The pain of *mastoiditis* accompanying an obvious case of otitis media is usually felt behind the ear in the vicinity of the mastoid antrum and tip. The physician should also watch for the possible breakdown of cellular partitions and for the appearance of an abscess between the mastoid cortex and its periosteum—a subperiosteal abscess, which is recognized as a tender and painful postauricular swelling. A clue that mastoiditis is developing is swelling of the skin of the superior and posterosuperior walls of the osseous portion of the external auditory canal, otherwise known as sagging of the canal wall skin. This condition must be differentiated from a circumscribed otitis externa and must be treated surgically.

Some patients continue to complain of ear pain despite an apparent resolution of the otitis media and return of the drumhead to a normal or nearly normal appearance. These children have developed a sequestered infection of the mastoid known as the *aditus block syndrome:* The narrow communication between the middle ear and mastoid segments has become blocked by mucosal edema. This diagnosis is made by demonstrating radiologic changes consistent with mastoiditis.

Masked mastoiditis is due to an incomplete suppression of the infection of the middle ear and mastoid segment. It may be due to inadequate treatment, to the partial effectiveness of a bacteriostatic antimicrobial, or to the fact that the child has an inadequate immune system (resulting from an immunodeficiency state, diabetes, or suppression of immunity by corticosteroids being administered for an unrelated disorder). A child with masked mastoiditis may have no otologic symptoms or signs until the antibiotic has been discontinued, when the symptoms and signs of otitis media and mastoiditis recrudesce (Chap. 22).

When complications of *tympanomastoiditis* occur, the nature of the pain may change and additional symptoms and signs may appear. Meningitis will become manifest by a generalized headache, signs of meningeal irritation, and the appearance of severe toxicity. A sigmoid sinus thrombophlebitis will be marked by the appearance of mastoid pain and manifestations of septicemia. Brain abscesses and encephalitis, after a quiescent stage, are heralded by severe headache and profound neurologic changes. The pain of Gradenigo syndrome (periapical meningitis) is felt in the ear and behind the ipsilateral eye and is accompanied by diplopia due to a neuritis of the sixth cranial nerve (Chap. 23).

Tumors of the ear, such as rhabdomyosarcoma, lymphoma and leukemic infiltration, may also cause ear pain and must be differentiated from otitis media (Chap. 27).

The ear may become involved by *histiocytosis* X.

Wegener granulomatosis, which may sometimes be seen in older pediatric patients, is heralded by what appears to be a common otitis media (Karmody, 1978). The physician should suspect Wegener granuloma when otitis media does not respond to myringotomy and vigorous antibiotic therapy. The diagnosis is made by submitting mastoid tissue for pathologic examination, or it may be made clinically if the patient develops concomitant involvement of the respiratory tract (granulomatous changes in the nose, nasopharynx, larynx, trachea, or lungs).

OTALGIA REFERRED VIA THE
TRIGEMINAL NERVE

The auriculotemporal branch of the mandibular division of the trigeminal nerve supplies sensory innervation to the anterior part of the auricle, the tragus, anterior and superior canal walls, and anterior portion of the tympanic membrane (Fig. 12–1). According to the principle of referred pain, diseases affecting structures innervated by the mandibular division, as well as those involving structures innervated by the maxillary and ophthalmic divisions, may result in pain referred to areas innervated by the mandibular division. Under most circumstances, pain is referred to other sites only when the irritation persists for more than several minutes.

In order to be guided as to where to search for pain referred via the trigeminal nerve, one must consider the areas of the head and neck, besides the ear, that are innervated by the sensory branches of the trigeminal nerve (Warwick and Williams, 1973g). Because these are many, the search for trigeminal nerve–mediated referred otalgia must be extensive.

Dental Disorders

Dental diseases, such as carious teeth, periapical infections, impacted teeth, unerupted teeth, and disorders of the gingivae, irritate trigeminal fibers of the mandibular or maxillary divisions and hence may cause referred otalgia. A consultation with a dentist may be required to evaluate patients with this problem. Infants and young children with such otalgia may give no clue that would direct the attention of the parents to the mouth: They fuss instead with their ears. If there has been a past problem with otitis media, the parents naturally assume that the present episode is another attack of otitis media (Chaps. 48 to 50).

Disorders Involving the Jaw

Inflammatory and neoplastic disorders, as well as disorders of unknown cause such as histiocytosis X, may involve the jaws, giving rise to referred otalgia. The diagnosis may require appropriate radiographs of the mandible and maxilla, including dental films, to demonstrate the alveolar processes to the best advantage.

Temporomandibular Joint

Disorders of the temporomandibular joint and its associated muscles are among the most common forms of referred otalgia in children as well as in adults. True arthritic disorders of this joint are uncommon and are usually seen only in patients with a background of a systemic arthritis such as rheumatoid arthritis. Other types of intrinsic joint disease that are also uncommon include posttraumatic alterations and septic arthritis. The more common disorders, which are somewhat inaccurately categorized under the heading of "tem-

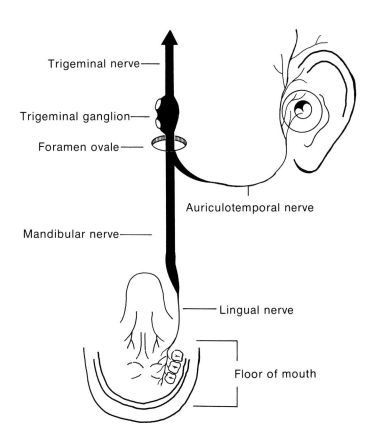

Figure 12–1. Referred otalgia mediated by the trigeminal nerve may be caused by intraoral disorders such as carious teeth, impacted wisdom teeth, and a calculus in the duct of the submandibular salivary gland.

poromandibular joint syndrome," involve the muscles and ligaments associated with the temporomandibular joint. These structures, under certain conditions, may cause pain as a result of being abused, stretched, and irritated. The situation is entirely analogous to the muscular pain that occurs in other parts of the body when a muscle is contracted excessively (as in muscle tension headaches).

In children, these periarticular structures may be irritated by bruxism, excessive gum chewing, dental malocclusion, and sometimes merely as a result of clenching of the teeth. The history may suggest that the otalgia is aggravated by movement of the jaw. The diagnosis is made by eliciting tenderness of the temporomandibular joint in front of the tragus and through the anterior cartilaginous external canal wall. Painful spasm of the pterygoid muscle can be diagnosed by palpating these muscles intraorally between the zygomatic arch and the coronoid process of the mandible. The forward excursion of the mandibular condyle may be reduced on the side with otalgia (Chap. 51).

Oral Cavity

The diagnosis of disorders of the oral cavity that cause referred otalgia should be straightforward. Such lesions may include herpetic stomatitis, inflammatory and traumatic lesions of the tongue and floor of the mouth, and embedded foreign bodies. Malignant tumors of the hard and soft palate may also cause otalgia (Chap. 55).

Salivary Gland Disorders

Whereas disorders of the submandibular and sublingual glands are not common in children, diseases of the parotid gland are seen frequently. The most common disorder besides mumps is that of recurrent parotitis due to sialectasia (chronic punctate parotitis). Although the pathologic ectasia of the ductal system is usually bilateral, the clinically apparent, recurrent parotid swelling with pain in and around the ear is often unilateral. The diagnosis is based upon the results of sialography, which usually demonstrates ectasia of the major and minor intraglandular ducts and pooling of contrast material in them. The episodes of parotid inflammation tend to decrease in frequency as the child gets older. Some of these children subsequently develop systemic autoimmune disorders, such as Sjögren's disease, and therefore must be observed over an extended period of time (Chap. 57).

Paranasal Sinuses

The paranasal sinuses are innervated by the trigeminal nerve, principally the maxillary division. Inflammatory disease and, less commonly, neoplastic disorders in children can result in otalgia. The otalgia is due to two mechanisms that sometimes act jointly: otalgia may be referred via the trigeminal nerve, or otalgia may be due to an intrinsic aural disease that is secondary to the primary sinus disorder. An example of the latter is tubotympanitis caused by infectious secretions from the maxillary sinus as they pass over the torus tubarius in the nasopharynx (Chap. 37).

Other

Before the trigeminal nerve is discounted as the cause of referred otalgia, the physician must consider the possibility that the trigeminal roots or ganglion are being irritated intracranially by a tumor, an anomalous artery, or a demyelinating process. Therefore, careful neurologic evaluation must be performed in such cases.

REFERRED OTALGIA MEDIATED BY THE FACIAL NERVE

Although the facial nerve is primarily a motor nerve, there exists evidence that it contains several somatic sensory elements that innervate the posterior portion of the tympanic membrane and part of the posterior wall of the external auditory canal (Warwick and Williams, 1973c, d).

Bell palsy, or idiopathic facial paralysis, is usually accompanied by pain in the ear or, more commonly, behind the ear in the area of the tip of the mastoid process. The otoscopic findings are usually negative. Occasionally, an imminent idiopathic facial paralysis may be preceded for several days by postauricular pain. Keeping in mind this possibility, the physician should reevaluate children with otalgia of undetermined cause after a period of a few days.

Tumors involving the facial nerve in its intracranial course or in its temporal bone course may also cause pain in and around the ear. Such tumors are uncommon in the pediatric population.

Herpes zoster oticus, or the *Ramsay Hunt syndrome*, is a viral neuritis of the facial nerve that may also involve the fifth and eighth cranial nerves. Patients with this disorder have severe otalgia and vesicular eruption in the ear canal. Once the acute inflammatory changes have subsided and the vesicles have disappeared, otalgia may persist for many weeks. In obscure cases of otalgia, a history should be sought about a vesicular eruption in and about the ear. Chorda tympani nerve function and stapedius muscle function should be checked (Chap. 17).

REFERRED OTALGIA MEDIATED BY THE GLOSSOPHARYNGEAL NERVE

The ninth, or glossopharyngeal, cranial nerve exits from the base of the skull through the jugular foramen in company with the vagus and spinal accessory nerves. It subsequently is distributed to the tonsils, pharynx, eustachian tube, and posterior third of the tongue (Warwick and Williams, 1973e). A branch ascends into the middle ear as the nerve of Jacobson, ramifies on the promontory, and exits from the anterior part of the middle ear as the lesser superficial petrosal nerve (Warwick and Wiliams, 1973h). The latter reaches the otic ganglion and supplies preganglionic, special visceral motor fibers to the parotid gland. The nerve provides general somatic sensory fibers to the posterior portion of the external auditory meatus and canal and to the posterior portion of the external surface of the drumhead. The glossopharyngeal nerve also probably supplies most of the sensory innervation of the mucosa of the middle ear, mastoid air cells, and eustachian tube. The glossopharyngeal nerve is one of the most common mediators of deep ear pain referred from the pharynx (Fig. 12–2).

Tonsillar Diseases

In pediatric patients, inflammatory diseases of the tonsils, mainly acute tonsillitis, peritonsillitis, and peritonsillar abscess, are the main causes of referred otalgia mediated by the ninth cranial nerve. The diagnosis of this type of referred ear pain is made readily upon inspection of the pharynx. Referred otalgia is very common after tonsillectomy. Therefore, patients should be advised to expect it, so they do not confuse posttonsillectomy otalgia with a bout of otitis media. Referred otalgia is not as commonly seen after adenoidectomy alone (Chap. 53).

Oropharyngeal Diseases

Because of the widespread sensory distribution of the glossopharyngeal nerve, pharyngeal disorders other than those involving the tonsils also may cause referred otalgia. These include lingual tonsillitis, retropharyngeal abscess, and foreign bodies embedded in either the tongue base or other portions of the pharynx. These diagnoses can be made by careful pharyngeal examination aided by a lateral radiograph of the neck. Tumors of the pharynx, another potential cause of otalgia referred via the glossopharyngeal nerve, fortunately are uncommon in the pediatric age group. An uncommon cause of otalgia is an infection in the pharyngeal end of a branchial cyst or fistula. Glossopharyngeal tic, a cause of severe otalgia in adults, is rare in the pediatric age group (Chap. 52).

Nasopharyngeal Sources of Referred Otalgia

The nasopharynx derives its sensory innervation partly from the glossopharyngeal nerve and partly from the maxillary division of the trigeminal nerve (Warwick and Williams, 1973f). Both of these nerves, as has already been pointed out, can mediate referred otalgia. The nasopharynx must be examined in cases of obscure otalgia, although it is not a common source of otalgia in children.

Nasopharyngeal disorders that might cause otalgia include nasopharyngitis, adenoiditis, a foreign body lodged in the nasopharynx, and, rarely, a neoplasm such as a lymphoma, epithelial malignancy, or mes-

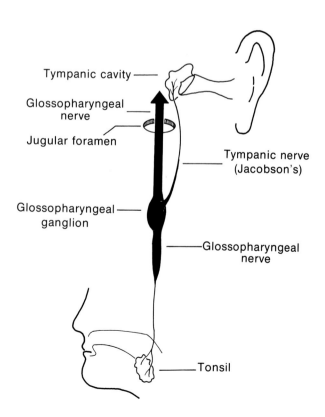

Figure 12–2. Referred otalgia mediated by the glossopharyngeal nerve may be caused by tonsillitis, peritonsillar abscess, or neural irritation after tonsillectomy.

enchymal tumor. A hypertrophic adenoid may occasionally produce otalgia when it causes intermittent obstruction of the eustachian tube, which results in negative middle-ear pressure. When such an adenoid becomes infected as part of a pharyngitis it may result in a salpingitis or tubotympanitis, which in turn causes otalgia.

REFERRED OTALGIA MEDIATED BY THE VAGUS NERVE

In the ear, the sensory fibers of the vagus nerve are distributed by the nerve of Arnold. They supply a portion of the cavum conchae, posterior wall of the external auditory canal, and posterior portion of the external surface of the drumhead (Fig. 12–3). The vagus nerve also supplies the sensory innervation of the entire larynx, esophagus, trachea, and thyroid gland (Warwick and Williams, 1973*i*). According to the principles of referred pain, disorders in these structures may be a source of pain that is referred to the ear. In general, vagus nerve–mediated causes of otalgia are not seen as commonly in pediatric patients as they are in adults. When they occur, the local manifestations usually predominate over referred otalgia, which tends to be a secondary symptom.

Laryngeal Disorders

Laryngeal injuries and foreign bodies of the larynx of pyriform sinus may be a source of otalgia. The diagnosis is made by laryngoscopic examination aided by radiographs. Otalgia is usually found in patients with epiglottitis and epiglottic abscess, but the laryngeal symptoms dominate the clinical picture (Chap. 67).

Esophageal Disorders

Pediatric esophageal disorders with referred otalgia include impacted foreign bodies and burns of the esophageal mucosa. As in the case of laryngeal disorders, the local esophageal symptoms predominate over the otalgia.

Thyroiditis

The thyroid gland receives its sensory innervation via the vagus nerve. An occasional cause of occult otalgia is the occurrence of thyroiditis (usually de Quervain thyroditis), which causes symptoms of throat and neck discomfort and otalgia as a prominent symptom. The diagnosis is often a clinical one based upon the finding of a tender, somewhat swollen thyroid gland, which upon palpation usually evidences otalgia. Childhood thyroiditis must also always be considered as possible cause of recurrent throat discomfort, often misdiagnosed as pharyngitis or tonsillitis. Such patients

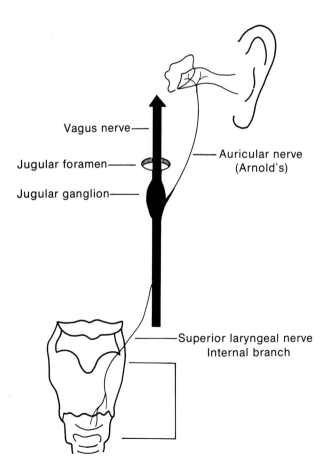

Figure 12–3. Referred otalgia mediated by the vagus nerve may be caused by such laryngopharyngeal disorders as retropharyngeal abscess, epiglottis, esophagitis around an impacted foreign body, and a sharp foreign body in the pyriform sinus.

should be referred to a pediatric endocrinologist (Chap. 85).

REFERRED OTALGIA MEDIATED BY CERVICAL NERVES

The upper cervical nerves, especially the great auricular nerve, supply a significant somatic sensory distribution to the external ear and postauricular area. These nerve endings are distributed in the posterior half of the lateral aspect of the auricle and some of the skin of the cavum conchae (Warwick and Williams, 1973a, b). These cervical nerves also innervate the skin and muscles of the neck and spine. Therefore, they can mediate pain referred to the ear from a variety of disorders of the neck and cervical spine.

When a patient has otalgia referred from a disease affecting a structure innervated by the sensory fibers of the cervical plexus, the otalgia is usually only one component of a constellation of symptoms. Nevertheless, the parents tend to emphasize the otalgia component of the symptoms and minimize the other symptoms that would indicate the neck as a source of the ear pain.

Lymph Nodes

Cervical lymphadenitis, in addition to causing local neck discomfort, may also cause referred otalgia. This is most commonly seen in the case of inflamed nodes in the upper neck, including the jugulodigastric area, parotid nodes, and postauricular and occipital nodes. The management of such pain, of course, rests in pursuing the cause of the lymphadenitis and treating it (Chap. 88).

Infected Cysts of the Neck

Infected branchial cysts, including those of the second arch and preauricular sinuses, may cause otalgia. The management of such pain depends on appropriate treatment of the cyst (Chap. 87).

Cervical Spine

Injuries, infections, and tumors of the cervical spine are possible but relatively uncommonly seen causes of referred otalgia in children.

A condition that is occasionally seen in children is the Grisel syndrome (Martin, 1942), which consists of painful torticollis due to subluxation of the atlantoaxial joint. The condition follows upper respiratory tract infections and adenoidectomy and is thought to be due to an inflammatory softening of the perivertebral ligaments. These children present with torticollis, a lateral cervical "mass," and pain in the ear. The condition, which may be confused with cervical lymphadenitis,

can be diagnosed by obtaining an anteroposterior radiograph of the upper cervical spine and identifying a lateral shift of the atlas relative to the axis and odontoid process.

Neuralgias

Neuralgias involving the occipital nerves are uncommon causes of otalgia in the pediatric age group.

MISCELLANEOUS

Migraine

Migraine headaches may occur in children. Ear pain is usually a nondominant component of the constellation of symptoms characterizing the various forms of cranial migraine in children. As has been mentioned in several places in this chapter, parents are sometimes so fearful of ear disease that they may overemphasize the otalgia component of the symptoms that turn out on careful evaluation to represent migraine or some other disorder.

Aural Neuralgia

In attempting to diagnose obscure cases of otalgia, the physician should consider an uncommon form of ear pain, intrinsic aural neuralgia (Ballantyne and Groves, 1971). This ailment presents as a ticlike, brief, sharp pain localized deep in the ear without radiation beyond the ear. The cause of this condition, as with most other tic syndromes, is not known. The author has made this diagnosis once in 25 years of practice. As suggested by Golding-Wood (Ballantyne and Groves, 1971) this patient, aged 9 years, was relieved of the pain by a tympanic neurectomy.

SUMMARY

The diagnosis of the cause of otalgia is one of the most challenging in the area of diseases of the head and neck. Nevertheless, the pursuit of the cause of ear pain can be systematized by an understanding of the sensory neuroanatomy of the ear and by logic evaluation on this basis. In this manner, the precise cause of intrinsic or referred otalgia can be discovered in the majority of patients presenting with this symptom.

REFERENCES

Ballantyne, J., and Groves, J. 1971. Tympanic plexus neuralgia. In Diseases of the Ear, Nose and Throat, Vol. 3, 3rd ed. Philadelphia, J. B. Lippincott Co., pp. 335–338.
Hayden, G. F., and Schwartz, R. H. 1985. Characteristics of earache

among children with acute otitis media. Am. J. Dis. Child. 139:721.

Karmody, C. S. 1978. Wegener's granulomatosis: Presentation as an otological problem. Trans. AAOO, July–August.

Martin, R. C. 1942. Atlas-axis dislocation following cervical infection. J.A.M.A. *118*:874.

Saunders, R. L., and Weider, D. 1985. Tympanic membrane sensation. Brain 108:387.

Tremble, G. E. 1965. Referred pain in the ear. AMA Arch. Laryngol. 81:57.

Warwick, R., and Williams, P. L. 1973*a*. Auricle innervation. *In* Gray's Anatomy, 35th British ed. Philadelphia, W. B. Saunders Co., p. 1136.

Warwick, R., and Williams, P. L. 1973*b*. Cervical plexus. *In* Gray's Anatomy, 35th British ed. Philadelphia, W. B. Saunders Co., pp. 1034–1036.

Warwick, R., and Williams, P. L. 1973*c*. Facial nerve, sensory portion. *In* Gray's Anatomy, 35th British ed. Philadelphia, W. B. Saunders Co., p. 1012.

Warwick, R., and Williams, P. L. 1973*d*. Facial nerve, cutaneous fibres. *In* Gray's Anatomy, 35th British ed. Philadelphia, W. B. Saunders Co., p. 1015.

Warwick, R., and Williams, P. L. 1973*e*. Glossopharyngeal nerve. *In* Gray's Anatomy, 35th British ed. Philadelphia, W. B. Saunders Co., pp. 1017–1019.

Warwick, R., and Williams, P. L. 1973*f*. Pharyngeal innervation. *In* Gray's Anatomy, 35th British ed. Philadelphia, W. B. Saunders Co., p. 1249.

Warwick, R., and Williams, P. L. 1973*g*. Trigeminal nerve. *In* Gray's Anatomy, 35th British ed. Philadelphia, W. B. Saunders Co., pp. 1001–1010.

Warwick, R., and Williams, P. L. 1973*h*. Tympanic and mastoid innervation. *In* Gray's Anatomy, 35th British ed. Philadelphia, W. B. Saunders Co., pp. 1145–1146.

Warwick, R., and Williams, P. L. 1973*i*. Vagus nerve. *In* Gray's Anatomy, 35th British ed. Philadelphia, W. B. Saunders Co., pp. 1019–1023.

White, J. C., and Sweet, W. H. 1969. Intermedius, vagoglosso-pharyngeal, and upper cervical neuralgias. *In* White, J. C., and Sweet, W. H.: Pain and the Neurosurgeon. Springfield, IL, Charles C Thomas.

Chapter 13

OTORRHEA

Melvin D. Schloss, M.D.

Otorrhea, or discharge from the ear, indicates a disturbance in normal ear function. The clinical approach to this problem is of utmost importance in determining its cause, and the following observations should be made when examining a patient presenting with otorrhea.

FEATURES OF OTORRHEA

Apparent Source

Adequate visualization of the external auditory canal and the tympanic membrane is imperative. An aural discharge may be secondary to disease of the external ear, middle ear, or inner ear. Purulent discharge is usually secondary to disease involving the external or middle ear, whereas a clear discharge usually indicates pathologic conditions within the inner ear (Chap. 8).

Presence of Pulsation

A pulsating discharge is usually due to a disease involving the middle ear or, rarely, the inner ear. Pulsating otorrhea secondary to pathologic conditions of the external auditory canal is unusual.

Odor of the Discharge

A foul-smelling discharge is indicative of infection. Otorrhea, which is nonfoul-smelling, may be inflammatory or noninflammatory in nature.

Associated Signs and Symptoms

PAIN. A painful discharge is generally associated with disease of the external ear. The pain of acute suppurative otitis media is relieved when the tympanic membrane perforates spontaneously or following myringotomy, and the discharge that follows is painless. Pain and otorrhea associated with middle-ear disease suggest that a complication, either otologic or intracranial, is present.

LOCAL SIGNS. Swelling of the auricle or external auditory meatus may suggest an otitis externa. Of course, one must always be aware that an underlying neoplastic process frequently causes swelling as well.

Protrusion of the auricle, swelling and tenderness over the mastoid bone, and sagging of the posterosuperior bony meatal wall, in addition to persistent otorrhea, are signs of acute coalescent mastoiditis.

Regional lymphadenitis is usually present with inflammatory processes of the external or middle ear.

SIGNS AND SYMPTOMS OF A COMPLICATION. There are essentially two major categories of complications that result from middle-ear infections—otologic and intracranial. Persistent fever, pain, vertigo, drowsiness, headache, diplopia, and facial nerve paresis are indicative of a complication (Chaps. 22 and 23).

Most complications are amenable to medical or surgical therapy, but results of therapy are usually in direct proportion to the speed with which these are recognized. Thus, ensuring proper medical therapy as soon as possible is essential.

Character of the Discharge

Only by careful examination of the discharge can the cause of otorrhea be diagnosed. The easiest method is to collect the discharge in a clear glass tube. The discharge should be examined first with the naked eye and then, if possible, under the microscope. Essentially five types of discharges may be seen: (1) serous, (2) mucoid, (3) bloody, (4) purulent, and (5) clear (Paparella, 1976). All except the clear discharge (which is usually cerebrospinal fluid) are results of pathologic conditions of the external and middle ear.

By analyzing the type of discharge, the clinician should be able to establish the correct etiology of the otorrhea, and since the character of the otorrhea is so readily established at the time of examination, this step is an efficient way to establish the differential diagnosis of otorrhea.

Each of the five types of fluid will be discussed separately.

SEROUS FLUID

Clinically, this fluid is a pale yellow transudate resembling serum. It is clear, with no mucous strands present.

MUCOID FLUID

Clinically, this is a white, cloudy exudate. This fluid may be tenacious, resembling glue; thus, the term "glue ear" is used to describe this condition. Numerous mucous strands are present, accompanied by some cells, mostly phagocytes.

Serous and mucoid fluids have been proposed to be closely related to other conditions (Paparella and Shumrick, 1980): (1) adenoid hypertrophy, (2) cleft palate, (3) tumors, (4) barotrauma, (5) inflammation and antibiotics, (6) allergy, (7) iatrogenic effects (inadequate antibiotic therapy, radiation therapy, or trauma), (8) immunologic deficiencies, and (9) metabolic disturbance.

Serous and mucoid fluids are usually seen at the time of paracentesis of a middle-ear effusion, and rarely are they a spontaneous discharge. The causes of these types of otorrhea are multiple (Table 13–1).

PURULENT FLUID

A purulent aural discharge is the type of otorrhea most commonly encountered.

This type of fluid is the result of an inflammatory process affecting the external or middle ear (Table 13–1). Examination of the fluid reveals many neutrophils with mucous strands and a moderate number of cellular remnants. The determination of the bacteriologic components of the fluid is worthwhile in most cases presenting with purulent otorrhea (Healy and Teele, 1977).

Although purulent discharge resulting from infections of the external ear is usually secondary to gramnegative bacilli, routine cultures are unnecessary except for infections resistant to the usual therapy.

In middle-ear infections, cultures are accurate if proper aspiration is done and if the external ear canal has been properly cleansed. These cultures are particularly important for infections resistant to the standard therapy and for those individuals who are compromised hosts (e.g., those with immunologic deficiencies).

Diseases of the External Ear

Purulent otorrhea is caused by purulent inflammatory processes or inflammation secondary to other pathologic conditions of the external auditory canal (Table 13–1). Pain associated with a purulent discharge is almost always secondary to inflammation involving the external auditory canal, and pain produced by pressure to the external auditory canal, pulling on the auricle, or pressing on the tragus indicates disease of the external auditory canal.

Purulent otorrhea may be present as a result of infection of a congenital anomaly. For instance, a fistula of the first branchial cleft may be presented to the physician as a draining ear (Work, 1972).

The fissures of Santorini, which are fibrous channels in the cartilaginous portion of the external auditory canal, may transmit infection between the parotid gland and the external canal (Chap. 20).

Diseases of the Middle Ear

These are by far the most common causes of purulent otorrhea (Table 13–1) (Chaps. 21 and 22).

Acute Suppurative Otitis Media

In the stage of suppuration, the tympanic membrane may be perforated spontaneously or by myringotomy. There is characteristically a copious drainage of hemorrhagic or serosanguineous fluid that soon assumes a mucopurulent character. It is usually odorless and is accompanied by loss of pain. The otorrhea will continue until the inflammation of the middle ear has settled; as a rule the acute processes resolve within several weeks. If the disease progresses to acute coalescent mastoiditis, the discharge will persist longer than two or three weeks and will become more profuse and foul-smelling.

Pain and persistent discharge following a simple mastoidectomy usually signify acute petrositis (Shambaugh, 1980).

Otorrhea is the most common complication following insertion of tympanostomy tubes. The reported incidence is between 15 and 34 per cent (Cummings, 1986).

A foul-smelling discharge devoid of mucus is often the first symptom of acute, necrotizing otitis media (Shambaugh, 1980).

Chronic Suppurative Otitis Media

With chronicity, the suppuration produces irreversible damage to the middle-ear mucosa and underlying bone. This results clinically in otorrhea that is scanty or profuse, painless, and usually accompanied by some hearing impairment. Pain in middle-ear disease is a sign of a complication, in contrast to disease of the external auditory canal, of which pain is an early symptom. Because the onset of chronic otitis media is often insidious, the patient may not consult the otologist until the symptoms of a complication occur.

By careful examination and documentation of the otorrhea, the state of the chronic ear disease can be ascertained (Paparella and Shumrick, 1980), an essential step in planning the proper therapy. The active state of chronic disease is characterized by a steady purulent discharge; the quiescent, or inactive, state is

TABLE 13–1. Causes of Otorrhea

A. SEROUS, MUCOID, AND PURULENT
1. congenital anomalies
   a. first branchial cleft fistula
   b. salivary flow through fissures of Santorini
2. inflammatory
   a. external ear
      i. keratosis obturans
      ii. benign necrotizing osteitis of the meatus
      iii. foreign bodies
      iv. otitis externa
         1. furunculosis
         2. diffuse otitis externa
      v. otomycosis
      vi. otitis externa haemorrhagica (bullous myringitis)
      vii. herpes zoster oticus
      viii. herpes simplex
      ix. seborrheic dermatitis
      x. neurodermatitis
   b. middle ear
      i. acute otitis media
         1. acute suppurative otitis media
         2. acute necrotizing otitis media
         3. acute mastoiditis
         4. acute petrositis
      ii. chronic otitis media
         1. chronic suppurative otitis media
            a. tubotympanic disease
               i. permanent perforation syndrome
               ii. persistent mucosal disease
            b. atticoantral disease
         2. tuberculous otitis media
         3. syphilis of the ear
         4. histiocytosis X
      iii. iatrogenic
         1. after-insertion of tympanostomy tubes
3. tumors
   a. external ear
      i. benign
         1. adenoma
            a. sebaceous adenoma
            b. ceruminoma
         2. osteoma
         3. exostoses
      ii. malignant
         1. squamous cell carcinoma
         2. basal cell carcinoma
         3. adenocarcinoma
         4. metastatic
   b. middle ear
      i. benign
         1. adenoma
         2. neurofibroma
         3. glomus jugulare tumors
      ii. malignant
         1. squamous cell carcinoma
         2. metastatic

B. BLOODY
1. congenital anomalies
   a. high, dehiscent jugular bulb
   b. anomalous internal carotid artery
2. inflammatory
   a. external ear
      i. otitis externa
         1. furunculosis
         2. diffuse otitis externa
      ii. otitis externa haemorrhagica (bullous myringitis)
   b. middle ear
      i. acute otitis media
      ii. chronic otitis media
3. traumatic
   a. temporal bone fractures
   b. self-inflicted (e.g. cotton swab injuries)
   c. foreign body
   d. iatrogenic
      1. myringotomy
      2. tympanocentesis
      3. curetting to remove wax
4. tumors (e.g., glomus tympanicum, rhabdomyosarcoma)
5. coagulation defects (e.g., leukemia)

C. CLEAR (PERILYMPH FISTULA)
1. congenital anomalies
   a. without associated temporal bone or extracranial anomalies
      i. isolated stapes footplate fistula
   b. with associated temporal bone or extracranial anomalies
      i. Mondini dysplasia
      ii. Klippel-Feil syndrome
      iii. Pendred's syndrome
      iv. craniosynostosis
      v. widely patent cochlear aqueduct
2. acquired
   a. iatrogenic, poststapedectomy
   b. traumatic
      i. direct—penetrating wound in the ear
      ii. indirect—blunt injury to the head
      iii. barotrauma
         1. explosive—alteration in cerebrospinal fluid pressure
         2. implosive—alteration in tubotympanic pressure
   c. erosion of bone
      i. luetic
      ii. cholesteatoma
      iii. neoplasm (intracranial, extracranial)
3. combined

characterized by intermissions between discharges; and the healed state is the period during which the perforation of the tympanic membrane is healed or repaired.

It is of utmost importance to determine whether the ear being examined has "dangerous" or "benign" mid-dle-ear disease (Paparella and Shumrick, 1980). "Dangerous" means that the chronic ear disease could produce early complications. If the ear disease is potentially dangerous, urgent surgical intervention is indicated.

"Benign" middle-ear disease is due to pathologic

conditions involving the eustachian tube and the middle ear cleft. It is helpful to divide this "benign" disease into two stages.

Permanent perforation is a persistent perforation of the pars tensa of the tympanic membrane (Ballantyne and Groves, 1979). The margins of the perforation are completely covered with healed epithelium, and the ear may remain dry for long periods or may discharge intermittently because of water entering the middle-ear cleft via the external auditory canal. Another route for the infection to spread to the middle ear is via the eustachian tube after blowing the nose. The discharge is profuse and mucoid or mucopurulent, and has no odor.

Chronic tubotympanic mucositis is a more active disease state within the middle ear. There may be a prolonged or even persistent mucoid or mucopurulent discharge, which becomes profuse with an upper respiratory infection. On careful examination of the ear, there is a large, nearly total defect of the tympanic membrane. The exposed mucosa is thickened and red. Polyps may be present, owing to marked swelling of the tympanic mucosa.

"Dangerous" chronic ear disease is due to a pathologic condition extending into the attic and antrum (Ballantyne and Groves, 1979). This usually signifies a congenital cholesteatoma, primary acquired cholesteatoma, or occlusion of the attic floor by a chronic noncholesteatomatous process. The otorrhea is often not profuse, and usually there is a foul odor to the discharge. A bloody discharge may occur from trauma to the granulation tissue or polyps.

Tuberculous Otitis Media

Tuberculous involvement of the middle ear produces a scanty, thin, odorless and purulent otorrhea, but the discharge is generally less copious than that seen in chronic suppurative otitis media. Tuberculous otitis media is generally painless, although it is associated with surrounding lymphadenopathy. The involved ear occasionally demonstrates a profound hearing loss, with otorrhea being a late sign in this disease. Otoscopy reveals multiple minute tympanic membrane perforations with little surrounding reaction (Chap. 21).

Other Specific Diseases of the Middle Ear

Syphilis and histiocytosis X may present with otorrhea. These diseases are rare but must be included in the differential diagnosis of a purulent aural discharge (Chap. 27).

BLOODY FLUID

There are many causes of bleeding from the ear.
1. It may be secondary to lacerations or abrasions of the skin of the external auditory canal. The trauma causing the injury may be self-inflicted, for instance by a cotton swab, secondary to foreign bodies, or iatrogenic (as by a wax curette).

2. Tumors of the external auditory canal and middle ear, for instance glomus tympanicum, may present with a bloody aural discharge (Chap. 27).

3. Bleeding from the ear can be secondary to acute inflammatory processes of the external auditory canal and middle ear. Bloody otorrhea is commonly seen secondary to bullous myringitis.

4. Profuse bleeding may occur following a myringotomy and tympanocentesis. This is possible in cases involving a congenital vascular anomaly within the middle ear (e.g., with a high, dehiscent jugular bulb and anomalous internal carotid artery), with tumors in the middle ear (as mentioned), or with coagulation defects (as in leukemia).

5. Bleeding from the ear is one of the most frequent symptoms of middle-ear damage from head injury. Hough has described a triad of signs characteristic of a temporal bone fracture (Hough and Stuart, 1968): Hearing loss, bleeding from the ear, and unconsciousness. If temporal bone fractures are characterized as transverse or longitudinal, it is the longitudinal type that results in bleeding from the ear. Bleeding may last for a short time or for days and may be from the mouth or nose, owing to flow through the eustachian tube. The bleeding most often ceases spontaneously (Chap. 26).

CLEAR FLUID

A clear discharge from the ear is assumed to be cerebrospinal fluid until it is proved otherwise (Shambaugh, 1980).

Skull trauma resulting from a temporal bone fracture is the most common cause of clear otorrhea. Surgical defects following mastoidectomy or posterior craniotomy are less common. Intracranial or extracranial tumors and congenital anomalies are uncommon causes of clear otorrhea.

Trauma

To locate the site of leakage secondary to skull trauma is a diagnostic challenge. A detailed history and a physical examination are the cornerstones in diagnosis and are aided by relatively simple office or bedside procedures. Since cerebrospinal fluid has a high glucose concentration, there is a strongly positive reaction with simple glucose oxidase test paper. Occasionally, cerebrospinal fluid otorrhea presents as rhinorrhea, the transit from the ear to the nasopharynx being via the eustachian tube, in which case the positive reaction with simple glucose oxidase test paper may be invalid because of the reducing substance in lacrimal gland secretions.

High-resolution computed tomography (CT) scanning with a bone algorithm is the radiologic study of choice to evaluate potential fractures of the skull base.

A leak from the middle or posterior cranial fossa may be evaluated with nuclear medical techniques. Intrathecal injection of fluorescein or radioactive carrier substance may be useful when a cerebrospinal fluid leak is suspected directly from the external auditory canal or eustachian tube (Cummings, 1986). Metrizamide, a water-soluble agent, when injected into the subarachnoid space and followed by rapid serial CT scanning, has proved useful in determining the site of a cerebrospinal fluid fistula (Margaret et al., 1984).

Perilymphatic Fistulas

Spontaneous clear otorrhea has been described as a result of perilymphatic fistulas. Classification of perilymphatic fistulas has been proposed by Grundfast and Bluestone (1978) and Althaus (1981). This classification includes congenital and acquired conditions (Table 13–1) (Chap. 19).

It is generally accepted that rupture of the labyrinthine window membrane may be the result of rapid alterations in perilymphatic fluid pressure. If the cochlear aqueduct is patent, alterations in cerebrospinal fluid pressure are transmitted via this pathway to the inner ear perilymph-containing compartment (Grundfast and Bluestone, 1978).

Explosive and implosive mechanisms resulting in perilymphatic fistulas have been described (Goodhill et al., 1973). The explosive mechanism is the result of increased cerebrospinal fluid pressure (due to physical exertion). This pressure is transmitted from the subarachnoid space via the cochlear aqueduct or the laminae cribrosa of the inner ear. The implosive mechanism is the result of sudden alteration in middle-ear pressure (barotrauma) acting directly on the middle-ear side of the round window membrane, at the annular ligament of the oval window, or both.

A spontaneous perilymphatic fistula resulting in recurrent meningitis is most commonly secondary to an underlying congenital anomaly of the middle or inner ear (Parisier and Birken, 1976). A perilymph leak should always be suspected in a patient having congenital footplate fixation (Farrior and Endicott, 1971; Glasscock, 1973); spontaneous perilymphatic fistulas have been reported without any surgical intervention (Chap. 19).

An uncommon cause of clear otorrhea is discharge through the fissures of Santorini connecting the parotid gland and the external auditory canal.

SUMMARY

In summary, otorrhea is an important sign of ear disease. There are basically five types of aural discharge: (1) serous, (2) mucoid, (3) bloody, (4) purulent, and (5) clear. A combination of two or more types is the usual clinical presentation. If otorrhea is approached by the clinician in an organized manner, a correct diagnosis will be established and the proper therapy will be instituted.

SELECTED REFERENCES

Glasscock, M. E. 1973. The stapes gusher. Arch. Otolaryngol. 98(2):82.
   This is an excellent review of spontaneous cerebrospinal fluid otorrhea. It is an article related specifically to congenital abnormalities.
Paparella, M. 1976. Middle ear effusions: Definitions and terminology. Ann. Otol. Rhinol. Laryngol. (Suppl. 25) 15(2):8.
   Clearly outlines and defines fluid in the middle ear.
Hough, J. V. D., and Stuart, W. D. 1968. Middle ear injuries in skull trauma. Laryngoscope 78:899.
   Classic reference for skull trauma related to middle-ear injuries.

REFERENCES

Althaus, S. R. 1981. Perilymph fistulas. Laryngoscope 91:538.
Ballantyne, J., and Groves, J. 1979. Scott-Brown's Diseases of the Ear, Nose and Throat, 3rd ed. London, Butterworth's.
Cummings, C. W. 1986. Otolaryngology—Head and Neck Surgery, Vol. IV, Sec. B. St. Louis, The C. V. Mosby Co.
Farrior, J. B., and Endicott, J. H. 1971. Congenital mixed deafness: Cerebrospinal fluid otorrhea. Ablation of the aqueduct of the cochlea. Laryngoscope 81(5):684.
Glasscock, M. E. 1973. The stapes gusher. Arch. Otolaryngol. 98(2):82.
Grundfast, K. M., and Bluestone, C. D. 1978. Sudden or fluctuating hearing loss and vertigo in children due to perilymph fistula. Ann. Otol. Rhinol. Laryngol. 87:761.
Goodhill, V., Brackman, S. J., Harris, J., et al. 1973. Labyrinthine window ruptures. Ann. Otol. Rhinol. Laryngol. 82:2.
Healy, G. B., and Teele, D. W. 1977. The microbiology of chronic middle ear effusions in children. Laryngoscope 87:1472.
Hough, J. V. D., and Stuart, W. D. 1968. Middle ear injuries in skull trauma. Laryngoscope 78:899.
Margaret, A. W., Reede, D. L., Meisler, W., et al. 1984. CT of the base of the skull. Radiol. Clin. North Am. 22(1).
Paparella, M. 1976. Middle ear effusions: Definitions and terminology. Ann. Otol. Rhinol. Laryngol. (Suppl. 25) 15(2):8.
Paparella, M., and Shumrick, D. A. 1980. Otolaryngology, Vol. 2, Sec. 4. Philadelphia, W. B. Saunders Co.
Parisier, S. C., and Birken, E. A. 1976. Recurrent meningitis secondary to idiopathic oval window CSF leak. Laryngoscope 86:1503.
Shambaugh, E., Jr. 1980. Surgery of the Ear, 3rd ed. Philadelphia, W. B. Saunders Co.
Work, W. P. 1972. Newer concepts of first branchial cleft defects. Laryngoscope 82:1581.

Chapter 14

HEARING LOSS

Kenneth M. Grundfast, M.D.

Much of a child's learning is dependent on information received from listening to speech and other sounds in the environment. As children grow and develop, they continually acquire and refine their communicative skills, cognitive abilities, and skills in social interaction. Because hearing is so important in the process of developing these skills, significant impairment in a child's hearing ability may affect various related aspects of development.

In light of the importance of hearing in the context of a child's overall development, it can be seen that a child who is suspected of having a hearing loss needs thorough evaluation. To delay and temporize can be detrimental, whereas an evaluation that leads to a finding of normal hearing either may allay a parent's fears about possible deafness or may lead to the conclusion that there is dysfunction somewhere in the nervous system other than in the auditory portion.

Depending on the age of the child, an evaluation to determine if manifest symptoms are due to hearing impairment can be difficult. In the sense that hearing is perceptual, involving psychoacoustic phenomena, there is an element of subjectivity inherent in the meaningful perception of auditory stimuli. Although inferences can be made from observing a child's response to auditory stimuli, only the child is actually aware of the type of information that is ultimately received from auditory stimuli. Younger children are less able than older children to verbalize about abnormalities in the perception of sound and to cooperate for behavioral audiometric tests. However, the availability of nonbehavioral (objective) audiometric testing makes it feasible at least to estimate the hearing ability of young children and even of newborn infants (Chap. 9). *No child is too young to be tested or too young to be evaluated when there is the suspicion that hearing ability may be impaired.*

Because it is not always easy to know where to begin an evaluation for the symptom of hearing loss, an orderly approach is helpful. The complete process of evaluation and management can be subdivided into the initial phase of collecting core information and then proceeding with four tasks that are undertaken in a sequential, stepwise fashion. As a memory aid, the initial phase and succeeding tasks are all described with words beginning with the letter C; thus, the five Cs constitute the rudiments of evaluation and management for a child with hearing impairment.

EVALUATION AND TASKS

- CORE information. Information gleaned from history taking and physical examination combined with results of appropriate laboratory and radiographic studies constitutes core information.
- CONFIRM. Establish that hearing impairment exists.
- CHARACTERIZE. Ascertain the type of hearing impairment (e.g., conductive, sensorineura, and mixed), and quantify the degree of impairment.
- CAUSE. Attempt to discover the pathophysiologic process that caused the hearing impairment.
- CARE. Formulate a plan for habilitation or rehabilitation, education, and periodic reassessment of the hearing-impaired child.

Collecting the core information (i.e., establishing the data base) is fairly routine and is done in much the same way for children in all age groups. However, the method to be chosen for accomplishing the succeeding four tasks depends on the age of the child. Audiometric test techniques, diagnostic possibilities, and management modalities utilized for the neonate with suspected hearing loss differ markedly from those that are appropriate for a preadolescent child who develops difficulty in hearing. Regarding the symptom of hearing loss, then, it must be realized that the pediatric population is somewhat heterogeneous. Conceptually dividing the childhood years into five age categories makes it possible to develop several different approaches, each of which is more or less specifically suited for use with children in a certain age category. The age categories utilized in this chapter are (1) neonate, birth to 4 weeks; (2) infant, 4 weeks to 2 years; (3) preschool age, 2 to 5 years; (4) school age, 5 to 10 years; and (5) preadolescent, 10 to 14 years.

Keeping in mind these arbitrary age categories and the sequential tasks previously mentioned, one is able to develop an age-specific, task-oriented approach to the evaluation and management of hearing loss in children. To demonstrate how this approach is utilized, the five "C" tasks are described, and then methods for accomplishing the tasks are discussed for each of the five age categories. Because the method of acquiring core information is much the same for children of all ages, separate descriptions are not given in each age category. Rather, the detailed description of a method for acquiring core information is intended to be utilized for children in all age categories. Methods for accomplishing the remaining tasks (i.e., *confirm, characterize, cause,* and *care*) are considered in subsequent separate sections corresponding to the five arbitrary age categories.

Core Information—Data Base

Whereas hearing impairment manifesting during the later adult years usually is the result of degenerative processes, hearing impairment during childhood can be caused by any of a number of factors. Therefore, significant unilateral or bilateral hearing impairment discovered during childhood should be viewed as a specific pathologic process involving one sensory system. Childhood hearing loss may be the result of a common disorder such as otitis media with effusion, or it could represent the initially discovered manifestation that leads to later diagnosis of a syndromal or neurologic disorder. To commence the evaluation of a child with hearing impairment, a detailed history and physical examination are warranted, as well as certain appropriate diagnostic studies.

Confirm

Not all children who are suspected of having hearing loss actually have impairment of hearing ability. The importance of early detection has been widely publicized; consequently, many types of screening programs have been developed. Even where screening programs are nonexistent, parents, educators, and day care center personnel have become sufficiently cognizant of the importance of early detection to notice young children who may possibly have hearing impairments. As a result, it is becoming common for neonates, infants, and children to be referred to a physician, medical center, or audiologist for further evaluation of hearing ability. Depending on the accuracy and specificity of a given screening procedure, a proportion of children initially identified as possibly hearing impaired will ultimately be found to have normal hearing. This being the case, the first task is to confirm the presence of and measure the amount of hearing loss with a test procedure that is appropriate for the chronologic age and developmental level of the child (Chap. 9).

Characterize

Next, it is important to characterize the type of hearing impairment as being one of the following.

CONDUCTIVE. Impairment of hearing by air conduction can be due to any condition that interferes with transmission of sound through the external auditory canal or transmission of vibrations from the tympanic membrane through the ossicular chain to the oval window.

SENSORINEURAL. When hearing by bone conduction is impaired, the malfunction is in the cochlea, the cochlear portion of the eighth cranial nerve, or both. In the purist sense, if the impairment of function is solely in the cochlea, then the hearing loss should be termed sensory, and if the abnormality is only in the cochlear nerve, then it should be termed neural hearing loss. Practically speaking, these distinctions are rarely made, and it is usually considered adequate to identify a hearing loss as being sensorineural.

MIXED. When hearing by both air and bone conduction is impaired, the loss is termed mixed. The malfunction in such cases is in the middle ear transformer mechanism and in the cochlea or the cochlear nerve, or at some or all of these sites.

RETROCOCHLEAR. A retrocochlear hearing loss involves impaired neuronal transmission somewhere in the cochlear nerve, brain stem auditory pathways, or both, with presumably normal function in the cochlea.

CENTRAL. When a hearing loss is central in nature, the middle-ear transformer mechanism, the cochlea, and the cochlear nerve function properly, but there is abnormal processing of auditory signals within the brain.

Determining the type of hearing impairment that a child has helps localize the portion of the auditory system that is not functioning normally. In turn, this helps in the diagnosis and management of the hearing impairment.

Cause

An attempt should be made to discover the pathophysiologic process that has caused hearing impairment. Because severe hearing impairment can be such a devastating handicap for a child, attention is often focused on the hearing threshold itself rather than considering the hearing loss as a symptom that requires a complete evaluation to discover the pathophysiologic mechanisms involved. If a child has difficulty hearing, some portion of the auditory pathway is not functioning properly. Although hearing loss in adults can usually be attributed to degenerative changes in the cochlea, such is not the case with children. The child with sensorineural hearing impairment should be viewed as a child with a significant pathologic process in one sensory system. Then, further investigation is warranted to determine the etiologic factors involved and to determine whether other sensory systems or even other organ systems also may have been affected by a common etiologic factor. There may be an inherent abnormality in a single portion or several portions of the auditory system, or there may have been an inflammatory, degenerative, neoplastic, metabolic, or traumatic process that affected some aspect of the auditory system (Chap. 18).

In a broad sense, childhood hearing impairment may be thought of as being congenital, acquired, or of unknown etiology. A detailed history and thorough medical evaluation combined with audiometric tests and laboratory and radiographic studies yield the information that is necessary for formulating a reasonable hypothesis of causality. Because hearing impairment can be an isolated abnormality or can be associated with other abnormalities, it is important to attempt to uncover any associated findings. A questionnaire may be helpful in discovering subtle but significant findings associated with hearing loss (Fig. 14–1).

Finally, even though inferences regarding causality can be based on certain information and observations, a greater understanding of the cause of a given hearing impairment can be achieved by histopathologic examination of the involved temporal bone. That is, the damaged or malfunctioning portion of the auditory pathway may involve the ossicles, the basilar membrane, the hair cells, the eighth nerve, the temporal lobe, or any other area in the complex sensory system that enables meaningful perception of auditory stimuli. Because biopsy of middle-ear and inner-ear structures is not really feasible, there is a need to locate the temporal bones of people who have had hearing impairment during childhood so that histopathologic examinations can be made and the pathophysiology of childhood hearing impairment can be elucidated. Many major medical centers throughout the world have temporal bone laboratories where detailed examinations can be made on temporal bone specimens that have been donated.

Care

After a child's hearing impairment has been characterized and quantified and an attempt has been made to discover the etiology, a plan must be established for helping the child function optimally despite the hearing handicap. Depending on the severity of the hearing impairment, a child may require a hearing aid, preferential seating in school, or some special type of education. The cochlear implant may be helpful for children who are postlingually deaf and for some children who are congenitally deaf (House et al., 1987; Kirk and Hill-Brown, 1985; Berliner and Eisenberg, 1985; Miyamoto et al., 1986). In addition, an implantable bone-conduction hearing aid may be helpful for some children. It may be necessary to provide the child with assistance in developing communication skills. The child may require assistance in making various psychologic and social adjustments. The family of a child newly diagnosed with significant hearing impairment will need assistance in making adjustments. Resources are available to assist parents in making choices (Schwartz, 1987; Terry, 1980). Genetic counseling for the parents may be advisable (Chap. 97).

The child with impaired hearing will require frequent assessments of hearing ability to make sure that the hearing is not worsening. There will also be a continual need for otologic evaluation.

METHOD FOR ACQUIRING CORE INFORMATION—APPLICABLE TO ALL AGES

An appropriate physical examination and relevant history taking are essential. The most common cause of hearing loss in children is otitis media with effusion. When there is a history of frequent ear "infections" and it seems probable that persistent middle-ear effusion could be causing a conductive hearing loss, it is important to determine the nature and frequency of prior ear "infections." In doing this, the term infection must be defined. Often a parent may report that the child has had four or five "ear infections" in the past several months. When questioned further, it becomes evident that the child has had no fever or otalgia, but a physician who periodically examines the child has noticed fluid in the child's ear and the parent was told that the child had an "infection" (Grundfast and Carney, 1987). Rather than using the term infection, it is helpful to decide from the history whether the otologic problem is frequent acute otitis media, persistent otitis media with effusion, or chronic suppurative otitis media (Chaps. 21 and 22).

When there is no history suggestive of frequent or persistent otitis media with effusion and it is suspected that the hearing impairment is sensorineural, history taking should attempt to discover causative perinatal or genetic factors (Chap. 24).

Gestational History

It is important to identify the factors that may have acted during fetal development to cause impaired hearing after birth. The human embryo is most susceptible to factors that can cause major morphologic abnormalities from about 3 weeks through 10 weeks of gestation; until 20 weeks of gestation, certain physiologic defects and minor morphologic abnormalities may occur (Moore, 1977). Prenatal infections, such as rubella, toxoplasmosis, influenza, cytomegalovirus infection, and syphilis, can cause changes in the embryo that will ultimately result in some form of hearing impairment (Bergstrom and Stewart, 1971; Bergstrom, 1974). Subclinical rubella infection in the mother can cause rubella embryopathy; this can occur even if the mother has had a previous attack of rubella, as immunity is not necessarily permanent (Karmody, 1968). Although the evidence is not entirely conclusive, it is probable that certain medications taken during pregnancy can have a deleterious effect on portions of the developing inner ear. Streptomycin, especially in the dihydro form, quinine, and chloroquine phosphate all have been described as causing sensorineural hearing

1. Are the external ears malformed?
   No.
   Yes. Describe: _____

   _____

   Consider:
   _____ Microtia
2. Are the ear canals extremely narrow or completely closed?
   No.
   Yes. Describe: _____

   Consider:
   _____ Treacher Collins syndrome (mandibulofacial dysostosis)
   _____ Goldenhar syndrome (eye, ear, spine deformities)
   _____ Atresia/microtia, absent or deformed ear canals
   _____ Hemifacial microsomia (small half face)
3. Are there pits or skin appendages in front of the ears and has there been drainage from openings in front of the ears or on the neck?
   No.
   Yes. Describe: _____

   _____

   Consider:
   _____ Otofaciocervical syndrome, branchio-oto syndrome, or branchio-oto-renal syndrome
4. Is vision poor, are strong eyeglasses required?
   No.
   Yes. Describe: _____

   _____

   Consider:
   _____ Stickler syndrome (myopia, retinal detachment, cleft palate, joint enlargements)
   _____ Marshall syndrome (myopia, cataract, saddle nose)
5. Has there been progressive loss of vision?
   No.
   Yes. Describe: _____

   _____

   Consider:
   _____ Usher syndrome (retinitis pigmentosa and sensorineural hearing loss)
   _____ Refsum syndrome (retinitis pigmentosa, neuropathy)
   _____ Cockayne syndrome (retinal degeneration, senile appearance)
6. Has there been severe irritation or infection in the eyes?
   No.
   Yes. Describe: _____

   _____

   Consider:
   _____ Cogan syndrome (nonsyphilitic keratitis)
7. Have there been cataracts or corneal problems?
   No.
   Yes. Describe: _____

   _____

   Consider:
   _____ Harboyan syndrome
   _____ Marshall syndrome (myopia, cataract, saddle nose)
8. Do the whites of the eyes have a blue color?
   No.
   Yes.
   Consider:
   _____ Osteogenesis imperfecta (blue sclerae, brittle bones, large skull)
9. Is there an unusually broad flat nose?
   No.
   Yes. Describe: _____

   _____

   Consider:
   _____ Craniometaphyseal dysplasia (large coarse facial structure)
   _____ Mohr syndrome (orofaciodigital syndrome type II) (cleft lip, small midface, extra fingers, and toes often fused)
   _____ Otopalatodigital (cleft palate, large brows, flat face, deformed fingers and toes)
   _____ Waardenburg syndrome (widely spaced eyes, white forelock)
10. Is there a receding chin or other unusual facial features?
    No.
    Yes. Describe: _____

    _____

    Consider:
    _____ Treacher Collins syndrome (mandibulofacial dysostosis, downward slopping face, deformed low-set ears)
    _____ Micrognathia (receding chin)

_____ Apert syndrome (craniosynostosis, fusion of fingers and toes)
_____ Pierre Robin sequence (small chin, big tongue)
_____ Crouzon syndrome (craniofacial dysostosis: small midface, large chin)
_____ Pfeiffer syndrome (craniosynostosis, broad thumb and toes)
11. Has there been abnormal growth?
    No.
    Yes. Describe: _____

    _____

    Consider:
    _____ Hurler syndrome (mucopolysaccharidoses)
12. Were there any skeletal, extremity, or facial abnormalities at birth, or developing after birth?
    No.
    Yes. Describe: _____

    _____

    Consider:
    _____ Klippel-Feil sequence (no neck)
    _____ Cleidocranial dysplasia (short collar bone)
    _____ Marfan syndrome (anachnodactyly, tall thin, spiderlike, hypermobile joints)
13. Is there a spot of white hair on the forehead (white forelock)?
    No.
    Yes. Describe: _____

    _____

    Consider:
    _____ Waardenburg syndrome (widely spaced eyes, different color eyes, white forelock)
14. Is there lack of pigment in skin, white hair, and pink eyes?
    No.
    Yes. Describe: _____

    _____

    Consider:
    _____ Albinism
15. Are there white areas, brown areas, or other pigmentation abnormalities on the skin?
    Describe the general area of the spots, whether they have always been present or have developed, and if so, at what age.

    _____

    _____

    Consider:
    _____ Café-au-lait spots (von Recklinghausen)
    _____ Multiple lentigines (Leopard syndrome)
    _____ White spots (vitiligo)
16. Is there unusual skin texture?
    No.
    Yes. Describe the condition. _____

17. Is there kidney disease?
    No.
    Yes. Describe present severity of disease, any treatment given for it, and at what age it developed. _____

    _____

18. Have tests ever revealed abnormal substances in the urine?
    No.
    Yes. Describe: Was it one of the following substances. Specify what you have been told about the substances and any treatments.
    Proline _____
    Protein _____
    Phosphate _____
    Alanine _____
    Amino acids _____
    Others
19. Has there been a thyroid problem?
    No.
    Yes. Describe: State whether thyroid extract or any other medication has been prescribed for this and give dosages if known.

    _____

    Consider:
    _____ Referral to clinical geneticist if there are any indications of kidney or thyroid disease, or abnormal skin.
20. Is there sickle cell anemia?
    No.
    Yes.

Figure 14–1. The Associated System Abnormalities Questionnaire. (With permission from Grundfast, K. M., The role of the audiologist and etologist in the identification of the dysmorphic child. Ear Hear. 4(1):24—30, © by Williams & Wilkins, 1983.)

loss by damaging neural elements in the developing ear of the embryo. Thalidomide embryopathy, on the other hand, is due to a widespread involvement of the auditory apparatus, including the auricles and osseous structures of the middle and inner ear (Partsch and Maurer, 1963; Rosendal, 1963; Kittel and Saller, 1964).

Finally, there have been reports that endocrine diseases of the mother, such as pseudohypoparathyroidism (Hinojosa, 1958) or diabetes mellitus (Kelemen, 1960; Jørgensen, 1961) may predispose the children to congenital hearing loss.

Thus, the prenatal history must be reviewed for any factor, infectious or otherwise, that may have had a deleterious effect on the developing middle or inner ear in the embryo.

Perinatal History

Certainly, the birth process and the adaptation to extrauterine life can be stressful for the neonate. Intrapartum asphyxia and anoxia may lead to hearing loss through toxic damage to the cochlear nuclei, as well as through the production of hemorrhages into the inner ear (Fisch, 1955; Hall, 1964). There is some evidence that the auditory system is selectively vulnerable to brief episodes of asphyxia at birth (Hall, 1964). Early injury to brain stem auditory pathways can interfere with the development of normal auditory processing and can cause impaired language development. Kernicterus may also cause damage to the cochlear nuclei or other central auditory pathways (Kuriyama et al., 1986; Haymaker et al., 1961). Although there is no definite evidence, it is logical to assume that events such as intrauterine hemorrhage, placenta previa, prolonged labor, instrument delivery, and possibly cesarean section may cause damage to the middle ear, inner ear, or central auditory pathways of the newborn. In addition to these factors, it has been observed that a relatively high number of premature infants develop hearing impairment.

Family History

Approximately half of all congenital deafness discovered during childhood is caused by genetic factors (Nance and Sweeney, 1975). Of the inherited types of deafness, 75 to 88 per cent are recessively inherited, and about 10 per cent are dominantly inherited (Chung and colleagues, 1959). Inherited sensorineural hearing loss can be present and manifest at birth, it may be discovered later in childhood, or it may not be discovered until adult life. The hearing loss that is inherited in a dominant manner tends to worsen progressively, whereas the recessively inherited hearing loss usually remains stable. There are more than 50 types of hereditary hearing impairment that are characterized according to the type of hearing loss, age at onset, severity, genetic mode of transmission, and associated clinical findings (Rose et al., 1976). Despite the mul-

tiplicity of named syndromes, the great majority of cases of sensorineural hearing loss due to single-gene mendelian inheritance, whether dominant or recessive, are clinically undifferentiated (Fraser, 1976). That is, the hearing impairment does not constitute part of a recognizable syndrome in which it is associated with visible malformations or in which other organs and body systems are involved.

The family history provides information concerning the mode of inheritance. When two or more siblings are affected and the parents and other relatives are not, recessive inheritance is probable, although when the children with hearing loss are exclusively males, it may be difficult to differentiate the X-linked from the autosomal variety. When the parents are consanguineous, it can be presumed that inheritance is autosomal recessive, and this is true whether there is only one or several affected children. When one or more siblings are affected and, in addition, relatives such as parents, uncles, aunts, grandparents, or cousins are deaf, identification of a specific mode of inheritance may be extremely difficult. However, the presence of unilateral or mild bilateral sensorineural hearing loss in relatives is suggestive of dominant inheritance.

Even though one is persistent in acquiring information about family members who developed hearing impairment early in life, it may be difficult to construct a meaningful pedigree. Hearing impairment can be defined in social as well as biologic terms, and persons who are mildly or unilaterally affected may not consider themselves hearing impaired, or they may even be totally unaware of the hearing impairment. As audiometric test methods improve and as mandatory screening tests become more prevalent, children will be discovered who are labeled as having significant sensorineural hearing impairment, although the same degree of hearing impairment in their parents or in previous generations may have remained undetected throughout life. In fact, it is not uncommon for such mild hearing loss in parents and other relatives to be identified for the first time during the family investigation initiated because of the failure of a child to pass a school screening test (Fraser, 1976).

No examples are known of conductive autosomal recessive deafness that is not part of a syndrome. Therefore, familial conductive hearing loss that is not part of an obvious syndrome is likely to be inherited in an autosomal dominant or, more rarely, X-linked recessive manner. The most common type of dominant, clinically undifferentiated conductive hearing loss is otosclerosis, but this usually does not affect young children.

Physical Examination

Significant abnormalities detected during a physical examination may indicate that an observed hearing loss is part of a syndrome. In Table 14–1, physical abnormalities are listed with their corresponding syndromes or diseases and the type of associated hearing

TABLE 14–1. Physical Abnormalities and Their Associated Syndromes Related to Hearing Loss

PHYSICAL EXAMINATION	PHYSICAL ABNORMALITY	DISEASE OR SYNDROME	TYPE OF HEARING LOSS
Skull	Macrocephaly	Osteopetrosis (Albers-Schönberg disease)	PSN or PC
		Osteogenesis imperfecta	PSN or PC
	Abnormal shape	Apert syndrome	CC
		Crouzon disease	CC and/or CSN
		Craniostenosis	CC
		Craniometaphysial dysplasia (Pyle disease)	CSN and/or CC
		Cranial clefts	CC
		Osteitis deformans (Paget disease)	PSN or PC
	Failure of fontanelle to close	Cleidocranial dysostosis	CSN
Hair	White forelock	Waardenburg syndrome	CSN
	Low posterior hairline	Turner, and Klippel-Feil syndrome	CC
	Twisted hair	Recessive pili torti	CSN
Face	Hemifacial atrophy	First branchial arch syndrome	CC
		Goldenhar syndrome	CC
	Facial clefts		CC
	Leonine facies	Generalized cortical hyperostosis (Van Buchem syndrome)	PSN
		Osteopetrosis	PSN or PC
	Dysplasia of supraorbital ridges	Frontometaphysial dysplasia (Gorlin-Hart syndrome)	CSN and CC
	Prominence of frontal bone and coarse facial features	Hurler syndrome	CC
	Frontal bossing	Otopalatodigital syndrome	CC
	Narrow face in region of orbits and flattening of midface	Otofacial cervical syndrome	CC
	Flattened cheeks and coloboma of eyelids	Treacher Collins syndrome	CC
	Facial paralysis	Möbius syndrome	CC
Eyes	Strabismus	Möbius syndrome	CC and/or CSN
		Duane syndrome	CC
	Hypertelorism		CC
	Eyelid abnormalities		
	Coloboma of eyelids, slant, epicanthal fold, ptosis		CC and CSN
	Lateral displacement of medial canthi	Waardenburg syndrome	CSN
	Adherent	Cryptophthalmus	CC
	Microphthalmus		CSN
	Coloboma	CHARGE Association	CSN
	Cornea		
	Dystrophy	Fehrs dystrophy	PSN
	Clouding or keratoconus		CC and CSN
	Sclera		
	Epibulbar dermoids	Oculoauriculovertebral dysplasia (Goldenhar syndrome)	CC
	Blue	Osteogenesis imperfecta	PSN or PC
	Iris		
	Heterochromia	Waardenburg syndrome	CSN
	Lens		
	Cataracts	Congenital rubella	CSN
		Flynn-Aird syndrome	PSN
	Fundus abnormalities	Usher syndrome	CSN, PSN
	Blindness	Norrie disease	PSN
		Primary testicular insufficiency	PSN
Ears	Pinna malformations		CC
	Atresia		CC and CSN
	Preauricular sinuses (dominant)		CSN
Nose	Saddle	Congenital lues	CSN
		Marshall syndrome	CSN
	Bifid	Medial facial cleft	CC
	Cleft lip, nose		CC

TABLE 14–1. Physical Abnormalities and Their Associated Syndromes Related to Hearing Loss *Continued*

PHYSICAL EXAMINATION	PHYSICAL ABNORMALITY	DISEASE OR SYNDROME	TYPE OF HEARING LOSS
Mouth	Midline cleft lip	Orofaciodigital syndrome (Mohr II)	CC
	Microstomia	Otopalatodigital syndrome	CC
		Trisomy 18 syndrome	CSN, CC
Teeth	Pegged incisors	Congenital lues	CSN and PSN
	Abnormal dentine	Osteogenesis imperfecta	PSN and/or PC
	Coniform teeth and dominant onychodystrophy		CSN
	Abnormal dental crown morphology		CSN
Palate	Cleft palate	Otopalatodigital syndrome	CC
		Pierre Robin syndrome	CC and/or CSN
		Other syndromes	CC
	Bifid uvula		CC
Neck	Goiter (recessive)	Pendred syndrome	CSN
	Goiter (recessive) and stippled epiphyses		CSN
	Short (torticollis)	Klippel-Feil syndrome	CSN and/or CC
		Wildervanck syndrome	CSN and/or CC
	Absent clavicles	Cleidocranial dysostosis	CC
	Narrowing of shoulders	Otofaciocervical syndrome	CC
	Webbing	Turner syndrome	CSN and/or CC
Chest	Pigeon breast	Goiter and stippled epiphyses	CSN
		Trisomy 18	CSN and/or CC
		Marfan syndrome	CSN and/or CC
Lungs	(None)		
Heart	Murmur	Ventricular septal defect with congenital rubella	CSN
	Murmur of congenital pulmonary stenosis	Lewis syndrome	CSN
	Murmur of mitral insufficiency	Forney syndrome	CC
Abdomen	Hepatomegaly	Wilson disease	CSN
Extremities			
Hands	Knuckle pads and leukonychia		CSN and/or CC
	Small fissured nails	Dominant onychodystrophy and coniform teeth	CSN
	Small fissured nails	Recessive onychodystrophy and strabismus	CSN
Hands and feet	Congenital flexion contractions of fingers and toes	"Hand-hearing" syndrome	CSN
	Clubfoot	Diastrophic dwarfism	CSN
	Split hand-foot	Wildervanck syndrome	CSN
	Flexion contracture of fingers	Hurler syndrome	CC
	Absent joint of fingers	Symphalangism and strabismus syndrome	CC
	Exaggerated space between thumb and index fingers	Otopalatodigital syndrome	CC
	Lobster claw hands and feet	Cockayne syndrome	CC
	Stiff joints	Arthrogryposis	CC
Legs	Short lower legs	Absence of tibia	CSN
	Bowing of legs	Osteogenesis imperfecta	CSN and/or CC
Arms	Limited elbow motion	Frontometaphysial dysplasia	CSN
	Limited radial abduction of arm and hand	Madelung deformity	CC
Spine	Scoliosis		CC
Dwarf	Achondroplasia		CC and/or CSN
Skin	Albinism-dominant		CSN
	Small hyperpigmented lesion, especially head and neck	Dominant lentigines	CSN
	Hypopigmentation spots, especially head and arms	Hereditary piebaldness	CSN
	Keratitis, ichthyosis	KID syndrome	CSN
	Leopardlike spots of hypo- and hyperpigmentation	Sex-linked pigmentary abnormalities	CSN
	Ichthyosis of arms but not legs	Recessive atypical atopic dermatitis	CSN

Table continued on following page

TABLE 14–1. Physical Abnormalities and Their Associated Syndromes Related to Hearing Loss *Continued*

PHYSICAL EXAMINATION	PHYSICAL ABNORMALITY	DISEASE OR SYNDROME	TYPE OF HEARING LOSS
Skin (*Continued*)	Inability to sweat	Dominant anhidrosis (ectodermal dysplasia)	CSN
	Xeroderma pigmentosum (with neurologic disease)	DeSanctis-Cacchione syndrome	CSN
	Urticaria, nephritis, and amyloidosis	Muckle-Wells syndrome	PSN
	Ota nevus		
	Neurofibromatosis	von Recklinghausen disease	PSN and CC
Neurologic			
Epilepsy	Photosensitive epilepsy	Hyperprolinemia Type I (major part)	
		Herrmann syndrome	PSN
	Progressive familial myoclonic epilepsy and progressive cerebral degeneration (minor part)	Unverricht disease	PSN
Mental status			
Retardation from birth	And ataxia and hypogonadism	Richards-Rundle syndrome	CSN
	And coarse facies and spine and digit bone changes	Hurler syndrome	
	And muscular wasting and recessive retinal detachment	Small syndrome	CSN
	And hyperprolinemia Type I (minor part)	Shäfer syndrome	
	And hereditary nephritis, epilepsy, diabetes	Herrmann syndrome	PSN
	And retinitis pigmentosa and obesity and polydactyly	Laurence-Moon-Biedl syndrome	CSN
	And retinal malformation	Norrie disease	PSN
	And homocystinuria (one case)		
Mental deterioration	And retinitis pigmentosa and dwarfism	Cockayne syndrome	PSN
	And myopia	Flynn-Aird syndrome	CSN
	And encephalopathy, subcortical	Schilder disease	
Motor abnormalities	Cerebral palsy		CSN
	Spasticity and optic atrophy	Opticocochleodentate degeneration	CSN
	Ataxia	Spinocerebellar degeneration (Friedreich ataxia)	PSN
		Richards-Rundle syndrome	CSN
		Herrmann syndrome	PSN
		Vestibulocerebellar and retinitis pigmentosa (Hallgren syndrome)	CSN
		Hyperuricemia and renal insufficiency (dominant in Rosenberg progressive ataxia)	PSN
	Childhood Huntington chorea (rare part)		CSN and PSN
Sensory neuropathy	Dominant sensory radicular neuropathy		PSN
Motor neuropathy	Polyneuropathy, ichthyosis, and retinitis pigmentosa	Refsum syndrome	PSN
	Peripheral neuropathy and skeletal anomalies and dominant myopia	Flynn-Aird syndrome	CSN
	Familial polyneuropathy (resembling Charcot-Marie-Tooth disease) with nerve deafness seen with optic atrophy, or nephritis, or neurofibromatosis, or achalasia		
	And mental deficiency and ataxia	Richards-Rundle syndrome	CSN
Myopathy	And growth failure and chronic lactic acidemia		
	Muscle wasting and retinal detachment and mental retardation	Small syndrome	CSN
	Facioscapulohumeral dystrophy associated with nerve deafness		

TABLE 14–1. Physical Abnormalities and Their Associated Syndromes Related to Hearing Loss *Continued*

PHYSICAL EXAMINATION	PHYSICAL ABNORMALITY	DISEASE OR SYNDROME	TYPE OF HEARING LOSS
Endocrine	Goiter	Pendred syndrome	CSn
	Hypogonadism and blindness		CSN
	Obesity and diabetes, retinal degneration	Alström syndrome	CSN
	Obesity and polydactyly and retinitis pigmentosa	Laurence-Moon-Biedl syndrome	CSN
Multiple Physical Changes		Trisomy 13–15 (Patau syndrome, trisomy D₁)	CSN and CC
No Physical Findings		Trisomy 18 (trisomy E)	CSN and CC

CC, Congenital conductive; PC, progressive conductive; CSN, congenital sensorineural; PSN, progressive sensorineural.
Modified and reprinted with permission from Jaffe, B. F. (ed.) 1977. Hearing Loss In Children: A Comprehensive Text. Baltimore, University Park Press.

loss. In examining the ears, the external canals should first be cleansed of debris, then inspected. It is best to use a pneumatic otoscope to test eardrum mobility and to gain information about the presence or absence of fluid in the middle ear (Pransky and Grundfast, 1987). In addition, the examiner should be aware that there are anatomic differences between the eardrum of a neonate and that of an older child (Chap. 8).

Laboratory Studies

Although several investigators (Bergstrom, 1974; Jaffe, 1977) have analyzed the problem of defining an appropriate test battery, there is really no specific set of tests that has proved to be of exceptional diagnostic value in the evaluation of all children with hearing losses. Most often, a laboratory test will tend to confirm or negate a tentative diagnosis. It is better to order whatever specific studies seem to be appropriate than to attempt to discover an underlying etiology with a battery of tests. The following laboratory studies may be helpful.

TORCHS STUDIES. TORCHS is an acronym used to describe the group of specific IgM antibody assays for toxoplasmosis, others, rubella, cytomegalovirus, herpes simplex, hepatitis B, and syphilis. Usually, an immunoassay for syphilis is done along with the TORCHS study. Results are reported as titer values, and it is important to know the normal titers for the laboratory where the serum was analyzed. The TORCHS studies can help determine whether or not an intrauterine infection may have caused a hearing impairment in a neonate.

In infants with congenital rubella, hemagglutination inhibition (HAI) and complement fixation (CF) titers remain elevated during the first few years of life, because these include fetally produced antibodies (IgM). In unaffected infants, serial rubella titers show a decline and disappearance at about 6 months of age, as the majority of the antibody is maternally produced IgG. In congenital rubella, the virus may be cultured from the infant as old as 3 years of age in spite of the presence of rubella antibodies (Michaels, 1969).

In evaluating a congenitally deaf child for intrauter-

ine infection, serial antibody studies are necessary. If a hearing loss is diagnosed or suspected shortly after birth, blood should be obtained for serum gamma-globulin determinations and for specific hemagglutination inhibition and complement fixation antibody titers to suspected agents. If the IgM levels are elevated, specific fluorescent antibody tests should be done if available. Although an elevated IgM level is highly suggestive of intrauterine infection, a normal level does not exclude it. Cultures for rubella and cytomegalovirus may also be obtained from the urine, nasopharynx, and throat. At 10 to 12 months of age, these titer determinations should be repeated. Persistent elevation is highly suggestive of an intrauterine infection.

It is possible that the rubella vaccine may aid in the late diagnosis of congenital rubella as a cause of hearing loss. It has been reported that about 19 per cent of children with known congenital rubella have no demonstrable antibody titer by 5 years of age (Florman et al., 1970). When these children are given the rubella vaccine, only 10 per cent reconvert to seropositive. Although more work needs to be done in this area, the failure of a deaf child to develop antibodies after receiving the rubella vaccine may suggest rubella as the etiology of the hearing loss (Bergstrom and Stewart, 1971).

VDRL (VENEREAL DISEASE RESEARCH LABORATORY) AND FTA-ABS (FLUORESCENT TREPONEMAL ANTIBODY ABSORPTION) TESTS. Although the VDRL test provides a good method for screening a population for syphilis, the VDRL test result may not be positive in individuals who have congenital syphilis. Therefore, the FTA-ABS test is necessary when congenital syphilis is the suspected cause of deafness or hearing impairment occurring in early childhood. Because many laboratories will not proceed to the FTA-ABS test until a VDRL test has been done, when attempting to rule out congenital syphilis as the cause of an infant's or a neonate's hearing impairment, one should note clearly that the FTA-ABS test, not the VDRL, is *required*.

URINALYSIS. Protein found in the urine may indicate that hearing impairment is part of a syndrome such as Alport syndrome (hereditary nephritis and progressive sensorineural hearing loss) or Muckle-Wells syndrome (nephritis with recurrent urticaria and deafness). Because hearing loss can occur in children with mucopolysaccharide abnormalities, a urine screen for inborn errors in metabolism can be helpful if a metabolic or mucopolysaccharide abnormality is suspected.

THYROID FUNCTION TESTS. An abnormal thyroxine (T_4) uptake may help confirm the suspicion that hearing loss is part of Pendred syndrome (congenital defective binding of iodine by the thyroid gland associated with sensorineural hearing loss).

ELECTROCARDIOGRAM (ECG). A prolonged QT interval, when associated with syncopal episodes and congenital sensorineural hearing loss, is indicative of Jervell and Lange-Nielsen syndrome. ECG abnormalities, such as increased PQ interval, nodal and auricular extrasystoles, and alteration in the QRS complex, are seen in about a third of children with Refsum syndrome (retinitis pigmentosa, hypertrophic peripheral neuropathy, and sensorineural hearing loss) (Richterich et al., 1965). In some cases of Friedreich ataxia (ataxia, speech impairment, lateral curvature of the spinal column, peculiar swaying and irregular mannerisms, and paralysis of muscles, especially of the lower extremities), both sensorineural hearing loss and cardiomyopathy may be present.

VESTIBULAR FUNCTION TESTS. In evaluating the child with sensorineural hearing loss, the testing of vestibular function can be problematic. Depending on the age of the child, obtaining sufficient cooperation to complete test procedures can be difficult, and the acquisition of data that can be meaningfully interpreted sometimes is nearly impossible. However, when vestibular function is accurately assessed, analysis of the data can confirm that the labyrinth as well as the cochlea is affected by an underlying disorder. Tests of vestibular function appropriate for children include caloric tests, torsion swing, simple and computerized rotating chair studies, and electroposturography. Abnormal caloric responses have been found in children with cretinism (Costa et al., 1964), Hallgren syndrome, Klippel-Feil malformation (Proctor and Proctor, 1967), onychodystrophy (Feinmesser and Zelig, 1961), Pendred syndrome (Black et al., 1971), unilateral congenital deafness (Black et al., 1971), Waardenburg syndrome (Matalon et al., 1970), and the cervicooculoacusticus syndrome of Wildervanck (Black et al., 1971), and in 26 of 33 ears of children with various disorders reported by Valvassori and associates (1969). Electronystagmography (ENG) can be done in children as young as 6 years of age. Electronystagmographic abnormalities reportedly have been detected along with congenital deafness in three patients with familial hyperuricemia and ataxia (Rosenberg et al., 1970). In addition, electronystagmographic abnormalities have been reported in one patient with rubella and central nervous system involvement (Bergstrom and Stewart, 1971). Absent vestibular function was found in two rubella patients in whom electronystagmograms were obtained (Alford, 1968). This suggests pathologic change more extensive than the classic cochleosaccular degeneration traditionally reported in rubella.

Results of vestibular tests can help distinguish dominant from recessive congenital severe deafness. It is advisable to test vestibular function in children with sensorineural hearing impairment who are having difficulty in walking or maintaining their equilibrium. Although it has never been proved, it has been suspected that young children with middle-ear effusions may, at times, develop difficulties with equilibrium and postural control. When parents of a child with hearing impairment remark that the child seems excessively clumsy, awkward, or intermittently unable to maintain an upright posture, some assessment of vestibular function is warranted (Chap. 11).

OTHER TESTS. Additional tests, such as chromosomal analysis, dermatoglyphics, electroretinography, amino acid screen, blood urea nitrogen determination, platelet count, serum pyrophosphate determination, and uric acid assay, may be of diagnostic value in certain instances, especially in confirming the tentative diagnosis of a syndromal type of hearing impairment.

Radiographic Studies

In most cases of childhood hearing impairment, radiographic studies do not provide information that is essential for decision making. Further, normal findings on radiographic studies do not exclude the possibility that congenital middle-ear or inner-ear malformations exist because minor abnormalities may not be radiographically demonstrable even with modern polytomographic techniques. Several types of radiographic studies can be used for evaluating otologic disorders. The mastoid series can be of value in determining whether or not cholesteatoma is present and in assessing the extent of bone erosion involving the lateral wall of the epitympanum (scutum) or the ossicles. Transorbital views of the internal auditory canals enable a screening type of comparative measurement of size of the right and left internal auditory canals. Because eighth nerve tumors can cause bone erosion, a difference in width between the internal auditory canals can be indicative of a vestibular schwannoma (acoustic neuroma). Computed tomography (CT) scanning demonstrates the minute anatomic structures of the temporal bone. The ossicles, semicircular canals, facial nerve canal, oval and round windows, and internal auditory canals can be visualized.

In cases of sensorineural hearing impairment, a CT scan can aid in assessing relative development of the cochlea so that malformations involving the optic capsule can be categorized. In cases of conductive hearing impairment, especially those with external canal atresia, temporal bone CT can be extremely helpful in determining the status of the ossicular chain and in assessing the suitability of a given ear for reconstructive surgery. In addition, CT scanning is helpful in locating the position of the facial nerve in the child who will be operated on for reconstruction of the middle ear. When the diagnosis of vestibular schwannoma is being considered, CT of the temporal bone provides the best noninvasive method for detecting characteristic widening of an internal auditory canal. If a perilymph fistula is considered the probable cause of a sensorineural hearing loss, radiographic studies may demonstrate abnormalities within the otic capsule or a widely patent cochlear aqueduct (Wtodyka, 1978; Dorph et al., 1973), both of which are known sometimes to be associated with perilymph fistulae (Grundfast and Bluestone, 1978) (Chap. 10).

AGE–SPECIFIC TASKS

Utilizing the age-specific, task-oriented approach to the evaluation of hearing loss, the seemingly awesome challenge of evaluating a neonate who is suspected of having impaired hearing is considered first (Chap. 9).

Neonate

Confirm

For those who believe that early detection and intervention are key factors in enabling a child to cope successfully with a hearing handicap, the ultimate goal is detection of significant hearing impairment at birth. Accordingly, it is logical to attempt to test the hearing ability of neonates soon after birth and before discharge from the hospital in which the neonate was born. In a sense, while neonates are still in the hospital, they are part of a captive population, whereas when they are discharged to their respective homes, it becomes more difficult to identify and test those children suspected of having hearing impairment. Thus, much attention has been focused on in-hospital hearing screening programs for neonates.

Although there is general agreement that such screening is worthwhile, several methods are available for identifying neonates who have impaired hearing. Some experts have thought that all newborn infants should undergo a screening procedure that is designed to identify hearing loss. Indeed, several such procedures were developed, including tests that monitor the neonate's reflexive body movements, blink, or altered respiratory or heart rate in response to a sound stimulus of specific intensity. Although such all-encompassing screening procedures were in vogue for a while, results of large-scale programs appeared to indicate that testing all neonates was not an efficient, cost-effective way of identifying newborn children with hearing impairments. Rather, in an attempt to identify those newborns who are most likely to have impaired hearing, it is now becoming common to define and utilize a so-called high risk register. This registry is composed of neonates who manifest any or all of a list of characteristics that are likely to be associated with hearing impairment in neonates.

When infants in the high-risk category are identified, they are tested by some screening method. Evidence that there is now a trend toward more selective screening procedures lies in the recommendation of the Joint Committee on Infant Hearing. This Committee was established in 1969 by the American Speech and Hearing Association, the American Academy of Ophthalmology and Otolaryngology, and the American Academy of Pediatrics. In 1974, the Committee stated that there was not yet available any satisfactory mechanized technique to screen the hearing of all newborn infants reliably (Northern and Downs, 1978; ASHA report, 1974). Further, the Committee recommended that infants at risk for hearing impairment be identified by history and physical examination.

In 1982, the Joint Committee on Infant Hearing elucidated on and further expanded recommendations regarding detection of hearing impairment in neonates and infants. The Joint Committee position statement (1982) follows:

I. IDENTIFICATION
  A. Risk criteria
  Factors that identify those infants who are at risk for having hearing impairment include the following:
  1. Family history of childhood hearing impairment
  2. Congenital perinatal infection (e.g., cytomegalovirus, rubella, herpes, toxoplasmosis, syphilis)
  3. Anatomic malformations involving the head or neck (e.g., dysmorphic appearance including syndromal and nonsyndromal abnormalities, overt or submucous cleft palate, morphologic abnormalities of the pinna)
  4. Birth weight <1500 gm
  5. Hyperbilirubinemia at level exceeding indications for exchange transfusion
  6. Bacterial meningitis, especially *Haemophilus influenzae*
  7. Severe asphyxia, which may include infants with Apgar scores of 0 to 3 or who fail to institute spontaneous repiration by ten minutes and those with hypotonia persisting to 2 hours of age
  B. Screening procedure
  The hearing of infants who manifest any item on the list of risk criteria should be screened, preferably under the supervision of an audiologist, optimally by 3 months of age but not later than 6 months of age. The initial screening should include the observation of behavioral or electrophysiologic response to sound. (The Committee has no recommendations at this time regarding any specific device.) If consistent electrophysiologic or behavioral responses are detected at appropriate sound levels, then the screening process will be considered complete except in those cases in which there is a probability of a progressive hearing loss; e.g., family history of delayed onset or degenerative disease, or history of intrauterine infection. If results of an initial screening of an infant manifesting any risk criteria are equivocal, then the infant should be referred for diagnostic testing.
II. DIAGNOSIS FOR INFANTS FAILING SCREENING
  A. Diagnostic evaluation of an infant 6 months of age should include:
  1. General physical examination and history including:
      a. Examination of the head and neck
      b. Otoscopy and otomicroscopy

      c. Identification of relevant physical abnormalities
      d. Laboratory tests such as urinalysis and diagnostic tests for perinatal infections
    2. Comprehensive audiologic evaluation:
      a. Behavioral history
      b. Behavioral observation audiometry
      c. Testing of auditory evoked potentials, if indicated
  B. After the age of 6 months, the following are also recommended:
    1. Communication skills evaluation
    2. Acoustic immittance (impedance) measurements
    3. Selected tests of development

III. MANAGEMENT OF HEARING-IMPAIRED INFANT

Habilitation of the hearing-impaired infant may begin while the diagnostic evaluation is in process. The Committee recommends, however, that whenever possible, the diagnostic process should be completed and habilitation begun by the age of 6 months. Services to the hearing-impaired infant younger than 6 months of age include:

  A. Medical management
    1. Reevaluation
    2. Treatment
    3. Genetic evaluation and counseling when indicated
  B. Audiologic management
    1. Ongoing audiologic assessment
    2. Selection of hearing aid(s)
    3. Family counseling
  C. Psychoeducational management
    1. Formulation of individualized educational plan
    2. Information about implications of hearing impairment

After the age of 6 months, the hearing-impaired infant becomes easier to manage in a habilitation plan but he or she will require the services listed above.*

A clever mnemonic that can be used to help remember some of the perinatal risk factors has been described (Downs and Silver, 1972). It is called the ABCD'S of congenital deafness: A, affected family member; B, bilirubin (greater than 15 mg per 100 ml); C, congenital rubella or other intrauterine infection; D, defects of ear, nose, and throat; S, small at birth (weight less than 1500 gm).

Although neonates can be screened for hearing impairment with mechanized crib devices, the auditory brain stem evoked response (ABR) test is becoming a useful and reliable method for identifying neonates with hearing impairment (Sanders et al., 1985; Levi et al., 1983; Bradford et al., 1985). With the use of ABR tone pips and clicks, even the frequencies involved can be approximated when testing young infants (Hyde, 1985).

Even though the use of established risk criteria helps select the infants at highest risk for having hearing impairment, using the risk factors for selection of infants to be tested is not a foolproof method. A review by Stein and colleagues (1983) has shown that

one quarter of infants ultimately diagnosed with some type of hearing impairment did not manifest any of the risk criteria delineated in the 1982 Joint Committee position statement.

When it has been determined that a newborn child is at risk of having impaired hearing or when a parent or referring physician has the impression that a child has a hearing impairment, further evaluation is warranted.

The first step is to *confirm* the impression that there is impairment of hearing and to assess the degree of hearing loss. Not long ago, it was nearly impossible to test a neonate's hearing reliably. However, nonbehavioral (objective) tests such as the stapedial reflex test, electrocochleography, and the auditory brain stem evoked response test are available (Chap. 9). Although these may not actually be tests of hearing per se, they are helpful indicators of significant functional impairment in the neural pathways serving the auditory system. As for quantifying hearing loss, it is virtually impossible to measure precise hearing thresholds in the neonate. Despite this, nonbehavioral tests can be used to estimate a relative magnitude of hearing impairment. That is, test results can be interpreted as being nearly normal, indicative of significant hearing impairment, or indicative of moderate to severe hearing impairment. Although such information may not be precise, it can be helpful in identifying newborn children who will need close follow-up, further evaluation, and possibly early hearing amplification.

Characterize

Unless there is obvious ear canal atresia or other aural deformity, it is extremely difficult to differentiate conductive and sensorineural hearing impairment in the neonate. Observations made on ABR test patterns can be helpful (Chap. 9). Delayed appearance of the first wave with normal interwave latencies may be indicative of a conductive type of hearing loss. Elevated thresholds without a delay in the appearance of the first wave and with normal interwave latencies indicate that sensorineural impairment is probable. When interwave latencies are abnormal, some central nervous system abnormality may be responsible for the hearing impairment. Again, these are helpful diagnostic indicators, but they are not as precise or reliable as a battery of sophisticated behavioral tests. However, in dealing with neonates, it is of primary importance to know whether a significant hearing impairment is present; characterization of the type of hearing loss is of secondary importance. After it has been established that a neonate has poor hearing, further testing and evaluation during the first 2 years of life will usually elicit the information that is needed to proceed with proper diagnosis and management.

Cause

Hearing impairment that is discovered during the neonatal period is most probably the result of some

---

*Reproduced by permission of Pediatrics, Vol. 70, page 496, copyright 1982.

untoward circumstance that occurred during fetal development or at birth. Hereditary factors need to be considered, and a detailed family history should be obtained. A thorough physical examination should reveal abnormalities characteristic of one of the previously described syndromes with which hearing loss is associated (see Table 14–1). TORCHS studies and the VDRL or FTA-ABS tests are helpful in determining whether intrauterine infection may have been a causal factor. A urine sample tested for protein and inborn errors in metabolism may be helpful in diagnosing syndromes that include nephritis or abnormalities of mucopolysaccharide metabolism. If thyroid enlargement is apparent, Pendred syndrome should be considered, and a T_4 uptake test is indicated. If there is a family history of Usher syndrome or if the neonate appears to have eye abnormalities, electroretinography may be of diagnostic value. An electrocardiogram is probably not often helpful, although the Jervell and Lange-Nielsen syndrome can be diagnosed early in life when profound congenital deafness is found in association with a prolonged QT interval. Routine mastoid films and temporal bone CT scan are probably not warranted in the evaluation of neonates with hearing impairment because radiographic findings will be of little value in formulating plans for management of the neonate with impaired hearing.

After information has been gathered and analyzed, it may be possible to discover the cause of a neonate's hearing impairment. Of course, to recognize syndromal types of hearing impairment, one must have some familiarity with the syndromes that include hearing loss. Syndromes that can include hearing impairment are listed in Tables 14–2, 14–3, and 14–4.

Even though it is possible to conceive of numerous factors that may cause hearing impairment in the neonate, it may be difficult to detect specific etiology in individual cases unless the neonate has a clear family pedigree of inherited hearing loss or unless there are obvious abnormalities characteristic of a nonmendelian malformation syndrome known to include morphologic or functional aberrations in the auditory system. Further, making a differentiation between truly congenital hearing loss (i.e., that which is present at birth) and acquired hearing loss is extremely difficult during the neonatal period. Fraser (1976) has succinctly summarized the problem of determining the cause of neonatal hearing loss as follows.

> It is clear that the relationship between perinatal problems and subsequent deafness is an exceedingly complicated one and, while in some cases a specific circumstance, such as hemorrhage into the inner ears as a result of birth injury, the administration of ototoxic drugs, or kernicterus due to Rhesus incompatibility, may be identified as the proximate cause of hearing loss, in many others multiple factors must be taken into consideration; these may arise as a result of interaction between both genetic and environmental variables.

Thus, it can be seen that finding the cause of hearing

loss detected in a neonate may be a complex and difficult problem. Nonetheless, an attempt should be made to find the factors that are most likely to have caused an observed hearing impairment.

Care

Once it has been established that a neonate has impaired hearing, management must be planned. Otologic surgery is not warranted during the neonatal period, and usually the infant must be more than 2 months old before he or she can be considered for fitting of a hearing aid. Early steps will have to be taken to assist the child with a congenital hearing loss to learn speech and language. It is most important to help the parents understand and adjust to the problem of having a hearing-impaired child. In addition, if the family is indigent or inadequately covered by medical insurance, it will be necessary to involve appropriate agencies so that the family can continue to provide the medical care and special education that the child may require.

Infant

Confirm

After a child is beyond the neonatal period, concerns about hearing ability usually come from a parent or an observant primary care physician. The parent or another family member initially tends to become concerned when the infant appears not to respond in an appropriate way to sounds in the environment. A parent will remark that the infant is not startled by loud noises or that the infant does not awaken or appear disturbed when a sibling in the same room is crying loudly. Parents may be concerned that the child of about 2 years is not speaking words while they remember that an older sibling was saying three-word phrases by the age of 18 months. If an infant has had meningitis or a severe infection that required the administration of potentially ototoxic medications, the astute pediatrician or family physician may want to have the infant's hearing evaluated.

Even though an infant is brought for evaluation by parents who seem overly impatient about speech development, it is not advisable simply to perform rudimentary tests of hearing in the office, then attempt to reassure the parents that their child's hearing is normal. In the present era of advanced medical technology, observing an infant's response to the loud clapping of hands cannot be considered the definitive test for determining the presence or absence of hearing impairment. When a pediatrician, family physician, or anyone who knows an infant well becomes concerned about an infant's hearing ability, a full evaluation, including audiometric testing, is warranted.

The infant from 2 through 24 months of age progressively becomes easier to condition for play audi-

TABLE 14–2. Skeletal and Cranial Defects Associated with Hearing Impairment

SYNDROME	CHARACTERISTICS	MODE OF INHERITANCE	TYPE OF HEARING LOSS SN	Conductive	Mixed
Osteogenesis imperfecta	Brittle bones Blue sclerae	Recessive	X	X	X
Hurler syndrome	Mental retardation, cloudy corneas, blindness, thick eyebrows, onset of skeletal deformities after first year of life	Recessive (X-linked form is known as Hunter syndrome)	X	X	
Morquio disease	Dwarfism, normal-sized head, long extremities, short trunk	Recessive			
Otopalatodigital syndrome	Frontal bossing, prominent occiput, ocular hypertelorism, antimongoloid slant of eyes, fish mouth, pseudowinged knobby scapulae, broad distal phalanges of hands and feet, cleft palate	Recessive		X	
Albers-Schönberg syndrome	Brittle bones, intermittent facial palsy, optic atrophy, hydrocephalus, ocular nystagmus, exophthalmos	Recessive	X	X	X
Klippel-Feil syndrome	Fused cervical vertebrae, low posterior hairline; spina bifida and external canal atresia may be present	Recessive	X	X	X
Cervicooculoacusticus syndrome	Fused neck vertebrae, spina bifida occulta, abducens palsy of eye, possible radiographic evidence of underdevelopment of the cochlea or labyrinth	Recessive	X		
Crouzon disease	Synostosis of cranial sutures, shallow orbits with secondary proptosis (frog eyes), hypoplasia of maxilla with relative prognathism, parrot nose, possible atresia of external auditory canal	Dominant	X	X (Usually conductive)	X
Cleidocranial dysostosis	Fontanelles fail to close, facial bones underdeveloped, high arched palate, absence of clavicles	Dominant	X		
Treacher Collins syndrome	Malformations of malar and other facial bones, antimongoloid slant of eyes with notching of lids (colobomas), high palate, external auditory canal and pinna malformations, middle-ear ossicular abnormalities	Dominant	X	X	
Pierre Robin syndrome	Cleft palate, small mandible, glossoptosis; may have atresia of ear canal, microtia of auricles, middle-ear anomalies, or digital abnormalities	Dominant	X	X	
Apert syndrome	Acrocephaly (tower skull), fused digits (lobster claw hands), shallow orbits, underdeveloped maxillas, fixation of stapes footplate	Dominant		X	
Achondroplasia	Dwarfism with normal-sized trunk, large head and shortened extremities, saddle nose, and frontal mandibular bone protrusions	Dominant	X	X*	X
Marfan syndrome	Long, spidery fingers, scoliosis, hammer toe, pigeon breast, dolichocephaly, low hairline, tall, thin body structure	Dominant	X	X	X

TABLE 14–2. Skeletal and Cranial Defects Associated with Hearing Impairment *Continued*

SYNDROME	CHARACTERISTICS	MODE OF INHERITANCE	TYPE OF HEARING LOSS SN	Conductive	Mixed
Branchial anomalies (Karmody-Feingold)	Cervical fistulas, malformed external ears, preauricular pits, preauricular appendages	Dominant	X	X	X
Myositis ossificans	Formation of true osseous tissue in skeletal muscles, microdactyly of great toes, shortened thumbs	Dominant	X	X	X
Symphalangism	Fusion of proximal and middle phalanges of fingers and toes giving characteristic "stiff finger and toe" appearance, prominence on medial and lateral sides of foot at level of navicular and fifth metatarsal bones	Dominant		X	

*Due to middle ear effusions.

Modified from Black, F. O., Bergstrom, L., Downs, M., et al. 1971. Congenital Deafness: A New Approach to Diagnosis Using a High Risk Register. Boulder, CO, Colorado Associated University Press.

ometry. Whereas audiometric testing in the neonate necessarily relies on nonbehavioral test methods, it becomes increasingly feasible to utilize behavioral techniques as the child grows and develops during infancy. About the age of 1 year, an infant develops the ability to localize sound, and this enables the use of visual reinforcement audiometry. Beyond the age of 1 year, development of the bony tympanic ring makes the ear canal less pliable and more rigid. This means that tympanometry can more readily be utilized to provide accurate information about physical properties of the eardrum and the middle ear.

A more detailed discussion of methods for audiometric testing in infants can be found in Chapter 9. It should be emphasized here, however, that methods are available for identifying hearing thresholds in infants. Although some audiologists may not have the requisite equipment or specific skills for testing infants, there is usually some nearby medical or diagnostic facility where the testing can be done. Whenever there is a suspicion that an infant has a hearing impairment, it is imperative that the infant undergo appropriate audiometric testing. There is no reason for delaying such tests until the later childhood years.

TABLE 14–3. Eye Abnormalities Associated with Hearing Impairment

SYNDROME	CHARACTERISTICS	MODE OF INHERITANCE	TYPE OF HEARING LOSS SN	Conductive	Mixed
Usher syndrome	Retinitis pigmentosa, vestibulocerebellar ataxia, mental retardation	Recessive	X		
Cockayne syndrome	Retinal atrophy, motor disturbances, mental retardation, dwarfism	Recessive	X		
Alström syndrome	Obesity, diabetes mellitus, retinal degeneration	Recessive	X		
Hallgren syndrome	Retinitis pigmentosa, vestibulocerebellar ataxia, nystagmus, sometimes mental retardation	Recessive	X		
Laurence-Moon-Biedl-Bardet syndrome	Retinitis pigmentosa, polydactyly, hypogenitalism, obesity, mental retardation	Recessive	X		
Refsum syndrome (heredopathia atactica polyneuritiformis)	Retinitis pigmentosa, cerebellar ataxia, polyneuritis, electrocardiographic abnormalities, ichthyosis-type skin disorder	Recessive	X		
Duane syndrome	Ocular palsy (congenital fibrous replacement of rectus muscle), auricular malformations, meatal atresia, cervical rib, torticollis, cervical spina bifida	Recessive		X	
Möbius syndrome	Facial diplegia; lateral and/or medial rectus palsy bilaterally; auricular malformation; micrognathia; absence of hands, feet, fingers, or toes; tongue paralysis; mental retardation	Recessive	X	X	X

Modified from Black, F. O., Bergstrom, L., Downs, M., et al. 1971. Congenital Deafness: A New Approach to Diagnosis Using a High Risk Register. Boulder, CO, Colorado Associated University Press.

TABLE 14–4. Pigmentary Abnormalities Associated with Hearing Impairment

SYNDROME	CHARACTERISTICS	MODE OF INHERITANCE	TYPE OF HEARING LOSS SN	Conductive	Mixed
Albinism-deafness syndrome	Fair skin and hair; absence of pigment in iris, sclera, and fundus	Recessive or X-linked	X		
	Fair skin, fine hair; eyes not affected (blue irides)	Dominant	X		
Partial albinism or piebaldness	Areas of skin depigmentation, light-blue clumps of pigment throughout the retina, good vision	Dominant	X		
Waardenburg syndrome	Heterochromic irides, broad nasal root, thick eyebrows, lateral displacement of medial canthi, white forelock, dappling of skin	Dominant	X		

Modified from Black, F. O., Bergstrom, L., Downs, M., et al. 1971. Congenital Deafness: A New Approach to Diagnosis Using a High Risk Register. Boulder, CO, Colorado Associated University Press.

Characterize

As the infant becomes older and able to be tested with behavioral techniques, it becomes possible to perform the audiometric tests that will help characterize the type of hearing impairment.

Conductive, sensorineural, and mixed hearing losses are the types that will most often be discovered during infancy. Although it is conceivable that auditory brain stem evoked response audiometry may help in the early diagnosis of central and retrocochlear types of hearing loss, such hearing difficulties are relatively rarely discovered during infancy. At one time, it may have been sufficient merely to detect hearing impairment during infancy. However, with the newer audiometric test techniques that are available, it is imperative to attempt to determine the nature of the hearing impairment.

Auditory brain stem response testing, tympanometry, and acoustic reflex testing can be helpful in characterizing the type of hearing loss.

When considering the types of hearing loss that can be seen in infancy, conductive hearing loss due to otitis media with effusion deserves specific mention. When otitis media with effusion is discovered in the infant who has been referred for evaluation of hearing impairment, it should not be assumed that effusion in the middle ear is the sole reason for the hearing loss. Audiometric tests should be obtained to determine whether or not a previously undetected sensorineural hearing loss is also present. Further, if tympanostomy tubes are inserted as treatment for a chronic effusion, a repeat audiogram several weeks after myringotomy should be obtained when the middle ear is aerated (i.e., when no effusion is present). If it was possible to obtain an air-conduction and bone-conduction pure-tone audiogram prior to insertion of a tympanostomy tube, then a repeat audiogram following the tube insertion should reveal air-conduction thresholds that have returned to normal. If a conductive hearing loss persists after the insertion of a tympanostomy tube with aeration of the middle ear, the infant may have a congenital ossicular abnormality. If it was not possible to obtain an air-conduction and bone-conduction au-

diogram prior to insertion of the tympanostomy tube, then a persistent hearing loss following insertion of the tube may be entirely sensorineural or mixed, or the residual conductive loss may be associated with an ossicular abnormality. It has been discovered that children with Down syndrome not only are prone to developing otitis media with effusion but also may have congenital middle-ear ossicular abnormalities (Balkany et al., 1979).

The ABR test combined with myringotomy and insertion of tympanostomy tubes under general anesthesia may help differentiate the type of hearing loss an infant has. Comparing characteristics of the ABR pattern before and after the insertion of a tympanostomy tube gives helpful clues about the type of hearing loss that is present. There is no doubt that as more experience is gained with electrocochleography and ABR testing, their usefulness in evaluating infants with hearing loss will be expanded.

Although it may not always be possible to characterize an infant's hearing loss accurately, some attempt should be made to discover the type of hearing loss that is present. Certainly, the diagnostic possibilities and plans for management will vary according to the type of hearing impairment that is discovered.

Cause

Hearing loss discovered during infancy can be thought of as being either congenital or acquired. Cases of congenital hearing loss that were not discovered during the neonatal period will often become manifest during the infant years. Of course, where the high-risk register and selective neonatal hearing screening programs are utilized, there is less likelihood that a neonate will leave the hospital where he or she was born with an undetected congenital hearing impairment.

When evaluating an infant with hearing loss, it is advisable to obtain copies of the medical record from the hospital where the infant was born. The records can then be reviewed to see if excessive jaundice for a prolonged period, infection, or ototoxic medications could have been factors in the pathogenesis of the hearing impairment.

Next, it is helpful to question the parents carefully about how the suspicion of hearing loss arose. Some helpful questions follow.

1. Do you think that your child was born with normal hearing?

2. When did you first become suspicious that your infant has difficulty in hearing?

3. What has it been that gives you the impression that your child has a hearing loss?

4. Did your baby babble and coo? Has the babbling activity ceased? If so, when? What is the level of the infant's speech development?

5. Did meningitis, measles, a high fever, seizures, an exanthematous disease, a viral infection, or any other disorder immediately precede the noticeable hearing problem?

6. Have there been frequent bouts of otitis media? If so, what characterized each episode, and how were they treated?

Answers to these questions may help determine whether the hearing loss is congenital or whether it is causally related to some other event. Often, the infant born with a severe hearing impairment will experiment with verbalization, making several speech sounds; then at about 8 months of age, lacking the reinforcement of hearing his or her voice and lacking the stimulation of hearing others speak, the infant will eventually stop experimenting with speech. Thus, language development sometimes offers a clue about the time of onset of hearing impairment.

In contrast to the difficulty of uncovering the cause of congenital hearing loss, when it can be determined that the hearing loss was acquired after birth, a more direct cause-and-effect relationship may be discernible. For example, bacterial meningitis is a common cause of sensorineural hearing impairment acquired after the perinatal period (Teng et al., 1962; Nadol, 1978). Obviously, if an infant appeared to be developing speech normally and then hearing difficulty was noticed after the occurrence of bacterial meningitis, it can reasonably be assumed that meningitis was a factor in causing the hearing loss, especially if there had been no suspicion of a hearing loss preceding the meningitis infection. Although parents often recall that a high fever, a viral syndrome, or some minor head trauma immediately preceded the noticeable hearing loss, it is difficult to prove that such common entities actually are the cause of hearing loss. Still, it is worthwhile to ask the questions and find out what the parents think was the time of onset and cause of their infant's hearing loss. Understanding the parents' concept of the cause for their infant's hearing loss can be of help in counseling the parents and in mollifying the lingering sense of guilt that they may harbor. Further, it is worthwhile to collect whatever information seems relevant so that a retrospective analysis can be undertaken and relative probability of causality can be ascribed to events that appear to have caused the hearing loss. As the pathogenesis of childhood hearing loss is

elucidated, it may be discovered that certain seemingly unrelated factors play a role in the pathogenesis of hearing impairment.

Physical examination adds additional information that can be helpful in determining the cause of hearing loss. Subtle abnormalities that were not noticed at birth may become evident when the infant with a hearing loss undergoes a thorough examination. Special attention must be directed to examining the pinnae, ear canals, eardrums, the retinae, the facial bones, and the neck, and to testing of the cranial nerves. Many of the laboratory studies suggested for the evaluation of the neonate (see subsection entitled Cause, under section on age-specific tasks) are useful for evaluation of nonsyndromal infants with a hearing loss of unknown etiology. Radiographic studies are usually not warranted during infancy.

As already mentioned (see section on method for acquiring core information), otitis media with effusion cannot always be assumed to be the sole cause of a confirmed significant hearing impairment.

If it appears that genetic factors are not responsible for the hearing impairment, then a hypothesis should be formulated based on review of all collected information. In many cases, there will be no clear cause to explain the hearing loss discovered during infancy.

Care

When a significant hearing impairment is discovered during infancy, habilitative measures can be taken. If persistent bilateral otitis media with effusion is discovered, the hearing may be improved simply by aspirating the fluid and inserting tympanostomy tubes. Almost all infants born with cleft palate have abnormal eustachian tube function and a consequent tendency to develop recurrent or persistent otitis media with effusion. The palate deformity itself makes it difficult for these infants to learn speech. Therefore, every attempt must be made to provide them with keen auditory acuity so that they will be able to hear clearly the subtleties of speech enunciation that they will try so hard to imitate. Early insertion of tympanostomy tubes is advisable and may conveniently be done in conjunction with the first plastic surgery repair of a cleft lip deformity or as a brief surgical procedure for the infant born with an isolated cleft palate deformity.

When an infant without a craniofacial defect is found to have hearing impairment because of frequently recurring or persistent middle-ear effusions, the decision to perform a myringotomy with insertion of tympanostomy tubes should be based on the severity and duration of a measurable hearing loss and the inability to eradicate the effusions with medical therapy. In some instances, it will be advisable to insert tympanostomy tubes more as a means of diminishing a sizable conductive hearing loss than as a therapeutic measure aimed at reducing the frequency of middle-ear infections.

When all available evidence seems to indicate that there is a significant conductive hearing loss being caused by a factor other than middle-ear effusion, therapeutic measures should be aimed at providing amplification of sound and assistance in learning speech. Surgical procedures to improve hearing deficits due to malformations or fixation of the ossicles usually are not undertaken during infancy. Rather, ossicular reconstruction of the congenitally malformed ear is better undertaken later in childhood.

If the hearing impairment is more sensorineural than conductive, the infant should undergo complete developmental and neurologic evaluation. The infant discovered to have a moderate or severe sensorineural hearing impairment may also have other previously undetected impairment of central nervous system function. That is, it is important to determine whether the sensorineural hearing loss is an isolated problem or whether it is occurring along with visual impairment, mental retardation, or delayed motor development. If the hearing impairment is an isolated problem, early sound amplification and speech training should be provided. If the sensorineural hearing impairment is one of a constellation of problems, the benefit to be derived from early hearing amplification will have to be considered in relation to the child's capabilities and other handicaps. However, it is best not to consider an infant too young or unsuitable for a hearing aid until after the infant has been seen and evaluated by a skilled audiologist (Whetnall and Fry, 1964). In fact, when formulating a plan for the management of a severely hearing-handicapped infant, it is best to make sure that a pediatrician, otolaryngologist, audiologist, and a social worker all are involved initially and that each is kept informed of the infant's progress.

It is important to realize that young children can experience serious deficiency in language and communicative skills even if an intensive preschool program is initiated by age 3 years. For maximal effectiveness, intervention should be achieved before age 3 years, at which time the child with normal hearing is attuned to the sound environment and has become a functionally communicative individual, able to express desires and exchange ideas (Horton, 1975). Therefore, the infant years before age 3 years should be viewed as a critical time for effecting change in the course of development of children with severe sensorineural hearing impairment. During these all-important infant years, training in a structured classroom situation or even an informal nursery-kindergarten setting is not appropriate. It is the parents, the child's natural teachers, who can provide the best educational experience. Parents should be taught methods of capitalizing on the innumerable ways in which auditory training and language acquisition can occur on a daily basis in the child's own home.

The fundamental assumptions that the people most important to a young child are his or her parents and that the place most important to the child is the home have led some speech and hearing centers to institute programs focusing on the role of the parents in the home (Horton, 1975). While some centers send specially trained teachers into the child's home on a regular basis to provide instruction to the parents, others have developed a "model home" for all families to utilize. The model home enables concurrent parent teaching, audiologic assessment, and the use of videotape and sophisticated audiovisual equipment to facilitate parent teaching while closely monitoring the child's development.

In summary, the primary concern in management of a severely hearing-impaired infant should be the acquisition of communicative skills and the inculcation of a positive attitude toward learning. As the child develops during the infant years, his or her potential will become manifest. Some hearing-handicapped children will show a remarkable ability to function nearly normally, whereas others will have difficulty in communicating. By the time a hearing-impaired child reaches 3 years of age, the parents and educators should be able to determine the educational mode that will most suit the child. Essentially, the alternatives for education will be a school for the deaf, a special class in a regular public school, or an ordinary public school class. The more information that is accrued during the infant years regarding a child's capabilities, the more appropriate will be the choice of an educational program for future learning. Further, the earlier that special training is begun and the more sophisticated and intensive the training, the greater will be a child's chance for integration into a regular public school system. Early aggressive appropriate intervention yields the best results.

Preschool Child

The main difference between the preschool child and the infant is that a child aged 2 to 5 years old is able to complain of difficulty in hearing. Moreover, preschool-age children begin to become involved in group play and social interactions in which auditory acuity is important.

Confirm

It is becoming common for state and local health agencies to encourage or require screening hearing tests for nursery school children and children about to enter elementary school. As a result, increasing numbers of young children are being referred for otologic examination and confirmative audiometric testing. Of the children who fail screening tests, some actually have hearing impairment, whereas others do not. In an attempt to identify the children who have significant hearing impairment, the following questions should be asked:

1. Was the screening test merely a tympanogram or was it a pure-tone audiogram?

2. Was the screening test administered to several children simultaneously in a classroom, or was each child tested individually in a soundproof booth?

3. Did the child have an upper respiratory tract or

ear infection at the time that the screening test was administered or within the week prior to the test?

4. Prior to failing the screening test, was there any suspicion of the child's having abnormal hearing?

5. Is there a history of frequently recurring acute otitis media or persistent otitis media with effusion?

With the information gained from the answers to these questions, it is possible to formulate an impression quickly regarding the validity and meaningfulness of the screening procedure in each case. Pneumatic otoscopy can then be performed to gain additional information about the status of the eardrum and the middle ear. Tuning fork tests may be helpful in older preschool children, but often young children find it difficult to comprehend the instructions they are given for comparing the relative loudness of tuning fork tones. Obviously, the definitive way of confirming an apparent hearing loss is to obtain a complete air-conduction and bone-conduction pure-tone audiogram, to test speech reception thresholds, and possibly to obtain tympanograms.

Surprisingly often, repeat audiometric tests reveal normal hearing in a child who has been referred for having failed a screening test. There are several reasons for this. First, the screening examinations may have been done where noise conditions were less than optimal and where children could be distracted or tempted to trick the examiner. Second, the child may have had an upper respiratory tract infection accompanied by a transient otitis media with effusion at the time that the screening test was administered; such children may have essentially normal hearing as soon as the infection resolves. Children with mild forms of eustachian tube dysfunction often tend to develop an otitis media with effusion when they have an upper respiratory tract infection. Thus, a child who recently failed a hearing screening test and then appears to have normal hearing when a more complete audiogram is obtained may have borderline abnormal eustachian tube dysfunction. Third, it should be realized that screening programs utilizing only tympanometry are not testing hearing per se. Such programs are supposedly designed to identify children who have previously undiagnosed otitis media with effusion. Because the tympanogram is really measuring acoustic impedance rather than hearing, children with normal hearing and various eardrum or middle-ear pressure abnormalities are likely to be identified as "abnormal" and referred for further evaluation. Thus, when an abnormal tympanogram was the main reason for referral, obtaining a reliable air-conduction and bone-conduction audiogram along with speech reception thresholds should differentiate children with significant hearing problems from those who have innocuous types of tympanogram abnormalities.

Characterize

When it has been established that a preschool child has a significant hearing impairment, a variety of audiometric tests can be utilized to determine the type of hearing loss that is present. About the age of 2 years, it becomes possible to condition children to respond to pure-tone signals. In addition, because the normal 2-year-old child has developed some receptive and expressive language skills, it is possible to explain and have the child follow simple, explicit instructions. Both speech and pure-tone testing can be utilized. Children can be asked to identify familiar pictures as the loudness is varied for the words describing the pictures. Audiometers are available that route a speech signal to a bone vibrator so that a bone-conduction speech threshold can be obtained.

Although speech testing in younger children may differentiate conductive from sensorineural hearing loss, pure-tone testing is required to yield information about hearing ability at specific frequencies. Usually, an air-conduction and bone-conduction audiogram can be obtained when a child is able to be conditioned to respond to a pure-tone signal by dropping an object into a box, placing rings on a peg, or performing some other simple task. Further information about the type of hearing impairment can be gained with the ABR test. With a cooperative child, the ABR test can be done awake. In children who are not cooperative, sedation or general anesthesia can be used. Tympanometry (sometimes referred to as immittance or impedance testing), of course, can be useful in assessing the functional status of the eardrum and ossicular chain.

Thus, it should be possible to characterize a hearing impairment in the young child as being conductive, sensorineural, or mixed. From the test results it might be difficult to distinguish a retrocochlear type of hearing loss from a sensorineural one, but analysis of the ABR test pattern, word discrimination scores (if obtainable), and other clinical information should be helpful in making the differentiation. Although retrocochlear lesions such as vestibular schwannomas (acoustic neuromas) are rarely seen in young children, they can occur in this age group.

Cause

Otitis media with effusion is the most common cause of conductive hearing loss in preschool-age children. Mild to moderate conductive hearing losses due to congenital ossicular chain abnormalities may also be discovered in children of this age.

Children with congenital bilateral severe sensorineural hearing losses are usually identified before 2 years of age, but in some cases the hearing impairment may go unnoticed until the third year of life. When a bilateral moderate to severe sensorineural hearing loss is first discovered in a child between ages 2 and 3 years, the question often arises as to whether the child was born with poor hearing or whether hearing progressively worsened in the first few years of life. A clue to the time of onset of the hearing loss lies in the child's ability to speak. Children who were born with little or no hearing ability usually have considerable difficulty in learning to speak, whereas those who could hear initially tend to have better speech.

Whether the hearing impairment was present at birth or developed in the first years of life, genetic factors may be the cause. There are at least 16 types of hereditary hearing loss with no associated abnormalities (Konigsmark and Gorlin, 1976). In the early-onset type of inherited hearing loss, the auditory impairment can begin during the preschool years. The family pedigree, shape of the audiogram, severity of the hearing loss, and age at onset of hearing impairment help separate one type of inherited hearing loss from another when there are no associated abnormalities to aid in identifying a genetic or other etiologic factor.

The three most common inherited syndromes that include hearing loss are Pendred, Usher, and Jervell and Lange-Nielsen syndromes. Because all three syndromes can first occur during the preschool years, it is worthwhile to look specifically for goiter, retinitis pigmentosa, or electrocardiographic abnormalities in young children who are being evaluated for sensorineural hearing losses.

If it appears that hereditary factors are not responsible for the hearing loss, the search for an identifiable (acquired) etiologic factor begins with a careful prenatal and perinatal history. A history of meningitis or any other severe infection during infancy may be significant. If the child had been hospitalized for any reason, it is worthwhile to obtain the hospital records to see if ototoxic medications were administered. Review of the family history may reveal a hereditary hearing problem. After the physical examination has been completed, FTA-ABS tests and urinalysis should be ordered. Results of thyroid function studies and an electrocardiogram may also be helpful. Routine mastoid films are sufficient for demonstrating the presence or absence of the cochlea, but temporal bone polytomography is necessary for the diagnosis of certain ossicular chain abnormalities and malformations of the otic capsule.

Care

Conductive and sensorineural hearing losses require different types of management. Hearing impairments discovered in children of preschool age are usually conductive and tend to be less severe than sensorineural hearing impairments. There is no consensus on management of the child who has unilateral or bilateral middle-ear effusion with associated conductive hearing loss. Audiologists, educators, and medical practitioners hold variant opinions on the timing and the types of intervention that are warranted (Chap. 21). Divergent opinions notwithstanding, it should be realized that impairment of hearing may adversely affect language development and cognitive function in young children (Hanson and Ulvestad, 1979; Klein, 1984). To avoid or minimize the adverse effect, a child with middle-ear effusion and concomitant hearing loss should be seen frequently and should undergo sequential audiometric

tests. If it is determined that the child has hearing significantly worse than normal (speech receptional threshold greater than 20 dB in both ears) most of the time, measures should be taken to improve hearing. Although decongestant medication is often prescribed to promote and quicken the resolution of otitis media with effusion, the efficacy of such medication for this purpose has never been scientifically proved. Tympanocentesis with aspiration of fluid from the middle-ear space can provide quick disappearance of the conductive hearing loss caused by a middle-ear effusion. Insertion of tympanostomy tubes is widely accepted as a method of ensuring that an aspirated middle-ear effusion will not recur. Although there may be controversy regarding the efficacy of tympanostomy tubes in reducing the frequency of bouts of acute otitis media, it should be realized that myringotomy and insertion of tympanostomy tubes is one effective method of removing middle-ear effusion, preventing its recurrence, and abolishing the conductive hearing loss associated with the effusion (Grundfast and Carney, 1987; Gates et al., 1985; Luxford and Sheehy, 1984). If for some reason it is deemed inappropriate to utilize tympanostomy tubes, use of a hearing aid can be considered.

While the goal in managing children who have hearing losses due to otitis media with effusion is eradication of the hearing deficit, for those children with entirely sensorineural or predominantly sensorineural mixed hearing losses, management is directed more toward finding optimal ways of coping with a given hearing impairment. When a significant sensorineural hearing loss is discovered in a preschool child, attention is focused on methods for enabling the child to develop communicative skills, and plans must be made for selecting an appropriate educational environment.

The preschool years are exceptionally important in a child's overall development. It is a time during which the child develops concept formation and methods for problem solving. The child's natural curiosity and eagerness to explore the environment make the preschool years most fertile for educational experiences. The nurture and reinforcement—or seeming neglect—of the child's earliest attempts to interact with others constitute the experiences that form the child's impression of the world. Pleasant experiences enable the child to trust himself or herself and others in the competitive business of everyday life with siblings, playmates, and adults. The quality of parent-child interaction and the timing and intensity of parental responses to the young child's activities combine to determine whether the child will realize full potential in developing social skills and intellectual prowess or will regress to more immature behavior because of frustration and feelings of inadequacy (Erikson, 1963; Mowrer, 1960).

Because much of the learning experience for the preschool child is derived from activities at home with the family, parental participation is of utmost importance in fostering optimal development for the hearing-impaired child. Therefore, once it is established that a preschool child has hearing impairment, a comprehensive program should be undertaken to counsel and provide guidance and teaching for the parents. Emotional and psychologic support is often warranted to help parents cope with the concept of having a handicapped child and to aid in resolving feelings of guilt. Parents need to be taught how to utilize maximally a child's residual hearing for linguistic stimulation during play and other home activities. If the child has no residual hearing, the parent must learn the methods of communicating with the deaf child that will enable behavior management and lead to the child's developing a sense of self-reliance through the acquisition of daily living skills. In addition, parents require factual information regarding sources for financial assistance, local and regional education centers for hearing-impaired children, and special preschool nursery school programs suited for hearing-impaired children. Parents should be made aware that special laws have lowered or eliminated the minimal age for enrollment in publicly funded special education programs (Ebenson, 1963).

In 1975, Public Law 94-142 was passed. This statute acknowledged and protected the right of handicapped children to free public education. Under the provisions of P.L. 94-142, state and local education agencies were required to develop and administer suitable programs for these children. The age specifications of P.L. 94-142 varied for the different provisions of the law.

A major innovation of P.L. 94-142 was the requirement that an individualized education program be prepared for each child identified as handicapped and that this plan be monitored and updated annually (Palfrey et al., 1978). In a sense, the legislation virtually ensured that a hearing-handicapped child could attend a regular public school, provided that a suitable individualized educational program could be developed and annual evaluations indicated that the child was learning adequately.

In 1986, Public Law 99-457 covering education for the handicapped was passed. There are three main sections to P.L. 99-457. Title I, often referred to as the "handicapped infants and toddlers section," established a discretionary program calling for states to create comprehensive systems for providing early intervention services to disabled infants from birth until their third birthday. Title II requires states by 1992 to provide free and appropriate public education and related services to disabled children over the age of 3 years. Effectively, this section of P.L. 99-457 replaces the earlier P.L. 94-142. Title III of P.L. 99-457 reauthorizes discretionary programs such as services for deaf-blind children. Physicians and other professionals who work with severely hearing-impaired infants and young children should be familiar with certain aspects of P.L. 99-457. Importantly, the law represents the first time that the federal government stated a commitment to provide funds for provision of *early intervention* services from the time of birth for disabled children. Compared with the earlier P.L. 94-142, the more recent P.L. 99-457 is designed to foster better cooperation between health care professionals and educators as well as placing a greater emphasis on needed services for the families of affected children.

Thus, the options for educating a child with significant hearing impairment have been expanded. As a result, the matter of selecting an appropriate educational setting has become somewhat controversial. In the past, it was traditional for severely hearing-impaired and deaf children to attend schools that were specifically equipped and staffed to educate these children (deaf schools) instead of the "regular" public schools. However, some parents and educators are in favor of having children with severe hearing impairments educated in the regular public school system. This concept of integrating hearing-impaired children and children with normal hearing is known as mainstreaming. Proponents of mainstreaming believe that the earlier a hearing-impaired child is surrounded by people with normal hearing, the earlier he or she will learn to cope with real-life problems. They believe that proper assistance and preparation will enable the hearing-impaired child to receive a solid education without having to attend a special school. Opponents of the mainstreaming concept believe that the hearing-impaired child's total education and general sense of well-being may suffer when the hearing-impaired child, surrounded by normal-hearing children, is forced to try to learn from teachers who are not specifically trained in methods of educating the hearing-impaired.

There is probably no single best way of educating a severely hearing-impaired child. The child should be placed in the educational setting that best accommodates his or her individual capabilities and needs. In general, children born with severe hearing impairments or total deafness require more specialized types of training. When a severe hearing impairment is discovered late in the preschool years and the child has not yet developed a facility with communication skills, attempts to have the child attend a regular public school may be ill advised. On the other hand, when the hearing impairment was discovered early and specific habilitative measures were undertaken, the child may have developed receptive and expressive skills sufficient to enable his or her placement in a regular classroom with children who have normal hearing.

Thus, the most important aspect of management when dealing with a preschool child who has significant sensorineural hearing impairment is education. After an appropriate hearing aid has been provided, attention should be focused on development and preservation of language skills. The decision regarding where and how the child will receive an education is one that should be made with liberal advice from an audiologist, a psychologist, parents, educators, and others.

Additional services that are important in such cases are genetic counseling for parents and maintenance of otologic care for the hearing-impaired child. When the child's hearing impairment is clearly hereditary, the parents should be apprised of the probabilities that another offspring will be hearing-impaired. Children who utilize hearing aids need frequent otologic and audiometric reevaluation to make sure that the hearing aid functions properly and that the ear mold is not causing skin excoriation or ulceration and to detect changes in hearing thresholds or to uncover symptoms of intermittent middle-ear disorders that could superimpose a conductive hearing loss on the sensorineural impairment already present.

School-Age Child

Confirm

Hearing tests are almost universally required, either prior to school enrollment or during the first school year. When questions arise as to a child's hearing ability, the parents are informed, and it is usually requested that the child be evaluated by an audiologist, a medical practitioner, or both. Thus, large numbers of children are being referred for further evaluation after having "failed" a school screening audiogram.

With the increasing awareness of hearing problems in children, the likelihood is diminishing that significant hearing impairment in a school-age child will go undetected. In fact, many of the hearing screening test procedures are designed to have high sensitivity and only moderately high specificity. The underlying philosophy is that it is better to accept that some children with entirely normal hearing will be referred for further testing than to allow the risk of not identifying all children with significant hearing impairment.

Almost all school-age children are able to cooperate for some type of behavioral audiometric test that will enable an accurate assessment of hearing ability. However, there are some children who are frightened by earphones or the soundproof booth or generally are uncooperative in other ways. These children who are slightly difficult to test may have failed a screening procedure done in a test situation where time allotted, space, and personnel did not accommodate the child's specific needs. Children with slightly lower than normal intelligence or those who are emotionally immature may not perform well on a screening hearing test, but then when the child is tested individually in more optimal surroundings, it can be determined that hearing actually is not impaired.

When a child fails a screening hearing test but is found on later testing to have normal hearing, it is advisable to obtain additional information about the child's hearing. A history of frequent otalgia and otitis media probably means that the child has some form of eustachian tube dysfunction with variations in middle-ear pressure and possibly intermittent otitis media with effusion. At the time of the screening test, the child may have had otitis media with effusion, which then resolved spontaneously prior to further evaluation and more definitive audiometric tests. When there is suspicion that variations in middle-ear pressure or

effusion are causing intermittent hearing difficulty, it is best to have the child return for audiometric tests in 1 or 2 months and to instruct the parent to return with the child whenever it seems that the child is having difficulty in hearing.

Children who appear to have difficulty in learning in school should undergo hearing evaluation. Children who are having difficulty with reading may have subtle hearing deficits. Aware of the importance of auditory acuity in the learning process, many educators and specialists in developmental psychology are now referring children for hearing evaluation as part of a total evaluation for learning disability. When assessing these children, it is important to bear in mind that a child's ability to respond to pure-tone signals at normal threshold levels does not entirely rule out auditory pathway problems as a contributing factor in the learning disability; it may be necessary to obtain tests of central auditory processing. Moreover, children who seem to have difficulty in hearing, especially children who manifest most of their hearing or listening problems in school, need to be evaluated for attention deficit disorders (ADD). Attention deficit disorders can mimic mild to moderate sensorineural hearing loss in a school-age child!

Characterize

Most school-age children are able to cooperate for the behavioral and impedance tests that will enable assessment of the severity and diagnosis of the type of hearing impairment that is present. Many of the tests used for adults are adapted for use with children. A pure-tone audiogram and speech reception thresholds can be obtained with conditioning and play audiometry. Simple word lists can be used to assess hearing discrimination ability. As more attention is focused on learning disabilities, newer tests are being developed for assessing central auditory function in children. Thus, once it is confirmed that a school-age child has a hearing impairment, tests are available to characterize and quantify the hearing loss.

Hearing impairment that is newly discovered during the early school years usually will be conductive or of the mild sensorineural type. Children with more severe types of hearing impairment often have difficulty with language development, which usually leads to recognition of the hearing deficit prior to the child's reaching school age. On the other hand, children with unilateral moderate to severe sensorineural hearing losses may learn to speak without difficulty and appear to have normal hearing until the time that they enter school. Then a screening test may uncover the hearing deficit, or difficulty in listening to the teacher may make the child aware of the hearing impairment.

Cause

CONDUCTIVE. Most of the inherited forms of conductive hearing impairment will be discovered before a child enters school. A large proportion of children who develop hearing impairment during the school years have eustachian tube dysfunction or middle-ear disorders, such as effusion, negative pressure, or both. As the child who has been prone to developing otitis media with effusion gets older, the tendency to develop effusions usually diminishes, and hearing tends to improve. However, some children develop sequelae that adversely affect hearing. Children who have had chronic middle-ear effusions and numerous bouts of acute otitis media can develop a nonhealing eardrum perforation, tympanosclerosis, erosion of portions of the ossicular chain, or even cholesteatoma. The lenticular process of the incus is the portion of the ossicular chain that is most vulnerable to damage from acute and chronic types of otitis media. Trauma must also be considered as an etiologic factor. School-age children may poke objects in the ear canal, causing damage to the eardrum, the ossicles, or even the inner ear. Blunt head trauma, as in an automobile accident, can cause dislocation of the ossicles and can result in a conductive hearing loss. Tumors involving the temporal bone are rare. Benign neoplasms such as osteomata or fibrous dysplasia can affect hearing, depending on the location of the lesion, or malignant lesions such as rhabdomyosarcoma may cause hearing loss when portions of the auditory system are destroyed.

SENSORINEURAL. When it is discovered that a school-age child has a sensorineural hearing impairment, it must be established whether the loss is stable or progressive, and an attempt must be made to discover the etiology. Even though sensorineural hearing impairment is not detected in the first 5 years of life, genetic factors cannot be excluded when attempting to discover the cause of such a hearing loss. There is a type of dominant, high-frequency, progressive sensorineural hearing loss that begins to appear after age 5 years and rapidly worsens up to the third decade (Huizing et al., 1966). A list of other types of inherited progressive sensorineural hearing losses with no associated anomalies follows (Konigsmark and Gorlin, 1976).

1. Dominant, autosomal, low-frequency hearing loss—onset of hearing loss can be in infancy; but progression is not usually seen until adulthood.

2. Dominant, mid-frequency hearing loss—onset of hearing loss in childhood with early progression.

3. Dominant, autosomal, progressive, early-onset sensorineural hearing loss—moderate to severe hearing loss by adolescence, considerable variation in expressivity.

4. Recessive, early-onset neural hearing loss—onset early in childhood with progression to a plateau of marked severity by mid to late childhood.

5. X-linked, early-onset neural hearing loss—progressive deafness after attainment of speech.

6. X-linked, moderate hearing loss—slowly progressive hearing loss in males.

Nongenetic causes of sensorineural hearing loss in school-age children include infections, such as syphilis (congenital), meningitis, or mumps. Administration of ototoxic medications can cause sensorineural hearing loss. All the aminoglycoside antibiotics can affect the inner ear. Dihydrostreptomycin and kanamycin mostly affect the auditory system, whereas streptomycin and gentamicin mostly affect the vestibular system. Neomycin affects both systems about equally. Diuretics such as furosemide and ethacrynic acid can affect hearing, and salicylates can cause a reversible type of hearing impairment. It has been reported that the intravenous administration of erythromycin lactobionate can be associated with reversible sensorineural hearing loss (Karmody and Weinstein, 1978).

Perilymph Fistula

Children can develop fistulas at the oval or round window membrane with leakage of perilymphatic fluid and associated sensorineural hearing impairment (Grundfast and Bluestone, 1979). Usually, the children who have a perilymphatic fistula have some history of barotrauma, blunt head trauma, or predisposing conditions such as a widely patent cochlear aqueduct or an anomaly involving the temporal bone. Classically, the patient with a perilymph fistula has sudden onset of fluctuating hearing loss and ataxia. However, in recent years, there have been reports of patients with fluctuating and progressive sensorineural hearing loss who have been found to have perilymph fistulas of the oval and round windows. Petroff and associates (1986) have reported the case of a 2½-year-old child with bilaterally symmetric, progressive sensorineural hearing loss who was found to have bilateral oval and round window fistulas. They also reported on a child who presented originally with an unexplained unilateral sensorineural hearing loss. After hearing deteriorated in the opposite ear several years later, a perilymph fistula was suspected and confirmed by tympanotomy. Based on information from these cases, the authors describe what they call "emerging perilymph fistula syndromes." Further, they suggest that children who are believed to have "congenital" hearing impairment may really have a "predisposition" to fistulas, and the hearing impairment may be secondary to fistulas that have developed. Consistent with reports by other authors, Petroff and associates (1986) state that repair of a perilymph fistula is more likely to "stabilize" a progressive sensorineural hearing loss than to restore normal hearing. Weider and Musiek (1984) have reported bilateral congenital oval window microfistulas in a mother and a son. The boy demonstrated a slowly progressive, bilateral and symmetric sensorineural hearing loss closely resembling a hearing loss that had previously been manifested by the mother. The authors stress that "so-called cases of hereditary, progressive sensorineural hearing loss" should be carefully evaluated for the possibility of perilymphatic fistulas. They also suggest that a fistula may exist over a long period of time with little change in hearing level. Then, when the hearing change occurs, it can be slow and progressive. Balance may be minimally affected, if at all.

Kanzaki (1986) has reported on 24 cases of idiopathic

sudden progressive deafness in which worsening of sensorineural hearing loss after initial examination was confirmed by serial audiometric tests. Exploratory tympanotomy was performed in 10 of 24 patients and perilymphatic fistulas were found in four patients. Kanzaki found that perilymphatic fistulas were confirmed in 40 per cent of the patients who had exploratory tympanotomy. In the remaining patients, it was not clear whether there was a natural closure of the fistula, the fistula was inadvertently overlooked, or a fistula had never existed. The more severe hearing impairments at the higher frequencies and the configuration of the audiogram suggested to Kanzaki that there was a lesion such as a break in Reissner membrane in the basal turn of the cochlea. Gussen (1981) has reported a rupture of Reissner membrane in the region of the junction of the ductus reuniens and the cochlear duct on the cecum vestibulare side of the cochlea in patients who have experienced sudden hearing loss associated with rupture of an inner-ear membrane.

Even though progressive sensorineural hearing impairment can be a devastating disorder, the otologic surgeon would be well advised to view cautiously recent claims that suggest that there is a large population of patients with many different types of fluctuating and progressive sensorineural hearing loss caused by perilymph fistulas. The paucity of pathognomonic findings, the lack of reliable diagnostic studies, and the extreme subtlety of confirmatory intraoperative findings combine to make the ultimate diagnosis of perilymphatic fistula, in some ways, the artifactual self-fulfilling prophecy of a well-meaning otologic surgeon attempting to offer some hope and assistance to a patient who is losing or has lost hearing in an affected ear. This having been said, it would seem that more scientific studies are necessary before the judicious otologic surgeon should accept the notion that perilymphatic fistula is a commonly overlooked diagnosis and frequent underlying pathologic condition in patients who have progressive sensorineural hearing loss. Further, even if the perilymphatic fistula is occurring more commonly than had previously been recognized in patients with progressive or fluctuating sensorineural hearing loss, it must be remembered that well-designed randomized controlled studies have not yet been done to prove sufficiently that surgical intervention offers the patient any better chance for "stabilizing" the hearing loss or improving the hearing than observation alone (Grundfast, 1988).

If the family history gives no clues as to the cause of a hearing loss and if the child has no history of exposure to ototoxic agents that could have caused an observed sensorineural hearing loss, it may be worthwhile to test the urine for protein. If there is a palpably enlarged thyroid, thyroid function studies are indicated. Transorbital views of the internal auditory canals will be helpful if there is retrocochlear-type hearing impairment and an acoustic neuroma is suspected. Then, if transorbital views of the internal auditory canal show an abnormality, CT scan or even posterior

fossa myelography may be of diagnostic value. When a perilymph fistula is suspected as the cause of the hearing loss, it is worthwhile to perform the fistula test as well as to obtain electronystagmography, including positional tests.

Finally, it should be emphasized that the diagnosis and management of a sudden or fluctuating sensorineural hearing loss are different from those of a stable or slowly progressive sensorineural loss. In general, otologists view sudden-onset and fluctuating hearing losses as potentially treatable disorders. Although there are numerous approaches to treatment of a patient with sudden hearing loss, no single therapeutic regimen is universally effective. Similarly, no single approach to the management of patients with fluctuating hearing losses has been shown to be optimal. Despite the lack of a proven therapeutic regimen, it is advisable immediately to pursue complete evaluation of any child who suddenly develops a sensorineural hearing loss or who has documented variations in sensorineural hearing.

Care

Management of the school-age child with a hearing loss depends on the type and severity of the hearing impairment. The discussion concerning management of preschool children with middle-ear disorders pertains as well to school-age children. However, while younger children are prone to develop otitis media, the incidence of middle-ear disease decreases as a child grows older. Hence, the child who has had frequent middle-ear disease as a young child with sequelae of impaired conductive hearing may be a candidate for tympanoplasty with ossicular reconstruction as an older child. Reconstructive otologic surgery is best undertaken whenever it appears that problems with otitis media and inadequate ventilation of the middle ear have subsided.

At one time, children with unilateral hearing impairment were thought to require minimal, if any, special care. Classically, advising "preferential seating" in school was all that would be done for children with unilateral hearing loss—even if the hearing impairment was profound in the single involved ear. However, reports demonstrate that unilateral hearing impairment of varying severity can represent a *significant* handicap for a child (Bess and Tharpe, 1984; Bess, 1985; Keller and Bundy, 1980).

When a child develops a bilateral moderate to severe sensorineural hearing loss during the school years, a hearing aid may be necessary, and sometimes measures may have to be taken to ensure that loss of auditory feedback does not result in deterioration of the child's ability to articulate and enunciate properly.

Although sensorineural hearing loss is generally considered not to be reversible with otologic surgery, sensorineural hearing loss associated with a perilymphatic fistula may be an exception. Reports have appeared describing restoration of hearing following identification and surgical repair of a perilymphatic fistula (Healy et al., 1978; Petroff et al., 1986).

Preadolescent

Confirm

Preadolescence can be a turbulent time emotionally. It is a time during which endocrinologic changes occur, and there tends to be an increased sense of body awareness. In contrast to younger children, the preadolescent child is more likely to complain of difficulty in hearing rather than to have an unnoticed hearing deficit uncovered through screening testing. With younger children, the task of confirming a suspected hearing loss involves selection of an audiometric test procedure that will manifest the hearing deficit. A cooperative preadolescent child should be entirely capable of providing valid responses to air-conduction and bone-conduction pure-tone signals and to speech and discrimination testing. However, it is sometimes necessary to consider the use of tests for nonorganic or functional types of hearing loss in the process of evaluating the preadolescent child.

Another point to remember is that the preadolescent child may be subject to noise-induced temporary threshold shifts. With many children listening to or participating in rock bands, the possibility arises that a hearing loss may be induced by acoustic trauma. In confirming the presence of a hearing loss, it may be important to consider that certain types of hearing impairment can be transient.

Characterize

Audiometric testing for a preadolescent child should be a relatively straightforward matter. Air-conduction and bone-conduction pure-tone audiograms with speech reception threshold tests are sufficient in most cases. Where retrocochlear pathologic change is suspected, discrimination tests and other sites-of-lesion audiometric tests may be warranted. When nonorganic hearing loss is suspected, acoustic reflex testing and such tests as the Stenger, Doerfler-Stewart, or delayed auditory feedback test may be indicated.

Cause

By the time they reach the preadolescent years, most children have outgrown troublesome middle-ear disorders. Ossicular damage or adhesive changes caused by early childhood middle-ear disease can cause conductive hearing loss that persists into a child's later years. Otospongiosis, an early form of otosclerosis, can cause conductive hearing loss in children approximately 11 to 14 years of age.

Although unusual, it is possible for an inherited sensorineural hearing loss to become manifest in a preadolescent child. Endolymphatic hydrops (Ménière disease) can account for a sensorineural hearing loss when associated with tinnitus and vertigo (Meyerhoff et al., 1978; Hausler et al., 1987). Multiple sclerosis can cause transient sensorineural hearing loss as well as vertigo during adolescence (Molteni, 1977). Inadequately treated or previously undiagnosed congenital syphilis can cause sensorineural hearing loss in late childhood. Acoustic trauma should also be considered as a possible cause of sensorineural hearing loss. Although the sensorineural hearing loss from bacterial meningitis is generally thought to be stable approximately 2 years after resolution of the meningitis, reports suggest that additional hearing loss can occur many years after the episode of meningitis (Silkes and Chabot, 1985).

When sensorineural hearing loss develops in late childhood and no etiology is apparent, acoustic neuroma must be considered, especially if inordinately poor discrimination scores are obtained.

Other than serologic tests for syphilis, urinalysis, and possibly temporal bone radiographs, special studies are not usually helpful in the evaluation of sensorineural hearing loss that occurs late in childhood. Unless there have been syncopal episodes, an electrocardiogram will probably be superfluous. Unless there is a palpably enlarged thyroid gland and a family history of goiter, thyroid function tests will probably not be helpful. When a child has had middle-ear disease early in childhood and then developed a conductive hearing loss, temporal bone CT scan can be helpful in assessing the status of the ossicles or the location of cholesteatoma. At times, the CT scans can provide information that is helpful in choosing an operative approach or planning reconstruction of the middle ear. Finally, when there is a question of a retrocochlear pathologic condition or a demyelinating disorder, the ABR test can provide helpful information.

Care

In comparison to the potentially devastating effect of hearing loss in early childhood, the hearing loss of later childhood tends to present fewer problems in management. By the time a child has reached the preadolescent years, language and communication skills are well developed. Although it is usually inadvisable to attempt ossicular reconstruction during a child's younger years, when otitis media with effusion is most prevalent, during adolescence there is diminution of the tendency to develop otitis media with effusion, and it is reasonable to attempt otologic surgery that may improve certain conductive hearing deficits. For children who develop a sensorineural loss late in childhood, hearing amplification, speech preservation training, and counseling are appropriate.

REFERENCES

Alford, B. R. 1968. Rubella—la bete noire de la medecine. Laryngoscope 88:1623.

American Speech and Hearing Association, American Academy of

Ophthalmology and Otolaryngology, and American Academy of Pediatrics. 1974. Supplementary statement of Joint Committee on Infant Hearing Screening. ASHA 16:160.

Balkany, T. J., Downs, M. P., Jafek, B. W., et al. 1979. Hearing loss in Down's syndrome. A treatable handicap more common than generally recognized. Clin. Pediatr. 18(2):116.

Bergstrom, L. 1974. Hearing loss in children. In Northern, J. L., and Downs, M. P. (eds.): Hearing in Children. Baltimore, Williams & Wilkins Co.

Bergstrom, L., and Stewart, J. 1971. New concepts in congenital deafness. Otolaryngol. Clin. North Am. 4(2):431.

Berliner, K. I., and Eisenberg, L. S. 1985. Methods and issues in the cochlear implantation of children: An overview. Ear Hear. 6:65.

Bess, F. H. 1985. The minimally hearing-impaired child. Ear Hear. 6:43.

Bess, F. H., and Tharpe, A. M. 1984. Unilateral hearing impairment in children. Pediatrics 74:206.

Black, F. O., et al. 1971. Congenital Deafness: A New Approach to Early Detection of Deafness Using a High Risk Register. Boulder, CO, Associated University Press.

Bradford, B. C., Baudin, J., Conway, M. J., et al. 1985. Identification of sensorineural hearing loss in very preterm infants by brainstem auditory evoked potentials. Arch. Dis. Child. 60:105.

Chung, C. S., Robinson, O. W., and Morton, N. E. 1959. A note on deaf mutism. Ann. Hum. Genet. 23:357.

Conference on Hearing Screening Services for Preschool Children. Columbus, Ohio, 1977. Maternal and Child Health Bureau, HEW, Washington, D.C.

Costa, A., Cottino, F., Mortara, M., et al. 1964. Endemic cretinism in Piedmont. Panminerva Med. 6:250.

Dorph, S., Jensen, J., and Olgaard, A. 1973. Visualization of canaliculus cochleae by multidirectional tomography. Arch. Otolaryngol. 98:121.

Downs, M. P., and Silver, H. K. 1972. The ABCD's to H.E.A.R.: Early identification in nursery, office, and clinic of the infant who is deaf. Clin. Pediatr. 11:563.

Ebenson, A. 1963. Legal change for the handicapped through litigation. State-Federal Clearinghouse for Exceptional Children. The Council for Exceptional Children, Arlington, VA.

Erikson, E. 1963. Childhood and Society. New York, W. W. Norton.

Feinmesser, M., and Zelig, S. 1961. Congenital deafness associated with onychodystrophy. Arch. Otolaryngol. 74:507.

Fisch, L. 1955. The etiology of congenital deafness and audiometric patterns. J. Laryngol. 69:479.

Florman, A. L., et al. 1970. Response to rubella vaccine among seronegative children with congenital rubella. American Pediatric Society Abstracts, First Plenary Session, May.

Fraser, G. R. 1976. The causes of profound deafness in childhood. Baltimore, Johns Hopkins University Press.

Gates, G. A., Wachtendorf, C., Hearne, E. M., et al. 1985. Treatment of chronic otitis media with effusion: Results of tympanostomy tubes. Am. J. Otolaryngol. 6:249.

Grundfast, K. M. 1983. The role of the audiologist and otologist in the identification of the dysmorphic child. Ear Hear. 4:24.

Grundfast, K. M. 1988. Progressive sensorineural hearing loss. In Harker, L. (ed.): Otolaryngology—Head and Neck Surgery—Clinical Update. St. Louis, C. V. Mosby Co.

Grundfast, K., and Bluestone, C. D. 1978. Sudden or fluctuating hearing loss and vertigo in children due to perilymph fistula. Ann. Otol. Rhinol. Laryngol. 87:761.

Grundfast, K. M., and Carney, C. 1987. Ear Infections In Your Child. Hollywood, FL. Compact Books.

Gussen, R. 1981. Sudden hearing loss associated with cochlear membrane rupture. Arch. Otolaryngol. 107:598.

Hall, J. 1964. Cochlea and cochlear nuclei in asphyxia. Acta Otolaryngol. (Stockh.) Suppl. 194.

Hanson, D. G., and Ulvestad, R. F. 1979. Otitis media and child development—speech, language, and education. Ann. Otol. Rhinol. Laryngol. 88, Suppl. 60 (5).

Hausler, R., Toupet, M., Guidetti, G., et al. 1987. Meniere's Disease in Children. Am. J. Otolaryngol. 8:187.

Haymaker, et al. 1961. Pathology of Kernietenic and Postleteric Encephalopathy; Kernicterus. Springfield, IL, Charles C Thomas, pp. 22–230.

Healy, G. B., Friedman, J. M., and DiTrola, J. 1978. Ataxia and hearing loss secondary to perilymphatic fistula. Pediatrics 61:238.

Hinojosa, R. 1958. Pathohistological aural changes in the progeny of a mother with pseudohypoparathyroidism. Ann. Otol. Rhinol. Laryngol. 67:964.

Horton, K. B. 1975. Early intervention through parent training in sensorineural hearing loss in children. Otolaryngol. Clin. North Am. 8:143.

House, W. F., Berliner, K. I., and Eisenberg, L. S. 1983. Experiences with the cochlear implant in preschool children. Ann. Otol. Rhinol. Laryngol. 92:587.

House, W. F., Berliner, K. I., and Luxford, W. M. 1987. Cochlear implants in deaf children. Curr. Probl. Pediatr. 17:345.

Huizing, E. H., Van Bolhuis, A. H., and Odenthal, D. W. 1966. Studies on progressive hereditary perceptive deafness in a family of 335 members. Acta Otolaryngol. 61:35.

Hyde, M. L. 1985. Frequency-specific BERA in infants. J. Otolaryngol. 14:19.

Jaffe, B. F. 1977. Hearing Loss in Children—A Comprehensive Text. Baltimore, University Park Press.

Joint Committee on Infant Hearing, American Academy of Pediatrics. 1982. Position statement. Pediatrics 70:496.

Jørgensen, M. B. 1961. Influence of maternal diabetes on the inner ear of the foetus. Acta Otolaryngol. (Stockh.) 53:49.

Kanzaki, J. 1986. Idiopathic sudden progressive hearing loss and round window membrane rupture. Arch. Otorhinolaryngol. 243:158.

Karmody, C. S. 1968. Subclinical maternal rubella and congenital deafness. N. Engl. J. Med. 278:809.

Karmody, C. S., and Weinstein, L. 1978. Reversible sensorineural hearing loss with intravenous erythromycin lactobionate. Ann. Otol. Rhinol. Laryngol. 87:761.

Kelemen, G. 1960. Maternal diabetes. Changes in the hearing organ of the embryo: Additional observation. Arch. Otolaryngol. 71:921.

Keller, W. D., and Bundy, R. S. 1980. Effects of unilateral hearing loss upon educational achievement. Child Care Health Dev. 6:93.

Kirk, K. I., and Hill-Brown, C. 1985. Speech and language results in children with a cochlear implant. Ear Hear. 6(Suppl. 3):36S.

Kittel, G., and Saller, K. 1964. Ohrmissbildungen in Beziehung zu Thalidomid. Z. Laryngol. Rhinol. 43:469.

Klein, J. O. 1984. Otitis media and the development of speech and language. Pediatr. Infect. Dis. 3:389.

Konigsmark, B. W., and Gorlin, R. J. 1976. Genetic and Metabolic Deafness. Philadelphia, W. B. Saunders Co.

Kuriyama, M., Konishi, Y., and Mikawa, H. 1986. The effect of neonatal hyperbilirubinemia on the auditory brainstem response. Brain Dev. 8:240.

Levi, H., Tell, L., Feinmesser, M., et al. 1983. Early detection of hearing loss in infants by auditory nerve and brainstem responses. Audiology 22:181.

Luxford, W. M., and Sheehy, J. L. K. 1984. Ventilation tubes: Indications and complications. Am. J. Otol. 5:468.

Mandel, E. M., Bluestone, C. D., Paradise, J. L., et al. 1984. Efficacy of myringotomy with and without tympanostomy tube insertion in the treatment of chronic otitis media with effusion in infants and children. In Lim, D. J., Bluestone, C. D., Klein, J. O., et al. (eds.): Recent Advances in Otitis Media with Effusion. Toronto, B. C. Decker, pp. 308–312.

Matalon, R., Jacobson, C. B., and Dorfman, A. 1970. Prenatal diagnosis of the mucopolysaccharidoses by a chemical method. American Pediatric Society Abstracts, First Plenary Session, May.

Meyerhoff, W. L., Paparella, M. M., and Shea, D. 1978. Meniere's disease in children. Laryngoscope 88:1504.

Michaels, R. H. 1969. Immunologic aspects of congenital rubella. Pediatrics 43:339.

Miyamoto, R. T., Myres, W. A., Pope, M. L., et al. 1986. Cochlear implants for deaf children. Laryngoscope 96:990.

Molteni, R. 1977. Vertigo as a presenting symptom of multiple sclerosis in childhood. Am. J. Dis. Child. 131:553.

Moore, K. L. 1977. The Developing Human: Clinically Oriented Embryology. Philadelphia, W. B. Saunders Co.

Mowrer, O. H. 1960. Learning Theory and Behavior. New York, John Wiley & Sons.

Nadol, J. 1978. Hearing loss as a sequela of meningitis. Laryngoscope 88:739.

Nance, W. E., and Sweeney, A. 1975. Genetic factors in deafness of early life in sensorineural hearing loss in children: Early detection and intervention. Otolaryngol. Clin. North Am. 8:1.

Northern, J. L., and Downs, M. P. 1978. Hearing in Children. Baltimore, Williams & Wilkins Co.

Palfrey, J. S., Mervis, R. C., and Butler, J. A. 1978. New directions in the evaluation and education of handicapped children. N. Engl. J. Med. 298:819.

Partsch, J., and Maurer, H. 1963. Zur formalen Genese von Ohrmissbildungen bei der Thalidomid—Embriopathis. Arch. Ohr-Nas-Ukelk-Heilk 182:594.

Petroff, M. A., Simmons, F. B., and Winzelberg, J. 1986. Two emerging perilymph fistula "syndromes" in children. Laryngoscope 96:498.

Pransky, S., and Grundfast, K. M. 1987. Pneumatic otoscopy. J. Respir. Dis. 8:61.

Proctor, C. A., and Proctor, B. 1967. Understanding hereditary nerve deafness. Arch. Otolaryngol. 85:23.

Richterich, R., Van Mechelen, P., and Rossi, E. 1965. Refsum's disease (heredopathia atactica polyneuritiformis). Am. J. Med. 39:230.

Rose, S. P., Conneally, P. M., and Nance, N. E. 1976. Genetic analysis of childhood deafness. In Bess, F. H. (ed.): Childhood Deafness. New York, Grune & Stratton.

Rosenberg, A. L., Bergstrom, L., Troost, B. T., et al. 1970. Hyperuricemia and neurologic deficits—a family study. N. Engl. J. Med. 282:992.

Rosendal, T. 1963. Thalidomide and aplasia-hypoplasia of the otic labyrinth. Lancet 1:724.

Sanders, R., Durieu-Smith, A., Hyde, M., et al. 1985. Incidence of hearing loss in high-risk and intensive-care nursery infants. J. Otolaryngol. 14:28.

Sarno, C. N., and Clemis, J. D. 1980. A workable approach to the identification of neonatal hearing impairment. Laryngoscope 90:1313.

Schwartz, S. 1987. Choices in Deafness: A Parent's Guide. Kensington, MD, Woodbine House. Trade paperback.

Silkes, E. D., and Chabot, J. 1985. Progressive hearing loss following Haemophilus influenzae meningitis. Int. J. Pediatr. Otolaryngol. 9:249.

Stein, L., Clark, S., and Kraus, N. 1983. The hearing-impaired infant: Patterns of identification and habilitation. Ear Hear. 4:232.

Teng, Y. C., Liu, J. H., and Hsu, Y. H. 1962. Meningitis and deafness. Clin. Med. J. 81:127.

Terry, L. L., 1980. Support of programs for the communicatively disadvantaged child: Role of the private foundation. Ann. Otol. Rhinol. Laryngol. [Suppl.] 89(5 Pt. 2 Suppl. 74):5.

Valvassori, G. E., Naunton, R. F., and Lindsay, J. R. 1969. Inner ear anomalies: Clinical and histopathological considerations. Ann. Otol. Rhinol. Laryngol. 78:929–938.

Weider, D. J., and Musiek, F. E. 1984. Bilateral congenital oval window microfistulae in a mother and son. Laryngoscope 94:1455.

Whetnall, E., and Fry, D. B. 1964. The Deaf Child. Springfield, IL, Charles C Thomas, pp. 14–31.

Wtodyka, J. 1978. Studies on cochlear aqueduct patency. Ann. Otol. Rhinol. Laryngol. 87:22.

Chapter 15

VERTIGO

Sidney N. Busis, M.D.

Dizziness and disturbed balance are not infrequent complaints in childhood. Although the symptoms may seem to be frivolous and insignificant, they are of concern to the patient and the family, and they may be due to organic disease. Therefore, every child with these complaints deserves thoughtful evaluation. Vague symptoms of this nature may be attributable to anxiety, peripheral vestibular disorder, or central nervous system disease (Harrison, 1962; Busis, 1976; Beddoe, 1977).

True vertigo may be described as a hallucination consisting of an illusion of motion, which is usually rotatory but may be linear, and a sensation of disorientation in space. Lesions within the labyrinth of the inner ear produce this "true" vertigo, whereas lesions elsewhere may produce a variety of symptoms such as lightheadedness, swimming sensation, presyncope, disturbed consciousness, headache, pressure in the head, or poor balance called dysequilibrium. The latter suggests the possibility of a lesion along the eighth nerve.

Vertigo of labyrinthine origin is characterized by recurrent acute episodes with postural vertigo (vertigo produced by changing position) between attacks. On the other hand, sensations of dizziness and disturbance of balance due to central nervous system disease are likely to be persistent and progressive (Chap. 11).

The evaluation of the child complaining of dizziness should include history, physical examination, and tests of hearing and balance. Following the basic examination, further special studies, such as auditory evoked brain stem response (ABR) testing, imaging, and pediatric or neurologic consultation, may be considered (Chap. 9).

A detailed history is invaluable but, at times, difficult to obtain, especially when dealing with very young children. However, it is important to try to extract a subjective report from the child and to acquire an objective description of the child's problem from the family. Although specific symptoms are frequently difficult to elicit because even older children may be shy and vague, at times the child's account can be quite vivid and detailed. The parents may then be able to elaborate on the symptoms outlined by the patient. If the parents have witnessed few, if any, of the episodes of dizziness, they should be advised to try to record future episodes in detail, and they should be instructed as to how to observe the child for nystagmus during an episode of dizziness.

Historical data are helpful in deciding whether the child has an organic lesion. The following symptoms or observations suggest the presence of one.

1. Obvious fright, alarm, pallor, perspiration, nausea, or vomiting during an attack.

2. Objective alteration of balance with ataxia or falling.

3. Alteration in the level of consciousness or loss of consciousness. If there is confirmed loss of consciousness, the lesion is located in the central nervous system.

4. The presence of seizures or bizarre turning or circling movements suggests temporal lobe disease.

5. Abnormal tilting of the head or twisting of the neck in infants suggests the possibility of paroxysmal torticollis, which may be due to vestibular dysfunction.

6. Abnormal eye movements during an attack of dizziness, as witnessed by the family, suggest nystagmus indicative of organic disease.

Other data that are less specific but still helpful in determining the etiology of the dizziness include the following:

1. Chronology of symptoms: Are they progressive, increasing, or decreasing in frequency and intensity? Has the child had any similar complaints in the past that cleared spontaneously?

2. Headache or pain may be reflections of tension but may also suggest vascular or central nervous system disease.

3. Is there a family history of migraine?

4. Recurrent ear symptoms, such as hearing loss, tinnitus, autophony, or ear infections, suggest the possibility of an otologic etiology.

5. Physical trauma, drugs, and exposure to toxic fumes or chemicals could cause dizziness.

6. The general state of health of the child and her or his family is important to ascertain. There may be similar symptoms in other members of the family, suggesting that an environmental factor is present or that the symptoms represent a hereditary disorder.

7. Interpersonal relationships and the child's performance in school and behavior at home should be

explored, because problems in these areas frequently cause anxiety in the patient and family.

8. Another factor to consider is any litigation or possible litigation connected with the child's case. If such exists, the physician should be aware that this may influence the symptoms.

The physical examination includes a complete otorhinolaryngologic examination and a scan of the cranial nerves (Busis, 1973). Hearing should be tested by tuning forks and by complete audiologic evaluation. Auditory evoked brain stem response testing may be helpful. Considering that a cerebral cortical disorder may be present, it has been suggested that all children with vertigo have an electroencephalogram (Eviatar and Eviatar, 1977).

The vestibular examination includes examination for nystagmus in various directions of gaze and in different head and body positions, as well as the testing of balance by the Romberg test and the evaluation of gait. Tests of vestibular function should be performed. A young child, even an infant held in a parent's lap, may be turned in a rotating chair to evaluate the vestibular system. The presence of postrotatory nystagmus indicates vestibular activity. Electric recording of nystagmus by electronystagmography (ENG) may be accomplished in school-age children and in many preschool children as well. Most children will cooperate well enough to allow recording of pursuit movements by visually following a pendulum, optokinetic drum, or both. In addition, recordings can be made to determine whether there is any spontaneous nystagmus in various directions of gaze or whether there is nystagmus elicited by changing position. Caloric testing with recording of the induced nystagmus can usually be performed, even in the young child. Children normally have calorically induced nystagmus that is somewhat dysrhythmic and of wider amplitude and slower velocity than that found in adults. Examples of these patterns are pictured in Figures 15–1 and 15–2. This response may be due to incomplete maturation of central nervous system pathways, perhaps with incomplete myelination. Posturography (Black et al., 1977; Peeters et al., 1984; Norré et al., 1987), which consists of computer analysis of the Romberg test on a posture platform, may also be helpful in evaluating the child experiencing dizziness.

Dizziness may be the primary symptom or may accompany the following: middle-ear disease, benign paroxysmal vertigo of childhood, perilymph fistula, Ménière disease, disturbance of the vestibular cortex, paroxysmal torticollis in infancy, trauma, migraine, multiple sclerosis, and other diagnostic considerations.

Middle-Ear Disease

Eustachian tube dysfunction, with or without otitis media with effusion (secretory or serous otitis media), is perhaps the most common cause of vestibular disturbance in children. Children with otitis media with effusion, which is usually characterized by an auditory disorder, seldom complain of distinct vertigo. However, they frequently have abnormal balance as evidenced by awkwardness, clumsiness, and occasional falling (Chap. 21).

These symptoms are due to altered middle-ear pressure caused by eustachian tube dysfunction. Because this abnormality can be documented most consistently by tympanometry (Bluestone et al., 1973; Cantekin et al., 1977), every child who has any apparent vestibular disturbance should undergo this test. If the result is normal on the initial examination, the test should be repeated in a few weeks if symptoms persist. The symptoms of otitis media with effusion or negative pressure can be relieved by medical or surgical treatment. If medical treatment is unsuccessful, indwelling ventilating tympanostomy tubes are usually effective.

Acute or chronic purulent otitis media may produce secondary serous labyrinthitis with associated vestibular symptoms. In these patients, if response to medication is not prompt or spontaneous drainage is not adequate, a wide myringotomy should be performed. If there are signs or symptoms of an associated mastoiditis, the patient should have a mastoidectomy. Rarely, purulent otitis media may be followed by purulent labyrinthitis, which is accompanied initially by vertigo with subsequent complete loss of auditory and vestibular function (Chaps. 22 and 23).

The occurrence of a cholesteatoma is not uncommon in children. Although the cholesteatoma is often invasive, it seldom produces a fistula into the labyrinth, which would cause balance disturbance. However, in the vertiginous child with a chronically discharging ear, the possibility of a fistula must be considered, and careful microscopic examination, including a fistula test, should be performed. If a cholesteatoma is found, aggressive surgical removal is essential.

Benign Paroxysmal Vertigo of Childhood

Benign paroxysmal vertigo of childhood is a distinct entity that frequently causes dizziness in children. It usually occurs in early childhood and in preschool or early elementary school–age children, but also may occur in the older child and young teen-ager. The attacks that are often mistaken for seizures (Gomez and Klass, 1972; Eeg-Olofsson et al., 1982) are most probably due to vestibular dysfunction. Spontaneous complete recovery from the vertiginous episodes usually takes place over a period of several months to a year or two.

As initially described (Basser, 1964; Koenigsberger et al., 1970; Chutorian, 1972), and later discussed (Koehler, 1980; Eeg-Olofsson et al., 1982; Mira et al., 1984 a and b; Lanzi et al., 1986), the clinical features of benign paroxysmal vertigo include sudden abrupt attacks of dizziness that only last for a few seconds to a few minutes. These episodes, in which the child may cry out and lose balance, cause the child great fright and alarm. Concomitant autonomic symptoms, such as pallor and vomiting, may occur. Some children are

RIGHT COLD

LEFT COLD

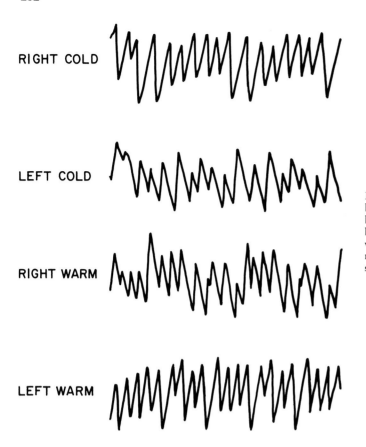

RIGHT WARM

LEFT WARM

Figure 15–1. Electronystagmographic recording of an alternate bithermal caloric test in an adult. The order of stimuli, top to bottom, is right cold (left-beating nystagmus); left cold (right-beating nystagmus); right warm (right-beating nystagmus); left warm (left-beating nystagmus). This is a normal tracing with regular, equal, and symmetric responses from each ear. The slow-phase velocity averages 42 degrees/second.

vivid in their descriptions of sensations of rotation and turning. Nystagmus may be present and discernible to an observer; the parents should be told about this possibility so that they can look for nystagmus in subsequent episodes and thus help confirm the diagnosis.

Children with benign paroxysmal vertigo have normal hearing, normal electroencephalograms, and normal imaging studies of the head. It had initially been reported that vestibular testing indicated decreased sensitivity of one vestibular system. Koenigsberger and colleagues (1970) compared a group of affected children with control subjects and found that there was a consistent bilateral or unilateral decrease of caloric response. Koehler (1980), using ice-cold water caloric tests without recording, also reported unilateral reduced response in one child and bilateral reduced response in two children in a series of eight patients. However, other investigators (Eeg-Olofsson et al., 1982; Mira et al., 1984a; Lanzi et al., 1986), using electronystagmography with bithermal caloric stimulation and rotation tests, did not find unilateral vestibular hypoactivity. The only ENG abnormality was positional nystagmus indicating vestibular dysfunction (Eeg-Olofsson et al., 1982).

Based on several factors, including a positive family history for migraine, associated autonomic dysfunction with vascular instability, a positive response to headache provocation tests (Mira et al., 1984a and b), the prior occurrence of paroxysmal torticollis of infancy (Eeg-Olofsson et al., 1982), and the subsequent development of true migraine (Koehler, 1980; Finkelhor

and Harker, 1987), it has been postulated that benign paroxysmal vertigo of childhood is a migraine equivalent or a migraine precursor.

The diagnosis of benign paroxysmal vertigo of childhood is based on the history as previously described and normal results of otologic, audiologic, and neurologic examination. Every child suspected of having this disorder should have vestibular tests because the test results, such as the finding of nystagmus, may confirm that the child has vestibular dysfunction. Clinical management consists primarily of reassuring the patient's family that there is no evidence of serious disease and that the symptoms are self-limited. However, if the patient and the family are not coping, then vestibular suppressant medication (dimenhydrinate) should be considered for relief of symptoms.

Perilymph Fistula

It is well recognized that perilymph fistulas can account for hearing loss and dizziness in adults. Fistulas have been demonstrated as the cause of dizziness and ataxia, as well as hearing loss, in children in a number of instances (Stroud and Calcaterra, 1970; Grundfast and Bluestone, 1978; Supance and Bluestone, 1983; Petroff et al., 1986). Therefore, it is important to be aware of this possibility when making a diagnosis in the child experiencing dizziness (Chap. 19).

Labyrinthine membrane ruptures may occur not only at the inner ear–middle ear interface, producing

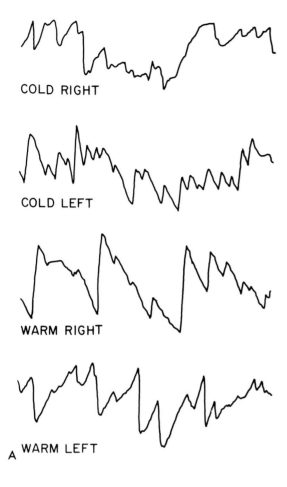

COLD RIGHT

COLD LEFT

WARM RIGHT

A WARM LEFT

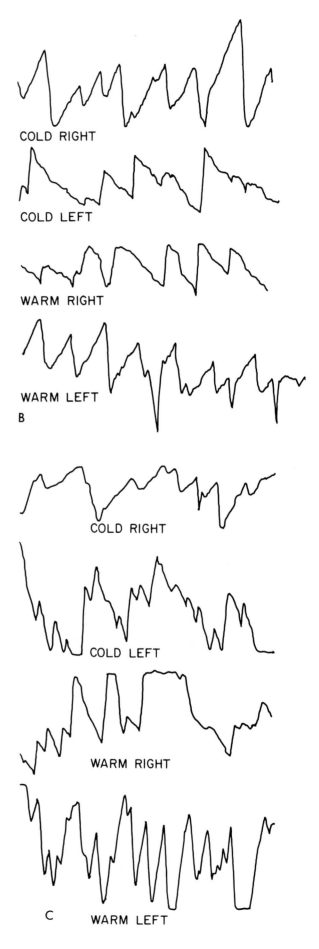

COLD RIGHT

COLD LEFT

WARM RIGHT

WARM LEFT

B

COLD RIGHT

COLD LEFT

WARM RIGHT

C   WARM LEFT

Figure 15–2. *A*, Four-year-old boy complaining of recurrent dizziness. This caloric test result, in contrast to the normal adult tracing in Figure 15–1, demonstrates somewhat dysrhythmic responses of wide amplitude and slower velocity. This tracing, which indicates equal response from each ear, is considered to be within normal limits for a child. *B*, Similar tracing demonstrating the same wide amplitude and slower velocity in a 6-year-old boy. *C*, A 6-year-old child complaining of vertigo. In this tracing, in addition to the pattern noted above, there is decreased sensitivity of the right vestibular labyrinth, indicating an organic vestibular lesion.

a fistula (usually of the oval or round window), but also within the labyrinth itself, probably in Reissner membrane and possibly in the basilar membrane. Breaks within the labyrinth most probably account for hearing loss by allowing a mixing of endolymph and perilymph to occur (Goodhill et al., 1973; Simmons, 1978). A leak of perilymph into the middle ear may cause balance disturbance, ataxia, and vertigo and possibly hearing loss.

A fluctuating sensorineural hearing loss may be explained on the basis of repeated, small, intralabyrinthine breaks that heal spontaneously. On the other hand, persistent balance disturbance (with or without hearing loss) may be explained on the basis of a continuous leakage of perilymph into the middle ear.

Membrane ruptures may occur spontaneously or may follow physical strain or stress (Goodhill, 1971) in which an increase in intralabyrinthine pressure occurs. This may be attributable to an increase in pressure either within the cranial cavity or within the middle-ear space. The former, described as "explosive" (Goodhill et al., 1973), may follow elevated cerebrospinal fluid pressure, which causes an increase in perilymphatic pressure, or elevated cranial venous pressure. The latter, caused by increased middle-ear pressure, described as "implosive" (Goodhill et al., 1973), may follow an alteration in middle-ear pressure, such as that occurring in barotrauma (Knight, 1977).

There may be at least two routes for transmission of cerebrospinal fluid pressure to the perilymph. Some pressure transmission may take place through the internal auditory canal, but the primary route for transmission of pressure is through the cochlear aqueduct. It has been demonstrated that the infantile cochlear aqueduct is larger and more patulous than the adult cochlear aqueduct; thus, it is understandable that, in some children, pressure differentials will enhance the probability of a membrane rupture within the labyrinth as a result of increased cerebrospinal fluid pressure. Because a great many children are subjected to frequent great physical stresses and suffer no ill effects, there must be an individual predisposition (such as a congenital abnormality of the ear) to account for the formation of fistulas in certain children.

Dizziness due to a labyrinthine fistula may occur alone, as episodes of vertigo and balance disturbance, or with an associated sensorineural hearing loss. Supance and Bluestone (1983) reported that in a series of 33 infants and children on whom exploratory tympanotomies for fistula were performed, ten had histories of vertigo prior to tympanotomy. Of these, four were found to have a fistula, and all of these children had relief of vertigo. However, of the six who did not have a fistula, three also reported relief of vertigo.

There are no symptoms pathognomonic of a perilymph fistula; however, several features of the history are suggestive.

1. A history of head injury, physical strain or stress, exposure to sudden alterations in environmental pressure (e.g., diving or flying), or marked alteration in middle-ear pressures (e.g., violent sneezing, laughing, or blowing a wind instrument).

2. Continuous dizziness, which may be increased by postural change, or continuous poor balance or ataxia, especially following any of the preceding.

3. A sensorineural hearing loss that fluctuates in degree, that is progressive, or both (Petroff et al., 1986).

4. "Sudden" sensorineural hearing loss; however, the suddenness may be difficult to define, because children frequently are unable to express a specific onset or time frame.

5. A sensation of a "pop" in the ear followed by hearing loss or dizziness.

6. A prior history of recurrent meningitis, convulsions, or aural discharge suggestive of cerebrospinal fluid otorrhea.

7. The complaint that loud sounds produce dizziness. This may be explained on the basis of the stapedial reflex increasing an oval window leak.

Certain physical findings are suggestive of the diagnosis of perilymph fistula.

1. Continuous vestibular dysfunction as evidenced by the following: (a) persistent spontaneous nystagmus noted with eyes open or on ENG recording with eyes closed; nystagmus produced by position change, and (b) poor balance, ataxia, or both on physical examination (Healy et al., 1978). The patient may demonstrate an abnormality on the Romberg or tandem Romberg test or on gait testing. With a labyrinthine disorder, the patient tends to fall to one side and has more difficulty in maintaining balance in the dark. In cerebellar ataxia, the tendency to fall in one direction and the influence of darkness are less marked. Ataxia due to proprioceptive dysfunction may be similar to labyrinthine ataxia. However, in the former, there is usually some other manifestation of a proprioceptive deficit, such as disturbed position sense.

2. An unexplained sensorineural hearing loss that may be moderate in degree and associated with poor speech discrimination (if testable) or a profound loss of auditory function.

3. An abnormal fistula test result can be elicited by using a pneumatic otoscope or a tympanometer with ENG recording of eye movements. To be considered abnormal, a fistula test response must include not only the patient's report of dizziness but also the occurrence of eye movements following ear canal pressure change. The detection of these eye movements can be facilitated by electronystagmography. Occasionally, head movements may also occur following a pressure change in the external auditory canal. Fistula tests are not definitive, and there may be false-positive or false-negative results. Therefore, they are of questionable diagnostic value.

4. Congenital abnormalities of the head or imaging studies (tomography, computed tomography scan, or magnetic resonance imaging) that reveal congenital abnormalities of the temporal bone. Supance and Bluestone (1983) report that Mondini or Mondini-like inner-ear dysplasia possibly predisposes to the development of perilymph fistulas.

5. Caloric testing responses recorded by ENG may

demonstrate a decreased response of one vestibular labyrinth. If this unilateral depression of vestibular function is combined with spontaneous and positional nystagmus, the likelihood of a fistula is greater, but not certain.

If a sudden-onset perilymph fistula is suspected after physical exertion or barotrauma, the immediate treatment is complete bed rest with the head elevated and careful observation. Hearing may return to normal, and vertigo may gradually subside. If this occurs, no further treatment is necessary. However, if this does not occur, exploratory tympanotomy should be considered.

If there is suspicion of a perilymph fistula based on the risk factors previously described, an exploratory tympanotomy should also be considered. Petroff and associates (1986) pointed out that a normal exploration result does not mean that a fistula does not exist. Fistulas may be intermittent, and therefore a second exploratory tympanotomy should be considered in certain cases. Closure of a perilymph leak may control the dizziness, but it is less probable that it will improve hearing. In 44 operated ears, Supance and Bluestone (1983) reported improved hearing in 5 per cent but poorer hearing in 9 per cent with surgical closure.

Ménière Disease

Ménière disease may occur in children (Meyerhoff et al., 1978; Filipo and Barbara, 1985; Hausler et al., 1987). Although there are several reports of its occurrence in preschool and early elementary school–age children, it is more likely to occur in children over the age of 10 years. In a small percentage of patients, the disease may be bilateral (Kitahara et al., 1978).

As in adults, Ménière disease in children is characterized by a triad of symptoms: dizziness, hearing loss, and tinnitus. The dizziness occurs in clusters of acute attacks, each marked by severe vertigo, frequently accompanied by autonomic symptoms of pallor, perspiration, nausea, or vomiting. Between these acute episodes, the patient may have vague symptoms of disturbed balance.

The hearing loss is a sensorineural loss, frequently accompanied by paracusis (distorted hearing) and diplacusis (hearing a different pitch in each ear). The hearing loss characteristically fluctuates in degree. It has been reported that a difference between Ménière disease in children and that in adults may be that children are more likely to recover auditory function than are adults.

Tinnitus is usually low pitched and roaring, frequently likened to the sound of a seashell held against the ear. The tinnitus may change in pitch or intensity prior to an attack and so serve as an aura preceding vertigo. This is not usually reported by children.

Objective evidence, if attainable, includes a flat, low-tone, sensorineural hearing loss on audiologic examination, with the results of special tests indicating a cochlear disorder. Vestibular testing by electronystag-mography may reveal spontaneous nystagmus and decreased function of one vestibular labyrinth. These abnormalities may not be present and are not essential for the diagnosis. Vestibular dysfunction is manifested by the presence of nystagmus during an attack of vertigo. The child's family and teacher should be alerted to the possibility of nystagmus, because it is unlikely that the physician will have the opportunity to observe the child during an attack.

Filipo and Barbara (1985) reported five cases of Ménière disease in children (aged 9 to 17 years), representing 7 per cent of all of their cases of Ménière disease. They emphasized the importance of dehydration procedures (glycerol test) in confirming the diagnosis and believed that the glycerol test is more helpful in children than it is in adults.

Hausler and associates (1987) reported on 14 children (7 to 14 years of age) studied in four neurootologic centers. Nine of these children had what the authors classified as idiopathic Ménière disease, whereas the remaining five children were classified as having "secondary Ménière's syndrome" because their initial hearing losses followed a specific event such as mumps, meningitis, and temporal bone fracture. These 14 children represented 1 per cent of all of Hausler and associates' patients with idiopathic or secondary Ménière disease in the previous 5 years. Their patients met the requirements for diagnosis of the Committee on Hearing and Equilibrium of the American Academy of Otolaryngology (Pearson and Brackmann, 1985). In regard to etiology, they postulated that, as occurred in their five cases of "secondary Ménière's syndrome," an insult to the ear is the etiologic factor and that, because the time between this insult and the first symptom of Ménière disease can be lengthy, the relationship may not be recognized. They concluded that Ménière disease in childhood is indistinguishable from the condition in adults and that the incidence in children is about 100 times less than in adults.

Medical management consists of reassuring the patient and the family, treatment of any associated systemic disorder, and medication (dimenhydrinate) in graduated doses according to age. Filipo and Barbara (1985) considered the use of diuretics to be the most effective medical management. In some instances, vertiginous episodes may continue and become incapacitating. In these patients, Meyerhoff and coworkers (1978) have reported gratifying results with endolymphatic mastoid shunt operations. Before considering surgery, the child should be completely reevaluated pediatrically, neurologically, and radiologically, as well as otologically, to validate the diagnosis.

Disturbance of the Vestibular Cortex

Although there may be additional cortical vestibular representation on the inferior part of the postcentral gyrus, the main vestibular projection area appears to be on the anterior end of the supratemporal gyrus of the temporal lobe. Therefore, cortical dysfunction in this area may be associated with vertiginous symptoms. The dysfunction may be due to epilepsy, tumor, or concussion.

In a detailed study of 666 patients with temporal lobe epilepsy, Currie and colleagues (1971) reported that 12 per cent of those studied were under the age of 10 years and 14 per cent were under the age of 15 years; the youngest patient was 1 year old. The incidence of vertigo as an associated symptom in the total series was 19 per cent, but as an isolated symptom it occurred much less frequently.

The diagnosis of temporal lobe epilepsy, complex partial seizures, in a child experiencing dizziness is suggested by the presence of other symptoms or signs. More than 75 per cent of these patients have loss of consciousness during seizure, and others have altered consciousness with disturbance in thinking. There is a high incidence of associated visceral complaints, such as abdominal discomfort. Special sensory symptoms, such as visual or auditory hallucinations (or both) and unpleasant olfactory or gustatory sensations, frequently occur. There may also be motor phenomena, speech disorders, and emotional upsets. The results of electroencephalography may be helpful in making the diagnosis. However, a child with temporal lobe epilepsy may have a normal electroencephalogram (EEG). Nystagmus is not a feature of temporal lobe epilepsy, which is due to a primary abnormal cortical discharge and does not involve the brain stem directly. On the other hand, vestibulogenic epilepsy, in which epileptiform attacks are precipitated by stimulation of the labyrinth, is accompanied by nystagmus because the brain stem is involved. Idiopathic vestibulogenic temporal lobe seizures are rare. They may follow vestibular testing. Sherman and Easton (1976), in a discussion of the differential diagnosis of syncope, pointed out that akinetic seizures, brief attacks of unconsciousness with loss of muscle tone, occur primarily in children and may be confused with syncope.

In the study of Currie and colleagues (1971), 9.5 per cent of all children with temporal lobe epilepsy were found to have tumors. Schneider and coworkers (1968) and Schneider (1978), in a study of 46 patients who were operated on for the treatment of intractable temporal lobe seizures, found 12 temporal lobe tumors. Seven of the patients who had tumors had vertigo either as a presenting complaint or as a conspicuous symptom. In several cases, the vertigo had begun in early childhood. These young patients frequently exhibited bizarre turning patterns and associated auditory and visual hallucinations. Some experienced altered consciousness with trancelike states, memory impairment, and aphasia. Because vertigo may be a prominent symptom early in the course of a temporal lobe tumor, it is important to consider this possibility, especially if there is any suggestion of other temporal lobe dysfunction as described previously.

Head injury, particularly a blow to the occiput, may produce a contrecoup injury to the temporal lobe vestibular cortex as it strikes the sphenoid ridge (Schneider et al., 1968). This may account for postcon-

cussion syndrome vertigo. In the series of Currie and colleagues (1971), 7 per cent were found to have a significant head injury, which was considered to have some etiologic relationship to the problem. The possibility of temporal lobe concussion is being recognized more frequently by specialists in sports medicine, and it is suggested that clinical traumatic syndromes that include dizziness may, at times, be neurologic rather than otologic in origin.

Paroxysmal Torticollis in Infancy

Paroxysmal torticollis is an unusual syndrome occurring in infants and may be due to vestibular dysfunction (Gourley, 1971). There are episodes in which the infant holds the head tilted to one side or the other, frequently rotating it to the opposite side. At the onset, there may be vomiting and pallor, and the baby may appear to be quite agitated, especially when an attempt is made to straighten the head. The episodes are brief and self-limited and may recur over a period of several months or, in some children, a few years. Aside from torticollis, physical examination reveals no other abnormalities.

Snyder (1969) reported a series of 12 cases in which the attacks lasted from 10 minutes to 14 days, recurring for varying lengths of time. In children in whom the attacks lasted until speech was present, four complained that they were dizzy and that the "house was turning."

It has been suspected that this ailment is in some way related to benign paroxysmal vertigo that occurs later in childhood. Mira and associates (1984a) postulated that both paroxysmal torticollis in infancy and benign paroxysmal vertigo in childhood may be migraine equivalents or migraine precursors. It has been suggested that these episodes are vascular in origin (Mira et al., 1984a; Eeg-Olofsson et al., 1982), and it has further been suggested that as the brain stem develops there is a progression from paroxysmal torticollis to benign paroxysmal vertigo to migraine.

However, it has also been reported that paroxysmal torticollis may be related to gastroesophageal reflux and hiatal hernia (Sandifer syndrome) (Ramenofsky et al., 1978). In infancy, reflux of gastric contents into the esophagus may occur in a significant number of infants. Normally the pH of the esophagus is neutral, thus acid stomach contents entering the esophagus are irritating, and it is postulated that this stimulus in the esophagus and in the pharynx may reflexively produce torticollis. In consideration of this possibility, in the patient with suspected paroxysmal torticollis, a pH determination of the upper esophagus should be obtained to ascertain whether there is significant acidity.

Trauma

Head trauma may cause perilymph fistula, temporal lobe concussion, temporal bone fracture, or labyrinthine concussion.

Fractures of the temporal bone may be longitudinal or transverse. Any temporal bone injury can cause initial acute vertigo followed by postural dizziness. Longitudinal fractures are usually accompanied by a conductive hearing impairment without loss of cochlear function. Transverse fractures, on the other hand, may involve the cochlea, producing a profound sensorineural hearing loss (Chap. 26).

Vartiainen and associates (1985) studied 61 children (age 16 years or younger) who had experienced blunt head injuries. Although spontaneous nystagmus, positional nystagmus, or both were found on ENG recording in almost half the children, few complained of dizziness immediately after the injury; after 6 months only 1.5 per cent had dizziness. Vartiainen and coworkers noted that Meran and colleagues (1978) had reported that 76 per cent of their adult patients had vestibular symptoms 6 months after head injury. Vartiainen and associates (1985) concluded that after head injury children appear to have as frequent objective signs of injury but much fewer symptoms. It was also their impression that "psychosocial factors" play a significant role in the occurrence of late vestibular symptoms in adults but not in children (Vartiainen et al., 1985). It is also recognized that compensation from vestibular injury occurs much more rapidly in children than in adults. Vartiainen and coworkers (1985) also noted that their findings indicated that high-frequency hearing loss and vestibular disorders caused by head injury seem to be independent of each other. None of the control group patients in this study had any spontaneous or positional nystagmus or canal paresis.

Because labyrinthine concussion may be present without a discernible fracture or other abnormalities on physical examination, tests of vestibular function should be performed on the child complaining of dizziness following head trauma. Electronystagmography performed with the eyes closed or in a darkened room may reveal spontaneous or positional nystagmus or both and hypoactivity of one vestibular labyrinth. Vartiainen and associates (1985) reported that shortly after head injury, about 20 per cent of patients had reduced caloric response on one side on ENG recording. Six to 12 months after the injury, this percentage dropped to 6 to 7 per cent. Rotation testing may also indicate abnormalities in the vestibular system. Testing of the vestibular system is especially important if litigation is a possibility.

Migraine

Migraine has been reported to occur in children much more frequently than was originally suspected (Gomez and Klass, 1972; Watson and Steele, 1974; Saper, 1978). Because vertigo may be a feature of classic migraine or migraine equivalent, the diagnostic possibility of migraine should be considered in the child experiencing dizziness. Classic migraine is accompanied by headache, whereas migraine equivalent may not be (Chap. 33).

Watson and Steele (1974) studied 286 children with migraine, of whom 66 experienced true vertigo. Of these, 43 had accompanying headache and other neurologic signs and symptoms of classic migraine, and 23 had migraine equivalents without headache. Over half of these children with classic migraine had basilar artery migraine accompanied by signs and symptoms of brain stem dysfunction. These included weakness and paresthesias of the extremities, diplopia, and other visual disturbances.

The diagnosis of vertigo due to migraine without headache is tenable if the patient has accompanying transient neurologic abnormalities, such as weakness of the extremities, slurred speech, sensory changes, or hallucinations. Episodes of dizziness, which may be abrupt, lasting several minutes, are associated with prostration, pallor, nausea and vomiting, and frequently abdominal pain. A family history of migraine is strongly supportive of this diagnosis in the child.

The symptom complex of migraine equivalent may be similar to that of temporal lobe epilepsy. With epilepsy, there is more likely to be altered consciousness, whereas with migraine there may be a strong family history. Motor phenomena may occur with either.

Because there is also similarity between these episodes and benign paroxysmal vertigo of childhood, migraine equivalent may be related to or may be a cause of benign paroxysmal vertigo (Koehler, 1980; Mira et al., 1984a).

Multiple Sclerosis

Vertigo may be a presenting symptom of multiple sclerosis. Molteni (1977) reported that in a series of 14 cases of childhood multiple sclerosis, vertigo was a presenting symptom in four. When combined with the findings of others, this suggests that the incidence of vertigo as the presenting symptom in multiple sclerosis is approximately 20 per cent. In the evaluation of the child with unexplained dizziness, the possibility of multiple sclerosis should be considered.

Vertigo in multiple sclerosis is due to an area of demyelination or plaque formation in the region of the vestibular nuclei. Nystagmus and ataxia are likely to accompany vertigo; however, they more frequently occur independently. Because of the exacerbation and remission pattern characteristic of multiple sclerosis, the episodes of vertigo may be relatively brief, sporadic, and isolated and are likely to be attributed to other causes. This type of vertigo is not accompanied by hearing loss or tinnitus, but associated syncope or convulsions may occur.

Although multiple sclerosis is a rare diagnosis in pediatric practice, childhood onset of this disease has been estimated to occur in 0.4 to 10 per cent of all cases of multiple sclerosis (Molteni, 1977). Physicians should be alert to the possibility that an isolated episode of dizziness without associated symptoms or signs could be the first evidence of this disease.

Other Diagnostic Considerations

In children, especially in the school-age child, dizziness may be a manifestation of anxiety, tension, hyperventilation, or drug intoxication.

Children are frequently under great pressure at home and at school (Fried, 1980). There are many divorces, single-parent families, two-career families, and day care centers, all of which can produce tension in a child. There are also parental and teacher demands to achieve and to excel. This buffeting of a child can cause great anxiety, manifested by dizziness as well as other symptoms.

Certain classes of drugs, such as aminoglycosides, are ototoxic. Barbiturates frequently cause nystagmus and anticonvulsive medication, such as phenytoin, may cause ataxia. The older child may be using street drugs that may produce vestibular disturbances. Therefore, the evaluation of every child with dizziness should include questions about possible drug ingestion, and, if there is uncertainty about this possibility, blood levels for specific drugs can be obtained.

In the child with disturbed balance without clear-cut episodes of dizziness, the possibility of familial ataxia, pontine tumor, or cerebellar disease should be considered. In addition, balance disturbance may be present in hydrocephalus. In these patients, Painter (1978) notes that there may be pressure on the cerebellar afferent pathways as they sweep around the lateral horns (Chap. 27). Epidemic vertigo on a viral basis has been reported by Williams (1963).

Children wearing hearing aids may experience dizziness owing to an excessively high sound pressure level. This is likely to occur if amplification is about 120 dB in an ear with a sensory hearing impairment.

There has been considerable interest and publicity about the relationship between vestibular disturbance and learning disabilities or attention deficit disorder (ADD). Silver (1986) presented an excellent review of this entire subject. He described the origin of the terms minimal brain damage, minimal cerebral dysfunction, minimal brain dysfunction, dyslexia, dyscalculia, dysgraphia, and the currently recommended terms learning disability or specific learning disability. Children formerly called hyperactive, hyperkinetic, or distractable are now included under attention deficit disorder (ADD). These two conditions are frequently seen in the same child.

Silver (1986) described the generally acceptable therapies and those that are controversial. Those that are considered acceptable are special education, psychostimulants, and psychologic treatment. The controversial therapies include two classes of treatment: neurophysiologic retraining and orthomolecular medicine. Vestibular therapy is one of the methods of neurophysiologic retraining. The others described are patterning and optometric visual training. In his discussion of vestibular dysfunction, Silver (1986) recognized that investigators have suggested that vestibular system dysfunction is the cause of learning disabilities in certain children. Silver (1986) discussed the re-

ported investigations, reviewed the literature, and concluded that, in regard to learning disabilities, "at this time there is no evidence supportive of the vestibular theories nor of the proposed treatment approaches."

SELECTED REFERENCES

Currie, S., Heathfield, K. W. G., Henson, R. A., et al. 1971. Clinical course and prognosis of temporal lobe epilepsy. Brain 94:173.

Extensive survey of 660 patients, mostly adults, with temporal lobe epilepsy. Clinical features, including the types of components of seizures, electroencephalographic findings, etiologic factors, management, and outcome are discussed.

Koenigsberger, M. R., Chutorian, A. M., Gold, A. P., et al. 1970. Benign paroxysmal vertigo of childhood. Neurology 20:1108.

A study of 17 children with paroxysmal vertigo and a control group. A thoughtful review of the literature and discussion of an entity that is clinically recognizable but perhaps not as frequent as originally thought.

Schneider, R. C., Calhoun, H. D., and Crosby, E. C. 1968. Vertigo and rotational movement in cortical and subcortical lesions. J. Neurol. Sci. 6:493.

A pioneering clinical study that emphasizes the importance of considering possible temporal lobe disease in patients with vertigo and balance disturbance. In 26 patients operated on for intractable temporal lobe seizures, 12 were found to have temporal lobe tumors. Of these, seven had vertigo either as a presenting complaint or as a prominent symptom. Temporal lobe trauma as a possible cause of postconcussion vertigo is also discussed. An important article stressing the relationship between cortical dysfunction and balance disturbances.

Silver, L. B. 1986. Controversial approaches to treating learning disabilities and attention deficit disorder. Am. J. Dis. Child. 140:1045.

An excellent update on learning disabilities and attention deficit disorder. He discusses with great clarity the definitions of these diagnoses, generally accepted therapies, and controversial therapies. The generally accepted therapies are special education, psychostimulants, and psychologic treatment. There are two classes of controversial therapies, neurophysiologic retraining and orthomolecular medicine. Neurophysiologic retraining includes patterning, optometric visual training, and vestibular dysfunction. Orthomolecular medicine includes megavitamins, trace elements, and hypoglycemia. This article is a "must" for those interested in learning disabilities and attention deficit disorder.

Supance, J. S., and Bluestone, C. D. 1983. Perilymph fistulas in infants and children. Otol. Head Neck Surg. 91:663.

Based on the experience with 33 infants (44 ears) operated on over a 6-year period, Supance and Bluestone present current thinking in regard to perilymph fistulas. They discuss classification, pathogenesis, diagnostic measures, and management.

Watson, P., and Steele, J. C. 1974. Paroxysmal dysequilibrium in the migraine syndrome of childhood. Arch. Otolaryngol. 99:177.

A study of 286 children with migraine, 66 of whom experienced true vertigo. Of these, 43 had accompanying headache and other neurologic signs and symptoms of classic migraine, and 23 had migraine equivalents without headaches. An excellent review of migraine in children.

REFERENCES

Basser, L. S. 1964. Benign paroxysmal vertigo of childhood. Brain 87:111.

Beddoe, G. M. 1977. Vertigo in childhood. Otolaryngol. Clin. North Am. 10:139.

Black, F. O., O'Leary, D. P., Wall, C., III, et al. 1977. The vestibulospinal stability test: Normal limits. Trans. Am. Acad. Ophthalmol. Otolaryngol. 84:549.

Bluestone, C. D., Beery, Q. C., and Paradise, J. L. 1973. Audiometry and tympanometry in relation to middle ear effusions in children. Laryngoscope 83:594.

Busis, S. N. 1973. Diagnostic evaluation of the patient presenting with vertigo. Otolaryngol. Clin. North Am. 6:3.

Busis, S. N. 1976. Vertigo in children. Pediatr. Ann. 5:478.

Cantekin, F. I., Bluestone, C. D., Saez, C. A., et al. 1977. Normal and abnormal middle ear ventilation. Ann. Otol. Rhinol. Laryngol. 86:1.

Chutorian, A. M. 1972. Benign paroxysmal vertigo of childhood. Dev. Med. Child Neurol. 14:513.

Currie, S., Heathfield, K. W. G., Henson, R. A., et al. 1971. Clinical course and prognosis of temporal lobe epilepsy. Brain 94:173.

Eeg-Olofsson, O., Odkvist, L., Lindskog, U., et al. 1982. Benign paroxysmal vertigo in childhood. Acta Otolaryngol. 93:283.

Eviatar, L., and Eviatar, A. 1977. Vertigo in children: Differential diagnosis and treatment. Pediatrics 59:833.

Filipo, R., and Barbara, M. 1985. Juvenile Meniere's disease. J. Laryngol. Otol. 99:193.

Finkelhor, B. K., and Harker, L. A. 1987. Benign paroxysmal vertigo of childhood. Laryngoscope 97:1161.

Fried, M. P. 1980. The evaluation of dizziness in children. Laryngoscope 90:1548.

Gomez, M. R., and Klass, D. W. 1972. Seizures and other paroxysmal disorders in infants and children. Curr. Probl. Pediatr. 2:3.

Goodhill, V. 1971. Sudden deafness and round window rupture. Laryngoscope 81:1462.

Goodhill, V., Brockman, S. J., Harris, I., et al. 1973. Sudden deafness and labyrinthine window ruptures. Ann. Otol. Rhinol. Laryngol. 82:2.

Gourley, I. M. 1971. Paroxysmal torticollis in infancy. Can. Med. Assoc. J. 105:504.

Grundfast, K. M., and Bluestone, C. D. 1978. Sudden or fluctuating hearing loss and vertigo in children due to perilymph fistula. Ann. Otol. Rhinol. Laryngol. 87:761.

Harrison, M. S. 1962. Vertigo in childhood. J. Laryngol. 76:601.

Hausler, R., Toupet, M., Guidetti, G., et al. 1987. Meniere's disease in children. Am. J. Otolaryngol. 8:187.

Healy, G. B., Friedman, J. M., and DiTroia, J. 1978. Ataxia and hearing loss secondary to perilymphatic fistula. Pediatrics 61:238.

Kitahara, M., Matsubara, T., Takeda, T., et al. 1978. Bilateral Meniere's disease. Abstracts, Barany Society Ordinary Meeting in Uppsala, Sweden, June 1–3, pp. 39–40.

Knight, N. J. 1977. Severe sensorineural deafness in children due to perforation of the round-window membrane. Lancet 2:1003.

Koehler, B. 1980. Benign paroxysmal vertigo of childhood: A migraine equivalent. Eur. J. Pediatr. 134:149.

Koenigsberger, M. R., Chutorian, A. M., Gold, A. P., et al. 1970. Benign paroxysmal vertigo of childhood. Neurology 20:1108.

Lanzi, G., Ballottin, U., Fazzi, E., et al. 1986. Benign paroxysmal vertigo in childhood: A longitudinal study. Headache 26:494.

Meran, A., Rohner, Y., and Pfaltz, C. 1978. Zur Symptomatologie und Diagnostik der vestibularen Funktionstorungen nach Schadelhirntrauma. HNO 26:41.

Meyerhoff, W. L., Paparella, M. M., and Shea, D. 1978. Meniere's disease in children. Presented at the Southern Section of the American Laryngological, Rhinological and Otological Society Inc., Houston, TX, January 13.

Mira, E., Piacentino, G., Lanzi, G., et al. 1984a. Benign paroxysmal vertigo in childhood: A migraine equivalent. ORL Otorhinolaryngol. Relat. Spec. 56:97.

Mira, E., Piacentino, G., Lanzi, G., et al. 1984b. Benign paroxysmal vertigo in childhood. Acta Otolaryngol. [Suppl.] (Stockh.) 406:271.

Molteni, R. A. 1977. Vertigo as a presenting symptom of multiple sclerosis in childhood. Am. J. Dis. Child. 131:553.

Norre, M. E., Forrez, G., and Beckers, A. 1987. Benign paroxysmal positional vertigo. Clinical observations by vestibular habituation training and by posturography. J. Laryngol. Otol. 101:443.

Painter, M. J. 1978. Personal communication regarding balance disturbance associated with hydrocephalus.

Pearson, B. W., and Brackmann, D. E. 1985. Committee on Hearing and Equilibrium guidelines for reporting treatment results in Meniere's disease. Otolaryngol. Head Neck Surg. 93:579.

Peeters, H., Breslau, E., Mol, J., et al. 1984. Analysis of posturographic measurements on children. Med. Biol. Eng. Comput. 22:317.

Petroff, M. A., Simmons, F. B., and Winzelberg, J. 1986. Two emerging perilymph fistula "syndromes" in children. Laryngoscope 96:498.

Ramenofsky, M. L., Buyse, M., Goldberg, M. J., et al. 1978. Gastroesophageal reflux and torticollis. J. Bone Joint Surg. 604:1140.

Saper, J. R. 1978. Migraine. J.A.M.A. 239:2380.

Schneider, R. C. 1978. Personal communication regarding temporal lobe concussion.

Schneider, R. C., Calhoun, H. D., and Crosby, E. C. 1968. Vertigo and rotational movement in cortical and subcortical lesions. J. Neurol. Sci. 6:493.

Sherman, D. G., and Easton, J. D. 1976. Syncope. J. Fam. Pract. 3:419.

Silver, L. B. 1986. Controversial approaches to treating learning disabilities and attention deficit disorder. Am. J. Dis. Child. 140:1045.

Simmons, F. B. 1978. Fluid dynamics in sensorineural hearing loss. Otolaryngol. Clin. North Am. 11:55.

Snyder, C. H. 1969. Paroxysmal torticollis in infancy. Am. J. Dis. Child. 117:458.

Stroud, M. H., and Calcaterra, T. C. 1970. Spontaneous perilymph fistulas. Laryngoscope 80:479.

Supance, J. S., and Bluestone, C. D. 1983. Perilymph fistulas in infants and children. Otolaryngol. Head Neck Surg. 91:663.

Vartiainen, E., Karjalainen, S., and Karja, J. 1985. Vestibular disorders following head injury in children. Int. J. Pediatr. 9:135.

Watson, P., and Steele, J. C. 1974. Paroxysmal dysequilibrium in the migraine syndrome of childhood. Arch. Otolaryngol. 99:177.

Williams, S. 1963. Epidemic vertigo in children. Med. J. Aust. 2:660.

Chapter 16

TINNITUS IN CHILDREN

F. Owen Black, M.D.   David J. Lilly, Ph.D.

> Why is it that the buzzing in the ears ceases if one makes a sound? Is it because the greater sound drives out the less?
> *Hippocrates*

The word tinnitus has been used to describe a variety of sounds of unknown origin. Although a clinician may be able to hear some of these sounds (objective tinnitus) through direct or mediate auscultation (Glanville et al., 1971; Huizing and Spoor, 1973), most are audible only to the patient (subjective tinnitus). Some clinicians have added additional modifiers to indicate whether the sensation fills the patient's head (tinnitus cerebri) or is localized to the ears (tinnitus aurium) (Douek, 1981).

The problem of tinnitus in adults is reviewed systematically in most standard otolaryngology reference works. In contrast, textbooks and monographs that focus on pediatric otorhinolaryngology (Jazbi, 1977), hearing in children (Jaffe, 1977; Northern and Downs, 1984), and pediatric audiology (Martin, 1978) provide little information regarding the incidence, prevalence, etiology, evaluation, and management of tinnitus in children. In consequence, the primary goals of this chapter are to summarize work that addresses specifically tinnitus in children, to contrast these reports with parallel material for adults, and to direct the reader to germane publications.

CLASSIFICATION

Clinical description, scientific description, and associated teaching all will benefit if tinnitus can be classified in a standard way. This desirable goal has been addressed (Evered and Lawrenson, 1981). The outline below is based on their recommendation. It has, however, been modified somewhat to meet the needs of pediatric otolaryngologists, who, in contrast to those who manage adults, must usually seek the complaint of tinnitus in the child.

Classification by Described Characteristics

This classification is dependent completely on the child's ability to characterize his or her tinnitus verbally. Obviously, its value is related directly to the age of the patient and to his or her rate of language acquisition (Lenneberg, 1967). Still, if the child can describe the "sounds" perceived in the ears or in the head, the classification can serve as a framework for the case history.

I. INITIAL CLASSIFICATION. How many different sounds does the child hear?

II. FURTHER CLASSIFICATION. Each sound perceived, or at least the most troublesome sensations, should be classified with respect to the following:

A. *Loudness.* Is the sound faint (i.e., not interfering with communication), moderately loud, or very loud (i.e., interfering with communication)?

B. *Pitch.* Is the pitch medium or high? If the sound does not have a spontaneously discernible pitch, the child should be asked to compare the tinnitus with other familiar sounds in the environment. Does the pitch of the sound remain steady or does it warble?

C. *Temporal Characteristics.* Is the tinnitus continuous or intermittent? If intermittent, how long is it present? How long are the silent intervals? Does the sound pulsate in synchrony with respiration or with pulse rate? What causes the sound to occur, or what makes the sound worse?

D. *Localization.* Is the sound perceived to be in one ear only, in both ears, throughout the head, or "outside" of the head?

E. *Annoyance.* Is the sound annoying to the child? If so, is the annoyance judged to be mild, moderate, or severe? Does the sound prevent the child from getting to sleep? Does it ever waken him or her? What makes the sound tolerable or causes the sound to go away?

F. *Affective (Psychologic) Component.* What nonphysical conditions exacerbate the tinnitus? What nonphysical conditions produce remission? Are any characteristics of the sound affected by stress or by relaxation?

G. *Effect of Environmental Noise.* How do environmental sounds affect the tinnitus? Is the sound suppressed, masked, unchanged or worsened by environmental noise?

240

Classification According to the Psychophysical Measurements

Evered and Lawrenson (1981) underscored the value of psychophysical measurements to help characterize tinnitus. Although the reliability and the accuracy of these measurements increase with the age of the child, pitch matching, loudness matching, and masking tests can be accomplished successfully by most children who give reliable responses during pure-tone audiometry. Moreover, instruments for tinnitus evaluations on adults often can be used even with young children to help them with judgments of sound quality.

Each classification category below is labeled with the name of the recommended test. The procedure then is outlined briefly.

I. QUALITY JUDGMENT OF TINNITUS. Pure tones, narrow bands of noise, and broad-band noise are presented in order to the child at a comfortable loudness level. The tinnitus is classified with respect to the external signal that has a similar quality.

II. PITCH MATCHING OF TINNITUS. If the tinnitus has a tonal quality, the frequency of an external pure tone or the center frequency of a noise band is varied systematically until the child obtains the closest match. The tinnitus is classified with respect to the external signal that produces the closest match. When this test is used with young children, it often is necessary to spend some time discussing the difference between pitch and loudness.

III. RELATIVE LOUDNESS OF TINNITUS. The sound pressure level (SPL) of the signal identified during the pitch-matching test is adjusted systematically until the child reports that the loudness of the test signal approximates the loudness of his or her tinnitus. For classification purposes, the loudness of the child's tinnitus is reported in decibels (dB) SPL or in decibels relative to the threshold of the external test signal (dB sensation level).

IV. MASKING OF TINNITUS. The SPL of the signal identified during the pitch-matching test next is increased until it covers completely (masks) the child's tinnitus. When possible, this test is repeated with a 500-Hz tone and with white noise. If the patient's tinnitus can be masked, the characteristics of effective, external maskers are reported. Feldmann (1971) has used the masking test results to establish a five-group classification scheme for tinnitus.

V. TEST OF RESIDUAL INHIBITION. In this test, the SPL of the most effective masker is increased by 10 dB. This signal then is turned on for 60 seconds. When the masker is turned off, the child is asked whether the tinnitus has changed. She or he may report that the tinnitus has disappeared. This observation is labeled total residual inhibition. The child may report that the loudness of the tinnitus has decreased (partial residual inhibition). She or he also may report that the tinnitus is unchanged or that its loudness has increased. The duration of total inhibition or partial inhibition should be measured from the cessation of the test signal and reported also.

VI. SUBJECTIVE ASSESSMENT OF TINNITUS. It is important to know the child's subjective assessment of the loudness of the tinnitus relative to its "usual loudness." This information is useful during the initial interview, during any period of partial residual inhibition, and following efforts to suppress tinnitus. A seven-point rating scale, where 0 indicates silence and 7 indicates a very loud sound, is recommended (Evered and Lawson, 1981). This concept is easier for children to grasp if the magnitude-estimation task is changed to one of magnitude production. More specifically, young children find it easier to slide a plastic ear along a horizontal continuum that has appropriate pictures or colors at each of the seven positions.

Classification by Probable Site

The traditional terms objective and subjective have been used to classify tinnitus in children (Leonard et al., 1983). This classification is valuable and still is used extensively in clinical reports. The current chapter expands this classification somewhat and takes the approach suggested by Evered and Lawrenson (1981). Specifically, the terms *peripheral*, *central*, *paraauditory*, and *unknown* are used to identify the putative structure or generation site for the tinnitus perceived by the child. These terms improve the resolution of site classification while still using categories that are familiar to clinicians who deal with ear disease in children.

I. PERIPHERAL TINNITUS often is subdivided further into conductive, sensorineural, and mixed categories.

A. *Conductive tinnitus* can accompany simple middle-ear effusions (Draper, 1967), acute and chronic otitis media (Shambaugh and Quie, 1973; Proctor, 1973), atelectasis (Bluestone and Klein, 1983), chronic mastoiditis and cholesteatoma (Parisier et al., 1984), granulomatous diseases of the middle ear (Lederer, 1973), and fixation of the stapes (Nager, 1947) or the lateral ossicular chain (Goodhill, 1979; Causse and Causse, 1984). In some cases, the tinnitus reported may reflect cochlear involvement owing to the relative permeability of the round-window membrane to toxic agents produced by inflammatory middle-ear diseases (Ronis, 1984) (Chap. 21).

Impacted cerumen and foreign bodies lodged in the external auditory meatus are not uncommon findings in pediatric otologic practice. When these problems produce conductive hearing losses, they also reduce the masking effects of environmental sounds. This attenuation of background noise can make tinnitus produced by sensorineural or by paraauditory structures distressingly loud to the child. Obviously, an explanation of this process can reduce anxiety for the parents who have been listening to the child's complaints of "strange noises" in his or her head.

Finally, obstruction of the external auditory meatus and many middle-ear disease processes produce an enhancement of hearing by bone conduction at low frequencies. This "occlusion effect" (Tortual, 1827; Wheatstone, 1827; Bing, 1891; Huizing, 1960) will increase the perceived loudness of tinnitus generated by paraauditory structures.

B. *Sensorineural tinnitus* originates within the cochlea or in the fibers of the auditory nerve. This subjective phenomenon typically is defined as "the sensation of sound in the absence of any relevant external stimulus; as such, it is a symptom, not a disease" (Mihail et al., 1988). Chapter 19 summarizes the primary congenital and postnatal conditions that produce sensorineural hearing impairment in children. Review of the literature suggests that tinnitus has been associated with virtually every one of these lesions. This review has highlighted at least ten additional generalizations:

1. Children rarely have a primary complaint of tinnitus (Leonard et al., 1983; Graham, 1987).

2. Although adult patients without measurable hearing loss may complain of tinnitus (Fowler, 1913; Seltzer, 1947; Heller and Bergman, 1953; Graham and Newby, 1962), the frequency of this complaint in the clinic and the severity of the perceived tinnitus both are related directly to the magnitude of the average pure-tone hearing loss (Weston, 1964). This same observation seems to hold for the pediatric population (Nodar, 1972), at least to the point at which loss of hearing becomes so severe that the child can be educated adequately only in a school for the deaf (Graham, 1987).

   The prevalence of tinnitus without some hearing impairment has been questioned (McFadden, 1982). The reduced frequency range and frequency resolution of most clinical audiometers can obscure a hearing problem that coexists with the patient's tinnitus (McFadden, 1982). More specifically, pure-tone audiometry with children normally is accomplished at octave intervals from 250 Hz through 8000 Hz. The onset of tinnitus, however, may signal the progression of disease at the basal end of the cochlea where the effects on hearing are for frequencies beyond the range of the audiometer. A common example involves the child who has received aminoglycosides (Fee, 1980). When questioned, the child may describe a high-pitched tinnitus; he or she may have a significant loss of hearing at 13,000 Hz but normal hearing at 8000 Hz and below (Fausti et al., 1984) (Chap. 24).

   Further, a child may have a focal cochlear lesion that produces tinnitus and a significant hearing loss for a restricted range of frequencies. If this range falls between two standard (octave) test frequencies, the audiogram will appear normal (Kemp, 1979; Wilson, 1980). These "notches" in the audiogram can be characterized best if the child is able to understand

and perform the task required for sweep-frequency Békésy audiometry (Wilson, 1986).

3. The histopathologic characteristics of congenital sensorineural lesions can be categorized as to whether the osseous labyrinth and the cochlear neuroepithelia are normal or abnormal (Ruben, 1983). In general, the presence of sensorineural tinnitus is a less common complaint from a child with an abnormal bony labyrinth than it is from a hearing-impaired child whose bony labyrinth is normal but whose organ of Corti presumably is abnormal.

4. It has been known for more than a century that some clinically useful drugs also are toxic to the auditory system, to the vestibular system, or to both systems (Schwabach, 1884; North, 1890). Over the last four decades (Schatz et al., 1944), however, there has been a proliferation of drugs that are potentially ototoxic. Review of the literature suggests that complaints of sensorineural tinnitus have been associated with the use of virtually all of these agents. This observation holds for analgesics (salicylates), antimalarials (quinine), "loop" diuretics (furosemide, ethacrynic acid), metallo compounds (mercurials, arsenicals), and antineoplastic drugs (*cis*-diamminedichloroplatinum) (DeBeukelaer et al., 1971; Hawkins, 1976; McCracken and Nelson, 1977). The greatest number of reports of tinnitus in children, however, has been associated with the neonatal administration of antibacterial aminoglycosides (gentamicin, kanamycin) and polypeptide antibiotics (viamycin, vancomycin) (Yow et al., 1962; Eichenwald, 1966; Elfving et al., 1973; Finitzo-Hieber et al., 1979).

   When a child complains of tinnitus, the clinician should question the parents carefully regarding the "medicines" the child has taken. If indicated, an effort also should be made to secure records of neonatal drug therapy. These records can be especially useful for children with a history of neonatal intensive care.

5. For some children, the existence of tonal tinnitus may lead to pure-tone audiometric findings that are inconsistent (Graham and Butler, 1984). This problem can be reduced, however, if an ascending method rather than a descending method is used to present the test tones (Graham, 1987).

6. Some children report that hearing-aid use can suppress or mask their tinnitus (Graham and Butler, 1984). This type of relief has been documented well for adult patients. Approximately 50 per cent of new hearing-aid wearers report partial or total relief from their tinnitus (Saltzman and Ersner, 1947; Surr et al., 1985). In contrast, a hearing aid that has excessive acoustic gain and inadequate limiting of its acoustic output can overstimulate structures on the child's organ of Corti. This problem can

produce temporary or permanent loss of hearing and provoke or exacerbate sensorineural tinnitus (Holmgren, 1939; Kinney, 1961; Macrae and Farrant, 1965; Ross and Lerman, 1967; Jerger and Lewis, 1975; Humes and Bess, 1981).

7. Most adults with acquired tinnitus report a constant auditory sensation (Hazell, 1981; Coles et al., 1981). In contrast, the majority of children with congenital deafness report intermittent tinnitus (Nodar and LeZak, 1984; Graham, 1987).

8. "Perilymph fistulas are reported in all age groups but, because of diagnostic difficulties, they are probably more common in the pediatric population than the literature would indicate. A moderately severe sensorineural hearing loss in a toddler may be assumed to be congenital. Vertiginous spells in young children may be diagnosed as nonspecific disorders like benign paroxysmal vertigo of childhood. We have no doubt that some of these disorders are fistulas that could be treated" (Parnes and McCabe, 1987). With this quotation, Parnes and McCabe (1987) open their discussion of a retrospective study of perilymph fistulas in 16 children. Symptoms and signs of cochleovestibular disease were observed in 26 ears of these 16 patients. For six of the children, radiologic studies revealed developmental abnormalities of the inner ear (Mondini dysplasia). A history of trauma was reported for six additional children. No discernible cause for the symptoms could be identified in the remaining four children. At exploratory tympanotomy, at least one perilymph fistula was found and repaired in at least one ear of each child. Preoperatively, 11 of the children (69 per cent) complained of tinnitus. Seven reported tinnitus following surgery.

The report of Parnes and McCabe (1987) reinforces clinical observation that, because of the variety and variability of signs and symptoms, perilymph fistulas can masquerade as many other inner-ear problems. This position is supported well in the literature (Healy et al., 1976; Thompson and Kohut, 1979; Goodhill, 1981; Supance and Bluestone, 1983). Still, perilymph fistula is one of the few pediatric inner-ear diseases that can be confirmed and treated successfully at surgery. For this reason, it should be included in the differential diagnosis for any child with sensorineural tinnitus.

9. Sensorineural hearing impairment, vestibular dysfunction, and tinnitus often accompany the various stages of congenital luetic disease (Karmody and Schuknecht, 1966; Fiumara and Lessell, 1970; Kerr et al., 1973; Hungerbuhler and Regli, 1978; Adams et al., 1983). Steckelberg and McDonald (1984) reported a complaint of tinnitus from 12 of 15 patients with congenital syphilis. Almost half of the patients in this series noted tinnitus at the onset of their ear disease. These patients frequently used terms like "roaring," "machinelike," and "waterfall" to describe the perceived sensation. The youngest patient in the group with congenital disease was 12 years old. The authors' experience in this area has led to the inclusion of the treponema-specific fluorescent treponemal antibody absorption (FTA-ABS) test when a child has sensorineural tinnitus and when the history supports the possibility of congenital syphilis.

10. Tinnitus is a common complaint. It is reported by 55 to 93 per cent of all adult patients with acoustic neurilemomas and other neoplasms that invade the cerebellopontine angle (Cushing, 1917; Lundborg, 1952; Hambley et al., 1964; Hitselberger and House, 1964; House and Brackmann, 1981). Tumors of cranial nerve VIII, occurring either as primary neurilemomas or in association with neurofibromatosis (von Recklinghausen disease), are rare in children. They should be considered in the differential diagnosis, however, if the child has other evidence of retrocochlear ear disease (Stam, 1983).

C. *Mixed tinnitus*, like mixed hearing loss, involves both conductive and sensorineural components. A common mixed configuration in children involves a patient with serous effusion who also is receiving aspirin. The course of salicylates has potential for producing both mild, temporary sensorineural hearing loss and tinnitus (McCabe and Dey, 1965; Myers and Bernstein, 1965; Mongan et al., 1973; McFadden and Plattsmier, 1982), while the conductive hearing loss attenuates environmental masking. This combination can increase the perceived loudness of the tinnitus for the child (Leonard et al., 1983).

II. *Central tinnitus*, like its audiologic counterpart central auditory dysfunction, is encumbered by speculation, controversy, and incomplete reports. There is little doubt that intracranial lesions that affect the central auditory nervous system can disrupt many aspects of auditory processing (Bocca and Calearo, 1963; Lynn et al., 1972; Jerger and Jerger, 1981). Moreover, these processing problems have been documented for children and for adults with normal hearing for pure tones (Goldstein et al., 1956; Goetzinger, 1972; Hodgson, 1972; Korsan-Bengtsen, 1973; Collard et al., 1986). It is difficult, however, to determine the prevalence of tinnitus within these groups. Although some investigators have documented the presence and type of tinnitus reported by their patients (Parker et al., 1968), this information is missing in most studies that focus on central auditory and central vestibular disease. Accordingly, the authors reviewed 48 published case reports. When all patients with evidence of peripheral ear disease were excluded, as well as all patients on medication that might induce tinnitus (Levin et al., 1987), tinnitus was a complaint for only about 16 per cent of patients with intracranial lesions and evidence of central auditory or central vestibular dysfunction. This value is about one fifth of the 83 per cent that House and Brackmann (1981) reported for a series of 500 patients with acoustic neuromas.

Tinnitus is a potential side effect for hundreds of drugs (Physician's Desk Reference, 1988). The authors' review has not addressed the reputed sensorineural or central mechanisms for these sources of tinnitus in children. The authors also have not addressed the role of central tinnitus in those cases in which there is an apparent sensorineural source. The preponderance of published evidence suggests that a central component may be associated with many forms of peripheral tinnitus. If this were not the case, (1) how could unilateral tinnitus be masked by signals presented at virtually the same level to *either* ear (Tyler and Conrad-Armes, 1984) and (2) how could tinnitus persist for some patients following complete transection of cranial nerve VIII (House and Brackmann, 1981)? Human and animal research that currently is underway ultimately may provide answers to these questions. For the present, however, one must consider the possibility of a central component in all peripheral tinnitus. Finally, from the pediatric point of view, it is difficult to distinguish between central tinnitus and bilateral sensorineural tinnitus in small children.

III. *Paraauditory* tinnitus also has been called "extraauditory" tinnitus (Evered and Lawrenson, 1981) and "nonauditory" tinnitus (Leonard et al., 1983). Paraauditory tinnitus can arise from any normal or abnormal bodily function capable of generating motions in the frequency range of auditory function. The most common type in this group is tinnitus arising from transmission of normal or abnormal vascular pulsations to the cochlea. Though the sound stimulus producing the tinnitus is arising outside the auditory system, a defect within the auditory system (e.g., a conductive hearing loss) can exacerbate or cause tinnitus.

Tinnitus of vascular origin has been divided by some researchers into two categories (Hentzer, 1968): (1) tinnitus caused by an anomaly within the arteries of the head and neck and (2) essential tinnitus, which constitutes a category for which no reasonable explanation can be found. It is believed by many investigators, however, that the cause of this latter type of tinnitus is to be searched for within the venous return from the head (Ward et al., 1975).

A. *Arterial Causes.* The more common causes of vascular tinnitus are listed in Table 16–1. Some examples of the conditions are described, as well as the management of the conditions and the eventual outcome following treatment (Hentzer, 1968). In most cases, according to Hentzer, the anomalies within the arterial system can be demonstrated by angiography.

B. *Essential Tinnitus.* This type of tinnitus may be characterized by a lack of distinctive symptoms and by the fact that it has been impossible to demonstrate a cause (Graf, 1952). Certain criteria should

TABLE 16–1. Causes of Vascular Tinnitus

Arterial aneurysms
Arterial malformations
Arteriovenous malformations
Stenosis of the carotid or other cerebral arteries
Arteriosclerosis of the basilar artery
Transmitted cardiac murmur
Inflammatory hyperemia of the ear
Hemangioma of the head and neck
Chemodectomas of the head and neck

After Hentzer, E., 1968. Objective tinnitus of the vascular type. Acta Otolaryngol. 66:273.

be fulfilled before a diagnosis of essential tinnitus can be made: The tinnitus must be of sudden onset and must be unrelated to any demonstrable disease or injury. The character of tinnitus can change in pitch and intensity. Essential tinnitus, however, should be persistent and unchanging for a year or more. There should be pronounced lateralization, and the sound should be synchronous with the arterial pulse.

Various factors indicate that the cause should be searched for within the venous system of the head and neck and, in keeping with the vascular nature of the condition, the tinnitus should have certain relations to altered head positions. Turning the head away from the side of the tinnitus typically increases the intensity of the sound, possibly owing to some internal jugular vein compression by the ipsilateral sternocleidomastoid muscle.

As previously stated, the condition has not been associated with any other disease or injury and, therefore, does not occur with increased intracranial pressure, pulsating exophthalmos, or abnormalities of extracranial arteries.

Less common causes have been described by Rossberg (1967), Wengraf (1967), Ward and associates (1975), and Tyler and Babbin (1986). Some of these are

1. Arteriovenous malformations between the branches of the occipital artery and the transverse sinus. These types of malformations are relatively more common in the posterior cranial fossa but may occur in the middle cranial fossa between the posterior branch of the middle meningeal artery and the greater petrosal sinus.
2. Abnormalities occurring between the internal maxillary artery and vein resulting from trauma or lesions in that region.
3. Cerebral or cervical angiomas and giant cell tumors of the mandible.

Also of serious importance are arteriovenous communications (fistulas) between the internal carotid artery and the cavernous sinus, which occur following head trauma. The pulsatile tinnitus associated with these vascular fistulas may often be detected by both the patient and the physician. Palpation of the eye often reveals a thrill, and on auscultation a bruit may be heard (see Table 16–2).

TABLE 16–2. Diagnostic Criteria for Essential (Objective) Tinnitus

Sudden onset, related to other disease or injury
Persistence, unchanged for more than a year
Pronounced lateralization
Synchrony with the pulse
Related to altered head position
No symptoms of increased intracranial pressure
No pulsation exophthalmos
No abnormalities of extracranial arteries
Normal cerebral angiogram

C. *Myogenic Causes of Nonauditory Tinnitus.* Tinnitus resulting from rhythmic contractions of the soft palate was first described by Politzer in 1878. Since then, tinnitus of myogenic origin has been described by many others and has been classified according to the three main muscle groups affected (Yamamoto, 1958): soft palate muscles, eustachian tube muscles, and intratympanic muscles.

1. *Palatal Myoclonus.* Palatal myoclonus occurs as involuntary rhythmic contractions of the soft palate and pharyngeal musculature, including the tensor veli palatini, levator veli palatini, salpingopharyngeus, and superior constrictor muscles. These pathologic contractions commonly affect younger people and are associated with an audible clicking. The patient may volunteer the information that he or she has rhythmic contractions occurring somewhere in the oropharynx or oral cavity and that they are associated with a disturbing sound.

   Examination of the mouth and pharynx in these cases reveals a rhythmically contracting pharyngeal musculature associated with an audible click. The contraction may not be present with the mouth widely open and may have to be viewed endoscopically. The symptoms are usually continuous and do not cease during sleep.

   Palatal myoclonus has been thoroughly reported (Heller, 1962; MacKinnon, 1968; Litman and Hausman, 1982; Toland et al., 1984; Tyler and Babbin, 1986), including a discussion of probable causes and the pathologic anatomy associated with the condition (Chadwick and MacBeth, 1953). In 1886, Spencer described "pharyngeal nystagmus" in a 12-year-old boy who had a tumor of the cerebellar vermis. Others have described the condition in association with cerebral and cerebellar pathologic changes (Grunwald, 1903; Pfeiffer, 1919). Pathologic correlation has been possible in other cases, and most of the lesions that were thought to have caused the condition were found in the pons, brain stem, and cerebellar regions (Klein, 1907; Graeffner, 1910; Wilson, 1928; Van Bogaert and Bertrand, 1928). The causative lesions are located in a triangular area within the midbrain bounded by the red nucleus, the inferior olivary and accessory nuclei, and the contralateral dentate nucleus (Guillain and Mollaret, 1931; Guillain et al., 1933). Palatal myoclonus has also been associated with brain stem infarctions, multiple sclerosis, brain stem tumors, trauma, syphilis, malaria, and other degenerative processes. Thus, it appears that any destructive lesion within this anatomic triangle can result in palatopharyngeal myoclonus (see Table 16–3).

   The cause of palatal myoclonus has been thoroughly explored. Despite this, however, the most common type is idiopathic, cases in which there is no obvious underlying cause.

2. *Tinnitus Arising from Abnormal Contraction of Intratympanic Muscles.* Intermittent tinnitus during recovery from facial paralysis due to facial nerve dysfunction has been reported (Watanabe et al., 1974). The tinnitus typically occurred in association with both voluntary or involuntary facial muscle contractions. The tinnitus in these eight cases was relieved by cutting the stapedial tendon. Williams (1980) has described posttraumatic facial-nerve synkinesis to the stapedius muscle and the resultant tinnitus.

   Rhythmic contractions of the tensor tympani are usually associated with palatal myoclonus. Among the many biologic factors considered to be related to this type of tinnitus are the following:

   a. Propagation of muscle contraction noise.
   b. Periodic vibration of the tympanic membrane.
   c. Stimulation of the tympanic plexus.
   d. Temporal variation of inner ear pressure or cochlear microphonic potentials.

   Each of these was considered (Watanabe et al., 1974), but a conclusion could not be reached concerning the genesis of the tinnitus.

3. Nasopharyngeal sounds may be transmitted via a patient's eustachian tube to the middle ear space. Occasionally, vascular tumors, such as nasopharyngeal angiofibromas, may transmit sounds to the auditory system via the eustachian tube or via bone conduction.

4. Nonauditory tinnitus may also arise from crepitation in the temporomandibular joint.

TABLE 16–3. Causes of Palatal Myoclonus

Moderate or severe cerebrovascular insufficiency
Myocardial infection and diabetes
Progressive cerebellar degeneration of multiple sclerosis
Brain stem tumors
Trauma
Syphilis
Malaria
Following surgical clipping or ligation of the posterior inferior cerebellar artery
Familial tremor associated with palatal myoclonus
Cerebellar tumors
Idiopathic

IV. *Unknown* was the word selected to classify tinnitus when the probability of identifying correctly the putative structure or generation site "is assessed at 50% or less" (Evered and Lawrenson, 1981). In the author's experience, this category is used more with young children than with adults because of problems associated with taking of the history, with describing the symptoms, and with testing. It also may be necessary to use the unknown category when the psychologic source of the tinnitus cannot be separated from the anatomic and physiologic sources (Fowler and Fowler, 1955; Reinhart, 1981).

EPIDEMIOLOGY

Definitive epidemiologic studies currently are not available. Stated differently, the prevalence and characteristics of tinnitus for most of the disease processes reviewed cannot be described. The published epidemiologic data for children are general in nature.

Nodar (1972) probably was the first to study the prevalence of tinnitus in school children. He administered questionnaires during audiometric screening sessions to more than 2000 children over a period of 3 years. These children ranged in age from 10 to 18 years. The presence of tinnitus was reported by 58.6 per cent of those children who passed the audiometric screening and by 13.3 per cent of those who failed. In response to the question, "When do you hear" these "noises in your ears?" the more common responses were related to (1) time ("late at night"); (2) emotional stress; (3) physical stress; (4) noise exposure; (5) illness, "colds," or "headaches"; (6) frequency ("all the time" or "whenever it's quiet"); and (7) location ("in the library" or "in bed").

Graham (1981) surveyed 74 children whose hearing losses were severe enough to require the use of hearing aids. These children ranged in age from 12 to 18 years. The main findings of this study follow:

1. 64% of the children had tinnitus.

2. Only two children had continuous tinnitus: in the rest it was intermittent.

3. In the small number (14) who had a hearing loss symmetrical between the two ears and unilateral aiding, the tinnitus was equally distributed between the aided and the unaided ears, so was not consistently related to the use of aids.

4. Tinnitus was commoner in a child's better hearing ear.

5. The degree of annoyance was considered to be disturbing in 40% of the children.

These epidemiologic findings have been supported generally in all subsequent studies (Nodar and LeZak, 1984; Graham and Butler, 1984; Graham, 1987).

SUMMARY

Because hearing loss is a common complaint in childhood, it is probable that the symptom of tinnitus is much more frequent in children than has previously been supposed, particularly because body-image consciousness is not fully developed in childhood. The most common cause of intermittent, fluctuating tinnitus in children occurs during conductive hearing losses associated with otitis media with middle ear effusions, especially if a child is taking aspirin. Continuous and persistent tinnitus is usually associated with loss of sensory or neural auditory function and may be associated with systemic nervous system diseases. If tinnitus is associated with nonauditory complaints or physical findings, the critical path to diagnosis may be simplified considerably. When vertigo and hearing loss occur with tinnitus, the patient's problem is most likely located within or near the temporal bone. If involvement of other cranial nerves, headaches, or other systemic symptoms are present, a search for central nervous system or general system disease, respectively, should be instituted.

SELECTED REFERENCES

Hazell, J. W. P. 1987. Tinnitus. Edinburgh, Churchill Livingstone, pp. 1–207.
   This current tinnitus handbook provides a clear summary of historical antecedents, theory, epidemiology, assessment, and drug therapy, together with surgical, nonsurgical, and psychologic management. Although the focus is not pediatrics, the chapter by Graham includes references to all major reports on tinnitus in children, along with a concise review of assessment and management.
Hentzer, E. 1968. Objective tinnitus of the vascular type. Acta Otolaryngol. 66:273.
   The author describes 24 cases of tinnitus of vascular origin and classifies them into two groups: those caused by arterial anomalies within the head and neck and those that probably arise within the venous system of the head and neck. He gives guidelines for the best form of treatment based on his extensive experience.
Shulman, A. (Chairman). 1979. Proceedings of the II International Tinnitus Seminar. J Laryngol. Otol. Suppl. 9:1.
   These seminar proceedings include contributions from 43 participants. In addition to the topics covered in the Hazell handbook (above), this compendium also addresses electric stimulation of the inner ear and additional techniques for objective evaluation, quantitative assessment, and measurement of tinnitus.
Tyler, R. S., and Babbin, R. W. 1986. Tinnitus. *In* Cummings, C. W., and Harker, L. A. (eds.): Otolaryngology—Head and Neck Surgery, Vol. IV, Ear and Skull Base. St. Louis, C. V. Mosby, pp. 3201–3217.
   This work is the counterpart for adults of the present chapter. The terminology in the two chapters is similar, and both have been prepared by an otolaryngologist and an audiologist working together. The Tyler and Babbin work provides good background for psychoacoustic measurements and electroacoustic measurements and their potential value in the characterization of tinnitus. Although some of the techniques described are not applicable to younger children, many of the sections on diagnosis, management, and surgery have value for all patients.

REFERENCES

Adams, D. A., Kerr, A. G., Smyth, G. D. L., et al. 1983. Congenital syphilitic deafness—a further review. J. Laryngol. Otol. 97:399.
Bing, A. 1891. Ein neuer Stimmgabelverscuh. Beitrag zur Differentialdiagnostik der Krankheiten des mechanischen Schalllei-

tungs-und des nervösen Hörapparates. Wien. Med. Blatter 41:637.

Bluestone, C. D., and Klein, J. O. 1983. Otitis media with effusion, atelectasis and eustachian tube dysfunction. In Bluestone, C. D., and Stool, S. E. (eds.): Pediatric Otolaryngology, Vol. 1. Philadelphia, W. B. Saunders Co., pp. 356–512.

Bocca, E., and Calearo, C. 1963. Central hearing processes. In Jerger, J. (ed.): Modern Developments in Audiology. New York, Academic Press, pp. 337–370.

Causse, J. R., and Causse, J. B. 1984. Otospongiosis as a genetic disease. Am. J. Otol. 5:211.

Chadwick, D. L., and MacBeth, R. 1953. Rhythmic palatal myoclonus. J. Laryngol. 67:301.

Collard, M. E., Lesser, R. P., Luders, H., et al. 1986. Four dichotic speech tests before and after temporal lobectomy. Ear Hear. 7:363.

Cushing, H. 1917. Tumors of the Nervus Acusticus and the Syndrome of the Cerebellopontine Angle. Philadelphia, W. B. Saunders Co., pp. 153–154.

DeBeukelaer, M. M., Travis, L. B., and Dodge, W. F. 1971. Deafness and acute tubular necrosis following parenteral administration of neomycin. Am. J. Dis. Child. 121:250.

Douek, E. 1981. Classification of tinnitus. Ciba Found. Symp. 85:4.

Draper, W. L. 1967. Secretory otitis media in children: A study of 540 children. Laryngoscope 77:636.

Eichenwald, H. F. 1966. Some observations on dosage and toxicity of kanamycin in premature and fullterm infants. Ann. N.Y. Acad. Sci. 132:984.

Elfving, R., Pettay, O., and Raivio, M. 1973. A follow-up study on the cochlear, vestibular and renal function in children treated with gentamicin in the newborn period. Chemotherapy 18:141.

Evered, D., and Lawrenson, G. (eds.). 1981. Tinnitus. Ciba Found. Symp. 85:300.

Fausti, S. A., Rappaport, B. Z., Schecter, M. A., et al. 1984. Detection of aminoglycoside ototoxicity by high-frequency auditory evaluation: Selected case studies. Am. J. Otolaryngol. 5:177.

Fee, W. E. 1980. Aminoglycoside ototoxicity in the human. Laryngoscope 90 Suppl. 24.

Feldman, H. 1971. Homolateral and contralateral masking of tinnitus by noise bands and pure tones. Audiology (Basel) 10:138.

Finitzo-Hieber, T., McCracken, G. H., Jr., Roeser, R. J., et al. 1979. Ototoxicity in neonates treated with gentamicin and kanamycin: Results of a four-year controlled follow-up study. Pediatrics 63:443.

Fiumara, N. J., and Lessell, S. 1970. Manifestations of late congenital syphilis: An analysis of 271 patients. Arch. Dermatol. 102:78.

Fowler, E. P. 1913. Determining factors in tinnitus aurium. Laryngoscope 23:182.

Fowler, E. P., and Fowler, E. P., Jr. 1955. Somatopsychic and psychosomatic factors in tinnitus, deafness, and vertigo. Ann. Otol. Rhinol. Laryngol. 64:29.

Glanville, J. D., Coles, R. R. A., and Sullivan, B. M. 1971. A family with high-tonal objective tinnitus. J. Laryngol. Otol. 85:1.

Glasscock, M. E., Dickins, J. R. E., Jackson, C. G., et al. 1980. Vascular anomalies of the middle ear. Laryngoscope 90:77.

Goetzinger, C. P. 1972. The Rush Hughes test in auditory diagnosis. In Katz, J. (ed.): Handbook of Clinical Audiology. Baltimore, Williams & Wilkins Co., pp. 325–333.

Goldstein, R., Goodman, A. C., and King, R. B. 1956. Hearing and speech in infantile hemiplegia before and after left hemispherectomy. Neurology 6:869.

Goodhill, V. 1979. Tinnitus. In Goodhill, V. (ed.): Ear Diseases, Deafness and Dizziness. Hagerstown, MD, Harper & Row, pp. 731–739.

Goodhill, V. 1981. Leaking labyrinth lesions, deafness, tinnitus and dizziness. Ann. Otol. Rhinol. Laryngol. 90:99.

Graeffner, A. 1910. Berl. Klin. Wschr. 47:1081.

Graf, W. 1952. Kraniala Blas Jud. Nord. Med 28:2499.

Graham, J. M. 1987. Tinnitus in hearing-impaired children. In Hazell, J. W. P. (ed.): Tinnitus. Edinburgh, Churchill Livingstone, pp. 131–143.

Graham, J. M., and Butler, J. 1984. Tinnitus in children. J. Laryngol. Otol. Suppl. 9:236.

Graham, J. T., and Newby, H. 1962. Acoustical characteristics of tinnitus—an analysis. Arch Otolaryngol. 75:162.

Grunwald, L. 1903. Hyperkinetic disturbances of the pharynx. In Atlas and Epitome of Diseases of the Mouth, Pharynx and Nose, 2nd ed. Philadelphia, W. B. Saunders Co., p. 186.

Guillain, G., and Mollaret, P. 1931. Deux cas de myoclonies synchrones et rhythmées velo-pharyngolaryngo-oculo-diaphragmatiques. Rev. Neurol. 2:545.

Guillain, G., Mollaret, P., and Bertrand, I. 1933. Sur la lesion responsable du syndrome myoclonique du troie cerebrae. Rev. Neurol. 2:666.

Hambley, W. M., Gorshenin, A. N., and House, W. F. 1964. The differential diagnosis of acoustic neuroma. Arch. Otolaryngol. 80:708.

Hawkins, J. E. 1976. Drug ototoxicity. In Keidel, W. D., and Neff, W. D. (eds.): Handbook of Sensory Physiology, Vol. 5. Berlin, Springer-Verlag, pp. 707–748.

Hazell, J. W. P. 1981. Patterns of tinnitus: Medical and audiologic findings. J. Laryngol. Otol. [Suppl.] 4:39.

Healy, G. B., Friedman, J. M., and Strong, M. S. 1976. Vestibular and auditory findings of perilymph fistula: A review of 40 cases. Trans. Am. Acad. Ophthalmol. Otolaryngol. 82:44.

Heller, M. F. 1962. Vibratory tinnitus and palatal myoclonus. Acta Otolaryngol. 55:292.

Heller, M. F., and Bergman, M. 1953. Tinnitus aurium in normally hearing persons. Ann. Otol. Rhinol. Laryngol. 62:73.

Hentzer, E. 1968. Objective tinnitus of the vascular type. Acta Otolaryngol. 66:273.

Hippocrates. c. 400 B.C. Book 32. Paragraph 961–A.

Hitselberger, W. E., and House, W. F. 1964. Tumors of the cerebellopontine angle. Arch. Otolaryngol. 80:720.

Hodgson, W. R. 1972. Filtered speech tests. In Katz, J. (ed.): Handbook of Clinical Audiology. Baltimore, Williams & Wilkins Co., pp. 313–324.

Holmgren, L. 1939. Can hearing be damaged by a hearing aid? Acta Otolaryngol. (Stockh.) 28:440.

House, J. W., and Brackmann, D. E. 1981. Tinnitus: Surgical Treatment. Ciba Found. Symp. 85:204.

Huizing, E. H. 1960. Bone conduction, the influence of the middle ear. Acta Otolaryngol. (Stockh.) Suppl. 155:1.

Huizing, E. H., and Spoor, A. 1973. An unusual type of tinnitus. Arch. Otolaryngol. 98:134.

Humes, L. E., and Bess, F. H. 1981. Tutorial on the potential deterioration in hearing due to hearing aid usage. J. Speech Hear. Res. 24:3.

Hungerbuhler, J. P., and Regli, F. 1978. Cochleovestibular involvement as the first sign of late syphilis. J. Neurol. 219;199.

Jaffe, B. F. (ed.). 1977. Hearing Loss in Children. Baltimore, University Park Press.

Jazbi, B. (ed.). 1977. Symposium on pediatric otorhinolaryngology. Otolaryngol. Clin. North Am. 10.

Jerger, J. F., and Lewis, N. 1975. Binaural hearing aids: Are they dangerous for children? Arch. Otolaryngol. 101:480.

Jerger, S., and Jerger, J. 1981. Auditory Disorders, A Manual for Clinical Evaluation. Boston, Little, Brown and Co., pp. 79–93.

Karmody, C. S., and Schuknecht, H. F. 1966. Deafness in congenital syphilis. Arch. Otolaryngol. 83:18.

Kemp, D. T. 1979. The evoked cochlear mechanical response and the auditory microstructure—evidence for a new element in cochlear mechanics. Scand. Audiol. Suppl. 9:35.

Kerr, A. G., Smyth, G. D. L., and Cinnamond, M. J. 1973. Congenital syphilitic deafness. J. Laryngol. Otol. 87:1.

Kinney, C. E. 1961. The further destruction of partially deafened children's hearing by the use of powerful hearing aids. Ann. Otol. Rhinol. Laryngol. 70:828.

Klein, H. 1907. Neurol. Zentrabl 26:245.

Korsan-Bengtsen, M. 1973. Distorted speech audiometry. Acta Otolaryngol. (Stockh.) Suppl. 310:7.

Lederer, F. L. 1973. Granulomas and other specific diseases of the ear and temporal bone. In Paparella, M. M., and Shumrick, D. A. (eds.): Otolaryngology, Vol. 2, Ear. Philadelphia, W. B. Saunders Co., pp. 161–184.

Lenneberg, E. H. 1967. Biological Foundations of Language. New York, John Wiley & Sons.

Leonard, G., Black, F. O., and Schramm, V. L. 1983. Tinnitus in children. In Bluestone, C. D., and Stool, S. E. (eds.): Pediatric Otolaryngology, Vol. 1. Philadelphia, W. B. Saunders Co., pp. 271–277.

Levin, V. A., Chamberlain, M. C., Prados, M. D., et al. 1987. Phase I–II study of eflornithine and mitoguazone combined in the treatment of recurrent primary brain tumors. Cancer Treat. Rep. 71:459.

Litman, R. S., and Hausman, S. A. 1982. Bilateral palatal myoclonus. Laryngoscope 92:1187.

Lundborg, T. 1952. Diagnostic problems concerning acoustic tumors. Acta Otolaryngol. Suppl. 99:28.

Lynn, G., Benitez, J., Eisenbrey, A., et al. 1972. Neuroaudiological correlates in cerebral hemisphere lesions. Audiology 11:115.

MacKinnon, D. M. 1968. Objective tinnitus due to palatal myoclonus. J. Laryngol. 82:369.

Macrae, J. H., and Farrant, R. H. 1965. The effect of hearing aid use on the residual hearing of children with sensorineural deafness. Ann. Otol. Rhinol. Laryngol. 74:409.

Martin, F. N. (ed.). 1978. Pediatric Audiology. Englewood Cliffs, NJ, Prentice-Hall.

McCabe, P. A., and Dey, F. L. 1965. The effect of aspirin upon auditory sensitivity. Ann. Otol. Rhinol. Laryngol. 74:312.

McCracken, G. H., and Nelson, J. D. 1977. Antimicrobial Therapy for Newborns. Practical Application of Pharmacology to Clinical Usage. New York, Grune & Stratton.

McFadden, D. 1982. Tinnitus Facts, Theories and Treatments. Washington, National Academy Press, p. 23.

McFadden, D., and Plattsmier, H. S. 1982. Aspirin can induce noise-induced temporary threshold shift. J. Acoust. Soc. Am. 71:S106.

Mihail, R. C., Crowley, J. M., Walden, B. E., et al. 1988. The tricyclic trimipramine in the treatment of subjective tinnitus. Ann. Otol. Rhinol. Laryngol. 97:120.

Mongan, E., Kelly, P., Nies, K., et al. 1973. Tinnitus as an indication of therapeutic serum salicylate levels. J.A.M.A. 226:142.

Myers, E. N., and Bernstein, J. M. 1965. Salicylate ototoxicity: A clinical and experimental study. Arch. Otolaryngol. 82:483.

Nager, F. R. 1947. Pathology of the labyrinthine capsule and its clinical significance. In Fowler, E. P., Jr. (ed.): Medicine of the Ear. New York, Thomas Nelson & Sons, Chap. VII.

Nodar, R. H. 1972. Tinnitus aurium in school-age children: A survey. J. Aud. Res. 12:133.

Nodar, R. H., and LeZak, M. H. W. 1984. Pediatric tinnitus (a thesis revisited). J. Laryngol. Otol. Suppl. 9:234.

North, A. 1890. Two cases of poisoning by the oil of chenopodium. Am. J. Otol. 2:197.

Northern, J. L., and Downs, M. P. 1984. Hearing in Children, 3rd ed. Baltimore, Williams & Wilkins Co.

Parisier, S. C., Chute, P. M., Kramer, M. S., et al. 1984. Tinnitus in patients with chronic mastoiditis and cholesteatoma. J. Laryngol. Otol. Suppl. 9:94.

Parker, W., Decker, R. L., and Richards, N. G. 1968. Auditory function and lesions of the pons. Arch. Otolaryngol. 87:228.

Parnes, L. S., and McCabe, B. F. 1987. Perilymph fistula: An important cause of deafness and dizziness in children. Pediatrics 80:524.

Pfeiffer, R. A. 1919. Mschr. Psychiat. Neurol. 45:96.

Physician's Desk Reference, 42nd ed. 1988. Oradell, NJ, Medical Economics Co.

Politzer, A. 1878. Lehrbuch der Ohren hal kunde, Stuttgart.

Proctor, B. 1973. Chronic otitis media and mastoiditis. In Paparella, M. M., and Shumrick, D. A. (eds.): Otolaryngology, Vol. 2, Ear. Philadelphia, W. B. Saunders Co., pp. 121–160.

Reinhart, J. B. 1981. The psychiatric aspects of ear, nose and throat disorders. Pediatr. Clin. North Am. 28:991.

Ronis, M. 1984. Inflammatory ear disease and tinnitus. J. Laryngol. Otol. Suppl. 9:203.

Ross, M., and Lerman, J. 1967. Hearing aid usage and its effect upon residual hearing. Arch. Otolaryngol. 86:639.

Rossberg, G. 1967. Pulsierende Ohrerausche bei anomalie der arteria carotis und arteria occipitalis externa. J. Laryngol. Rhinol. 46:79.

Ruben, R. J. 1983. Diseases of the inner ear and sensorineural

deafness. In Bluestone, C. D., and Stool, S. E. (eds.): Pediatric Otolaryngology, Vol 1. Philadelphia, W. B. Saunders Co., pp. 577–604.

Saltzman, M., and Ersner, M. 1947. A hearing aid for relief of tinnitus aurium. Laryngoscope 57:358.

Schatz, A., Bugie, E., and Waksman, S. A. 1944. Streptomycin, a substance exhibiting antibiotic activity against gram-positive and gram-negative bacteria. Proc. Soc. Exp. Biol. Med. 55:66.

Schwabach, D. 1884. Uber bleibende Storungen im Gehororgan nach chinin und salicylgebrauch. Dt. Med. Wschr. 10:163.

Seltzer, A. 1947. The problems of tinnitus in the practice of otolaryngology. Laryngoscope 57:623.

Shambaugh, G. E., and Quie, P. G. 1973. Acute otitis media and mastoiditis. In Paparella, M. M., and Shumrick, D. A. (eds.): Otolaryngology, Vol. 2, Ear. Philadelphia, W. B. Saunders Co., pp. 113–120.

Spencer, H. R. 1886. Pharyngeal and laryngeal "nystagmus." Lancet 2:702.

Stam, J. R. 1983. Tumors of the ear and temporal bone. In Bluestone, C. D., and Stool, S. E. (eds.): Pediatric Otolaryngology, Vol. 1. Philadelphia, W. B. Saunders Co., pp. 637–644.

Steckelberg, J. M., and McDonald, T. J. 1984. Otologic involvement in late syphilis. Laryngoscope 94:753.

Supance, J. S., and Bluestone, C. D. 1983. Perilymph fistulas in infants and children. Otolaryngol. Head Neck Surg. 91:663.

Surr, R. K., Montgomery, A. A., and Mueller, H. G. 1985. Effect of amplification on tinnitus among new hearing aid users. Ear Hear. 6:71.

Thompson, J. N., and Kohut, R. I. 1979. Perilymph fistulae: Variability of symptoms and results of surgery. Otolaryngol. Head Neck Surg. 87:898.

Toland, A.D., Porubsky, E. S., Coker, N. J., et al. 1984. Velopharyngo-laryngeal myoclonus: Evaluation of objective tinnitus and extrathoracic airway obstruction. Laryngoscope 94:691.

Tourtual, C. Th. 1827. Die Sinne des Menschen in den Wechselseitigen Beziehungen ihres psychischen und organischen Lebens. Ein Beitrag zur physiologischen Aesthetit. Munster, Friedrich Regensberg.

Tyler, R. S., and Babbin, R. W. 1986. Tinnitus. In Cummings, C. W., and Harker, L. A. (eds.): Otolaryngology—Head and Neck Surgery, Vol. IV, Ear and Skull Base. St. Louis, C. V. Mosby, pp. 3201–3217.

Tyler, R. S., and Conrad-Armes, D. 1984. Masking of tinnitus compared to the masking of pure tones. J. Speech Hear. Res. 27:106.

Van Bogaert, I., and Bertrand, I. 1928. Sur les myoclonies associees synchrones et rhythmiques par lesionsen foyer du trone cerebrale. Rev. Neurol 1:203.

Ward, P. H., Babin, R., Calcaterra, T. C., et al. 1975. Operative treatment of surgical lesions with objective tinnitus. Ann. Otol. Rhinol. Laryngol. 84:473.

Watanabe, I., Kumagami, H., and Tsuda, Y. 1974. Tinnitus due to abnormal contraction of stapedial muscle. Otorhinolaryngol. 36:217.

Wengraf, C. 1967. A case of objective tinnitus. J. Laryngol. 81:143.

Weston, T. E. T. 1964. Presbycusis—a clinic study. J. Laryngol. Otol. 78:273.

Wheatstone, C. 1827. Experiments on audition. Quart. J. Sci. Lit. Art. 67:67.

Williams, J. D. 1980. Unusual but treatable cause of fluctuating tinnitus. Ann. Otol. Rhinol. Laryngol. 89:239.

Wilson, J. P. 1980. Evidence for a cochlear origin for acoustic re-emissions, threshold fine-structure, and tonal tinnitus. Hear. Res. 2:233.

Wilson, J. P. 1986. Otoacoustic emissions and tinnitus. Scand. Audiol. Suppl. 25:109.

Wilson, S. A. K. 1928. Cases of palato-laryngeal nystagmus. Brain 51(1):119.

Yamamoto, T. 1958. Objective tinnitus. Otolaryngol. (Tokyo) 30:708.

Yow, M. D., Tengg, N. E., and Bangs, J. 1962. The ototoxic effects of kanamycin sulfate in infants and children. J. Pediatr. 60:230.

Chapter 17

FACIAL PARALYSIS IN CHILDREN

Mark May, M.D.

Because the most common cause of facial paralysis is a lesion within the temporal bone (Cawthorne, 1953), the otolaryngologist should best be able to handle problems of this nature. However, most clinicians have not had sufficient opportunities to deal with facial paralysis to accumulate a knowledgeable approach to these cases and must rely on scattered journal reports—frequently representing conflicting or controversial opinions on the subject—to formulate a plan of management of these patients.

This chapter presents the author's approach to facial paralysis, which has been developed during 22 years of evaluating and treating 1989 patients with this problem. Of these patients, 339 were 18 years old or younger (Table 17–1). With few exceptions, all the patients had complete medical otoneurologic evaluations and were followed for six months or longer.

TABLE 17–1. Causes of Facial Palsy in 339 Patients Between Birth and 18 Years of Age

CAUSES	NUMBER	%
Bell palsy	133	39
Herpes zoster cephalicus	13	4
Birth	62	18
Developmental (46)		
Traumatic (16)		
Traumatic	62	18
Accidental (33)		
Iatrogenic (24)		
Surgical (5)		
Infection	38	11
Acute otitis media (28)		
Chronic otitis media (4)		
Chickenpox (3)		
Mononucleosis (1)		
Mumps (1)		
Diphtheria (1)		
Tumor	19	6
Other	12	4
Melkersson-Rosenthal syndrome (4)		
Poliomyelitis (3)		
Guillain-Barré syndrome (1)		
Hypothyroidism (1)		
Sickle cell crisis (1)		
Myotonic dystrophy (1)		
Sarcoidosis (1)		
Total	339	

ANATOMY OF THE FACIAL NERVE

A fundamental knowledge of the anatomy of the seventh cranial nerve is essential for localizing the level of the lesion and is helpful in arriving at the diagnosis (Fig. 17–1; Table 17–2). Further, locating the site of the lesion is critical for the surgical approach in instances of nerve compression by infection, neoplasms, or fractures.

The course of the facial nerve, for the sake of this discussion, may conveniently be divided into three segments: supranuclear, nuclear, and infranuclear. The infranuclear segment is further subdivided into the

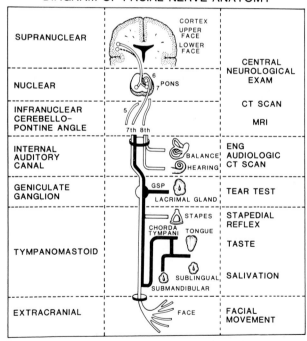

DIAGRAM OF FACIAL NERVE ANATOMY

Figure 17–1. The facial nerve may be divided into three segments for anatomic study: supranuclear, nuclear, and infranuclear. The infranuclear segments have been further divided (as shown in the left column). Each level can be identified by employing tests listed in the column on the right and signs detailed in Table 17–2. CT, Computed tomography; MRI, magnetic resonance imaging; ENG, electronystagmography; GSP, greater superficial petrosal nerve.

249

TABLE 17–2. Signs and Probable Diagnoses Resulting from Lesions of the Facial Nerve at Various Levels as Detailed in Figure 17–1

LEVEL	SIGNS	DIAGNOSIS
Supranuclear Cortex Internal capsule	Tone and upper face intact, loss of volitional movement with intact spontaneous expression, slurred speech (tongue weakness), hemiparesis (arm greater than leg) on side of facial involvement	Lesion of motor cortex or lateral capsule on opposite side of facial involvement. Paresis upper extremity (middle cerebral artery). Paresis lower extremity (another cerebral artery)
Extrapyramidal	Increased salivary flow, spontaneous facial movement impaired, volitional facial movement intact	Tumor or vascular lesion of basal ganglion
Midbrain	Involvement of face and oculomotor roots—loss of pupillary reflexes, external strabismus, and oculomotor paresis on opposite side of facial paresis	Unilateral Weber syndrome (vascular lesion)
	Bilateral facial paresis with other cranial nerve deficits, emotional lability, hyperactive gag reflex, marked hyperreflexia associated with hypertension	Pseudobulbar palsy—associated with multiple infarcts
Nuclear Nuclear pons	Involvement of cranial nerves VII and VI on side of lesion, with gaze palsy on side of facial paresis. Contralateral hemiparesis, ataxia, cerebellovestibular signs	Involvement of pons at level of cranial nerves VII and VI nuclei by pontine glioma, multiple sclerosis, encephalitis, infections, or poliomyelitis
	Cranial nerves VII and VI involved with other anomalies noted at birth	Congenital facial palsy, Möbius syndrome, and thalidomide toxicity
Infranuclear **Intracranial**	Involvement of cranial nerve VIII (decreased tearing and taste, stapes reflex decay, decreased discrimination), facial motor deficit (late sign)	Acoustic neuroma
Cerebellopontine angle	Cranial nerves VIII and VII involved in succession, beginning with facial pain or numbness. Computed tomography scan shows pathologic change, enhanced with contrast	Meningioma
	Cranial nerves VII and VIII involved successively, beginning with facial twitching, appearance of erosion or lysis on plain radiographs of temporal bone	Cholesteatoma arising in temporal bone
Skull base	Cranial nerves VII, VIII, IX, X, XI, and XII involved in succession; pulsatile tinnitus, purple-red pulsating mass noted bulging through tympanic membrane	Glomus jugulare tumor
	Same as above with cranial nerve involvement	Glomus jugulare tumor extending to petrous apex and involving middle fossa
	Conductive or sensorineural hearing loss, acute or recurrent Bell palsy, positive family history by skull radiograph	Osteopetrosis
	Multiple cranial nerves involved in rapid succession	Carcinomatous meningitis, leukemia, Landry-Guillain-Barré syndrome, mononucleosis, diphtheria, tuberculosis, sarcoidosis
Infranuclear **Transtemporal Bone**	Same as listed under Cerebellopontine angle	Same as listed under Cerebellopontine angle
Internal auditory canal	Ecchymoses around pinna and mastoid prominence (Battle sign); hemotympanum with sensorineural hearing loss by tuning fork (lateralizes to normal side); vertigo, nystagmus (fast component away from involved side); sudden, complete facial paralysis following head trauma	Transverse fracture of temporal bone
Geniculate ganglion	Dry eye, decreased taste, and decreased salivation; erosion of geniculate ganglion area or middle fossa as demonstrated by polytomography of temporal bone	Neurinoma, meningioma, cholesteatoma, ossifying hemangioma, arteriovenous malformation
	Pain, vesicles on pinna, dry eye, decreased taste and salivary flow; sensorineural hearing loss, nystagmus, vertigo, red chorda tympani nerve	Herpes zoster oticus (Ramsey-Hunt syndrome)
	Same as above without vesicles and no cause can be found (keep in mind, if no recovery in 6 months, dealing with tumor at geniculate ganglion, which may require exploration for confirmation)	Bell palsy (viral inflammatory-immune disorder)
	Ecchymoses around pinna and mastoid (Battle sign), hemotympanum; conductive hearing loss by tuning fork (lateralizes to involved ear, bone greater than air), no vestibular involvement	Longitudinal fracture of temporal bone. May be proximal or at geniculate ganglion (dry eye), or distal to geniculate ganglion (tears symmetrical)

TABLE 17–2. Signs and Probable Diagnoses Resulting from Lesions of the Facial Nerve at Various Levels as Detailed in Figure 17–1 *Continued*

LEVEL	SIGNS	DIAGNOSIS
Infranuclear **Transtemporal Bone** Tympanomastoid segment	Involvement at this level characterized by decreased taste and salivation and loss of stapes reflex. Tearing is normal. There is sudden onset of facial paralysis, which may be complete or incomplete and may progress to complete	
	Pain and vesicles present, red chorda tympani	Herpes zoster oticus
	Pain without vesicles, red chorda tympani	Bell palsy
	Red, bulging tympanic membrane, conductive hearing loss; usually a history of upper respiratory infection; lower face may be involved more than upper	Acute suppurative otitis media
	Foul drainage through perforated tympanic membrane; history of recurrent ear infection, drainage and hearing loss	Chronic suppurative otitis media, most likely associated with cholesteatoma
	Pulsatile tinnitus, purple-red pulsatile mass noted through tympanic membrane	Glomus tympanicum or jugulare
	Recurrent facial paralysis, positive family history, facial edema, fissured tongue; may present with simultaneous bilateral facial paralysis	Melkersson-Rosenthal syndrome
Extracranial	Incomplete involvement of facial nerve (usually one or more major branches spared); hearing, balance, tearing, stapes reflex, taste, and salivary flow spared	Penetrating wound of face; postparotid surgery; malignancy of parotid, tonsil, or oronasopharynx
	Uveitis, salivary gland enlargement, fever	Sarcoidosis (Heerfordt syndrome), lymphoma
Sites Variable	Facial paralysis, especially simultaneous bilateral facial paralysis with symmetric ascending paralysis, decreased deep tendon reflexes, minimal sensory changes. Abnormal spinal fluid (protein and few cells, albuminocytologic dissociation)	Landry-Guillain-Barré syndrome

Gratitude is extended to Richard Kasden, M.D., for his assistance in developing this table. (Material relating to signs of facial nerve involvement in supranuclear and nuclear regions based on Crosby, E. C., and De Jonge, B. R. 1963. Experimental and clinical studies of the central connections and central relations of the facial nerve. Ann. Otol. Rhinol. Laryngol. 72:735.)

cerebellopontine angle; internal auditory canal; and labyrinthine, tympanic, mastoid, and extracranial segments (Fig. 17–1). Pathologic conditions at any particular level may be diagnosed by special tests, detailed in Figure 17–1.

Supranuclear Segment

In the cortex, the tracts to the upper face are crossed and uncrossed. The tracts to the lower face are crossed only; therefore, the forehead is bilaterally innervated, and a lesion in the facial area on one side of the cortex would spare the forehead. However, one must not rely solely on sparing of the forehead to differentiate supranuclear from infranuclear lesions, because sparing of the forehead or other parts of the face can occur with lesions involving a more distal portion of the nerve. In addition to an intact upper face, characteristics of supranuclear lesions include the presence of facial tone, spontaneous facial expression, and loss of volitional facial movement. Most important, there are usually other neurologic signs of central nervous system involvement. The sparing of involuntary movement with supranuclear lesions is thought to be due to sparing of the extrapyramidal system, which is considered to be responsible for involuntary or emotional facial movement. With nuclear and infranuclear lesions, there is loss of both involuntary and voluntary movement.

Nuclear Segment

From its nucleus in the pons, the facial nerve begins a circuitous journey around the sixth nerve nucleus before emerging from the brain stem. Because of this relationship between the sixth and seventh cranial nerves, a lesion in the region of the pons that caused a facial paralysis of the peripheral type would most probably be accompanied by a sixth cranial nerve palsy and would result in inability to rotate the eye to the side of the facial paralysis.

Infranuclear Segment

Cerebellopontine Angle

At the cerebellopontine angle, the eighth cranial nerve joins the facial nerve, and they enter the internal auditory canal together. Lesions in this area would be associated with vestibular and cochlear as well as seventh nerve deficits. Large lesions filling the cerebellopontine angle might compress other cranial nerves and cause deficits of the fifth cranial nerve and later the ninth, tenth, and eleventh cranial nerves.

Internal Auditory Canal

The motor facial nerve and the intermedius nerve are loosely joined together as they enter the internal auditory meatus with the acoustic nerve. The acoustic nerve enters the internal auditory canal inferiorly, while the facial nerve runs superiorly along the roof of the internal auditory canal. The intracranial segment of the facial nerve from the brain stem to the fundus of the internal acoustic meatus is covered only by a thin layer of glia, which makes it quite vulnerable to any type of surgical manipulation but quite resistant to a slow process of stretching or compression. The facial nerve in this region can become quite elongated and spread out over the surface of a sizable but slow-growing vestibular nerve schwannoma without any gross evidence of facial weakness. Although it is unusual to see facial nerve motor involvement in this instance, there is often evidence of such involvement in disruption of tearing, taste, and salivary flow owing to compression of the intermedius nerve. If the intermedius nerve is considered part of the facial nerve, then the facial nerve is the most common cranial nerve involved with vestibular schwannomas.

Labyrinthine Segment

At the fundus of the internal auditory meatus, the facial nerve is physiologically "pressed" into the fallopian canal. The facial and intermedius nerves carry with them a continuation of the dura mater and periosteum from the internal acoustic meatus, and this dural continuation forms a well-defined and tough fibrous sheath that covers these nerves all the way to the terminal branches of the facial nerve in the face and neck. The portion of the facial nerve from its entrance into the fallopian canal to the geniculate ganglion is designated the labyrinthine segment because it runs between the cochlear and vestibular labyrinths. This segment lies beneath the middle fossa and is the shortest and narrowest part of the fallopian canal, averaging 5 mm in length and 0.68 mm in diameter (Fisch, 1977b). Because this is the narrowest part of the facial canal, it is reasonable to suspect that this is the most vulnerable part of the facial nerve when there are inflammatory changes within the canal. The facial nerve in the labyrinthine segment is further jeopardized by any process that causes further limitation of this narrow space because the blood supply to the nerve in this region is unique: This is the only segment of the facial nerve in which there are no anastomosing arterial arcades (Blunt, 1956).

The labyrinthine segment of the facial nerve includes the geniculate ganglion, from which arises the first branch of the facial nerve, the greater superficial petrosal nerve (Fig. 17–2). This nerve carries secretory motor fibers to the lacrimal gland. The second branch from the geniculate ganglion is a tiny thread that forms the lesser superficial petrosal as it is joined by fibers of the tympanic plexus, contributed by the ninth cranial nerve. This nerve carries secretory fibers to the parotid gland.

Tympanic Segment

At the geniculate ganglion the facial nerve makes a sharp angled turn backward, forming a knee, or genu, to enter the tympanic or horizontal portion of the fallopian canal. The proximal end of the tympanic portion is marked by the geniculate ganglion, from which point the facial nerve courses peripherally 3 to 5 mm, passing posterior to the cochleariform process and the tensor tympani tendon. The distal end of the tympanic segment of the facial nerve lies just above the pyramidal eminence, which houses the stapedius muscle. This segment is approximately 12 mm long. At the beginning of the tympanic segment, the fallopian canal forms a prominent, rounded eminence between the bony horizontal semicircular canal and the niche of the oval window. The tympanic wall of this part of the fallopian canal is thin and easily fractured. In addition, there are frequent dehiscences present, allowing contact between the nerve and the tympanic mucoperiosteum. In some patients, the uncovered nerve is prolapsed into the oval window niche, partly or completely concealing the footplate of the stapes, and therefore is subject to trauma during stapes surgery. (The surgeon must look for this anomaly when there is a congenital deformity of the incus and stapes superstructure. It is also worthwhile to palpate the horizontal segment of the facial nerve in performing surgery of the middle ear or tympanomastoid to determine whether the nerve is covered by bone or whether there is a dehiscence in the fallopian canal.)

Just distal to the pyramidal eminence, the fallopian aqueduct makes another turn downward, the second genu. The second genu is another area where the facial nerve may be injured during mastoid surgery. The nerve emerges from the middle ear between the posterior canal wall and the horizontal semicircular canal, just beneath the short process of the incus. In the presence of chronic infection, in which granulation tissue is present, one must be careful not to confuse a pathologic dehiscence of the facial nerve in this region with a mound of granulation tissue. The best way to avoid this is to identify the nerve proximal and distal to the area that looks suspicious. The facial nerve gives off its third branch, the motor nerve to the stapedius muscle, at the distal end of the tympanic segment.

Mastoid Segment

The fallopian canal aqueduct proceeds vertically down the anterior wall of the mastoid process to the stylomastoid foramen. The distance from the second genu to the foramen averages 13 mm.

The chorda tympani nerve, which is the fourth branch of the facial nerve and its last sensory branch and thus the terminal branch of the intermedius nerve, usually arises from the distal third of the mastoid segment of the facial nerve, runs upward and anteriorly over the incus and under the malleus, and crosses the tympanic cavity through the petrotympanic fissure to join the lingual nerve. The chorda tympani contains

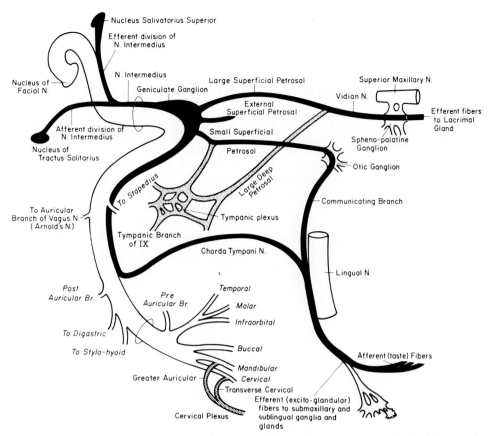

Figure 17–2. Diagram of facial nerve connections with other nerves. The facial nerve connects with the fifth cranial nerve through the large superficial and large deep petrosal nerves, which join the vidian nerve. The small petrosal passes through the otic ganglion. The chorda tympani joins the lingual nerve. The tympanic branch of the cranial nerve in the middle ear (Jacobson nerve) connects with the facial nerve. The auricular branch of the vagus (Arnold nerve) connects with the facial nerve. The cervical plexus connects with the peripheral branches of the facial nerve in the neck and lower face. (Modified from Warwick, R., and Williams, P. L. 1979. Gray's Anatomy, 36th ed. Philadelphia, W. B. Saunders Co.)

secretory motor fibers to the submaxillary and sublingual glands; it also contains sensory fibers from the anterior two thirds of the tongue (taste) and from the posterior wall of the external auditory meatus (pain, temperature, and touch).

Extracranial Segment

The facial nerve leaves the fallopian canal at the stylomastoid foramen, lateral to the styloid and vaginal processes. In newborns and in children up to 2 years of age, the facial nerve as it exits the skull is just deep to the subcutaneous tissue underlying the skin; after 2 years of age, as the mastoid tip and tympanic ring form, the facial nerve takes a deeper position up to 2 cm from the level of the skin.

Beyond the age of 2 years, the facial nerve is protected by the tympanic bone, the mastoid tip, the ascending ramus of the mandible, and the fascia between the parotid and cartilaginous external canal. In this region, there are branches from the occipital artery and a venous plexus, which account for brisk bleeding

when this area is entered in the process of approaching the facial nerve. (Meticulous hemostasis during surgery can be achieved without injuring the facial nerve, which lies deep to these vessels, by employing a bipolar cautery.) As the nerve exits the stylomastoid foramen, nerve branches to the digastric and stylohyoid and postauricular muscles are given off. The seventh nerve communicates with branches from the ninth and tenth cranial nerves, as well as with the auriculotemporal branch of the fifth nerve. In addition, there are anastomoses between the great auricular and lesser occipital branches of the cervical plexus (Fig. 17–2). After exiting the stylomastoid foramen, the facial nerve runs anteriorly for about 2 cm before bifurcating into an upper and lower division; both divisions run through the substance of the parotid gland, passing over the external jugular vein. After emerging from the parotid gland, the facial nerve passes over the fascia of the masseter muscle; although its course in this region is variable, there are some relationships that are relatively constant. There are communications between the upper and lower divisions in the majority of patients (Anson and Donaldson, 1973), which explains the faulty regeneration that sometimes follows injuries to the nerve in this region. (Symptoms of faulty regeneration include synkinesis, evidenced by mouth movement with blinking or eye closure with smiling.) This undesirable complication can be discouraged to a great extent by dividing and clipping these anastomotic branches during reanimation surgery.

In the newborn and the infant, the marginal mandibular nerve, which innervates the lower lip, courses over the mandible and is superficial and quite vulnerable to injury. This is in contrast to the course of this branch in the adult, in whom the nerve is up to 2 cm or more below the angle of the jaw (Sammarco et al., 1966).

The upper division of the facial nerve courses over the fascia covering the *zygomatic arch* and is anterior to the *superficial temporal artery and vein*. The branches to the midface cross over the buccal compartment and deep to the facial muscles. At this point, there is widespread intermingling of nerve fibers with duplication of fibers innervating the same areas. This duplication allows for injuries in the periphery to recover by peripheral sprouting without any noticeable deficit. In addition, it allows surgically for borrowing from the extra branches for cross-face reinnervation.

There are also free communications between the peripheral segments of each of the branches of the facial nerve with each of the divisions of the trigeminal nerve. This free intermingling between the fifth and seventh nerves has been proposed as a mechanism for spontaneous return of facial nerve function following unrepaired peripheral injuries to the nerve. Based on clinical and laboratory experiments, it is generally agreed that the only possible regenerative role of these anastomoses is providing available roots for the facial nerve to regrow through aberrant and communicating pathways, eventually to reach the denervated facial muscles. There has been no evidence to support the fifth nerve nucleus and its axonal extensions as an alternate system for facial mimicking and expressive functions.

PATHOPHYSIOLOGY OF INJURY AND CLASSIFICATION OF FACIAL FUNCTION RECOVERY

Sunderland (1978) described five possible degrees of injury that a nerve fiber might undergo. Figure 17–3 and Table 17–3 show the pathologic changes that occur in the nerve and the anticipated responses of the nerve to electric testing, as well as the type of recovery (House-Brackmann classification system) expected with the various types of injuries. The range of electric responses as well as recovery reflects the variations of degree of injury that might occur.

The five degrees of injury suggested by Sunderland describe the pathophysiologic events associated with all types of disorders that affect the facial nerve. The first three degrees of injury can occur with the viral

inflammatory immune disorders, such as Bell palsy and herpes zoster cephalicus. The fourth and fifth degrees of injury occur when there is disruption of the nerve, as in transection, which might occur during surgery, as a result of a severe temporal bone fracture, or from a rapidly growing benign or malignant tumor.

In a first-degree injury, referred to as neuropraxia, a physiologic neural block is created by increased intraneural pressure. The nerve will not conduct an impulse across the site of compression. Yet, the nerve will respond to electric stimulation applied distal to the lesion. If the compression is relieved, return of facial movement may begin immediately or within three weeks (Fig. 17–4).

A second-degree injury occurs if the compression is not relieved. The mechanism of injury is thought to be obstruction of venous drainage with increased intraneural pressure, further damming up of axoplasm with proximal and distal swelling, and eventual interruption of the flow of nutrients via the compressed arterioles. The result is loss of axons and myelin. If the process is reversed there will be complete recovery, although recovery will take longer than with a first-degree injury, beginning in 3 weeks to 2 months, because it takes time for the degenerated axons to regenerate. If it is a pure second-degree injury, recovery will be complete without any evidence of faulty regeneration. Because the lesions are rarely pure, second-degree injury usually has an element of third-degree injury and therefore recovery is usually marred by some faulty regeneration. There may be slight blink lag, asymmetry with smiling, or subtle evidence of synkinesis (Fig. 17–5).

Fortunately, the pathologic processes causing facial paralysis in patients with Bell palsy and herpes zoster cephalicus usually do not progress beyond first- or second-degree injury, which accounts for satisfactory recovery in most individuals.

A similar process is involved in facial paralysis due to acute suppurative otitis media, chronic otitis media associated with a cholesteatoma, slow-growing benign neoplasms, and temporal bone fractures. In each of these disorders, the nerve is usually not transected, but rather is compressed. In acute otitis media and trauma, compression may be sudden or slowly progressive, evolving over 5 to 10 days, just as noted with Bell palsy and herpes zoster cephalicus. However, unlike the process that occurs with Bell palsy or herpes zoster cephalicus, in these other disorders pressure is exerted on the nerve from without rather than from within the intraneural space; nevertheless, the results of compression of the nerve are the same. Eventually, axoplasm is dammed up; compression of venous drainage leads to further compression of the nerve, loss of axons, and eventually loss of endoneural tubes, which leads to third-degree injury. The type of recovery with this degree of injury is noted in Figure 17–6.

Fourth- or fifth-degree injury results from partial or complete transection of the nerve. Spontaneous recovery should not be expected from fourth- or fifth-degree injury to the nerve; the best results come with surgical

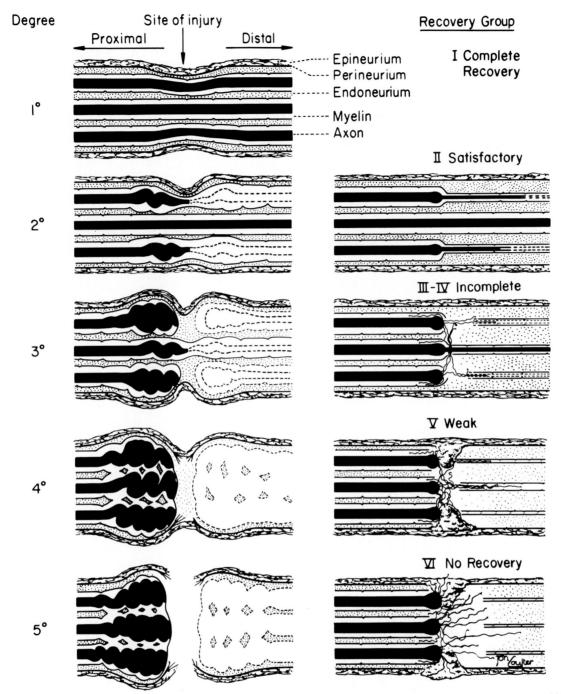

Figure 17–3. Facial nerve injuries may be classified (Sunderland, 1978) by the extent of the lesion from first degree (1°) to fifth degree (5°). First degree—Compression without loss of structure; recovery is complete. Second degree—Axon degeneration; regeneration is appropriate, and recovery is satisfactory. Third degree—Loss of endoneural tubes; recovery is incomplete with synkinesis. Fourth degree—Disruption of perineurium; recovery is poor. Fifth degree—Complete disruption; no recovery. Recovery is classified (House and Brackmann, 1985) from Grade I to Grade VI. (Reprinted by permission from May, M. [ed.]: *The Facial Nerve*, Thieme Medical Publishers, New York, 1985, p. 71.)

nerve repair at the earliest possible moment following injury. Because most or all of the endoneural tubes have been disrupted, as well as the perineurium in fourth-degree injuries and the perineurium and epineurium in fifth-degree injuries, recovery even under ideal conditions is never as good as with the first three degrees of injury.

PROGNOSTIC TESTS

Evaluation of the Intermediate Nerve of Wrisberg

Testing the autonomic and special sensory functions carried with the facial nerve is of limited topognostic

TABLE 17–3. Neuropathologic Findings and Spontaneous Recovery Correlated with Degree of Injury to the Facial Nerve

DEGREE OF INJURY	PATHOLOGIC FINDINGS	EEMG RESPONSE (% OF NORMAL)	NEURAL RECOVERY	CLINICAL RECOVERY BEGINS	SPONTANEOUS RECOVERY RESULT 1 YEAR POSTINJURY*
1	Compression, damming up of axoplasm; no morphologic changes (neuropraxia)	100	No morphologic changes noted	1–3 weeks	Grade I Complete, without evidence of faulty regeneration
2	Compression persists; increased intraneural pressure; loss of axons but endoneurial tubes remain intact (axonotmesis)	11–25	Axons grow into intact, empty myelin tubes at a rate of 1 mm/day, which accounts for longer period for recovery in second-degree compared with first-degree injuries; less than complete recovery is due to some fibers with third-degree injury	3 weeks to 2 months	Grade II Fair (some noticeable difference with volitional or spontaneous movement), minimal evidence of faulty regeneration
3	Intraneural pressure increases; loss of myelin tubes (neurotmesis)	0–10	With loss of myelin tubes the new axons have opportunity to get mixed up and split, causing mouth movement with eye closure (synkinesis)	2–4 months	Grade III to IV Moderate to poor (obvious incomplete recovery to crippling deformity) with moderate to marked complications (Fig. 17–6)
4	Above plus disruption of perineurium (partial transection)	0	In addition to problems caused by second- and third-degree injuries, now the axons are blocked by scars, impairing regeneration	4–18 months	Grade V Recovery poor, complications of faulty regeneration are not as noticeable because of marked facial weakness
5	Above plus disruption of epineurium (transection)	1	Complete disruption with scar-filled gap presents insurmountable barrier to regrowth and neuromuscular hook-up	None	Grade VI None

EEMG, Evoked electromyography.

*Classification by Grades I to VI modified from House and Brachmann (1985).

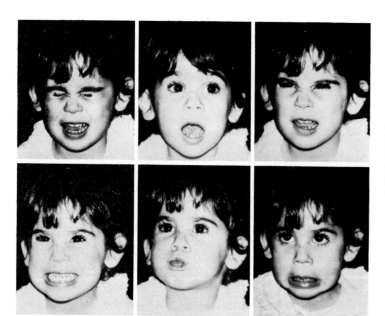

Figure 17–4. Example of fair recovery six months following Bell palsy. Upper photographs suggest complete recovery. Lower photographs taken at same time demonstrate incomplete recovery. This series of photographs stresses the importance of including pictures of facial movement that are exaggerated in order to give accurate evaluation.

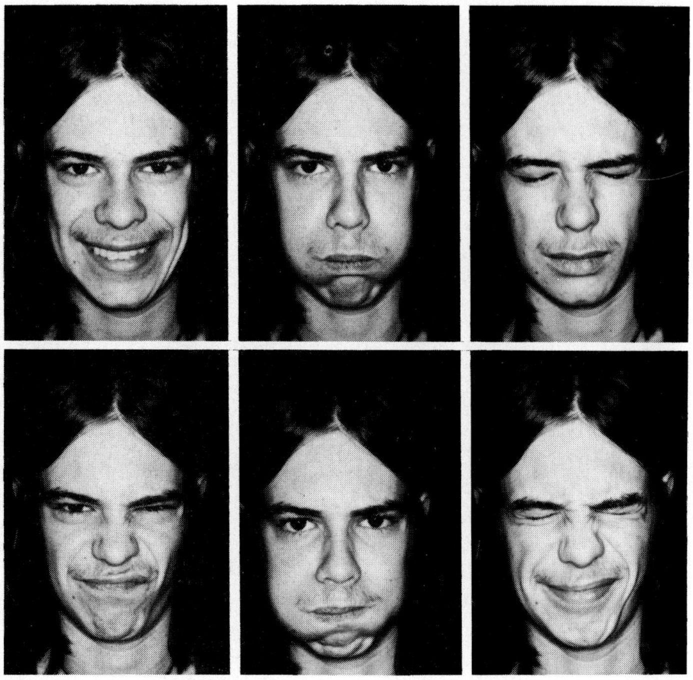

Figure 17–5. This figure shows recovery from a second-degree injury to the facial nerve (Grade II recovery according to House-Brackmann classification system).

or prognostic value in long-standing or slowly progressive facial palsy. The lack of correlation between test results and the location of the lesion is related to a number of variables: (1) the anatomy of the facial nerve and its branches is quite variable, allowing for a variety of alternate pathways for the axons to reach their terminations; (2) the lesion responsible for the paralysis may not be sharply localized to a particular level, as a lesion may affect different components of the nerve at various levels and with different degrees of severity; (3) recovery of the various components may occur at different times; and (4) the techniques used to measure

the various facial nerve functions may not be completely reliable. However, there are patients with acute facial palsy in whom the lesion is sharply defined and can be localized accurately by testing for hearing, submandibular salivary flow, and taste.

Tear Test

A marked reduction or absolute absence of tear production on the involved side is useful but not completely reliable as a topognostic and prognostic test in a patient with peripheral facial nerve paralysis.

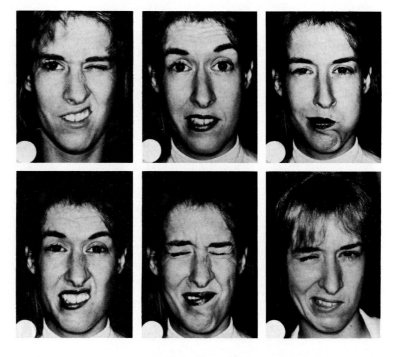

Figure 17–6. Example of poor recovery six months following Bell palsy. The injury in this case was third degree, and recovery was classified as House-Brackmann Grade IV. (Courtesy of Laryngoscope.)

The pathologic decrease or absence of tears on the involved side usually indicates a lesion at or proximal to the geniculate ganglion. Seventy-three per cent of patients with Bell palsy evaluated within 10 days of onset who had a reduction in tearing to 25 per cent or less had unsatisfactory recovery (May et al., 1985).

Tear production must be tested because a history of a dry eye is not reliable. Newborns and young children can be evaluated reliably by observing them during crying: absence of tear production on the involved side is a pathologic sign, and no further testing is required.

Evaluation of tear production may lead to erroneous results. An excess of tearing might often be more apparent than real, owing to the effects of the pathologic condition. For instance, Horner muscle, which dilates the lacrimal sac, may be paralyzed, or there may be outward displacement of the opening of the nasolacrimal duct owing to orbicularis oculi muscle weakness, which results in ectropion. Possibly, lack of muscle tone of the lower lid might allow it to fall slightly away from the globe, producing an increased volume of the inferior conjunctival cul-de-sac, or an excess of tears may be caused by irritation of the exposed eye. Finally, paralysis of the orbicularis oculi muscle causes a defect in the lacrimal pump, inactivating the fine slips of muscle that lie just under the skin along the upper and lower eyelids and that insert on the medial canthus and close the lid; this allows tears to pass across the edges of the lids toward the superior and inferior canaliculi. The opening and closing of the eyelids as a result of contraction and relaxation of the orbicularis oculi muscle dilate and contract the lacrimal sac, which is thought to be responsible for emptying the tears into the nose and then drawing the tears into the sac.

The method used by the author to quantify tearing was based on the nasolacrimal reflex. Filter paper strips (Schirmer test strips) can be purchased (Crookes-Barnes Laboratories, Inc., Wayne, NJ) or can be fashioned so that they are 3.5 cm long and 0.5 cm wide. These strips are folded at one end so that the folded tab can be placed over the lower lid, in the conjunctival sac, leaving 3 cm to absorb the tears produced. Placing the filter paper strip in the normal side first is advised. If the paper is placed in the paralyzed side first, the irritation of the paper will cause a reflex contraction on the normal side, leading to difficulty in placing the paper slip in the normal eye. These strong reflex contractions do not occur on the paralyzed side. It is important to empty the sacs with a piece of cotton prior to inserting the strips, to avoid erroneous results from pooled or excess tears that may be present in the involved side prior to the start of a test. After the strips are in place, the patient is asked to take a sniff of fresh spirits of ammonia, which sets up a nasolacrimal reflex. The filter paper strips are left in place for a period of three minutes or until one strip is completely moistened, at which time the strips are removed and the amount of liquid on each is noted. The test results are considered abnormal if the strip from the affected side has 10 per cent or less liquid than the strip from the normal side.

The tear test is most accurate if absolutely no tears are produced on the involved side over a period of three minutes. This is considered to represent a dry eye and portends a poor prognosis.

Salivation Test

The submandibular salivary flow test is no longer considered a useful prognostic indicator in cases of acute peripheral facial palsy. Reduction in salivary flow to 25 per cent or less of normal predicted an unsatisfactory recovery in 56 per cent of cases (May et al., 1985). Employing the House-Brackmann classification system of reporting results, approximately half the patients with reduced salivary flow exhibited Grades I and II recovery and the other half Grades III and IV. Following these observations, the salivation test has been discontinued as a prognostic test.

Evaluation of Facial Motor Fibers by Electric Tests

The problem for the clinician who sees a patient with facial paralysis of recent onset is to determine whether the involved nerve is mildly compressed and is in a state of first-degree injury from which it will recover spontaneously, or whether there is beginning second-degree injury that will go on to third-degree injury and involve the entire nerve trunk if pressure is not relieved. There are three electric tests that are useful clinically: the maximal percutaneous excitability test (MST), evoked electromyography (EEMG), and electromyography (EMG). The first two tests are capable of detecting early or ensuing degeneration, whereas the last test becomes useful after degeneration has occurred. The first two tests are useful in the two weeks following onset of facial nerve paralysis; the last test becomes useful by the 10th to the 21st day following the onset of paralysis.

Maximal Stimulation Test

The maximal stimulation test (MST) is based on the fact that a motor nerve will conduct in response to an electric stimulus applied distal to a lesion, even though the lesion blocks volitional movement, provided the nerve is morphologically intact distal to the lesion (i.e., the injury is first degree). When the injury is second degree, causing damage to the axon, an increase in the intensity of the stimulus is required to cause a muscle twitch. If the myelin and axon distal to the lesion have degenerated, as with a third-degree injury, then no conduction will occur no matter how intense the stimulus. It has been shown that a completely sectioned nerve may continue to conduct distal to the section for as long as 48 to 72 hours after the injury. For this reason, the MST has limited value until 48 to 72 hours after the onset of the paralysis. In addition, MST is only of value as long as the nerve remains intact. After the nerve degenerates and response to electric excitability is lost, the test is no longer useful. Duchenne (1872), who first suggested the excitability test, stated that when excitability is lost after degeneration, it returns in only a minority of cases, even if there is recovery and return of volitional movement. Another limitation of this test is the need to compare the results of the involved side with those of the normal side, which acts as a control. Thus, in cases of recurrent palsy or alternating bilateral involvement the test has limited value.

The excitability test can be performed with any electric stimulus in which the strength and duration can be varied. The Hilger nerve stimulator is especially designed to test the facial nerve. (Model 2r with a rechargeable battery is favored by the author: the instrument is conveniently portable, allowing for bedside consultation, and testing can be performed in several minutes without discomfort to the patient.) The test is performed by setting the intensity at 5 ma, or the highest setting tolerated by the patient without undue discomfort. An area of the patient's skin between the sideburns and the eyebrow and extending down over the cheek, jaw, and neck is wiped with electrode conduction paste. Then the stimulating probe is passed slowly over this area. The responses over the forehead, eye, nose, mouth, lower lip, and neck are noted and recorded as equal, decreased, or absent on the involved side, as compared with those on the normal side. The test is repeated by stimulating at the area of the stylomastoid foramen, between the mastoid tip and the ascending ramus. Because degeneration proceeds from proximal to distal, evidence of degeneration might be detected a day or two earlier by testing at the site where the facial nerve exits the temporal bone. The nerve is tested more peripherally to evaluate each major branch, which cannot be done by testing only in the area of the stylomastoid foramen.

Results of the maximal stimulation test, as described, were more reliable and became altered earlier than did those of the minimal percutaneous electric stimulation test, which depends on looking for a 3.5 ma difference in excitability between the two sides (May et al., 1971). The maximal stimulation test, although quite useful, was not completely accurate in predicting the patient's ultimate degree of recovery. When the response to maximal stimulation was equal, 12 per cent of the patients had incomplete return, and, when the response to MST was decreased, 73 per cent of the patients had incomplete return of facial function. The test was most accurate when MST was lost: in this case all patients had incomplete return with marked evidence of faulty regeneration (May et al., 1976a).

The rationale for testing each major facial motor area supplied by the nerve is that certain fibers can be affected more than others, depending on the nature, location, and severity of the lesion. (The author has observed a first-degree injury in one part of the face and a third-degree injury in another part.) This has been noted in acute cases as well as during the phase of recovery. In acute involvement of the facial nerve, as with paralysis following trauma or infection, ideally the electric test should be repeated daily until the response to MST becomes abnormal or return of volitional facial movement is noted.

Evoked Electromyography

EEMG is the recording of evoked summation potentials. This test was popularized and referred to by Fisch and Esslen (1972) as electroneurography (ENOG). In principle, it is similar to the maximal stimulation test except that instead of depending on muscle twitch elicited, evoked summating potentials (SP) are recorded on a graph produced by a sophisticated electrodiagnostic apparatus, the direct recording electromyograph. The amount of degeneration is related to the difference in amplitude of the measured SPs on the normal and involved sides.

The great advantage of EEMG over the simple observation of facial movements as described under maximal stimulation is the precise quantitative assessment of the response available with EEMG.

Fisch (1977b) recommended surgical exposure of the intratemporal portion of the facial nerve (1) in traumatic lesions when the amplitude of the SP became reduced to 10 per cent or less of that of the normal side within 6 days after the onset of the palsy; (2) in idiopathic (Bell) palsy as soon as the SP became reduced to 10 per cent or less of that of the normal side within 2 weeks of onset of the palsy or in the presence of a lesser reduction when inner ear symptoms are present; and (3) in acute otitis media when there is a reduction to 10 per cent or less in spite of paracentesis and antibiotic treatment.

EEMG is a welcome contribution to help document accurately the electric changes in an injured nerve, but unfortunately it has the same disadvantages as have been noted with MST. Furthermore, waiting until the SPs become reduced to 10 per cent of normal values may preclude intervention at an appropriate time to reverse nerve damage.

Electromyography (EMG)

After degeneration occurs, EMG is indispensable as a measure of damage to the nerve. A denervated muscle, being hyperirritable, produces spontaneous electric potentials, referred to as fibrillation potentials, which can be measured. Usually, these fibrillation potentials do not appear until 10 to 21 days after degeneration occurs. Although the time delay is a major limitation in the application of EMG, EMG is the most reliable test to determine nerve degeneration because it samples motor unit activity. When the motor unit is intact, a motor unit potential can be detected with volitional movement. When this is demonstrated following trauma, nerve transection can be ruled out. Further, reappearance of motor unit potentials in acute facial palsies in which response to EEMG is absent indicates a deblocking phenomenon and, in spite of loss of response to EEMG, indicates that the acute process impairing nerve function is abating.

Other Prognostic Indicators

Prognostic evaluation of a particular case of facial paralysis must be based on the history of onset, the duration of palsy, and the completeness of the paralysis, in addition to electric test results. The progression of paresis to complete paralysis over a period of three to ten days is a poor prognostic sign. Seventy-five per cent of the patients with this type of history developed degeneration with incomplete return of function (May et al., 1976a). The maintenance of some facial movement, or the early return of facial movement within the first two weeks of onset, indicates a favorable prognosis for spontaneous recovery in spite of the presence of abnormal prognostic indicators, such as abnormal electric test results.

The most useful application of EEMG is predicting outcome in acute facial paralysis. By studying the results of EEMG and evaluating the completeness of the palsy, the patient's prognosis for recovery of facial function can be predicted with a high degree of accuracy. Ninety per cent of patients will have a satisfactory recovery if the palsy is incomplete and response to evoked electromyography remains greater than 10 per cent of normal response beyond the first 14 days after onset. However, patients with a complete palsy and response to EEMG of 10 per cent or less of that of the normal side within the first 14 days have a 50 per cent chance of an unsatisfactory recovery. This latter group requires the greatest attention in terms of treatment directed toward improving the natural history of facial palsy and preventing complications of nerve degeneration. At the moment surgical treatment, including treatment of compression of the meatal segment (the most proximal portion of the fallopian canal reached through a middle fossa approach), remains investigational. Patients that fall into the poor prognostic group can be advised that recovery of facial function may not occur for two to four months from the time of onset and are offered guidelines for eye care.

MANAGEMENT OF FACIAL PARALYSIS: GENERAL PRINCIPLES

The patient with facial paralysis or his or her family usually asks three questions: (1) What caused the facial paralysis? (2) When can recovery be expected? (3) What can be done to bring about recovery at the earliest possible time? These three questions can be translated into the medical tasks of (1) making a diagnosis, (2) determining the prognosis, and (3) recommending treatment.

Diagnosis

The diagnosis can be made in a majority of cases by a careful history and physical examination, as well as by neurootologic evaluation. It should be emphasized that *Bell palsy is a diagnosis of exclusion* and should be used only when all other causes of facial paralysis have been eliminated.

Facial paralysis due to acute and chronic suppurative infection usually can be diagnosed by the presence of ear pain and by a bulging, red tympanic membrane in acute suppurative otitis media and a fetid mucoid discharge or evidence of a *cholesteatoma* in chronic otitis media (Chap. 22).

Facial paralysis associated with a closed head injury is diagnostic of a *temporal bone fracture*. Tuning forks can distinguish between a conductive and a sensorineural hearing loss: a conductive hearing loss usually indicates a longitudinal fracture with sparing of the otic capsule, whereas a sensorineural hearing loss is diagnostic of a transverse fracture with violation of the otic capsule (Chap. 26).

A tumor as a cause of facial paralysis should be suspected if (1) the paralysis is slowly progressive beyond three weeks; (2) the paralysis is recurrent on the same side; or (3) there is no recovery from an acute facial paralysis after six months. Examination of the nasopharynx, tonsil, parotid, and neck, as well as of the area between the ascending ramus and mastoid tip, might discover a neoplasm that could involve the facial nerve.

The presence of vesicles on the pinna, face, or oral mucosa suggests herpes zoster oticus, which may also be associated with dysequilibrium and a sensorineural hearing loss. The onset of a simultaneous bilateral facial paralysis suggests Guillain-Barré syndrome, bulbar palsy, sarcoidosis, or some other systemic disorder. A detailed, general neurologic examination usually reveals other neurologic signs in such patients.

Pregnancy, especially in the third trimester, is significant in the evaluation of facial paralysis. Facial paralysis of the Bell palsy type has a three times higher incidence among pregnant women, particularly those in the third trimester, than in nonpregnant women of the same age group (Hilsinger et al., 1975).

Recurrent facial paralysis occurs in 10 per cent of patients with Bell palsy, but when it recurs on the same side the presence of a tumor must be considered. Melkersson-Rosenthal syndrome is a rare noncaseating granulation disease of undetermined etiology. It is characterized by the presence of facial edema (usually eyelid or lips), recurrent alternating, seventh nerve palsy, positive family history, migraine, and headaches (Alexander and James, 1972).

Bell palsy is the likely diagnosis when other causes have been excluded and in those patients with one or more of the following: (1) a positive family history of facial paralysis; (2) a viral prodrome; or (3) the presence of a red chorda tympani nerve. Of the author's patients, 13 per cent who were diagnosed as having Bell palsy had a positive family history for that illness; 60 per cent had had a viral prodrome; and a red chorda tympani nerve was noted in 40 per cent of those patients whose chorda tympani nerve was visible (May, 1974).

Although Bell palsy has been thought of as a mononeuropathy, there is clinical evidence that many nerves are involved (May and Hardin, 1978). This impression is supported by decreased or lost corneal sensation; presence of pain or numbness over the side of the head, ear, face, neck, and shoulder; and numbness of the tongue in patients with Bell palsy (Fig. 17–7). The loss of corneal sensation may be due to direct involvement of the fifth nerve endings innervating the conjunctiva or due to exposure hypesthesia. The changes in sensation may be explained by involvement of nerves that connect with the facial nerve. These include branches of the cervical plexus, ninth nerve, tenth nerve, and fifth nerve (see Fig. 17–2).

The presence of intact, symmetric upper facial movements has been noted with acute suppurative otitis media, temporal bone fractures, and lower motor neuron lesions such as Bell palsy and therefore is not an exclusive diagnostic sign of a central lesion (May and Hardin, 1978).

Prognosis

After the diagnosis has been established, the prognosis can be made with 90 per cent accuracy, within the first 10 days after onset of facial paralysis.

The presence or absence of taste or pain has not been of prognostic value. The presence of a stapes reflex is a favorable sign, provided the lesion is not distal to the pyramidal segment of the facial nerve, as

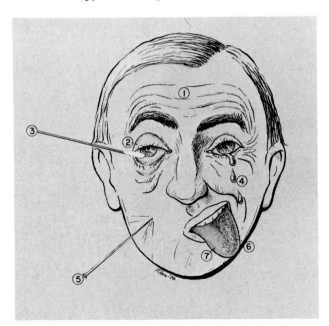

Figure 17–7. Misleading signs associated with Bell palsy: (1) intact forehead, (2) Horner syndrome (constricted pupil and ptosis of upper eyelid), (3) loss of corneal sensation, (4) tearing only on uninvolved side, (5) loss of skin sensation, (6) apparent tongue deviation, (7) loss of taste papillae. (Courtesy of Laryngoscope.)

noted with trauma or tumor involving the facial nerve in the vertical segment or in the extratemporal bone region. Loss of stapes reflex did not have prognostic significance, as it was commonly lost in patients with complete loss of facial movement and half of these patients had complete recovery without treatment.

After the first few days, electric tests become valuable. Although results usually become altered by the third day in a transected nerve, they may not become altered until the fifth to the tenth day in a dynamic, slowly progressive lesion, such as is noted with Bell palsy, or a slowly compressive lesion due to infection or following trauma. When the response to maximal stimulation, evoked electromyography, or both becomes reduced to 10 per cent or less of that of the normal side, 80 per cent of patients will have an unsatisfactory recovery (House-Brackmann Grade III or IV).

The natural history of Bell palsy, the most common type of facial paralysis, has been established. Peitersen (1982) reported the natural history of Bell palsy in over 1000 subjects. In 84 per cent of these patients recovery was satisfactory (Grade I or II). The other 16 per cent of patients had incomplete recovery of facial function, but sequelae were crippling in only 4 per cent. These results have been confirmed by others (Olsen, 1975; May et al., 1976b).

The time that recovery is first noted is one of the most useful late prognostic indicators: (1) if recovery begins between the tenth day and the third week, with few exceptions, recovery will be complete (Grade I); (2) if recovery does not begin until after three weeks but before two months, the majority of these patients will have a satisfactory recovery of function (Grade II); and (3) if recovery does not begin until the second to the fourth month, recovery will be poor (Grade III or IV).

Progression and completeness of palsy during the first three weeks after onset have been found to have prognostic significance. There are four distinct patterns of facial motor involvement exhibited by patients with Bell palsy. Patients may fall about equally into: (1) those with complete paralysis at onset, who have a 50 per cent chance of having incomplete recovery; (2) those with incomplete paralysis at onset and whose palsy does not progress, who will recover completely; (3) those with incomplete paralysis that progressed (but not to complete paralysis), who will have complete recovery; and finally (4) those that have incomplete paralysis that progresses to complete paralysis, who have a 75 per cent chance of incomplete recovery.

These guidelines, which were derived from treating patients with Bell palsy, have been found to be just as valid for other disorders that cause compressive lesions of the facial nerve.

Treatment

Contrary to the opinion of most primary physicians, who see only an occasional case of facial paralysis that resolves without treatment, facial paralysis is a potential medical-surgical emergency. On occasion a patient with a facial paralysis has an underlying, life-threatening disorder, and others spend their lives as facial cripples because treatment was not offered until death of the facial nerve was established by electric tests. In chronic otitis media with cholesteatoma, nerve death may occur between the fifth and tenth day after onset of paralysis, and in most severe cases denervation may occur as early as the first or second day. Treatment can be effective only if the compressive lesion is treated at the earliest possible moment following onset of the paralysis. Therefore, facial paralysis in such an instance is truly an emergency.

The rationale for treatment and expected results for the various lesions causing facial paralysis is based on the existing neuropathologic findings in each case (see Fig. 17–3; Table 17–3).

Eye

Considerations for management of the eye in patients with facial paralysis were discussed in detail by Levine (1974, 1979). There are two major problems that result when eye closure is impaired: the eye becomes irritated owing to exposure, and this irritation is significantly compounded when tear production is impaired. Treatment is thus directed toward protecting the eye from exposure and drying. This can be accomplished by having the patient instill artificial tears every hour during waking hours and a bland ointment at night. The eye may also be protected by a moisture chamber* that either may be secured with a band or may fit on the eyeglasses. A half-moon cutout of skin-tone micropore surgical tape acts as an effective splint for the upper eyelid: it should be placed with the dome toward the fold in the upper eyelid and the base along the eyelash margin. This often allows the patient to overcome the pull by the superior levator muscle and affords natural protection for the eye.

Eye care should be continued until return of spontaneous eye closure. Patients with acute facial paralysis who have a favorable prognosis can be managed adequately by the conservative treatment suggested. On rare occasions, surgical measures are necessary for patients who are developing eye complications in spite of conservative treatment, and especially when the prospects for recovery are poor. The surgical techniques used involve reestablishing eye closure as well as tightening up the sagging lower eyelid.

Pain

Patients with pain, particularly that associated with herpes zoster oticus or Bell palsy, often require analgesic medication for the first week sometimes longer.

Depression

The emotional impact of facial palsy can be significant, particularly in the first few weeks, and must not be neglected. Reassurance may be offered to those patients who are expected to have a complete or satisfactory recovery, but if the prognosis is unfavorable, the patient should be advised of this possibility so that he or she does not develop an attitude of denial that leads him or her to deal unrealistically with residual deformity.

It is reassuring to patients with facial palsy of the acute compressive type, such as Bell, herpes zoster oticus, or acute otitis media, to learn that the face will not remain completely paralyzed, as some recovery is expected even in the most severe cases. The depression that accompanies the onset of the facial paralysis is often relieved by the prediction of a favorable outcome, as well as an indication of when the recovery may be noted. Occasionally, temporary treatment with sedatives is helpful. Reassurance and support can be offered by arranging for the patient to share experiences with another person who had facial paralysis. If the depression persists in spite of this counseling, psychiatric consultation should be considered.

Medications

Medications, such as vitamins or antihistamines, have no efficacious influence on the natural history of Bell palsy but may serve as psychologic support. Patients often feel better when they know that they are taking a medication rather than relying on the physician's predictions alone. The author's preference is to prescribe vitamins to patients with a favorable prognosis. Steroids have no place in the management of facial paralysis, may cause serious complications, and often delay appropriate management. Table 17–4 summarizes the studies that demonstrate that the administration of steroids to patients with Bell palsy did not have any influence on recovery of facial function.

Surgery

To date no randomized, stratified, controlled clinical trial with a sufficient number of patients for meaningful statistical analysis has shown that surgical exploration and decompression of the facial nerve is effective in relieving facial paralysis due to any pathologic condition that does not interrupt the nerve. Thus, the benefit of surgery has not been established for idiopathic (Bell) palsy, herpes zoster cephalicus, acute suppurative otitis media, necrotizing external otitis, or facial paralysis following iatrogenic or external temporal bone trauma.

However, facial paralysis due to an ongoing process such as chronic suppurative otitis media, with or without cholesteatoma, can only be relieved by eradicating the primary process. In this case, surgery should be performed prior to electric denervation to give the

---

*Pro-Optics, 317 N. Woodwork Lane, Palatine, Illinois 60067. Large with band (adult), small with band (child), clip-on left or right for use with eyeglasses.

TABLE 17–4. Steroids Ineffective for Bell Palsy

REFERENCE	PATIENTS	STEROID DOSE (14 DAYS)	RECOVERY COMPLETE*		COMMENTS
			Steroids	Controls	
Peitersen (1977)	Consecutive 778	—	—	70%	Results represent natural history
May et al. (1976b)	Double blind, randomized 51	400 mg	60%	65%	Difference not statistically significant
Wolf et al. (1978)	Randomized 239	760 mg	88%	80%	Difference not statistically significant
Devriese (1977)	Consecutive 76	570 mg	66%	—	Results not significantly better than achieved without treatment

*Studies quoted were controlled; patients were evaluated within 7 days, the majority within 3 days; and complete recovery was defined similarly as full volitional activity and absence of distortion at rest or on volitional movement.

most satisfactory facial function recovery and must not be delayed if the palsy has progressed from incomplete to complete over a period of hours or days and if the response to EEMG is less than 25 per cent of normal or is dropping precipitously after the third day following onset.

In addition, there are two situations in which surgery is absolutely indicated in managing facial nerve disorders: facial nerve transection and tumor infiltration. Further, there are times when nerve transection or tumor infiltration can only be established by surgical exploration, in particular when the temporal bone has fractured or a tumor is suspected.

Surgical Treatment of Transected Nerve

If the nerve has been interrupted by tumor or trauma, a variety of approaches are available. The decision to use any approach is based on the cause and location of the lesion, the status of hearing, and the length of time since paralysis was first noted (Fisch, 1977b).

The ideal technique for facial reanimation achieves facial symmetry at rest and spontaneous facial expression with mouth movement and eye closure. The techniques include, in order of preference, (1) end-to-end anastomosis; (2) cable interposition grafts; (3) crossover graft from normal facial nerve to the paralyzed nerve (Samii, 1977; Fisch, 1977a; Anderl, 1977); (4) grafting the hypoglossal or spinal accessory nerve to the paralyzed nerve (Fisch, 1977b; Conley, 1977a, 1977b); (5) muscle-nerve pedicle grafting from the ansa hypoglossal nerve (Tucker, 1977); (6) free-muscle grafting with neural or neurovascular anastomosis (Thompson, 1971; Thompson and Gustavsson, 1976; Anderl, 1977; Hakelius, 1977); (7) temporalis or masseter muscle swings (Conley and Gullane, 1978; Rubin, 1976); (8) facial suspension; or (9) combinations of the preceding.

Tucker (1978) discussed the management of extracranial facial nerve injuries and proposed pertinent considerations in the choice of an approach to the repair of such injuries.

SPECIAL CONSIDERATIONS IN MANAGING FACIAL PARALYSIS IN YOUNG CHILDREN

The principles involved in managing facial paralysis are the same for patients of all ages, perhaps excepting young children (newborn to age 5 years). Facial paralysis noted at birth can be due to trauma or to a developmental anomaly. The distinction is important because the prognosis and treatment of each differ (Bergman et al., 1986). Traumatic paralysis may require immediate surgical decompression or nerve repair, whereas the congenital type presents no urgency. Isolated involvement of the marginal mandibular branch of the facial nerve, noted at birth, might be associated with other congenital anomalies as reported by Pape and Pickering (1972). These authors stress that asymmetric crying facies, as evidenced by the lack of pulling down of the lower lip on the involved side, may signal the presence of congenital anomalies in the skeletal, genitourinary, respiratory, or cardiovascular systems.

Isolated unilateral paralysis, as noted with involvement of the marginal mandibular branch in a young child, may be associated with acute, suppurative otitis media (Fig. 17–8) and should be treated by myringotomy and administration of an appropriate antibiotic.

Prepubescent children, particularly those under 5 years of age, rarely are reliable in relating historical factors, such as alterations in sensation, hearing, balance, taste, or tear production or the presence of vesicles, all of which may be helpful in making a diagnosis. This information might be obtained by questioning the parents, but it is interesting that even the most concerned parents are not always reliable historians. This observation is supported by evaluating young children with mild facial weakness that was not noted by the parents but was picked up by friends or teachers. However, some parents can provide useful information and must be questioned carefully regarding the time of onset of the crooked cry or whether tears formed on the involved side during crying. This is quite helpful in dating the onset of the paralysis as well as in assessing the involvement of tear production.

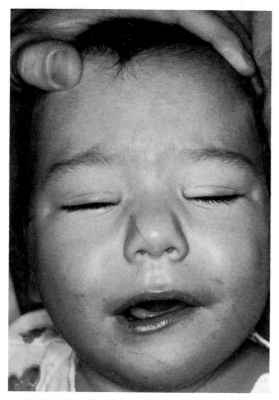

Figure 17–8. Palsy of left lower lip associated with acute suppurative otitis media involving the left ear.

Old photographs are another aid in documenting the presence of facial asymmetry that was previously unnoticed.

Tests requiring subjective responses, such as audiometry and taste perception, may not be reliable in the young child. Measurement of evoked auditory brain stem potentials, however, may help to overcome these problems because the measurements depend on objective responses.

Evaluation of facial motor function is possible with children as young as 2 years of age who are very expressive and who will mimic facial expressions (Fig. 17–4). Although most require observation while spontaneous emotions are displayed, play therapy, tickling, and at times provoking crying, such as might occur with electric testing, are quite useful in the evaluation of facial motor function and of tear production.

Taste testing may not be a reliable method of evaluating the integrity of the chorda tympani nerve in the young child. However, because the taste papillae in children are prominent, one may easily note by inspection if the papillae have atrophied on the involved side, which implies that the chorda tympani nerve has been interrupted. A lesion involving the chorda tympani nerve that causes atrophy of the taste papillae may be the result of a disorder located anywhere between the middle ear and the brain stem.

Electric tests may be used if the stimulus is kept below the pain threshold. Usually a stimulus in the range of 2 to 3 ma is tolerated by young children.

Maximal stimulation, EEMG, and electromyographic testing have not been used successfully in young children without sedation or general anesthesia.

Eye care is usually not required in children. The exact reason for this is not known, but children born with facial paralysis who are unable to close the eye, and even those who suffer loss of tear production, rarely develop eye complications even without additional moisture or protection for the eye. It is interesting to note that young children (those between birth and age 5 years) blink infrequently and that the ratio of the area of the iris to that of the sclera is greater in the younger than in the older child; thus, perhaps something is unique in the tear content or production of young children that allows them to avoid most eye problems associated with facial paralysis in adults.

ETIOLOGY

Infection

Acute otitis media is not a rare cause of facial paralysis in children; it was the second most common cause in the author's series. Paralysis due to acute otitis media is not benign, as 7 of 19 children had incomplete recovery of facial function, and one of the seven had an extremely poor return of function.

Acute Otitis Media

PATHOPHYSIOLOGY. The pathophysiology of facial paralysis associated with acute otitis media was described by Tschiassny (1944) and included thinness of the outer wall of the fallopian canal as it bends around the oval window; persistence of dehiscences of the fallopian canal, which are normally present only during the first year of life; anatomic connections of the nerve with the tympanic cavity; and pathways into the fallopian canal from the stapedius nerve, the chorda tympani, and the posterior tympanic artery. Further, because the facial nerve is enclosed in a bony fibrous conduit, it is vulnerable to increases in its volume as a result of exudate, edema, congestion, or hemorrhage. Toxins, as well as osteitis of the mastoid associated with acute infection, may be additional factors in facial paralysis.

Botman and Jongkees (1955) reported that facial paralysis complicating acute otitis media increases in severity when there is osteitis surrounding the nerve.

MEDICAL TREATMENT. Antibiotics and myringotomy are the recommended treatments of choice for acute otitis media and are thought to be effective in the great majority of cases. It was of interest to note that four patients treated for acute suppurative otitis media with an appropriate antibiotic developed complete peripheral facial paralysis two to five days following the start of the antibiotics. Facial nerve function in four patients degenerated following antibiotic and myringotomy therapy. Each of these had incomplete recovery, and in one of these the final return of facial nerve function was poor.

These observations suggest that in some cases the infectious process progresses to damage the facial nerve in spite of medical therapy. For this reason, prognostic tests must be employed to determine if the facial nerve is being threatened. In this way surgery can be carried out at the earliest appropriate moment, ideally before there is degeneration.

SURGICAL FINDINGS AND RESULTS. Suppurative mastoiditis was confirmed in 10 of 19 patients operated on. The surgical findings consisted of granulation tissue lying against an exposed nerve in the horizontal segment in five ears; in three patients there was soft, osteitic bone around the vertical segment in addition to the granulation tissue found in the horizontal segment. In two ears the findings were limited to osteitic bone around the vertical segment. In each of these cases, the nerve was exposed and the sheath opened. Twelve patients had complete recovery (Grade I), six had good recovery (Grade II), and one had poor recovery of facial nerve function (Grade III).

Two patients were initially treated with penicillin and myringotomy and operated on after electric response was lost. One had complete recovery and the other had Group II recovery of facial nerve function.

Chronic Otitis Media

There is little controversy regarding treatment for facial paralysis associated with chronic otitis media and mastoiditis, particularly when it is associated with cholesteatoma. Whereas conservative treatment is advised for acute suppurative otitis media, surgical intervention at the earliest possible moment is recommended for facial paralysis associated with chronic infection. The mechanism in chronic infection is extraneural compression from cholesteatoma, usually in the region of the cochleariform process. This is the only point in the middle ear where cholesteatoma can impinge on the facial nerve and this process. The pathophysiologic events in chronic infection are less acute, and the results, provided the surgery is done prior to the loss of electric response and within the first 24 to 48 hours after onset, have been uniformly excellent (Chap. 22).

Trauma

Traumatic facial paralysis occurred in 62 (18 per cent) of the patients in the author's series, as shown in Table 17–1.

Birth

Facial paralysis noted at birth can be traumatic or congenital in origin (see discussion of congenital causes below). There are factors that aid in differentiating one from the other (Table 17–5). The presence of other congenital anomalies, facial diplegia, or upper face palsy suggests a congenital cause, whereas the absence of these signs and the presence of a history of a prolonged labor in a primipara mother, high-forceps delivery, evidence of forceps marks over the area of the ear, or a hemotympanum suggest birth trauma. Congenital facial paralysis does not improve, whereas paralysis due to birth trauma may. With recovery following trauma, there is usually some evidence of faulty regeneration such as a tic, synkinesis, or spasm. This does not occur with paralysis of the congenital type.

Patients must be evaluated within a few days of birth for traumatic causes of facial paralysis to be documented, as the clues suggesting trauma disappear quickly.

The differentiation of traumatic from developmental causes of neonatal facial palsy is occasionally difficult despite an adequate history, physical examination, and radiographic studies. Electrophysiologic testing performed sequentially during the first days of life is often capable of unequivocally resolving this problem. Results of facial nerve conduction studies are usually abnormal immediately at birth with developmental anomalies, whereas with traumatic injuries conduction studies are normal at birth and become abnormal three to seven days after birth. Infants with congenital facial palsy of uncertain cause should, therefore, have electrophysiologic testing performed sequentially starting from two days after birth or sooner. Based on a study by Bergman and associates (1986), a conservative approach for neonatal traumatic facial palsy is recommended. This is because (1) more than 90 per cent of infants with this injury recover spontaneously; (2) there are no controlled studies demonstrating an improved outcome in this condition following surgical exploration and decompression of the facial nerve; (3) surgical exploration may produce iatrogenic injury to the vestibular or cochlear apparatus, as well as to the facial nerve itself.

However, this recommendation does not preclude surgical exploration in all cases. Children who do not recover spontaneously are left with a significant lifelong functional and cosmetic disability, which might have been ameliorated by relatively early surgical repair of a lacerated or transected facial nerve. Surgical exploration of the facial nerve is considered an option in newborns who meet the following criteria: (1) unilateral complete paralysis present at birth, (2) hemotympanum and displaced fracture of the petrous bone, (3) electrophysiologic studies demonstrating absence of voluntary and evoked motor unit responses in all muscles innervated by the facial nerve by three to five days after birth, and (4) no return of facial nerve function clinically or electrophysiologically at 5 weeks of age. This period of observation minimizes the chance of unnecessary surgery, and, although nerve repair is best accomplished immediately after the injury, a good repair can still be effected five weeks following the injury.

Temporal Bone Fractures

INCIDENCE. Mitchell and Stone (1973) reported the incidence of facial paralysis among 1015 children with

TABLE 17–5. Facial Palsy at Birth—Differential Diagnosis

CHARACTERISTICS OF CONGENITAL CAUSES	METHOD OF DIFFERENTIATION	CHARACTERISTICS OF TRAUMATIC CAUSES
Illness in first trimester No recovery of facial function after birth Family history of facial and other anomalies	History	Total paralysis at birth with some recovery noted subsequently
Other anomalies, facial diplegia (bilateral palsy)	Physical examination	Hemotympanum, ecchymoses, tics, syskinesis
Anomalous (external, middle, or inner ear)	Radiograph of temporal bone	Fracture
Response reduced or absent without change	MST EEMG	Normal at birth, then decreasing response may be lost
Reduced or absent response, no evidence of degeneration	EMG	Normal at birth, then loss of spontaneous motor units and fibrillations 10 to 21 days later

MST, Maximal stimulation test; EEMG, evoked electromyography; EMG, electromyography.

head injuries over a two-year period. Of the total, 71 patients had temporal bone fractures, and 21 per cent of these had facial paralysis.

PATHOPHYSIOLOGY. A longitudinal fracture, the most common type of temporal bone fracture, usually courses along the long axis of the pyramid, down the squamous bone, across the mastoid cortex, and through the posterior canal wall and involves the facial nerve at the second genu; or if the fracture crosses the mastoid tegmen, the facial nerve is usually compressed or torn in the area of the geniculate ganglion. This type of fracture is usually associated with a hemotympanum and may cause disruption of the ossicular chain. An excellent review of injuries to the middle ear with skull trauma was reported by Hough and Stuart (1968). There may or may not be a tear of the tympanic membrane. Vertigo will be present along with spontaneous nystagmus if the stapes is subluxed into the vestibule. Longitudinal fractures usually involve the middle ear, and facial paralysis occurs in approximately 25 per cent of these patients. Cerebrospinal fluid leaks are associated with longitudinal fractures but are more common with transverse fractures.

Transverse fractures are caused by a more severe injury than are longitudinal fractures, and loss of consciousness is common. The fracture is usually across the occiput and up the posterior wall of the pyramid, through the internal auditory canal and the otic capsule. Facial paralysis occurs in 50 per cent of such cases and rarely spares the inner ear.

DIAGNOSIS. Peripheral facial paralysis following a head injury usually indicates a fractured temporal bone. The fracture may be longitudinal, transverse, or a combination of these two. The types can be differentiated by the use of a tuning fork. A conductive hearing loss usually indicates a longitudinal fracture, and a profound sensorineural hearing loss indicates a transverse fracture.

Location of the fracture can be determined by tear testing. Loss of tearing indicates that the fracture is at or proximal to the geniculate ganglion, whereas the injury is usually distal to the geniculate ganglion if tearing is normal. Testing for tearing and responses to

tuning forks have been found to be more accurate for defining the type of fracture and its location than have sophisticated radiographic techniques such as polytomography of the temporal bone. Further, tuning fork tests can differentiate a hemotympanum from an ossicular dissociation. If the Weber test response lateralizes to the injured ear but air conduction is greater than bone conduction with a 512-Hz tuning fork, an ossicular chain disruption is unlikely.

MANAGEMENT. After the status of the patient's central nervous system and general condition have been stabilized, attention is directed toward injuries within the temporal bone. These include, in the order of priority, vertigo, facial paralysis, cerebrospinal fluid leak, a tear of the tympanic membrane, and ossicular discontinuity. Schneider and Boles (1968) discussed the neurosurgical and neurootologic problems in head trauma. The following discussion will be limited to facial paralysis.

Otologic consultation is encouraged as soon as possible following a head injury when there is associated facial paralysis. Surgical exploration for total facial paralysis is indicated if there is evidence of disruption or severe compression, both to confirm the injury and to repair it if possible. If the onset of facial palsy after temporal bone fracture is delayed or slowly progressive, and response to evoked electromyography remains greater than 10 per cent of normal through the fifth day, surgery is not indicated. However, if the paralysis is sudden and complete and response to evoked electromyography is lost by the fifth day, it is presumed that the injury to the nerve is severe and surgical exploration should be considered. One of the most definitive signs of nerve transection is marked disruption of bone fragments through the fallopian canal. If transmastoid exploratory surgery is indicated, it should be performed as soon as the patient's general condition permits, as the results of nerve repair are directly related to the immediacy of repair. Unnecessary delay may occur if the attending physician assumes that spontaneous recovery will occur without otologic intervention. Another factor that leads to delay is the assumption that the nerve is not severely injured because the child can close the eyelids on the paralyzed side. However, this is a misleading sign because children may maintain excellent facial tone even with a transected nerve, and, when the child is lying down so that gravity is eliminated, the eyelids may approximate even when the nerve is transected.

Although the history of delayed onset of the palsy is a contraindication to surgery, this history may be false. The impression that the paralysis was delayed may be based on noting the facial nerve involvement for the first time a day or so after the injury. The deficit could well have been present immediately but was not appreciated for a number of reasons. If the patient was severely injured and comatose, the trauma team may have been too engaged in lifesaving measures to assess facial function accurately until several days later when the patient's general condition was more secure. Further, eliciting facial movement in an unconscious patient, and particularly one who may have facial soft tissue and bony injuries, is extremely challenging. Bilateral traumatic facial palsy is also difficult to evaluate, as facial weakness is best detected when one side is compared with the other. In the last case, if the patient is unconscious, a painful stimulus (pushing on the supraorbital rim or pinching the skin over the clavicle) may be presented; if facial grimacing results and is equal bilaterally, facial nerve function is probably grossly intact. However, if no movement is noted it may be assumed that the reflex was not elicited because of a central deficit, when in fact the facial nerve may have been injured bilaterally.

SURGICAL APPROACH. The surgical approach selected is dependent on the status of hearing (Fig. 17–9). A transmastoid approach is indicated for a patient with intact hearing, and a translabyrinthine approach is recommended for patients with profound sensorineural hearing loss. Surgical exploration of the facial nerve in temporal bone fractures must include the entire fallopian canal segment from the stylomastoid foramen to the labyrinthine portion. One cannot depend on topognostic tests to be certain of the location of the injury. This recommendation is based on the frequency of involvement at the level of the geniculate ganglion or proximal to the geniculate ganglion in the author's experience, as well as that reported by Fisch (1974). Facial nerve surgery for managing facial paralysis due to a fractured temporal bone is most challenging. The surgeon not only must be capable of exploring the facial nerve through its entire transtemporal course but must be prepared to reconstruct the ossicular chain, repair a torn tympanic membrane, seal a cerebrospinal fluid leak, or take a donor nerve from the neck or leg to place a nerve graft between the freshened ends of a transected facial nerve.

Iatrogenic Causes of Facial Paralysis

Otologic Surgery

Facial nerve injuries in otologic surgery continue to occur, even with the most experienced surgeons. The

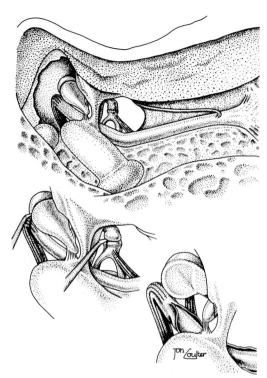

Figure 17–9. Transmastoid, extralabyrinthine, subtemporal approach to the right facial nerve can reach the labyrinthine segment while avoiding a middle fossa craniotomy. Top drawing illustrates posterior tympanotomy looking at the mastoid and tympanic segment of the facial nerve. The bottom two drawings show that by disarticulating the incus and rotating it forward with its attachment to the fossa incudis, the surgeon can reach the geniculate ganglion and labyrinthine segment of the facial nerve. The incus is replaced in its anatomic position at completion of the procedure.

facial nerve runs through the temporal bone between the middle ear and the mastoid, and congenital anomalies as well as distortions due to chronic infection, tumors, and trauma make the facial nerve vulnerable to injury during surgery. The possibility of an injury to the facial nerve must always be included as part of informed consent whenever surgery is performed on any part of the temporal bone or parotid gland. Positive identification of the facial nerve during all stages of surgery is the best method of avoiding injury. Anatomic landmarks that help to identify the facial nerve in the temporal bone have been described by Rulon and Hallberg (1962) and by Glasscock (1971).

Temporal Bone Surgery

NONSURGICAL TREATMENT. The author suggests that facial paralysis following a temporal bone procedure does not require reexploration if the nerve (1) was positively identified, (2) was purposely decompressed proximal and distal to where it was exposed, and (3) responded to direct electric stimulation prior to completion of the procedure. Nothing can be gained by exploring the nerve that is intact. The only reason for reexploring the facial nerve in such a case would be to rule out traumatic interruption of the nerve. Immediate paralysis following an otologic procedure can be due to the influence of the local anesthesia, but this should not last beyond two hours. The postoperative dressing might put pressure against an exposed nerve and should be removed in the event that postoperative facial paralysis is noted.

SURGICAL TREATMENT. If unexpected facial paralysis follows a surgical temporal bone procedure and the nerve was not identified, exploration of the nerve is mandatory.

This can best be performed the following day when the surgeon is free from fatigue and stress and the patient and family have been fully advised of the situation. This time period also allows for careful reevaluation to confirm that there is total facial paralysis. Further, this allows an opportunity for consultation.

If the nerve is intact, then only decompression above and below the area of involvement is necessary. If the sheath is frayed but the endoneural contents are grossly intact, then reapproximation is better than a graft. If the nerve is transected, the ends should be freshened, and an interposition graft should be placed. The anticipated results can be predicted by the degree of injury (see Fig. 17–3; Table 17–3). With an intact nerve, the injury can be of first- to third-degree severity; if the nerve is frayed or transected, then the injury is usually of the fourth- to fifth-degree level.

Parotid Surgery

PREVENTION. Surgery in or around the parotid gland in the young child is hazardous. The nerve fibers are extremely small and often require magnification for identification. Benign lesions, such as hemangiomas or cystic hygromas, frequently send out fingerlike projections that envelop the facial nerve, making dissection difficult and placing the facial nerve fibers in great jeopardy. These benign lesions should thus be managed conservatively.

In the event that surgery in this region becomes necessary, great experience and skill are required not to injure the facial nerve. Not only is the use of the microscope helpful, but identification of the major branches of the facial nerve as they emerge from the parotid gland over the masseter fascia also may be useful to follow the nerve branches back into the tumor region. In some instances it is helpful to identify the facial nerve in the temporal bone and follow it out to the parotid substance. Surgery of the parotid gland requires positive identification of the facial nerve to avoid injuring it; the adage "if you don't see it, you won't injure it" is not only untrue but also dangerous. Familiarity with the anatomic variations of the facial nerve in the young child is essential to avoid injuring the facial nerve. The lack of development of the mastoid tip, the narrow tympanic ring, and lack of subcutaneous tissue in young children place the main trunk of the facial nerve just beneath the skin as it emerges from the temporal bone in the young child. As compared with its much deeper position in the adult, the lower division of the facial nerve in the

young child runs over the mandible and is quite superficial. It is in these two locations, the exit site from the temporal bone and over the mandible, that the facial nerve is most often injured by an incorrectly placed incision.

MANAGEMENT. Ideally, injury to the facial nerve should be avoided, but in the event that it is injured the nerve should be treated as outlined in the discussion of surgical treatment of facial nerve injury in temporal bone surgery. The facial nerve should be identified during the procedure and stimulated when the procedure is completed prior to closing the wound at its most proximally exposed segment. This is usually near its exit from the temporal bone. If all parts of the face move, the surgeon can be certain that the nerve is intact. Even if the patient awakens with facial paralysis, no further treatment is required, and recovery can be expected. On the other hand, if the face does not respond to stimulation following this procedure, the fibers should be followed out to their termination in an effort to locate the area of injury. If the nerve is still intact, then nothing further need be done. The injury is due to stretching, and recovery, although it may be delayed two to four months, is usually satisfactory. In the event that branches have been severed, they should be repaired. If part of the nerve has been removed and the ends cannot be approximated, an interposition graft should be placed. The grafting technique consists of fascicular anastomosis with the aid of the otomicroscope. Nylon 10–1 sutures are used. The epineurium is trimmed back, and the sutures are placed through the perineurium and endoneurium, approximating the ends of the fascicles of the donor and recipient nerves. Immediate grafting will yield excellent results (Chap. 57).

Facial Wounds

Injuries to the extracranial segment of the facial nerve should be explored as soon after the injury as possible so that one can use the nerve stimulator to find the distal branches. These branches will continue to respond to stimulation up to three days following transection. If the wound is clean, primary repair or interposition grafting should be carried out. In case the wound is contaminated, such as occurs with a shotgun injury, the distal ends of the nerve should be tagged with nonabsorbable sutures. The proximal end can always be found as it emerges from or within the temporal bone. The wound should be drained and allowed to granulate and heal. Secondary repair of the nerve can be accomplished within three weeks with practically the same results as one might achieve with immediate repair.

Congenital Causes of Facial Paralysis

Many authors discuss congenital causes of facial paralysis (Paine, 1957; Harrison and Parker, 1960; Parker, 1963; Masaki, 1971; Garcin et al., 1976).

In the author's series of patients with facial palsy, 18 patients (12 per cent) were born with facial paralysis. The paralysis was congenital in 11 and traumatic in 7. The diagnosis was established in each case by employing the factors listed in Table 17–5 (Chap. 18).

Associated Anomalies

The most common finding associated with congenital facial paralysis was the presence of one or more other anomalies. This was noted in 9 of the 11 patients. There were five patients with an anomaly of the maxilla, making this the most common site of defect. A cleft palate was noted in two, a hypertrophied maxilla in one, a hypoplastic maxilla in another, and an accessory palate containing teeth and a tonguelike structure was present in the maxilla in one patient.

Three patients had skeletal deformities: two involved the cervical spine and one had spina bifida. One patient had a gastrointestinal anomaly, and another had a cardiac defect.

Multiple Anomalies

Eight patients had multiple congenital anomalies. Multiple congenital anomalies were noted in two of three patients with paralysis of the lower lip on one side. One of these two patients eventually died as a result of the multiple anomalies.

There were three patients with a hearing loss: two with a sensorineural type and one with a congenital conductive defect.

Two patients had an anomaly of the external pinna on the paralyzed side, but both patients had normal hearing.

Family History

There were two patients with a positive family history of congenital facial paralysis. One involved nine members of the same family covering three generations. Each member of this family who had facial paralysis had identical facial involvement as well as the same congenital defects. The defects consisted of hypertrophy of the maxilla, hypertelorism, and a congenital conductive hearing loss. The other patient with a positive family history of congenital facial paralysis had an older brother with an identical anomaly involving the same side of the face and associated malformation of the nares on the involved side.

Möbius Syndrome

Four of the patients in this series had Möbius syndrome. One had involvement of the sixth and seventh nerves bilaterally and lacked tear production. Another had involvement of only the seventh nerve with preservation of taste papillae and tear production. A third had bilateral involvement of the seventh and sixth nerves, as well as unilateral 12th nerve involvement, a cleft palate, and absence of tearing. The fourth had bilateral involvement of the sixth and seventh nerves, cervical fusion, an anomaly of the external pinna, a nasoorbital sinus, and an accessory palate. A report by Rubin (1976) is recommended for an excellent discussion of Möbius syndrome.

Significance of Lower Lip Involvement

There were two patients with multiple congenital anomalies with involvement of only the lower lip on one side. It is important to look for other anomalies in the presence of congenital facial paralysis, even if the paralysis involves only the lower lip (Pape and Pickering, 1972). Lower lip involvement is significant in assessing the patient for other, more serious anomalies; the one patient who died as a result of serious multiple anomalies was one with facial nerve involvement of the lower lip only.

Management of Congenital Facial Paralysis

The presence of nerve and muscle must be determined prior to planning facial rehabilitation surgery. This can be ascertained by the presence of spontaneous movement or by electromyography determinations. In the absence of spontaneous movement or electric evidence of the presence of muscle, the muscle should be explored and samples should be obtained for histologic evaluation.

Improvement of facial function may be accomplished in patients with a congenital facial paralysis by careful analysis of the defect and by the use of appropriate surgical approaches.

Tumors

Although tumors are an unusual cause of facial paralysis in children, they did account for facial paralysis in 19 patients (6 per cent) in the author's series. A tumor involving the facial nerve should be considered in patients regardless of age if there is one or more of the following findings: (1) facial paralysis does not resolve after six months; (2) paralysis progresses slowly beyond three weeks; (3) paralysis recurs on the same side; (4) there is facial weakness associated with twitching; or (5) there is facial paralysis associated with other neurologic signs (Chap. 27).

The 19 patients exemplified each of these presentations that are classic for tumors involving the facial nerve, and yet there was a significant delay between onset of symptoms and appropriate diagnosis and treatment. A plea is made to evaluate carefully all patients with facial nerve disorders so that the natural history of the causative disease can be arrested and the patient can be treated with a minimum of morbidity.

REFERENCES

Alexander, R. W., and James, R. B. 1972. Melkersson-Rosenthal syndrome. J. Oral Surg. 30:599.

Anderl, R. 1977. Cross-face nerve grafting up to twelve months of seventh nerve disruption. *In* Rubin, I. R. (ed.): Reanimation of the Paralyzed Face. St. Louis. C. V. Mosby Co., pp. 241–277.

Anson, B. J., and Donaldson, J. A. 1973. Surgical Anatomy of the Temporal Bone and Ear, 2nd ed. Philadelphia, W. B. Saunders Co., pp. 363–364.

Bergman I., May, M., Wessel, H. B., and Stool, S. E. 1986. Management of facial palsy caused by birth trauma. Laryngoscope 96:381.

Blunt, M. J. 1956. The possible role of vascular changes in etiology of Bell's palsy. J. Laryngol. Otol. 70:701.

Botman, J. W. N., and Jongkees, L. B. W. 1955. Results of intratemporal treatment of facial palsy. Pract. ORL 17:80.

Cawthorne, T. 1953. Surgery of the temporal bone. Hunterian Lecture. J. Laryngol. Otol. 67:437.

Conley, J. 1977a. Hypoglossal crossover—122 cases. Trans. Am. Acad. Ophthalmol. Otolaryngol. 84:763.

Conley, J. 1977b. Panel on rehabilitation of the face. *In* Fisch, U. (ed.): Facial Nerve Surgery. Birmingham, AL, Aesculapius Publishing Co., pp. 241–243.

Conley, J., and Gullane, P. J. 1978. Facial rehabilitation with temporal muscle—new concepts. Arch. Otolaryngol. 104:423.

Crosby, E. C., and De Jonge, B. R. 1963. Experimental and clinical studies of the central connections and central relations of the facial nerve. Ann. Otol. Rhinol. Laryngol. 72:735.

Devriese, P. P. 1977. Prednisone in idiopathic facial paralysis (Bell's palsy). ORL 39:257.

Duchenne, G. B. 1872. De I Electrisation Localisée, 3rd ed. Paris, France, Baillere, pp. 864–870.

Fisch, U. 1974. Facial paralysis in fractures of the temporal bone. Laryngoscope 84:2141.

Fisch, U. (ed.) 1977a. Special techniques of facial nerve repair; Rehabilitation of the face by seventh nerve substitute; New concepts in rehabilitation of the long standing facial paralysis. *In* Fisch, U. (ed.): Facial Nerve Surgery. Birmingham, AL, Aesculapius Publishing Co, pp. 204–226, 227–250, 251–284.

Fisch, U. 1977b. Total facial nerve decompression and electroneurography. *In* Silverstein, H., and Norrell, H. (eds.): Neurological Surgery of the Ear. Birmingham, AL, Aesculapius Publishing Co.

Fisch, U., and Esslen, E. 1972. Total intratemporal exposure of the facial nerve; pathologic findings in Bell's palsy. Arch. Otolaryngol. 95:335.

Garcin, M., Magnan, F. X. L., and Bremond, G. 1976. Facial paralysis in children, review of 82 cases. J. Franc. Oto-rhino-laryngol. 25:435.

Glasscock, M. E. 1971. Unusual facial nerve problems. Some thoughts on identifying the nerve in the temporal bone. Laryngoscope 81:8669.

Hakelius, L. 1977. Free muscle and nerve grafting in the face. *In* Rubin, L. R. (ed.): Reanimation of the paralyzed face. St. Louis, C. V. Mosby Co., pp. 278–293.

Harrison, M., and Parker, N. 1960. Congenital facial diplegia. Med. J. Aust. 1:650.

Hilsinger, R. L., Jr., Adour, K. K., and Doty, H. E. 1975. Idiopathic facial paralysis, pregnancy in the menstrual cycle. Ann. Otol. Rhinol. Laryngol. 84:433.

Hough, J. V. D., and Stuart, W. D. 1968. Middle ear injuries in skull trauma. Laryngoscope 78:899.

House, J. W., and Brackmann, D. E. 1985. Facial nerve grading system. Otolaryngol. Head Neck Surg. 93:146.

Levine, R. E. 1974. Management of the eye in facial paralysis. Otolaryngol. Clin. North Am. 7:531.544.

Levine, R. E. 1979. Management of the eye after acoustic tumor surgery. *In* House, W. F., and Laetje, C. M. (eds.): Acoustic Tumors, Vol. II, Management. Baltimore, University Park Press, pp. 105–149.

Masaki, S. 1971. Congenital bilateral facial paralysis. Arch. Otolaryngol. 74:259.

May, M., Harvey, J. E., Marovitz, W. F., et al. 1971. The prognostic accuracy of the maximal stimulation test compared with that of the nerve excitability test in Bell's palsy. Laryngoscope 81:931.

May, M. 1973. Anatomy of the facial nerve (spatial orientation of fibers in the temporal bone). Laryngoscope 83:1311.

May, M. 1974. Red chorda tympani nerve and Bell's palsy. Laryngoscope 84:1507.

May, M. 1976. Red chorda tympani nerve and herpes zoster oticus. Laryngoscope 86:1572.

May, M., Harvey, J. E., Marovitz, W. F., et al. 1976. The prognostic accuracy of the maximal stimulation test compared with that of the nerve excitability test in Bell's palsy. Laryngoscope 81:931.

May, M., Hardin, W. B., Sullivan, J., et al. 1976a. Natural history of Bell's palsy; The salivary flow test and other prognostic indicators. Laryngoscope 86:704.

May, M., Hardin, W. B., Sullivan, J., et al. 1976b. The use of steroids in Bell's palsy: A prospective controlled study. Laryngoscope 86:1111.

May, M., and Hardin, W. B. 1978. Facial palsy: Interpretation of neurologic findings. Laryngoscope 88:1352.

May, M., Klein, S. R., and Taylor, F. H. 1985. Idiopathic (Bell's) facial palsy: Natural history defies steroid or surgical treatment. Laryngoscope 95:406.

Mitchell, D. P., and Stone, P. 1973. Temporal bone fracture in children. Can. J. Otolaryngol. 2:156.

Olsen, P. Z. 1975. Prediction of recovery in Bell's palsy. Acta Neurol. (Suppl. 6) 52:1.

Paine, R. S. 1957. Facial paralysis in children. Review of the differential diagnosis and report of ten cases treated with cortisone. J. Pediatr. 19:303.

Pape, R. E., and Pickering, B. 1972. Asymmetric crying facies: An index of other congenital anomalies. J. Pediatr. 81:21.

Parker, N. 1963. Dystrophia myotonica presenting as congenital facial diplegia. Med. J. Aust. 2:939.

Peitersen, E. 1982. The natural history of Bell's palsy. Am. J. Otol. 4:107.

Rubin, L. R. 1976. The Möbius syndrome: Bilateral facial diplegia. Clin. Plast. Surg. 3:625.

Rulon, J. T., and Hallberg, O. E. 1962. Operative injuries to the facial nerve. Explanation for its occurrence during operations on the temporal bone and suggestions for its prevention. Arch. Otolaryngol. 76:131.

Samii, M. 1977. Panel on rehabilitation of the face. *In* Fisch, U. (ed.): Facial Nerve Surgery. Birmingham, AL, Aesculapius Publishing Co., pp. 243–245.

Sammarco, J. G., Ryan, R. F., and Longenecker, C. G. 1966. Anatomy of the facial nerve in fetuses and stillborn infants. Plast. Reconstr. Surg. 37:566.

Schneider, R. C., and Boles, R. 1968. Combined neurootologic and neurosurgical problems in head trauma. Laryngoscope 78:955.

Sunderland, S. 1978. Nerve and nerve injuries, 2nd ed. London, Churchill Livingston, pp. 88–89, 96–97, 133.

Thompson, N. 1971. Autogenous free grafts of skeletal muscle. Plast. Reconstr. Surg. 48:11.

Thompson, N., and Gustavsson, E. H. 1976. The use of neuromuscular free autografts with microneural anastomosis to restore elevation of the paralyzed angle of the mouth in cases of unilateral facial paralysis. Chir. Plastics (Berlin) 3:165.

Tschiassny, K. 1944. Facial palsy, when complicating a case of acute otitis media, indicative for immediate mastoid operation? Cincinnati J. Med. 25:262.

Tucker, H. M. 1977. Selective reinnervation of paralyzed facial muscles by the nerve muscle pedicle technique. *In* Fisch, U. (ed.): Facial Nerve Surgery. Birmingham, AL, Aesculapius Publishing Co., pp. 276–284.

Tucker, H. M. 1978. The management of facial paralysis due to extra-cranial injuries. Laryngoscope 88:348.

Wolf, S. M., Wagner, J. H., Davidson, S., et al. 1978. Treatment of Bell's palsy with prednisone; a prospective randomized study. Neurology 28:158.

Chapter 18

CONGENITAL ANOMALIES OF THE EXTERNAL AND MIDDLE EAR

Isamu Sando, M.D., D.Med.Sc.   **Yoshihiro Shibahara, M.D., D.Med.Sc.**

Raymond P. Wood, II, M.D.

We owe a great debt for our knowledge of congenital anomalies of the ear to the early students of otohistopathology and their successors. Guild, Nager, Reudi, and Lindsay stand out in any list of distinguished investigators in temporal bone pathology. At the time when much of their work was done, the surgical techniques for correction of middle-ear anomalies did not exist. The period of rapid development of otosurgical techniques that began in the early 1950s has continued to the present. Although much of this work has been focused on the treatment of chronic infectious disease, an important result of such study has been the development of procedures applicable to the correction of middle-ear anomalies.

From studying the temporal bones of patients who suffered from many varied diseases, we know that congenital anomalies of the ear may be caused by genetic (familial) factors, chromosomal alterations *in utero*, and maternal infectious diseases. Agents that are related to the production of congenital anomalies may have an effect either on genetic material or directly upon the developing otocyst anlagen. In many cases, congenital anomalies are of unknown origin, but by comparing the nature and extent of the anomaly and the normal embryonic development of the ear, we can in some cases determine the point in gestation at which the insult occurred.

The clinician must be cognizant of the association of certain anomalies with others. When one congenital anomaly is found, others must be sought. The use of a high-risk register for deafness is helpful in this regard.

For the otologic surgeon, knowledge of the associated occurrence of structural anomalies is imperative. Failure to realize that in an ear with an anomaly the presence of a normal fallopian canal on tomographic radiographs does not mean that the facial nerve lies within the canal has resulted in many surgical disasters.

The purpose of this chapter is to make the physician aware of the possibility of encountering anomalies of the external and middle ear during examinations and surgery. To do this, the anomalies are reviewed and discussed by grouping them according to their etiology (Classification I) and according to the anatomic structures involved (Classification II). A brief section is devoted to the current surgical techniques for correction of anomalies of the external and middle ear and hearing improvement. In certain cases, most notably Down syndrome, our failure to achieve satisfactory hearing improvement surgically probably reflects our imperfect understanding of the factors involved in the hearing loss rather than the absence of appropriate surgical techniques.

CLASSIFICATION OF DISEASES WITH ANOMALIES OF THE EXTERNAL AND MIDDLE EAR BY THEIR ETIOLOGIC FACTORS (CLASSIFICATION I)

The diseases associated with anomalies of the external and middle ear can be classified by their origins into five divisions.

DISEASES OF UNKNOWN ETIOLOGY
DISEASES WITH HEREDITARY CHARACTERISTICS
DISEASES ASSOCIATED WITH PRENATAL INFECTIONS
DISEASES OF IATROGENIC OTOTOXICITY
DISEASES ASSOCIATED WITH ENVIRONMENTAL FACTORS

Each of these classifications will be dealt with in turn.

Table 18–1 is a list of the diseases by eponym and pathologic name to assist the reader.

TABLE 18–1. Diseases with Anomalies of the External and Middle Ear Listed by Their Pathologic Defects and by Their Traditional Names

EPONYM	PATHOLOGIC NAME
(11) *Turner syndrome	Gonadal aplasia
(12) Goldenhar syndrome	Oculoauriculovertebral dysplasia
(13) Potter syndrome	Renal agenesis, bilateral
(14) Patau syndrome	Trisomy 13–15 syndrome
(15) Edwards syndrome	Trisomy 18 syndrome
(16) Down syndrome	Trisomy 21 syndrome
(21) Apert syndrome	Acrocephalosyndactyly
(24) Klippel-Feil syndrome	Brevicollis
(26) Pierre Robin syndrome	Cleft palate, micrognathia, and glossoptosis
(28) Möbius syndrome	Congenital facial diplegia
(30) Crouzon disease	Craniofacial dysostosis
(31) Pyle disease	Craniometaphyseal dysplasia
(33) Duane syndrome	Duane retraction syndrome
(35) Hurler syndrome	Gargoylism
(39) Treacher Collins syndrome	Mandibulofacial dysostosis
(41) Fanconi syndrome	Multiple congenital anomalies
(42) Mohr syndrome	Orofaciodigital syndrome II
(43) Paget disease of bone	Osteitis deformans
(44) Melnick-Needles syndrome	Osteodysplasty
(45) Van der Hoeve syndrome	Osteogenesis imperfecta
(46) Albers-Schönberg disease	Osteopetrosis
(52) DiGeorge syndrome	Third and fourth pharyngeal pouch syndrome

*The number in parentheses indicates the disease as it is listed in the classification system in the first section of this chapter.

DISEASES OF UNKNOWN ETIOLOGY

1. Without Associated Anomalies

External-Ear Anomaly

(1)* CRYPTOTIA (E)⁺ (SILCOX, 1967)**

Cryptotia is of unknown etiology and is present at birth. It may be observed alone. This anomaly is rare. The auricle demonstrates fusion of the superior portion with the scalp.

(2) MACROTIA (E) (SILCOX, 1967)

Macrotia is of unknown etiology and may be observed alone. This anomaly is uncommon. Associated anomalies are rare.

Middle Ear Anomaly

(3) ANOMALIES OF OSSICLES (M) (*KOIDE ET AL., 1967)§

This is a disorder of unknown etiology, although some cases are reported to be autosomally dominant. This is considered a rare condition and is present at birth.

---

*The numbers in parentheses are the numbers of the diseases as we have designated them throughout the chapter.

⁺The following notations are used throughout the chapter:
(D) Dominant hereditary disease;
(R) Recessive hereditary disease;
(E) Anomalies observed in the external ear;
(M) Anomalies observed in the middle ear;
(I) Anomalies observed in the inner ear;
(O) Anomalies observed in other parts of the body.
(Some diseases have more than one etiologic factor or more than one mode of hereditary transmission. Only one representative description is selected for each disease.)

**Some of the information listed for the diseases in Classifications I and II may not be annotated by the reference listed. Only one recent, representative reference was permitted for each category of disease and anatomic structural anomaly; selected papers with the latest literature review were added in some cases.

§The asterisk (*) before an author indicates that there are reports that describe the temporal-bone histopathology in this disease.

Ossicular anomalies can be observed alone. Malleolar anomalies include absence of the malleus, deformed malleolar head, triple bony union of the malleolar handle with the long process of the incus and head of the stapes, and bony fusion of the incudomalleolar joint. Incudal anomalies include absence of the incus, bony fusion of the short process of the incus with the horizontal semicircular canal wall, shortening of the long process of the incus, malformed long process of the incus, absence of the incudostapedial joint, bony fusion of the incudostapedial joint, and fibrous union of the incudostapedial joint. Stapes anomalies include absence of the stapes, absence of the head and crura of the stapes, small or fetal form of the stapes, a columella-type stapes, bony fusion of the stapes head to the promontory, and stapes footplate fixation.

The major anomalies of the middle ear associated with ossicular anomalies include facial nerve anomalies and absence of the stapedial muscle, stapedial tendon, and pyramidal eminence. It may be worthwhile to note that in cases of a congenitally fixed stapes footplate, an abnormally patent cochlear aqueduct may be present, which results in a geyser of cerebrospinal fluid if the footplate is removed at surgery.

Audiometric testing of individuals with ossicular anomalies reveals a unilateral or bilateral, nonprogressive, moderate to severe, flat type of conductive hearing loss.

(4) ABERRANT FACIAL NERVE (M) (*BASEK, 1962)

The etiology of an aberrant facial nerve is unknown. This condition is felt to be rare and present at birth. It may be observed alone.

Many anomalies of the facial nerve have been reported. The nerve may be displaced anteroinferiorly, with or without the fallopian canal, and pass through the middle ear on either side of the stapes. It may run in a canal on the promontory inferiorly from the geniculate ganglion. Also, the nerve may be seen to split into two or three branches that continue separately in the descending (mastoid) portion of the nerve; this condition is frequently associated with hypoplasia of the nerve. Stapes anomalies, atresia of the external auditory canal, malformations of the auricle, and other anomalies may be seen with anomalies of the facial nerve.

There are no specific audiometric findings in cases of facial-nerve aberrations.

(5) ANOMALOUS INTERNAL CAROTID ARTERY IN MIDDLE EAR (M) (RUGGLES AND REED, 1972)

This is a disorder of unknown origin. It is rare; six cases have been described—five in females and one in a male—and it is present at birth. The condition is usually unilateral.

The middle ear shows a vascular mass in the inferior portion of the tympanum behind the tympanic membrane. There are no associated anomalies.

Clinical findings include pulsatile tinnitus with a bruit heard in the external auditory canal. The carotid arteriogram shows a small internal carotid artery coming up through the posterior hypotympanum, turning abruptly forward beneath the stapes and the fallopian canal to head toward the area of the eustachian tube. Tomograms do not show a normal carotid canal, and indentations are seen on the promontory. A conductive or mixed type of hearing loss may be present.

This condition may be confused with an aneurysm of the carotid artery.

(6) INTERNAL CAROTID ARTERY ANEURYSM (M) (STALLINGS AND McCABE, 1969)

This is a disorder of unknown etiology and unknown prevalence; however, it is rare. It presents as a pulsatile smooth mass in the anterior inferior portion of the tympanic cavity. There are no known associated anomalies. It is sometimes symptomatic, with the patient complaining of pulsatile tinnitus. The diagnosis is aided by carotid arteriograms with subtraction studies. No specific treatment is required.

(7) HERNIATION OF JUGULAR BULB (M) (STEFFEN, 1968)

This is a disorder of unknown origin and unknown prevalence. This anomaly is present at birth as a jugular bulb in the middle ear, occurring just below the oval window through the dehiscent floor of the middle ear. There are no associated anomalies and no audiometric findings. There is no specific treatment.

(8) CONGENITAL ABSENCE OF ROUND WINDOW (M) (HARRISON ET AL., 1966)

This anomaly is of unknown origin and is rare. It is present at birth and can be observed alone. The audiometric configuration of round window closure by itself is indistinguishable from that observed with oval window closure; there is a nonprogressive, moderate, flat, conductive hearing loss.

2. With Associated Anomalies

(9) CONGENITAL CHOLESTEATOMA OF THE MIDDLE EAR (EPIDERMOID OF MIDDLE EAR) (E,M,O) (HOENK ET AL., 1969)

This is a lesion of unknown origin that is usually acquired but is occasionally congenital.

The findings in the middle ear include an epidermoid mass. The ossicles and bony walls of the tympanum may be eroded by this growth. Cholesteatoma has been described in connection with atresia, appearing behind an atretic bony plate, and also in association with cup-ears.

Mastoid radiographs and petrous pyramid tomograms show areas of bony erosion by cholesteatoma. A conductive hearing loss may result from involvement of the tympanic membrane or ossicles.

(10) CONGENITAL HEART DISEASE (M,I,O) (*EGAMI ET AL., 1979)

Congenital heart disease is of unknown origin but is frequently found associated with trisomies 13–15, 18, and 21, although no regular relationship between the chromosomal and cardiac anomalies has yet been established. Any major congenital heart defect may be associated with ear anomalies. Findings are present at birth. Anomalies of the external and middle ear include a bulky incus, wide angle of the facial genu, persistence of the stapedial artery, a high jugular bulb, dehiscence of the facial canal, and remnants of mesenchymal tissue present in the middle ear.

Anomalies of the inner ear observed include a shortened cochlea, thickened trabecular bone at the cribriform base of the cochlea, absence of the helicotrema, patent utriculoendolymphatic valve, complete absence of all semicircular canals, and simple outpouching of the lateral semicircular canal.

Other associated anomalies include scleral dermoid, cleft of the soft palate, Meckel diverticulum, duodenal atresia, absence of the spleen, supernumerary pulmonary lobulation, and absence of the kidney.

(11) GONADAL APLASIA (TURNER SYNDROME) (E,M,O) (SZPUNAR AND RYBAK, 1968)

Turner syndrome is a chromosomal aberration in which the patients are sex chromatin–negative in 80 per cent of the cases with a chromosomal configuration of XO. The prevalence is 1 in 5000 live births.

Anomalies of the external and middle ear include low-set ears with large lobes, poor development of the mastoid air cell system, and developmental malformation of the stapes.

Other anomalies and clinical findings include short stature, disturbance of the organs of sight, webbing of the neck, various bony dysplasias, malformations of the heart, and deformed kidney.

Hearing loss of a sensorineural or mixed type may be present.

(12) OCULOAURICULOVERTEBRAL DYSPLASIA (GOLDENHAR SYNDROME) (E,M,I,O) (DIJKSTRA, 1977; BERGSMA, 1979; FISHER ET AL., 1982; PHELPS ET AL., 1983; *WELLS ET AL., 1983; *SANDO AND IKEDA, 1986)

Although this is a disorder of unknown origin, it is possibly secondary to a vascular abnormality during fetal life. This syndrome affects the development of mostly first and second branchial arch derivatives. The findings in the external and middle ear include preauricular tags, deformity of the auricle, atresia of the external auditory canal, malformation or absence of ossicles, hypoplasia of the oval window, hypoplasia of the facial nerve, absence of the chorda tympani nerve, straightened tensor tympani tendon running past the absent cochleariform process, and poor development of the stapedius muscle. Anomalies of the inner ear include dysplasia and shortening of the lateral and superior semicircular canals, and narrowing and shortening of the internal auditory meatus.

Other anomalies include unilateral facial hypoplasia, dermoids, lipodermoids, lipomas of the eyes, colobomas of the upper eyelid, and vertebral abnormalities.

(13) RENAL AGENESIS, BILATERAL (POTTER SYNDROME) (E,M,I,O) (BERGSMA, 1979; *SAITO ET AL., 1982)

Although this syndrome was reported in two sisters, no hereditary factor has been defined. In this syndrome, renal agenesis is accompanied by findings in the external and middle ear, including low-set ears with deficient auricular cartilages, a hypoplastic external auditory canal, absence of auditory ossicles, atresia of the oval window, and abnormal course of the facial nerve. Findings in the inner ear include hypoplasia of the basal turn of the cochlear membranous labyrinth.

Other associated anomalies and clinical findings include redundant and dehydrated skin, wide-set eyes, prominent fold arising at inner canthus of each eye, "parrot-beak" nose, receding chin, facial expression of an older infant, "no urine output," and bilateral absence of kidneys. The patient may have multiple malformations, including bilateral pulmonary hypoplasia, gastrointestinal malformations, genital organ abnormalities, single umbilical artery, and major deformities of the lower part of the body or of the lower limbs.

(14) TRISOMY 13–15 SYNDROME (PATAU SYNDROME) (E,M,I,O) (*SANDO ET AL., 1975)

Trisomy 13–15 is a chromosomal aberration in which the somatic cells have an extra chromosome in the 13–15 group. The lesions are present at birth. The prevalence of this syndrome is 0.45 per 1000 births.

Findings in the external and middle ear include low-set, malformed ears, stenotic external auditory canal, small tympanic membrane, thick manubrium of the malleus, distorted incudostapedial joint, deformed stapes, small facial nerve, wide angle of the facial genu, absence of the stapedial muscle and tendon, persistence of the stapedial artery, dehiscence of the facial canal, absence of the pyramidal eminence, absence of the antrum, a small antrum, and a small mastoid.

Anomalies of the inner ear include a distorted and shortened cochlea, absence of the hook portion of the cochlea, malformed apical turn of the cochlea, absence of the modiolus, underdevelopment of the modiolus, malformed Rosenthal canal, scala communis between apical and middle cochlea turns, scala communis between middle and basal cochlea turns, underdevelopment of the osseous spiral lamina, malformed scala vestibuli with moderately small space in the basal turn, displacement and encapsulation of the tectorial membrane, large and patent cochlear aqueduct, unusual shape of the macule of the utricle, shortened utriculoendolymphatic valve, direct communication between the utricle and saccule, partial absence of the lateral limb of the superior semicircular canal, partial absence of the membranous superior semicircular canal, wide bony lateral semicircular canal, large ampulla of the membranous lateral semicircular canal, nearly flat crista of the membranous lateral semicircular canal, narrow lumen of the bony posterior semicircular canal, short and straight endolymphatic duct, shallow and wide internal auditory canal, spiral ganglion cells serving the basal turn located in the fundus of the internal auditory canal, and the singular nerve entering the otic capsule from the posterior fossa via a separate canal.

Individuals with trisomy 13–15 syndrome may have other associated anomalies: microcephaly, arhinencephaly, multiple eye anomalies, hypertelorism, cleft lip and palate, intraventricular septal defect, abnormal palm print, simian creases, and hyperconvexity of the nails.

The diagnosis is proved by the karyotype, which shows 47 chromosomes with an extra chromosome in the 13–15 group. It arises as a result of nondisjunction of the chromosomes.

(15) TRISOMY 18 SYNDROME (EDWARDS SYNDROME) (E,M,I,O) (*SANDO ET AL., 1970)

The symptoms of trisomy 18 syndrome are due to the presence of an extra chromosome in the 16–18 group. The findings are present at birth. The prevalence is 0.23 to 2 per 1000 births. It appears to be more common in infants born of older mothers.

Anomalies of the external and middle ear include low-set, deformed ears, atretic external auditory canals, deformed malleus and incus, malformed stapes of the columella type or of a fetal form, a split tensor tympani muscle in separate bony canals, exposed stapedial muscle in the middle-ear cavity, absence of the stapedial tendon, underdevelopment of the facial nerve, abnormal course of the facial and chorda tympani nerves, and absence of the pyramidal eminence.

Anomalies of the inner ear include incompletely developed modiolus, scala communis between apical and middle turns, underdeveloped cystic stria vascularis, absence of the utriculoendolymphatic valve, absence of the lateral limb of the superior semicircular canal and crista, absence of the lateral limb of the lateral semicircular canal, a flat, maculalike crista of the lateral semicircular canal, an enlarged endolymphatic duct, and a double singular nerve.

Other associated anomalies include ptosis of the eyelids, a high arched palate, micrognathia, flexion deformities, such as the index finger overlapping the third finger, and hypertrophy of the pancreatic tissue. These patients generally show failure to thrive, mental retardation, and hypertonicity and have a very poor prognosis.

Audiometric testing shows a failure to respond to sound.

(16) TRISOMY 21 SYNDROME (DOWN SYNDROME) (E,M,I,O) (*IGARASHI ET AL., 1977, *BALKANY ET AL., 1979, *HARADA AND SANDO, 1981)

The trisomy 21 syndrome is due to a chromosomal aberration in which the somatic cells have an extra chromosome in the 21–22 group. The findings are present at birth. The prevalence is 0.1 to 1.0 per 1000 births.

The findings in the external and middle ear include low-set ears, deformed stapes, slightly distorted crura of the stapes, and poor development of the mastoid air cells.

Associated anomalies in the inner ear include a shortened cochlea, absence of the utriculoendolymphatic valve, hypogenesis of the posterior semicircular canal, and an enlarged bony posterior canal ampulla.

Other associated anomalies include hypertelorism, epicanthic fold, slanting eyes, strabismus, narrowing of the nasal space, impaired development of the paranasal sinuses, protruding tongue, a high palate, and cardiovascular malformations, such as a ventricular atrial septal defect, patent ductus arteriosus, and situs inversus.

Audiometric tests show the presence of a sensorineural, mixed, or conductive hearing loss.

(17) TRISOMY 22 SYNDROME (E,M,I,O) (*ARNOLD ET AL., 1981)

Trisomy 22 syndrome is due to an extra chromosome, which is derived from two identical segments of chromosome 22 consisting of satellites, the entire short arm, the centromere, and a tiny piece of the long arm.

Findings in the external and middle ear include low-set ears, aural atresia, nonpneumatization of the middle ear, absence of the stapes and oval window, and bony closure of the round window niche. Anomalies of the inner ear include a shortened cochlea, incompletely developed modiolus, rudimentary osseous spiral lamina, and short and wide lateral semicircular canal.

Other associated anomalies include mild mental deficiency; mild hypertelorism; down-slanting palpebral fissures; inferior coloboma of the iris, choroid, retina, or all three; micrognathia; preauricular pits, tags, or both; cardiac defects; renal agenesis; and anal atresia.

(18) VATER SYNDROME (M,I,O) (*SAKAI ET AL., 1986)

This syndrome is of unknown origin, but the most probable possibility is a single primary defect in the germinal center of disk morphogenesis, leading to disorganization of the primitive streak and thus migration of early caudal mesoderm.

Anomalies in the middle ear include hypoplasia of the facial nerve, chorda tympani nerve, and greater superficial petrosal nerve; marked reduction of cells in the geniculate ganglion; anteriorly curved superstructure of the stapes; and hypertrophic anterior annular ligament.

Anomalies of the inner ear observed include irregular course of the lateral semicircular canal and duct; superiorly positioned utricle; abnormally high location of the saccule; large endolymphatic sinus, duct, and sac; and reduction in the population of spiral ganglion cells.

Other anomalies and clinical findings include vertebral defects, anal atresia, tracheoesophageal fistula with esophageal atresia, renal defects, radial limb dysplasia, large fontanelles, cardiac defects, single umbilical artery, and genital anomalies.

DISEASES WITH HEREDITARY CHARACTERISTICS

1. Without Associated Anomalies

(19) OTOSCLEROSIS (D,M) (LARSSON, 1962; *SCHUKNECHT, 1974)

Otosclerosis is a disorder inherited as an autosomal dominant trait. The penetrance appears to be 40 to 50 per cent, with a clinically apparent prevalence of 1 in 500 persons in the United States. According to pathologic studies of the temporal bone, the prevalence is 1 in 8 among white adult females and 1 in 15 among white adult males; it is much less common in Asians and blacks. The clinical onset is usually postpubertal (average age 20 to 25 years), and the disease is exacerbated by pregnancy. The main surgical finding is fibrous or bony fixation of the stapedial footplate to the otic capsule owing to invasion by the otosclerotic focus. Both ears are affected in the majority of patients.

Histopathologically, abnormal changes are first seen in the enchondral bone of the otic capsule, in which the normal bone is replaced by a network of newly formed weblike bone. This bone has a mosaic pattern. The sites of predilection are the oval window and round window areas. A primary focus may be present in the stapes footplate. The physical examination is usually normal, although there may be a pinkish color to the promontory as seen through the intact tympanic membrane (Schwartze sign). Otosclerosis has been related to van der Hoeve disease and Paget disease, but the characteristics of these diseases are in fact quite different.

The audiometric findings in individuals with otosclerosis include a low-frequency conductive loss sometimes associated with a sensorineural loss. Uncommonly, a sensorineural hearing loss alone is seen (cochlear otosclerosis). Caloric tests are usually normal. The treatment is usually surgical (stapedectomy), but these patients frequently obtain good results from hearing aids.

2. With Associated Anomalies

(20) ACHONDROPLASIA (CHONDRODYSTROPHIA FETALIS) (D,M,I,O) (*SCHUKNECHT, 1967)

Achondroplasia is a hereditary dominant disorder with many sporadic cases and is probably the result of mutation. It is also seen as a recessive trait in rare instances. The onset of the anomalies occurs in fetal life. The disorder occurs in 1 of 10,000 newborn infants and 1 of 50,000 in the general population.

Anomalies of the middle ear associated with achondroplasia include fusion of the ossicles to the surrounding bony structures and the appearance of dense, thick trabeculae without islands of cartilage in the endochondral bone and periosteal bone.

Associated anomalies of the inner ear include a deformed cochlea and thickened intercochlear partitions. Other associated anomalies include dwarfism due to imperfect ossification within the cartilage of the long bones, which results in shortening of the extremities, with the proximal bones being more affected than the distal bones. Many of these patients die at birth or shortly thereafter. The hearing loss associated with this disorder has been described as being either conductive or mixed.

(21) ACROCEPHALOSYNDACTYLIA (APERT SYNDROME, ACROBRACHYCEPHALY, AKROKRANIODYSPHALANGIE, SPHENAKROKRANIOSYNDAKTYLIE, ACRODYSPLASIA) (D,M,I,O) (*LINDSAY ET AL., 1975)

This disorder is apparently transmitted as an autosomal dominant trait. It appears to be associated with a high mutation rate and has been related to increasing parental age. The malformation occurs in 1 in 100,000 to 1 in 160,000 live births, and the manifestations are present at birth. There are no reports of external-ear anomalies. The middle-ear anomaly associated with this disorder is fixation of the stapedial footplate. Inner-ear anomalies include a patent cochlear aqueduct, an enlarged internal auditory canal, and an unusually large subarcuate fossa that connects to the middle fossa dura.

Other associated anomalies reported include craniofacial dysostosis, brachiocephaly, hypertelorism, bilateral proptosis, saddle nose, high arched palate, spina bifida, ankylosis of the joints, and syndactyly.

The audiometric findings are usually those of a flat conductive hearing loss, although a sensorineural component is suspected in some cases.

(22) ANENCEPHALY (R,E,M,I,O) (*ALTMANN, 1957; *FRIEDMANN ET AL., 1980)

This anomaly is a hereditary recessive disorder and consists of complete or incomplete absence of the forebrain and midbrain. Anencephaly accompanies acrania, which is described as holocrania or meroacrania on the basis of the degree of the osseous changes. The prevalence of this disease is 1 in 1000 births.

Anomalies of the external and middle ear include a small stapes footplate, exposed facial nerve, hypoplasia of the intratympanic muscles, a persistent stapedial artery, dehiscence of the facial canal, and a small oval window.

Inner-ear anomalies include a shortened cochlea, an underdeveloped modiolus, scala communis between middle and basal cochlea turns, communication between the bony lateral canal and the posterior canal, and an unusually narrow or wide internal auditory canal.

Other associated anomalies reported are spina bifida and amelia.

(23) ATRESIA AURIS CONGENITA (D,E,M,I,O) (*HIRAIDE ET AL., 1974)

Atresia is inherited as an autosomal dominant trait and is present at birth. It can be either unilateral or bilateral, partial or complete, and with or without deformities or absence of the auricle.

Middle-ear anomalies associated with atresia include a misshapen tympanic membrane, replacement of the tympanic membrane by a bony plate, absence of the malleus and incus, fused malleus and incus, misshapen malleus and incus, lack of an incudostapedial connection, absence of the stapes head and crura, a deformed stapes and crura, stapes footplate fixation, anomalous course of the chorda tympani nerve, absence of the lesser superficial petrosal nerve, hypoplastic and displaced tensor tympani muscle, persistent stapedial artery, a hypoplastic tympanic cavity, and absence of the tympanic cavity.

Inner-ear anomalies include all degrees of deformity of the cochlea, vestibule, semicircular canals, and internal auditory meatus.

Associated conditions include epilepsy, mental retardation, internal hydrocephalus, posterior choanal atresia, mandibulofacial dysostosis, and cleft palate.

Audiometric testing shows the presence of a nonprogressive maximum conductive loss with variable degrees of sensorineural loss, including total absence of hearing.

(24) BREVICOLLIS (KLIPPEL-FEIL SYNDROME) (R,E,M,I,O) (*McLAY AND MARAN, 1969; RICHARDS AND GIBBIN, 1977)

Brevicollis is a hereditary disorder that appears to be due to a recessive gene. Females are predominantly affected, and the disease is rare. Anomalies of the external and middle ear include microtia, presence of a preauricular appendage, atresia of the external auditory canal, narrowing of the external auditory canal, a slitlike malleoincudal joint, short process of the incus fused to the floor of the attic, long process of the incus attached to the stapes by fibrous tissues without any sign of a lenticular process, an elongated stapes with its anterior crus fused to the cochleariform process, and fistula of the stapes footplate.

Inner-ear anomalies include a rudimentary cochlea (a short, curved, single tube extending from the vestibule), a rudimentary modiolus, a poorly developed and shallow internal auditory canal, internal auditory canal more superiorly positioned than normal, absence of statoacoustic nerve in the internal auditory canal, and a vestigial inner ear.

Associated anomalies include congenital deformity of the cervical spine due to a fusion or reduction in the number of cervical vertebrae, spina bifida, and Sprengel scapular deformity. There is a very short, almost immobile neck with prominent soft tissue and the hairline going down to the back.

Deafness is the second most common finding in this disorder and is of the sensorineural or mixed type. There is frequently an absence of vestibular function.

(25) CHEMODECTOMA OF THE MIDDLE EAR (NONCHROMAFFIN TYMPANOJUGULAR PARAGANGLIOMA, GLOMUS TYMPANICUM AND JUGULARE TUMOR, CAROTID BODY TUMOR) (D,M,O) (ROSEN, 1952)

Chemodectoma of the middle ear is a hereditary autosomal dominant tumor with low penetrance and variable expressivity. It is uncommon, and 70 per cent of these middle-ear tumors occur in women. The tumor becomes clinically evident in adulthood, frequently quite late.

Middle-ear anomalies include a fleshy red tumor of the middle ear arising from the jugular bulb or from the tympanic plexus (Jacobson nerve) on the promontory. The tumor is sometimes seen to fill the middle-ear space and to surround the ossicles. The lesion may be associated with ipsilateral or contralateral carotid body tumors of the neck. These middle-ear tumors do not produce epinephrine. The lesion bleeds easily and blanches on compression with a pneumatic otoscope (Brown sign). The patient may report pulsatile tinnitus.

Diagnostic studies include retrograde jugular venography and carotid arteriography with subtraction studies.

The audiometric findings are those of a conductive hearing loss when the tumor impairs tympanic membrane mobility or the function of the ossicular chain. The ice-cold water caloric response may be decreased. Treatment is usually excision of the tumor after controlling the blood supply.

(26) CLEFT PALATE, MICROGNATHIA, AND GLOSSOPTOSIS (PIERRE ROBIN SYNDROME) (D,E,M,I,O) (*IGARASHI ET AL., 1976)

This is a hereditary disorder that may also result from an intrauterine insult in the first trimester. If it is hereditary, the syndrome is probably inherited as an autosomal dominant trait with variable penetrance. The prevalence is 1 in 30,000 live births. The findings are present at birth.

Anomalies of the external ear include cup-ears and low-set ears. Anomalies of the middle ear include thickened stapes crura and footplate, a small facial nerve, dehiscence of the facial canal, and absence of the middle ear.

Inner-ear anomalies observed are a scala communis between the apical and middle cochlear turns, an underdeveloped modiolus, an abnormally narrow communication between the crus commune and the utricle, superior dislocation of the crus commune and the posterior semicircular canal, and a small internal auditory canal.

Other associated findings include mental retardation, hydrocephalus, microcephaly, microphthalmia, myopia, congenital cataracts, esotropia, retinal detachment, sixth nerve palsy, Möbius syndrome, cleft palate, hypoplasia of the mandible, the tongue being displaced backward and downward, congenital heart anomalies, spina bifida, hip dislocation, syndactylia, and clubfoot.

A conductive hearing loss has been found to be associated with this disorder.

(27) CLEIDOCRANIAL DYSOSTOSIS (D,E,M,O) (FØNS, 1969)

This is a hereditary autosomal dominant disorder. The findings are present at birth.

Anomalies of the external and middle ear include a small auricle, atresia of the external auditory canal, a narrow external auditory canal, small ossicles, absence of the manubrium of the malleus, absence of the long process of the incus, fixation of the stapes footplate, and a small tympanic cavity.

Associated anomalies include aplasia of the clavicle, overdevelopment of the transverse diameter of the cranium, and retardation of ossification of the fontanelles.

Audiometric tests may reveal a sensorineural hearing loss.

(28) CONGENITAL FACIAL DIPLEGIA (MÖBIUS SYNDROME) (D,E,M,I,O) (LIVINGSTONE AND DELAHUNTY, 1968; *SAITO ET AL., 1981)

This is a disorder that may be either genetic or nongenetic in etiology; on a genetic basis it appears to be of the autosomal dominant type. Parental consanguinity and the possibility of recessive inheritance have also been suggested. Most patients have no family history of the disease. It is rare.

Anomalies of the external ear include microtia and slight atresia of the external auditory canal. Some form of auricular malformation is seen in 15 per cent of patients. Anomalies of the middle ear include an ossicular mass without a clearly identifiable stapes, oval window, or round window at surgical exploration, and absence of the facial nerve in the horizontal segment.

Anomalies of the inner ear that have been observed radiologically include a dilated vestibule and canal system.

Other associated anomalies are absence of the abductors of the eye, aplasia of the brachial and thoracic muscles, anomalies of the extremities, and involvement of the cranial nerves, especially of the oculomotor, trigeminal, facial, and hypoglossal nerves.

Audiometrically, deafness has been reported in 15 per cent of individuals with this syndrome.

(29) CONGENITAL HEART DISEASE, DEAFNESS, AND SKELETAL MALFORMATION (D,E,M,O) (FORNEY ET AL., 1966)

This disorder is inherited as an autosomal dominant trait. Its prevalence is unknown. Anomalies of the external and middle ear include a narrowed and oblique external auditory canal and fixation of the stapes footplate to the oval window. Associated anomalies and clinical findings include fusion of the carpal and tarsal bones and mild to moderate mitral insufficiency. Audiometric tests show a moderate congenital conductive hearing loss.

(30) CRANIOFACIAL DYSOSTOSIS (CROUZON DISEASE) (D,E,M,O) (*KONIGSMARK AND GORLIN, 1976)

Craniofacial dysostosis is a hereditary autosomal dominant disorder. It is a rare condition. The main features of this disease consist of skull deformity, hypoplasia of the maxilla, ocular malformations, and aural malformations.

Anomalies of the external ear reported to be associated with this disease are atresia and stenosis of the external auditory canal. Anomalies of the middle ear include absence of the tympanic membrane, ankylosis of the malleus to the outer wall of the epitympanum, a deformed stapes with bony fusion to the promontory, distortion and narrowing of the middle-ear space, a narrow round window niche, underdevelopment of the periosteal portion of the labyrinth, and a greatly reduced periosteal layer of the petrous bone.

This disease includes anomalies of the skull with exophthalmos; craniosynostosis involving the coronal, sagittal, and lambdoidal sutures; small maxillae; a hypoplastic mandible; and facial abnormalities with ocular hypertelorism, a parrot-beaked nose, a short upper lip, and mandibular prognathism.

Audiometric findings reveal that approximately one third of the patients with this syndrome have a hearing loss that is usually nonprogressive and conductive in nature.

(31) CRANIOMETAPHYSEAL DYSPLASIA (PYLE DISEASE) (D,M,I,O) (KONIGSMARK AND GORLIN, 1976)

This hereditary autosomal disorder is quite rare; some cases have appeared to be inherited as an autosomal recessive trait. The disorder becomes evident clinically in early childhood and is progressive.

Anomalies of the middle ear include encasement of the malleus in bone from the promontory, a deformed incus fixed by bone to the promontory, a stapes head in an oval window filled with bone, and enlargement of the chorda tympani nerve.

The inner-ear anomaly most frequently observed is constriction of the internal auditory meatus.

Associated anomalies and clinical findings include hypertelorism, deformity of the nasal dorsum, saddle nose, prognathism, posterior choanal atresia, defective dentition, metaphyseal widening of the long bones, nystagmus, optic atrophy, seventh nerve palsy, narrowing of the nasal passage, obliteration of the paranasal sinus, and obstruction of the nasolacrimal duct.

Audiometric tests have shown a sensorineural, high-frequency sloping loss with an associated large conductive loss. No results of vestibular tests on such individuals have been reported.

(32) DOMINANT PROXIMAL SYMPHALANGISM AND HEARING LOSS (D,E,M,O) (VASE ET AL., 1975)

This disease is inherited as an autosomal dominant trait with variable penetrance. Anomalies of the external and middle ear include stenotic external auditory meatus, an elongated long process of the incus, and fusion of the stapes to the petrous bone.

Associated anomalies include symphalangism involving the proximal interphalangeal joints, most marked at the ulnar digits. Audiometric tests reveal a conductive hearing loss.

(33) DUANE RETRACTION SYNDROME (DUANE SYNDROME) (D,E,M,O) (PFAFFENBACH ET AL., 1972; TACHIBANA ET AL., 1984)

This syndrome involves autosomal dominant inheritance, but some cases seem to be inherited recessively and to be X-linked. Thalidomide has also been implicated in the etiology of this disorder. Anomalies of the external and middle ear include microtia, atresia of the external auditory canal, fusion of the ossicles, lack of contact of the fused ossicles with the oval window, closure of the oval window by a thin membrane, and an ossicular mass that does not connect to the stapes.

Also seen in this disorder are limitation or absence of abduction, restriction of adduction, retraction of the globe upon adduction, and narrowing of the palpebral fissure on adduction. The condition is usually unilateral. It is more frequent in females and most often occurs on the left side. The hearing loss is said to be conductive.

(34) EAR MALFORMATION, CERVICAL FISTULAS OR NODULES, AND MIXED HEARING LOSS (D,E,M,I,O) (*FITCH ET AL., 1976; *LINDSAY AND HINOJOSA, 1978)

This is a hereditary autosomal dominant disease. Anomalies of the external and middle ear include a preauricular sinus, a preauricular appendage, malformations of the auricle, an enlarged incus, a bony mass in place of the ossicles, and an inferiorly located tympanic cavity. Anomalies of the inner ear include a broad base of the modiolus, deformed stria vascularis, a deformed vestibule, a large vestibular aqueduct, a misshapen utricular macula, a large endolymphatic duct, a wide nonampullated end of the superior semicircular canal, an underdeveloped lateral semicircular canal, and an absence of the common crus.

Other associated anomalies include cervical fistulas or nodules and renal dysplasia. Audiometric tests reveal a mixed hearing loss.

(35) GARGOYLISM (HURLER SYNDROME) (R,E,M,O) (*KELEMEN, 1966a; *FRIEDMANN ET AL., 1985)

Gargoylism is inherited as an autosomal recessive, sometimes X-linked, disorder and was the first of the genetic mucopolysaccharidoses to be recognized. The clinical findings become manifest by 1 year of age.

The external-ear anomaly usually included in this syndrome is low-set ears. Anomalies of the middle ear include absence of the incudomalleolar joint, deformed stapes, fibrous tissue invasion into the otic capsule with the presence of "gargoyle cells," multiple bony outgrowths into the middle ear, a small middle-ear space filled with mesenchymal tissue, obliteration of the oval window and round window areas by mesenchymal tissue, a small mastoid antrum, poor development of the mastoid air cell system, and hypertrophy of the mucosa.

Other associated anomalies and clinical findings include dwarfism, hepatosplenomegaly, corneal clouding, and mental deficiency. These patients frequently have large, deformed heads with hypertelorism, prominent eyebrows, a saddle nose, wide nostrils, a long mouth, a high palate, thick lips and tongue, widely spaced teeth, and a prominent chin. Also seen are optic nerve atrophy, hypertrichosis, a short neck, a deformed thorax, lumbar kyphosis, a prominent abdomen, hernia, limitation of joint movements, and broad hands with stubby fingers.

The diagnosis is made on the basis of the presence of mucopolysaccharides (chondroitin sulfate B and heparitin sulfate) in the urine. These same substances may be seen in the tissues. In the autosomal recessive type, deafness is seen in 5.2 per cent of individuals. In the X-linked recessive type, which is rare, deafness is seen in 43 per cent of individuals.

(36) HALLUX SYNDACTYLY—ULNAR POLYDACTYLY—ABNORMAL EAR LOBE SYNDROME (D,E,O) (GOLDBERG AND PASHAYAN, 1976)

This disorder is inherited as an autosomal dominant trait. External-ear anomalies associated with this syndrome include a deep horizontal groove or a nodule on the ear lobe.

Other associated anomalies include webbed toes, partial toe syndactyly, and absence of the middle phalanx. Neither audiometric nor vestibular test results have been reported in such cases.

(37) LETTERER-SIWE DISEASE (R,E,M,I,O) (COHN ET AL., 1970)

This is a hereditary autosomal recessive disorder of unknown prevalence, although it is uncommon. The onset is early in childhood. Findings in the external and middle ear include bony destruction of the external auditory canal; partial destruction of the ossicles, fallopian canal, and tympanic membrane; the occurrence of remnant ossicles; and the middle ear being filled by tissue containing many histiocytes.

Associated anomalies in the inner ear include destruction of the bony cochlea and internal auditory canal. Hydrops of the scala media, rolling of the tectorial membrane into the inner sulcus, spiral ganglion cell loss, and replacement of the inner-ear spaces by either growth or fibrous tissue are other inner-ear findings reported.

Associated findings include ulcerative tonsillitis, stomatitis, hepatosplenomegaly, diffuse lymph node enlargement, anemia, thrombocytopenia, and leukopenia.

The hearing loss is of either the conductive or the mixed type, and vestibular function is depressed or absent.

(38) KNUCKLE PADS, LEUKONYCHIA, AND DEAFNESS (D,M,O) (BART AND PUMPHREY, 1967)

This disease is inherited as an autosomal dominant trait. The knuckle pad manifestation appears in childhood. Anomalies of the middle ear include absence of the ossicles and facial nerve, a high jugular bulb, and absence of the facial canal. Audiometric and vestibular examinations reveal sensorineural and mixed hearing losses and hypoactive vestibular responses.

(39) MANDIBULOFACIAL DYSOSTOSIS (TREACHER COLLINS SYNDROME) (D,E,M,I,O) (*SANDO ET AL., 1968; KONIGSMARK AND GORLIN, 1976)

Mandibulofacial dysostosis is a hereditary disorder. It is of dominant inheritance by a gene or group of genes and is present at birth.

Anomalies in the external ear include various auricular deformities and atresia or stenosis of the external auditory canal. Anomalies of the middle ear include replacement of the tympanic membrane by a bony plate, and deformities of the malleus, incus, and stapes. Other anomalies are absence of the tensor tympani muscle, stapedius muscle, tendon of the stapedius muscle, pyramidal eminence, cochleariform process, and mastoid antrum. The facial nerve has been seen to course directly lateral in this disorder with no tympanic or mastoid portions. The chorda tympani, and superficial petrosal nerves also have been reported to be absent. The epitympanum and sometimes the mesotympanum are said to be small, irregular, and filled with fibrous tissue.

Anomalies of the inner ear include a huge cochlear aqueduct and a blind-pouch horizontal canal.

Other associated anomalies include antimongoloid slant of the eyes with colobomas of the lower lids, absence of eyelashes medially, micrognathia, a short palate, and hypoplasia of the malar bones and intraorbital rims. Cleft lip and cleft palate are sometimes present. Clinodactyly and sternal deformities have also been reported.

Audiometric tests show sensorineural and nonprogressive conductive hearing losses that involve the high frequencies especially.

(40) MIXED HEARING LOSS, LOW-SET MALFORMED EARS, AND MENTAL RETARDATION (R,E,M,O) (MENGEL ET AL., 1969)

This very rare disorder is inherited as an autosomal recessive trait. Anomalies of the external and middle ear are present at birth and include a low-set, malformed auricle; a single ossicle shaped like a malleus and placed posteriorly; absence of the incus, stapes superstructure, and footplate; and absence of the round window niche.

Associated anomalies and clinical findings include mental retardation, a high arched palate, a systolic murmur, and small stature.

The hearing loss is mainly of the conductive type, with some sensorineural loss. Vestibular tests may be normal.

(41) MULTIPLE CONGENITAL ANOMALIES WITH HYPOPLASTIC ANEMIA (FANCONI SYNDROME) (R,E,M,O) (McDONOUGH, 1970; HARADA ET AL., 1980)

Fanconi syndrome consists of congenital abnormalities and aplastic anemia. This is a hereditary autosomal recessive disorder.

External-ear anomalies include atresia of the external ear. Anomalies of the middle ear include fixation of the stapedial footplate. Inner-ear anomalies include hypodevelopment of the hook portion of the cochlea and reduced overall length of the cochlear duct. Other associated anomalies include skin pigmentation, skeletal deformities, renal anomalies, and mental retardation.

(42) OROFACIODIGITAL SYNDROME II (MOHR SYNDROME) (R,M,O) (RIMOIN AND EDGERTON, 1967)

This is a hereditary autosomal recessive disorder. Its prevalence is unknown.

Anomalies of the middle ear include blunting of the long process of the incus and absence of the incudostapedial joint.

Associated anomalies include facial deformities with widely spaced medial canthi, a flat nasal ridge, a high arched palate, a hypoplastic body of the mandible, a lobulated tongue, and digital abnormalities, including polydactyly, syndactyly, and brachydactyly. Audiometric tests reveal a conductive hearing loss.

(43) OSTEITIS DEFORMANS (PAGET DISEASE OF BONE) (D,E,M,I,O) (*LINDSAY AND SUGA, 1976)

Osteitis deformans is inherited as an autosomal dominant trait with variable penetrance. The onset of symptoms occurs in middle age, and the disease is seen in 3 per cent of those older than 40 years of age.

The external-ear anomaly usually reported is narrowing of the external bony auditory canal. Anomalies of the middle ear observed are pagetic bone growth in the epitympanum, pagetic changes in the stapes superstructure, thickening of the stapes footplate, footplate fixation, ossification of the stapedial tendon, and vascular spaces in the periosteal layer. These mosaic (pagetic) bony changes may involve any part of the temporal bone, the endochondral bone being most resistant.

Associated anomalies in the inner ear include loss of spiral ganglion cells, atrophy of the organ of Corti, atrophy of the stria vascularis, sarcomatous degeneration, and fractures of the temporal bone.

Other features include an enlarged skull, progressive kyphosis with shortening of stature, and pagetic involvement of the spine, femur, and fibula. Headaches are one of the most common and constant features of this disease, and vertigo is likewise a common complaint.

Radiographs originally show osteolytic lesions that are succeeded in several years by osteoblastic lesions. The semicircular canals and labyrinth are more visible on radiographic examination than usual. Audiometric findings show an early conductive loss, which progresses to a mixed loss that may become profound. Responses to vestibular testing range from normal to those representative of canal paresis.

(44) OSTEODYSPLASTY (MELNICK-NEEDLES SYNDROME) (D,E,M,O) (SELLARS AND BEIGHTON, 1978)

This is a hereditary autosomal dominant disorder. The anomalies of the external ear include small and distorted pinnae and narrow external auditory canals. Anomalies of the middle ear include absence of a round window and mastoid sclerosis.

Other associated anomalies include late closure of fontanelles; dense base of skull; small facial bones with prominent eyes; full cheeks; lag in paranasal sinus development; small mandible; short upper arms; short distal phalanges; bowing radius and tibia; flaring of distal humerus, tibia, and fibula; and coxa valga.

(45) OSTEOGENESIS IMPERFECTA (D,M,I,O) (*BERGSTROM, 1977)

Osteogenesis imperfecta is a hereditary autosomal dominant disease. It is present at birth, but symptoms of the tarda form (van der Hoeve syndrome) appear later in childhood. It is characterized by defective synthesis of connective tissue, including bone matrix. Anomalies of the middle ear include an abnormally shaped stapes head and crura; they may be very delicate and are sometimes replaced by fibrous tissue. The remainder of the temporal bone may show areas of skeinlike bone throughout its structure.

Other associated anomalies and clinical findings include blue sclerae (in 95 per cent of patients), skeinlike bone replacing lamellar bone throughout the body, multiple bone fractures, weak joints, prominence of the occiput, and abnormal tooth dentin with caries and dental fractures. Deformities such as kyphoscoliosis and pectus excavatum are common, and internal hydrocephalus, nerve root compression, cardiovascular and platelet lesions, and thin and atrophic skin also occur with this syndrome.

The audiogram usually shows a conductive hearing loss, although a sensorineural loss may occur in the high frequencies.

(46) OSTEOPETROSIS (ALBERS-SCHÖNBERG DISEASE) (R,M,O) (KONIGSMARK AND GORLIN, 1976)

Osteopetrosis is a hereditary disorder that is usually recessive but occasionally dominant. The onset is in early infancy or fetal life. Anomalies of the middle ear include a stapes of fetal form with an abnormal malleus and incus, persistence of the stapedial artery, a small middle-ear space, lack of pneumatization of the antrum, and abnormally basophilic enchondral bone.

Associated deformities and clinical findings include macrocephaly, blindness due to optic nerve atrophy, absence of the paranasal sinuses, choanal atresia, facial paralysis, hepatosplenomegaly, bone fractures due to brittleness of the bones, and severe anemia.

The hearing loss is mainly of a sensorineural type.

(47) OTOPALATODIGITAL SYNDROME (R,M,I,O) (KONIGSMARK AND GORLIN, 1976; *SHI, 1985)

This is a hereditary autosomal recessive disorder. The middle-ear anomalies associated with this syndrome include crudely shaped ossicles that resemble their fetal forms, fixed stapes, and no round window. Anomalies of the inner ear include a defect of the modiolus.

Associated deformities include a characteristic facies consisting of frontal and occipital bossing, hypertelorism, a broad nasal root, a small mandible, and cleft palate. Mild dwarfism and skeletal abnormalities, including retardation of ossification in the carpal and tarsal centers, also occur. There are abnormalities of the hands with widely spaced first and second digits and a shortened first digit. Mental retardation may also be associated with this disease.

The hearing loss is of the conductive type.

(48) RECESSIVE MICROTIA, MEATAL ATRESIA, AND HEARING LOSS (R,E,M,O) (KONIGSMARK ET AL., 1972)

This is an autosomal recessive disorder. Anomalies of the external and middle ear include microtia, atresia of the external auditory canal, and malformed ossicles.

Associated anomalies include pectus excavatum and duplication of the thumb.

The hearing loss associated with this syndrome is said to be conductive.

(49) RECESSIVE RENAL, GENITAL, AND MIDDLE-EAR ANOMALIES (R,E,M,O) (WINTER ET AL., 1968)

This is a hereditary autosomal recessive condition. Anomalies of the external and middle ear include small, low-set ears with a stenotic external ear canal, fixation of the malleus and incus in the attic, and a deformed or absent incus. Also a part of this syndrome is renal agenesis or atresia and variable involvement of the genital system, occasionally with atrophic ovaries, tubes, or vagina. The hearing loss is reported to be conductive in nature.

(50) SICKLE CELL DISEASE (D,M,O) (*MORGENSTEIN AND MANACE, 1969)

Sickle cell disease is a hereditary dominant disorder. It is said that it affects 7 to 8 per cent of African blacks.

Anomalies of the middle ear include resorption of the body and long process of the incus and the head of the stapes.

Other associated anomalies include hemolytic anemia, extramedullary hemopoiesis, and hyperplastic bone marrow.

Audiometric tests may reveal a sensorineural hearing loss.

(51) THICKENED EAR LOBULE AND INCUDOSTAPEDIAL MALUNION (D,E,M) (ESCHER AND HIRT, 1968)

This is a hereditary dominant, non–X-linked autosomal anomaly of rare occurrence. It is present at birth. Anomalies of the external and middle ear include a hypertrophic, thickened ear lobule, malformation of the long process of the incus, absence of the lenticular process of the incus, presence of a fibrous connection from the stapes to the incus, and absence of the stapes head.

A conductive hearing loss should be present. No vestibular studies have been reported.

(52) THIRD AND FOURTH PHARYNGEAL POUCH SYNDROME (DiGEORGE SYNDROME, PARTIAL DiGEORGE SYNDROME) (R,E,M,I,O) (*ADKINS AND GUSSEN, 1974a,b; *BLACK ET AL., 1975; *OHTANI AND SCHUKNECHT, 1984)

This is a hereditary autosomal recessive defect. The anomalies are present at birth. The prevalence of this syndrome is quite low. Anomalies of the external and middle ear include a malformed, low-set auricle; atresia of the external auditory canal; absence of the malleus, incus, and stapes; a small facial nerve; absence of the stapedial muscle; partial atresia of the tympanic cavity; and absence of the oval window. Anomalies of the inner ear include absence of the apical portion of the modiolus, absence of the horizontal semicircular canal, and hypoplastic seventh and eighth cranial nerves.

Other anomalies include absence or hypoplasia of the thymus, abnormalities of the aortic arch, patent ductus arteriosus, agenesis of the thyroid, acrania, microcephaly, and micrognathia.

DISEASES ASSOCIATED WITH PRENATAL INFECTIONS

(53) CONGENITAL RUBELLA SYNDROME (M,I,O) (*HEMENWAY ET AL., 1969; *GUSSEN 1981)

Maternal rubella is an infectious viral disorder. Its manifestations are present at birth. Anomalies of the middle ear include a small area of malleus head fixation on one side; an absence of the medial component of the posterior incudal ligament; an anomalous stapes with a rudimentary thickened head, neck, crura, and footplate; cartilaginous fixation of the stapes footplate; and persistence of fetal mesenchymal tissue in the middle ear.

Associated features in the inner ear include depression of the Reissner membrane, cystic dilatation of the stria vascularis, rolling of the tectorial membrane into the inner sulcus, hair cell degeneration, spiral ganglion cell loss, and collapse of the saccular membrane with adherence to the saccular macula.

Other associated anomalies and clinical findings are mental retardation, microcephaly, microphthalmia, retinitis, congenital cataracts, thrombocytopenia, cardiovascular deformities, and deformities of the lower extremities. Confirmatory tests include the presence of fluorescent antibodies in the serum, serum hemagglutination, and positive viral cultures of the stool and throat.

Audiometric testing reveals sensorineural and conductive hearing losses.

(54) CONGENITAL SYPHILIS (M,I,O) (*KARMODY AND SCHUKNECHT, 1966)

Congenital syphilis is an infection of the fetus by *Treponema pallidum* that passes the placenta. Symptoms may begin in childhood, but 50 per cent of individuals first develop symptoms between the ages of 25 and 35 years. The middle-ear findings reported are thickening of the malleus as a result of bony hyperplasia, fusion of the malleolar head to the body of the incus, spongy appearance of the long process of the incus, and abnormalities of the stapes. Histopathology of the temporal bones reveals primary osteitis with mononuclear leukocytic infiltration and obliterative endoarteritis of the otic capsule with secondary labyrinthitis characterized by endolymphatic hydrops and degeneration of the membranous labyrinth end-organs. Other associated findings are a perforated nasal septum, interstitial keratitis, and Hutchinson teeth.

The diagnosis is made by the history and verifying tests, including serum and cerebrospinal fluid tests for syphilis. However, these tests are not always positive. Audiometric findings include a typical sensorineural type of hearing loss with a flat audiometric curve in 38 per cent of the patients with congenital syphilis. Sometimes, the curve shows a conductive component if the middle ear is involved. The onset of hearing loss in childhood is usually sudden, bilaterally symmetric, severe to profound, and unaccompanied by marked vestibular symptoms. In adults, deafness begins abruptly, and a partial, asymmetric, flat, sensorineural hearing loss is accompanied by episodes of vertigo. Tinnitus may be present. Treatment involves the administration of large doses of penicillin and steroids.

DISEASES OF IATROGENIC OTOTOXICITY

(55) THALIDOMIDE OTOTOXICITY (E,M,I,O) (*JØRGENSEN ET AL., 1964)

Thalidomide ototoxicity is an iatrogenic, drug-induced congenital disorder that occurs following the administration of thalidomide to a pregnant woman. The probability of malformation following exposure is unknown. Twenty per cent of the children suffering from thalidomide-induced anomalies show ear anomalies. Anomalies of the external and middle ear include a deformed or absent auricle, complete or partial atresia of the external auditory canal, a deformed tympanic membrane, a fixed malleus, a displaced long process of the incus, absence of the stapes, absence of the facial nerve and chorda tympani nerve, persistence of the stapedial artery, a slit-shaped tympanic cavity, and absence of the oval window. Inner-ear anomalies include aplasia of the inner ear and absence of the facial nerve and statoacoustic nerve in the internal auditory canal.

Associated anomalies include shortening, deformity, or absence of the long bones; capillary hemangiomas of the forehead, nose, and lips; colobomas; microphthalmia; congenital heart disease; intestinal atresia; and renal hypoplasia or agenesis.

Approximately 75 per cent of the infants affected can be expected to have a moderate to profound sensorineural hearing loss, and 25 per cent have a maximal conductive hearing loss. Absence of vestibular function has also been reported.

DISEASES ASSOCIATED WITH ENVIRONMENTAL FACTORS

(56) ENDEMIC CRETINISM (M,I,O) (WARKANY, 1971)

This disease is caused by environmental factors. Anomalies of the external and middle ear associated with endemic cretinism include plump ossicles, thickened periosteal parts of the stapes, a small mastoid process, and thickened periosteal layers of the otic capsule.

Other anomalies include a brachiocephalic cranium, brachydactyly with shortness of the thumb, and abnormal hip joint. These individuals often have a hearing loss.

CLASSIFICATION OF THE EXTERNAL AND MIDDLE-EAR ANOMALIES BY THEIR INVOLVED ANATOMIC STRUCTURES (CLASSIFICATION II)

In order to enhance the reader's understanding of anomalies of the external and middle ear, the various kinds of anomalies that occur in the external and middle ear are classified according to the anatomic structures that are involved in the anomaly.

CONGENITAL EXTERNAL EAR ANOMALIES

(A) **Auricular Anomalies** (1)**, (2), (9), (11)–(16), (22)–(24), (26)–(28), (33)–(36), (39), (40), (44), (48), (49), (51), (52), (55)

    1. AURICULAR ANOMALIES (IN GENERAL) (1), (2), (9), (11)–(16), (22)–(24), (26)–(28), (33)–(35), (39), (40), (44), (48), (49), (52), (55)

      a. Absence of auricle—anotia (Altmann, 1951a)
      b. Superior portion of the auricle buried in the scalp—cryptotia (Altmann, 1951a)
      c. Double ear (Altmann, 1951a)
      d. Auricle smaller than normal—macrotia (Altmann, 1949)
      e. Auricle larger than normal—macrotia (Altmann, 1951a)
      f. Auricle located on the upper anterior cervical region near the midline of the neck—synotia (Black et al., 1973)
      g. Ear located on the cheek—melotia (Altmann, 1951a)

**Numbers in parentheses refer to the diseases listed in Classification I.

    h. Lack of aural ascent due to underdevelopment of the mandibular area—low-set ear (Altmann, 1957)
    i. Other (Altmann, 1951a)

2. LOBULAR ANOMALIES (36), (51)

    a. Absence of lobule (Altmann, 1951a)
    b. Adherent lobule (Altmann, 1951a)
    c. Split lobule (Altmann, 1951a)
    d. Deep horizontal groove on the lobule (Goldberg and Pashayan, 1976)
    e. Hypertrophic and thickened lobule (Escher and Hirt, 1968)
    f. Nodule on the lobule (Goldberg and Pashayan, 1976)

3. HELIX ANOMALIES

    a. Auricle folded forward and downward in varying degrees from above and behind—cat's ear (Altmann, 1951a)
    b. Helix with sharp angle on its tip portion—*Cercopithecus* ear (Altmann, 1951a)
    c. Small projection from the descending part of the helix—Darwin tubercle (Altmann, 1951a)

4. ANTHELIX ANOMALIES (9)

    a. Absence of anthelix (Hoenk et al., 1969)
    b. Poor development of the anthelix—lop ear (Converse et al., 1955)
    c. Small projection from the descending part of the helix—Darwin tubercle (Altmann, 1951a)
    d. Enlarged portion of the anthelix connecting with the helix—Mozart ear (Altmann, 1951a)
    e. Crus extending from the helix to the cymbae—Stahl ear (Altmann, 1951a)

5. TRAGUS ANOMALY (23)—RUDIMENTARY TRAGUS (ALTMANN, 1949)

6. CONCHAL ANOMALY—VERTICAL CARTILAGINOUS RIDGE IN THE CONCHA—CRUS CYMBAE (ALTMANN, 1951a)

7. APPENDAGE (24), (34)

    a. Numerous appendages—Polytia (Altmann, 1951a)
    b. Preauricular appendage (Altmann, 1951a)

8. FISTULA (34)

    a. Colloaural fistula (Altmann, 1951a)
    b. Preauricular fistula (Altmann, 1951a)
    c. Postauricular fistula (Altmann, 1951a)
    d. Prehelical pit (Melnick et al., 1975)

(B) External Auditory Meatus Anomalies (9), (11)–(15), (17), (22)–(24), (26)–(30), (32), (33), (39), (41), (43), (44), (48), (49), (52), (55)

    a. *Atresia auris (Altmann, 1949) (Fig. 18–1)
      i. *membranous atresia*
      ii. *bony atresia*
    b. *Stenotic external auditory meatus (Kelemen, 1966a)
    c. *Short bony external auditory meatus (Altmann, 1957)
    d. Long bony external auditory meatus (Stratton, 1965)

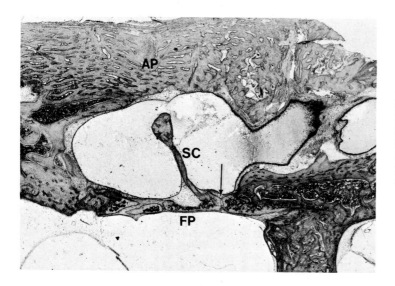

Figure 18–1. Horizontal section of the left temporal bone from a patient with Treacher Collins syndrome with the following middle-ear anomalies: columella-type stapes (SC) with a single crus attached to an underdeveloped footplate (FP), which was partially ankylosed anteriorly (arrow); absence of the malleus and incus, which were probably included in the bony atresia plate (AP), which replaced the area of the typmpanic membrane (H & E, × 22).

CONGENITAL ANOMALIES OF THE MIDDLE EAR

(A) **Tympanic Membrane Anomalies** (9), (14), (23), (30), (34), (39), (55)

    a. *Tympanic membrane replaced by bony plate (Sando et al., 1968)
    b. Tympanic membrane replaced by fibrous tissue (Schuknecht, 1974)
    c. *Small tympanic membrane (Bordley and Hardy, 1969)
    d. *Distorted tympanic membrane (Sando et al., 1970)

(B) **Ossicular Anomalies** (3), (9)–(24), (26)–(35), (37)–(43), (45)–(56)

    1. OSSICULAR ANOMALIES IN GENERAL (20), (28), (33), (34), (37), (47)

        a. *Remnant ossicle (Cohn et al., 1970)
        b. *Fusion of three ossicles (Hough, 1963)
        c. Thickening of ossicles (Buran and Duvall, 1967)

    2. MALLEUS ANOMALIES (3), (9), (12)–(15), (23), (24), (27), (30), (31), (38)–(40), (46)–(49), (52)–(56)

      a. Absence of:
          i. *malleus (Ruedi, 1954) (Fig. 18–1)
          ii. manubrium (Herberts, 1962)
          iii. lateral process (Hoenk et al., 1969)
          iv. head (Herberts, 1962)
      b. Bony fusion of:
          i. *malleolar head to epitympanic wall (Ritter, 1971)
          ii. anterior malleolar ligament to tympanic ring (McGrew and Gregg, 1971)
      c. Other anomalies:
          i. *displacement of malleus (Ruben et al., 1969)
          ii. long manubrium (Hough, 1963)
          iii. shortening of manubrium (Buran and Duvall, 1967)
          iv. cartilaginous fusion between malleus and Meckel cartilage (Zonis, 1969)

    3. INCUS ANOMALIES (3), (10), (12)–(15), (23), (24), (27), (31), (32), (34), (35), (38)–(40), (42), (46)–(52), (54)–(56)

      a. Absence of:
          i. *incus (Sando et al., 1968) (Fig. 18–1)

      ii. long process (Fons, 1969)

      iii. *lenticular process (McLay and Maran, 1969)

   b. Bony fusion of:

      i. *incus to malleus (Altmann, 1949)

      ii. incudomalleolar joint (Maran, 1965)

      iii. *short process to floor of aditus ad antrum (McLay and Maran, 1969)

      iv. short process to horizontal canal wall (Koide et al., 1967)

   c. Other anomalies

      i. *displacement of incus (Ruben et al., 1969)

      ii. shortening of short process (Jaffee, 1968)

      iii. shortening of long process (Maran, 1965)

      iv. *dislocation of long process (Sando et al., 1970)

      v. resolution of body and long process (Morgenstein and Manace, 1969)

4. STAPES ANOMALIES (3), (9), (11)–(19), (21)–(24), (26)–(32), (35), (38)–(43), (45)–(48), (50)–(56)

   a. Absence of:

      i. stapes (Fernandez and Ronis, 1964)

      ii. *incudostapedial joint (Altmann, 1955)

      iii. *head (Altmann, 1955)

      iv. suprastructure (Isenberg and Tubergen, 1980)

      v. *crus (Altmann, 1957)

      vi. *footplate (Jørgensen et al., 1964)

   b. Rudimentary form of stapes

      i. *columellar-type stapes (Kelemen, 1966b) (Fig. 18–1)

      ii. *doughnut-type stapes (Hough, 1963)

      iii. *thickening of stapes (Sando et al., 1970)

      iv. *two-layer footplate (Lindsay et al., 1960)

   c. Bony fusion of:

      i. incudostapedial joint (Hough, 1958)

      ii. head to promontory (Hough, 1963)

      iii. *head to facial canal (Altmann, 1949)

      iv. *crus to cochleariform process (McLay and Maran, 1969)

      v. *crus to oval window bony wall (Altmann, 1955)

      vi. *crus to promontory (Jørgensen et al., 1964)

      vii. crus to pyramidal eminence (Buran and Duvall, 1967)

      viii. *footplate to otic capsule (Altmann, 1957)

   d. Other anomalies

      i. adherence of stapes to facial nerve (Durcan et al., 1967)

      ii. *fibrous connection of incudostapedial joint (McLay and Maran, 1969)

      iii. displacement of incudostapedial joint (Black et al., 1971)

      iv. *resolution of head (Morgenstein and Manace, 1969)

      v. degeneration of crus into fibrous threads (Opheim, 1968)

      vi. *small bone on footplate (Bergstrom et al., 1972)

      vii. *Cartilaginous primordium of the stapes (Sando and Ikeda, 1986) (Fig. 18–2)

      viii. *Cartilaginous fixation of footplate to the otic capsule (Sando and Ikeda, 1986) (Fig. 18–2)

(C) Nerve Anomalies (4), (10), (12)–(15), (18), (22), (23), (25), (26), (31), (34), (38), (39), (52), (55)

1. FACIAL NERVE ANOMALIES (4), (10), (12)–(15), (18), (22), (26), (34), (38), (39), (52), (55)

   a. *Absence (Jørgensen et al., 1964)

   b. *Poor development (Henderson, 1939; Kodama, 1982)

   c. Abnormal course

      i. In general (Jahrsdoerfer, 1981)

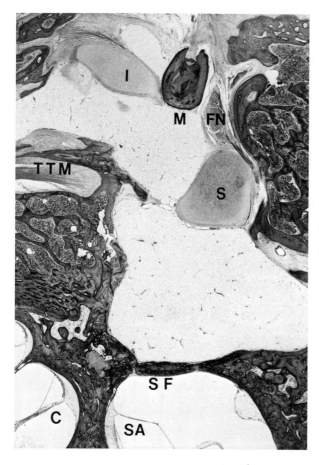

Figure 18–2. Horizontal section of the right temporal bone from a 6-month-old patient with Goldenhar syndrome, showing anomalous bony and cartilaginous masses, presumably malleus (M), incus (I), and primordium of stapes (S). No connection between primitive stapes footplate (SF) and primordium of stapes. C, cochlea; FN, facial nerve; SA, sacccule; TTM, tensor tympani muscle (H & E, × 18).

    ii. *wide angle of facial genu (Egami et al., 1979)
   iii. *runs laterally from geniculate ganglion and leaves temporal bone immediately (Sando et al., 1968)
   iv. runs inferiorly from geniculate ganglion (Caparosa and Klassen, 1966)
    v. *runs more inferiorly than normal (Adkins and Gussen, 1974a; Willis, 1977; Winther and Elbrønd, 1977)
   vi. *absence of second genu (Sando et al., 1970)
  vii. facial nerve located medial to stapedial muscle (Sando et al., 1970)
  d. Other—*exposed facial nerve (Altmann, 1957)

2. CHORDA TYMPANI NERVE ANOMALIES (12), (15), (18), (23), (31), (39), (55)

  a. *Absence (Sando et al., 1968)
  b. Abnormal course
    i. *runs out of temporal bone (Altmann, 1949)
   ii. runs from the area of the geniculate ganglion (Fowler, 1961)
   iii. *runs more vertically than normal (Sando et al., 1970)
   iv. bifurcation (Durcan et al., 1967)
  c. Other anomalies
    i. enlargement (Hough, 1958)
   ii. chorda tympani with bony sleeve at posterior edge of external auditory meatus (Kraus and Ziv, 1971)

3. SUPERFICIAL PETROSAL NERVE ANOMALIES (18), (23), (39)

  a. *Absence of greater superficial petrosal nerve (Sando et al., 1968)
  b. *Absence of lesser superficial petrosal nerve (Altmann, 1949)

4. JACOBSON NERVE ANOMALY (25)—PARAGANGLIOMA (VAN DER BORDEN, 1967)

(D) Intratympanic Muscular Anomalies (12), (14), (15), (22), (23), (39), (43), (52)

1. TENSOR TYMPANI MUSCLE AND TENDON ANOMALIES (12), (22), (23), (39)

    a. Absence of muscle and tendon (Sando et al., 1968)
    b. Abnormal course
       i. abnormal course without connection to cochleariform process and malleus (Ruben et al., 1969)
       ii. abnormal course without connection to cochleariform process (Hiraide et al., 1974)
       iii. *split in muscle (Kos et al., 1966)

2. STAPEDIUS MUSCLE AND TENDON ANOMALIES (12), (14), (15), (22), (39), (43), (52)

    a. *Absence of muscle and tendon (Sando et al., 1968)
    b. *Huge muscle exposed in the middle ear (Sando et al., 1970)
    c. Two muscles (Wright and Etholm, 1973)
    d. Absence of tendon (Jaffee, 1968)
    e. Atrophy of tendon (Tabor, 1961)
    f. Ossification of tendon (Hough, 1958)
    g. Tendon attached to lenticular process (Pou, 1963; Isenberg and Tubergen, 1980)
    h. Tendon attached to head or posterior crus (Hough, 1958)

3. OTHER ANOMALIES (14)—*SUPERNUMERARY OR ECTOPIC MUSCLES (DRUSS, 1952)

(E) Vascular Anomalies (5)–(7), (10), (14), (22), (23), (38), (46), (55)

1. INTERNAL CAROTID ARTERY ANOMALIES (5), (6)

    a. Existence in middle ear (Goldman et al., 1971)
    b. Existence of aneurysm in the middle ear (Steffen, 1968)

2. STAPEDIAL ARTERY ANOMALY (10), (14), (22), (23), (46), (55)—*Persistence (Altmann, 1945; Marion et al., 1985) (Fig. 18–3)

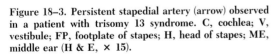

Figure 18–3. Persistent stapedial artery (arrow) observed in a patient with trisomy 13 syndrome. C, cochlea; V, vestibule; FP, footplate of stapes; H, head of stapes; ME, middle ear (H & E, × 15).

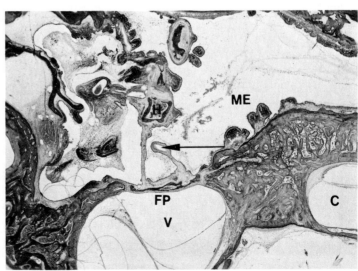

3. JUGULAR BULB ANOMALIES (7), (10), (38)

    a. Herniation of jugular bulb into the middle ear (Steffen, 1968)
    b. *High jugular bulb (Egami et al., 1979) (Fig. 18–4)

(F) Tympanic Cavity Anomalies (9), (10), (12), (14), (15), (22)–(24), (26), (27), (30), (34), (35), (37)–(39), (46), (52), (55)

    a. Absence of:
        i. tympanic cavity (Gnanapragasam, 1975)
        ii. *cochleariform process (Sando et al., 1968)
        iii. *facial canal (Altmann, 1957)
        iv. *pyramidal eminence (Sando et al., 1970)
    b. Dehiscence of:
        i. *facial canal (Altmann, 1957) (Fig. 18–5)
        ii. floor (Steffen, 1968)
        iii. *tegmen tympani (Sando et al., 1968)
    c. Rudimentary form:
        i. *small tympanic cavity (Jørgensen et al., 1964)
        ii. *small tympanic cavity with fetal connective tissue (Jørgensen et al., 1964)
    d. *Bony mass in promontory (Sando et al., 1968)
    e. Others:
        i. *congenital cholesteatoma (Hoenk et al., 1969)
        ii. *H-shaped tympanic cavity (Ruben et al., 1969)
        iii. large facial canal (Fernandez and Ronis, 1964)

(G) Window Anomalies (8), (12), (13), (17), (22), (28), (30), (40), (44), (46), (52), (55)

1. OVAL WINDOW ANOMALIES (12), (13), (17), (22), (28), (52), (55)

    a. *Absence (Jørgensen et al., 1964; Jahrsdoerfer, 1977; Harada et al., 1980)
    b. *Calcification of annular ligament (Davis, 1968)
    c. *Filled with fetal connective tissue (Kelemen, 1966a)
    d. Thin membranous window (Livingstone and Delahunty, 1968)
    e. *Small (Sando et al., 1968)

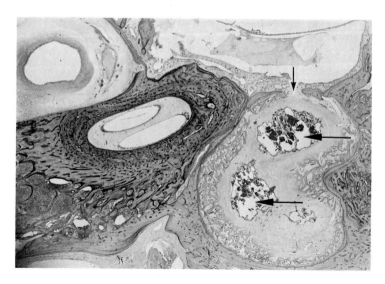

Figure 18–4. High jugular bulb (large arrows), accompanied by dehiscence (small arrow) of the medial bony wall of the tympanic cavity (H & E, × 11).

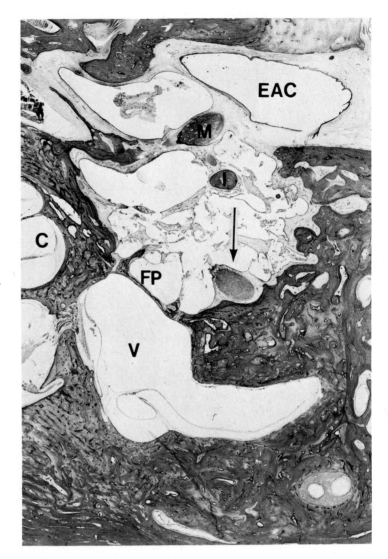

Figure 18–5. Several dehiscences of the facial canal (arrow) in a patient with congenital heart anomalies. C, cochlea; EAC, external auditory canal; FP, footplate of stapes; I, incus; M, malleus; V, vestibule (H & E, × 10.5).

2. ROUND WINDOW ANOMALIES (8), (17), (28), (30), (40), (44), (47)

    a. Absence (Hough, 1963)
    b. Round window partitioned by bony bar (Livingstone and Delahunty, 1968)
    c. Displacement of round window (Hough, 1958)
    d. Absence of niche (Hough, 1958)
    e. Connective tissue obstruction of niche (Ruedi, 1954)
    f. Narrow niche (Baldwin, 1968)

(H) Otic Capsule Anomalies (19), (20), (30), (35), (43), (45), (46), (54), (56)

    a. *Achondroplasia (Schuknecht, 1967)
    b. *Fibrous resorption focus in two external layers due to gargoylism (Kelemen, 1966a)
    c. *Osteitis due to syphilis (Goodhill, 1939)
    d. *Osteitis deformans (Davis, 1968)
    e. *Osteogenesis imperfecta (Altmann, 1962)
    f. *Osteopetrosis (Myers and Stool, 1969)
    g. *Otosclerosis (Schuknecht, 1974)
    h. Thickened periosteal layer due to endemic cretinism (Warkany, 1971)
    i. *Underdevelopment of periosteal layer due to craniofacial dysostosis (Baldwin, 1968)

(I) Mastoid Anomalies (11), (14), (16), (17), (35), (39), (44), (56)

    a. *Absence of mastoid antrum (Sando et al., 1968)
    b. *Poor development of mastoid antrum (Ruedi, 1954)
    c. *Poor development of mastoid air cells (Ruedi, 1954)
    d. *Small mastoid process (Ruedi, 1954)

(J) Eustachian Tube Anomalies (23)

    a. Absence (Altmann, 1951b)
    b. Abnormally narrow (Altmann, 1949)
    c. Diverticula of eustachian tube (Von Kostanecki, 1887, quoted by Altmann, 1951b)
    d. Congenital tumor (polyp) (Henke, 1924, quoted by Altmann, 1951b)

DISCUSSION

Anomalies of the external and middle ear are of major importance to both the patient and the otologist. When they are bilateral and associated with significant hearing loss from birth, they result in poor speech and language development or failure of such development. Children thus afflicted are sometimes mistakenly classified as being mentally retarded and are needlessly condemned to a lifetime of institutionalization and intellectual deprivation. Also, cosmetic anomalies of the external ear may produce severe psychologic trauma in children. Early correction of deformities is essential in ensuring normal development of speech and is also helpful to the psychologic development of the patient who is affected by the anomaly. Correction of congenital anomalies represents a challenge to the surgical ingenuity of the otologist, but the fact that a hearing loss is frequently correctible by modern otomicrosurgical techniques should be encouraging to the patient, his or her family, and the otologist. As has been mentioned, surgical misadventures may result from encountering unexpected anatomic variations. A study of the nature of the anomaly often provides the otologist with some clue as to the period of embryonic development during which the insult occurred and, thus, to what other anomalies might be encountered during corrective surgery.

From a review of the literature on this subject and from study of temporal bones, certain trends are evident.

1. Anomalies of the external and middle ear that occur in the absence of associated anomalies usually are of unknown origin and occur in the absence of any family history of anomalies.

2. Anomalies of the external and middle ear that occur with other anomalies usually are of known etiology or are associated with a positive family history.

3. Of the middle-ear anomalies that occur without other anomalies, those most frequently encountered include ossicular anomalies and anomalies of the facial nerve. There is a tendency for middle-ear anomalies to occur together, such as facial nerve and ossicular anomalies, especially those involving the stapes. This,

of course, reflects their interdependent embryonic development.

4. In the case of anomalies of the external and middle ear associated with other anomalies, the association of branchial arch anomalies with anomalies of the external and middle ear is clear. Because of the small number of histopathologic reports available regarding the temporal bone, it is not yet possible to compile a comprehensive list of associated anomalies.

5. Routine audiometric testing does not provide any clue as to the nature of the anomaly.

Some findings do provide us with diagnostic clues.

1. A positive family history of congenital malformations is important.

2. A maternal history of infectious disease during pregnancy and drug ingestion or exposure to ionizing irradiation before or during pregnancy should be sought.

3. A history of a nonprogressive, usually unilateral, conductive hearing loss present since birth suggests an anomaly of the external auditory meatus or ossicles, or both.

4. A history of retarded or absent speech development suggests a congenital hearing loss.

5. The presence of any other congenital anomalies makes imperative a complete physical and audiometric examination (Chaps. 8 and 9).

In studying suspected congenital anomalies of the external and middle ear, we would make the following suggestions.

1. A careful family history must be taken, with emphasis on congenital anomalies, ear infections, hearing aid use, and hearing loss.

2. The maternal history of drug ingestion, exposure to ionizing radiation, or utilization of chelating agents or antimetabolites before or during pregnancy as well as a history of infectious diseases, especially viral, during pregnancy is important.

3. For differential diagnosis, a history of postnatal infections, perinatal trauma, or postnatal injury or surgery may provide information as to the origin of the anomaly.

4. Polytomographic studies may reveal anomalies of the external auditory meatus, middle ear, and inner ear (Chap. 10).

5. The result of testing a child with an anomaly with the acoustic impedance bridge may make possible a differential diagnosis between ossicular fixation and ossicular discontinuity.

6. Chromosomal analysis may be helpful in making a differential diagnosis.

7. Surgical exploration, aided by radiographic findings, provides the only definitive diagnosis and also the treatment for these conditions.

8. During surgery to correct conductive hearing losses of unknown origin, extreme care must be exercised in order to avoid injuring anatomic structures, such as the facial nerve, that may be located in other than their usual locations in anomalous ears. A knowledge of embryology provides the surgeon with some information as to where these structures are likely to be found when they are not in their normal locations.

An intensive campaign should be carried out to obtain the temporal bones from all patients with known anomalies of the ear, other associated anomalies, or conductive and sensorineural hearing loss of unknown origin so that histopathologic studies of the temporal bone can be carried out.

TREATMENT AND REHABILITATION OF PATIENTS WITH CONGENITAL ANOMALIES OF THE EXTERNAL AND MIDDLE EAR

The variety and seriousness of anomalies of the external and middle ear range from minor variations from the normal and no functional disability to total absence of identifiable structures and of hearing. Even within any one disease category, the degree of abnormality and the nature of the anomaly (i.e., the structures affected) may vary widely.

Consequently, such patients cannot be managed by a "cookbook" approach. Because many of the anomalies found at surgery are unsuspected preoperatively (many of them occurring without any other associated anomalies) or the surgeon encounters hitherto undescribed anatomic variations in the middle ear, it is necessary to understand the *principles* of correction and to have a broad knowledge of the myriad of possibilities for creating a satisfactory mechanism for conducting sound to the cochlea. In some instances, surgical correction of an anomaly simply will not be possible.

Many of the conditions discussed are associated with mild to severe or even total sensorineural hearing losses. At the present time, no satisfactory medical or surgical treatment exists for a sensorineural hearing loss, except perhaps in the case of otosclerosis (Shambaugh and Causse, 1974). There are some as yet unpublished reports on the stabilization of progressive sensorineural hearing losses in patients with Mondini-type (shortened cochlea) cochlear deformities using the endolymphatic shunt operation. Direct electrical stimulation of the cochlear nerve by cochlear electrode implantation, which is currently under investigation, may be beneficial to patients in whom there is essen-

tially total sensory hearing loss but the fibers of the cochlear nerve are intact.

The role of any physician who undertakes the care of patients with congenital anomalies is to remedy their problems in whatever manner is feasible. When dealing with anomalies of the ear, this includes restoration of hearing or at least improvement of hearing to as nearly normal levels as possible and the prevention or correction of any speech and language disorders that may accompany the hearing loss. The physician's responsibility goes beyond that, however, and now includes the determination and remediation of any learning disabilities that may be associated with the hearing loss and its resultant speech and language disorders.

The process of treatment must begin with a determination of the extent of the disability. In many medical centers, in addition to the routine neonatal examination that will, hopefully, discover many visible congenital anomalies, a high-risk register (Northern and Downs, 1978) for hearing loss is used to determine which babies should receive neonatal hearing screening; determinations are based upon family history, prenatal history, conditions surrounding the birth, and early neonatal history. Some centers do routine hearing screening on all newborn infants.

Once an infant has been placed in the high-risk category by virtue of the register criteria, repeated physical examinations and hearing screening are performed in the first few months of life until it is determined that the hearing is normal.

For children in whom a hearing loss is strongly suspected or proved, remediation is begun at once. It is the policy at the University of Colorado Medical Center to fit any infant suspected of having a hearing loss greater than 20 dB bilaterally with a hearing aid. The earliest fittings have been at about 1 month of age. Air-conduction aids are used whenever possible; in cases of external atresia, bone conduction aids are used. Very close follow-up with frequent hearing retesting is carried out until accurate estimations of the hearing can be obtained. Speech and language development are closely observed, and special education is provided when necessary. In cases of multiple anomalies in which mental and motor retardation may be present, it is difficult to determine the child's developmental potential early in the course.

In cases in which the association between certain anomalies and hearing loss is very high (e.g., cleft palate and middle-ear effusion), a myringotomy will be performed and middle-ear ventilation tubes placed as soon as possible (Paradise, 1975).

In other cases, as soon as the nature and severity of the hearing loss (i.e., conductive, sensorineural, or mixed loss) have been determined, a course of action is decided upon. The children with sensorineural losses will continue to use hearing amplification. When a conductive loss is accompanied by a middle-ear effusion, a myringotomy is performed, and ventilating tubes are placed. The hearing must be carefully monitored after tube placement, since the first clue to an otherwise unsuspected middle-ear anomaly frequently is the failure of hearing to improve after tube placement. (Normally, if a hearing loss is caused by a middle-ear effusion, hearing will improve quickly following myringotomy.)

Patients who are known to have anomalies, such as aural atresia, and those with severe conductive and mixed hearing losses are further studied using polytomographic studies of the temporal bone to evaluate the condition of the external ear canal, the presence of an atretic bony plate, the size and condition of the middle-ear space and ossicular chain, and the cochlea, vestibule, semicircular canals, and internal auditory meatus. The locations of the carotid artery, sigmoid sinus, and fallopian canal are also determined by these studies.

Following these studies, a decision is made as to the feasibility of surgery to improve hearing and to correct cosmetic deformities.

THE SURGICAL CORRECTION OF CONGENITAL ANOMALIES OF THE EXTERNAL EAR AND MIDDLE EAR

Auricle

Surgery to correct anomalies of the auricle has been carried out for many years; however, there has been a difference of opinion as to the efficacy of different types of surgical management of some of the anomalies. It is generally agreed that minor deformities of the auricle can be repaired surgically with quite acceptable cosmetic results, but severe deformities with few normal structures frequently still appear distinctly abnormal, even to casual view, after multiple operative procedures. In such cases, the question arises as to whether or not a better alternative might not be excision of the minor skin tags and fitting with a good cosmetic prosthesis rather than the trauma of multiple operations resulting in an equivocal cosmetic result (Jensen and Terkildson, 1967; Lowenstein, 1966).

The simplest auricular anomaly to correct is an outstanding (protruding) auricle. With the exception of failure of formation of the anthelical rim and sometimes an exceptionally deep concha, the auricle is well-formed. Although the standard surgical procedures (Becker, 1952; Converse et al., 1955) for correcting such deformities yield excellent results in the best of hands, the cartilaginous incisions can result in unpleasant, sharp demarcations that are visible from the anterior and lateral aspects. In recent years, we have instead used the simpler technique of Mustarde (1963).

Next in complexity is the repair of cryptotia. In this disorder, the superior portion of auricular cartilage is buried beneath the scalp. Usually a relatively simple operative procedure to release the buried cartilage framework and overlying skin from the side of the head and to place a split-thickness graft to the posterior aspect of the auricle and postauricular area will yield a satisfactory result. Some minor revisions may be necessary (Pollock, 1969).

Far more serious problems are encountered in the correction of anotia and microtia. These conditions represent a continuum of deformity ranging from total absence of any identifiable auricular structures (anotia), to the presence of primordial hillocks (microtia Type III) barely recognizable as auricular structures, to the existence of a curving elevation representing a deformed helix (microtia Type II), and finally to the presence of a small auricle that is deformed but possesses the essential structures (microtia Type I) (Fig. 18–6). In all these anomalies, the structures may be displaced downward and anterior to their usual locations. Although many surgical procedures have been described for the correction of these conditions, it is the authors' opinion that anotia and Type III microtia are better handled by excision of any vestigial tags and fitting of a good cosmetic prosthesis.

Microtia Types I and II may be repaired by the procedures described by Converse (1964), sometimes with very acceptable results.

External Auditory Meatus and Middle Ear

For those interested in the well-being and development of the child with bilateral congenital atresia of the external auditory meatus, there is a moral and medical dilemma. Although there are mild forms of this condition, manifested only by abnormally narrow external auditory meatuses without any associated conductive hearing loss and requiring no correction or only minor treatment (such as frequent cleaning or canaloplasty), the more serious forms involve total or partial absence of the external canal. These are normally accompanied by a maximum conductive hearing loss in the range of 60 to 70 dB. This is compounded by the inability to fit an air-conduction hearing aid and, frequently, lack of an auricle or the presence of a deformed or misplaced auricle. Also associated are anomalies of the middle ear ranging from minor anomalies of the ossicles to absence of the mastoid and middle-ear cleft. There may also be anomalies of the inner ear ranging from minor malformations of the labyrinth to absence of the inner ear. The surgical correction of the more serious anomalies presents a risk to hearing and facial nerve function.

The presence of anomalies of the auricle and the external auditory meatus makes imperative a careful examination of the patient to determine the extent of the deformities. This involves first a physical examination to determine if other anomalies are present. Next, audiometric testing must be performed in a center that is equipped to do neonatal testing. Even in the immediate postnatal period, reasonably accurate behavioral test results may be obtained. Localization, however, may be difficult to determine. Next, radiographic studies must be performed. In planning the surgical correction of atresia, anteroposterior and lateral polytomographic roentgenograms of the external auditory meatus, mastoid, middle ear, inner ear, and internal auditory meatus are mandatory. In order to

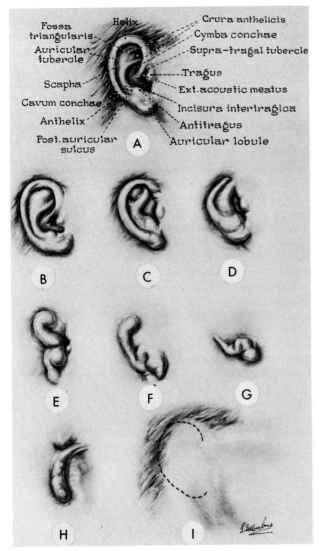

Figure 18–6. Examples of auricular malformations. *A*, Normal adult pinna. *B*, Example of a minor malformation. The pinna reveals regular overall dimensions and position but incomplete differentiation. *C* and *D*, Examples of microtia Type I: The auricle is smaller, rudimentary, and often located in an abnormal position. The different parts of the pinna are still discernible. *E* and *F*, Examples of microtia Type II: The auricle, besides being smaller and often in an abnormal position, is represented by a vertical curving ridge, resembling a primitive helix. *G* and *H*, Examples of microtia Type III: The rudiment of the auricle has no resemblance to any portion of the pinna. *I*, Example of anotia. (From Nager, G. T., and Levin, L. S. 1980. *In* Paparella, M. M., and Shumrick, D. A. [eds.]: Otolaryngology, Vol. 2, 2nd ed. Philadelphia, W. B. Saunders Co., p. 1314.)

obtain adequate data from these tests in infants, general anesthesia is frequently necessary (Chap. 10).

Once these studies are completed, a plan may be formulated for the surgical management of the patient's deformities. It is the authors' opinion that if the atresia is unilateral and the hearing is normal in the opposite ear, *no* surgical correction is indicated other than cosmetic until the patient reaches the age of consent so that he or she may decide whether to undertake the risk inherent in surgical correction of severe mal-

formations. In the case of bilateral atresia, there is a question as to which ear should be operated on. Before any operation, it should be determined that the patient has hearing in the opposite ear so that the patient would have functional hearing should there be a sensorineural hearing loss secondary to the surgery.

Evaluation of the polytomograms includes establishing the presence of a normal internal auditory canal and cochlea. Next, the presence of a middle-ear cleft and mastoid air cell system must be determined. The condition of the ossicular chain must be evaluated, and the presence of a fallopian canal may be determined on lateral views. (It must be remembered, however, that the presence of the bony canal *does not* mean that the nerve is lying within it.) If possible, the canal is traced to its point of exit from the temporal bone. (It must be remembered that, in normal infants, the nerve exits laterally behind and below the external auditory meatus because the mastoid tip is not yet developed.) The location and the condition of the oval window niche, round window, and the horizontal semicircular canal are determined. The examiner must also look for replacement of the tympanic membrane by a bony atresia plate. Last, the external auditory meatus is examined to determine if the atresia is made up of soft tissue or bone and to establish the relative position of the mandibular condyle, which may be displaced posteriorly, occupying the normal position of the external auditory meatus.

The more normal ear should be operated on first. Then, if an auricular deformity has occurred in addition to the canal deformity, the staging of surgery must be decided with whoever will operate to correct the external deformity. Usually, the middle ear and canal correction will be done first to locate the new ear canal, although there are differences of opinion on this aspect. The auricle can then be relocated to place it over the canal.

The surgical procedure to correct ear deformities has several goals. The first is to create a patent external auditory meatus and is accomplished by removing the stenotic soft tissue of the existing canal. If the medial portion of the canal is bony, this must be drilled away to create a large meatus, which is then lined with a split-thickness graft. Next, if a bony atresia plate is present, this must be drilled away carefully so as not to transmit unnecessary trauma to the stapes. Most authors recommend disarticulating the incus and stapes prior to drilling in this region. It is desirable to create a shelf of bone approximating the annulus onto which one can lay the drum prosthesis. In some cases, the posterior position of the mandibular condyle will drastically alter the position of the external auditory meatus (Figs. 18–7, 18–8, and 18–9).

The condition of the ossicular chain is then ascertained; fixation of the malleus and incus to the bony atretic plate is not uncommon. If this is the case, it must be determined if the ossicles can be salvaged or if they must be sacrificed. It is best to save them if possible, but if the risk of refixation seems great, they must be removed. The condition of the stapes

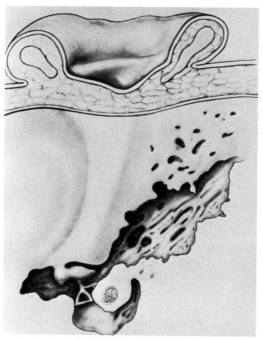

Figure 18–7. Sagittal section of the temporal bone illustrating absent bony external auditory meatus with malleus-incus complex fused to bony atresia plate. (From Jahrsdoerfer, R. A. 1978. Congenital atresia of the ear. Laryngoscope, 88, Suppl. 13.)

superstructure and footplate is then determined. Most important, mobility of the footplate must be established.

The recreation of the sound-conducting mechanism is the next step. If the middle-ear ossicles are relatively normal and mobile, a fascia graft is placed beneath the manubrium of the malleus in the usual fashion. If not, grafting may be accomplished with fascia or with a homograft tympanic membrane–ossicular prosthesis. We believe that the homograft will become more commonly used in time. The attachment to the stapes may be carried out at the first operation or in a later reconstruction, depending upon the situation encountered. In the absence of an incus, either a homograft ossicle or an alloplastic strut may be used. Our personal experience with alloplastic struts in middle-ear reconstruction has not been entirely favorable, and hence we prefer to use autograft or homograft ossicles.

Last, the external auditory meatus is lined with a split-thickness skin graft. Preferably, no external canal stent is used, as we believe this may cause further stenosis.

The results of surgery for congenital atresia have not been uniformly good (or else there would have been considerably more enthusiasm for it); however, recent reports have been encouraging. The chief problems have been damage to the facial nerve, stenosis of the external auditory meatus, poor hearing results (for unknown reasons), and sensorineural hearing loss. For a complete review of the problem, its analysis, and treatment, we refer readers to the excellent articles by Jahrsdoerfer (1978) and Crabtree (1968).

Middle Ear

The exact nature of anomalies of the middle ear is seldom known prior to surgical exploration. In children in the early years of life, when middle-ear effusions and recurrent suppurative otitis media are common, and in those with a predisposition to eustachian tube malfunction (e.g., those with cleft palates), one would anticipate poorer surgical results than in patients whose eustachian tube function is normal. Consequently, the surgeon must weigh the possibility of complications resulting from impaired eustachian tube function against the benefits of early improvement in hearing. Entering into this is the frequent refusal of some children to wear hearing aids.

Owing to the diverse nature of anomalies of the middle ear, there is no single operative procedure for the restoration of hearing. In some circumstances, no feasible way of improving hearing may be found.

It is beyond the purview of this text to discuss all the possible methods for re-creation of the sound-conducting mechanism of the middle ear; however, some examples will be given. The principle involved is to create a mobile ossicular chain with good contact between a mobile tympanic membrane and a mobile stapes footplate (Figs. 18–10, 18–11, and 18–12) (Tabor, 1971). In turn, for this system to be effective, there must be a normal round window membrane. In rare instances (where an oval window niche is not

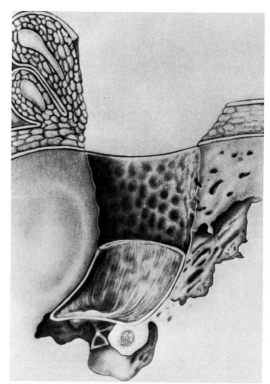

Figure 18–8. Drawing illustrating newly created bony external auditory meatus, with a fascia graft placed over the ossicular chain and the facial ridge, lining a portion of the external canal walls. (From Jahrsdoerfer, R. A. 1978. Congenital atresia of the ear. Laryngoscope, 88, Suppl. 13.)

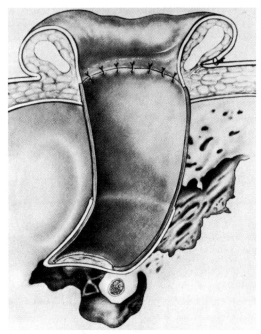

Figure 18–9. In this drawing, a split-thickness skin graft with a hole over the neotympanum graft has been placed to line the bony external auditory meatus. (From Jahrsdoerfer, R. A. 1978. Congenital atresia of the ear. Laryngoscope, 88, Suppl. 13.)

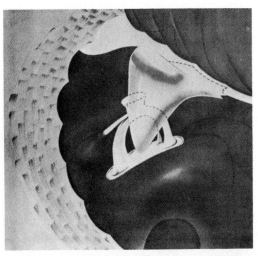

Figure 18–11. Drawing illustrating transposition of the incus with the short process on the stapes footplate between the superstructure and the promontory. The articular surface of the incus is placed medial to the malleus manubrium. (From Tabor, J. R. 1971. Methods of Ossiculoplasty. Courtesy of Charles C Thomas, Publisher, Springfield, Illinois.)

present or is covered by an aberrant facial nerve), sound must be conducted to other than the stapes footplate; usually the horizontal semicircular canal is fenestrated in such cases (Shambaugh, 1967).

The most straightforward operative procedure for the treatment of a congenital conductive hearing loss is the performance of a stapedectomy to correct the effects of otosclerosis. In this instance, the fixed footplate and stapes are removed, the oval window is covered by a tissue graft such as perichondrium, and a wire is placed from the incus to the oval window to transmit sound (Fig. 18–13).

Summary

Minor abnormalities of the auricle can usually be corrected by simple operative procedures that give quite acceptable cosmetic results. Where only vestigial auricular structures are present, surgical reconstruction through many operative procedures frequently yields unacceptable cosmetic results. In these cases, a well-made auricular prosthesis is preferable.

When a child presents with atresia in which there is considerable distortion of the normal anatomy of the external auditory meatus, middle ear, and sometimes inner ear, sophisticated roentgenographic studies must be made to determine the feasibility of reconstructing the existing ear. Care must be exerted to avoid damage

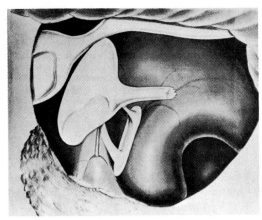

Figure 18–10. Drawing illustrating transposition of the incus between the malleus long process and the stapedial head, with the incudal head flat on the stapedial head. (From Tabor, J. R. 1971. Methods of Ossiculoplasty. Courtesy of Charles C Thomas, Publisher, Springfield, Illinois.)

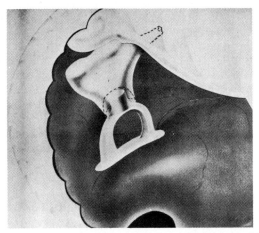

Figure 18–12. Drawing illustrating incus transposition in which a cup that has been drilled in the short process of the incus is placed over the head of the stapes. The long process of the incus is placed beneath the medial aspect of the malleus manubrium. (From Tabor, J. R. 1971. Methods of Ossiculoplasty. Courtesy of Charles C Thomas, Publisher, Springfield, Illinois.)

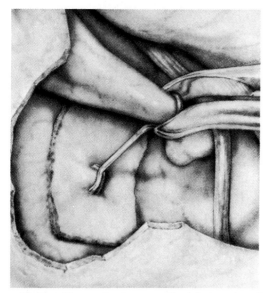

Figure 18–13. A House wire stapes prosthesis being crimped over the long process of the incus. The loop is resting upon tissue (compressed fat, vein, fascia, perichondrium) that seals the oval window. (From Goin, D. W. 1976. *In* English, G. M. [ed.]: Otolaryngology, a Textbook. Hagerstown, MD, Harper & Row, p. 154.)

to the facial nerve and cochlea, which would result in a sensorineural hearing loss. Ultimately, one of the most difficult problems encountered in this type of reconstruction is in the prevention of postoperative external meatus stenosis.

Anomalies of the middle ear sound-conducting mechanism may very frequently be corrected by modern otomicrosurgical techniques. The exact nature of the anomaly is almost never known until surgical exploration is carried out. At that time, hitherto unsuspected anomalies, such as those of the facial nerve and carotid artery or a persistent stapedial artery, may be encountered. Nowhere is the experience and flexibility of the otologic surgeon of greater import than in the correction of these anomalies: Using accepted surgical principles, he or she must often remedy previously undescribed conditions.

The responsibility of the otologist does not end with the surgical correction of otic anomalies. This practitioner must be aware of the social, psychologic, and educational consequences of these anomalies and the speech and language delays that may result from the associated hearing loss. It is incumbent on the physician to be responsible for seeing that the appropriate rehabilitative measures are instituted. Likewise, in those cases of sensorineural hearing loss or conductive hearing loss that are not amenable to surgical correction, it is the responsibility of the otologist to oversee an appropriate amplification treatment program (Chap. 96).

SELECTED REFERENCES

Crabtree, J. A. 1968. Tympanoplastic techniques in congenital atresia. Arch. Otolaryngol. 88:89.
This article is particularly valuable for its explanation of the surgical approach to congenital atresia.

Hough, J. V. D. 1958. Malformations and anatomical variations seen in the middle ear during the operation for stabilization of the stapes. Laryngoscope 68:1337.
This report on anomalies and variations in middle-ear structures encountered during stapes surgery is valuable, especially for its description of a number of interesting cases and for the colored photomicrographs and illustrations that accompany these descriptions.

Jahrsdoerfer, R. A. 1978. Congenital atresia of the ear. Laryngoscope 88, Suppl. 13.
This article gives an excellent, complete review of the problem, analysis, and treatment of congenital atresia of the ear.

Konigsmark, W., and Gorlin, R. J. 1976. Genetic and Metabolic Deafness. Philadelphia, W. B. Saunders Co.
This textbook is a valuable reference source for information on many types of hereditary hearing losses.

Schuknecht, H. F. 1974. Pathology of the Ear. Cambridge, MA, Harvard University Press.
This textbook should be extremely helpful to both researchers and clinicians who concern themselves with the function of hearing in association with anomalies of the external and middle ear.

Tabor, J. R. 1971. Methods of Ossiculoplasty. Springfield, IL, Charles C Thomas Co.
This textbook discusses clearly and concisely the principles of ossicular chain reconstruction in various situations that may be encountered in the middle ear.

REFERENCES

Adkins, W. Y., Jr., and Gussen, R. 1974a. Oval window absence, bony closure of round window, and inner ear anomaly. Laryngoscope 84:1210.

Adkins, W. Y., Jr., and Gussen, R. 1974b. Temporal bone findings in the third and fourth pharyngeal pouch (DiGeorge) syndrome. Arch. Otolaryngol. 100:206.

Altmann, F. 1947. Anomalies of the internal carotid artery and its branches. Laryngoscope 58:313.

Altmann, F. 1949. Problem of so-called congenital atresia of the ear. Arch. Otolaryngol. 50:759.

Altmann, F. 1951a. Malformations of the auricle and the external auditory meatus (A Critical Review). Arch. Otolaryngol. 54:115.

Altmann, F. 1951b. Malformations of the Eustachian tube, the middle ear, and its appendages (A Critical Review). Arch. Otolaryngol. 54:241.

Altmann, F. 1955. Congenital atresia of the ear in man and animals. Ann. Otol. Rhinol. Laryngol. 64:824.

Altmann, F. 1957. The ear in severe malformations of the head. Arch. Otolaryngol. 66:7.

Altmann, F. 1962. The temporal bone in osteogenesis imperfecta congenita. Arch. Otolaryngol. 75:486.

Arnold, W., Schuknecht, H. F., and von Voss, H. 1981. Felsenbeinbefunde bei der Trisomie 22. Laryngol. Rhinol. Otol. 60:545.

Baldwin, J. L., 1968. Dysostosis craniofacialis of Crouzon. Laryngoscope 78:1660.

Balkany, T. J., Mischke, R. E., Downs, M. P., et al. 1979. Ossicular abnormalities in Down's syndrome. Otolaryngol Head Neck Surg 1979; 87:372.

Bart, R. S., and Pumphrey, R. E. 1967. Knuckle pads, leukonychia and deafness. A dominantly inherited syndrome. N. Engl. J. Med. 276:202.

Basek, M. 1962. Anomalies of the facial nerve in normal temporal bones. Ann. Otol. Rhinol. Laryngol. 71:382.

The authors are grateful to Professor Bruce Jafek, M.D., Department of Otolaryngology, University of Colorado Medical Center, for the use of the Center's cases for some of the figures in this chapter.

The authors wish to express their deep gratitude to Professor E. N. Myers, M.D., Department of Otolaryngology, University of Pittsburgh School of Medicine, for encouraging them to study this subject and for giving helpful criticism during the preparation of this chapter.

The authors are also grateful to Mrs. Ruth Anderson for her assistance.

Becker, O. J. 1952. Correction of protruding deformed ear. Brit. J. Plast. Surg. 5:187.

Bergsma, D. 1979. Birth defects compendium. *In* Bergsma, D. (ed.): Birth Defects Compendium. New York, AR Liss, Inc.

Bergstrom, L. 1977. Osteogenesis imperfecta. Otologic and maxillofacial aspects. Laryngoscope 87, Suppl. 6.

Bergstrom, L., Hemenway, W. G., and Sando, I. 1972. Pathological changes in congenital deafness. Laryngoscope 82:1777.

Black, F. O., Myers, E. N., and Rorke, L. B. 1973. Aplasia of the first and second branchial arches. Arch. Otolaryngol 98:124.

Black, F. O., Sando, I., Wagner, J. A., et al. 1971. Middle and inner ear abnormalities, 13–15 (D₁) trisomy. Arch. Otolaryngol. 93:615.

Black, F. O., Spanier, S. S., and Kohut, R. I. 1975. Aural abnormalities in partial DiGeorge syndrome. Arch. Otolaryngol. 101:129.

Bordley, J. E., and Hardy, J. M. B. 1969. Laboratory and clinical observations on prenatal rubella. Ann. Otol. Rhinol. Laryngol. 78:917.

Buran, D. J., and Duvall, A. J. 1967. The oto-palato-digital (OPD) syndrome. Arch. Otolaryngol. 85:394.

Caparosa, R. J., and Klassen, D. 1966. Congenital anomalies of the stapes and facial nerve. Arch. Otolaryngol. 83:420.

Cohn, M., Statloff, J., and Lindsay, J. R. 1970. Histiocytosis X (Letterer-Siwe disease) with involvement of the inner ear. Arch. Otolaryngol. 91:24.

Converse, J. M. 1964. Reconstructive Plastic Surgery: Principles and Procedures in Correction, Reconstruction and Transplantation. Vol. 3. Philadelphia, W. B. Saunders Co.

Converse, J. M., Nigro, A., Wilson, F. A., et al. 1955. A technique for surgical correction of lop ears. Plast. Reconstr. Surg. 15:411.

Crabtree, J. A. 1968. Tympanoplastic techniques in congenital atresia. Arch. Otolaryngol. 88:89.

Davis, D. G. 1968. Paget's disease of the temporal bone. Acta Otolaryngol. (Stockh.) Suppl. 24.

Dijkstra, B. K. S. 1977. Goldenhar's syndrome, oculo-auricular malformation, in a Bantu girl. O. R. L. 39:101.

Druss, J. G. 1952. Supernumerary muscle of middle ear. Arch. Otolaryngol. 55:206.

Durcan, D. J., Shea, J. J., and Sleeckx, J. P. 1967. Bifurcation of the facial nerve. Arch. Otolaryngol. 86:619.

Egami, T., Sando, I., and Myers, E. N. 1979. Temporal bone anomalies associated with congenital heart disease. Ann. Otol. Rhinol. Laryngol. 88:72.

Escher, F., and Hirt, H. 1968. Dominant hereditary conductive deafness through lack of incus-stapes junction. Acta Otolaryngol. (Stockh.) 65:25.

Fernandez, A. O., and Ronis, M. L. 1964. Congenital absence of the oval window. Laryngoscope 74:186.

Fisher, S. R., Farmer, J. C., and Baylin, G. 1982. Bilateral congenital absence of the stapes and cervical spine anomaly. Am. J. Otol. 4:166.

Fitch, N., Lindsay, J. R., and Srolovitz, H. 1976. The temporal bone in the preauricular pit, cervical fistula, hearing loss syndrome. Ann. Otol. Rhinol. Laryngol. 85:268.

Føns, M. 1969. Ear malformations in cleidocranial dysostosis. Acta Otolaryngol. (Stockh.) 67:483.

Forney, W. R., Robinson, S. J., and Pascoe, D. J. 1966. Congenital heart disease, deafness, and skeletal malformations: A new syndrome? Pediatr. 68:14.

Fowler, E. P., Jr. 1961. Variations in the temporal bone course of the facial nerve. Laryngoscope 71:937.

Friedmann, I., Spellacy, E., Crow, J., et al. 1985. Histopathological studies of temporal bones in Hurler's disease [Mucopolysaccharidosis (MPS)IH]. J. Laryngol. Otol. 99:29.

Friedmann, I., Wright, J. L. W., and Phelps, P. D. 1980. Temporal bone studies in anencephaly. J. Laryngol. Otol. 94:929.

Gnanapragasam, A. 1975. Bilateral symmetrical maldevelopment of the external ear and middle ear cleft with pharyngeal and soft palate defects. J. Laryngol. Otol. 89:845.

Goldberg, M. J., and Pashayan, H. M. 1976. Hallux syndactyly–ulnar polydactyly–abnormal ear lobes: A new syndrome. Birth Defects 12(5):255.

Goldman, N. C., Singleton, G. T., and Holly, E. H. 1971. Aberrant internal carotid artery. Arch. Otolaryngol. 94:269.

Goodhill, V. 1939. Syphilis of the ear: A histopathologic study. Ann. Otol. Rhinol. Laryngol. 48:676.

Gussen, R. 1981. Middle and inner ear changes in congenital rubella. Am. J. Otolaryngol. 2:314.

Harada, T., Black, F. O., Sando, I., et al. 1980. Temporal bone histopathologic findings in congenital anomalies of the oval window. Otolaryngol. Head Neck Surg. 88:275.

Harada, T., and Sando, I. 1981. Temporal bone histopathologic findings in Down's syndrome. Arch. Otolaryngol. 107:96.

Harada, T., Sando, I., Stool, S. E., et al. 1980. Temporal bone histopathologic features in Fanconi's anemia syndrome. Arch. Otolaryngol. 106:275.

Harrison, W. H., Shambaugh, G. E., Jr., and Derlacki, E. L. 1966. Congenital absence of the round window: Case report with surgical reconstruction by cochlear fenestration. Laryngoscope 76:967.

Hemenway, W. G., Sando, I., and McChesney, D. 1969. Temporal bone pathology following maternal rubella. Arch. Klin. Exp. Ohr. Nas. Kehlk. Heilk. 193:287.

Henderson, J. L. 1939. The congenital facial diplegia syndrome: Clinical features, pathology and aetiology. A review of sixty-one cases. Brain 62:381.

Herberts, G. 1962. Otological observations on the "Treacher Collins syndrome." Acta Otolaryngol. (Stockh.) 54:457.

Hiraide, F., Nomura, Y., and Nakamura, K. 1974. Histopathology of atresia auris congenita. J. Laryngol. Otol. 88:1249.

Hoenk, B. E., McCabe, B. F., and Anson, B. J. 1969. Cholesteatoma auris behind a bony atresia plate. Arch. Otolaryngol. 89:470.

Hough, J. V. D. 1958. Malformations and anatomical variations seen in the middle ear during the operation for mobilization of the stapes. Laryngoscope 68:1337.

Hough, J. V. D. 1963. Congenital malformations of the middle ear. Arch. Otolaryngol. 78:335.

Igarashi, M., Filippone, M. V., and Alford, B. R. 1976. Temporal bone findings in Pierre Robin syndrome. Laryngoscope 86:1679.

Igarashi, M., Takahasi, M., Alford, B. R., et al. 1977. Inner ear morphology in Down syndrome. Acta Otolaryngol. (Stockh.) 83:175.

Isenberg, S. F., and Tubergen, L. B. 1980. An unusual congenital middle ear ossicular anomaly. Arch. Otolaryngol. 106:179.

Jaffee, I. S. 1968. Congenital shoulder-neck-auditory anomalies. Laryngoscope 78:2119.

Jahrsdoerfer, R. A. 1977. Congenital absence of the oval window. Trans. Am. Acad. Ophthalmol. Otolaryngol. 84:904.

Jahrsdoerfer, R. A. 1978. Congenital atresia of the ear. Laryngoscope 88, Suppl. 13.

Jahrsdoerfer, R. A. 1981. The facial nerve in congenital middle ear malformations. Laryngoscope 91:1217.

Jensen, P. V., and Terkildson, K. 1967. Prosthetic reconstruction of external ear defects. Acta Otol. 64:492.

Jørgensen, M. B., Kristensen, H. K., and Buch, N. H. 1964. Thalidomide-induced aplasia of the inner ear. J. Laryngol. Otol. 78:1095.

Karmody, C. S., and Schuknecht, H. F. 1966. Deafness in congenital syphilis. Arch. Otolaryngol. 83:18.

Kelemen, G. 1966a. Hurler's syndrome and the hearing organ. J. Laryngol. Otol. 80:791.

Kelemen, G. 1966b. Rubella and deafness. Arch. Otolaryngol. 83:520.

Kodama, A., Sando, I., Myers, E. N., et al. 1982. Severe middle ear anomaly with underdeveloped facial nerve. Arch. Otolaryngol. 108:93.

Koide, Y., Kato, I., Yamasaki, H., et al. 1967. Congenital anomalies of the ossicles without deformities of the external ear. Jap. J. Otol. 70:1358.

Konigsmark, W., Nager, G. T., and Haskins, H. L. 1972. Recessive microtia, meatal atresia and hearing loss. Arch. Otolaryngol. 96:105.

Konigsmark, W., and Gorlin, R. J. 1976. Genetic and Metabolic Deafness. Philadelphia, W. B. Saunders Co.

Kos, A. O., Schuknecht, H. F., and Singer, J. D. 1966. Temporal bone studies in 13–15 and 18 trisomy syndromes. Arch. Otolaryngol. 83:439.

Kraus, P., and Ziv, M. 1971. Incus fixation due to congenital anomaly of chorda tympani. Acta Otolaryngol. (Stockh.) 72:358.

Larsson, A. 1962. Genetic problems in otosclerosis. *In* Schuknecht, H. (ed.): Henry Ford Symposium on Otosclerosis. Boston, Little, Brown, and Co., pp. 109–118.

Lindsay, J. R., Sanders, S. H., and Nager, G. T. 1960. Histopathologic observations in so-called congenital fixation of the stapedial footplate. Laryngoscope 70:1587.

Lindsay, J. R., Black, F. O., and Donnelly, W. H. 1975. Acrocephalo-syndactyly (Apert's syndrome). Temporal bone findings. Ann. Otol. Rhinol. Laryngol. 84:174.

Lindsay, J. R., and Hinojosa, R. 1978. Ear anomalies associated with renal dysplasia and immunodeficiency disease. Ann. Otol. Rhinol. Laryngol. 87:10.

Lindsay, J. R., and Suga, F. 1976. Paget's disease and sensorineural deafness. Temporal bone histopathology of Paget's disease. Laryngoscope 86:1029.

Livingstone, G., and Delahunty, J. E. 1968. Malformation of the ear associated with congenital ophthalmic and other conditions. J. Laryngol. Otol. 82:495.

Lowenstein, H. 1966. Long-term observations on ear and nose prostheses. Br. J. Plast. Surg. 19:385.

Maran, A. G. D. 1965. Persistent stapedial artery. J. Laryngol. Otol. 79:971.

Marion, M., Hinojosa, R., and Khan, A. A. 1985. Persistence of the stapedial artery: A histopathologic study. Otolaryngol. Head Neck Surg. 93:298.

McDonough, S. R. 1970. Fanconi anemia syndrome. Arch. Otolaryngol. 92:284.

McGrew, R. N., and Gregg, J. B. 1971. Anomalous fusion of the malleus to the tympanic ring. Ann. Otol. Rhinol. Laryngol. 80:138.

McLay, K., and Maran, A. G. D. 1969. Deafness and the Klippel-Feil syndrome. J. Laryngol. Otol. 83:175.

Melnick, M., Bixler, D., Sil, K., et al. 1975. Autosomal dominant branchio-oto-renal dysplasia. Birth Defects 11(5):121.

Mengel, M. C., Konigsmark, B. W., Berlin, C. I., et al. 1969. Conductive hearing loss and malformed low-set ears, as a possible recessive syndrome. J. Med. Genet. 6:14.

Morgenstein, K. M., and Manace, E. D. 1969. Temporal bone histopathology in sickle cell disease. Laryngoscope 79:2172.

Mustarde, J. C. 1963. The correction of prominent ears using simple mattress sutures. Br. J. Plast. Surg. 16:170.

Myers, E. N., and Stool, S. E. 1969. The temporal bone in osteopetrosis. Arch. Otolaryngol. 89:460.

Northern, J. L., and Downs, M. P. 1978. Hearing in Children. Baltimore, Williams & Wilkins Co., pp. 204–211.

Ohtani, I., and Schuknecht, H. F. 1984. Temporal bone pathology in DiGeorge's syndrome. Ann. Otol. Rhinol. Laryngol. 93:220.

Opheim, O. 1968. Loss of hearing following the syndrome of van der Hoeve–De Kleyn. Acta Otolaryngol. (Stockh.) 65:337.

Paradise, J. L. 1975. Middle ear problems associated with cleft palate. Cleft Palate J. 12:17.

Pfaffenbach, D. D., Cross, H. E., and Kearns, P. K. 1972. Congenital anomalies in Duane's retraction syndrome. Arch. Ophthalmol. 88:635.

Phelps, P. D., Lloy, G. A. S., and Poswillo, D. E. 1983. The ear deformities in craniofacial microsomia and oculo-auriculo-vertebral dysplasia. J. Laryngol. Otol. 97:995.

Pollock, W. J. 1969. Technique for correction of cryptotia. Plast. Reconstr. Surg. 44:501.

Pou, J. W. 1963. Congenital absence of the oval window. Laryngoscope 73:384.

Richards, S. H., and Gibbin, K. P. 1977. Recurrent meningitis due to congenital fistula of stapedial footplate. J. Laryngol. Otol. 91:1063.

Rimoin, D. L., and Edgerton, M. T. 1967. Genetic and clinical heterogeneity in the oral-facial-digital syndrome. J. Pediatr. 71:94.

Ritter, F. N. 1971. The histopathology of the congenital fixed malleus syndrome. Laryngoscope 81:1304.

Rosen, S. 1952. Glomus jugulare tumor of middle ear with normal drum: Improved biopsy technique. Ann. Otol. Rhinol. Laryngol. 61:448.

Ruben, R. J., Toriyama, M., Dische, M. R., et al. 1969. External and middle ear malformations associated with mandibulo-facial dysostosis and renal abnormalities: A case report. Ann. Otol. Rhinol. Laryngol. 78:605.

Ruedi, I. 1954. The surgical treatment of atresia auris congenita: A clinical and histological report. Laryngoscope 64:666.

Ruggles, R. L., and Reed, R. C. 1972. Symposium on ear surgery. V. Treatment of aberrant carotid arteries in the middle ear: A report of two cases. Laryngoscope 82:1199.

Saito, H., Kishimoto, S., and Furuta, M. 1981. Temporal bone findings in a patient with Möbius syndrome. Ann. Otol. Rhinol. Laryngol. 90:80.

Saito, R., Takata, N., Matumoto, N., et al. 1982. Anomalies of the auditory organ in Potter's syndrome. Arch. Otolaryngol. 108:484.

Sakai, N., Igarashi, M., and Miller, R. H. 1986. Temporal bone findings in VATER syndrome. Arch. Otolaryngol. Head Neck Surg. 112:416.

Sando, I., Bergstrom, L., Wood, R. P., II, et al. 1970. Temporal bone findings in trisomy 18 syndrome. Arch. Otolaryngol. 91:552.

Sando, I., Hemenway, W. G., and Morgan, W. R. 1968. Histopathology of the temporal bones in mandibulofacial dysostosis. (Treacher Collins syndrome). Trans. Am. Acad. Ophthalmol. Otol. 72:913.

Sando, I., and Ikeda, M. 1986. Temporal bone histopathological findings in oculo-auriculo-vertebral dysplasia (Goldenhar syndrome). Ann. Otol. Rhinol. Laryngol. 95:396.

Sando, I., Leiberman, A., Bergstrom, L., et al. 1975. Temporal bone histopathological findings in trisomy 13 syndrome. Ann. Otol. Rhinol. Laryngol. 84, Suppl. 21.

Schuknecht, H. F. 1967. Pathology of sensorineural deafness of genetic origin. *In* McConnell, F., and Ward, P. H. (eds.): Deafness in Childhood. Nashville, Vanderbilt University Press, pp. 69–90.

Schuknecht, H. F. 1974. Pathology of the Ear. Cambridge, MA, Harvard University Press.

Sellars, S. L., and Beighton, P. H. 1978. Deafness in osteodysplasty of Melinick and Needles. Arch. Otolaryngol. 104:225.

Shambaugh, G. E., Jr. 1967. Surgery of the Ear. Philadelphia, W. B. Saunders Co., p. 525.

Shambaugh, G. E., and Causse, J. 1974. Ten years experience with fluoride in otosclerotic (otospongiotic) patients. Ann. Otol. Rhinol. Laryngol. 83:635.

Shi, S. R. 1985. Temporal bone findings in a case of otopalatodigital syndrome. Arch. Otolaryngol. 111:119.

Silcox, L. 1967. The ear. *In* Rubin, A. (ed.): Handbook of Congenital Malformation. Philadelphia, W. B. Saunders Co., pp. 229–247.

Stallings, J. O., and McCabe, B. F. 1969. Congenital middle ear aneurysm of internal carotid. Arch. Otolaryngol. 90:39.

Steffen, T. N. 1968. Vascular anomalies of the middle ear. Laryngoscope 78:171.

Stratton, H. J. M. 1965. Gonadal dysgenesis and the ears. J. Laryngol. Otol. 79:343.

Szpunar, J., and Rybak, M. 1968. Middle ear disease in Turner's syndrome. Arch. Otolaryngol. 87:34.

Tabor, J. R. 1961. Absence of the oval window. Arch. Otolaryngol. 74:515.

Tabor, J. R. 1971. Methods of Ossiculoplasty. Springfield, IL, Charles C Thomas Co.

Tachibana, M., Hoshino, A., Oshima, W., et al. 1984. Duane's syndrome associated with crocodile tear and ear malformation. Arch. Otolaryngol. 110:761.

Van der Borden, J. 1967. Bilateral non-chromaffin tympano-jugular paraganglioma. J. Laryngol. Otol. 81:445.

Vase, P., Prytz, S., and Pedersen, P. S. 1975. Congenital stapes fixation, symphalangism and syndactylia. Acta Otolaryngol. (Stockh.). 80:394.

Warkany, J. 1971. Congenital Malformations: Notes and Comments. Chicago, Year Book Medical Pub., pp. 401–416.

Wells, M. D., Phelps, P. D., and Michaels, L. 1983. Oculo-auriculo-vertebral dysplasia. A temporal bone study of a case of Goldenhar's syndrome. J. Laryngol. Otol. 97:689.

Willis, R. 1977. Conductive deafness due to malplacement of 7th nerve. J. Otolaryngol. 6:1.

Winter, J. S. D., Kohn, G., Mellman, W. J., et al. 1968. A familial syndrome of renal, genital and middle ear anomalies. J. Pediatr. 72:88.

Winther, L. K., and Elbrønd, O. Congenital anomaly of the facial nerve. J. Laryngol. Otol. 91:349.

Wright, J. L. W., and Etholm, B. 1973. Anomalies of the middle ear muscles. J. Laryngol. Otol. 87:281.

Zonis, R. D. 1969. Meckel's cartilage remnant. Laryngoscope. 79:2012.

Chapter 19

PERILYMPHATIC FISTULAS IN INFANTS AND CHILDREN

James S. Reilly, M.D.   George A. Modreck, M.A., C.C.C.-A

Linda Bond, M.S.

There are many well-known causes of sensorineural hearing loss in infants and young children, and these can be divided, arbitrarily in some cases, into either congenital or acquired conditions. These specific syndromes and diseases are described more completely in other chapters in this book.

What is most important to remember, however, is that many factors potentially have an effect on hearing and that, even when the best clinical investigations are undertaken, the source of sensorineural hearing loss in infants and children remains unknown in about 50 per cent of cases (Fraser, 1976). Careful scrutiny must therefore be given to patterns of clinical symptoms or signs that may further unravel the unsolved mysteries of hearing loss in infants and children (Fig. 19–1).

Congenital perilymphatic fistulas (PLFs) are abnormal spontaneous leaks of perilymph (cerebrospinal fluid) into the middle ear or mastoid air cell system caused by a congenital weakness or defect in the temporal bone (Nenzelius, 1951). The PLF leaks may be observable or occult and can be persistent or intermittent. Acquired PLF can also occur; generally is a direct result of trauma to any area of the temporal bone, especially the middle ear; and should be included in the differential diagnosis when there is a history suggestive of trauma (e.g., head trauma or middle ear surgery).

The physician will develop better understanding of these occult congenital PLFs with a brief historical review of the patterns of associated symptoms.

Detectable PLF

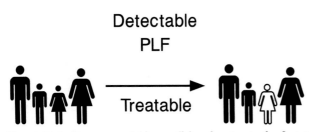

Treatable

Figure 19–1. How many children will lose hearing in the first 6 years of life is unknown.

HISTORICAL PERSPECTIVE

The evolution of knowledge of congenital PLF and of associated cerebrospinal fluid (CSF) leaks, meningitis, temporal bone defects, and deafness began over 90 years ago with the earliest description of a young girl with a spontaneous CSF otorrhea (Escat, 1897). Fifteen years later, a distinct association was first reported among gross CSF otorrhea, temporal bone abnormalities, severe meningitis, and death in a second case involving a young child. Post-mortem examination of the child's temporal bone revealed a large communication between the middle ear and the brain through a defect of the petrous apex of the mastoid (Canfield, 1913).

The existence of spontaneous, occult CSF leaks within the middle ear was not recognized for almost 40 years until a middle ear exploration was undertaken to determine the cause of recurrent meningitis in a young deaf girl. The middle ear was grossly abnormal, with a malformed cochlea and semicircular canals. This child was the first to survive this condition because a craniotomy was performed and the temporal bone defect sealed (Nenzelius, 1951). As this association of deafness, occult CSF leaks, and recurrent meningitis became more widely recognized, prompt middle ear explorations were undertaken to successfully repair and correct this condition (Barr, 1965).

Spontaneous decreases in hearing, without meningitis, was the next recognized mechanism of occult PLF and resulted in a progressive sensorineural hearing loss in both adults (Simmons, 1968) and children (Goodhill, 1973). Could these "leaks" be occurring every day in normal children with unexplained progressive sensorineural hearing loss? Is recurrent meningitis or gross CSF otorrhea still required to make the diagnosis?

During a period of 18 months, five children with fluctuating, progressive sensorineural hearing loss were confirmed by middle ear surgery to have PLF as a sole explanation (Grundfast and Bluestone, 1978). These investigators both challenged the rarity of this condition and postulated congenital PLF as a not uncommon minor defect in temporal bone structure.

305

The spectrum of temporal bone abnormalities that is associated with congenital PLF is quite varied. Previous generations of physicians relied solely on temporal bone specimens to define the leaks from the CSF pathway. Malformations of the round window together with a large cyst of the cochlear aqueduct have been noted (Bauer, 1962). More commonly, there was deficient ossification of the footplate of the stapes and a congenital PLF was observed. Because this footplate area is exclusively dependent on the otic capsule for mineralization, isolated defects in this area can occur (Rice and Waggoner, 1967).

Prompt radiologic examination of the temporal bone has permitted clues to hidden temporal bone defects. Basal cysternography demonstrated that radiopaque contrast material was able to pass from the internal auditory canal through the vestibule and into the middle ear preoperatively in a child with congenital PLF (Stool et al., 1967). Polytomographic examination of the temporal bone first demonstrated dysgenesis of the labyrinth and a Mondini-type deformity in cases of otitic meningitis (Biggers et al., 1973). The importance of radiographic demonstration of abnormal anatomy of the temporal bone as an important marker for congenital PLF of children has been emphasized in several large studies (Supance and Bluestone, 1982; Pappas, 1988). Fluid (presumed CSF) was noted by computed tomography (CT) scan in one child with unilateral, documented PLF (Zalzal et al., 1986).

However, unexplained fluctuations of hearing, particularly with documented progression of sensorineural hearing loss, should never be ignored and merit exploratory tympanotomy to rule out congenital PLF, even in the presence of normal temporal bone anatomy. A prospective study of 244 children with documented sensorineural hearing loss identified 15 children (6 per cent) with congenital PLF (Fig. 19–2). Seventy-five per cent of the children had deterioration of hearing as the primary symptom (Reilly, 1989). Congenital PLF must be included in the differential diagnosis of unexplained sensorineural hearing loss in children (Fig. 19–3).

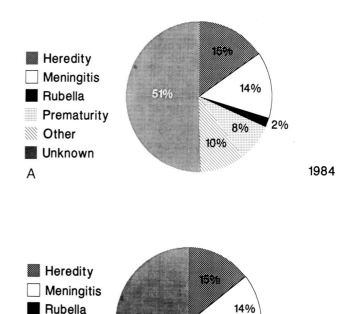

Figure 19–3. Distribution of causes of sensorineural hearing loss (SNHL). (Modified from Schildroth, A. 1986. Hearing impaired children under age 6. Am. Ann. Deaf 131[2]:85–90.)

EVALUATION

Infants and children who are suspected of having unexplained progression of hearing loss should be evaluated thoroughly. A complete birth and developmental history must be taken. Questions must be directed toward any history of viral or bacterial infections, birth or head trauma, exposure to teratogens, ototoxic drugs, or a history of prematurity. A comprehensive questionnaire is regularly used by the authors.

Physical examination is also extremely important. Any craniofacial anomalies must be noted and are compared with known syndromes that have associated sensorineural hearing loss (e.g., Waardenburg or Treacher Collins syndromes). Otitis media, eustachian tube dysfunction, or both may be present and must be treated and eliminated as a cause of any recent hearing change.

Complete audiologic evaluation includes conventional audiologic testing via both sound field and headphone. In very young infants, or poorly cooperative children, serial auditory brain stem evoked response (ABR) may be necessary to confirm deterioration in hearing. All previous audiologic test results should be obtained and thoroughly reviewed for documentation. Significant deterioration of hearing (greater than 20 dB in speech reception thresholds) is frequently seen to affect primarily one ear in children with PLF.

The young child should also have examination by a

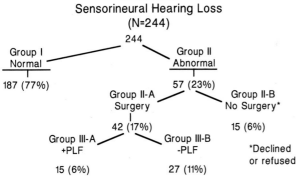

Figure 19–2. Distributions of children evaluated for unexplained sensorineural hearing loss, demonstrating 15 children (6 per cent) with perilymphatic fistula. (Modified from Reilly, J. S. 1989. Congenital perilymphatic fistula, a prospective study in infants and children. Laryngoscope 99:393–397.)

speech therapist. The level of language skills can be compared with that of normally hearing children. Good language acquisition suggests that hearing was preserved during the first couple of years of life and that any deterioration of hearing may be of recent onset. This is helpful, as audiograms may not be available.

Imaging of the temporal bone is the next critical step. CT scanning is the most useful technique at present. A thorough study, using thin (1.5 mm) sections obtained through both axial and coronal planes, is important. Bony detail is enhanced by proper windowing programs (Fig. 19–4).

The images must be carefully and critically evaluated by a skilled radiologist familiar with temporal bone anatomy. Malformations of the cochlea may be visualized and will include loss of partitioning between interscalar septa (Mondini deformity); development of a common cavity or complete aplasia (Michel deformity) can be seen in extreme cases. The vestibule may be enlarged, and the horizontal semicircular canal may be foreshortened and rudimentary. The internal auditory canal and vestibular aqueduct may be dilated and asymmetric (Chap. 9).

A review of a large series of children who had documented sensorineural hearing loss and evaluation of the temporal bone by conventional polytomes or CT scan illustrated a spectrum of malformations of the cochlea and semicircular canals (Jackler et al., 1987). Interestingly, the authors were able to correlate the state of the labyrinth with the week of arrested embryogenesis of the temporal bone. Severe abnormalities occur during the fourth week and more subtle changes occur at the seventh week (Jackler et al., 1987) (Fig. 19–5).

Vestibular function evaluation for vertigo or dysequilibrium has been useful in a small number of cases. Generally, this has been only when a degenerative neurologic abnormality is the cause of the instability. The classic fistula test employs a sweep of -400 mm H_2O to $+400$ mm H_2O pressure in the ear canal, and

monitoring for eye movements with electrodes has not been useful. This fistula test did not detect a congenital PLF in any of 15 affected children (Reilly, 1989).

After all testing has been completed, the information should be thoroughly reviewed by physicians, audiologists, and other caretakers. The results should be explained to the family, who are often extremely anxious and hopeful. Careful follow-up and monitoring of speech and hearing are important. Many children must be screened, and PLF occur in only about 1 of 20 of children with sensorineural hearing loss.

CLINICAL PRESENTATION

It has been suggested that two different syndromes of congenital PLF may be discernible (Petroff et al., 1986). The first involves young infants with bilateral congenital PLF whose hearing deteriorates in the first 2 to 3 years of life and has frequently been misdiagnosed and labeled congenital or hereditary. Only auditory brain stem evoked response, performed promptly at a young age, can document the presence of useful hearing. The second, and more common, occurs in children with unilateral hearing loss who experience deterioration of hearing in the good ear over months or years (Petroff et al., 1986). The authors agree with these findings.

The second type of syndrome is easier for the physician to diagnose and appears to occur more frequently. When a congenital PLF is identified, the contralateral ear appears to be at risk in about half (Reilly, 1989) to less than one third (Pappas, 1987; Seltzer and McCabe, 1986) of the children. Unless the hearing is normal in the unexplored ear, surgery should be considered to rule out a second PLF in the contralateral ear.

The degree of hearing loss experienced by the child with congenital PLF can vary from mild to severe (22 to 14 per cent loss). The hearing loss was asymmetric in about half of the children. No specific pattern of hearing impairment was regularly seen. However, a predominant low-frequency loss was occasionally observed in children with better hearing. Numerous children have been reported with serial decreases in hearing over periods of months to years prior to surgical identification and repair (Weider and Musiek, 1984; Petroff et al., 1986).

Vertigo and tinnitus are two symptoms that are more commonly elicited from adults with PLF but are only rarely noted in children. Of 244 children evaluated, 27 children (11 per cent) exhibited vertigo (Reilly, 1989). Over one half of these children (15 of 27) had vertigo as the sole complaint. Only two children with persistent vertigo had middle ear exploration, and congenital PLF was not identified. Other series of children have noted PLF to be present with vertigo and to improve following repair (Seltzer and McCabe, 1986; Parrell and Burke, 1986). In both these studies, the patients had history of trauma as the probable

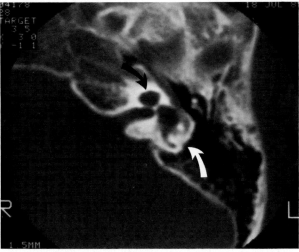

Figure 19–4. CT scan in axial plane demonstrating Mondini dysplasia. Black arrow shows dilated cochlea; white arrow, the enlarged vestibule.

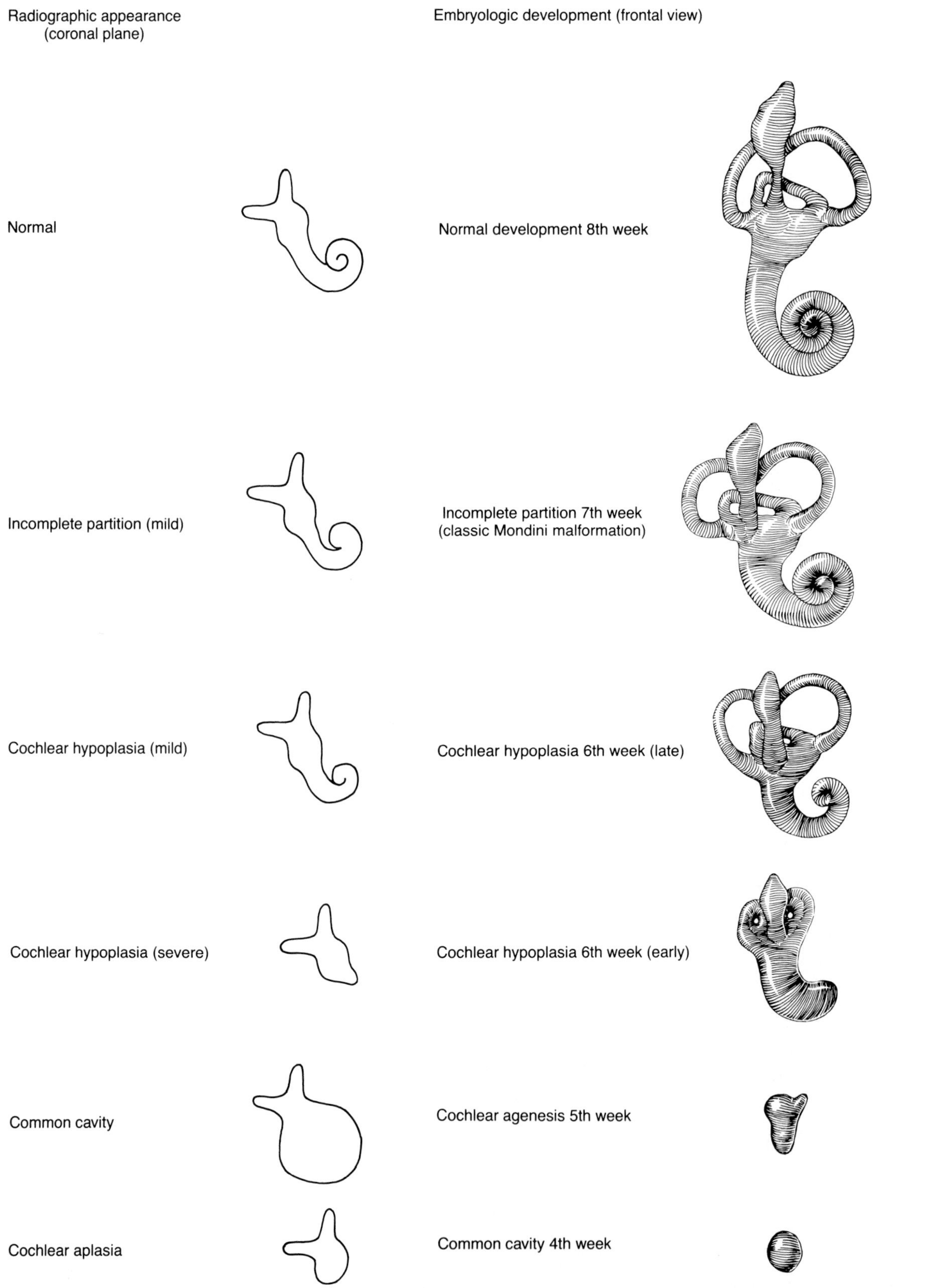

Radiographic appearance
(coronal plane)

Embryologic development (frontal view)

Normal

Normal development 8th week

Incomplete partition (mild)

Incomplete partition 7th week
(classic Mondini malformation)

Cochlear hypoplasia (mild)

Cochlear hypoplasia 6th week (late)

Cochlear hypoplasia (severe)

Cochlear hypoplasia 6th week (early)

Common cavity

Cochlear agenesis 5th week

Cochlear aplasia

Common cavity 4th week

Figure 19–5. Correlation of arrested inner ear development and radiographic abnormalities. (Adapted from Jackler, R. K., Luxford, W. M., and House, W. F. 1987. Congenital malformations of the inner ear: A classification based on embryogenesis. Laryngoscope 97:2.)

TABLE 19–1. Audiologic Follow-up of Children with Sensorineural Hearing Loss

	PRESENCE OF PLF						ABSENCE OF PLF					
	Better		Same		Worse		Number of Patients	Better		Same		Worse		Number of Patients
Supance and Bluestone, 1982	1	(5%)	19	(86%)	2	(9%)	22	1	(6%)	11	(73%)	2	(13%)	14
Pappas et al., 1988	1	(25%)	1	(25%)	2	(50%)	4	2	(6%)	20	(62%)	10	(31%)	32
Reilly, 1989†	5	(23%)	13	(59%)	3	(14%)	22	2	(6%)	24	(75%)	5	(16%)	32
Totals	7	(15%)	33	(69%)	7	(15%)	48	5	(6%)	55	(71%)	17	(22%)	78

*Eight ears with no follow-up.
†Two ears with no follow-up.

cause (Seltzer, 1986), but it is more common in adults (Parell, 1986).

TREATMENT

The treatment of persistent PLFs that are clinically suspected and associated with any symptoms (e.g., hearing loss, recurrent meningitis, vertigo, tinnitus, and fullness of the ear) is surgical control of the fistula. Most PLFs are controlled satisfactorily through a middle ear exploration and packing of the fistula site. Material used for packing includes fat and perichondrium (Glasscock et al., 1987), although others prefer temporalis muscle (Reilly, 1989) or subcutaneous aureole tissue (Seltzer and McCabe, 1986). The most common site of PLF is the oval window alone, followed by the round window and both windows in about equal percentage of cases.

When the PLF results in copious and persistent CSF leaks despite middle ear packing, a stapedectomy and prosthesis and tissue graft can be used. If there is no serviceable hearing, the vestibule may have to be packed completely to seal the leak. When these methods are not successful, the exploratory craniotomy is necessary.

Although rare, additional sites of temporal bone PLF have been reported. These include petrosquamous suture, the epitympanic space, Hyrtl fissure, and the mastoid antrum. In most series of children, however, PLFs have almost always been explored through the middle ear exclusively when associated with fluctuating hearing loss.

HEARING OUTCOME

There is widespread agreement among otologists that PLF must be identified and repaired. In the most severe cases, recurrent meningitis is controlled or eliminated. Unexplained or persistent vertigo seems to be improved also when the proper tissue repair of a PLF is achieved.

Perhaps the most important outcome for children is stabilization and improvement of hearing. Sudden or progressive sensorineural hearing loss is a frightening symptom that brings children to medical attention. Isolated case reports have documented dramatic improvements in hearing in some cases. However, this

is generally not the result. Only three studies of PLF in children have provided audiologic follow-up (Table 19–1). Although the numbers are small, they suggest that hearing is improved in about 15 per cent of children. Deterioration of hearing occurs less frequently in children with PLF (15 per cent) compared with non-PLF children (22 per cent). About 70 per cent of children have their hearing remain unchanged. One series reported approximately 48 per cent improvement of hearing (Seltzer and McCabe, 1986). This dramatic result has not been observed in other studies.

Most investigators agree that the sooner that the PLF is identified and repaired, the better the chance of hearing improvement is (Seltzer and McCabe, 1986). Each series varies in methodology, but the average age of detection of PLF in the author's patients was 6 years of age.

There may well be multiple other abnormalities of the cochlea in addition to window defects that may seriously impair hearing and prevent recovery. A study of 100 temporal bones of children with congenital anomalies showed numerous abnormalities of temporal bone structures in children that had not been previously recognized (Sando et al., 1988). Cochlear anomalies were present in 44 per cent, with 16 different types of deformities noted. Vestibular abnormalities were even more common. The vestibule was generally enlarged (in 18 per cent), and the lateral semicircular canal was absent or foreshortened.

SUMMARY

Congenital PLFs are abnormalities of the temporal bone that occur in about 6 per cent of children with unexplained, asymmetric sensorineural hearing loss. These leaks can be associated with fluctuating or deteriorating hearing, vertigo, fullness of the ear, tinnitus, and even recurrent meningitis in severe cases. Repair of the fistula is essential and generally is accomplished by an exploratory tympanotomy. Hearing improvement can occur but should be expected in only about 15 per cent of cases.

SELECTED REFERENCES

Althaus, S. 1981. Perilymph fistulas. Laryngoscope 91:538.
This author gives the most complete and detailed survey of

perilymphatic fistulas and includes both congenital and acquired for us. It is important to read this for proper understanding of this complex condition.

Grundfast, K. M., and Bluestone, C. D. 1978. Sudden or fluctuating hearing loss and vertigo in children due to perilymph fistula. Ann. Otol. Rhinol. Laryngol. 87:761.

This is the first series to look critically at a small group of children with both acquired and congenital PLF. Detailed case histories are presented.

REFERENCES

Barr, B., and Wersall, J. 1965. Cerebrospinal otorrhea with meningitis in congenital deafness. Arch. Otolaryngol. 81:26.

Bauer, E. 1962. Spontane oto-lequorrhoe auf grundeiner kongenitalen missbildung des aquaeductus cochleae. Laryngol. Rhinol. Otol. 41:704.

Biggers, W. P., Howell, N. N., Fischer, N. D., et al. 1973. Congenital ear anomalies associated with otic meningitis. Arch. Otolaryngol. 97:399.

Canfield, R. B. 1913. Some conditions associated with the loss of cerebrospinal fluid. Ann. Oto. Rhinol. Laryngol. 22:604.

Escat, E. 1897. Ecoulement spontane de liquide cephalorachidien parle conduit auditif externe; fistule congenitale probable. Arch. Int. Laryngol. 10:653.

Fraser, G. R. 1976. The Causes of Profound Deafness in Childhood. Baltimore, Johns Hopkins University Press, pp. 20–30.

Glasscock, M. E., McKennan, K. X., and Levine, C. C. 1987. Persistent traumatic perilymph fistulas. Laryngoscope 97:860.

Goodhill, V., Harris, I., Brockman, S. J., et al. 1973. Sudden deafness and labyrinthine window ruptures. Audiovestibular observations. Ann. Otol. Rhinol. Laryngol. 82:2.

Grundfast, K. M., and Bluestone, C. D. 1978. Sudden or fluctuating hearing loss and vertigo in children due to perilymph fistula. Ann. Otol. Rhinol. Laryngol. 87:761.

Jackler, R. K., Luxford, W. M., and House, W. F. 1987. Congenital malformations of the inner ear: A classification based on embryogenesis. Laryngoscope 97(Suppl. 40):2.

Nenzelius, C. 1951. On spontaneous cerebrospinal otorrhea due to congenital malformations. Acta Otolaryngol. 39:314.

Pappas, D. G., Simpson, L. C., and Godwin, G. H. 1988. Perilymphatic fistula in children with pre-existing sensorineural hearing loss. Laryngoscope 98:507.

Parell, G. J., and Berke, G. D. 1986. Results of repair of inapparent perilymph fistula. Otolaryngol. Head Neck Surg. 95:344.

Petroff, M. A., Simmons, F. B., and Winzelbert, J. 1986. Two emerging perilymph fistula syndromes in children. Laryngoscope 96:498.

Reilly, J. S. 1989. Congenital perilymphatic fistula, a prospective study in infants and children. Laryngoscope 99:393.

Rice, W. J., and Waggoner, L. G. 1967. Congenital cerebrospinal fluid otorrhea via a defect in the stapes footplate. Laryngoscope 77:341.

Sando, I., Shigahara, Y., Takagi, A., et al. 1988. Frequency and localization of congenital anomalies of the middle ear and inner ears: A human temporal bone study. Int. J. Pediatr. Otorhinolaryngol. 16:1.

Seltzer, S., and McCabe, B. 1986. Perilymph fistula: The Iowa experience. Laryngoscope 94:37.

Simmons, F. B. 1968. Theory of membrane breaks in sudden hearing loss. Arch. Otolaryngol. 88:41.

Stool, S. E., Leeds, N. E., and Shulman, K. 1967. The syndrome of congenital deafness and otitis meningitis: Diagnosis and management. J. Pediatr. 71:547.

Supance, J. S., and Bluestone, C. D. 1982. Perilymph fistulas in infants and children. Otolaryngol. Head Neck Surg. 91:663.

Weider, D. J., and Musiek, F. E. 1984. Bilateral congenital oval window microfistulae with mother and son. Laryngoscope 94:1455.

Zalzal, G. H., Shott, S. R., Towbin, R., and Cotton, R. T. 1986. Value of CT scan in the diagnosis of temporal bone diseases in children. Laryngoscope 96:27.

Chapter 20

DISEASES OF THE EXTERNAL EAR

LaVonne Bergstrom, M.D.

ANATOMY AND PHYSIOLOGY

Certain features of form and function are important to an understanding of diseases of the external ear.

The external ear is composed of a flexible, potentially mobile auricle and attached external auditory canal formed of fibrous tissue and elastic cartilage. These elements are in continuity with the osseous external canal, which medially ends in a tympanic ring incomplete superiorly. It contains the annular, or tympanic, sulcus into which the tympanic membrane inserts. The mobile, lateral one third of the canal inserts by fibrous bands on the external surface of the osseous canal. The cartilaginous canal contains slitlike fissures of Santorini, which communicate with the parotid gland. An inconstant hiatus may occur in the floor of the osseous canal (Anson and Donaldson, 1967; Hollinshead, 1968). Over this skeletal framework the skin is applied tightly, especially over the lateral surface of the pinna, where the skin is immobile. It is thin over the pinna where blood vessels are superficial, and it is unprotected by a layer of fat except for small amounts on the mastoid surface where the skin is slightly mobile. The skin becomes thicker over the meatus and cartilaginous canal, where there are coarse hairs in the auditory meatus and, just within the meatus, modified sweat, or cerumen, glands. Medially, the skin becomes very thin and inseparable from the periosteum over the osseous canal, and it contains no skin adnexae. Finally its squamous layer continues on over the lateral tympanic membrane surface (Hollinshead, 1968).

In later childhood and in adult life, the osseous canal constitutes about two thirds of the depth of the canal. However, in infancy, the bony canal consists only of the tympanic ring and hence is very shallow. Furthermore, the ring, into which the tympanic membrane inserts, is nearly horizontal when the infant is held erect so that the membrane is nearly horizontal (Hollinshead, 1968). Its superior portion is quite close to the external meatus; thus, an ear speculum that is too small may touch or nearly touch this important area of the drumhead, exposing it to possible damage.

The vascular supply to the external ear is ample, coming from the posterior auricular, superficial temporal, and deep auricular branches of the external carotid circulation (Hollinshead, 1968). The terminal arterioles of these vessels supply skin, subcutaneous tissue, and perichondrium, but cartilage itself is avascular, extracellular fluid being replaced by solid cartilaginous matrix (Ham, 1957).

The venous drainage is via the superficial temporal, the posterior auricular, and the mastoid emissary veins to the external and internal jugular veins and sigmoid sinus. Lymphatic channels go to the preauricular parotid nodes, superficial cervical nodes along the external jugular vein, and postauricular nodes (Hollinshead, 1968).

The normal external canal is longer anteriorly to inferiorly in both infant and adult to accommodate to the obliquely inward slant of the drum membrane. The anterior osseous canal bulges, sometimes prominently, and thus serves somewhat to obscure the view of the anterior drum margin and adjacent external canal sulcus.

Cerumen varies both qualitatively and quantitatively. Most whites have wet, sticky, brown cerumen, which is considered to be a dominant genetic trait, whereas most Mongoloid races, including the American Indian, have dry, brittle, light-gray, "rice-bran" cerumen. Wet cerumen contains one third as much protein as the dry type but three times as much lipid. Dry cerumen occurs frequently in individuals who have Down syndrome, or "mongolism." Preliminary work suggests that dry cerumen is higher in lysozyme than wet cerumen and that there may be differences in immunoglobulin content, but this has been contested (Matsunaga, 1962; Hyslop, 1971; Petrakis et al., 1971). Studies using the scanning electron microscope suggest that the mode of cerumen secretion is both apocrine and eccrine (Main and Lim, 1976).

The squamous epithelium of the tympanic membrane and external canal skin desquamates keratin, but in the normal ear the epithelium migrates centrifugally so that keratin debris is mobilized out of the ear canal together with cerumen (Litton, 1963).

The normal flora of the external canal consists of *Staphylococcus epidermidis*, *Corynebacterium* species ("diphtheroids"), *Micrococcus* species, and occasionally *Staphylococcus aureus* and *Streptococcus viridans*. The contributory factors that may initiate the process that renders the skin of the canal vulnerable to infection are excessive wetness (swimming, bathing, or increased environmental humidity), excessive dryness (previous infection, dermatoses, or insufficient cerumen), and trauma (digital or foreign body). Once the preinflammatory stage has been set, endogenous bacteria assume pathogenic characteristics, or virulent exogenous bacteria may propagate in the canal (Chap. 21).

CERUMEN IMPACTION

In some individuals, spontaneous cerumen removal does not occur. Ultimately, physical discomfort and conductive hearing loss bring the person to the doctor. Chandler studied obstruction of the human ear canal experimentally and established that the perception of high-frequency sound is affected first, and even after lower frequencies are involved the loss is greater in higher frequencies (Chandler, 1964). Predisposing factors in cerumen impaction may include small or collapsing ear canals, unusual properties of the cerumen itself, increased production of cerumen, or a combination of these factors (Peterkin, 1974). However, in most patients, cerumen impaction results from ill-advised attempts at removal by the patient or from nervous digital ear canal manipulation, which shoves the bolus of cerumen deeper into the osseous canal. Children may introduce foreign bodies into the ear canal, thus pushing cerumen deeper.

Cerumen removal may be accomplished in a variety of ways. In preschool children in whom a small, firm plug partly obscures the view of the tympanic membrane, it may be removed quickly, deftly, and unobtrusively during the ear examination with head mirror and hand-held speculum, thus obviating some of the fears and objections that often occur if the ear loop or curet is displayed and an explanation is offered. However, if the ear canal is completely obstructed, a simple, step-by-step explanation is given and the child is positioned under the microscope for removal. In skilled hands, the otoscope or head mirror and hand-held speculum may be substituted for the microscope. For a somewhat apprehensive but inquisitive child, allowing him or her a preliminary opportunity to look through the microscope or otoscope at the examiner's hand or the parent's ear may then permit uneventful cerumen removal, which is accomplished using suction for soft cerumen and the curet, loop, or small cup forceps. The noise of the suction must be explained and demonstrated before introducing it into the ear canal because it is fairly loud and frightening there. Skilled help to steady the child's head is essential, as is the reassuring presence of the parent nearby where the child can see him or her.

Mechanical cerumen removal is preferred when the ear is symptomatic, as in cases of a documented hearing loss or when the ear is painful. Such removal should be accomplished, if at all possible, when the patient first presents. However, under circumstances in which the ear examination is for routine purposes and immediate removal proves difficult or in which the child

is incapable of cooperation, it is better to take a more leisurely course, which may involve using mineral oil or oily otic drops at home until the cerumen comes out spontaneously or can be removed easily. It may be possible to use body temperature irrigation to remove the cerumen, but it is this author's preference not to use this at the first examination of a patient, as instances have been known in which pain occurred owing to an unforeseen tympanic membrane perforation. In one instance, concurrent transient facial palsy occurred. A suitable irrigation solution is one containing lactated Ringer's solution mixed in equal parts of isopropyl alcohol, but a variety of other solutions are satisfactory, provided the ear is carefully dried afterward. Commercial detergents for removing cerumen may be quite irritating or may provoke an allergic response in the skin of the ear canal and probably should be used, if at all, only in adults. After cerumen removal, the canal should be inspected carefully for minor skin abrasions. If there has been any canal wall trauma, medicinal otic drops should be used for a few days (Chap. 8).

SPECIFIC INFLAMMATORY DISORDERS OF THE EXTERNAL EAR

External otitis may be divided into five types: (1) acute diffuse, (2) acute circumscribed, (3) chronic, (4) eczematous, and (5) malignant. In the pediatric age group, acute external otitis and eczematous otitis externa are the most commonly seen.

ACUTE OTITIS EXTERNA. Acute otitis externa may be divided into bacterial and fungal types. Bacterial otitis externa usually occurs as a result of getting and retaining water in the external ear canal, frequently when swimming and more frequently in hot, humid weather. At first, the ear itches, and the patient scratches, traumatizing the ear canal and introducing organisms into macerated skin. The superficial epithelium absorbs moisture and desquamates to expose a raw wet surface that is easily infected. The pH of the ear canal changes from a normal pH of 5 to 7 to alkaline. The ear canal fills with wet debris, itself a good culture medium. Pus exudes; edema of the ear canal and mild perichondritis of the ear canal may ensue, causing the ear to become quite painful when touched or manipulated or during chewing. Foul-smelling or sour-smelling exudate is noted by the patient or the parents. On physical examination, frank pus may be seen, and the canal may be very edematous or even closed, possibly making cleaning and culture difficult or impossible initially (Senturia, 1957, 1973). *Pseudomonas* species are found in one half to two thirds of instances. Other organisms seen include *Proteus* species, *Escherichia coli, Staphylococcus epidermidis, S. aureus,* streptococci, diphtheroids, *Enterobacter aerogenes, Klebsiella pneumoniae,* and *Citrobacter.* In patients younger than 21 years of age, the proportion of those with severe involvement is greater than in any other age group. There is a correlation between severity of external otitis and the organisms found: Gram-negative organisms tend to be found in severe infections, and gram-positive organisms are found in milder infections. Gram-negative organisms are found in 74 per cent of affected patients younger than 21 years of age as compared with 64 per cent in the older age group, and *Pseudomonas* species account for most of the positive bacterial cultures (Cassisi et al., 1977).

Probably the most important aspect of management of acute diffuse external otitis is thorough cleaning of the ear canal to remove all debris. This can be done with suction, gentle wiping with small, soft cotton pledgets, or irrigation with a solution at body temperature. Appropriate irrigants include 3 per cent saline, alcohol in a spray bottle attached to compressed air so that the canal can be dried, boro-alcohol solution, or a solution made up of alcohol and acetic acid, 3 to 5 per cent. If the ear canal is too swollen to permit cleaning, then a wick soaked in steroid-containing medication should be inserted gently into the canal. All these procedures are painful, and the usual local anesthetic block of the ear may not be successful because the pH change of infection does not allow the chemical reaction of local anesthetic agents in the tissues to occur. A field block around the pinna might be helpful, but often it is as efficacious to explain that the procedure will be uncomfortable briefly but will help make the ear feel better shortly. The ear should be cleaned and medicated daily. Drops containing neomycin or polymyxin and steroid in an acid vehicle can be administered as soon as the ear canal opens. Tampons or cotton pledgets medicated with cream containing similar compounds can be inserted into the ears of older children or adolescents, but this generally causes too much discomfort or apprehension in younger children. In children who wear hearing aids or who need pressure-equalizing tubes placed in the tympanic membrane, the need for prompt control and prevention is especially urgent. Prevention of otitis externa may involve abstaining from swimming or placing Domeboro or VōSol drops containing an acetic acid solution in the ear immediately after swimming (McLaurin, 1973; Senturia, 1973; Templer, 1976; Cassisi et al., 1977).

Other forms of acute diffuse otitis externa include erysipelas, which usually involves only the pinna; bullous myringitis, in which hemorrhagic bullae involve the canal and tympanic membrane skin; herpes simplex, which involves primarily the pinna and responds to 10 per cent carbamide peroxide in anhydrous solution; and herpes zoster oticus (Shambaugh, 1967; McLaurin, 1973; Templer, 1976).

Acute fungal otitis externa or otomycosis occurs in fewer than 10 per cent of patients in the United States (McLaurin, 1973) and may occur as part of generalized or regional fungal disorders. Otomycosis is said to occur most frequently in tropical climates and is usually due to *Aspergillus*, *Phycomycetes*, *Rhizopus*, *Actinomyces*, *Penicillium*, or yeasts. Hyphae may be seen in the ear canal as a dark or greenish-yellow mass (Beneke, 1970). *Aspergillus* causes about 90 per cent of

the fungal infections. Fungi may find a more favorable environment where tissues are rich in glucose, as in patients with uncontrolled diabetes. It is even possible that ordinarily saprophytic *Mucor* species of the *Phycomycetes* group, residing in the external ear, may infect the middle ear and mastoid of patients with diabetes (Bergstrom et al., 1970). Patients receiving immunosuppressive medications such as steroids or azathioprine, those who have been receiving long-term antibiotic therapy, or those who are immunodeficient may also be subject to fungal otitis externa. An interesting disorder is mucocutaneous candidiasis, found in immunodeficient children. The infecting organism is *Candida albicans*. The pinna, external canal, and even the middle ear may be infected (Fig. 20–1). Nails, skin, mouth, pharynx, larynx, trachea, bronchi, and esophagus may also be infected. Other fungal infections of adjacent skin and scalp may also involve the pinna and external canal, but this is extremely rare.

The causative organism can often be identified from

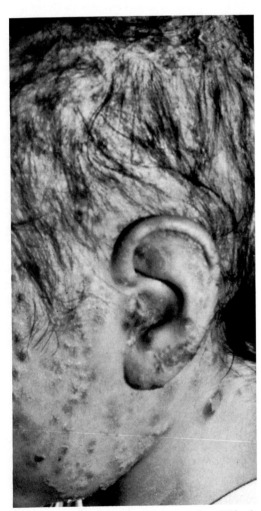

Figure 20–1. The affected scalp and pinna of a child who has chronic mucocutaneous candidiasis. The patient is immunodeficient, has similar lesions in the external auditory canal, and has otitis media as well. The last condition may be due to monilial nasopharyngitis that also involves the contiguous oropharynx, mouth, hypopharynx, and larynx.

scrapings or aspirated material on a 20 per cent potassium hydroxide preparation. At times, culture on Sabouraud's medium or even biopsy may be needed to establish the diagnosis (Beneke, 1970).

Treatment may consist of topical medications such as nystatin, amphotericin B, 1 per cent gentian violet, 1 per cent iodine, or 10 per cent resorcin; gentian violet and iodine may be unacceptable because of their staining properties (Beneke, 1970). Systemic agents such as griseofulvin or even amphotericin B may rarely be indicated. The usual measures of ear cleaning and aural hygiene are essential, and general improvement of health, control of diabetes, and discontinuing or lowering the doses of systemic antibiotics and immunosuppressants (when possible) should also be tried. If amphotericin B is used, the patient must be pretested for sensitivity and renal function must be monitored closely. If the fungus is deeply seated or if the patient requires, but cannot tolerate, amphotericin B, surgery may be indicated to remove diseased tissue (Bergstrom et al., 1970).

Actinomycosis and blastomycosis cause granulomatous lesions of the pinna that may need to be biopsied or drained but that respond to chemotherapy (McLaurin, 1973).

ACUTE CIRCUMSCRIBED EXTERNAL OTITIS. Acute circumscribed external otitis is synonymous with furuncle. These lesions, which are usually small, are pustules associated with a hair follicle, and the infecting organism is usually *Staphylococcus*. The pain is severe. Local heat and systemic antibiotics will usually lead to resolution of the problem, although incision and drainage may be necessary. Often an ointment-impregnated wick will provide some symptomatic relief and possibly protect the rest of the ear canal from infection. Frank cellulitis of the ear canal, usually due to streptococci or staphylococci, can be treated with penicillin or similar appropriate systemic antibiotics.

CHRONIC EXTERNAL OTITIS. Chronic external otitis seldom occurs in children, but when it does occur it may be quite stubborn. The author treated one young school-age patient who had cleft palate and a considerable conductive hearing loss resulting from persistent serous otitis media and nearly constant debris in the ear. Itching was a severe problem. After six months of frequent ear cleanings, a variety of topical and systemic medications, rigid adherence to aural hygiene and, fortunately, having a most cooperative patient and mother, the condition cleared and cultures, which had grown out *Pseudomonas*, cleared. The hearing loss was still significant, and middle-ear ventilating tubes were successfully placed. Frequent visits were essential to keep the ears clear of debris that seemed to cause considerable itching. The tubes remained patent, the middle ear was free of infection, and the tubes were still in place after more than a year had elapsed, without complications. Presumably in stubborn cases, surgery, such as the Proud procedure, might be required (Proud, 1967). It would also be important to rule out underlying systemic disease.

Other forms of chronic external otitis are granulo-

matous, such as tubercular (Sinha, 1969), luetic, and that due to yaws, leprosy, or sarcoidosis (McLaurin, 1973).

ECZEMATOUS OTITIS EXTERNA. Eczematous otitis externa may accompany typical atopic eczema, but it also occurs in association with seborrheic dermatitis, psoriasis, lupus erythematosus, neurodermatitis, sensitivities to topical medications, contact dermatitis, purulent otitis media, and infantile eczema. The pinna is often involved, and fissuring, weeping, and inflammation are seen in the various crevices and creases, particularly in the postauricular sulcus. Pruritus is extreme, and secondary infection is common. In the canal scaling, crusting, oozing, vesicles, and even hives may be seen. Nervous or emotionally disturbed children and adolescents greatly worsen the situation or even provoke it by unnecessary rubbing and scratching of the area. The specific cause is usually found by taking a history and by using the visual recognition so essential to dermatologic diagnosis. At times, biopsy or patch testing may be valuable. Oral antipruritics, antihistamines, analgesics, or tranquilizers are useful as general measures. Various topical agents, including solutions of aluminum acetate 8 per cent, lead subacetate 5 per cent and 5 per cent glycerin in water, acetic acid 2 per cent in aluminum acetate buffered to an acid pH, or Burrow's solution for acute oozing or weeping, are followed by steroid creams, lotions, or ointments as the acute phase abates. Occasionally, boric acid powder can be helpful. However, only topical preparations specifically suited for the ear canal should be used there. Eliminating from use around the ear common contact irritants such as spray colognes, hair sprays, certain shampoos, or soaps is essential but needs to be tailored to the particular patient. It may be necessary to keep gloves on the patient at night to lessen scratching and contamination with organisms found under the fingernails (McLaurin, 1973; Templer, 1976).

NECROTIZING "MALIGNANT" EXTERNAL OTITIS. "Malignant" external otitis is generally considered a disease of elderly, diabetic, or debilitated adults (Chandler, 1968, 1977). However, cases have been reported in children (Giguere and Rouillard, 1976). "Malignant" external otitis in children must be differentiated from a virulent otitis media, at times caused by *Pseudomonas* that has secondarily infected the external canal. Such a distinction can readily be made if the ear canal is carefully cleaned first (Chandler, 1977).

Malignant external otitis does not respond to measures generally successful for the usual varieties of external otitis. The usual infecting organism is *Pseudomonas*, which in this instance gains access to the deeper tissues of the ear canal and causes a localized vasculitis, thrombosis, and necrosis of the tissues. The bone and cartilage of the external ear canal, parotid gland, mastoid, facial nerve, regional lymph nodes, and skin are often involved by direct extension. Malignant external otitis can spread to the middle ear, sigmoid sinus, jugular bulb, cranial nerves in the jugular foramen, bone of the petrous pyramid, and adjacent base of the skull or to the meninges, brain, and brain stem substance. The external canal will often show granulation tissue at the junction of the osseous and cartilaginous canals, and the mastoid process may be red, tender, and swollen. Multiple cranial nerves may be involved, and the onset of symptoms may be delayed (Dinapoli and Thomas, 1971). Widespread central nervous system involvement and death may ensue. Permanent facial paralysis is frequent (Chandler, 1977). Bilateral malignant external otitis necessitating multiple hospital admissions and surgical explorations occurred in a 10-year-old girl; the course of the disease covered nearly one year and resulted in permanent diabetes insipidus and permanent unilateral facial palsy. She had apparently been healthy prior to the onset of the illness (Giguere and Rouillard, 1976).

Successful treatment requires hospitalization, supportive measures, work-up for underlying systemic disease, ear cleaning and debriding of devitalized tissue, topical and systemic treatment with gentamicin and carbenicillin intravenously for 4 to 6 weeks or longer, careful monitoring of renal function, and, in some instances, mastoidectomy, facial nerve decompression, removal of the infected clot from the affected dural sinuses, ligation of the internal jugular vein, removal of the jugular bulb, and removal of sequestra of osteomyelitic bone. The blood levels of antibiotics need to be followed closely; a sensitive organism will probably respond to a concentration of gentamicin of 1 μg per ml or less and of less than 32 μg per ml of carbenicillin, although sensitivity may need to be reassessed by tube dilution methods if the patient is not responding satisfactorily (Chandler, 1977). Vestibular and auditory baseline and follow-up testing should be done. Caloric tests using water are contraindicated in the presence of external otitis, but iced ear drops or air calorics might be substituted. Audiometric thresholds may need to be tested by bone conduction only or freefield testing, as pain, swelling, and drainage may preclude the use of earphones unless they are hand-held. The ear canal should have been cleaned just before audiometry to minimize the amount of conductive hearing loss. Vestibular function can to some degree be followed by having the patient stand with feet in a heel-to-toe position or by using posturography, where that is available; at present, it is still a research tool with limited availability.

The most difficult aspect of treatment is keeping the patient in the hospital for weeks of antibiotic treatment after ear pain and drainage have ceased. However, the recurrence rate after inadequate treatment is 100 per cent, and the mortality rate is significant.

OTHER INFLAMMATORY CONDITIONS OF THE EXTERNAL EAR

A potentially serious complication of external otitis, surgical procedures on the ear, hematoma, trauma to the ear, frostbite, or burns is perichondritis of the pinna, sometimes extending into the cartilaginous external auditory canal. Perichondritis at its most severe results in suppurative destruction of ear cartilage, which in turn finally causes a deformed ear, sometimes leaving but a nubbin of pinna. The pinna first becomes exquisitely tender and swollen and, if untreated, fluctuation and spontaneous but inadequate drainage occurs. Causative organisms are usually gram-negative, commonly *Pseudomonas*, but *Staphylococcus* may also be a cause (Martin et al., 1976).

After culture, treatment should be begun without waiting for fluctuation, using through-and-through irrigation of the area. Small catheters or open Penrose drains should be threaded just superficial to the cartilage through stepladder incisions on both the anterior and the posterior surfaces; the incisions should be concealed in creases and under ridges of the pinna as well as possible (Fig. 20–2). The irrigation solution may be acetic acid in propylene glycol diacetate, benzethonium chloride, or sodium acetate. Systemic antibiotics may be required as well. This treatment must continue for several weeks to be efficacious. Sometimes removal of necrotic cartilage is required (Wanamaker, 1972; McLaurin, 1973; Templer, 1976; Martin et al., 1976).

Recently, acupuncture in or near the pinna has been used as a treatment for deafness, tinnitus, and obesity. Perichondritis has occurred as a complication (Baltimore and Moloy, 1976).

A peculiar type of problem, the pathogenesis of which is uncertain, occurs in patients who have the autosomally recessive syndrome of diastrophic dwarf-

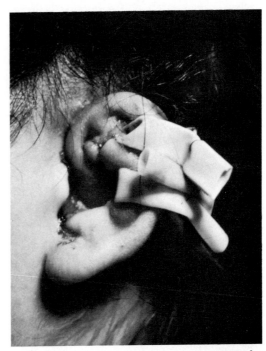

Figure 20–2. This teenager underwent a tympanomastoidectomy via a postauricular incision. Perichondritis caused by *Pseudomonas aeruginosa* developed in the postoperative period. It gradually resolved after intensive treatment, which included irrigations with topical gentamicin along the Penrose drains.

ism (diastrophic nanism syndrome). In early infancy the pinnae develop cystic swellings, thought to represent a hemorrhagic phase because from these swellings serosanguineous fluid can be aspirated. The condition is apparently painless, but the ears become deformed, with calcification and eventual ossification (Fig. 20–3) (McKusick, 1972; Gorlin et al., 1976; Smith, 1976). Mesomelic dwarfism, deformed extremities, and scoliosis are other prominent features. Conductive hearing loss, probably not directly related to the pinna degeneration, has been observed.

Relapsing polychondritis is another disorder included in the differential diagnosis of perichondritis. It is of uncertain etiology but probably is an autoimmune disorder, since tests for antinuclear antibody and rheumatoid factor are positive in some patients, and it has been observed in association with connective tissue disorders (McKenna et al., 1976; McCaffrey et al., 1978). Inflammatory degeneration of various cartilages occurs, including those of the pinna, ribs, and joints and the nasal, laryngeal, tracheal, and eustachian tube cartilages. Systemic symptoms also may occur (Schuknecht, 1974). Persons in their late teens have been afflicted with this disorder (McCaffrey et al., 1978). The ear may be the first visible area involved (Odkvist, 1970), and hence the exact nature of the problem may not at first be apparent. The pinna becomes painful, erythematous, and edematous, but the pain is not as excruciating as in bacterial perichondritis. In some instances, pain is not present, but the ear may be tender. Hemolytic complement factor may be decreased in fluid aspirated from the pinna (McKenna et al., 1976). Eventually, the ear may acquire a cauliflower configuration. Conductive hearing loss

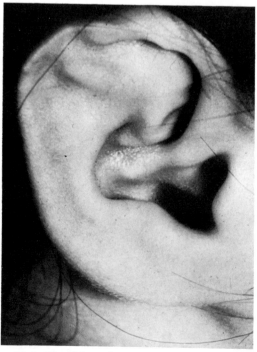

Figure 20–3. The deformed pinna of a young child who has diastrophic dwarfism. This represents fairly minimal involvement.

due to damage to the eustachian tube may occur; sensorineural hearing loss and vertigo are also reported. The pathogenesis of this disease is unknown (Schuknecht, 1974).

Frost bite injury to the pinna responds to fairly rapid rewarming using wet, sterile cotton pledgets warmed to 38 to 42°C. The ear should be stabilized during this procedure to minimize pain. Hot compresses can injure the already compromised ear. Systemic antibiotics are necessary only if there is cellulitis or perichondritis. Sulfadiazine silver or other antibiotic ointment should cover the deepithelialized or cartilage-exposed ear. Dressing may be required. Obviously, necrotic areas should be débrided, but months may go by before the viability of some areas may be evident. Only after complete healing should reconstruction be started (Templer, 1976).

Burns of the external ear occur in 90 per cent of patients with facial burns. Injury results from direct thermal injury or from suppurative chondritis. Direct tissue loss is treated with excision and skin grafting with the patient under general anesthesia. Second-degree burns are débrided and treated topically with Sulfamylon (mafenide) cream or silver nitrate. Topical therapy, including antibiotic iontophoresis, is more effective than systemic antibiotics, since the blood supply to the ear is poor. Pressure on the ear and bending of the ear will promote chondritis. Reconstruction may be accomplished by using autogenous cartilage grafts and local flaps. In some severe burns of a child's ears, it might be better after healing to prepare the site for a prosthesis. If the tissue at the site is tenuous and likely to break down, it might be better to suggest a long hair style to conceal the severely burned ear (Hammond and Ward, 1983). Superficial stenosis of the meatus of the ear canal is also a potential problem. Gentle stenting with Telfa smeared with Sulfamylon on the outside and tubed in the canal with Gelfoam or cottonoids in the lumen of the Telfa tube may be helpful.

Ear piercing is occasionally complicated by mild inflammation, cellulitis, or abscess. Because ear piercing is done in infancy in some cultures, infection is possible and is made even more probable should otitis media with otorrhea occur. Sometimes, infection recurs every time the earrings are reinserted. It is alleviated by topical or systemic antibiotics or changing to earrings of a different metal. Eventually, if desired, the earring holes can be closed surgically, although the cosmetic problem is not significant.

Posttraumatic healing after a sharp or blunt injury to the ear may result in keloid formation in darker-skinned patients (Figure 20–4A and B). The keloid should be removed sharply, with fine nylon suture 5-0 or 6-0 used for suturing. The incision should be gently infiltrated with a suitable steroid preparation, and reinjections should be done twice weekly. Reexcision one or more times may be necessary, followed by steroid injection. Low-dose radiation has been advocated.

Hepatitis may complicate either acupuncture or ear

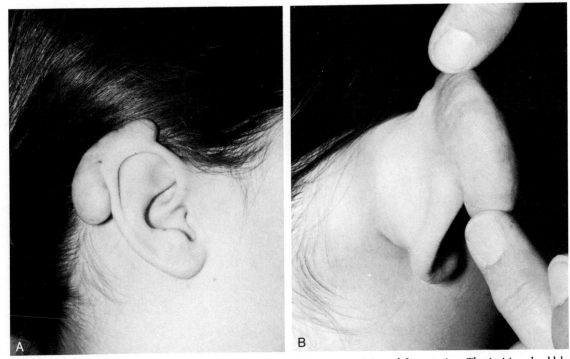

Figure 20–4. The keloid should be removed sharply, with fine nylon suture 5-0 or 6-0 used for suturing. The incision should be gently infiltrated with a suitable steroid preparation, and reinjections done twice weekly. Reexcision one or more times may be necessary, with use of steroid injection. Low-dose radiation has been advocated.

piercing (Johnson et al., 1974; Baltimore and Moloy, 1976).

Irradiation of the head and neck area, pituitary, or brain stem may include the external, middle, and inner ears in the field. Fairly commonly, the skin and its appendages within the ear canal may show inflammatory changes, some apparently permanent (Schuknecht, 1974). However, necrosis and breakdown of ear canal skin occur less frequently with cobalt 60 and other newer types of radiation than was true with orthovoltage radiation (Borsanyi et al., 1961). The production of cerumen ceases; the canal wall becomes edematous; the skin is dry and flaky; and material collects in the external canal, with resulting pruritus and at times secondary bacterial infection due to scratching. Telangiectatic skin changes may be seen in the pinna.

Leprosy may affect the external ear. The great auricular nerve may be thickened in the patient with tuberculoid leprosy. Lepromatous leprosy presents with vague, slightly hypopigmented or erythematous macules or papules. Arclike plaques may form on the helices and ear lobes in bilateral symmetry. In dimorphous or borderline leprosy, unilateral ear lobe lesions may be found. Ear deformities also present in lepromatous leprosy as gross ulcerations that give a "rat-eaten" appearance, or diffuse infiltrations may be seen. Oral 4,4'-diaminodiphenyl sulfone (dapsone) is the standard medical treatment. Rifampin is added to decrease drug resistance in dimorphous and lepromatous cases. Surgical reconstruction can be performed. Affected patients should be referred to the U.S. Public Health Hospital in Carville, Louisiana, where they will receive expert consultation and treatment (Brazin, 1982).

DERMATOSES AFFECTING THE PINNA

Some of the allergic and scaly dermatoses have already been mentioned, as they contribute to chronic external otitis. However, other disorders may produce other manifestations in or on the external ear.

Epidermolysis bullosa simplex produces cutaneous and mucosal blisters as early as birth. The condition is due to autosomal recessive inheritance. Stenosis of the ear canal may occur but apparently responds surprisingly well to surgical excision, canal drill-out, and skin grafting (Thawley et al., 1977). Another bullous lesion, pemphigoid or benign pemphigus, may also cause discrete rather than diffuse lesions in the ear canal and may occur in young persons (Rook et al., 1968).

Lipoid proteinosis of the skin and mucosa is a recessively inherited disease affecting the larynx, pharynx, mouth, lips, tongue, nose, and skin. On the pinna, waxy, hyperkeratotic deposits occur, and the pinna may lose its normal contours. The lesions are apparently neither painful nor pruritic, but those on the mucosa of the upper airway and mouth can cause considerable disruption of function (MacKinnon, 1968).

Acquired canal stenosis is more common than the congenital variety and generally results from surgery, trauma, or infection. It may occur as a complication of chronic external otitis (Proud, 1967), perichondritis, bullous lesions (Thawley et al., 1977), chronic otitis media, tuberculosis of the pinna and external auditory canal (Sinha, 1969), irradiation, and relapsing poly-chrondritis. Surgical excision alone or with the addition of a long-term stent postoperatively is the treatment of choice unless the patient's general condition does not permit it. However, surgery should be deferred until the causative lesion is inactive or as quiescent as possible. Surgery on young children for this problem would preferably be deferred, but upon suspicion of cholesteatoma behind the obstruction it might need to be done sooner.

THE EXTERNAL EAR AND CANAL IN SYSTEMIC DISEASE

Gardner syndrome, an autosomal dominant disorder, is characterized by gastrointestinal polyps and multiple skin lesions, including epidermal inclusion cysts, fibromas, desmoids, and osteomas that occur primarily in craniofacial bones. They may occur in the external auditory canal, and keratin debris may become trapped behind them when they are large, leading to canal infection (McKusick, 1975; Smith, 1976).

In Osler-Weber-Rendu disease (hereditary telangi-ectasia), mild forms may occur with only mild cutaneous telangiectasia. The pinna is a common site.

In alkaptonuria or ochronosis of recessive inheritance, cartilages and other tissues of collagen origin turn black. In the pinna, the cartilage is just under the skin, and the black color shines through. A characteristic laboratory finding is that urine turns dark when alkaline and left standing (McKusick, 1975).

SELECTED REFERENCE

Senturia, B. H. 1957. Diseases of the External Ear. Springfield, IL, Charles C. Thomas.

This small book, although 32 years old, is still the classic work to which all others refer. Senturia's completeness and synthesis of material relating to these common but often poorly managed problems has not been surpassed.

REFERENCES

Anson, B. J., and Donaldson, J. A. 1967. The Surgical Anatomy of the Temporal Bone and Ear, 1st ed. Philadelphia, W. B. Saunders Co.

Baltimore, R. S., and Moloy, P. J. 1976. Perichondritis of the ear as a complication of acupuncture. Arch. Otolaryngol. 102:572.

Beneke, E. S. 1970. Human Mycoses. Kalamazoo, MI, Upjohn Co., pp. 17–20, 38–41.

Bergstrom, L., Hemenway, W. G., and Barnhart, R. A. 1970. Rhinocerebral and otologic mucormycosis. Ann. Otol. Rhinol. Laryngol. 79:70.

Borsanyi, S., Blanchard, C. L., and Thorne, B. 1961. The effects of ionizing radiation on the ear. Ann. Otol. Rhinol. Laryngol. 70:255.

Brazin, S. A. 1982. Leprosy (Hansen's Disease). In Kornblut, A. D. (ed.): Symposium on Granulomatous Disorders of the Head and Neck. Otolaryngolic Clinics of North America. 15. Philadelphia, W. B. Saunders Co., pp. 600–603.

Cassisi, N., Cohn, A., Davidson, T., et al. 1977. Diffuse otitis externa, clinical and microbiologic findings in the course of a multicenter study on a new otic solution. Ann. Otol. Rhinol. Laryngol. 86, Suppl. 39.

Chandler, J. R. 1964. Partial occlusion of the external auditory meatus: Its effect upon air and bone conduction hearing acuity. Laryngoscope 74:22.

Chandler, J. R., 1968. Malignant external otitis. Laryngoscope, 78:1257–1294.

Chandler, J. R. 1977. Malignant external otitis: Further considerations. Ann. Otol. Rhinol. Laryngol. 86:417.

Damiani, J. M. 1979. Relapsing polychondritis—report of ten cases. Laryngoscope 89:929.

Dinapoli, R. P., and Thomas, J. E. 1971. Neurologic aspects of malignant external otitis: Report of three cases. Mayo Clin. Proc. 46:339.

Giguere, P., and Rouillard, G. 1976. Otite externe maligne bilatérale chez une fillette de 10 ans. J. Laryngol. 5:159.

Gorlin, R. J., Pindborg, J. J., and Cohen, M. M. 1976. Diastrophic dwarfism. In Gorlin, R. J., et al. (eds.): Syndromes of the Head and Neck, 2nd ed. New York, McGraw-Hill Book Co., pp. 250–252.

Ham, A. W. 1957. Histology, 3rd ed. Philadelphia, J. B. Lippincott Co., pp. 250–253, 860–866.

Hammond, J. S., and Ward, C. G. 1983. Burns of the head and neck. In Maniglia, A. J. (ed.): Symposium on Trauma to the Head and Neck. Otolaryngolic Clinics of North America 16. Philadelphia, W. B. Saunders Co., p. 6.

Hollinshead, W. H. 1968. Anatomy for Surgeons, Vol. 1, 2nd ed. New York, Hoeber Medical Division, Harper and Row, pp. 183–192.

Hoshino, T. 1978. Sudden deafness in relapsing polychondritis. Acta Otolaryngol. (Stockh.) 86:418.

Hoshino, T. 1980. Temporal bone findings in a case of sudden deafness in relapsing polychondritis. Acta Otolaryngol. (Stockh.) 90:257.

Hyslop, N. E., Jr. 1971. Ear wax and host defense. N. Engl. J. Med. 284:1099.

Johnson, C. J., Anderson, H., Spearman, J., and Madson, J. 1974. Ear piercing and hepatitis: Nonsterile instruments for ear piercing and subsequent onset of viral hepatitis. J.A.M.A. 227:1165.

Litton, W. B. 1963. Epithelial migration over tympanic membrane and external canal. Arch. Otolaryngol. 77:254.

MacKinnon, D. M. 1968. Hyalinosis cutis et mucosae (lipoid proteinosis). Acta Otolaryngol. (Stockh.) 65:403.

Main, T., and Lim, D. 1976. The human external auditory canal secretory system—an ultrastructural study. Laryngoscope 86:1164.

Martin, R., Yonkers, A. J., and Yarington, C. T. 1976. Perichondritis of the ear. Laryngoscope 86:664.

Matsunaga, E. 1962. The dimorphism in human normal cerumen. Ann. Hum. Genet. 25:273.

McCaffrey, T. V., McDonald, T. J., and McCaffrey, L. A. 1978. Head and neck manifestations of relapsing polychondritis. "A review of 29 cases." Trans. Am. Acad. Ophth. Otolaryngol. 86:473.

McKenna, C. H., Luthra, H. S., and Jordon, R. E. 1976. Hypocomplementemic ear effusion in relapsing polychondritis. Mayo Clin. Proc. 51:495.

McKusick, V. A. 1972. Heritable Disorders of Connective Tissue, 4th ed. St. Louis, The C. V. Mosby Co., pp. 772–775.

McKusick, V. A. 1975. Mendelian Inheritance in Man, 4th ed. Baltimore, The Johns Hopkins Press, pp. 272–273, 343–344.

McLaurin, J. W. 1973. Trauma and infections of the external ear. In Paparella, M. M., and Shumrick, D. A. (eds.): Otolaryngology, Vol. II. Philadelphia, W. B. Saunders Co., pp. 24–32.

Odkvist, L. 1970. Relapsing Polychondritis. Acta Otolaryngol. (Stockh.) 70:448.

Peterkin, G. A. G. 1974. External otitis. J. Laryngol. Otol. 88:15.

Petrakis, N. L., Doherty, M., Lee, R. E., et al. 1971. Demonstration and implications of lysozyme and immunoglobulins in human ear wax. Nature (Lond.) 229:119.

Proud, G. O. 1967. Surgical treatment of chronic otitis externa. Pac. Med. Surg. 75:186.

Rabuzzi, D. D. 1970. Relapsing polychondritis. Arch. Otolaryngol. 91:188.

Rogers, P. H. 1973. Relapsing polychondritis with insulin resistance and antibodies to cartilage. Am. J. Med. 55:243.

Rook, A., Wilkinson, D. S., and Ebling, F. J. G. 1968. Textbook of Dermatology, Vol. II. Oxford, Blackwell Scientific Publications, pp. 1183–1188.

Rothstein, J., Adams, G. L., Galliani, C. A., et al. 1985. Relapsing polychondritis in a 30-month-old child. Otolaryngol. Head Neck Surg. 93:680.

Schuknecht, H. G. 1974. Pathology of the Ear. Cambridge, MA, Harvard University Press, pp. 266–267, 311–312, 187–188.

Senturia, B. H. 1957. Diseases of the External Ear. Springfield, IL, Charles C. Thomas Co.

Senturia, B. H. 1973. External otitis, acute diffuse. Evaluation of therapy. Ann. Otol. Rhinol. Laryngol. 82, Suppl. 8.

Shambaugh, G. E., Jr. 1967. Surgery of the Ear, 2nd ed. Philadelphia, W. B. Saunders Co., pp. 229–232.

Sinha, S. N. 1969. Lupus vulgaris of the pinna and soft palate. Eye, Ear, Nose, Throat Monthly 48:471.

Smith, D. W. 1976. Recognizable Patterns of Human Malformation, 2nd ed. Philadelphia, W. B. Saunders Co., pp. 202–203.

Templer, J. W. 1976. Infections and inflammatory diseases of the external ear and external auditory canal. In English, G. M. (ed.): Otolaryngology. New York, Harper and Row, pp. 122–125.

Templer, J. W. 1976. Trauma to the pinna and external auditory canal. In English, G. M. (ed.): Otolaryngology, A Textbook. Hagerstown, MD, Harper and Row, p. 138.

Thawley, S. E., Black, M. J., Dudek, S. E., et al. 1977. External auditory canal stricture secondary to epidermolysis bullosa. Arch. Otolaryngol. 103:55.

Valenzuela, R., Cooperrider, P. A., Gogate, P., et al. 1980. Relapsing polychondritis. Immunomicroscopic findings in the cartilage of ear biopsy specimens. Hum. Pathol. 11:19.

Wanamaker, H. H. 1972. Suppurative perichondritis of the auricle. Trans. Am. Acad. Ophth. Otol. 76:1289.

Chapter 21

OTITIS MEDIA, ATELECTASIS, AND EUSTACHIAN TUBE DYSFUNCTION

Charles D. Bluestone, M.D.   Jerome O. Klein, M.D.

Otitis media is the most frequent diagnosis recorded for infants and children who visit physicians because of illness. Children exhibit not only the signs and symptoms of the acute episode but also the sequelae of infection of the middle ear, most important of which is persistent effusion. There is a wealth of new information from otolaryngologists, pediatricians, epidemiologists, biochemists, microbiologists, immunologists, and physiologists that has increased understanding of the disease and its most appropriate management. This chapter summarizes the results of recent investigations, integrates this information with that available previously, assesses the current state of the art, and considers optimal choices for management of the various stages of otitis media.

DEFINITIONS, TERMINOLOGY, AND CLASSIFICATION

During the past century, a multitude of terms have been used to describe various inflammatory conditions of the middle ear. This has resulted in confusion and misunderstanding among clinicians and investigators in their attempt to evaluate published reports, as interpretation of the results of these investigations depends on definition of the specific disease entity being studied. In defense of our well-meaning predecessors, the natural history, etiology, and pathogenesis of otitis media are better understood today than in the past. In an effort to eliminate ambiguity, the authors employ terminology that they believe meets current understanding of the disease process (Senturia et al., 1980a; Bluestone, 1984) and organizes the information in a manner that will aid the clinician's understanding of otitis media. The terminology used is defined, and a classification of otitis media and its complications and sequelae is presented.

Terminology and Definitions

Otitis media is an inflammation of the middle ear without reference to etiology or pathogenesis.

Otitis media with effusion is an inflammation of the middle ear in which a collection of liquid is present in the middle-ear space. (No perforation of the tympanic membrane is present.)

Middle-ear effusion is liquid in the middle ear. The effusion may be *serous*, a thin, watery liquid; *mucoid*, a thick, viscid, mucuslike liquid; or *purulent*, a puslike liquid, or a combination of these.

Atelectasis of the tympanic membrane, which may or may not be associated with otitis media, is collapse or retraction of the tympanic membrane. Collapse implies passivity, whereas retraction implies active pulling inward of the tympanic membrane, usually from negative middle-ear pressure.

A *retraction pocket* is a localized area of atelectasis of the tympanic membrane.

Otorrhea is a discharge from the ear.

Classification

The following classification is derived from present knowledge of the disease, but it is often difficult to determine by history and visual inspection of the tympanic membrane the specific type and stage of otitis media confronting the clinician (Paradise, 1987). The physician usually arrives at a presumptive diagnosis of the variety of otitis media present in the individual patient from limited data, but a more definitive diagnosis can be determined by the following:

1. Knowledge of the condition of the middle ear prior to onset of the present illness differentiates acute, subacute, and chronic forms. A child may have signs and symptoms of acute otitis media, but whether or not the middle ear was effusion free prior to the onset of the current episode may not be known.

2. Tympanocentesis determines the characteristics of the middle-ear effusion (i.e., serous, mucoid, or purulent), and appropriate cultures of the effusion establish the microbiologic origin.

3. Biopsy of the middle-ear mucosa, although rarely necessary for care of the patient in the clinical setting, defines the middle-ear pathologic state.

Otitis Media Without Effusion

In certain cases, only inflammation of the middle-ear mucous membrane and tympanic membrane will be present, without any evidence of a middle-ear effusion. The appearance of the tympanic membrane by pneumatic otoscopy will reveal only *myringitis*, in which there is usually erythema and opacification of the eardrum but relatively normal mobility to applied positive and negative pressure. Blebs or bullae may be present when the disease is acute. Otitis media without effusion is usually present in the early stages of acute otitis media but may also be found in the stage of resolution of acute otitis media or may even be chronic. Evidence for the existence of this type of otitis media has been provided by the examination of histopathologic specimens of temporal bone. The absence of a middle-ear effusion when a myringotomy is performed in the presence of otitis media has provided clinical proof that this condition exists in certain cases.

Acute Otitis Media

The rapid and short onset of signs and symptoms of inflammation in the middle ear is termed acute otitis media. Synonyms such as acute *suppurative* or *purulent* otitis media are acceptable (Table 21–1). One or more local or systemic signs are present: otalgia (or pulling of the ear in the young infant), otorrhea, fever, recent onset of irritability, anorexia, vomiting, or diarrhea. The tympanic membrane is full or bulging, is opaque, and has limited or no mobility to pneumatic otoscopy—indicative of a middle-ear effusion. Erythema of the eardrum is an inconsistent finding (Schwartz et al., 1981*d*). The acute onset of ear pain, fever, and a purulent discharge (otorrhea) through a perforation of the tympanic membrane (or tympanotomy tube) would also be evidence of acute otitis media. A middle-ear effusion that persists for longer than 3 months following an episode of acute otitis media is termed chronic otitis media with effusion.

Otitis Media with Effusion

The presence of a relatively asymptomatic middle-ear effusion has many synonyms, such as secretory, nonsuppurative, or serous otitis media (see Table 21–1), but the most acceptable term is *otitis media with effusion*. Because the effusion may be serous (transudate), the term *secretory* may not be correct in all cases. Likewise, the term *nonsuppurative* may not be correct, as asymptomatic middle-ear effusion may contain bacteria and may even be purulent. The term *serous* otitis media is appropriate if an amber or bluish effusion can be visualized through a translucent tympanic membrane; however, the most frequent otoscopic finding is opacification of the tympanic membrane, which prevents assessment of the type of effusion (e.g., serous, mucoid, or purulent). Pneumatic otoscopy will frequently reveal either a retracted or convex tympanic membrane in which the mobility is impaired. However, fullness or even bulging may be visualized. In addition, an air-fluid level, bubbles, or both may be observed through a translucent tympanic membrane. The duration (not the severity) of the effusion can be *acute* (less than 3 weeks), *subacute* (3 weeks to 2 to 3 months), or *chronic* (longer than 2 to 3 months). The most important distinction between this type of disease and acute otitis media (acute "suppurative" otitis media) is that the signs and symptoms of acute infection are lacking in otitis media with effusion (e.g., otalgia and fever), but hearing loss may be present in both conditions.

Atelectasis of the Tympanic Membrane–Middle Ear

Atelectasis of the tympanic membrane is not strictly a type of otitis media but is a related condition. It may be present prior to, concurrent with, or after an episode of otitis media with effusion. It also may be present in some patients without evidence of otitis media, and, if persistent and progressive, it can lead to complications or sequelae commonly attributed to otitis media, such as hearing loss, ossicular chain discontinuity, and cholesteatomas.

Complications and Sequelae

The complications and sequelae of otitis media are divided into those that occur within the middle ear and temporal bone (Chap. 22) and those that occur within the intracranial cavity (Chap. 23). It should be noted that these conditions are considered complications and sequelae of otitis media, but they also may develop from causes other than otitis media. For example, ossicular chain discontinuity may occur, among other possible means, as the result of trauma to the middle ear. On the other hand, several conditions may be complications or sequelae not of otitis media but of a related condition. An example of this situation would be the presence of atelectasis of the tympanic membrane without otitis media in which a discontinuity of the ossicular chain occurs or an acquired cholesteatoma develops (Bluestone et al., 1977*b*, 1978). There has been some confusion concerning *chronic suppurative otitis media*. For example, an acquired cholesteatoma may have a purulent discharge due to inflammation within the confines of the saclike structure, but the middle ear is not inflamed; therefore, the term chronic suppurative otitis media would be inaccurate. On the other hand, a cholesteatoma that is present in association with inflammation of the middle ear would be defined as chronic suppurative otitis media with cholesteatoma.

EPIDEMIOLOGY

Epidemiology is the study of disease in population groups rather than in individuals. *Incidence* is the frequency of occurrence of new or separate episodes of illness in a defined population over a specific period of time. New cases of otitis media in children observed in a physician's practice in 1 year would be representative of an incidence study. *Prevalence* is the fre-

TABLE 21–1. Synonyms Commonly Used in the Past for Otitis Media

ACUTE OTITIS MEDIA	OTITIS MEDIA WITH EFFUSION
Purulent	Serous
Suppurative	Secretory
Bacterial	Allergic
	Catarrhal
	Nonsuppurative
	Mucoid
	Secondary
	Tubotympanic catarrh
	Hydrotubotympanum
	Exudative catarrh
	Tubotympanitis
	Tympanic hydrops
	Glue ear
	Fluid ear
	Middle-ear effusion

quency of illness in a defined population at a given time. A survey of children for middle-ear disease in a school or village performed by a team in one or a few days would exemplify a prevalence study. Longitudinal studies provide information about children over a period of time and are an excellent source of information about the epidemiology of otitis media. These include a study of middle-ear disease in Alaskan Eskimo children (Kaplan et al., 1973; Reed et al., 1967); studies by Howie and Ploussard of Huntsville, Alabama, of the natural history of otitis media in children seen in their office practice (Howie, 1975; Howie et al., 1975); a prospective study of otitis media in 2565 children observed from birth in the greater Boston area (Teele et al., 1989); studies of respiratory disease in children attending a day-care project (Henderson et al., 1982; Loda et al., 1972; Sanyal et al., 1980); a prospective study of 2404 children born in Malmo, Sweden, in 1977 (Lundgren et al., 1984); studies of Finnish children and adults (Pukander et al., 1982; Pukander, 1982); and a study of 210 Nashville children observed from birth to 2 years of age (Wright et al., 1985). The results of these longitudinal studies and selected data from other reports are the basis for this review of the epidemiology of otitis media in children.

Historical Perspective

It is likely that humans have always had acute infection of the middle ear and its suppurative complications. Studies of 2600-year-old Egyptian mummies reveal perforations of the tympanic membrane and destruction of the mastoid (Lynn and Benitez, 1974). Evidence of middle-ear disease was also apparent in skeletal material from a prehistoric Iranian population (1900 to 800 B.C.) (Rathbun and Mallin, 1977). Prior to the introduction of antimicrobial agents, otitis media either resolved spontaneously (via central perforation of the tympanic membrane or evacuation of the middle-ear contents through the eustachian tube) or came to the attention of a physician who drained the middle ear by means of myringotomy. Purulent otitis media was a frequent reason for hospital admission. In 1932, purulent otitis media accounted for 27 per cent of all pediatric admissions to Bellevue Hospital (Bakwin and Jacobinzer, 1939). Mastoiditis and intracranial complications were common. The introduction of sulfonamides in 1935 and subsequent antibacterial drugs limited the course of otitis media and reduced the incidence of suppurative complications. Otitis media in children from developing countries today resembles the disease seen in the United States and Western Europe before the era of chemotherapy.

Incidence of Otitis Media

Acute Otitis Media

Otitis media is one of the most common infectious diseases of childhood. A survey of the office practices

TABLE 21–2. Proportion of Visits Attributable to Disease of the Middle Ear*

PURPOSE OF VISIT†	MEAN NUMBER OF VISITS	PERCENTAGE OF VISITS FOR OR WITH MIDDLE-EAR DISEASE
First Year of Life (2176 child-years of observation)		
Illness	2.19	34.0
Follow-up illness	1.18	69.9
Well-baby visit	4.73	5.7
Totals	8.10	22.7
Second Year of Life (1720 child-years of observation)		
Illness	2.10	34.7
Follow-up illness	1.10	75.7
Well-baby visit	1.77	7.1
Totals	4.96	33.9
Third Year of Life (1317 child-years of observation)		
Illness	1.75	29.5
Follow-up illness	0.77	74.1
Well-baby visit	1.07	5.7
Totals	3.58	34.6
Fourth Year of Life (660 child-years of observation)		
Illness	1.84	35.4
Follow-up illness	1.00	76.6
Well-baby visit	0.71	9.6
Totals	3.55	41.8
Fifth Year of Life (529 child-years of observation)		
Illness	1.39	34.2
Follow-up illness	0.66	72.1
Well-baby visit	0.59	9.0
Totals	2.64	38.1

*Children from greater Boston, 1975 to 1982.
†According to parents.
With permission from Teele, D. W., et al., 1983. Burden and the practice of pediatrics: Middle ear disease during the first five years of life. J.A.M.A. 249:1026–1029. Copyright 1983, American Medical Association.

of physicians who provide medical care to children showed that otitis media was the most frequent diagnosis for illness and the most frequent reason, after well-baby and -child care, for office visits (Koch and Dennison, 1974). A survey of the frequency of infectious diseases during the first year of life in 246 Rochester children indicated that otitis media was second only to the common cold as a cause of infectious illness (Hoekelman, 1977). Otitis media was the most frequent diagnosis (22 per cent) for visits of children to the Medical Emergency Clinic at Children's Hospital in Boston in a 6-week survey from March through April 1960 (Bergman and Haggerty, 1962). A review of the causes of visits to the Ambulatory Clinic of the Boston City Hospital in the fall of 1973 revealed that 19 per cent of children between 4 and 24 months of age had otitis media (Klein and Bratton, 1973). In addition to visits for acute episodes of otitis media, those for observation subsequent to a diagnosis of otitis media add substantially to the number of visits to physicians for the child. Investigators for the United States Food and Drug Administration found that approximately one half of the courses of antibiotics prescribed for children less than 10 years of age in 1986 were administered for otitis media; 44.5 million courses were prescribed and 42 per cent of the prescriptions were for otitis media (Nelson et al., 1987).

The proportion of office visits of young children for otitis media was further elucidated by Teele and colleagues (1983) (Table 21–2). Disease of the middle ear accounted for a large proportion of visits during the first 5 years of age, rising from 22.7 per cent in the first year to approximately 40 per cent in years 4 and 5; about one visit in three made for illness of any kind resulted in the diagnosis of middle-ear disease; approximately three quarters of all visits to follow up any illness were made to follow up disease of the middle ear; and either acute otitis media or asymptomatic middle-ear effusion was diagnosed at 5 to 10 per cent of all well-child visits.

Howie and colleagues (1975) found that two thirds of children seen in their office practice had had at least one episode of otitis media by their second birthday, and one in seven children had experienced more than six episodes. The Boston study showed similar trends: 71 per cent of children had had one or more episodes, and 33 per cent had had three or more episodes of otitis media by 3 years of age (Teele et al., 1989) (Table 21–3). In a study of Danish children followed from birth to age 9 years, the incidence of otitis media was 22 per cent during the first year of life, 15 per cent in the second year, 10 per cent for the third and fourth, and only 2 per cent by the eighth year (Stangerup and Tos, 1986).

These studies suggest that by 3 years of age children may be categorized into three groups of approximately equal size relative to acute infections of the middle ear. One group is free of ear infections, a second group may have occasional episodes of otitis, and a third group is "otitis prone," subject to repeated episodes of acute middle-ear infections.

Persistent and Asymptomatic Middle-Ear Effusions

The incidence or prevalence of otitis media with effusion that is apparently asymptomatic and unrecognized by parents (and therefore not brought to medical attention) has been the subject of studies in

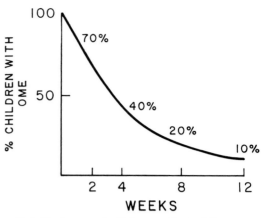

Figure 21–1. Persistence of middle-ear effusion following onset of acute otitis media. (Modified from Teele, D. W., et al. 1980. Epidemiology of otitis media in children. Ann. Otol. Rhinol. Laryngol. 89[68]:5–6.)

the United States and in Scandinavia. Persistence of middle-ear effusion for weeks to months after onset of acute otitis media was frequent in Boston children (Teele et al., 1989): 70 per cent of children still had effusion at 2 weeks, 40 per cent had effusion at 1 month, 20 per cent had effusion at 2 months, and 10 per cent had effusion at 3 months (Fig. 21–1). The means of periods of time spent with middle-ear effusion after the first, second, and third episode of acute otitis media were almost identical, ranging from 39 to 44 days. Age at time of diagnosis was inversely associated with duration of middle-ear effusion after first episode of acute otitis media. Similar results of persistent middle-ear effusion after an episode of acute otitis media have been noted in recent studies from other centers (Table 21–4), except for the study by Kaleida and coworkers (1987). They included recurrent acute otitis media in their study, which occurred in 50 per cent of subjects, and the point prevalence of middle-ear effusion ranged between about 40 per cent at 30

TABLE 21–3. Incidence of Acute Otitis Media

AGE (MONTHS)	CUMULATIVE PERCENTAGE OF CHILDREN OBSERVED WITH INDICATED NUMBER OF EPISODES OF OTITIS MEDIA*		
	≥ 1	≥ 3	≥ 6
12	62	17	1
36	81	46	16
60	91	65	30

*2565 Boston children enrolled at birth.

With permission from Teele, D. W., Klein, J. O., Rosner, B., and the Greater Boston Otitis Media Study Group. 1989. Epidemiology of otitis media during the first seven years of life in children in greater Boston: A prospective, cohort study. J. Infect. Dis. (in press).

TABLE 21–4. Percentage of Children with Persistent Middle-Ear Effusion After Initiating Antibiotic Treatment for Acute Otitis Media

INVESTIGATORS	ANTIBIOTICS	PERCENTAGE WITH MIDDLE-EAR EFFUSIONS AFTER Weeks				
		1.5–2	4	6	8	12
Puhakka et al., 1979		58	29			
Teele et al., 1980c		70	40		29	10
Thomsen et al., 1980	Ampicillin*	50	33			25
Schwartz et al., 1982		50	23		12	8
Mandel et al., 1982	Amoxicillin	56		33		
	Cefaclor	41		31		
Marchant et al., 1984a	Cefaclor	84	73			
	Trimethoprim-sulfamethoxazole	85	67			
Odio et al., 1985	Cefaclor	72	48		29	7
	Amoxicillin + clavulanic acid	70	44		13	5
Kaleida et al., 1987†	Cefaclor	45	39		34	25
	Amoxicillin + clavulanic acid	33	43		30	22

*Ampicillin in all but small numbers of children who received various alternative regimens.

†Includes otitis media with effusion, acute otitis media, and otorrhea.

days and 23 per cent at 90 days after the onset of the initial attack.

Surveys of healthy Danish children for presence of middle-ear fluid have identified a surprisingly high incidence of apparently asymptomatic middle-ear effusion (Fiellau-Nikolajsen et al., 1977; Lous and Fiellau-Nikolajsen, 1981; Poulson and Tos, 1978; Sly et al., 1980; Tos, 1980; Tos et al., 1978, 1979) (Table 21–5). All surveys used tympanometry to assess the status of the middle ear. The prevalence of effusion varied with age and the time of year. Incidence of effusion peaked during the second year of life and was more prevalent in winter than in summer months. Repeated examinations revealed that the middle-ear fluid cleared spontaneously in most children within a few months (Lous and Fiellau-Nikolajsen, 1981; Sly et al., 1980; Tos, 1980).

In Pittsburgh children 2 to 6 years of age observed monthly over a 2-year period, approximately two thirds of the episodes of otitis media with effusion cleared within a month (Casselbrant et al., 1985). In a similar study of 126 school children 5 to 12 years of age, the incidence of otitis media with effusion was found to be much lower in children 6 years of age and older (Casselbrant et al., 1986). In many children, the duration of effusion may be as short as one or several days; a novel investigation of daily impedance screening of children 3 to 6 years of age in a day-care center revealed that many children had tympanometric evidence of effusion (B curves) for 1 day only (Birch and Elbrønd, 1985). Some children, however, had fluid for 6 months or longer, and it often was seen first in one

ear and then in the other on subsequent examinations. Thus, asymptomatic middle-ear effusion is relatively frequent in healthy children but usually resolves without medical or surgical intervention, and the incidence decreases after age 5 years.

Age

Newborn

In the newborn infant otitis media may be an isolated infection, or it may be associated with sepsis, pneumonia, or meningitis. The incidence of otitis media in newborn infants is uncertain, but the few available studies suggest that the incidence is high in both normal infants and infants with underlying factors, such as prematurity, that place them in intensive care units. Otitis media with effusion was identified in 24 of 70 Cleveland infants (34 per cent) recruited from normal newborn nurseries observed at or before 2 months of age. Approximately half of the children at 2 months of age with otitis media with effusion were asymptomatic (Marchant et al., 1984b). Warren and Stool (1971) consecutively examined 127 infants whose birth weights were under 2300 gm, and they found three with infections of the middle ear (at 2, 7, and 26 days). Jaffe and associates (1970) examined 101 Navajo infants within 48 hours of birth and identified 18 with impaired mobility of the tympanic membrane. Balkany and coworkers (1978) identified effusion in the middle ear of 30 per cent of 125 consecutively examined infants

TABLE 21–5. Prevalence of Otitis Media with Effusion and High Negative Pressure*

INVESTIGATORS	AGE	MONTHS OF EVALUATION	PRESENCE OF NEGATIVE PRESSURE (%)	PRESENCE OF MIDDLE-EAR EFFUSIONS (%)
Poulsen and Tos, 1978	2–4 days	Jan 1977	10.6	—
	3 months	Apr 1977	17.9	—
	6 months	Jul 1977	36.9	1.3
Tos et al., 1979	9 months	Oct 1978	48.3	4.2
	12 months	Jan 1978	46.6	13.1
Tos and Poulsen, 1979	2 years	Nov 1977	39.4	12.0
		Feb 1978	38.5	14.6
		May 1978	36.7	77.3
		Aug 1978	29.7	7.2
Fiellau-Nikolajsen, 1979	3 years	Jan 1978	27.4	9.8
		Aug 1978	22.1	8.2
Thomsen and Tos, 1981		Feb 1979	39.0	11.0
Tos et al., 1982	4 years	Feb 1979	48.6	14.2
		May 1979	47.4	11.3
		Aug 1979	51.2	10.2
		Nov 1979	53.8	14.4
		Feb 1980	56.2	18.1
Lous and Fiellau-Nikolajsen, 1981	7 years	Aug–Sep 1978	15.0	5.7
		Nov–Apr 1979	20.0	9.0
		May–June 1979	18.0	6.0
		Aug 1979	9.0	2.4

*Children of ages 0 to 7 years in Denmark.

who were admitted to a neonatal intensive-care unit; the clinical diagnosis was corroborated by aspiration of middle-ear fluid. Nasotracheal intubation for more than 7 days was correlated with presence of effusion (Balkany et al., 1978). Pestalozza (1984) observed 970 newborn infants, 2 to 25 days of age, who were on the neonatal pathology ward; 205 infants (21.1 per cent) were diagnosed to have otitis media by otoscopy, corroborated in two consecutive visits within 48 hours.

Infants and Toddlers

Otitis media is common in infants beyond the neonatal period (after 28 days of age). In a study of children in Boston, 9 per cent had at least one episode of otitis media by 3 months of age, and 25 per cent had one or more episodes by 6 months of age. By 1 year of age, 67 per cent of children had one or more episodes of acute otitis media; by 3 years of age, experience with acute otitis media rose to 81 per cent (Table 21–3). The highest age-specific incidence for all episodes of acute otitis media (first and subsequent episodes) occurred between 6 and 13 months of age. Similar results were identified in Nashville children observed from birth; by 3 months of age 7 per cent had an episode of acute otitis media, and the peak incidence of middle-ear infection was 7 to 9 months of age (Wright et al., 1985). In a recent study from Finland, of 3189 infants 34.5 per cent had one or more episodes of acute otitis media during their first year of life, 24.8 per cent had one or two episodes, and 9.7 per cent had three or more attacks (Kero and Piekkala, 1987).

School-Age Children and Adults

The incidence of otitis media declines with age after the first year of life, except for a limited reversal of the downward trend between 5 and 6 years of age, the time of entrance into school. Otitis media is less common in children 7 years of age and older. Although the incidence of acute otitis media is limited in adults, a 1970 survey found that there are almost 4 million visits by adults each year to private physicians for this infection (NDTI Review, 1970). Approximately 20 per cent of young Swedish adult males (20 to 30 years old) and 30 per cent of older males (50 to 60 years old) had pathologic changes of the tympanic membrane; most with serious pathologic findings had histories of otitis and otorrhea of long duration (Rudin et al., 1985).

Age at First Episode and Recurrent Acute Otitis Media

Age at first episode of acute otitis media is significantly associated with recurrent episodes. In the Boston study, the peak incidence for first episodes of acute otitis media occurred at 6 months of age (Teele et al., 1980c). Age at first episode of acute otitis media was significantly and inversely associated with risk for one or more or two or more episodes of acute otitis media

in the 12 months after initial diagnosis. Cleveland infants with onset of otitis media with effusion before age 2 months had a mean of 3.5 total months of bilateral effusion, compared with 1.2 months for those with later onset (Marchant et al., 1984b). Bilateral middle-ear effusion in these infants at age 2 months was highly predictive of subsequent bilateral persistent otitis media with effusion (effusion for a continuous period of 3 months or longer) (Marchant et al., 1984b). Of 3189 infants in Finland, the mean age at the time of the first episode was 7.5 months; first episode occurred before the age of 6 months in 25 per cent, before the age of 8 months in 50 per cent, and before the age of 10 months in 75 per cent of infants who experienced acute otitis media in the first year of life (Kero and Piekkala, 1987). In another Finnish study that involved 1642 urban infants followed from birth to 18 months of age, 56.7 per cent had at least one episode of acute ear infection; 29.8 per cent had three or more (Sipilä et al., 1987).

Navajo infants with otitis media during the first months of life had more recurrences than those infants free of disease early in life (Jaffe et al., 1970). Alaskan Eskimo children who had onset of disease during the first 2 years of life had many more middle-ear infections in later life than did children who escaped middle-ear infections early in life (Kaplan et al., 1973). Howie and colleagues (1975) called children with two or more episodes in the first year of life "otitis-prone"; the children had twice as many subsequent episodes of otitis media as children who had no or one episode in the first year. The reasons that children with episodes of acute otitis media early in life are at risk for recurrent disease are uncertain. These children may have an underlying anatomic or physiologic predisposition to middle-ear infection, most likely due to the structure or function of the eustachian tube. Alternatively, infection early in life may cause changes in the mucosa of the middle-ear system that make children more susceptible to subsequent infection.

Age and Middle-Ear Effusion

The age-specific incidence of otitis media with effusion parallels that of acute infection; the peak was at ages 6 to 13 months in Boston children (Teele et al., 1980c) and 10 to 12 months in Nashville children (Wright et al., 1985). Persistent effusions of the middle ear were more likely in young children. Pelton and associates (1977) found that approximately 50 per cent of children 2 years of age or younger had effusions that lasted for 4 weeks or more after an episode of acute otitis media, whereas only 20 per cent of children older than 2 years had effusions of this duration. Asymptomatic middle-ear effusion identified in surveys of healthy children is more frequent in children 1 to 4 years of age than in children aged 7 years and older (see Table 21–5).

Sex

In most studies the incidence of acute episodes of otitis media was not significantly different in boys and girls. However, in the Boston study, males had significantly more single and recurrent (three or more) episodes (Teele et al., 1989). Finnish males had significantly more episodes than did females in eight communities studied in a 1-year period beginning June 1978 (Pukander et al., 1982). In another study from Finland, more male than female babies had acute otitis media during their first year of life (Kero and Piekkala, 1987). Males have more myringotomies and tympanoplasties than do females, suggesting that chronic or severe infections of the middle ear may be more common among males (Solomon and Harris, 1976).

Race

Studies of American Indians and Alaskan and Canadian Eskimos indicate that there is an extraordinary incidence of infection of the middle ear and that the disease is severe in these groups. Otorrhea is frequent, but chronic otitis and persistent effusion are uncommon. The following examples illustrate the extent and severity of ear disease in these populations. Zonis (1968) performed a prevalence study of an Apache community of 500 people of all ages; evidence of present or past ear infection was found in 23 per cent (draining ear, 5.6 per cent; perforation, 2.8 per cent; healed perforation, tympanosclerosis, or both, 13.1 per cent; serous otitis, 1 per cent; and acute otitis media, 0.4 per cent). Investigators found a high rate of otorrhea in Alaskan Eskimo children. By 1 year of age, 38 per cent had at least one episode and 20 per cent of all children had two or more episodes; by 4 years of age, 62 per cent of children had one or more episodes of otorrhea and 40 per cent of the children had two or more episodes (Reed et al., 1967). Ling and colleagues (1969) found that 31 per cent of Canadian Eskimo children 10 years of age or younger living on Baffin Island had draining ears at the time of examination; none of the children were febrile or had evidence of acute otitis media. In a study of 142 3- to 8-year-old children (mostly Inuits) in Greenland, 6 per cent had chronic suppurative otitis media (Pedersen and Zachau-Christiansen, 1986).

The severity of middle-ear infection has also been noted in African children and in Australian aboriginal children. Perforated eardrums are common. The prevalence of perforated eardrums in an aboriginal settlement in Queensland was 25 per cent in children 4 to 12 months of age and approximately 10 per cent in children 6 to 12 years of age (Dugdale et al., 1982). A prevalence survey in a Nigerian village identified wet or dry perforation in 4.2 per cent of 170 children under 15 years of age (Miller et al., 1983). In a prevalence study of children and adults in Micronesia, approximately one half of the infants under 1 year had otitis media with effusion, and 4 per cent of ears examined of persons aged 2 months to 25 years had a perforation (Dever et al., 1985). A form of the disease, termed necrotizing otitis media, is seen in these children that is rarely seen in children living in developed areas.

An episode of acute middle-ear infection progresses to perforation of the tympanic membrane with profuse discharge. Necrosis of the tympanic membrane follows, leaving a large central perforation that may persist for many years. This ear is called a "safe ear" because the perforation allows for drainage of the middle-ear infection, and intracranial complications rarely occur, even without use of antimicrobial agents. However, there may be destruction of the ossicular chain and deafness may result (Clements, 1968; Dugdale et al., 1978; Pisacane and Ruas, 1982). Parents in these areas accept otorrhea as a way of life.

Timmermans and Gerson (1980) described a more indolent form of otitis media in Inuit Eskimo children that they termed chronic granulomatous otitis media. After one or more episodes of acute otitis media (usually treated with antimicrobial agents), there is a sudden onset of otorrhea without pain or fever. The discharge may persist for years, interspersed with periods of variable length in which the ear is dry. A large central perforation of the tympanic membrane is present, and granulomatous tissue fills the middle-ear cavity. Resolution occurs with a scarred tympanic membrane and a mild to moderate hearing deficit.

Thus, the studies of children in different geographic and climatic areas suggest that the severity of disease represented by chronic otorrhea, destruction of the tympanic membrane and ossicles, and other forms of a necrotizing process in the middle ear is much more frequent (at present, almost unique) in underdeveloped areas.

American black children appear to have less disease due to middle-ear infection than do white American children. The incidence of pathologic ear disorders and hearing impairment was higher in white children than in black children aged 6 months through 11 years who lived in Washington, DC (Kessner et al., 1974). Ear disease was noted in 35 per cent of 112 white children and 18 per cent of 2031 black children. Hearing was tested in children 4 to 11 years of age; 20 per cent of 82 white children and 6 per cent of 1545 black children had significant impairment of hearing. The predominance of ear disease in white children was not readily explained. The results may be related to the relatively small size of the sample of white children or to socioeconomic factors unique to the white children living in a predominantly black community. In a second study in the Washington, DC, area, investigators observed a tenfold difference in the incidence of acute otitis media in white and black children. The disease rate in children less than 15 years of age with at least one encounter for acute otitis media was 155 per 1000 children attending a clinic in an affluent, predominantly white suburb; it was 15 per 1000 children attending a clinic in a blue-collar area of northeast Washington, DC, in which nearly all of the patients were black. Acute otitis media during the first year of life occurred in significantly more white (38 of 44 [86 per cent]) than black (16 of 26 [62 per cent]) Cleveland children observed in a uniform protocol (Marchant et al., 1984b). In a study of persistence of middle-ear effusions after acute episodes of otitis media, Pelton and coworkers (1977) also noted a higher incidence of persistent effusions in white or Hispanic children than in black children (21 per cent of 42 black children and 51 per cent of 51 white children).

The higher incidence of ear disease in white children (or lower incidence in black children) is not readily explained. Of interest are the studies of Doyle (1977) of the position of the bony eustachian tube in skulls of American blacks, Americans of Caucasian ancestry, and American Indians. Significant differences among the racial groups were present in the length, width, and angle of the tube in the groups, implicating an anatomic basis for racial predisposition to, or protection from, otitis media.

Further information about possible mechanisms was provided by Beery and associates (1980), who studied eustachian tube function in Apache Indians living in Arizona. The results of inflation-deflation tests indicated that American Indians had lower forced opening pressures than had been measured previously in a group of Caucasians (with perforations due to chronic otitis media). The eustachian tube of the American Indian was functionally different from that of the Caucasians previously studied and was characterized by comparatively abnormal, low passive tubal resistance, which may be considered to facilitate ventilatory activity but to impair the protective function of the tube. These investigators speculated that the difference may account for the high prevalence of otitis media with perforation (and the low incidence of cholesteatoma) in this population. Todd and Bowman (1985) who studied Apache Indians in Arizona, at two periods 16 years apart, arrived at similar conclusions.

Few interracial studies have been done, and therefore it is not possible to evaluate fully the significance of the extent and severity of ear disease in different racial groups. Poverty is a common factor among many of the nonwhite populations that have been studied. Other variables include extremes of climate (temperature, humidity, altitude), crowding in the homes, inadequate hygiene, poor sanitation, and lack of medical care. Although disparities in disease incidence for different racial groups may be real, other explanations must be considered, including differences in the perception of signs of ear infection by parents, the basis for visits to the physician, the basis of payment for medical services, and the diagnostic acumen or style of the physicians (Bush and Rabin, 1980).

Social and Economic Conditions

Cambon and associates (1965) noted a strong relationship between middle-ear disease and poor social conditions among American Indians of British Columbia. The specific reasons for the high incidence and severity of disease were not identified. Factors suggested include crowded living conditions, poor sanitation, and inadequate medical care. "The running ear is the heritage of the poor" (Cambon et al., 1965) may

be true today as in the past, but the reasons for the high incidence and marked severity of disease among the underprivileged are still not understood.

Children living in households with many members are more likely to have otitis media than are children living in smaller households. Canadian Eskimo children living in camps have less disease than do children living in villages and towns (Schaefer, 1971). Finnish children living in rural areas have fewer episodes of acute otitis media than do children living in towns (Pukander, 1982). These same investigators also noted an increased incidence in young children who had several siblings living in the same household (Pukander et al., 1985). Another study from Finland showed that babies in the lowest and middle socioeconomic classes were more likely to have acute otitis media during their first year of life than young infants in the highest class (Kero and Piekkala, 1987).

Day-Care Centers

The number of American children who receive some form of day care is large and growing. Current estimates are that more than 11 million children receive full or part-time day care. More than 50 per cent of mothers who have children younger than 6 years of age work outside the home. Day-care centers vary in size from small groups in the responsibility of one or two adults to large, organized group centers. Similarly, some facilities have adequate room and ventilation, whereas others are crowded and poorly ventilated. In the day-care setting, coughing and sneezing at close range are common. Rhinovirus and respiratory syncytial virus (RSV) can remain infective for hours to days in moist or dried secretions on nonporous materials such as toys, and the organisms can survive for more than 30 minutes on cloth or paper tissues saturated with secretions. Epidemics of disease due to respiratory viruses are common. There is ample opportunity for spread of respiratory tract infections among children in day care and for higher incidence of infection in children attending day care than in children who receive care at home.

In urban areas of Finland, community day-care centers are common and children have a higher incidence of otitis than do children living in the Finnish countryside, who are more likely to be cared for in their homes (Pukander et al., 1984). Similarly, Danish children cared for outside the home have shown a history of otitis media that is 25 per cent higher than that for children cared for in the home; in addition, effusion, identified by tympanometry, occurs more frequently in children cared for outside the home than at home (Vinther et al., 1982). Approximately three or more episodes of otitis media occurred in 10 per cent of 150 Swedish children aged 6 to 24 months in family day care (42 children) or in day-care centers (108 children) and in none of 57 children who received care at home (Strangert, 1977).

Although the data suggest that the incidence of otitis

media is higher in children who attend day care, problems of bias are present that may account for all or part of the difference in incidence. The estimate of acute otitis media in children cared for at home may be low. Parents of children in day care may seek medical attention for illness at a lesser degree of severity because of concern for loss of time at work if the parents need to stay home to care for a sick child. Alternately, the higher incidence of febrile illnesses in children in day care may result in more examinations by physicians and more observations of ears. Only the study by Wald and colleagues followed children prospectively from birth to determine the incidence of acute otitis media in various types of day care. Children in group day care (seven children or more) had many more episodes of otitis media than did children in home care. Myringotomy and tube placements were performed by the second year of life in 21 per cent of children in group day care and only 3 per cent of children in home care (Wald et al., 1988).

Season

The seasonal incidence of infections of the middle ear parallels the seasonal variations of upper respiratory tract infections. Acute episodes peak during the winter but are also frequent in the fall and spring; they are least frequent in the summer. In observations during 3 years in the Boston study, 27 per cent of children had an episode of otitis in the summer, compared with 48 per cent in the spring and fall and 51 per cent in the winter (Teele et al., 1984). The incidence of episodes of otitis media also increases during outbreaks of viral infections of the respiratory tract in children; these are most likely to occur in the winter and spring (Henderson et al., 1982).

The prevalence of middle-ear effusion in asymptomatic children of various ages has been determined by use of tympanometry combined, in some cases, with physical examination. In New Orleans, 4- to 5-year-old children had different prevalence of middle-ear effusion in winter and fall: 29 per cent of children tested in February and 6 per cent of those tested in September had effusion (Sly et al., 1980). Examination of Pittsburgh preschool-age children attending a day-care center identified a prevalence of zero for otitis media with effusion in August, 7 per cent in September, and 25 per cent in January and February (Casselbrant et al., 1984). A 1-year study of 389 7-year-old Danish schoolchildren used tympanometry on 8 to 10 occasions during the year to test for the presence of middle-ear effusions (Lous and Fiellau-Nikolajsen, 1981). Twenty-six per cent of the children had evidence of middle-ear effusion on one or more tests during the year. The prevalence varied from 5.7 per cent in August to 9 per cent in November through April and returned to 2.4 per cent in August. Middle-ear effusion occurring in the winter months persisted longer than effusion occurring in the summer months (Lous and Fiellau-Nikolajsen, 1981).

Smoking

Although investigators have presented evidence that passive exposure to maternal cigarette smoke may have important effects on the development of pulmonary function in children (Tager et al., 1983), the data are less certain about an effect of exposure to cigarette smoke on disease of the middle ear. Kraemer and colleagues (1983) evaluated risk features in children admitted to hospital for tympanostomy tube insertion and a control group of children admitted for other types of surgery. Household cigarette smoke exposure occurred more frequently in children with chronic ear disease. Relative risk of ear disease increased directly with the number of household smokers and the amount of cigarette use.

Parental smoking in the home may be a predisposing factor in development of otitis media in infants and children. Of 471 2- to 3-year-old children who lived in two cities in Finland, 202 had parents who smoked and 269 did not. Sixty-five per cent of children whose parents smoked had one or more attacks compared with only 49 per cent in those whose parents did not. However, Vinther and colleagues (1979) found no association between parental smoking history and the occurrence of otitis media. Even though controversy exists over so-called passive smoking as a risk factor for otitis media, elimination of smoking may be preventive. More information about the duration and intensity of exposure and inclusion in a model of multivariable analysis is needed to identify the importance of cigarette smoke exposure in etiology of disease of the middle ear.

Genetic Factors

Genetic predisposition to middle-ear infection was suggested by data from the Boston study (Teele et al., 1989) and by a study of Apache children living on a reservation as well as those who were adopted and living outside the Indian community (Spivey and Hirschhorn, 1977). Children enrolled in the Boston study who had single or recurrent episodes of otitis media were more likely to have siblings with histories of significant middle-ear infections than were children who had had no episodes of otitis media. Adopted Apache children had more episodes of acute otitis media than did their non-Apache siblings, and they had an illness rate similar to that of Apache children who remained on the reservation.

Hagerman and coworkers (1987) evaluated retrospectively 30 prepubertal boys with fragile X syndrome and found a significantly greater number of episodes of otitis media in them as compared with their normal male siblings and a group of unrelated, cytogenetically normal controls. The pathogenesis of the increased incidence in this group remains undefined at this time.

Low responses to pneumococcal polysaccharides were associated in some adults with lack of certain genetic markers of immunoglobulins (Ambrosino et al., 1985, 1986). Immunoglobulin allotypes were investigated in children with recurrent episodes of acute otitis media and in their parents (Prellner et al., 1985); the results did not identify differences among children with recurrent otitis media and controls for markers of genetic loci involved in antibody responses to pneumococcal polysaccharide antigens. The epidemiologic data suggest that genetic susceptibility to middle-ear disease does exist and that further investigation of genetic markers is likely to yield useful information.

Breast-Feeding

Breast-feeding has been suggested as an important factor in prevention of respiratory and gastrointestinal infections in infancy. Does breast-feeding prevent otitis media? Various investigators have attempted to answer the question in different geographic areas and different cultural populations. Schaefer (1971) surveyed Canadian Eskimo children in five areas, including an urban center (Frobisher Bay), village settlements, and hunting camps. There was an increase in the incidence of middle-ear disease in children who lived in urban centers, compared with those living in villages or camps, but in each area there was an inverse relationship of incidence of middle-ear disease and duration of breast-feeding. Children who were breast-fed for 12 months or more had significantly less frequent ear disease related to otitis media than did infants who were bottle-fed at birth, or within the first month.

Timmermans and Gerson (1980) conducted a prevalence study of ear disease in a small Inuit Eskimo community in Labrador. The number of children with evidence of otitis media (defined as acute otitis media, or wet or dry perforation) was inversely related to the age at onset of bottle-feeding. History of infant feeding was obtained by interview of the mother at the time of the prevalence study. Children who were bottle-fed at or soon after birth had significantly more disease (67 of 160 children, 42 per cent) than did children who had been bottle-fed after 6 months of breast-feeding (0 of 21 children).

Chandra (1979) reported a significant decrease in episodes of otorrhea (observed or recorded by a nurse midwife) among 35 infants who lived in a rural community in India and were breast-fed for at least 2 months, when they were compared with 35 bottle-fed infants matched for socioeconomic status and family size.

Cunningham (1977) reviewed the medical records of infants who were born at the Mary Imogene Bassett Hospital in Cooperstown, New York, and who were seen regularly in the pediatric clinic in the first year of life. A significant difference in acute lower respiratory tract infections occurred in infants who were breast-fed for at least 4.5 months, when compared with infants who were bottle-fed. The incidence of otitis media was lower in the breast-fed infants, but the difference was not statistically significant.

These studies suggest that breast-feeding does have a protective effect against infections of the middle ear in some populations. However, results are not conclusive because one or more significant defects in design is present in each of the studies, including retrospective analysis of records, otoscopic examination at one point in time to determine prior disease history, lack of uniform criteria for diagnosis, lack of standardization, absence of multivariable analysis or failure to control adequately for other variables, and insufficient sample size to provide appropriate analysis of confounding variables.

Saarinen (1982) followed 256 healthy term infants from birth through the first 3 years of life. Breast-feeding was categorized as long (only source of milk until 6 months or more), intermediate (2 to 6 months), and little or none (2 months). The incidence of otitis media was inversely associated with the duration of breast-feeding. The differences persisted up to age 3 years. No differences were associated with other respiratory tract infections.

In the Boston study children were followed from birth, with frequent examinations and frequent assessments of the mode of feeding (Teele et al., 1989). A large number of children were studied (692), and multivariable analysis was performed; 31.2 per cent of children were breast-fed at some time. Breast-feeding was associated significantly with decreased risk of recurrent acute otitis media (three or more episodes) by age 1 year but not by 3 years of age. Because the first year of life appears to be the most critical period in which middle-ear disease contributes to morbidity, method of feeding may be important, as it alters the risk for recurrent disease during the first year of life.

These studies do not provide reasons for the effect of feeding method on disease resulting from middle-ear infection. Is breastfeeding beneficial, or is bottle-feeding harmful? A number of hypotheses have been suggested:

1. Immunologic factors of value are provided in breast milk, and these prevent various bacterial and viral infections. Breast milk contains important antiinfective agents, including immunoglobulins (secretory IgA and IgG), various leukocytes (B cells, T cells, macrophages, and neutrophils), and components of complement. Although there is an abundant literature about specific factors in breast milk that may protect against enteric infection, there is a paucity of information about materials in breast milk that might protect against respiratory tract infections. Colostrum and, to a lesser extent, breast milk have neutralizing activity to respiratory syncytial virus, but the clinical importance of this immune factor is uncertain (Downham et al., 1976).

2. Allergy to one or more components in cow's milk or formula may result in alteration of the mucosa of the eustachian tube and middle ear.

3. Nonimmune components in breast milk may also play a role, including antiviral factors (interferon) and antibacterial factors (lactoferrin and lysozyme). Breast milk prevents the attachment of pneumococci and

Haemophilus influenzae to epithelial cells. The antiattachment capability for pneumococci was identified in a high- and a low-molecular-weight fraction of breast milk without detectable antibody. These studies suggest that breast milk prevents adhesion of these organisms to respiratory mucosa, the initial factor in infection in the respiratory tract (Hanson et al., 1985).

4. The facial musculature of breast-fed infants develops differently from that of bottle-fed infants. The muscles may affect eustachian tube function and assist in promoting the drainage of middle-ear fluids.

5. Aspiration of fluids into the middle ear occurs during bottle-feeding because the bottle-fed infant is required to produce high negative intraoral pressure, whereas breast-feeding involves nipple massage and reflex "let-down" of milk.

6. The breast-fed infant is maintained in a vertical or semivertical reclining position, whereas the bottle-fed infant is placed in a reclining or horizontal position. The horizontal position may result in reflux of milk through the wide and horizontal eustachian tube. The practice of propping a bottle in bed has been criticized because fluids are forced under pressure into the oral cavity, with possible reflux into the middle ear.

The results of a study of children with cleft palate appear to diminish the importance of the positional advantage of breast-feeding (Paradise and Elster, 1984). None of the 222 infants fed formula only was free of ear effusion at any examination during the first 18 months of life; whereas, in 11 of 30 infants fed breast milk, one or both ears were free of effusion at one or more examinations. The results suggest that breast milk protected infants in spite of the severe anatomic disability. Because all feedings, of breast milk or formula, were given via an artificial feeder, the protection afforded the infants was more likely to be a quality of the milk rather than the mode of feeding.

Effect of Altered Host Defenses or Underlying Disease

Although the vast majority of children have no obvious defect responsible for chronic otitis media with effusion, a small number may have altered host defenses, including anatomic changes (cleft palate, cleft uvula, and submucous cleft), alteration of normal physiologic defenses (patulous eustachian tube or barotrauma), congenital or acquired immunologic deficiencies (immunoglobulin deficiencies or chronic granulomatous disease), or presence of malignancies or use of drugs that suppress immune processes. Active middle-ear disease is almost constant in children with cleft palate. Some patients may have disease states, such as nasopharyngeal tumors or connective tissue disorders, that lead to otitis media. An increased incidence of otitis media occurs in children with Down syndrome (Schwartz and Schwartz, 1978). These conditions are too infrequent to affect epidemiologic studies but should be considered in management of individual patients.

Local and systemic bacterial infections, including otitis media, are early manifestations of acquired immunodeficiency syndrome (AIDS) in infants. Recurrent episodes of acute otitis media are seen in 10 to 50 per cent of these infants (Ammann and Shannon, 1985). Data about pediatric AIDS are increasing with such rapidity that the interested physician requires current information.*

Various procedures in the nose, throat, or airway may increase susceptibility to infection in the middle ear. Nasotracheal intubation was identified as a factor in development of middle-ear effusion in neonates (Balkany et al., 1978). A similar observation was made in children 2 days to 5 years of age in an intensive-care unit; nasotracheal, but not nasogastric, intubation was associated with development of middle-ear effusion. Effusion was identified within 4 days of intubation and appeared earlier in the ear on the side of intubation than in the contralateral ear (Persico et al., 1985).

ANATOMY OF NASOPHARYNX–EUSTACHIAN TUBE–MIDDLE EAR SYSTEM

The middle ear is part of a system of contiguous organs, including the nose, nasopharynx, eustachian tube, middle ear, and mastoid (Fig. 21–2). Respiratory mucosa is continuous through the system. Thus, signs and effects of inflammation, infection, or obstruction in one area are likely to be reflected in other areas.

Nasopharynx

The nasopharynx lies behind the nasal cavities and above the soft palate. Unlike the oral cavity, it is

*The most valuable resource for such information is Morbidity and Mortality Weekly Reports prepared by the Centers for Disease Control, Atlanta, GA, available through the Massachusetts Medical Society C.S.P.O., Box 9120, Waltham, MA 02254-9120.

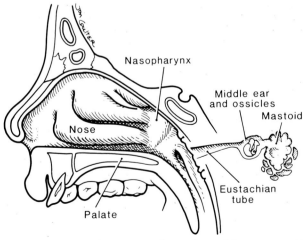

Figure 21–2. Nasopharynx–eustachian tube–middle ear–mastoid system.

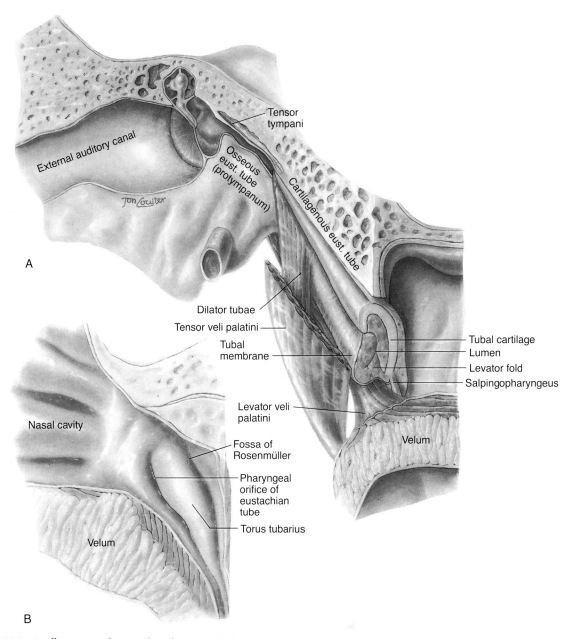

Figure 21–3. *A,* **Illustration of a complete dissection of the eustachian tube and middle ear. Especially evident are the relations of the eustachian tube, paratubal muscles, and cranial base, as well as the positioning of the juncture between the osseous portion of the eustachian tube and the middle ear.** *B,* **Appearance of the nasopharyngeal orifice of the eustachian tube. Note the large torus tubarius and its inferior continuation at the salpingopharyngeal fold.**

continually patent, communicating with the nasal cavities anteriorly via the paired choanae. The communication with the oral cavity is by means of the velopharyngeal port, which may be closed by elevation of the soft palate (its inferior boundary) and inward movement of the constrictor muscles of the oropharynx. On the lateral wall is a prominence, the torus tubarius, which protrudes into the nasopharynx. This prominence is formed by the abundant soft tissue overlying the cartilage of the eustachian tube. Anterior to this is the triangularly shaped nasopharyngeal orifice of the tube. From the torus a raised ridge of mucous membrane, the salpingopharyngeal fold, descends vertically. On the posterior wall lie the adenoids, or pharyngeal tonsil, composed of abundant lymphoid tissue.

Above the tonsil is a variable depression within the mucous membrane called the pharyngeal bursa. Behind the torus lies a deep pocket, extending the nasopharynx posteriorly along the medial border of the eustachian tube. This pocket, the fossa of Rosenmüller (Fig. 21–3), varies in height from 8 to 10 mm and in depth from 3 to 10 mm (Proctor, 1967). Adenoid tissue usually extends into this pocket, giving soft tissue support to the tube.

Eustachian Tube

In adults the tube lies at an angle of 45 degrees in relation to the horizontal plane, whereas in infants this

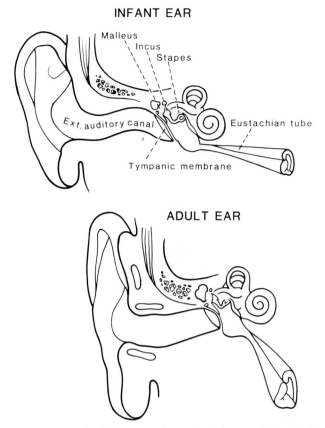

INFANT EAR

Malleus
Incus
Stapes
Ext. auditory canal
Eustachian tube
Tympanic membrane

ADULT EAR

Figure 21–4. The difference in the angle of the eustachian tube in infants and adults.

inclination is only 10 degrees (Proctor, 1967) (Fig. 21–4). The tube is longer in the adult than in the infant and young child, and its length varies with race; it has been reported to be as short as 30 mm (Speilberg, 1927) and as long as 40 mm (Bacher, 1912), but the usual range of length reported in the literature is 31 to 38 mm (Anson, 1967; Anson and Donaldson, 1967; Doyle, 1977; Goss, 1967; Macbeth, 1960; Proctor, 1967). It is generally accepted that the posterior third (11 to 14 mm) of the adult tube is osseous and the anterior two thirds (20 to 25 mm) is composed of membrane and cartilage (Graves and Edwards, 1944; Proctor, 1967).

The morphologic configuration of the eustachian tube and relation to other structures are presented in Figure 21–3A. The osseous eustachian tube (protympanum) lies completely within the petrous portion of the temporal bone and is directly continuous with the anterior wall of the superior portion of the middle ear. The juncture of the osseous tube and the epitympanum lies 4 mm above the floor of the tympanic cavity (Graves and Edwards, 1944). This relationship, although valid, is misrepresented in the more popular descriptions and depictions of the eustachian tube–middle ear juncture and is of some importance in the functional clearance of middle-ear fluids. As depicted in Figure 21–5, the course of the osseous tube is linear anteromedially, following the petrous apex and deviating little from the horizontal plane. The lumen is

roughly triangular, measuring 2 to 3 mm vertically and 3 to 4 mm along the horizontal base. The healthy osseous portion is open at all times, in contrast to the fibrocartilaginous portion, which is closed at rest and opens during swallowing or when forced open, such as during the Valsalva maneuver. The osseous and cartilaginous portions of the eustachian tube meet at an irregular bony surface and form an angle of about 160 degrees with each other. The medial wall of the bony portion of the eustachian tube consists of two parts: posterolateral (labyrinthine) and anteromedial (carotid), whose size, shape, and relations depend on the position of the internal carotid artery (Savic and Djeric, 1985). The average thickness of the anteromedial portion is 1.5 to 3 mm, and in 2 per cent of individuals the wall is absent, exposing the carotid artery.

The cartilaginous tube then courses anteromedially and inferiorly, angled in most cases 30 to 40 degrees to the transverse plane and 45 degrees to the sagittal plane (Graves and Edwards, 1944). The tube is closely applied to the basal aspect of the skull and is fitted to a sulcus tubae between the greater wing of the sphenoid bone and the petrous portion of the temporal bone. The cartilaginous tube is firmly attached at its posterior end to the osseous orifice by fibrous bands and usually extends some distance (3 mm) into the osseous portion of the tube. At its inferomedial end it is attached to a tubercle on the posterior edge of the medial pterygoid lamina (Anson and Donaldson, 1967; Bryant, 1907; Doyle, 1977; Graves and Edwards, 1944; Proctor, 1967; Rood and Doyle, 1982).

The cartilaginous tube has a crook-shaped mediolateral superior wall (Fig. 21–6). It is completed laterally and inferiorly by a veiled membrane (Terracol et al., 1949; Anson, 1967; Proctor, 1967), which serves as the site for the attachment of the fibers of the dilator tubae, or tensor veli palatini muscle (Bryant, 1907; Rood and Doyle, 1978). The tubal lumen is shaped like two cones joined at their apexes. The juncture of the cones is the narrowest point of the lumen and has been called the isthmus, and its position is usually described as at or near the juncture of the osseous and cartilaginous portions of the tube. The lumen at this point is approximately 2 mm high and 1 mm wide (Proctor, 1967). From the isthmus, the lumen expands to approximately 8 to 10 mm in height and 1 to 2 mm in diameter at the pharyngeal orifice (Rees-Jones and McGibbon, 1941). Tubal cartilage increases in mass from birth to puberty (Fig. 21–7), and this development has physiologic implications (Todhunter et al., 1984; Kitajiri et al., 1987) (see discussion of physiology, pathophysiology, and pathogenesis below, p. 342).

The cartilaginous eustachian tube does not follow a straight course in the adult but extends along a curve from the junction of the osseous and cartilaginous portions to the medial pterygoid plate, approximating the cranial base for the greater part of its course. The eustachian tube crosses the superior border of the superior constrictor muscle immediately posterior to

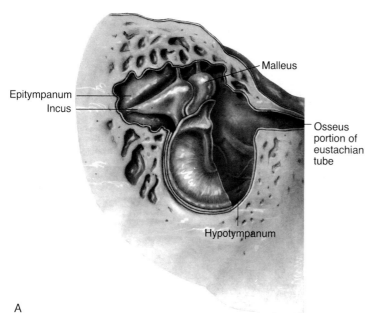

A

Figure 21–5. The anatomy of the aural portion of the eustachian tube as viewed from the external canal (upper). Note that the orifice of the eustachian tube is relatively high in the middle ear. Coronal section through middle ear (lower).

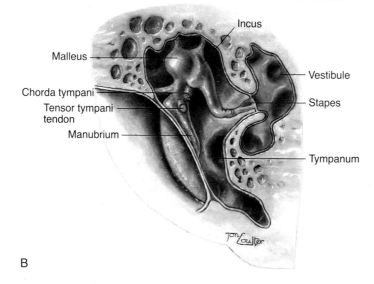

B

its terminus within the nasopharynx. The thickened anterior fibrous investment of the medial cartilage of the tube presses against the pharyngeal wall to form a prominent fold, the torus tubarius, which measures 10 to 15 mm in thickness (Proctor, 1967). The torus is the site of origin of the salpingopalatine muscle (Simkins, 1943) and is the point of origin of the salpingopharyngeal muscle, which lies within the inferoposteriorly directed salpingopharyngeal fold (Rosen, 1970) (see Fig. 21–3B).

The mucosal lining of the eustachian tube is continuous with that of the nasopharynx and middle ear and is characterized as respiratory epithelium. Structural differentiation of this mucosal lining is evident; mucous glands predominate at the nasopharyngeal orifice, and there is graded change to a mixture of goblet, columnar, and ciliated cells near the tympanum (Tos, 1984).

Muscles Associated with Eustachian Tube

Traditionally there are four muscles that are commonly cited as being associated with the eustachian tube: tensor veli palatini, levator veli palatini, salpingopharyngeus, and tensor tympani. Each has at one time or another been directly or indirectly implicated in tubal function (Anson, 1967; Brash, 1951; Bryant, 1907; Goss, 1967; Rood, 1973; Thomsen, 1957; Van Dishoeck, 1947).

Usually the eustachian tube is closed; it opens during such actions as swallowing, yawning, or sneezing and thereby permits the equalization of middle-ear and atmospheric pressures. Although controversy still exists as to the mechanism of tubal dilatation, most anatomic and physiologic evidence supports active dilatation induced solely by the tensor veli palatini muscle (Cantekin et al., 1979a; Honjo et al., 1979;

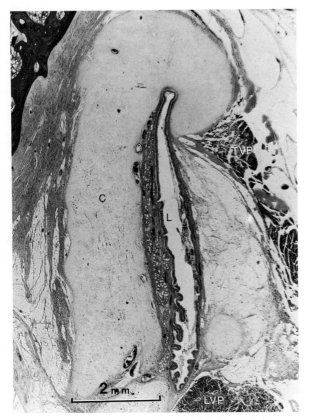

Figure 21–6. Midcartilaginous portion of normal eustachian tube of adult (vertical section). L, Tubal lumen; C, tubal cartilage; TVP, tensor veli palatini; LVP, levator veli palatini. (Courtesy of I. Sando, M.D.)

Rich, 1920*b*). Closure of the tube has been attributed to passive reapproximation of tubal walls by extrinsic forces exerted by the surrounding deformed tissues, by the recoil of elastic fibers within the tubal wall, or by both mechanisms. More recent experimental and clinical data suggest that, at least for certain abnormal populations, the closely applied internal pterygoid muscle may assist tubal closure by an increase in its mass within the pterygoid fossa; this increase applies medial pressure to the tensor veli palatini muscle and consequently to the lateral membranous wall of the eustachian tube (Cantekin et al., 1979*a*; Doyle et al., 1980*b*; Ross, 1971).

The tensor veli palatini is composed of two fairly distinct bundles of muscle fibers divided by a layer of fibroelastic tissue. The bundles lie mediolateral to the tube. The more lateral bundle (the tensor veli palatini proper) is of an inverted triangular design, taking its origin from the scaphoid fossa and entire lateral osseous ridge of the sulcus tubae for the course of the eustachian tube (see Fig. 21–3A). The bundles descend anteriorly, laterally, and inferiorly to converge in a tendon that rounds the hamular process of the medial pterygoid lamina about an interposed bursa (Fig. 21–8). This fiber group then inserts into the posterior border of the horizontal process of the palatine bone and into the palatine aponeurosis of the anterior portion of the velum (Fig. 21–9). The more posteroinferior

muscle fibers lack an osseous origin, extending instead into the semicanal of the tensor tympani muscle. Here, the latter group of muscle fibers receive a second muscle slip, which originates from the tubal cartilages and sphenoid bone. These muscle masses converge to a tendon that rounds the cochleariform process and inserts into the manubrium of the malleus (Fig. 21–10). This arrangement imposes a bipennate form to the tensor tympani muscle (Lupin, 1969; Rood and Doyle, 1978). The tensor tympani does not appear to be involved in the function of the eustachian tube (Honjo et al., 1983).

The medial bundle of the tensor veli palatini muscle lies immediately adjacent to the lateral membranous wall of the eustachian tube and is called the dilator tubae muscle (Goss, 1967; Rood and Doyle, 1978). It takes its superior origin from the posterior third of the lateral membranous wall of the eustachian tube. The fibers descend sharply to enter and blend with the fibers of the lateral bundle of the tensor veli palatini muscle. It is this inner bundle that is responsible for active dilatation of the tube by inferolateral displacement of the membranous wall (Rood, 1973; Rood and Doyle, 1978; Ross, 1971).

The levator veli palatini muscle arises from the inferior aspect of the petrous apex and from the lower border of the medial lamina of the tubal cartilage. The fibers pass inferomedially, paralleling the tubal carti-

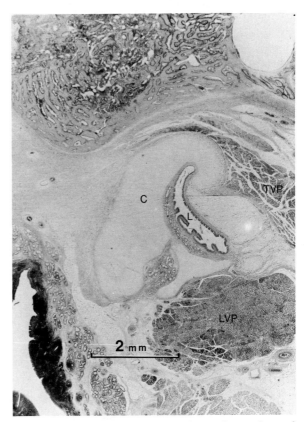

Figure 21–7. Midcartilaginous portion of normal eustachian tube of 1-day-old girl. Note size of cartilage (C) compared with that of adult (Fig. 21–6). L, Tubal lumen; TVP, tensor veli palatini; LVP, levator veli palatini. (Courtesy of I. Sando, M.D.)

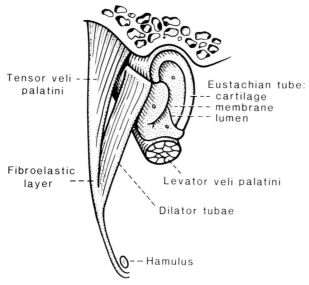

Figure 21–8. Diagrammatic representation of the relationship between the superficial muscle bundle (tensor veli palatini) and the deep bundle (dilator tubae) to the lateral wall of the eustachian tube.

lage and lying within the vault of the tubal floor (see Fig. 21–3A). They fan out and blend with the dorsal surface of the soft palate (Bryant, 1907; Graves and Edwards, 1944; Rood, 1973). Most investigators deny a tubal origin for this muscle and believe that it is related to the tube only by loose connective tissue (McMyn, 1940; Simkins, 1943). The levator is not an active opener of the tube but probably adds support (Cantekin et al., 1983a).

The salpingopharyngeal muscle arises from the medial and inferior borders of the tubal cartilage via slips

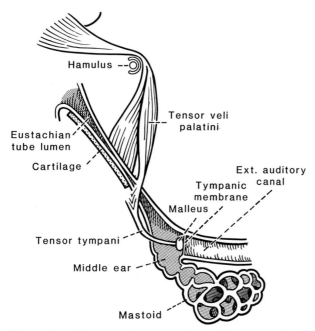

Figure 21–9. Diagrammatic representation of the tensor veli palatini muscle attachment along the lateral wall of the eustachian tube, its course around the hamulus of the pterygoid bone, and its attachment into the posterior margin of the hard palate.

of muscular and tendinous fibers (see Fig. 21–3A). The muscle then courses inferoposteriorly to blend with the mass of the palatopharyngeal muscle (Graves and Edwards, 1944; McMyn, 1940). Rosen (1970) examined ten hemisected human heads and identified the muscle in nine specimens. However, in all cases the muscle fibers were few in number and appeared to lack any ability to perform physiologically.

Blood Supply

Five arteries constitute the blood supply to the eustachian tube: the ascending palatine artery, the pharyngeal branch of the internal maxillary artery, the artery of the pterygoid canal, the ascending pharyngeal artery, and the middle meningeal artery. The venous drainage is via the pterygoid venous plexus (Graves and Edwards, 1944).

Lymph Supply

An extensive lymph network is maintained in the tunica propria of the submucosa of the eustachian tube, and it is more abundant in the cartilaginous portion than in the osseous portion. This network drains into either the retropharyngeal nodes medially or the deep cervical nodes laterally (Graves and Edwards, 1944). Early investigators (Gerlach, 1874, cited in Proctor, 1967) described a lymphoid mass within the tube of a 6-month-old infant. However, Wolff (1934), in an examination of 250 subjects, and Aschan (1954), in a histologic study of 39 eustachian tubes, failed to find such a structure. Further, in a study of the developmental anatomy of the tubal system, Rood and Doyle (1982) failed to find this lymphoid mass and concluded with Wolff and Aschan that this tubal tonsil was a rare pathologic abnormality.

Nerve Supply

The pharyngeal orifice of the eustachian tube is innervated by a branch from the otic ganglion, the sphenopalatine nerve, and the pharyngeal plexus. The remainder of the tube receives its sensory innervation from the tympanic plexus and the pharyngeal plexus. The glossopharyngeal nerve probably plays the predominant role in tubal innervation. Sympathetic innervation of the tube depends on the sphenopalatine ganglion, the otic ganglion, paired glossopharyngeal nerves, the petrosal nerves, and the caroticotympanic nerve (Proctor, 1967). Mitchell (1954) suggested that the parasympathetic nerve supply is derived from the tympanic branch of the glossopharyngeal nerve. Nathanson and Jackson (1976) provided experimental evidence for a secondary parasympathetic innervation via the vidian nerve from the sphenopalatine ganglion. Innervation of the tensor veli palatine is from the ventromedial part of the ipsilateral trigeminal motor nucleus through the trigeminal nerve (mandibular division), and the levator veli palatini muscle receives

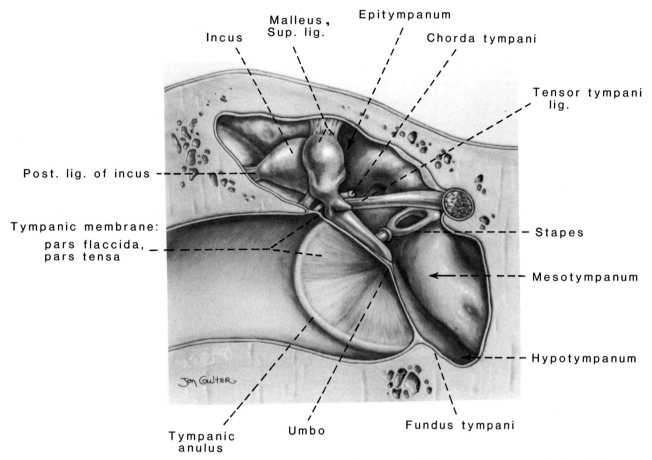

Figure 21–10. The tensor tympani inserts into the manubrium of the malleus as viewed from anterior to posterior in the middle ear.

its innervation from the nucleus ambiguus through the vagus nerve (Eden and Gannon, 1987; Ito et al., 1987).

Infant Eustachian Tube

The eustachian tube in the infant is about half as long as that in the adult; it averages about 18 mm. The cartilaginous tube represents somewhat less than two thirds of this distance, whereas the osseous portion is relatively longer and wider in diameter than it is in the adult. The height of the pharyngeal orifice of the infant eustachian tube is about one half that of the adult, but the width is similar. The ostium of the tube is more exposed in the infant than it is in the adult, as it lies lower in the shallower nasopharyngeal vault. The direction of the tube varies, from horizontal to an angle of about 10 degrees to the horizontal, and the tube is not angulated at the isthmus but merely narrows (Graves and Edwards, 1944) (see Fig. 21–4). Holborow (1975) demonstrated that in infants the medial cartilaginous lamina is relatively shorter because there is less tubal mass and stiffness in the infant tube than in that of the older child and adult (see Fig. 21–7). The tensor veli palatini muscle is less efficient in the infant.

Middle Ear

The middle ear is an irregular, laterally compressed, air-filled space lying within the petrous portion of the temporal bone between the external auditory canal and the inner ear (Fig. 21–11). This cavity can be considered to be divided into three parts superoinferiorly in relation to the tympanic membrane. The epitympanum, or attic, refers to that space lying above the superior border of the tympanic membrane. The mesotympanum lies opposite the membrane, and the hypotympanum lies below the membrane. At birth, the cavity and associated structures are of adult size. The vertical and anteroposterior diameters measure about 15 mm, whereas the transverse diameter measures 4 mm at the epitympanum, 2 mm at the mesotympanum, and 6 mm at the hypotympanum (Goss, 1967). Because of these dimensions, the middle ear has been termed a cleft or a narrow box.

Walls of Middle Ear and Contiguous Structures

The middle ear and its relation to contiguous structures are depicted in Figure 21–12. Superiorly, the cavity is bounded by a thin plate of bone, the tegmen tympani, which extends forward to cover the semicanal of the tensor tympani muscle and posteriorly to cover the attic, thereby isolating the middle ear from the middle cranial fossa. The floor of the cavity consists of a bony plate that separates the cavity anteriorly from the jugular fossa and the posterior wall of the ascending

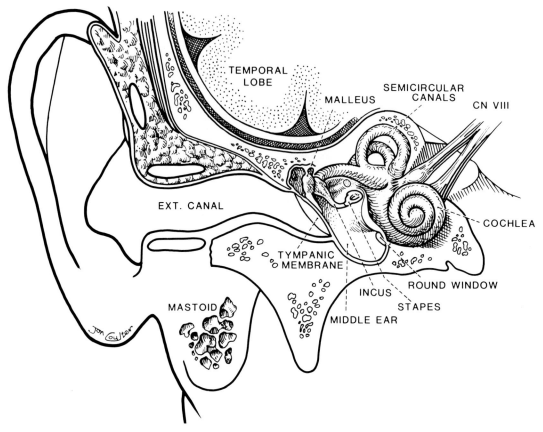

Figure 21–11. Illustration of relation of middle ear to external and inner ears. (From Bluestone, C. D., and Klein, J. O. 1988. Otitis Media in Infants and Children. Philadelphia, W. B. Saunders Co.)

portion of the carotid canal. Dehiscences are common in these bony structures occupying the floor of the middle ear.

Anteriorly, the floor of the middle ear cavity is raised to become continuous with that of the bony portion of the eustachian tube. Superiorly and beneath the tegmen tympani lies the cylindric semicanal for the tensor tympani muscle, which is separated from the eustachian tube by an upwardly concave thin bony septum, the cochleariform process. This process enters the middle ear along its superomedial margin to end just above the oval window, at which point it flares laterally. This termination of the cochleariform process serves as a pulley about which the tendon of the tensor tympani muscle makes a right-angled turn to proceed laterally to its insertion on the muscular process of the malleus.

The middle ear is bounded medially by the lateral surface of the bone covering the labyrinth of the inner ear. The bone is twice interrupted by areas of middle ear–inner ear communication (the oval window and the round window). The oval window is an opening leading from the middle ear into the vestibule of the inner ear. It is located at about the level of the superior border of the tympanic membrane. The raised facial prominence demarcating the position of the bony canal of the facial nerve is immediately superior to the oval window and curves vertically downward along its posterior border. The footplate of the stapes occupies the window and is tightly tied to the margin by an annular ligament. The round window is situated below and behind the oval window and is located within a funneled depression, the round window niche. The window is closed by the secondary tympanic membrane, which consists of three layers: a lateral mucosal layer derived from the middle-ear lining, an internal layer derived from the lining of the cochlea, and an intermediate fibrous layer. The membrane is drawn into the cochlea, giving it a concave appearance from the middle ear. A bulbous, hollowed prominence formed by the outward projection of the basal turn of the cochlea occupies the position between the oval and round windows. This structure, the promontory, is cross-hatched by the various branches of the tympanic plexus of nerves.

The lateral wall is formed by the tympanic membrane (eardrum), the tympanic ring, and a portion of the squamous temporal bone called the septum. The

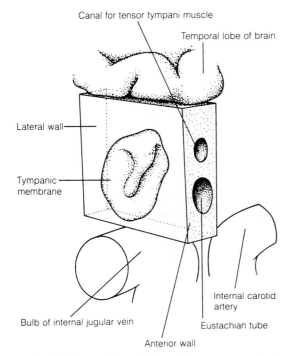

Figure 21–12. Relation of the middle ear to surrounding structures. (With permission from Klein, J. O., and Daum, R. S. The Diagnosis and Management of the Patient with Otitis Media. Copyright © Biomedical Information Corporation, New York, 1985.)

tympanic ring is superiorly incomplete, thereby forming the notch of Rivinus.

The posterior border of the middle ear is demarcated by the anterior wall of the mastoid cavity, pyramidal prominence, and mastoid antrum. The pyramidal prominence is a hollow, forward-projecting bony pyramid located behind the round window and anterior to the vertical portion of the facial nerve. It contains the stapedius muscle, whose tendon exits through a small hole in the apex of the pyramid. A small branch of the facial nerve pierces the pyramid to innervate the stapedius muscle. In the posterior part of the epitympanum is a small depression that lodges the short process of the incus.

Mucosa

The mucous membrane of the middle ear and mastoid is continuous with that of the nasopharynx via the eustachian tube. This membrane covers all structures within the middle ear, including the ossicles, vessels, and nerves. Examination of cells of the mucous membrane within the tympanic cavity reveals a gradual change from tall, columnar cells with interspersed goblet cells to shorter cuboid cells at the posterior portion of the promontory and aditus ad antrum (Fig. 21–13).

Nerve Supply

The tympanic cavity and contained structures are innervated by branches of the tympanic plexus of nerves. Jacobson nerve, a branch of the glossopharyngeal nerve, enters the cavity through its floor, divides, and ramifies about the promontory to contribute to the plexus (Fig. 21–14). The tympanic plexus has connections to the ventral subnucleus of ipsilateral nucleus of the solitary tract within the brain stem, which has been postulated to provide sensory input from middle-ear chemoreceptors, baroreceptors, or both, and thus is related to middle-ear aeration (Eden and Gannon, 1987).

Sympathetic innervation to the plexus is provided by the superior and inferior caroticotympanic nerves and parasympathetic fibers by the smaller superficial petrosal nerve. Oyagi and coworkers (1987) described sympathetic innervation of the middle-ear mucosa as arising from the ipsilateral superior cervical ganglion and not the stellar ganglion. In addition, they showed that parasympathetic fibers probably arise from the ipsilateral pterygopalatine ganglion.

Also contained within the middle-ear cavity is the chorda tympani nerve, which arises from the sensory part of the descending facial nerve. It enters the cavity through the iter chordae posterior, traverses the cavity by crossing the manubrium of the malleus and the long process of the incus, and exits via the iter chordae anterior. The tensor tympani muscle receives its innervation from the trigeminal nerve; the motor neurons are from an area just ventral to the ipsilateral trigeminal motor nucleus (Ito et al., 1987). The stapedius muscle derives its innervation from the facial nerve.

Tympanic Membrane

The eardrum is a thin, semitransparent membrane that separates the middle ear from the external-ear

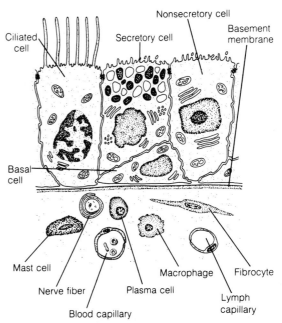

Figure 21–13. Mucosa of the middle ear. (Adapted with permission from Klein, J. O., and Daum, R. S. The Diagnosis and Management of the Patient with Otitis Media. Copyright © Biomedical Information Corporation, New York, 1985.)

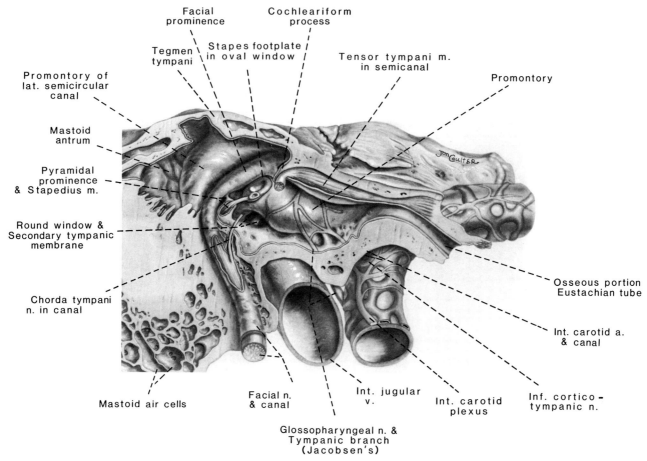

Figure 21–14. The innervation of the middle ear as depicted from lateral to medial.

canal. It measures about 8 to 10 mm in diameter and is positioned downward and inward. The outer margin is thickened and forms a fibrocartilaginous ring, the tympanic annulus, which is fitted into a sulcus in the bony tympanic ring. Superiorly, where the ring is deficient, the eardrum is lax and thin. This triangular region of the eardrum is called the pars flaccida, or flaccid part, and communication between the external and middle ears may occur in this area. The remaining eight ninths of the eardrum is called the pars tensa. The most depressed part of this concavity is called the umbo. The tympanic membrane has three layers. The most lateral layer is derived from the skin of the external-ear canal. The medial layer is derived from the mucous membrane of the middle ear. The intermediate fibrous layer consists of two sublayers: a radial layer with fibers diverging out from the manubrium like the spokes on a bicycle tire, and a circumferential layer with abundant fibers near the circumference and few fibers near the center.

Ossicles

Tiny bones, or ossicles, bridge the middle-ear cavity and provide a mechanical transmission of vibrations from the eardrum to the oval window and inner ear (Fig. 21–15). The most lateral of these is the malleus.

The malleus has a superior rounded head containing a posteriorly facing facet for articulation with the incus, a neck from which various processes are extended, and a manubrium, or handle, which is connected to the tympanic membrane on its internal surface. These ligaments attach to the processes arising from the neck, and they support the malleus within the cavity. The tendon of the tensor tympani muscle is inserted on a posteriorly directed muscular process. The middle ossicle is called the incus and has a body and two crura, or legs, which project at right angles to each other. The body is compressed transversely and pre-

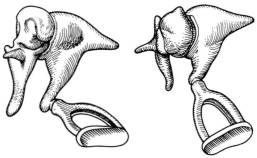

Figure 21–15. Middle-ear ossicles viewed from medial to lateral (left) and from above (right). (From Bluestone, C. D., and Klein, J. O. 1988. Otitis Media in Infants and Children. Philadelphia, W. B. Saunders Co.)

sents a concavoconvex facet on its anterior surface for articulation with the head of the malleus. The short crus projects backward and gives rise to a ligament that connects the incus to the fossa incudis of the epitympanic recess. The long crus descends vertically and bends medially to end in a small lens-shaped structure, the lenticular process, which provides an articulating surface for the stapes. The most medial ossicle is the stapes, which has a head, a neck, two crura, and a footplate. The small head presents a concavity at its termination for articulation with the lenticular process of the incus. Below the head, the stapes narrows to its neck, which provides insertion for the stapedius muscle tendon. From the neck the two crura diverge and are connected at their end to the flattened oval footplate. The footplate fills the oval window, to which it is affixed by an annular ligament.

Mastoid Air Space

Directly posterior to the epitympanum is a large air space called the mastoid antrum (see Fig. 21–2). The antrum serves as a patent communication between the middle ear and the mastoid air cells. The mastoid refers to that portion of the petrous temporal bone that lies posterior to the middle-ear cavity. In the adult, the mastoid is extended exteriorly and interiorly to form a process to which the sternocleidomastoid muscle is attached superficially. The mastoid cavity is partitioned by numerous air cells of variable size that intercommunicate in varying ways.

In the young infant, the mastoid process is small and the degree of pneumatization low. By between 5 and 10 years of age, the process of pneumatization is for the most part complete. Incomplete development of the air cell system has been associated with frequent bouts of otitis media in infancy and childhood.

PHYSIOLOGY, PATHOPHYSIOLOGY, AND PATHOGENESIS

The pathogenesis of acute otitis media is likely to occur with the following pattern in most children: the patient has an antecedent event (due to allergy or infection) that results in congestion of the respiratory mucosa throughout the respiratory tract, including the nasopharynx, eustachian tube, and middle ear; congestion of the mucosa in the eustachian tube results in obstruction of the narrowest portion of the tube, the isthmus; secretions of the mucosa of the middle ear have no egress and accumulate in the middle ear; microbial pathogens (bacteria in most cases) may be present in the middle ear and proliferate in the secretions, resulting in a suppurative and symptomatic otitis media. The acute onset of otitis media with effusion, although relatively asymptomatic in children, most likely has a similar sequence of events. For children with recurrent episodes of acute otitis media or otitis media with effusion, anatomic or physiologic abnor-

mality of the eustachian tube appears to be an important, if not the most important, factor. The child with such an underlying abnormality of the eustachian tube may be subject to recurrent episodes of otitis media or persistent fluid in the middle ear. The following discussion considers the physiology of the middle-ear system, including the nasal cavities, eustachian tube, middle ear, and mastoid air cells, and the pathophysiology and pathogenesis of acute otitis media and otitis media with effusion. The reader is also referred to a review of eustachian tube function and its role in otitis media (Bluestone and Doyle, 1985). Other features of physiology, pathophysiology, and pathogenesis are discussed with anatomy, epidemiology, microbiology, and immunology.

Abnormal function of the eustachian tube appears to be the most important factor in the pathogenesis of middle ear disease. This hypothesis was first suggested more than 100 years ago by Politzer (1862). However, later studies (Zollner, 1942; Suehs, 1952; Senturia et al., 1958; Sade, 1966) suggested that otitis media was a disease primarily of the middle-ear mucous membrane and was caused by infection or allergic reactions in this tissue, rather than by dysfunction of the eustachian tube. Related to this hypothesis is the concept that nasopharyngeal infection spreads up the mucosa of the eustachian tube. Figure 21–16 is an attempt to incorporate these hypotheses.

The vast majority of patients with otitis media and related conditions have (or have had in the past) abnormal function of the eustachian tube that may cause secondary mucosal disease of the middle ear, such as inflammation (Bluestone et al., 1972a). Infection results from reflux, aspiration, or insufflation of nasopharyngeal bacteria up the eustachian tube and into the middle ear (Bluestone and Beery, 1976). Inflammation due to infection or possibly allergy may also cause intrinsic mechanical obstruction of the eustachian tube (Bluestone et al., 1977a). Hematogenous spread of bacteria into the middle ear may also result in otitis media, but this is probably an uncommon event. A much smaller number of patients may have primary mucosal disease of the middle ear as a result of allergy (although this has not been proved) or, more rarely, an abnormality of cilia, such as in Kartagener syndrome (Fisher et al., 1978).

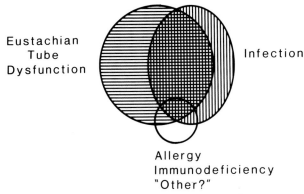

Figure 21–16. Pathogenesis of otitis media.

Physiology of Eustachian Tube and Pathophysiology of Eustachian Tube Dysfunction

The eustachian tube has at least three physiologic functions with respect to the middle ear (Fig. 21–17): (1) ventilation of the middle ear to equilibrate air pressure in the middle ear with atmospheric pressure; (2) drainage and clearance into the nasopharynx of secretions produced within the middle ear; and (3) protection from nasopharyngeal sound pressure and secretions. Even though the ventilatory function is the most important of these functions, the protective, drainage, and clearance functions are reviewed so that

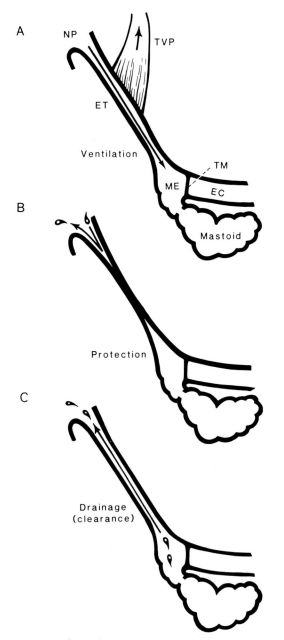

Figure 21–17. Three physiologic functions of the eustachian tube in relation to the middle ear. NP, Nasopharynx; ET, eustachian tube; TVP, tensor veli palatini muscle; ME, middle ear; TM, tympanic membrane; EC, external canal.

the reader will be better able to visualize and understand the ventilatory function; in the following discussion fluid flow through the tube includes gas (airflow) and liquid flow.

Clearance of secretions from the middle ear is provided by the mucociliary system of the eustachian tube and some of the middle-ear mucous membrane. In ideal tubal function, intermittent active opening of the eustachian tube, due only to contraction of the tensor veli palatini muscle during swallowing, maintains nearly ambient pressures in the middle ear (Cantekin et al., 1979a; Honjo et al., 1979; Rich, 1920b). Assessment of these functions has been helpful in understanding the physiology and pathophysiology of eustachian tube function, as well as in the diagnosis and management of children with middle-ear disease.

Protective, Drainage, and Clearance Functions

The clearance and drainage functions of the eustachian tube have been assessed by a variety of methods in the past. By means of radiographic techniques, the flow of contrast media from the middle ear (tympanic membrane not intact) into the nasopharynx has been assessed by Welin (1947), Aschan (1952, 1955), Compere (1960, 1970), Parisier and Khilnani (1970), Bluestone (1971), Bluestone and colleagues (1972a, 1972c), Ferber and Holmquist (1973), and Honjo and coworkers (1981). Rogers and associates (1962) instilled a solution of fluorescein into the middle ear and assessed the clearance function by subsequently examining the pharynx with an ultraviolet light. LaFaye and associates (1974) utilized a radioisotope technique to monitor the flow of saline solution down the eustachian tube. Bauer (1975) assessed clearance by observing methylene blue in the pharynx after it had been instilled into the middle ear. Elbrødn and Larsen (1976) assessed middle ear–eustachian tube mucociliary flow by determining the time that elapsed after saccharin had been placed on the mucous membrane of the middle ear until the subject reported tasting it. Unfortunately, all of these methods are qualitative and actually test eustachian tube patency rather than measure the clearance function of the tube quantitatively.

Even though abnormalities of the protective function are directly related to the pathogenesis of otitis media, this function has been assessed only by radiographic techniques (Bluestone, 1971; Bluestone et al., 1972a, 1972c) by a test that was a modification of a tubal patency test described by Wittenborg and Neuhauser (1963).

COMBINED RADIOGRAPHIC STUDIES

The protective and clearance functions of the eustachian tube have been assessed by a combined radiographic technique (Bluestone et al., 1972a, 1972c). Radiopaque material was instilled through the nose of patients so that the retrograde flow of the medium from the nasopharynx into the eustachian tube could be observed (Fig. 21–18). Patients were considered to have normal protective function when radiopaque material entered only the nasopharyngeal or isthmic portion of the tube and did not enter the bony portion of the tube or middle-ear cavity during swallowing. The normal eustachian tube protected the middle ear from the contrast material even when the liquid was under increased nasopharyngeal pressure during closed-nose swallowing (Fig. 21–19). If, during the retrograde study, contrast medium traversed the entire eustachian tube and refluxed into the middle ear during swallowing, the tube was considered to have increased distensibility and poor protective function (Fig. 21–20).

The effectiveness of the eustachian tube in clearing the radiopaque medium instilled into the middle ear was taken as an indication of the effectiveness of the eustachian tube in the clearance of secretions. Rapid and complete clearance of the medium into the nasopharynx was considered to indicate normal drainage function, whereas failure of the contrast material to drain from the middle ear into the nasopharynx indicated mechanical obstruction of the eustachian tube (Fig. 21–21), especially when contrast material also failed to enter the nasopharyngeal portion of the tube during the retrograde study (Fig. 21–22). These abnormal functions of the tube were found in patients with otitis media and were not found in a small group of normal subjects.

MODEL OF PROTECTIVE AND CLEARANCE FUNCTIONS

Understanding of these radiographic studies can be best shown by a model of the system (Bluestone and Beery, 1976). The eustachian tube, middle ear, and mastoid air cell system can be likened to a flask with a long, narrow neck (Fig. 21–23). The mouth of the flask represents the nasopharyngeal end; the narrow neck, the isthmus of the eustachian tube; and the bulbous portion, the middle ear and mastoid air chamber. Fluid flow through the neck would be dependent on the pressure at either end, the radius and length of the neck, and the viscosity of the liquid. When a small amount of liquid is instilled into the mouth of the flask, liquid flow stops somewhere in the narrow neck owing to capillarity within the neck and the relative positive air pressure that develops in the chamber of the flask. This basic geometric design is considered to be critical for the protective function of the eustachian tube–middle ear system. Reflux of liquid into the body of the flask occurs if the neck is excessively wide. This is analogous to an abnormally patent human eustachian tube, in which there is not only free flow of air from the nasopharynx into the middle ear but also free flow of nasopharyngeal secretions, which can result in "reflux otitis media." Figure 21–24 shows that a flask with a short neck would not be as protective as a flask with a long neck (Bluestone, 1985). Because infants have a shorter eustachian tube than adults, reflux is more likely to occur in the baby. The position of the flask in relation to the liquid is

another important factor. In humans, the supine position enhances flow of liquid into the middle ear; thus, infants might be at particular risk for developing reflux otitis media because they are frequently supine.

Reflux of a liquid into the vessel can also occur if a hole is made in the bulbous portion of the flask (Fig. 21–25B) because this prevents the creation of the slight positive pressure in the bottom of the flask that deters reflux; that is, in this situation the middle-ear and mastoid physiologic cushion of air is lost. This hole is analogous to a perforation of the tympanic membrane or the presence of a tympanostomy tube that could allow reflux of nasopharyngeal secretions as a result of the loss of the middle ear–mastoid air cushion. Similarly, following a radical mastoidectomy, a patent eustachian tube could cause troublesome otorrhea (Bluestone et al., 1978).

If negative pressure is applied to the bottom of the flask, the liquid is aspirated into the vessel (Fig. 21–25C). In the clinical situation represented by the model, high negative middle-ear air pressure could lead to the aspiration of nasopharyngeal secretions into the middle ear. If positive pressure is applied to the mouth of the flask, the liquid is insufflated into the vessel (Fig. 21–25D). Nose-blowing, crying, closed-nose swallowing, diving, or descent in an airplane could create high positive nasopharyngeal pressure and result in a similar condition in the human system.

One of the major differences between a flask with a rigid neck and a biologic structure such as the eustachian tube is that the isthmus (neck) of the human tube is *compliant*. Application of positive pressure at the mouth of a flask with a compliant neck distends the neck, enhancing fluid flow into the vessel. Thus, less positive pressure is required to insufflate liquid into the vessel. In humans, insufflation of nasopharyngeal secretions into the middle ear occurs more readily if the eustachian tube is abnormally distensible (has increased compliance). The effect of applied negative pressure in a flask with a compliant neck is shown in Figure 21–26; liquid flow through the neck does not occur until a negative pressure is slowly applied to the bottom of the flask. In this case, fluid flow occurs even if the neck is collapsed. If the negative pressure is applied suddenly, however, temporary locking of the compliant neck prevents flow of the liquid. Therefore, the speed with which the negative pressure is applied as well as the compliance in such a system appears to be a critical factor in the results obtained. Clinically, aspiration of gas into the middle ear is possible, because negative middle-ear pressure develops slowly as gas is absorbed by the middle-ear mucous membrane. On the other hand, sudden application of negative middle-ear pressure such as occurs with rapid alterations in atmospheric pressure (as in the descent in an airplane, in a descent after diving, or during an attempt to test the ventilatory function of the eustachian tube) could lock the tube, thus preventing the flow of air.

Certain aspects of fluid flow from the middle ear into the nasopharynx can be demonstrated by inverting

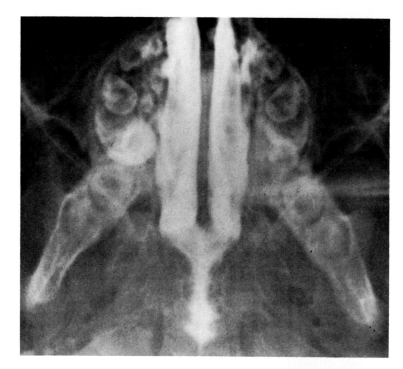

Figure 21–18. Submentovertex roentgenogram of a child without middle-ear disease. Radiopaque contrast material instilled into the nose and nasopharynx did not enter the eustachian tube when the subject did not swallow.

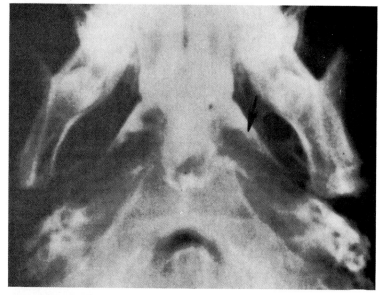

Figure 21–19. Normal retrograde function. During both open-nose and closed-nose swallowing, radiopaque contrast material filled the nasopharyngeal portion of the eustachian tube (arrow) of a child with normal tympanic membranes and a negative otologic history.

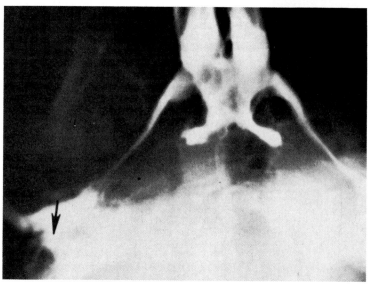

Figure 21–20. Retrograde reflux. Radiograph of a 6-year-old boy with recurrent otitis media with effusion. On open-nose swallowing, contrast material traversed the entire eustachian tube and refluxed into the middle ear and mastoid (arrow).

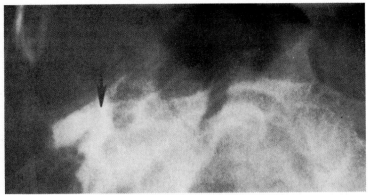

Figure 21-21. Roentgenogram showing prograde obstruction at the middle-ear end of the isthmus of the eustachian tube (arrow). Radiopaque contrast material failed to flow from the middle ear into the nasopharynx.

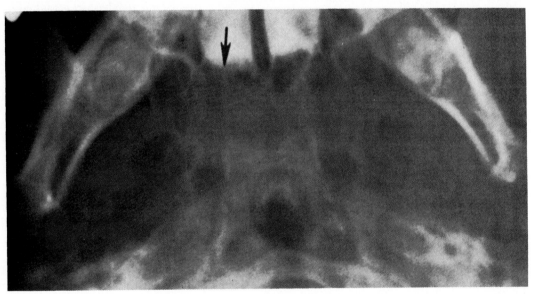

Figure 21-22. Retrograde obstruction. Radiograph of a 5-year-old boy with otitis media. Radiopaque medium failed to enter the nasopharyngeal portion of the eustachian tube during both open-nose and closed-nose swallowing. Note enlarged adenoids (arrow).

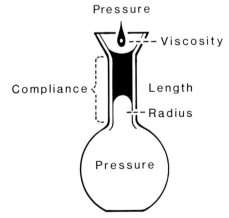

Figure 21-23. Flask model of eustachian tube–middle ear–mastoid air cell system, in which the mouth of the flask represents the nasopharyngeal end of the eustachian tube, the neck is the cartilaginous portion of the tube, and the bulbous portion represents the middle ear and mastoid air cells (see text).

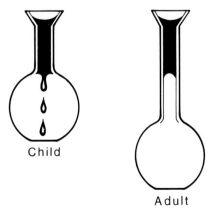

Figure 21-24. Flask model used to show how the shorter length of the eustachian tube can adversely affect the protective function in the child, as compared with the case in the adult.

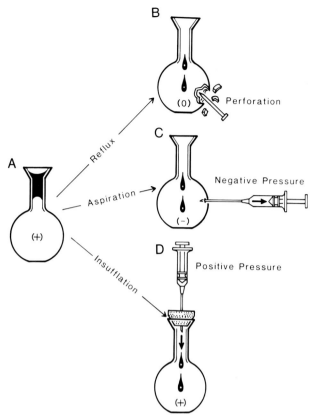

Figure 21–25. Fluid flow into a flask as a model for eustachian tube–middle ear function. *A*, Normal function. *B*, Effect of perforation. *C*, Effect of negative pressure on the bottom of the flask. *D*, Effect of positive pressure on the mouth of the flask.

the flask of the model (Fig. 21–27). In this case the liquid trapped in the bulbous portion of the flask does not flow out of the vessel because of the relative negative pressure that develops inside the chamber. However, if a hole is made in the vessel, the liquid drains out of the flask because the suction is broken. Clinically, these conditions occur in cases of middle-

ear effusion; pressure is relieved by spontaneous rupture of the tympanic membrane or by myringotomy. Inflation of air into the flask could also relieve the pressure, which may explain the frequent success of the Politzer or Valsalva method in clearing a middle-ear effusion.

The examples of fluid flow through a flask (see Figs. 21–23 through 21–27) present some of the mechanical aspects of the physiology of the human middle-ear system. Other factors that can affect flow of liquid and air through the middle ear include (1) the mucociliary transport system of the eustachian tube and middle ear (i.e., clearance) (Sade and Afula, 1967; Sade and Eliezar, 1970); (2) active tubal opening and closing, acting to pump liquid out of the middle ear (Honjo, 1981); and (3) surface tension factors.

The clearance function has been studied by insertion of foreign material into the middle ear of animal models (Albiin et al., 1983; Stenfors et al., 1985). Such material will flow toward the middle-ear portion of the eustachian tube. This movement is related to ciliary activity that occurs in the eustachian tube and parts of the middle ear; these ciliated cells in the middle ear are increasingly more active as their location becomes more distal to the opening of the eustachian tube (Ohashi et al., 1985; Ohashi et al., 1986). In a series of elegant experiments by Honjo (1981, 1985), the eustachian tube was shown to "pump" liquid out of the middle ear in both animal models and humans. However, when negative pressure was present within the middle ear, this function was impaired (Nozoe et al., 1984).

Several investigators have determined certain surface tension factors that could be involved with normal eustachian tube function. Birkin and Brookler (1972) isolated surface tension–lowering substances from washings of eustachian tubes of dogs. They postulated that these substances could act to enhance eustachian tube functions, similar to surfactant in the lung. Rap-

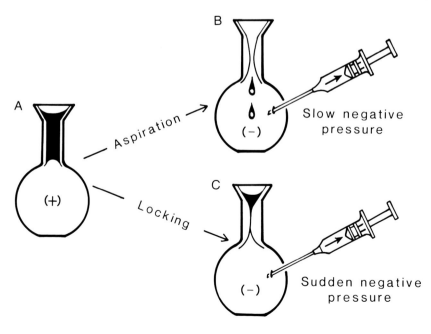

Figure 21–26. Fluid flow through a flask with a compliant neck as model for eustachian tube and middle-ear system. *A*, Fluid stopped in the neck of the flask. *B*, Effect of negative pressure applied slowly to the bottom of the flask. *C*, Effect of negative pressure applied suddenly to the bottom of the flask. (Modified from Bluestone, C. D., and Klein, J. O. 1988. Otitis Media in Infants and Children. Philadelphia, W. B. Saunders Co.)

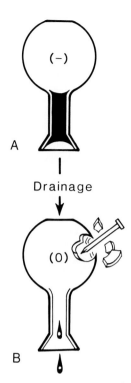

Figure 21–27. Fluid flow from an inverted flask as model for eustachian tube and middle-ear system. A, Fluid trapped by relative negative pressure in the chamber. B, Effect of perforation of the chamber. (Modified from Bluestone, C. D., and Klein, J. O. 1988. Otitis Media in Infants and Children. Philadelphia, W. B. Saunders Co.)

port and colleagues (1975) described a similar substance and demonstrated the effect of washing out the eustachian tube on the opening pressure in the experimental animal; others also have demonstrated a surfactantlike phospholipid in the middle ear and eustachian tube of animals and humans (Hagen, 1977; Hills, 1984a and b; Grace et al., 1987).

From these studies, it is apparent that the drainage and clearance functions of the eustachian tube–middle ear system are important in maintaining a healthy middle ear. Because otitis media is so common in humans, efficient removal of middle-ear effusions must depend, to a large extent, on these functions.

Ventilatory Function

From studies in children, the function of the eustachian tube has been postulated (Bluestone and Beery, 1976). The normal eustachian tube is functionally obstructed or collapsed at rest; there is probably a slight negative pressure in the middle ear. When the eustachian tube functions ideally, intermittent active dilatation (opening) of the tube maintains near-ambient pressures in the middle ear. It is suspected that when active function is inefficient in opening the eustachian tube, functional collapse of the tube persists, which results in negative pressure in the middle ear. When tubal opening does occur, a large bolus of air could enter the middle ear, which could eventually result in

even higher negative pressure (Cantekin et al., 1980b). This type of ventilation appears to be quite common in children, as moderate to high negative middle-ear pressures have been identified by tympanometry in many children who have no apparent ear disease (Beery et al., 1975b).

In an effort to describe normal eustachian tube function by using the microflow technique inside a pressure chamber (see p. 356), Elner and coworkers (1971d) studied 102 adults with intact tympanic membranes and apparently no history of otologic disorder. The patients were divided into four groups according to their abilities to equilibrate static relative positive and negative pressures of 100 mm H$_2$O in the middle ear (Table 21–6). The patients in Group 1 were able to equilibrate pressure differences across the tympanic membrane completely. Those in Group 2 equilibrated positive pressure, but a small residual negative pressure remained in the middle ear. The subjects in Group 3 were capable of equilibrating only relative positive pressure with a small residual remaining, but not negative pressure; those in Group 4 were incapable of equilibrating any pressure. These data probably indicate decreased stiffness of the eustachian tube in the subjects in Groups 2 to 4 when compared with those in Group 1. This study also showed that 95 per cent of normal adults could equilibrate an applied positive pressure and that 93 per cent could equilibrate applied negative pressure to some extent by active swallowing. However, 28 per cent of the subjects could not completely equilibrate either applied positive or negative pressure or both.

Children have less efficient eustachian tube ventilatory function than adults. Bylander (1980) compared the eustachian tube function of 53 children with that of 55 adults, all of whom had intact tympanic membranes and who were apparently otologically healthy. Employing a pressure chamber, Bylander reported that 35.8 per cent of the children could not equilibrate applied negative intratympanic pressure (-100 mm H$_2$O) by swallowing, whereas only 5 per cent of the adults were unable to perform this function. Children between 3 and 6 years of age had worse function than those of ages 7 to 12 years. In this study and a subsequent one conducted by the same research group (Bylander et al., 1983), children who had tympanometric evidence of negative pressure within the middle ear had poor eustachian tube function.

From these two studies, it can be concluded that even in apparently otologically normal children, eustachian tube function is not as good as in adults, which would contribute to the higher incidence of middle-ear disease in children.

Many children without apparent middle-ear disease have high negative ear pressure. However, in children eustachian tube function does improve with advancing age, which is consistent with the decreasing incidence of otitis media from infancy to adolescence (Bylander and Tjernstrom, 1983).

Another explanation for the finding of high negative middle-ear pressure in children is the possibility that

TABLE 21–6. Eustachian Tube Function Test Results of 102 Otologically Normal Adults with Intact Tympanic Membranes

TUBAL FUNCTION GROUP	NUMBER OF SUBJECTS (%)	EQUILIBRATION WHEN MIDDLE PRESSURE IS		TOYNBEE POSITIVE/ NO. TESTED (%)	VALSALVA POSITIVE/ NO. TESTED (%)
		+ 100 mm H_2O	− 100 mm H_2O		
1	74 (72)	Yes	Yes	67/69 (97)	63/73 (86)
2	21 (21)	Yes	Residual	7/18 (39)	16/21 (76)
3	2 (2)	Residual	No	0/2 (0)	2/2 (100)
4	5 (5)	No	No	0/5 (0)	5/5 (100)
TOTAL				74/94 (79)	86/101 (85)

Adapted from Elner, A., et al. 1971. The normal function of the eustachian tube: A study of 102 cases. Acta Otolaryngol. 72:320–328.

some individuals who are habitual "sniffers" actually create underpressure within the middle ear by this act (Falk and Magnuson, 1984). However, this mechanism is uncommon in children.

In studying the measurement of middle-ear pressure, Brooks (1969) determined by tympanometry that the resting middle-ear pressure in a large group of apparently normal children was between 0 and − 175 mm H_2O. However, pressures outside this range have been reported as normal for large populations of apparently asymptomatic children who were measured for middle-ear pressure by screening (Jerger, 1970). High negative middle-ear pressure does not necessarily indicate disease; it may indicate only physiologic tubal obstruction. Ventilation occurs, but only after the nasopharynx–middle ear pressure gradient reaches an opening pressure. It has been suggested that these children probably should be considered at risk for middle-ear problems until more is learned about the normal and abnormal physiology of the eustchian tube (Bluestone et al., 1973). In normal adults, Alberti and Kristensen (1970) obtained resting middle-ear pressures of between 50 and − 50 mm H_2O. Again, a pressure outside this range does not necessarily mean the patient has ear disease.

The *rate of gas absorption* from the middle ear has been reported by several investigators to be approximately 1 ml in a 24-hour period (Elner, 1972, 1977; Ingelstedt et al., 1967b; Riu et al., 1966). However, because values taken over a short period were extrapolated to arrive at this figure, the true rate of gas absorption over 24 hours has yet to be determined in humans.

In a study by Cantekin and coworkers (1980), serial tympanograms were obtained in rhesus monkeys to determine the gas absorption process. During a 4-hour observation period, the middle-ear pressure was approximately normal in alert animals, whereas when the animals were anesthetized and swallowing was absent, the middle-ear pressure dropped to − 60 mm H_2O and remained at that level. The experiment indicated that, normally, middle-ear gases are nearly in equilibrium with the mucosal blood-tissue gases or inner-ear gas pressures. Under these circumstances, the gas absorption rate is small because the partial pressure gradients are not great. In the normally functioning eustachian tube, the frequent openings of the tube readily equilibrate the pressure differences

between the middle ear and the nasopharynx with a small volume of air (1 to 5 µl) entering into the middle ear. However, an abnormally functioning eustachian tube may alter this mechanism.

The physiologic role of the *mastoid air cell system* in relation to the middle ear is not fully understood, but the current concept is that it acts as a surge tank of gas (air) available to the relatively smaller middle-ear cavity. During intervals of eustachian tube dysfunction, the compliance of the tympanic membrane and ossicular chain (which would affect hearing) would not be decreased owing to reduced middle-ear gas pressure because there is a reservoir of gas in the mastoid air cells. If this concept is correct, then a small mastoid air cell system could be detrimental to the middle ear if abnormal eustachian tube function is present.

Posture appears to have an effect on the function of the eustachian tube. The mean volume of air passing through the eustachian tube was found to be reduced by one third when the body was elevated 20 degrees to the horizontal, and by two thirds when in the horizontal position (Ingelstedt et al., 1967a). This reduction in function with change in body position was found to be the result of venous engorgement of the eustachian tube (Jonson and Rundcrantz, 1969).

A *seasonal variation* in eustachian tube function occurs in children (Beery et al., 1979). Children who had had tympanostomy tubes inserted for recurrent or chronic otitis media with effusion and were evaluated using serial inflation-deflation studies had better eustachian tube function in the summer and fall than in the winter and spring.

Classic Methods of Assessment

Until about 1960, most tests of the ventilatory function of the eustachian tube were in reality only assessments of the tubal patency. The classic methods of Valsalva, Toynbee, and Politzer for assessing the eustachian tube are still in use today, as is catheterization of the eustachian tube.

VALSALVA TEST. The effect of high positive nasopharyngeal pressures on the eustachian tube can be evaluated qualitatively by the Valsalva test. The test results are considered to be positive (i.e., normal) when the eustachian tube and middle ear can be inflated by a forced expiration (i.e., with the mouth closed and the nose held by the thumb and forefinger) (see Fig. 21–83). The amount of overpressure thus created is quite variable and may be as much as 2000 mm H_2O.

When the eardrum is intact, the overpressure in the middle ear can be observed as a bulging tympanic membrane by visual inspection of the tympanic membrane with a pneumatic otoscope or, more precisely, with the aid of the otomicroscope and a nonmagnifying Bruening or Siegle otoscope. The tympanic membrane moves inward when positive canal pressure is applied, but outward mobility in response to applied negative canal pressure is decreased or absent if positive pressure is present within the middle ear (Bluestone and Shurin, 1974).

The most accurate method of assessing changes in middle-ear pressure is by tympanometry, but because the positive pressure created in the middle ear for such a test may only be momentary—inflation followed by immediate equilibration prior to tubal closing—the alteration in middle-ear pressure may not be visualized or recorded by tympanometry. When the tympanic membrane is not intact, the sound of the air entering the middle ear can be heard with a stethoscope or with the Toynbee tube. However, these methods are outmoded, and measurements now are made with a manometric system, preferably one equipped with a strip chart recorder.

Unfortunately, regardless of the testing technique or method of assessment, the Valsalva test results are not reliable indicators of eustachian tube function. When positive, they indicate only an anatomically patent and probably distensible eustachian tube. Indeed, without inflation of the middle ear during this test, no useful information concerning tubal function is obtained. Elner and associates (1971*d*) found that 85 per cent of 101 adults with normal ears had positive results on the Valsalva test.

TOYNBEE TEST. In performing the Toynbee test, the subject is asked to swallow when the nose is manually compressed (Fig. 21–28). This maneuver usually creates a positive pressure within the nasopharynx, followed by a negative pressure phase (Perlman, 1951). If the eustachian tube opens during the test, the middle-ear pressure changes; the way in which it changes is determined by the timing of the tubal opening and the nasopharyngeal pressure gradient.

Change in middle-ear pressure is assessed on the Toynbee test in the same way that it is assessed on the Valsalva test. If negative pressure is present within the middle ear, the tympanic membrane will be retracted and will not move inward to applied positive pressure with the pneumatic otoscope. It will move outward to applied negative pressure if the pressure applied exceeds the negative pressure within the middle ear.

The test results are usually considered positive when there is an alteration in the middle-ear pressure. Negative middle-ear pressure after the Toynbee test or only momentary negative middle-ear pressure followed by ambient pressure usually indicates good tubal function, because it shows that the eustachian tube

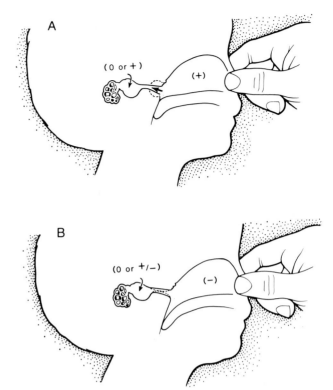

Figure 21–28. The Toynbee test of eustachian tube function. *A*, Positive phase. *B*, Negative phase. Closed-nose swallowing results in first positive pressure in the nose and nasopharynx, followed by a negative-pressure phase. When positive pressure is in the nasopharynx, air may enter the middle ear, creating positive pressure. During or after the negative-pressure phase, negative pressure may develop in the middle ear, or positive pressure may still be in the middle ear (no change in middle-ear pressure during negative phase), or positive pressure may be followed by negative middle-ear pressure, or ambient pressure will be present if equilibration takes place before the tube closes. If the tube does not open during either the positive or negative phase, no change in middle-ear pressure will occur (see text).

can open actively (the tensor veli palatini muscle contracts) and that the tubal structure is sufficiently stiff to withstand nasopharyngeal negative pressure (as noted by absence of temporary tubal locking). However, some abnormal eustachian tubes that are either patulous or have low tubal resistance may transfer gas from the middle ear into the nasopharynx during the Toynbee test (as they may with sniffing). The finding of only positive middle-ear pressure signifies tubal patency but does not have the same significance as does even transitory negative pressure.

Unfortunately, the absence of any alteration in middle-ear pressure during the Toynbee test does not indicate poor eustachian tube function. Zollner (1942) and Thomsen (1958*b*) reported that 30 per cent of the adults with negative ears that they examined had normal results on the Toynbee test. Elner and colleagues (1971*d*) reported that in 21 per cent of 94 normal adults, middle-ear pressure did not change during the Toynbee test. Cantekin and associates (1976) found that only 2 of 49 children with tympanostomy tubes inserted for otitis media with effusion could open their eustachian tubes during the Toynbee maneuver.

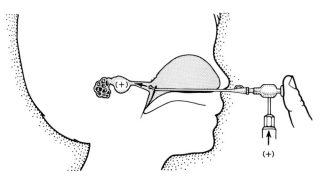

Figure 21–29. Catheterization of the eustachian tube to test patency of the tube.

POLITZER TEST. The Politzer test is performed by compressing one naris into which the end of a rubber tube attached to an air bag has been inserted while the opposite naris is compressed with finger pressure. The subject is asked to repeat the letter K or is asked to swallow to close the velopharyngeal port (see Fig. 21–84). When the test is positive, the overpressure that develops in the nasopharynx is transmitted to the middle ear, thus creating positive middle-ear pressure. Assessment of the middle-ear pressure and the significance of the test results are the same as with the Valsalva test in that an abnormal result indicates only tubal patency. However, both the Valsalva and Politzer methods can be of benefit as a treatment when effusion or high negative pressure is present within the middle ear if the child can successfully inflate the middle ear.

EUSTACHIAN TUBE CATHETERIZATION. Transnasal catheterization of the eustachian tube with the classic metal cannula has been used to assess tubal function for over a century (Fig. 21–29). Cannulation can be performed by blindly rooting for the orifice of the tube, by indirect visualization with a nasopharyngoscope, or via transoral right-angle telescope. Successful transferring of applied positive pressure from the proximal end of the cannula into the middle ear signifies only tubal patency. However, the use of this method as a test or treatment is limited in children, because it can be frightening and difficult to perform.

Tests of Ventilatory Function

The ventilatory function of the eustachian tube can be assessed by manometry, sonometry, and tympanometry. Not yet perfected, sonometry is available for investigation only in the laboratory, but the other two tests can be used in the clinical setting. Some of the manometric tests of eustachian tube function are technologically complicated and are available only in the laboratory; others are quite simple and are available to the clinician.

MANOMETRY

Manometric measurements of tubal function have been conducted for the past 100 years. The simplest techniques involve the placement of an ear canal catheter, with an airtight connection, between a pressure monitoring device and the middle-ear cavity. If the tympanic membrane is not intact, the middle-ear pressure is measured directly (intratympanic manometry); however, if the tympanic membrane is intact, then the middle-ear pressure must be inferred from the pressure change in the ear canal (extratympanic manometry). In both cases, it is a closed pneumatic system.

Recordings obtained by this method when the tympanic membrane is intact are of little value for assessing tubal function because atmospheric pressure changes, the system volume, and the effects of temperature on the system are much more significant than are the small volumes displaced by the tympanic membrane with changes in middle-ear pressure. On the other hand, this technique is a valuable tool for intratympanic applications when the tympanic membrane is not intact. In such cases, a middle-ear pressure application device, such as a syringe or an air pump, is connected to the ear canal through a valve. Using this arrangement, different levels of middle-ear pressure can be generated, and the equilibration capacity of the eustachian tube can be recorded directly as pressure drops after the subject swallows.

The first quantitative tubal function study performed by intratympanic manometry was the systematically conducted inflation-deflation test (Ingelstedt and Ortegren, 1963). Later, numerous investigators employed the same technique to determine tubal function (Miller, 1965; Holmquist, 1969a). The next improvement in this technique was the addition of a flow meter to the manometric system to involve pressure-flow relationships during eustachian tube function testing (Flisberg, 1966). The evaluation of tubal function was limited to the assessment of active function (owing to the contractions of the tensor veli palatini muscle) until Bluestone and coworkers (1972a, 1975a and b) introduced a modified inflation-deflation test by which passive function could also be described by variables such as forced opening pressure and closing pressure of the tube. Later, a device similar to the ear canal catheter was developed for use with the modified inflation-deflation test so that nasopharyngeal pressure could be measured (Cantekin et al., 1976). The forced-response test was developed to test eustachian tube function in the clinical setting when the tympanic membrane is not intact (Cantekin et al., 1979b). This technique seems to discriminate between normal and abnormal eustachian tube function without the overlap encountered in the inflation-deflation test. With the forced-response test, it has also been possible to make a distinction between tubal dysfunction that stems from inefficient active opening of the tube and that which is the result of structural properties of the eustachian tube.

Nonintact Tympanic Membrane
Inflation-Deflation Test. When a perforation of the tympanic membrane or a tympanostomy tube is present, inflation-deflation tests to measure the ventilatory function of the eustachian tube can be performed in

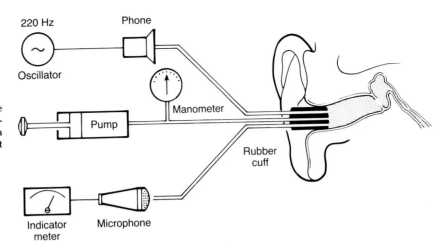

Figure 21–30. Electroacoustic immittance audiometer in which a pump-manometer system is employed for eustachian tube function tests when the tympanic membrane is not intact (see text).

the clinical setting with the pump-manometer portion of an electroacoustic immittance audiometer (Bluestone et al., 1972a) (Fig. 21–30) or a controlled syringe pump and manometer (Bluestone et al., 1977a) (Fig. 21–31).

Figure 21–32 is a simplified explanation of the combined passive and active function test when positive pressure is applied to the middle ear (inflation). This test is similar to ascending in an airplane until the eustachian tube opens passively. It involves the application of enough positive pressure to the middle ear to force the eustachian tube open. The pressure remaining in the middle ear after passive opening and closing is termed the *closing pressure*. Further equilibration of pressure is by swallowing (an active function), which is the result of contraction of the tensor veli palatini muscle (Rich, 1920b; Honjo et al., 1979; Cantekin et al., 1979a). When the muscle contracts, the lumen of the eustachian tube is opened and air flows down the tube. The pressures can be monitored on a strip chart recorder. The pressure remaining in the middle ear after passive and active function is termed the *residual positive pressure*.

Figure 21–33 shows the deflation phase of the study, which is similar to descent in an airplane. Low negative pressure is applied to the middle ear and is then equilibrated by active tubal opening. The pressure remaining in the middle ear after swallowing is termed the *residual negative pressure*.

In certain instances, the ability of the tube to open actively in response to applied low positive pressure is also assessed (Fig. 21–34). This is similar to ascent in an airplane to an altitude lower than a pressure that would force the eustachian tube open. The patient is asked to swallow in an attempt to equilibrate the pressure by active function.

Figure 21–35 shows the symbols employed and examples of results obtained in ventilation studies. Example *A* shows the results of a typical study in a patient with normal eustachian tube function. Following passive opening and closing of the eustachian tube during the inflation phase of the study, the patient was able to completely equilibrate the remaining positive pressure. Active swallowing also completely equilibrated applied negative pressure (deflation). Example *B* shows the results of a typical study in a child who had had otitis media with effusion. The eustachian tube passively opened and closed following inflation, but subsequent swallowing failed to equilibrate the residual positive pressure. In the deflation phase of the study, the child was unable to equilibrate negative pressure. Inflation to a pressure below the opening

Figure 21–31. Equipment employed to test inflation-deflation eustachian tube function when the tympanic membrane is not intact. A closed air pressure system is sealed into the external auditory meatus (ear canal) and into one naris by means of a double-lumen balloon catheter (modified Foley). A constant-speed syringe pump is used for inflation and deflation of the middle ear. The pump delivers constant airflow to the external canal. The volume of airflow is monitored by the piston displacement sensor. The rate of applied pressure is 20 to 30 mm H_2O/second, depending on the subject's middle ear–mastoid volume and the starting position of the pump piston. Middle-ear pressure is measured by a pressure transducer; nasopharyngeal pressure is measured simultaneously by another pressure transducer. Pressure signals are amplified and recorded onto heat-sensitive paper (Bluestone et al., 1977a and b). TM, Tympanic membrane; EC, external canal; ME, middle ear; M, mastoid; ET, eustachian tube; NP, nasopharynx.

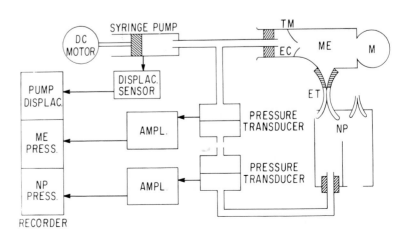

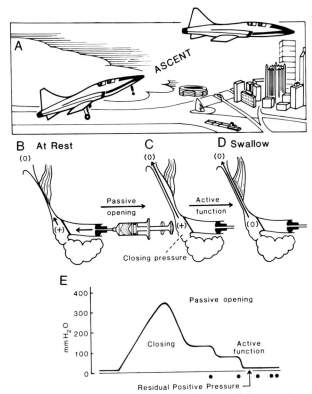

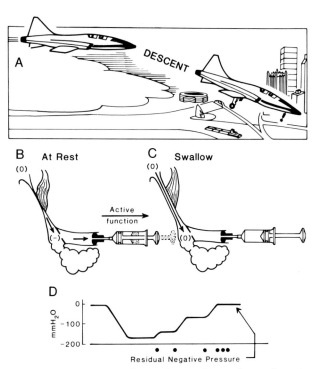

Figure 21–32. Test of passive and active function of the eustachian tube following application of positive middle-ear pressure. *A*, Analogous ascent in an airplane. *B*, Assessment of passive function. *C*, Closing pressure. *D*, Assessment of active function (swallowing). *E*, Strip chart recording showing an example of normal pressure tracing. Black circles represent swallows.

Figure 21–33. Deflation phase of eustachian tube testing. *A*, Analogous descent in an airplane. *B*, Application of low negative pressure to the middle ear. *C*, Equilibration by active tubal opening. *D*, Strip chart recording showing an example of a normal tracing. Black circles represent swallows.

pressure but above the closing pressure could not be equilibrated by the active swallowing function.

Failure to equilibrate the applied negative pressure indicates locking of the eustachian tube during the test. This type of tube is considered to have increased compliance or to be "floppy" in comparison with the tube with perfect function (Bluestone et al., 1972*a*; Bluestone and Shurin, 1974; Takahashi et al., 1987). A stiff tube will neither distend in response to high positive pressures nor collapse in response to negative pressures; however, a tube that lacks stiffness is collapsed, and this in turn results in functional tubal obstruction. The tube collapses even further and may lock entirely in response to negative pressures; it may not open in response to low positive pressure, but as pressure progressively increases, it opens and may ultimately distend.

The speed of the application of the positive and negative pressure is an important variable in testing eustachian tube function with the inflation-deflation test. The faster the positive pressure is applied, the higher the opening pressure is. During the deflation phase of the study, the faster the negative pressure is applied, the more likely it is that the locking phenomenon will occur.

Figure 21–36 illustrates elements of the procedure and the symbols used in recording the results of ventilatory studies in the clinical setting with an electroacoustic impedance bridge when a strip chart re-

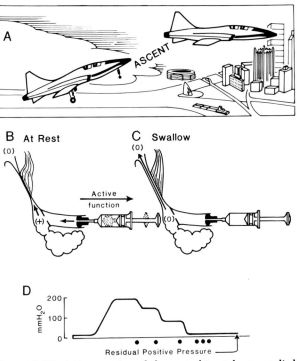

Figure 21–34. Active opening of the eustachian tube to applied positive pressure tested by inflation to a pressure below the opening pressure but above the closing pressure. *A*, Analogous ascent in an airplane. *B* and *C*, Attempt to equilibrate pressure by swallowing. *D*, Strip chart recording showing an example of a normal tracing. Black circles represent swallows.

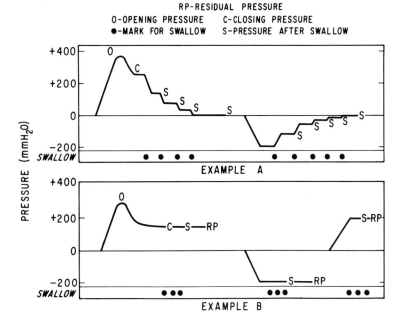

Figure 21–35. Examples of results of inflation-deflation ventilation studies that employed a strip chart recorder. *A,* Normal adult with a traumatic perforation. *B,* Four-year-old boy with a functioning tympanostomy tube who had had a persistent otitis media with effusion.

corder is not available (i.e., when the pressures are noted on the manometer). Example *A* in Figure 21–36 is similar to example *A* in Figure 21–35; in Figure 21–36, however, the tube did not open passively. Depending on the type of electroacoustic impedance bridge, the pump-manometer may not produce pressures greater than 400 mm H_2O. The mean opening pressure for apparently normal subjects with a traumatic perforation and negative otologic history re-

ported by Cantekin and coworkers (1977) was 330 mm H_2O (± 70 mm H_2O). Many eustachian tubes open at pressures above 400 mm H_2O, which is above the limit of the manometers used in the most commonly available bridges. Again, the opening pressure is dependent on the speed of the pump.

Example *B* in Figure 21–36 demonstrates functional obstruction of the eustachian tube. The diagnosis of total mechanical obstruction of the eustachian tube (air

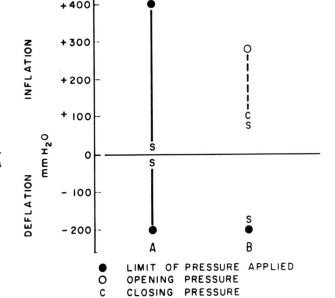

Figure 21–36. Procedure and symbols used in describing ventilatory (inflation-deflation) studies when a strip chart recorder is not employed. Two illustrative examples are shown *(A and B).*

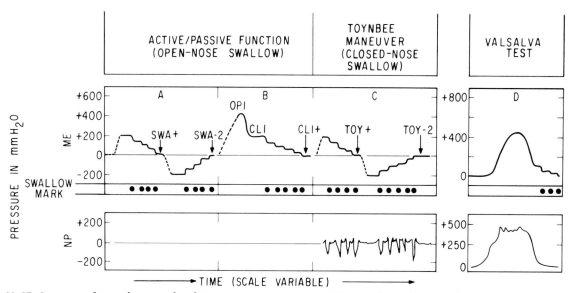

Figure 21–37. Sequence of procedures employed in assessing many aspects of the ventilatory function of the eustachian tube using the equipment shown in Figure 21–31. *A*, Active tubal function. After obtaining a hermetic seal in the ear canal, 200 mm H_2O pressure is applied in the middle ear (inflation). The subject is then instructed to swallow to equilibrate. The pressure remaining in the middle ear following five consecutive swallows without a pressure change is termed the residual positive pressure (SWA+). Then −200 mm H_2O is applied in the middle ear (deflation), and the patient is instructed to swallow. The pressure remaining in the middle ear following this test is termed the residual negative pressure (SWA-2). *B*, Passive and active tubal function. The middle ear is inflated with a constant flow of air until the tube spontaneously opens, at which time the syringe pump is manually stopped. The first passive opening of the eustachian tube by middle-ear overpressure is termed the opening pressure (OP1). Following discharge of air through the eustachian tube, the tube closes passively without a further decay in middle-ear pressure. This pressure is called the closing pressure (CL1). Then the patient is instructed to swallow for further equilibration. The residual pressure following passive closing and swallowing is termed CL1+. The minimal residual positive pressure (MIN+) is the lowest recorded pressure remaining in the middle ear after active and passive equilibration of middle-ear overpressure (lowest value of CL1+ and SWA+). *C*, The Toynbee test. Active function of the tube during closed-nose swallowing is assessed by applying a positive pressure of 200 mm H_2O in the middle ear and manually compressing the unattached naris. The opposite naris is connected to the pressure transducer to record the nasal pressure developed during closed-nose swallowing. The residual positive pressure remaining in the middle ear after closed-nose swallowing (TOY+) is determined. Next, the middle-ear pressure is reduced to −200 mm H_2O. The residual negative pressure remaining in the middle ear following closed-nose swallowing (TOY-2) is noted. *D*, Valsalva test. Passive opening of the eustachian tube by nasopharyngeal overpressure is observed by instructing the subject to blow against obstructed nares—the Valsalva maneuver—while the middle-ear pressure is ambient. The nasopharyngeal pressure corresponding to the first detectable change in middle-ear pressure is taken as the nasopharyngeal opening pressure of the eustachian tube. If a residual positive pressure remains in the middle ear after the termination of nasopharyngeal overpressure, equilibration is attempted by open-nose swallowing. Irrespective of eustachian tube opening, the maximal pressure achieved in the nasopharynx is also noted. ME, Middle ear; NP, nasopharynx.

cannot flow out of or into the middle ear) cannot be made if the pressures cannot be elevated above 400 mm H_2O.

During each equilibration, the time interval between each swallow should be approximately 20 seconds to avoid strain on the pharyngeal muscles. The subject should swallow "dry," but patients with reduced function of the eustachian tube may need water to swallow.

Figure 21–37 shows the procedures employed in assessing the ventilatory function of the eustachian tube with the equipment illustrated in Figure 21–31. The results are based on a four-part test in the following sequence: (1) active opening of the tube, (2) passive opening of the tube during open-nose swallowing, (3) active opening of the tube during closed-nose swallowing (Toynbee maneuver), and (4) the Valsalva test. These tests of ventilatory function are more complete and provide more information than the more simplified testing procedure.

Even though the inflation-deflation test of eustachian tube function is not strictly physiologic, the results are

helpful in differentiating normal from abnormal function. If the test results reveal passive opening and closing within the normal range, if residual positive pressure can be completely equilibrated by swallowing, and if applied negative pressure can also be equilibrated, the function of the eustachian tube can be considered to be normal. However, if the tube does not open to 1000 mm H_2O, one can assume that total mechanical obstruction is present. This pressure is not hazardous to the middle-ear or inner-ear windows if the pressure is applied slowly. An extremely high opening pressure (e.g., greater than 500 to 600 mm H_2O) may indicate partial obstruction, whereas a low opening pressure (e.g., less than 100 mm H_2O) would indicate a semipatulous eustachian tube. Inability to maintain even a modest positive pressure within the middle ear would be consistent with a patulous tube (i.e., open at rest). Complete equilibration by swallowing of applied negative pressure is usually associated with normal function, but partial equilibration or even failure to reduce any applied negative pressure may or may not be considered abnormal, because even a

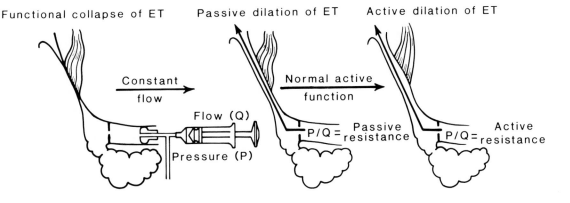

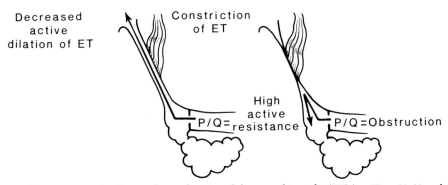

Figure 21–38. Forced-response test for the ventilatory function of the eustachian tube (ET) (see Figs. 21–39 and 21–40 for details of testing procedure).

normal eustachian tube will lock when negative pressure is rapidly applied. Therefore, inability to equilibrate applied negative pressure may not indicate poor eustachian tube function, especially when it is the only abnormal variable.

Forced-Response Test. Originally, the forced-response test was utilized to evaluate tubal function in the rhesus monkey animal model for normal and abnormal middle-ear ventilation (Cantekin et al., 1977); then the same procedure was used in the assessment of tubal function in human subjects (Cantekin et al., 1979b; Cantekin, 1984). The current

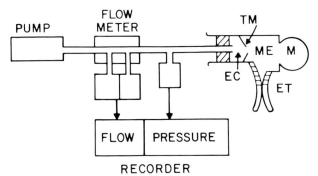

Figure 21–39. Equipment employed to conduct the forced-response test. EC, External canal; TM, tympanic membrane; ME, middle ear; M, mastoid; ET, eustachian tube.

equipment and method to test eustachian tube function in laboratories and clinics utilizes the forced-response. The tympanic membrane must be nonintact, and the middle ear should be dry.

Briefly, this method enables the investigator to study both passive and active responses of the eustachian tube. The active response is due to the contractions of the tensor veli palatini muscle, which displaces the lateral walls from the cartilage-supported medial wall of the tube. Thus, the clinician can determine if tubal dysfunction is due to the material properties of the tube or to a defective active opening mechanism. During this test, the middle ear is inflated at a constant flow rate, forcing the eustachian tube open. Following the forced opening of the tube, the pump continues to deliver a constant airflow, maintaining a steady stream of air through the tube. Then, the subject is instructed to swallow to assess the active dilatation of the tube.

The method is unique in that it eliminates the "mucous forces" in the eustachian tube lumen that may interfere with the results of the inflation-deflation test when an attempt is made to assess the active opening mechanisms and the compliance of the tube. In this test, the passive resistance is assessed, and the active resistance is determined during swallowing. Patients with nonintact tympanic membranes as a

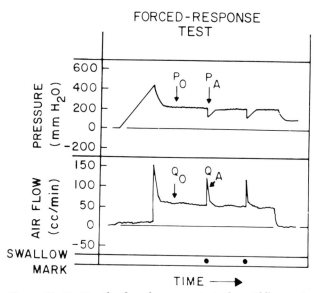

FORCED-RESPONSE TEST

Figure 21–40. For the forced-response test, the middle ear is inflated at a constant airflow rate until the eustachian tube is passively opened. Airflow is then maintained until steady states in airflow through the tube and in middle-ear pressure are observed. The child is induced to swallow, and the changes in steady state pressure and flow are recorded. The pump is then turned off, and the tube is allowed to close passively. In general, an attempt is made to define the values of the forced response for three rates of constant airflow: 12, 25, and 48 cc/minute. The *passive resistance* to airflow is determined by dividing the steady state pressure by the concurrent airflow through the tube. Similarly, *active tubal resistance* is determined by dividing the steady state pressure by the maximal airflow recorded during the induced tubal dilatations that accompany each swallow. P_O, Passive pressure; P_A, active pressure; Q_O, passive flow; Q_A, active flow.

result of chronic perforation or tympanostomy tubes can be distinguished from apparently normal subjects with traumatic perforations of the tympanic membrane and negative otologic histories. The ratio of the passive and active resistance correctly differentiates a normally functioning eustachian tube from an abnormally functioning one.

Figure 21–38 schematizes the forced-response test in a normal subject and compares the results with two response patterns that are commonly seen in association with defects in active dilatation. Figure 21–39 shows the equipment currently employed, and Figure 21–40 describes the testing procedure. Studies in a large number of patients with tympanostomy tubes in place or perforations due to otitis media revealed that all the abnormal ears either had poor active function (as demonstrated by weak or absent dilatation of the eustachian tube during swallowing activity) or constricted during swallowing. Constriction of the eustachian tube with swallowing was found to occur in most children with cleft palates (Doyle et al., 1980a) and has been attributed to opposing muscle force (Cantekin et al., 1979b). This test was also done with American Indians as subjects; they showed low resistance of the eustachian tube (Beery et al., 1980). The forced-response test result appears to be more indicative of the active function of the eustachian tube than is the inflation-deflation test outcome.

Intact Tympanic Membrane

Eustachian tube function in individuals with intact tympanic membranes may also be determined by manometry.

Pressure Chamber Technique. Middle-ear pressure is measured indirectly by the response to pressure changes in a pressure chamber. Decompression of the chamber creates relative positive pressure in the middle ear, whereas chamber compression results in relative negative pressure in the middle ear.

Investigation of eustachian tube function by means of pressure chambers dates back over a century to 1864, when Magnus first reported his findings on tubal function in a diving bell. By using rising external pressures, Magnus was able to make several observations: (1) he confirmed Toynbee's assumption that the eustachian tube is closed under normal conditions; (2) he realized the importance of deglutition for the opening of the tube; and (3) he noted that if the pressure difference between the middle ear and the bell became too pronounced (relative negative pressure in the middle ear), it could not be equilibrated by swallowing. These findings were confirmed by Mach and Kessel (1872), when they conducted experiments in a primitive pressure chamber. Their chamber consisted of a wooden box in which the pressure could be varied between -200 and -140 mm H_2O with the aid of an organ pump. Since that time, pressure chambers have been used to test the function of the eustachian tube.

Microflow Technique. Early volume displacement measurements of the tympanic membrane were done by means of closed manometry in the external ear, with simultaneous direct measurements of middle-ear pressure. This was abandoned as a clinical procedure because of the difficulties encountered in direct measurements, which were usually made by inserting a mandarin needle into the middle-ear cavity. More recently, however, tympanic membrane displacements have been recorded using microflow techniques. When the drum is moving, airflow is produced in the external ear canal. This flow is recorded by a flow meter and then is integrated to give quantitative measurements of volume displacement. Displacements as small as 1 μl have been recorded with up to 95 per cent accuracy.

The microflow method (Ingelstedt et al., 1967a and b; Elner et al., 1971a, b, and c) is the only method used to assess normal eustachian tube function quantitatively in adults. This technique permits continuous recording of the volume deviation of the tympanic membrane resulting from changes of ambient pressure and changes of pressure within the middle ear. During the test, the tympanic membrane is in permanent and free contact with ambient air.

Under an otomicroscope, the subject is fitted with a catheter through a rubber disc inserted in the bony part of the ear canal. The rubber disc maintains an airtight seal with the canal walls. The air cushion between the tympanic membrane and the disc is connected to a sensitive flow meter via the catheter; the other end of the flow meter is open to ambient air. An identical flow meter is connected to a reference volume simulating the air cushion volume between the tympanic membrane and the rubber disc seal. The signal from the reference flow meter is subtracted from that of the ear canal flow meter, compensating for the flow changes due to compression or expansion of air in the pressure chamber. This corrected airflow rate is integrated to obtain the volume displacement of the tympanic membrane. Then, by changing the ambient pressure in the chamber, the tympanic membrane displacement as a function of middle-ear pressure is obtained.

This procedure in a way calibrates the tympanic membrane as a pressure transducer so that after this measurement has been made the subjects can be tested for their abilities to equilibrate various middle-ear pressures created by changes in chamber pressure. Within the elastic limits of the tympanic membrane ($\pm$ 150 mm H_2O pressure differential between the middle ear and ear canal), an accurate inflation-deflation test can be conducted. However, because this technique requires a pressure chamber and sophisticated equipment, it is only practical for use in research centers.

Sonometry. Sound conduction through the eustachian tube was first reported by Politzer (1869). He observed that the sound of a tuning fork placed near the nose appeared to increase in amplitude during swallowing. He concluded that this sound must be traveling through the eustachian tube, which opens during swallowing. Politzer's findings were soon forgotten, and it was not until 1932 that sound conduction through the eustachian tube was reported again, this time by Gyergyay. He used various musical instruments to generate a sound that was introduced into the nose. He verified Politzer's experiments but concluded that the eustachian tube opens only intermittently during swallowing.

In 1939, Perlman studied sound conduction through the eustachian tube by introducing a 500-Hz tone through a tube to the nostril of his subjects. By placing a microphone in the ear canal of his subjects and recording the test sound, he was able to detect tubal opening. His results provided some information on tubal opening time but were too varied to be useful. Little work was done until 1951, when Perlman repeated his earlier studies. This time he reduced the tone frequency to 100 Hz, and by recording the output of the microphone he was better able to assess the duration of tubal opening. He observed increases in sound-pressure levels of up to 20 dB during swallowing. These measurements by Perlman were instrumental in the development of sonometry.

Elpern and associates (1964) used a 200-Hz tone as the sound source in experiments in eustachian tube conduction of sound. They catheterized the eustachian tube with a thin polyethylene tube to verify that the sound was presented to the tube only and were able to show that the sound indeed traveled through the eustachian tube during swallowing.

In 1966, Guillerm and colleagues repeated Perlman's procedure using a 100-Hz tone but made one important modification. They varied the pressure in the nasopharynx with the aid of an air pump and recorded the sound conduction and pressure change in the middle ear through a Foley catheter that was sealed at the external ear canal. If the eustachian tube opened during swallowing, both sound and pressure changes were recorded; conversely, if the tube did not open, neither was recorded. This procedure, known as sonomanometry, was used later by Venker (1973) and Pieraggi (1974).

Naunton and Galluser (1967) developed a eustachian tube analyzer that utilized a 200-Hz tone to analyze the theoretic vector of the response. Satoh and coworkers (1970) conducted experiments using 1930 Hz as the test frequency. Then, in 1975, Eguchi constructed a model of the eustachian tube and conducted similar tests using 2000 Hz.

The selection of the test frequency had been somewhat arbitrary up to this point; each experimenter had chosen a frequency believed to overcome the technical difficulties of the measurement, but little thought had been given to selecting the frequency (or frequencies) at which the maximal amount of sound would be transmitted through the open eustachian tube. All of the frequencies used were 2000 Hz or below.

In 1977, Virtanen conducted experiments using a wide set of frequencies. He chose single tones at 1-kHz intervals between 1 and 20 kHz and found that sound conduction through the eustachian tube appeared to be best at 6, 7, and 8 kHz. He also recorded the physiologic noise due to swallowing and found it to be significant up to 5 kHz. This led him to conclude that recordings of sound conduction using test frequencies below 5 kHz were invalid because they are distorted by the physiologic noise of swallowing.

Pilot studies were conducted using white noise as the stimulus (Murti et al., 1980). When white noise is used, no *a priori* assumptions are made about which test frequencies are most suitable. The results of these pilot studies were in agreement with those of Virtanen (1978). Based on these results, it appears that sound conduction may be a reliable test to indicate tubal function.

Figure 21–41 shows the system currently used in the authors' laboratories for testing eustachian tube function employing sonotubometry.

Tympanometry. Techniques for determining middle-ear pressure and acoustic impedance with electroacoustic impedance equipment were introduced more than 40 years ago (Metz, 1946). These same techniques have been used to perform tympanometry, which is the measurement of the acoustic driving-point admittance as a function of the static pressure in the canal. If low-frequency tones are used for the measurement, the static pressure that produces the maximal acoustic admittance is approximately equal to the pressure in the middle ear.

Thomsen (1958a) adapted the acoustic impedance method for use in a pressure chamber. He varied the chamber pressure and measured the percentage of absorption of a tone presented into the ear canal. He

ETF Sonometry System

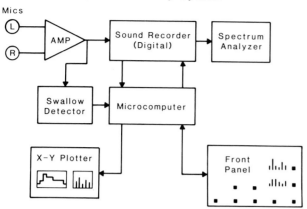

Figure 21–41. Equipment to perform tests of eustachian tube function (ETF) using sonometry. The system performs an evaluation of ETF based on passage of sound through the eustachian tube. The source of the sound used for the test is a small hand-held speaker connected to a tone generator. The tone generator produces either white noise or pure tones in the 3- to 10-kHz range. With tubal opening the sound passes through the nose and eustachian tube and to the external ear canal. Small microphones, which are placed in each external ear canal, receive the signal, which is then amplified and conditioned. The system detects an increase in sound level due to tubal opening and digitally records the sound in its computer memory. The plot of the recording shows the transmitted sound and the envelope of sound. These plots yield information on the duration and extent of tubal opening. Mics, Microphones; L, left; R, right; AMP, amplifier.

found that there was a fall in absorption as the pressure difference between the middle ear and the chamber was increased. The absorption reached a peak when the two pressures were identical.

Unfortunately, Thomsen's technique failed to account for the change in middle-ear pressure caused by the measurement procedure. As the pressure in the chamber is varied (in search of maximal loudness or absorption), the tympanic membrane moves from its original position to a new position, thus changing the volume of the middle-ear cavity. However, according to Boyle's law, as the volume of the cavity changes, the pressure must also change. Thus, by knowing the volume displacement and "measuring" the final pressure, the original pressure can be deduced.

Tympanometry has been widely used in clinical and basic research investigations. A variety of commercially available instruments allow this method to be used routinely in most clinical settings without a pressure chamber. However, an attempt was made to use tympanometry with a pressure chamber to evaluate eustachian tube function in normal children (Ingelstedt and Bylander, 1978; Bylander, 1980). In this method, the resting middle ear pressure is obtained from the initial tympanogram. Then, the chamber pressure is lowered to -100 mm H_2O relative to ambient pressure, and a second tympanogram is obtained, verifying the relative overpressure in the middle ear. Following this, after each deglutition of the subject, a tympanogram is recorded to determine middle-ear pressure. The same procedure is repeated with 100 mm H_2O relative overpressure in the chamber to assess the

subject's ability to actively equilibrate relative underpressure in the middle ear. Using this method, the inflation-deflation test was conducted on 50 children, and the results were compared with the results of tests that measured tubal function in adults. In this way, the first data base for tubal function in otologically normal children was established.

There are five methods for the clinical evaluation of eustachian tube function by tympanometry. Each of these methods is based on an indirect determination of middle-ear pressure under various conditions. The pressure is, of course, obtained by finding the peak in the tympanogram. It must be remembered, however, that only relative qualitative information can be obtained using these methods. If the subject fails to induce pressure changes in the middle ear, tubal function cannot be evaluated. Therefore, there is no truly satisfactory clinical test that is indicative of tubal function in subjects with intact tympanic membranes.

1. *Resting middle-ear pressure.* When the tympanic membrane is intact, tympanometry is a reliable method to determine the middle-ear pressure in the absence of a severely distorted tympanic membrane. Figure 21–42 is a tympanogram of a patient with normal middle-ear resting pressure. Figure 21–43 is a tympanogram of a patient with high negative middle-ear resting pressure, which is indicative of obstruction of the eustachian tube. (Such obstruction may be functional, mechanical, or both.) However, these determinations represent the middle-ear pressure only at one moment. A single measurement of normal resting middle-ear pressure does not necessarily indicate normal eustachian tube function, but a measurement of negative middle-ear pressure is presumptive evidence of eustachian tube dysfunction. Serial determinations are more indicative of the dynamics of tubal function in a single patient. Therefore, the chief drawback of this procedure is that it gives no indication of the ventilating capacity of the eustachian tube under various conditions of middle ear pressure. It is for this reason that the remaining four tests were developed.

2. *Toynbee and Valsalva tests.* The second method for measuring eustachian tube function, which involves the Toynbee and Valsalva tests, developed naturally as an extension of the first. This procedure gives a semiquantitative indication of the ability of the eustachian tube to equilibrate established overpressures and underpressures in the middle ear (Bluestone, 1975) (Fig. 21–44).

First, a tympanogram is obtained to determine the resting middle-ear pressure. Then the subject is asked to perform a Toynbee maneuver, which normally leads to negative pressure in the middle ear. The establishment of this negative middle-ear pressure is verified by a second tympanogram. If the second tympanogram fails to record a change in middle-ear pressure, the subject is classified as Toynbee negative, indicating possible tubal dysfunction. If the maneuver is successful in inducing negative middle-ear pressure, then the subject is asked to swallow in an attempt to equilibrate the negative pressure. A third tympanogram is re-

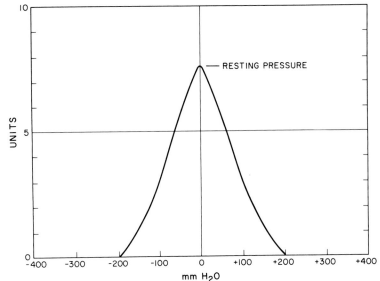

Figure 21–42. Tympanogram in which the resting middle-ear pressure is normal.

corded to determine whether the equilibration was successful and, if so, to what degree. If the equilibration was not complete, the subject is asked to swallow repeatedly. A tympanogram is recorded between each swallow to monitor the progressive equilibration. The pressure remaining in the middle ear after several swallows is termed residual negative pressure. A similar approach is used with the Valsalva (or Politzer air bag) maneuver to test for the tube's ability to equilibrate overpressure in the middle ear. Figure 21–45 illustrates the results of the Toynbee and Valsalva tests as they appear on a strip chart recorder.

These combined tests are most significant if the subject is able to develop negative pressure within the middle ear during the Toynbee test and then is able to equilibrate the negative pressure to the initial resting pressure. This indicates excellent function of the eustachian tube. However, inability to develop negative middle-ear pressure following the Toynbee test or positive intratympanic pressure after the Val-

salva test does not differentiate between normal and abnormal tubal function. One obvious problem with these tests is that it is impossible to control the relative amounts of overpressure and underpressure generated in each individual. (In fact, some individuals fail to generate negative pressure during the Toynbee maneuver.) To overcome this difficulty, three other tests were developed.

3. *Holmquist method.* The third test, developed principally by Holmquist (1969*b*, 1972), measures the ability of the eustachian tube to equilibrate induced negative middle-ear pressures. The test procedure involves five steps: (1) a tympanogram is recorded to determine the initial middle-ear pressure; (2) a negative pressure is created in the nasopharynx by a pressure device connected to the nose, and the subject is asked to swallow to establish a negative pressure of about -200 mm H_2O in the middle ear; (3) a second tympanogram is recorded to evaluate the exact negative middle-ear pressure achieved; (4) the patient is

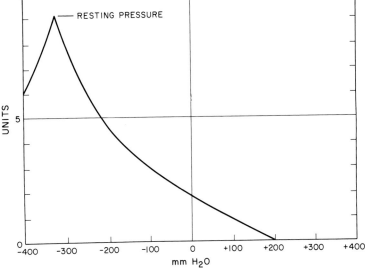
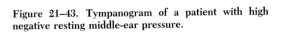

Figure 21–43. Tympanogram of a patient with high negative resting middle-ear pressure.

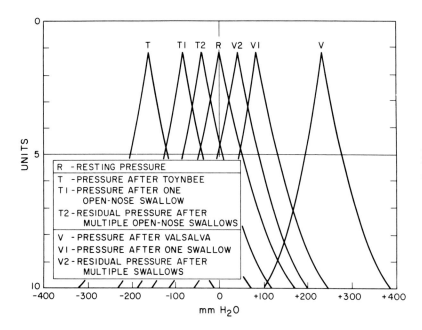

Figure 21–44. Tympanogram of the Toynbee and Valsalva tests of eustachian tube function when the tympanic membrane is intact.

told to swallow repeatedly (if the tube opens, the pressure is equalized); and (5) a third tympanogram is recorded to register the final middle-ear pressure.

Holmquist did not describe a similar procedure for testing equilibrating capacity with induced positive pressures. Siedentop and associates (1978) described the difficulties encountered in using this method to measure tubal function and concluded that many subjects could not be tested by this method even though they had normal tympanic membranes and negative otologic histories.

4. *Patulous eustachian tube test.* If a patulous eustachian tube is suspected, the diagnosis can be confirmed by tympanometry when the tympanic membrane is intact. One tympanogram is obtained while the patient is breathing normally, and a second is obtained while the patient holds his or her breath. The fluctuation in the tympanometric line should coincide with breathing (Fig. 21–46). The fluctuation can be exaggerated by asking the patient to occlude one nostril with the mouth closed during forced inspiration and expiration or by the Toynbee test (Fig. 21–47).

5. *Nine-step test.* Another method of measuring eustachian tube function, developed by Bluestone (1975), is also called an inflation-deflation test, although the applied middle-ear pressures are limited in magnitude. This test is currently used in our clinics to test eustachian tube function when the tympanic membrane is intact. The middle ear must be free of effusion. The nine-step tympanometry procedure (Fig. 21–48) may be summarized as follows:

(1) The tympanogram records resting middle-ear pressure.

(2) Ear canal pressure is increased to +200 mm H_2O with medial deflection of the tympanic membrane and a corresponding increase in middle-ear pressure. The subject swallows to equilibrate middle-ear overpressure.

(3) While the subject refrains from swallowing, ear canal pressure is returned to normal, thus establishing a slight negative middle-ear pressure (as the tympanic membrane moves outward). The tympanogram documents the established middle-ear underpressure.

(4) The subject swallows in an attempt to equilibrate negative middle-ear pressure. If equilibration is successful, airflow is from nasopharynx to middle ear.

(5) The tympanogram records the extent of equilibration.

(6) Ear canal pressure is decreased to −200 mm H_2O, causing a lateral deflection of the tympanic membrane and a corresponding decrease in middle-ear pressure. The subject swallows to equilibrate negative middle-ear pressure; airflow is from the nasopharynx to the middle ear.

(7) The subject refrains from swallowing while external ear canal pressure is returned to normal, thus establishing a slight positive pressure in the middle ear as the tympanic membrane moves medially. The tympanogram records the overpressure established.

(8) The subject swallows to reduce overpressure. If equilibration is successful, airflow is from the middle ear to the nasopharynx.

(9) The final tympanogram documents the extent of equilibration.

The test is simple to perform, can give useful information regarding eustachian tube function, and should be part of the clinical evaluation of patients with suspected eustachian tube dysfunction. In general, most normal adults can perform all or some parts of this test, but even some normal children have difficulty in performing it. However, if a child can pass some or all of the steps, eustachian tube function is considered good.

Eustachian Tube Dysfunction and Pathogenesis of Otitis Media and Certain Related Conditions

The major types of abnormal function of the eustachian tube that can cause otitis media appear to be

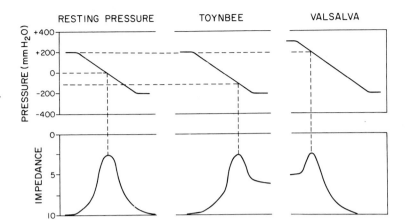

Figure 21–45. Strip chart tympanometric recording of the Toynbee and Valsalva tests of eustachian tube function when the tympanic membrane is intact.

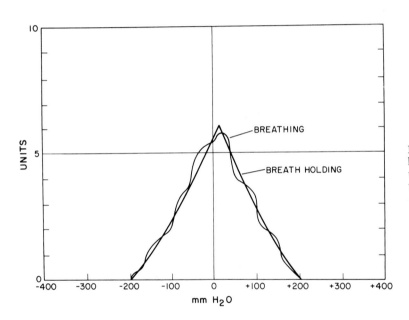

Figure 21–46. Tympanogram of a patient with a patulous eustachian tube. The wavy line was obtained while the subject was breathing; the steady line was recorded when the patient held his breath.

Figure 21–47. Tympanogram of the same patient as in Figure 21–46. Wide fluctuations were obtained when the patient swallowed several times with his mouth and nose closed (Toynbee test). The steady line was recorded when the patient held his breath.

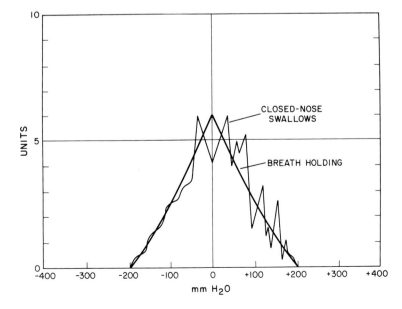

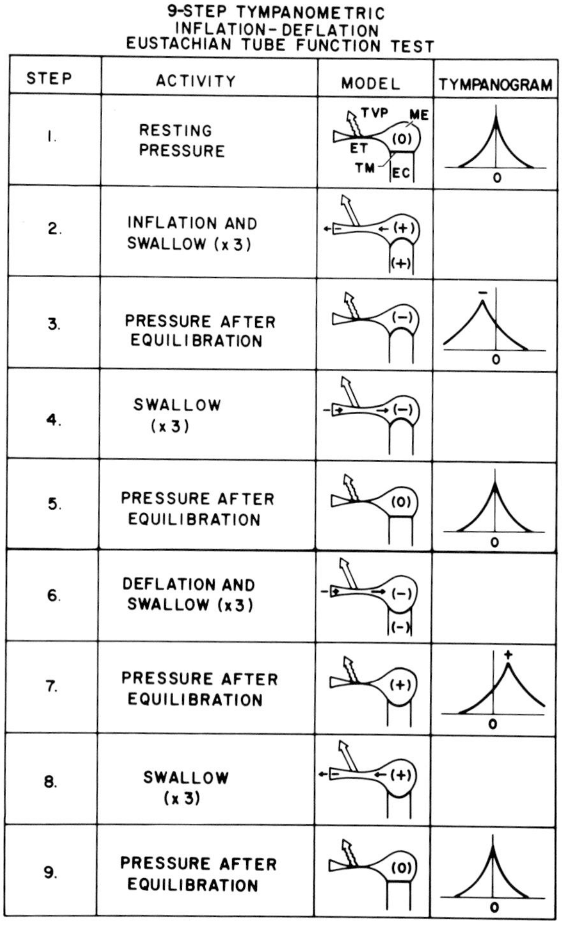

**9-STEP TYMPANOMETRIC
INFLATION-DEFLATION
EUSTACHIAN TUBE FUNCTION TEST**

STEP	ACTIVITY	MODEL	TYMPANOGRAM
1.	RESTING PRESSURE	TVP ME; ET (O); TM EC	
2.	INFLATION AND SWALLOW (x 3)	(+) (+)	
3.	PRESSURE AFTER EQUILIBRATION	(−)	
4.	SWALLOW (x 3)	(−)	
5.	PRESSURE AFTER EQUILIBRATION	(O)	
6.	DEFLATION AND SWALLOW (x 3)	(−) (−)	
7.	PRESSURE AFTER EQUILIBRATION	(+)	
8.	SWALLOW (x 3)	(+)	
9.	PRESSURE AFTER EQUILIBRATION	(O)	

Figure 21–48. Nine-step inflation-deflation tympanometric test. TVP, Tensor veli palatini muscle; ET, eustachian tube; ME, middle ear; TM, tympanic membrane; EC, ear canal. (From Bluestone, C. D., and Klein, J. O. 1988. Otitis Media in Infants and Children. Philadelphia, W. B. Saunders Co.)

cartilage support of the eustachian tube are less than in older children and adults. In addition, there appear to be marked age differences in the craniofacial base that render the tensor veli palatini muscle less efficient prior to puberty. In infants and young children, active tubal opening is probably impaired owing to lack of stiffness of the cartilage support during contraction of the tensor muscle (Bluestone et al., 1972a). *Mechanical obstruction* of the eustachian tube may be intrinsic or extrinsic. *Intrinsic* obstruction could be the result of abnormal geometry or intraluminal or mural factors that could compromise the lumen of the eustachian tube; the most common of these is inflammation due to infection or possibly to allergy. *Extrinsic* obstruction could be the result of increased extramural pressure, such as occurs when the subject is supine or when there is peritubal compression caused by a tumor or possibly an adenoid mass.

In extreme cases of abnormal patency of the eustachian tube, the tube is open even at rest (i.e., patulous tube). Lesser degrees of abnormal patency result in a semipatulous eustachian tube that is closed at rest but has low resistance in comparison with the normal tube. Increased patency of the tube may be due to abnormal tube geometry or to a decrease in the extramural pressure, such as occurs after weight loss or possibly as a result of mural or intraluminal factors.

Functional Eustachian Tube Obstruction

Figure 21–50 depicts the chain of events in the pathogenesis of otitis media with effusion when the eustachian tube is functionally obstructed. This type of obstruction may result in persistent high negative middle-ear pressure, and, when associated with marked collapse or retraction of the tympanic membrane, it has been termed *atelectasis*. This condition has been demonstrated in an experimental animal model (Cantekin et al., 1977). Following transection of the tensor veli palatini muscle posterior to the hamulus of the pterygoid bone in the rhesus monkey, temporary high negative middle-ear pressure and severe retraction of the tympanic membrane were noted to occur and persisted until the muscle healed. If ventilation occurs when there is high negative middle-

obstruction, abnormal patency, or both (Fig. 21–49). Eustachian tube obstruction can be functional or mechanical or a combination of these. *Functional obstruction* results from persistent collapse of the eustachian tube due to increased tubal compliance, an abnormal active opening mechanism, or both. Functional eustachian tube obstruction is common in infants and younger children, as the amount and stiffness of the

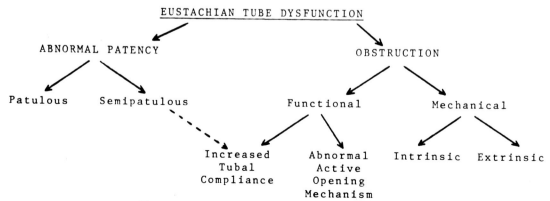

Figure 21–49. Various types of eustachian tube dysfunction.

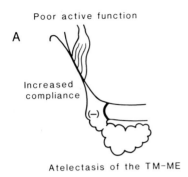

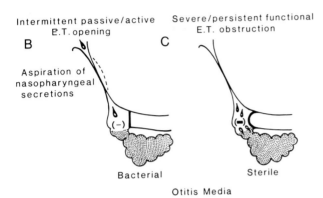

Figure 21–50. Mechanism by which functional obstruction of the eustachian tube can result in atelectasis of the tympanic membrane–middle ear *(A)* or a bacterial *(B)* or a sterile *(C)* otitis media with effusion. TM–ME, Tympanic membrane–middle ear; E.T., eustachian tube.

ear pressure, nasopharyngeal secretions can be *aspirated* into the middle ear and can result in an acute bacterial otitis media with effusion. To test this hypothesis, Cantekin and coworkers (1977) unilaterally transected the tensor muscle in the rhesus monkey. The result was persistent high negative middle-ear pressure without effusion; in the unoperated side, middle-ear pressure remained normal. Forty-eight hours after instillation of *Streptococcus pneumoniae* into the nasopharynx of the monkey, acute otitis media with effusion developed in the ear with the high negative middle-ear pressure but not in the unoperated side.

If ventilation does not occur, persistent functional eustachian tube obstruction could result in sterile otitis media with effusion. Cantekin and coworkers (1977) also reproduced this condition in the rhesus monkey by excision of the tensor muscle, which resulted in severe functional eustachian tube obstruction and the development of sterile otitis media with effusion shortly after the procedure. Development of otitis media with effusion at this stage might be dependent on the degree and duration of the negative pressure as well as middle-ear hypoxia or hypercapnia. Because tubal opening is possible in a middle ear with an effusion, aspiration of nasopharyngeal secretions might occur, thus creating the clinical condition in which persistent otitis media with effusion and recurrent acute bacterial otitis media with effusion occur together. Infants with unrepaired palatal clefts and chil-

dren with repaired cleft palates have otitis media with effusion as a result of functional obstruction of the eustachian tube (Bluestone, 1971).

Mechanical Eustachian Tube Obstruction

INTRINSIC MECHANICAL OBSTRUCTION. Intrinsic mechanical obstruction of the eustachian tube is most commonly the result of inflammation. Obstruction within the bony or protympanic portion of the tube is usually due to acute or chronic inflammation of the mucosal lining, which may also be associated with polyps or a cholesteatoma. Total obstruction may be present at the middle-ear end of the tube. However, these conditions are the result of eustachian tube dysfunction and not the initial cause. Stenosis of the eustachian tube has also been described but is a rare finding.

Figure 21–51 illustrates the sequence of events in which intrinsic inflammation of the cartilaginous portion of the eustachian tube may result in an abnormal middle-ear condition. Most ears at risk for developing atelectasis or otitis media with effusion when inflammation is present probably have a significant degree of functional obstruction. An upper respiratory tract infection in children with this condition has been shown to significantly decrease eustachian tube function (Bluestone et al., 1977a). Periods of upper respiratory tract infection may then result in atelectasis of the tympanic membrane–middle ear, bacterial otitis media with effusion, or sterile otitis media with effusion due to swelling of the eustachian tube lumen. The mechanisms are similar to those described for functional eustachian tube obstruction. Allergy as a cause of intrinsic mechanical eustachian tube obstruction has not been demonstrated (Bluestone, 1978). However, in adult volunteers, eustachian tube obstruction has been produced by a challenge with antigen inhaled into the nasal cavity (Friedman et al., 1983).

EXTRINSIC MECHANICAL OBSTRUCTION. Extrinsic mechanical obstruction of the eustachian tube may be the result of extrinsic compression by nasopharyngeal tumors, adenoids, or lesions of the base of the skull (Fig 21–52). In an attempt to improve criteria for the preoperative selection of children for adenoidectomy to prevent otitis media with effusion, Bluestone and colleagues (1972c) made radiographic studies of the nasopharynx and eustachian tube prior to and following adenoidectomy. The ventilatory function of the eustachian tube has also been studied by the inflation-deflation manometric technique both before and after adenoidectomy in a group of children with recurrent or chronic otitis media with effusion in whom tympanostomy tubes had been inserted (Bluestone et al., 1975a). The results of these studies indicated that following adenoidectomy eustachian tube function improved in some, remained the same in others, and in a few children worsened. Improvement was related to a reduction of extrinsic mechanical obstruction of the eustachian tube.

Figure 21–53 shows the possible mechanisms by

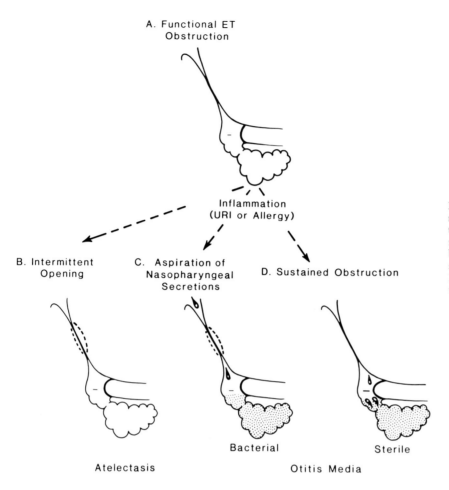

A. Functional ET
Obstruction

Inflammation
(URI or Allergy)

B. Intermittent
Opening

C. Aspiration of
Nasopharyngeal
Secretions

D. Sustained Obstruction

Bacterial

Sterile

Atelectasis

Otitis Media

Figure 21–51. Mechanism by which intrinsic mechanical obstruction of the eustachian tube that has functional obstruction *(A)* can result in atelectasis of the tympanic membrane–middle ear *(B)* or a bacterial *(C)* or a sterile *(D)* otitis media with effusion. ET, Eustachian tube; URI, upper respiratory tract infection.

which extrinsic obstruction may result in ear disease. Partial eustachian tube obstruction may result only in atelectasis of the tympanic membrane–middle ear or a bacterial otitis media with effusion, but more severe obstruction could result in a sterile otitis media with effusion. Otitis media with effusion has been produced in animal models when the eustachian tube was mechanically obstructed (Paparella et al., 1970).

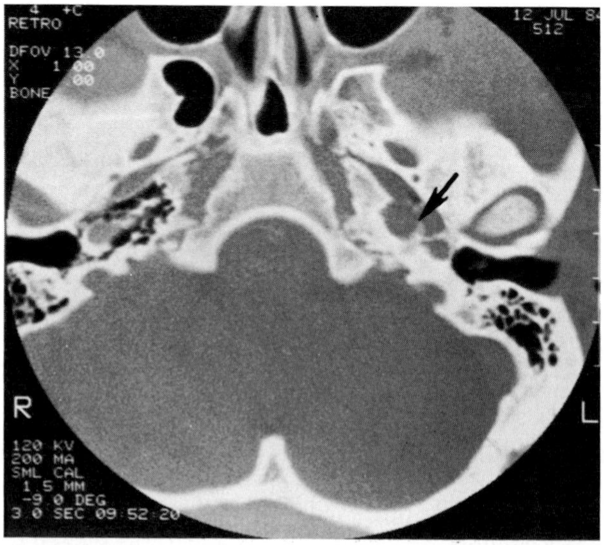

Abnormal Patency of the Eustachian Tube

Figure 21–54 depicts the possible sequence of events that can cause an otitis media with effusion when the eustachian tube is abnormally patent. A patulous eustachian tube usually permits air to flow readily from the nasopharynx into the middle ear, which thus remains well ventilated; however, unwanted nasopharyngeal secretions can also traverse the tube and result in *reflux otitis media*. A semipatulous eustachian tube may be obstructed functionally as the result of increased tubal compliance, and the middle ear may even have negative pressure, an effusion, or both. Because the tubal walls are abnormally distensible, nasopharyngeal secretions may readily be insufflated into the middle ear even with modest positive nasopharyngeal pressures (e.g., as a result of noseblowing, sneezing, crying (Fig. 21–55), or closed-nose swallowing). If active tubal opening (tensor veli palatini contraction) occurs, resulting in an abnormally patent tube, *reflux* or *insufflation* of nasopharyngeal secretions is also likely.

If the eustachian tube has lower resistance than normal but remains functionally obstructed even dur-

Figure 21–52. Example of total extrinsic mechanical obstruction: teen-ager who has had lifelong otitis media with effusion in the left ear. Computed tomogram shows two congenital cysts blocking the eustachian tube.

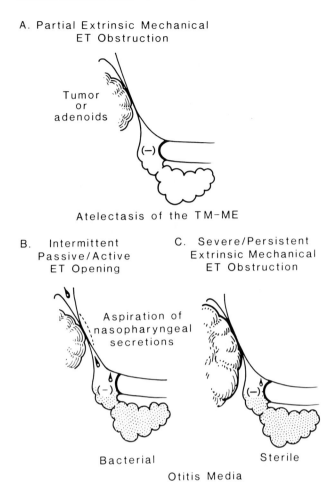

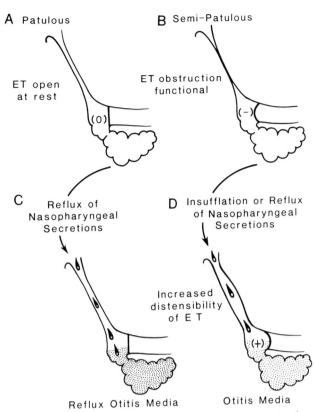

A. Partial Extrinsic Mechanical
ET Obstruction

Tumor
or
adenoids

Atelectasis of the TM-ME

B. Intermittent
Passive/Active
ET Opening

C. Severe/Persistent
Extrinsic Mechanical
ET Obstruction

Aspiration of
nasopharyngeal
secretions

Bacterial   Sterile

Otitis Media

Figure 21–53. Mechanism by which extrinsic mechanical obstruction of the eustachian tube can result in atelectasis of the tympanic membrane–middle ear (A) or bacterial (B) or sterile (C) otitis media with effusion. TM–ME, Tympanic membrane–middle ear; ET, eustachian tube.

A Patulous   B Semi-Patulous

ET open
at rest

ET obstruction
functional

C Reflux of
Nasopharyngeal
Secretions

D Insufflation or Reflux
of Nasopharyngeal
Secretions

Increased
distensibility
of E T

Reflux Otitis Media   Otitis Media

Figure 21–54. Abnormal patency of the eustachian tube. In the patulous condition (A), reflux of nasopharyngeal secretions can result in otitis media (B). If the eustachian tube is semipatulous (C), otitis media may occur following reflux, insufflation, or aspiration of nasopharyngeal secretions (D). ET, Eustachian tube.

ing attempts at active tubal opening, it is conceivable that nasopharyngeal secretions would enter the middle ear more readily than would air. American Indians have been shown to have tubal resistances that are lower than those of the average Caucasian (Beery et al., 1980). They seem to have an increased incidence of reflux of nasopharyngeal secretion into the middle ear and frequently experience recurrent acute otitis media that is often associated with perforation and discharge. However, American Indians have a low incidence of cholesteatoma. This type of eustachian tube function and middle-ear disease is different from the types of disease seen in individuals who have a cleft palate.

Nasal Obstruction Related to Eustachian Tube Function

Nasal obstruction may also be involved in the pathogenesis of otitis media with effusion. Swallowing when the nose is obstructed (owing to inflammation or obstructed adenoids) results in an initial positive nasopharyngeal air pressure followed by a negative-

pressure phase. When the tube is pliant, positive nasopharyngeal pressure might insufflate infected secretions into the middle ear, especially when the middle ear has a high negative pressure; with negative nasopharyngeal pressure, such a tube could be prevented from opening and could be further obstructed functionally, which was referred to as the Toynbee phenomenon (Bluestone et al., 1975a) (Fig. 21–56).

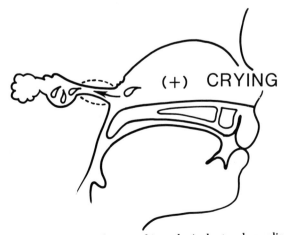

(+) CRYING

Figure 21–55. Because the eustachian tube is short and compliant in the infant, crying may insufflate nasopharyngeal secretions into the middle ear.

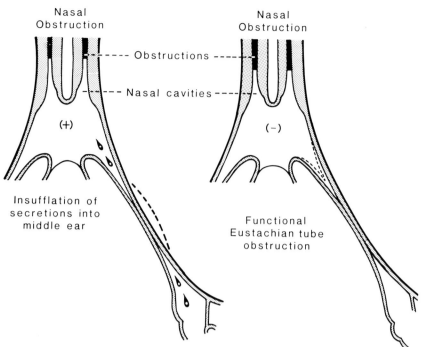

Figure 21–56. Toynbee phenomenon (see text).

Allergy and Eustachian Tube Function

Allergy is thought to be one of the etiologic factors in otitis media because otitis media occurs frequently in allergic individuals (Draper, 1967). The mechanism by which allergy might cause otitis media remains hypothetic and controversial. Figure 21–57 illustrates the role of allergy in the etiology and pathogenesis of otitis media by one or more of the following mechanisms: (1) middle-ear mucosa functioning as a "shock organ," (2) inflammatory swelling of the mucosa of the eustachian tube, (3) inflammatory obstruction of the nose, or (4) aspiration of bacteria-laden allergic nasopharyngeal secretions into the middle-ear cavity. In studies by Bernstein and coworkers (1984), a small percentage of children with proven allergy did have some evidence that the middle ear may be a shock organ, but they considered this condition to be rare. A more likely explanation for the role of allergy in otitis media is related to allergic inflammation of the eustachian tube (Fig. 21–58). Studies involving adult volunteers demonstrated a relationship among intranasal antigen challenge, allergic rhinitis, and eustachian tube obstruction (Ackerman et al., 1984; Doyle et al., 1984a; Friedman et al., 1983). It seems reasonable that children with signs and symptoms of allergy of the upper respiratory tract may have otitis media as a result of the allergic condition.

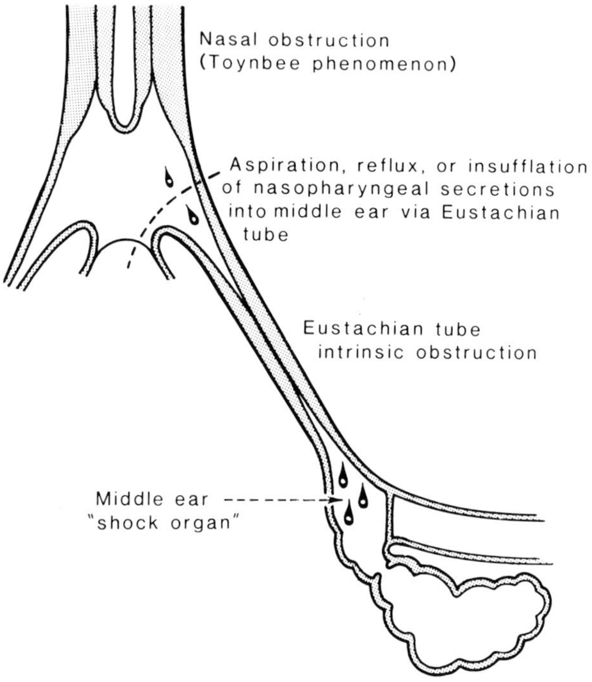

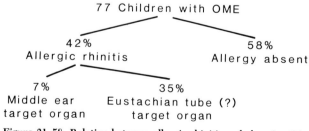

Figure 21–57. Four possible pathogenic mechanisms that could be involved in the relationship between allergy and otitis media.

Figure 21–58. Relation between allergic rhinitis and chronic otitis media with effusion (OME). Bernstein and coworkers (1983) showed that, of 77 children who had otitis media with effusion (OME), 42 per cent had allergic rhinitis but only 7 per cent of 77 children had any evidence that the middle ear was a target organ. (Modified after Bernstein, J. M., et al. 1983. The role of IgE mediated hypersensitivity in recurrent otitis media with effusion. Am. J. Otol. 5:66–69.)

Eustachian Tube Function Related to Cleft Palate

Otitis media with effusion is universally present in infants with an unrepaired cleft palate (i.e., functional obstruction of the eustachian tube) (Paradise et al., 1969; Stool and Randall, 1967) (Fig. 21–59). Palate repair appears to improve middle-ear status, but middle-ear disease nonetheless often continues or recurs even after palate repair (Paradise and Bluestone, 1974). Radiographic assessment has shown that infants and children with both unrepaired and repaired cleft palate have abnormal eustachian tube function. This suggests an abnormal opening mechanism in the infants with an unrepaired cleft palate (i.e., functional obstruction of the eustachian tube) (Bluestone, 1971; Bluestone et al., 1972d), and a persistent failure of the eustachian tube to open actively, increased distensibility of the eustachian tube, or both after repair of the soft palate (Bluestone et al., 1972b). Histopathologic temporal bone studies have confirmed that the eustachian tube of cleft palate patients is not anatomically obstructed, which would give credence to functional, as opposed to mechanical, obstruction as the underlying defect (Kitajiri et al., 1984) (see Fig. 21–51).

Inflation-deflation manometric eustachian tube function tests have shown that infants with unrepaired cleft palates have variable degrees of difficulty equilibrating increased middle-ear pressure and are unable to equilibrate negative pressure by active function (swallowing) (Bluestone et al., 1975a). Children with repaired cleft palates had either the same type of test results as did children with unrepaired palates or had lower opening pressures. Doyle and associates (1980a), employing the forced-response eustachian tube function test, found that the eustachian tubes of infants and children with cleft palates constricted instead of dilated during swallowing. Animal subjects in which the palate has been surgically split have developed otitis media with effusion (Doyle et al., 1980a, 1984b; Odoi et al., 1971).

All of these studies indicate that the eustachian tube is functionally obstructed in children with cleft palates, and this condition results in middle-ear disease characterized by persistent or recurrent high negative middle-ear pressure, effusion, or both. Cholesteatoma is a frequent sequela in such children; this is not the case in American Indians, in whom the eustachian tube has been shown to be abnormally patent (i.e., to have low tubal resistance).

Patients with a submucous cleft of the palate appear to have the same risk of developing middle-ear disease as those with an overt cleft. In addition, the presence of a bifid uvula has also been associated with a high incidence of otitis media (Taylor, 1972). Both of these conditions are probably associated with the same pathogenic mechanism for otitis media as is found in patients with overt cleft palates (i.e., functional obstruction of the eustachian tube).

Other Causes of Eustachian Tube Dysfunction

There are many other etiologic factors responsible for abnormal function of the eustachian tube. Inflammation of the nose–nasopharynx–eustachian tube–middle ear system has been presented as a major factor in the pathogenesis of otitis media, but there are congenital, traumatic, neoplastic, degenerative, metabolic, and idiopathic conditions that also can result in tubal abnormalities.

Because a cleft of the palate produces functional obstruction of the eustachian tube, any child with a craniofacial malformation that has an associated cleft palate will have otitis media or a related condition, one of the more common examples being Pierre Robin syndrome. However, children with craniofacial anomalies that do not include an overt cleft of the palate

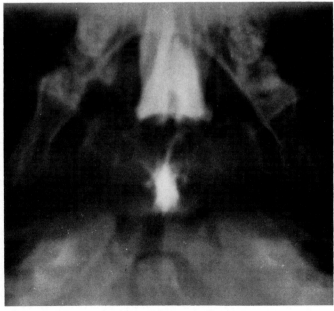

Figure 21–59. Submentovertex roentgenogram of infant with an unrepaired cleft palate showing retrograde obstruction of contrast material entering from the nasopharyngeal end of the eustachian tube.

also have an increased incidence of middle-ear disease. These anomalies include, among others, Down, Crouzon, Apert, and Turner syndromes. Even though there have been no reports of formal eustachian tube function studies in individuals with these and other anomalies, dysfunction of the eustachian tube is the most likely cause of such ear disease. Presumably, a defect related to the abnormal craniofacial complex influences the relation between the eustachian tube and the tensor veli palatini muscle.

Even in the absence of an obvious craniofacial malformation that is associated with otitis media, there is some evidence that children and adults with middle-ear disease have a congenital defect that results in a dysfunction of the tube. Such a dysfunction could be abnormal patency or functional obstruction of the tube that is the result of an abnormal relation between the eustachian tube and the tensor veli palatini muscle. Such an assumption is supported by apparent racial differences in the prevalence and incidence of otitis media: Eskimos and American Indians have a higher incidence of otitis media than do whites, whereas blacks have an incidence of otitis media that is half that in whites. There is also some evidence that otitis media is more prevalent in certain families. A familial tendency to otitis media has been found (Doyle, 1979).

It has also been observed that patients with dentofacial abnormalities may have otitis media or may develop middle-ear disease as a result of these abnormalities. Correction of the defect to relieve the eustachian tube dysfunction would appear to be indicated.

Congenital lesions can, on rare occasion, obstruct the eustachian tube. Figure 21–52 shows computed tomography (CT) scans of a teen-ager with total obstruction of the bony (intratemporal) portion of the eustachian tube due to congenital cholesteatoma.

In certain patients with a deviated nasal septum, impaired eustachian tube function has been reported. This dysfunction is especially apparent during attempts to equilibrate middle-ear pressure by the Valsalva maneuver during periods of wide fluctuations in barometric pressure, such as flying in an airplane or diving. In such cases, successful inflation of the middle ear by the Valsalva maneuver has been reported following repair of the deviated nasal septum (McNicoll and Scanlan, 1979; McNicoll, 1982).

Trauma to the palate, the pterygoid bone, the tensor veli palatini muscle, or the eustachian tube itself can also result in abnormal eustachian tube function. Injury to the trigeminal nerve or, more specifically, to the mandibular branch of this nerve, can result in either functional obstruction of the eustachian tube or a patulous tube, as the innervation of the tensor veli palatini is from this nerve (Perlman, 1951; Cantekin et al., 1979a). The trauma may be associated with surgical procedures, such as palatal or maxillary resection for tumor (Myers et al., 1984).

Neoplastic disease, either benign or malignant, that invades the palate, the pterygoid bone, or the tensor veli palatini muscle can interfere with tensor veli

palatini muscle function and can result in functional obstruction of the tube (Takahara et al., 1986; Myers et al., 1984) (Fig. 21–60). Functional obstruction or abnormal patency of the tube can also occur from involvement of the innervation of the tensor veli palatini muscle. Mechanical obstruction of the eustachian tube can result from direct invasion by neoplasm. Degenerative and metabolic diseases such as myasthenia gravis can alter the eustachian tube by affecting the tubal musculature or by changing the extramural or mural pressures in such a way as would occur with major shifts of extracellular fluids.

Finally, whenever eustachian tube dysfunction is diagnosed and the etiology is obscure, the dysfunction is usually termed idiopathic. Most patients with otitis media have been found to have idiopathic functional obstruction of the eustachian tube. It should not be forgotten, however, that the cause may be a congenital defect in the anatomy of the base of the skull.

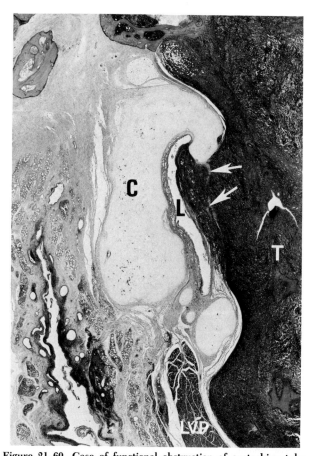

Figure 21–60. Case of functional obstruction of eustachian tube secondary to tumor invasion (× 12). Vertical section of middle of cartilaginous portion of left eustachian tube (H & E, original × 12). Tensor veli palatini (TVP) muscle is completely destroyed by tumor cells (T). Levator veli palatini (LVP) muscle is compressed by tumor medially, but tubal lumen (L) is still open. Only tendon of TVP muscle and surrounding connective tissue (arrows) remain intact. Top, superior; left, medial; right, lateral. C, Tubal cartilage. (With permission from Takahara, T., et al. 1986. Lymphoma invading the anterior eustachian tube: Temporal bone histopathology of functional tubal obstruction. Ann. Otol. Rhinol. Laryngol. 95:101.)

Eustachian Tube Function in Clinical Setting

The roentgenographic tests developed to assess the protective and clearance system of the eustachian tube–middle ear system have been helpful in understanding these functions but are not feasible in the usual clinical setting. However, methods to assess the ventilatory function of the system are readily available to the clinician and should be performed when indicated. The ventilatory function is the most important of the three functions, because adequate hearing depends on the maintenance of equal air pressure on both sides of the tympanic membrane. In addition, impairment of the ventilatory function can result not only in hearing loss but also in otitis media.

Prior to the examination of the patient, the presence of certain signs and symptoms may be helpful in determining if eustachian tube dysfunction is present. Conductive hearing loss, otalgia, otorrhea, tinnitus, or vertigo may be present with this disorder.

Otoscopy

Visual inspection of the tympanic membrane is one of the simplest (and oldest) ways to assess the functioning of the eustachian tube. The appearance of a middle-ear effusion, the presence of high negative middle-ear pressure, or both, as determined by the *pneumatic* otoscope (Bluestone and Shurin, 1974), is presumptive evidence of eustachian tube dysfunction, but the type of impairment, such as functional or mechanical obstruction, as well as the degree of abnormality, cannot be determined by this method. Moreover, a normal-appearing tympanic membrane cannot be considered to be evidence of normal functioning of the eustachian tube: for instance, a patulous or semipatulous eustachian tube may be present when the tympanic membrane appears to be normal. In addition, the presence of one or more of the complications or sequelae of otitis media (such as a perforation or atelectasis, as observed through the otoscope) may not correlate with dysfunction of the eustachian tube at the time of the examination, as eustachian tube function may improve with growth and development.

Nasopharyngoscopy

Indirect mirror examination of the nasopharyngeal end of the eustachian tube is also an old but still important part of the clinical assessment of a patient with middle-ear disease. For instance, a neoplasm in the fossa of Rosenmüller may be diagnosed by this simple technique. The development of endoscopic instruments has greatly improved the accuracy of this type of examination, but the function of the eustachian tube cannot be determined with the aid of currently available instruments (Jaumann et al., 1980).

Tympanometry

The use of an electroacoustic impedance instrument to obtain a tympanogram is an excellent way of determining the status of the tympanic membrane–middle ear system, and it can be helpful in the assessment of eustachian tube function (Bluestone, 1980) (see Fig. 21–71). The presence of a middle-ear effusion or high negative middle-ear pressure as determined by this method usually indicates impaired eustachian tube function; however, unlike the otoscopic evaluation, the tympanogram is an objective way of determining the degree of negative pressure present in the middle ear. Unfortunately, assessing the abnormality of values of negative pressure is not simple: high negative pressure may be present in some patients, especially children, who are asymptomatic and who have relatively good hearing, whereas in others, symptoms such as hearing loss, otalgia, vertigo, and tinnitus may be associated with modest degrees of negative pressure or even with normal middle-ear pressures. The middle-ear air pressure may depend on the time of day, season of the year, or condition of the other parts of the system, such as the presence of an upper respiratory tract infection. For instance, a young child with a common cold may have transitory high negative pressure within the middle ear while he or she has the cold but may be otherwise otologically normal (Casselbrant et al., 1985). The decision as to whether or not high negative pressure is abnormal or is only a physiologic variation should be made taking into consideration the presence or absence of signs and symptoms of middle-ear disease. If severe atelectasis or adhesive otitis of the tympanic membrane–middle ear system is present, the tympanogram may not be a reliable indicator of the actual pressure within the middle ear.

Therefore, a resting pressure that is highly negative is associated with some degree of eustachian tube obstruction, but the presence of normal middle-ear pressure does not necessarily indicate normal eustachian tube function; a normal tympanogram is obtained when the eustachian tube is patulous. The patulous tube tympanometric test and the nine-step inflation-deflation test can be easily performed in the office or clinic setting.

Manometry

The pump-manometer system of the electroacoustic impedance bridge is usually adequate to assess eustachian tube function clinically when the tympanic membrane is not intact. However, owing to the limitations of the manometric systems of all of the commercially available instruments, a controlled syringe and manometer (a water manometer will suffice) should be available when these limitations are exceeded (e.g., when eustachian tube opening pressure is in excess of $+400$ to $+600$ mm H_2O). The simple inflation-deflation test can be performed with this equipment. If mechanical obstruction is diagnosed, then the site of the obstruction must be investigated. The middle ear and nasopharynx should be examined.

Imaging

To determine if the site of the obstruction is within the temporal bone or adjacent structures, imaging should be obtained; computed tomograms will provide excellent information concerning the bone and soft tissue, but nuclear magnetic resonance imaging may also prove useful. If tumor is considered as a possible cause for mechanical or functional obstruction, or both, imaging can be helpful in determining the site and extent of the disease.

Clinical Indications for Testing Eustachian Tube Function

Diagnosis

One of the most important reasons for assessing eustachian tube function is the need to make a differential diagnosis in a patient who has an intact tympanic membrane without evidence of otitis media but who has symptoms that might be related to eustachian tube dysfunction (such as otalgia, snapping or popping in the ear, fluctuating hearing loss, tinnitus, or vertigo). An example of such a case would be a child or adolescent who has a complaint of fullness in the ear without hearing loss at the time of the examination, a symptom that could be related to abnormal functioning of the eustachian tube or could be due to an inner-ear disorder. A tympanogram that reveals high negative pressure (-50 mm H_2O or less) is presumptive evidence of tubal obstruction, whereas normal resting middle-ear pressure is not diagnostically significant. However, when the resting intratympanic pressure is within normal limits and the patient can develop negative middle-ear pressure following Toynbee test or can perform all or some of the functions in the nine-step inflation-deflation tympanometric test, the eustachian tube is probably functioning normally. Unfortunately, failure to develop negative middle-ear pressure during the Toynbee test or inability to perform the nine-step test does not necessarily indicate poor eustachian tube function, because many children who are otologically normal cannot actively open their tubes during these tests. Tympanometry is not only of value in determining if eustachian tube obstruction is present, it can also identify abnormality at the other end of the spectrum of eustachian tube dysfunction, and the presence of an abnormally patent eustachian tube can be confirmed by the results of the tympanometric patulous tube test.

Screening for the presence of high negative pressure in certain high-risk populations (i.e., children with known sensorineural hearing losses, developmentally delayed and mentally impaired children, children with cleft palates or other craniofacial anomalies, American Indian and Eskimo children, and children with Down syndrome) appears to be helpful in identifying those individuals who may need to be monitored closely for the occurrence of otitis media (Harford et al., 1978).

Tympanometry appears to be a reliable method for detecting the presence of high negative pressure as well as identifying otitis media with effusion in children (Beery et al., 1975b; Brooks, 1968). The identification

of high negative pressure without effusion in children is indicative of some degree of eustachian tube obstruction. These children as well as those with middle-ear effusions should have follow-up serial tympanograms, as they may be at risk of developing otitis media with effusion.

However, the best methods available to the clinician today for testing eustachian tube function are the nine-step test, when the eardrum is intact, or, when not intact, the inflation-deflation test. A perforation of the tympanic membrane or a tympanostomy tube must be present to perform the latter test. The test uses the simple apparatus described earlier, with or without the electroacoustic impedance bridge pump-manometer system. This test will aid in determining the presence or absence of a dysfunction, and the type of dysfunction (obstruction versus abnormal patency) and its severity when one is present. No other test procedures may be needed if the patient has either functional obstruction of the eustachian tube or an abnormally patent tube. However, if there is a mechanical obstruction, especially if the tube appears to be totally blocked anatomically, then further testing may be indicated. In such instances, computed tomography of the nasopharynx–eustachian tube–middle ear region can be performed to determine the site and cause of the blockage, such as by cholesteatoma or tumor. In most cases in which mechanical obstruction of the tube is found, inflammation is present at the middle-ear end of the eustachian tube (osseous portion), and this usually resolves with medical management or middle-ear surgery, or both. Serial inflation-deflation studies should show resolution of the mechanical obstruction. However, if no middle-ear cause is obvious, other studies should be performed to rule out the possibility of neoplasm in the nasopharynx.

Management

Ideally, patients with recurrent acute otitis media, chronic otitis media with effusion, or both should have eustachian tube function studies as part of their otolaryngologic workup, but for most of these children, one can assume eustachian tube function to be poor. However, patients in whom tympanostomy tubes have been inserted may benefit from serial eustachian tube function studies. Improvement in function as indicated by inflation-deflation tests might aid the clinician in determining the proper time to remove the tubes. Cleft palate repair (Bluestone et al., 1972a; Paradise and Bluestone, 1974), adenoidectomy (Bluestone et al., 1972b, 1975a), elimination of nasal and nasopharyngeal inflammation (Bluestone et al., 1977a), treatment of a nasopharyngeal tumor, or growth and development of a child (Holborow, 1970) may be associated with improvement in eustachian tube function.

Studies of the eustachian tube function of the patient with a chronic perforation of the tympanic membrane may be helpful in determining preoperatively the potential results of tympanoplastic surgery. Holmquist (1968) studied eustachian tube function in adults before and after tympanoplasty and reported that the operation had a high rate of success in patients with good eustachian tube function (i.e., those who could equilibrate applied negative pressure) but that, in patients without good tubal function, surgery frequently failed to close the perforation. These results were corroborated (Miller and Bilodeau, 1967; Siedentop, 1972), but other investigators (Cohn et al., 1979; Ekvall, 1970; Lee and Schuknecht, 1971; Virtanen et al., 1980) found no correlation between the results of the inflation-deflation tests and success or failure of tympanoplasty. Most of these studies failed to define the criteria for "success," and the postoperative follow-up period was too short. Bluestone and coworkers (1979a) assessed children prior to tympanoplasty and found that of 51 ears of 45 children, 8 ears could equilibrate an applied negative pressure (-200 mm H_2O) to some degree; in 7 of these ears, the graft took, no middle-ear effusion occurred, and no recurrence of the perforation developed during a follow-up period of between 1 and 2 years. However, as in the studies in adults, failure to equilibrate an applied negative pressure did not predict failure of the tympanoplasty.

The conclusion to be drawn from these studies is that if the patient is able to equilibrate an applied negative pressure, regardless of age, the success of tympanoplasty is likely, but failure to perform this difficult test will not help the clinician in deciding not to operate. However, the value of testing a patient's ability to equilibrate negative pressure lies in the possibility of determining from the test results if a young child is a candidate for tympanoplasty, when one might decide on the basis of other findings alone to withhold surgery until the child is older.

In children who have unilateral perforation of the tympanic membrane or tympanostomy tube in place and a contralateral tympanic membrane that is intact, the status of the intact side, observed for at least 1 year, can aid in determining whether tympanoplasty should be performed or a tube should be removed. Repair of the eardrum or removal of the tube is usually successful if the contralateral intact side has remained normal (i.e., no middle ear effusion or high negative pressure). Conversely, if the opposite ear has developed middle-ear disease during the previous year, tympanoplasty should be postponed, or, if a tympanostomy tube is in place, it should not be removed.

Even though the testing of eustachian tube function is not an exact science, the methods presently available provide useful information related to the diagnosis and management of otitis media in children.

Nonspecific Factors and Materials Present in Middle Ear

Tissue Factors

A variety of nonspecific factors are present in the middle ear that may play roles in defense against infection. The epithelium of the eustachian tube and middle ear is ciliated with mucus-producing cells that are equipped to trap and expel inhaled particles. The network of fibrin that is present in middle-ear effusions, particularly in mucoid and purulent effusions, restricts movement of organisms and facilitates phagocytosis. Destruction of white blood cells and cells lining the mucosa produces lactic acid and a decrease in pH sufficient to kill or inhibit growth of many bacteria.

Oxidative and Hydrolytic Enzymes

Biochemical studies of middle-ear fluids reveal the presence of a variety of oxidative and hydrolytic enzymes. Oxidative enzymes include lactic, malic, and succinic dehydrogenases. Hydrolytic enzymes include lysozyme, acid and alkaline phosphatases, nonspecific esterase, and leucine and alanine aminopeptidases. The enzymes in the middle-ear effusion may have a host cell origin derived from the blood or the inflamed mucosa. In some studies, concentrations of specific enzymes differed, depending on the quality (mucoid or serous) of the fluid. At present, most of the information about enzymes in middle-ear effusions is descriptive, but the increasing data may lead to hypotheses about the role of tissue and cell products in initiation and maintenance of the middle-ear effusion.

Lysozyme is a hydrolytic enzyme with bacteriolytic activity that is present in blood, urine, tears, middle-ear effusions, and other body fluids. Lysozyme is found in the lysosomes of neutrophils, monocytes, and phagocytic cells of the reticuloendothelial system. The bacteriolytic activity of lysozyme is the result of its ability to solubilize the rigid cell wall common to all bacteria. Lysozyme acts synergistically with complement and specific antibodies to achieve its antibacterial effect. High levels of lysozyme have been found in the middle-ear effusions of patients with otitis media with effusion (Juhn and Huff, 1976; Liu et al., 1975; Veltri and Sprinkle, 1973). Lysozyme concentrations in middle-ear effusions are higher than those in serum and are higher in mucoid than in serous effusions (Lang et al., 1976). The high concentration of this antimicrobial substance may explain the bactericidal and virucidal effects of middle-ear effusion identified by Siirala and colleagues (1952, 1961).

Significant concentrations in middle-ear effusions of lactic dehydrogenase, malate hydrogenase, leucine aminopeptidase, and alkaline phosphatase were identified by Juhn and Huff (1976). Lactic dehydrogenase is an intracellular enzyme liberated during the destruction of tissue. Malate dehydrogenase and the other dehydrogenases of the tricarboxylic acid (Krebs) cycle are believed to be bound to the inner mitochondrial membrane. In otitis media, proliferation of ciliated cells in the middle-ear mucosa occurs. The increase in number of cells and increase in mitochondria may result in higher activity of the enzyme in the middle-ear fluid than in serum (Juhn and Huff, 1976). Leucine aminopeptidase is a proteolytic enzyme that is present in various tissues and is concentrated in leukocytes. Histochemical studies of the location of the enzyme in the middle-ear mucosa show increased activity throughout the mucoperiosteum. The concentrations of all enzymes are higher in middle-ear effusions than they are in simultaneously obtained serum, and they are higher in mucoid than in serous middle-ear effusions. Glew and colleagues (1981) also found that there were higher concentrations of selected hydrolytic and oxidative enzymes in mucoid middle-ear fluids than there were in serous ones. The specific activity of alpha-glucosidase, alpha-mannosidase, beta-glucuronidase, hexosaminidase, acid phosphatase, beta-galactosidase, alkaline phosphatase, and lactic dehydrogenase was 3 to 10 times greater in the mucoid effusions.

Collagenase activity was identified in middle-ear effusions by Ganstrom and coworkers (1985). The enzyme had characteristics similar to those of granulocyte-derived collagenase. The authors hypothesized a role for the enzyme in tissue destruction and development of fluid in the middle ear.

Granulocyte proteases and protease inhibitors have been identified in middle-ear effusions (Carlsson et al., 1983). The proteases may play a role in enhancing the inflammatory response. Protease inhibitors, alpha$_1$-antitrypsin, alpha$_1$-antichymotrypsin, and alpha$_2$-macroglobulin, alone or in complex with proteases, were identified in middle-ear effusions of patients with acute otitis media and otitis media with effusion (Carlsson et al., 1983). The relative importance of the proteases and the inhibitors in the evolution and resolution of middle-ear effusion is uncertain.

Recently Described Factors with Possible Roles in Pathogenesis

The pathogenesis of acute otitis media and otitis media with effusion is not yet understood. The limited insight into modes of pathogenesis restricts rational and appropriate therapy. Therapy is now based on pragmatic responses; acute infection is treated with antimicrobial agents; persistent fluid is drained. Further understanding of the pathogenesis of middle-ear infection and its sequelae should yield more effective therapy.

In addition to the issues related to physiology, anatomy (defects in the integrity of the middle-ear system), epidemiology (genetic susceptibility), microbiology (products of microorganisms that elicit inflammation), and immunology (response to various antigens that lead to tissue injury), the following factors may play roles in the pathogenesis of middle-ear infection and its sequelae:

MUCOSAL DAMAGE. Damage to the epithelium of the upper respiratory tract, including nasal cavity, eustachian tube, and middle ear, may subject the individual to further damage from infectious or environmental agents. This theory suggests that early infection results in more disease because of damage caused by the agent, instead of genetic predisposition to disease that is identified by early infection.

CILIARY DYSKINESIA. Intact mechanical processes of the mucosa of the respiratory tract prevent particulate

antigens from reaching immunocompetent cells in the middle ear. Coordinated function of ciliated and secretory cells entraps and clears the airways of excess secretions, foreign particles, and cellular debris. A defect in ciliary activity may result in impairment of these functions. The ciliary defect may be genetic or may be due to acquired infectious or environmental factors. Children with the immotile cilia syndrome have recurrent pulmonary disease but also have chronic sinusitis and otitis media with effusion (Mygind and Pedersen, 1983). Infections by respiratory viruses are associated with transient abnormalities of cilia in nasal epithelium (Carson et al., 1985). Thus, antecedent viral infection may lead to compromise in mucociliary clearance, producing pooling of secretions in the middle ear and multiplication of bacteria, and resulting in acute suppurative infection in the middle ear.

BACTERIAL ADHERENCE. Biochemical factors of the mucosal membrane may inhibit or promote attachment of bacteria to respiratory mucosa. Preliminary studies of Jorgensen and colleagues (1984) identified increased receptivity for bacteria to nasopharyngeal epithelial cells in patients with acute otitis media, compared with healthy controls.

DRUG FACTORS. Drugs used for general or specific signs or symptoms may alter defense mechanisms and make the patient more or less prone to infection. Prostaglandins increase bronchial fluid secretions, whereas prostaglandin inhibitors decrease the output of serous and mucous cells. Salicylates, however, may also decrease lung mucociliary clearance and tracheal mucociliary transport rate (Gerrity et al., 1983). Similar mechanisms may occur in the eustachian tube and may result in development and persistence of effusion in the middle ear.

These factors are of speculative interest in developing pathogenic models for middle-ear infection. Future investigations will identify whether or not they are important.

MICROBIOLOGY OF OTITIS MEDIA

The microbiologic causes of otitis media have been documented by appropriate cultures of middle-ear effusions obtained by needle aspiration. Many bacteriologic studies of acute otitis media have been performed, and the results are remarkably consistent in demonstrating the importance of *Streptococcus pneumoniae* and *Haemophilus influenzae*. Investigations have identified an increased incidence of infection due to *Branhamella catarrhalis*. Studies of asymptomatic children with middle-ear effusion indicate that bacterial pathogens are also present in these fluids, suggesting that bacteria may be a factor in the development and persistence of the effusion. Epidemiologic evidence associates viral infection with otitis media, but viruses have been isolated or identified by detection of antigen in relatively few episodes of acute otitis media. *Chlamydia trachomatis* is responsible for some

TABLE 21–7. Bacterial Pathogens Isolated from Middle-Ear Aspirates in Infants and Children with Acute Otitis Media

| | PERCENTAGE OF CHILDREN WITH PATHOGEN | | | |
| | Prior to 1981* | | 1980–1987† | |
BACTERIAL PATHOGEN	Mean	Range	Mean	Range
Streptococcus pneumoniae	33	26–53	39	27–52
Haemophilus influenzae	21	14–31	27	16–52
Branhamella catarrhalis	3	0–4	10	2–15
Streptococcus, Group A	8	0.3–24%	3	0–11
Staphylococcus aureus	2	0–3	2	0–16
Miscellaneous bacteria	1	0–2	8	0–24
None or nonpathogens	31	2–47	28	12–35

*Twelve reports from centers in United States, Finland, and Sweden, 1952 to 1981: Bjuggren and Tunevall, 1952; Lahikainen, 1953; Mortimer and Watterson, 1956; Groonroos et al., 1964; Coffey, 1966; Feingold et al., 1966; Halstead et al., 1968; Nilson et al., 1969; Howie et al., 1970; Kamme et al., 1970; Howard et al., 1976; Schwartz, 1981.

†Nine reports from United States and Canada: Kaleida et al., 1986, 1987; Marchant et al., 1986; Harrison et al. 1985; Odio et al., 1985; Bergeron et al., 1987; Rodriguez et al., 1985; Carlin et al., 1987; Kenna et al., 1987.

Percentage greater than 100 per cent owing to multiple pathogens per middle-ear effusion.

episodes of otitis media in infants 6 months of age and younger. The results of these microbiologic studies are reviewed below, and various aspects of the infectious process in the middle ear are considered. The microbiology of complications of otitis media is discussed in Chapters 17 and 18.

Bacteria in Acute Otitis Media

The results of bacteriologic studies of acute otitis media in children from Sweden, Finland, and the United States during the period 1952 to 1981 are similar from country to country and over time. Table 21–7 compares these findings with those of studies that have been reported between 1981 and 1987 from the United States and Canada. The percentage of *S. pneumoniae* and *H. influenzae* is somewhat higher during the latter years, but the percentage of patients with *B. catarrhalis* has risen dramatically. Microbiologic testing results of middle-ear aspirates of Pittsburgh children with acute severe otitis media during the period 1981 to 1984 are presented in Figure 21–61. "Severe" was defined as body temperature greater than 38.5°C, acute otalgia, or headache and irritability.

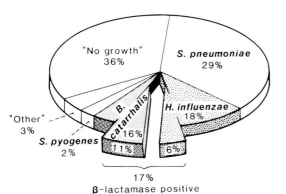

Figure 21–61. Microbiologic testing results of 247 middle-ear aspirates of infants and children with acute "severe" otitis media (From the Pittsburgh Otitis Media Research Center, 1981 to 1984). (From Bluestone, C. D., and Klein, J. O. 1988. Otitis Media in Infants and Children. Philadelphia, W. B. Saunders Co.)

Investigations in Japan (Sugita et al., 1983) and Colombia, South America (Trujillo et al., 1981) report similar bacteriologic results: *S. pneumoniae* and *H. influenzae* are the most frequent agents in all age groups. *B. catarrhalis*, Group A *Streptococcus*, *Staphylococcus aureus*, and gram-negative enteric bacilli are less frequent causes of otitis. No growth (or isolation of an organism considered to be a contaminant, such as *Staphylococcus epidermidis* or diphtheroids) occurs in approximately one third of effusions that are cultured for bacteria.

Streptococcus pneumoniae

Because *S. pneumoniae* is the most important cause of otitis media, investigators have carefully studied the types responsible for infections of the middle ear. The results of studies of 1837 episodes of acute otitis media due to *S. pneumoniae* indicate that relatively few types are responsible for most disease. The most common types in order of decreasing frequency are 19, 23, 6, 14, 3, and 18 (Austrian et al., 1977; Gray et al., 1979; Kamme et al., 1970) (Table 21–8). All are included in the currently available 23-type pneumococcal vaccine. Capsular polysaccharide antigens have been identified in most middle-ear fluids from which pneumococci can be cultured and also in some fluids that are sterile (Palva and Lehtinen, 1987). Detection of bacterial antigens is discussed below.

Studies of bacterial adherence of pneumococci to mucosal surfaces suggest mechanisms of pathogenicity for respiratory tract infections. Pneumococci isolated from patients with recurrent episodes of acute otitis media adhered in larger numbers to epithelial cells from the nasopharynx than did strains from cases of bacteremia or meningitis (Andersson et al., 1981). More bacteria attached to epithelial cells from patients with recurrent episodes of acute otitis media than to cells obtained from controls (Jorgensen et al., 1984).

A change in the ecology of *S. pneumoniae* is reflected in altered patterns of susceptibility to antimicrobial agents. The vast majority of strains of *S. pneumoniae* are susceptible to very small concentrations of penicil-

TABLE 21–8. Distribution of Serotypes of 1837 Strains of _Streptococcus pneumoniae_ Isolated from Middle-Ear Effusions of Children with Acute Otitis Media

SEROTYPE	PERCENTAGE OF STRAINS
1	2.1
3	8.5
4	3.4
6	12.0
7	2.3
8	1.5
9	2.9
14	10.3
18	5.8
19	23.0
23	12.5
Others	15.7

Data from Austrian et al., 1977; Gray et al., 1979; Kamme et al., 1970.

lin G; the minimal inhibitory concentration (MTC; least amount of drug required to inhibit growth of the organism) is less than 0.05 µg/ml. Multiresistant strains of _S. pneumoniae_ that are highly resistant to penicillin G (MIC more than 4 µg/ml) were first noted in South Africa (Appelbaum et al., 1977) and have remained restricted to that area. Few of these strains have been identified in the United States and Western Europe (Cates et al., 1978; Ward, 1981). However, many strains of _S. pneumoniae_ that have been isolated from more recent cases of otitis media have had decreased susceptibility to penicillin G (MIC 0.1 to 1.0 µg/ml) (Ward, 1981; Appelbaum, 1987).

Haemophilus influenzae

Otitis media due to _H. influenzae_ is associated with nontypable strains in the vast majority of patients. In approximately 10 per cent of cases due to _H. influenzae_ the isolate is Type b; some of these children appear to have severe infection, and about one quarter have concomitant bacteremia or meningitis (Harding et al., 1973). Cases of otitis due to types a, e, and f have been reported but are infrequent.

Until recently, no markers were available to distinguish among the nonencapsulated types of _H. influenzae_. It is now known that the group is heterogeneous and may be classified by biochemical and antigenic markers. Biochemical profiles have been used to classify strains of nontypable _H. influenzae_ isolated from middle-ear fluids; the majority of strains belong to two biotypes based on assays of indole, urease, and ornithine decarboxylase (DeMaria et al., 1984b). Current studies of outer membrane proteins also aim at a means of classifying the nonencapsulated strains; eight major proteins have been identified (Loeb and Smith, 1980). A serotyping system based on antigenic patterns of outer membranes has been suggested (Murphy and Apicella, 1985). Thus, outer membrane protein patterns may be used to evaluate the relatedness of nontypable _H. influenzae_ isolated from middle-ear fluids (Murphy et al., 1987).

H. influenzae was considered to be restricted in importance to otitis media occurring in preschool children; however, the organism is also a significant cause of otitis media in older children, adolescents, and adults. _H. influenzae_ was isolated from middle-ear fluids of 36 per cent of children, aged 5 to 9 years, with acute otitis media (Schwartz et al., 1977). _H. influenzae_ was the cause of otitis media in 33 per cent of 18 children aged 8 through 17 years (Schwartz and Rodriguez, 1981). _H. influenzae_ was also isolated from 15 of 45 patients over 16 years of age (Herberts et al., 1971). In a survey of cases of acute otitis seen in primary care hospitals in metropolitan Tokyo for the year beginning July 1979, 28 per cent of 31 bacteria isolated from middle-ear effusions of patients 10 to 15 years of age and 15 per cent of 76 bacteria found in patients 16 to 70 years of age were _H. influenzae_ (Sugita et al., 1983). Thus, the proportion of acute otitis media due to _H. influenzae_ is approximately the same in all age groups.

Fifteen to 33 per cent of nontypable strains of _H. influenzae_ isolated from middle-ear effusions of children with acute otitis media produce a beta-lactamase that hydrolyzes ampicillin, amoxicillin, and penicillins G and V. The incidence of beta-lactamase strains of nontypable _H. influenzae_ has risen in the Pittsburgh area and in 1986 had reached 30 per cent (Table 21–9).

Branhamella catarrhalis

Before 1983, _B. catarrhalis_ was isolated infrequently from purulent middle-ear fluids (Coffey et al., 1967), and many considered the organism a commensal with limited potential for causing disease. In 1983, reports from Pittsburgh (Kovatch et al., 1983) and Cleveland (Shurin et al., 1983) noted a marked increase in incidence; the organism was isolated from middle-ear fluids of 22 per cent and 27 per cent, respectively, of a consecutive series of children enrolled in studies of acute otitis media. In Dallas, during a similar time period, the incidence of _B. catarrhalis_ in middle-ear fluids was lower: 6 per cent of 150 children (Odio et al., 1985).

B. catarrhalis is a respiratory pathogen capable of causing acute otitis media. The data from Pittsburgh and Cleveland make it the third most likely bacterium

TABLE 21–9. Percentage of _Haemophilus influenzae_ and _Branhamella catarrhalis_ that Produce Beta-Lactamase

YEAR	H. INFLUENZAE		B. CATARRHALIS	
	Number	%	Number	%
1981	149	17	23	67
1982	103	21	46	80
1983	65	22	51	79
1984	70	36	33	68
1985	93	28	41	87
1986	113	34	74	82

From Pittsburgh Otitis Media Research Center, 1981–1986.
With permission from Bluestone, C. D. Management of otitis media in infants and children: Current role of old and new antimicrobial agents. Pediatr. Infect. Dis. J. 7:S129–136. © by Williams & Wilkins, 1988.

responsible for acute otitis media, behind *S. pneumoniae* and *H. influenzae* (Kaleida et al., 1986*b*, 1987; Marchant et al., 1986). Future studies will determine whether or not the Cleveland and Pittsburgh experiences were isolated or presage a uniform increase in importance of *B. catarrhalis* in otitis media.

Prior to 1970 almost all strains of *B. catarrhalis* were sensitive to penicillin and ampicillin. Most if not all strains of *B. catarrhalis* isolated from middle-ear fluids produce beta-lactamase in more recent studies (Table 21–9). The increased incidence of infection due to this organism may require a change in initial therapy from the ampicillins, which are susceptible to beta-lactamases. The proportion of cases of otitis media caused by beta-lactamase–producing *B. catarrhalis* and *H. influenzae* determines the need for a change in initial therapy.

Leinonen and colleagues (1981) provided serologic evidence for a pathogenic role of *B. catarrhalis* in children with acute otitis media. The presence of IgG and IgA antibodies to *B. catarrhalis* in serum, middle-ear fluid, or both was correlated with isolation of the organism from the middle ear. An increase in titer of antibodies to the organisms was found between acute and convalescent sera in 10 of 19 children with acute otitis media whose middle-ear fluid yielded *B. catarrhalis* alone, and no increase was seen in 14 children with acute otitis media whose middle-ear fluids yielded other pathogens.

Groups A and B Streptococci

During the preantibiotic era, otitis due to Group A streptococcus was frequently associated with scarlet fever and was often of a destructive form (Clarke, 1962). *Streptococcus hemolyticus* (presumably Group A streptococcus) was the most prevalent organism in cultures taken at myringotomy for acute otitis media and the most frequent cause of mastoid infection in patients undergoing mastoidectomy during 1934 (Page, 1935). More recently, Group A streptococcus has been a significant pathogen in some studies of otitis media from Scandinavia, but this has not been the case in most studies from the United States. Otitis media due to Group A streptococcus now seems to be less frequent and less virulent.

Group B streptococcus is, with *Escherichia coli*, the leading cause of sepsis and meningitis in the newborn infant, as reported by surveys in the United States and Western Europe (Klein and Marcy, 1983). Group B streptococci have been isolated from various body fluids, including middle-ear fluid in neonates with otitis media. Bacteremia is frequently associated with otitis media in these infants.

Staphylococcus aureus

S. aureus is an uncommon cause of acute otitis media; the organism was isolated in fewer than 3 per cent of samples of middle-ear fluids from children with acute infection (see Table 21–7). Studies from Japan indicate a higher incidence of middle-ear infection, approximately 10 per cent, due to *S. aureus* (Baba, 1985).

Staphylococcus epidermidis *and Diphtheroids*

The roles of coagulase-negative staphylococci (Feigin et al., 1973*b*) and diphtheroids in acute otitis media are uncertain. These organisms are considered commensals and are part of the skin flora of the external-ear canal. Isolation of pure cultures of coagulase-negative staphylococci from cases of purulent middle-ear effusions after adequate cleansing of the external canal suggest a pathogenic role in a limited number of cases. Nine different species of coagulase-negative staphylococci have been isolated from middle-ear fluids; *S. epidermidis* is the most common (Bernstein et al., 1984).

Specific antibody to diphtheroids was identified in middle-ear effusions and sera of children undergoing myringotomy for chronic otitis media with effusion (Lewis et al., 1979). Bernstein and colleagues (1980) found antibody-coated *S. epidermidis* and diphtheroids in the middle ears of children with otitis media with effusion. The fluids contained specific antibody, and, in several cases of otitis due to *S. epidermidis*, antibody was present in middle-ear fluid but absent from serum. These data indicate that diphtheroids and *S. epidermidis* may elicit an immune response in the middle ear. The role of these organisms in middle-ear disease, however, remains uncertain. It is possible that they are opportunistic bacteria that invade the middle ear only under certain circumstances, such as persistent effusion.

Gram-Negative Bacilli

Gram-negative bacilli are responsible for about 20 per cent of cases of otitis media in young infants, but these organisms are rarely present in the middle-ear effusions of older children with acute otitis media (Table 21–10). Gram-negative bacteria, particularly *Pseudomonas aeruginosa*, are frequently associated with chronic suppurative otitis media.

A report from Israel described 33 patients of varying ages with acute otitis media caused by gram-negative bacilli (Ostfeld and Rubinstein, 1980). *P. aeruginosa* was isolated from middle-ear fluids of 23 patients, and an indole-positive *Proteus* species was isolated from the fluids in six patients. Seven of the patients were 3 months of age or younger, 16 were 4 to 24 months of age, and 10 were 2 to 80 years of age. Four adult patients had diabetes mellitus, but there were no other patients with significant underlying diseases. The patients had a high rate of other disease manifestations due to the organism isolated from the middle-ear effusion; of these patients, five had acute mastoiditis, three had accompanying bacteremia, and four adult patients showed extensive osteomyelitis of the base of the skull. Culture material was obtained from purulent drainage from the middle ear in cases with perforated

TABLE 21–10. Bacterial Pathogens Isolated from 270 Neonates and Young Infants with Otitis Media During First 6 Weeks of Life

MICROORGANISM	INFANTS WITH PATHOGEN (%)
Respiratory Bacteria	
Streptococcus pneumoniae	18
Haemophilus influenzae	12
S. pneumoniae and *H. influenzae*	7
Staphylococcus aureus	8
Streptococcus, Groups A and B	3
Branhamella catarrhalis	6
Enteric Bacteria	
Escherichia coli	6
Klebsiella and *Enterobacter* species	5
Pseudomonas aeruginosa	2
Miscellaneous	6
None or Nonpathogens	32

Data from Berman et al., 1978; Bland, 1972; Shurin et al., 1978; Tetzlaff et al., 1977; Karma et al., 1987.

tympanic membranes, and the bacteriologic results may represent contaminants from the external ear. In addition, some patients had prolonged courses that might be better described as chronic suppurative otitis media. Nevertheless, this series indicates a potential danger of acute middle-ear infection due to gram-negative bacilli.

Anaerobic Bacteria

Improvements in techniques for isolation and identification of anaerobic bacteria have provided a better understanding of the anaerobic flora of humans and the roles of these organisms in disease. Brook and Schwartz (1981) identified a limited role for anaerobic bacteria in acute otitis media. Twenty-eight infants with acute infection were studied: aerobic bacteria were isolated from the middle-ear fluids of 20 children; cultures from two children yielded mixtures of aerobic and anaerobic bacteria. Brook (1987) has been able to isolate anaerobic bacteria in 12 per cent of culture-positive aspirates from ears of children with otitis media with effusion; predominant anaerobes were gram-negative cocci and *Bacteroides melaninogenicus*. Luotonen and coworkers (1982) failed to isolate anaerobic bacteria from 71 middle-ear aspirates from 59 subjects. These data suggest that anaerobic organisms are relatively uncommon in middle-ear effusions of children who have acute otitis media.

Mixed and Disparate Cultures

Disparate results of cultures of middle-ear fluids occur when cultures of the two ears in bilateral disease yield different information: effusion from one ear is sterile but a bacterial pathogen is isolated from the other ear, or a different bacterial pathogen is isolated from each of the two ears. Mixed cultures may also

occur: two types or two species of bacteria are found in the same middle-ear fluid. Groonroos and colleagues (1964) reported 31.6 per cent disparate results of cultures from children with bilateral otitis media. All children had *S. pneumoniae, H. influenzae,* or Group A streptococci in fluid from one middle ear and sterile fluid in the other. Van Dishoeck and colleagues (1959) found that 19 per cent of cultures from children with bilateral otitis media yielded different results. The majority of children had a pathogen recovered from one ear and sterile fluid in the other. Also included were six cases in which cultures of one middle-ear fluid yielded a single pathogen but, in the opposite middle-ear fluid, two pathogens were found. Austrian and associates (1977) recovered different serotypes of *S. pneumoniae* from middle-ear fluids in 18 children, which represented 1.5 per cent of the cases of bilateral pneumococcal otitis media. Pelton and coworkers (1980) cultured middle-ear fluid from both ears of 122 children with bilateral acute otitis media. Disparate results were found in 31 (25 per cent) of the children: in 25 children a pathogen was present in one ear and the fluid from the other ear was sterile or yielded a nonpathogen; in six children different pathogens (*H. influenzae* and *S. pneumoniae* in each case) were isolated from the two fluids. Howard and colleagues (1976) noted *S. pneumoniae* and *H. influenzae* together in 20 effusions (5 per cent of those studied).

These data indicate that investigative microbiologic studies of bilateral otitis media must include aspiration of both ears to determine the efficacy of methods of treatment (i.e., trials of antimicrobial agents) or prevention (i.e., evaluation of vaccines or drugs). In addition, the complete bacteriologic assessment of the middle ear for a child undergoing tympanocentesis for diagnostic purposes can only be accomplished by aspirating both middle-ear effusions when the disease is bilateral.

Sterile Cultures

In all studies of acute otitis media, a significant proportion (approximately one third) of middle-ear fluids are sterile after appropriate and usual cultures for bacteria have been made. The cause of these cases of otitis media may be one or more of the following:

1. A nonbacterial organism such as a virus, chlamydia, or mycoplasma.
2. A fastidious bacterial organism, such as an anaerobic bacterium, that is not isolated by usual laboratory techniques.
3. Bacterial antigens may be present in the absence of viable organisms indicating past or present bacterial infection and suppression of growth of the organism.
4. An immune response to a noninfectious agent such as pollen or other antigen.
5. Prior administration of an antimicrobial agent that would suppress growth of bacteria.
6. Presence of antimicrobial enzymes, such as lysozymes, alone or in combination with immunoglobu-

lins in middle-ear fluid, that would suppress growth of bacteria.

7. An acute illness in a child who has persistent middle-ear effusion from an episode of otitis media some time in the past. Because children may have middle-ear effusion for weeks to months after the onset of acute otitis media (Teele et al., 1980b), an illness due to a subsequent infectious episode, during the time spent with middle-ear effusion persisting from a prior episode of otitis, might be assumed by the physician to be a recurrence of acute otitis media.

Use of the Gram stain is of value in identification of fastidious bacterial organisms and may provide evidence of bacterial infection, although antibiotics or antimicrobial substances inhibit growth of bacteria. Techniques for identification of bacterial and viral antigens are also likely to decrease the number of episodes of otitis that are now categorized as "no growth."

Identification of Bacterial Antigens

Results of studies using techniques for identification of bacterial antigens provide insights into the infectious process. Counterimmunoelectrophoresis (CIE), latex agglutination, and enzyme-linked immunosorbent assay (ELISA) have been used to detect bacterial antigens such as capsular polysaccharides of *S. pneumoniae*, *H. influenzae* Type b, *Neisseria meningitidis*, and Group B streptococci in blood, urine, cerebrospinal fluid, and other body fluids. These methods are advantageous because of ease of performance, rapidity, specificity, sensitivity (as little as 0.2 ng of polysaccharide capsular antigens can be detected), and ability to identify bacteria that do not grow in culture media.

S. pneumoniae is identified by CIE in most middle-ear fluids in which the organism is cultured and in many specimens that have no bacterial growth (Luotonen et al., 1981; Ostfeld and Altmann, 1980). Luotonen and colleagues identified pneumococcal capsular polysaccharide in 83 per cent of middle-ear fluids from which *S. pneumoniae* was cultured and in about one third of middle-ear effusions from which no bacteria was grown. Type-specific pneumococcal antigens may persist for periods in excess of 6 months (Karma et al., 1985). Palva and Lehtinen (1987) found pneumococcus capsular polysaccharide antigen in 16 per cent of 108 middle-ear effusions from children who had otitis media with effusion, but in only 1 per cent was the pneumococcus isolated. Different serotypes have differing sensitivity of antigen detection. Thus, sensitivity for detection in culture-positive samples of Types 1, 15, and 19 was high, whereas sensitivity for Type 23 was low; the sensitivity for Type 6A was higher than that for 6B (Herva et al., 1984). These methods used to detect bacterial antigen add information about the large number of patients who have negative results of bacterial cultures.

Viruses in Acute Otitis Media

Epidemiologic data suggest that viral infection is frequently associated with acute otitis media. In a longitudinal study of respiratory illnesses and complications in children 6 weeks to 6 years of age attending a day-care and school program, Henderson and colleagues (1982) demonstrated a correlation between isolation of viruses from the upper respiratory tract and clinical diagnosis of otitis media. Concurrent or antecedent (within 14 days) viral infection was identified in 26.3 per cent of episodes of otitis media in children under 3 years of age. Viral outbreaks coincided with epidemics of otitis media. Otitis media was increased in the 14 days after upper respiratory tract isolation of respiratory syncytial viruses, adenoviruses (usually Types 1, 2, and 5), influenza virus Types A and B, parainfluenza and mumps viruses, and enteroviruses. Rhinoviruses were not significantly associated with the occurrence of otitis media.

Viruses are infrequently isolated from the middle-ear effusions of children with acute infection of the middle ear; a virus was isolated from only 4.4 per cent of 663 patients (Klein and Teele, 1976) (Table 21–11). Respiratory syncytial virus and influenza virus were isolated most frequently. The isolation of these two agents was usually made during periods of epidemic infection in the community. Isolation rates of viruses have not improved with current techniques. Howie and coworkers (1982) isolated viruses from 4 of 88 middle-ear fluids obtained from patients with acute otitis media: two specimens yielded adenovirus; influenza B virus and RSV were each present in one specimen. In a subsequent study, the investigators isolated viruses from 20 per cent of 84 children; influenza virus, enterovirus, and rhinovirus were the most common agents found (Chonmaitree et al., 1986).

Studies of viral antigens yield more information about their role in otitis media (Klein et al., 1982). Klein and colleagues (1982) found evidence of viral antigen by means of ELISA in middle-ear fluids obtained from approximately one quarter of children with acute otitis media. Of 13 children with viral antigen in the middle ear, RSV was most frequently identified (10 children); influenza virus (2 children) and rotavirus (1 child) were also identified but were uncommon. The ELISA measures viral antigens rather than replicating virions and may detect viral materials that grow poorly or not at all in tissue culture or animal systems. Failure to identify viruses in middle-ear fluids may be

TABLE 21–11. Isolation of Viruses in 663 Patients with Otitis Media*

VIRUS	NUMBER OF PATIENTS
Respiratory syncytial virus (RSV)	22
Influenza viruses	4
Coxsackievirus B4	1
Adenovirus 3	1
Parainfluenza 2	1
TOTALS	29 (4.4%)
No Growth	634

*622 patients had acute and 41 had chronic otitis media.
With permission from Klein, J. O., and Teele, D. W. 1976. Isolation of viruses and mycoplasmas from middle ear effusions: A review. Ann. Otol. Rhinol. Laryngol. 85 (Suppl. 25):140–144.

due to inadequate sensitivity of available techniques. During an epidemic of RSV, Sarkkinen and colleagues (1985) identified RSV antigen in the middle-ear effusions of 15 per cent of children with otitis media; adenovirus antigen was found in an additional 3 per cent of patients. Interferon was identified in four of eight middle-ear fluids that had positive results for RSV antigen (Salonen et al., 1984). Bacterial isolations were similar in middle-ear fluids, regardless of whether the results were positive or negative for viruses. Thus, antibacterial agents may successfully eradicate the bacterial agent from the middle-ear effusion, but signs of disease may persist because of the concurrent viral infection.

As in studies of isolation of viruses from middle-ear fluids, RSV antigen was identified in the majority of fluids, and other viral antigens were identified infrequently. Richman and colleagues (1984) believe that ELISA techniques have reached the limit of their sensitivity for identification of viral antigens and that rapid viral diagnosis will require new approaches. They discuss two useful techniques: detection of viral antigen by visual localization of virus-specific immunoenzyme staining, and detection of viral nucleic acids in clinical specimens by hybridization with nucleic acid probes (Richman et al., 1984).

Otitis media may accompany exanthematous viral infections, such as measles and infectious mononucleosis caused by Epstein-Barr virus (Sumaya and Ench, 1985). Invasion of the middle ear by smallpox virus has been demonstrated. Guarnieri bodies were present in the tympanic membrane of a 3-month-old Indian child who died of smallpox (Bordley and Kapur, 1972).

Viral studies of children with acute otitis media suggest an important role for RSV, a lesser role for adenoviruses and influenza viruses, but an uncertain role for other respiratory viruses. The small number of viruses other than RSV that have been isolated from middle-ear fluids may indicate that (1) viruses were present early in the course of the disease and were no longer present when the patients sought medical attention; (2) these viruses were present in low concentrations and not readily isolated from the ear fluids; (3) inhibitory materials such as antibody, interferon, or lysozymes prevented successful isolation; (4) viruses produced inflammatory changes in the upper respiratory tract but were not present in the effusion fluid; or (5) these viruses were not associated with many episodes of acute otitis media.

Mycoplasma

The isolation and identification of mycoplasma from secretions obtained from the upper respiratory tract are now readily accomplished in solid and liquid media. These organisms may have a role in otitis media: myringitis, associated with hemorrhage and bleb formation in the more severe cases, was observed in nonimmune volunteers inoculated with *Mycoplasma pneumoniae* (Rifkind et al., 1962). Bullous myringitis

in children may result from various bacterial pathogens responsible for otitis media; its presence does not indicate mycoplasma infection (Roberts, 1980). However, the middle-ear fluid of a large number of patients (771) has been studied (Klein and Teele, 1976), and *M. pneumoniae* was isolated in only 1 case (Sobeslavsky et al., 1965).

During an investigation of a community outbreak of pneumonia due to mycoplasma, 59 per cent of children with otitis media were shown (by isolation of the organism from the pharynx or by antibody responses) to have had an infection with *M. pneumoniae* (Jensen et al., 1967). Thus, it is likely that mycoplasma infection causes disease in all parts of the respiratory tract, including the middle ear. Patients with respiratory tract disease due to *M. pneumoniae* may have accompanying otitis media, but the organism appears to play a limited role in the overall picture of acute otitis media in children.

Chlamydia

C. trachomatis is the etiologic agent of a mild but prolonged pneumonitis in infants. Many infants with pneumonia due to *C. trachomatis* have otitis media (Schachter et al., 1979; Tipple et al., 1979). Tipple and coworkers (1979) isolated the organism from ear aspirates of 3 of 11 infants with chlamydial pneumonia. Chang and colleagues (1982) recovered *C. trachomatis* from the middle-ear effusions of 2 of 12 children with acute otitis media and 1 of 14 children with persistent middle-ear effusion. One of the children with acute infection was 10 months of age, but the report did not provide ages for the other two children. *C. trachomatis* was not isolated from middle-ear fluids obtained at the time of placement of tympanostomy tubes in 68 children, 9 months to 8 years of age (Hammerschlag et al., 1980). Thus, *C. trachomatis* is associated with acute respiratory tract infections, including otitis media, in young infants (under age 6 months).

Uncommon Microorganisms

Corynebacterium diphtheriae

Diphtheritic otitis may accompany diphtheritic croup and nasopharyngitis. Although many cases cannot be differentiated from other forms of purulent otitis, diphtheritic membranes may form and be recognized in the middle ear. Complications are frequent, including destruction of the tympanic membrane and ossicles and invasive infection of contiguous structures leading to necrosis of the mastoid process, temporal bone, and labyrinth (Downes, 1959; Drury, 1925). Two cases of otitis media due to *C. diphtheriae* were among 1741 cases reported to the Centers for Disease Control for the years 1959 and 1960 (Doege et al., 1962). Five cases of diphtheritic otitis occurred among 1433 cases of diphtheria seen at the Los Angeles

County Hospital during the 10-year period beginning June 1941 (Naiditch and Bower, 1954).

Mycobacterium tuberculosis

At the turn of the century, tuberculous otitis was an occasional cause of severe middle-ear disease, particularly in the very young. Turner and Fraser (1915) reported a series of cases at the Royal Infirmary in Edinburgh for the period 1907 to 1914; 51, or 2.8 per cent, were due to tuberculosis, and 84 per cent of these cases occurred in the first year of life. The disease is seen in underdeveloped areas of the world, but occasional cases occur in the United States: bovine tuberculosis was responsible for 29 cases of chronic otorrhea in children seen in Kampala between 1969 and 1972 (Raikundalia, 1975), 11 cases of tuberculous otitis were reported in Capetown children between 1967 and 1971 (Sellars and Seid, 1973), and 3 patients with tuberculous otitis were seen in Oklahoma City in the same period as the Capetown cases (MacAdam and Rubio, 1977). Tuberculous infection should be considered when chronic otorrhea occurs in recent immigrants from areas with high rates of infection. Skolnik and colleagues (1986) reviewed the literature of tuberculosis of the middle ear.

When otitis occurs as the only apparent focus of tuberculous infection, the disease is usually due to ingestion of infected cow's milk. The infection may also occur in patients with active pulmonary disease; the middle ear is infected from the upper respiratory tract.

Tuberculous otitis is characterized by a painless, watery otorrhea through single or multiple perforations of the tympanic membrane; enlarged periauricular lymph nodes; and a high incidence of facial paralysis and early hearing loss. Mastoiditis is a frequent complication (Mumtaz et al., 1983). The diagnosis of tuberculous otitis media is based on demonstration of acid-fast bacilli within granuloma in biopsy materials, with or without the culture of *M. tuberculosis* from the biopsy, aural drainage, or aspirate of middle-ear fluid. Chemotherapy shortens the course and severity of the disease, but persistent hearing loss is frequent.

Clostridium tetani

Otogenous tetanus usually occurs as a sequela of chronic otitis media. *C. tetani* multiplies in the purulent drainage in the external ear canal and may gain access to the middle ear (Deinard et al., 1980). The organism may be present also in the oropharynx, and it is possible that infection in the middle ear occurs via the eustachian tube. *C. tetani* was isolated from swabs of middle-ear fluid of eight children in Bangkok with otitis media, otorrhea, and trismus and other signs of tetanus (Fischer et al., 1977).

Ascaris lumbricoides

The only parasitic infection that has been associated with otitis media is *Ascaris lumbricoides*. Roundworms may be vomited through the mouth or nostrils, enter the eustachian tube, and produce an inflammatory reaction in the middle ear. The worm perforates the tympanic membrane and emerges through the external canal. A case report described infection in a 1.5-year-old child who was brought to a Bombay clinic with a worm emerging from the ear. A 7.5-cm-long roundworm, *A. lumbricoides*, was removed from the canal and middle ear (Shah and Desai, 1969).

Microbial Products in Middle-Ear Effusions

In addition to bacterial and viral antigens, other products such as endotoxin, interferon, and bacterial enzymes suggest the current or former presence of microorganisms.

Endotoxin

Endotoxin has been detected in middle-ear effusions that contain nontypable *H. influenzae*. Endotoxins are lipopolysaccharide complexes on the surface of gram-negative bacteria that have many biologic effects, including production of fever and inflammation. Physiologic activities persist after death of the organism. DeMaria and colleagues (1984d) detected endotoxin in 80 per cent of 89 middle-ear fluids obtained at placement of ventilating tubes. Endotoxin was not only present in all except one fluid from which *H. influenzae* was cultured but also was present (though in lesser concentrations) in fluids that had negative culture and fluids that cultured *S. pneumoniae* (which does not contain endotoxin). The source of endotoxin for the middle-ear fluids that did not contain endotoxin-producing microorganisms is unknown. Endotoxin may play a role in the pathogenesis of inflammation in the middle ear; purified endotoxin from killed *H. influenzae* induced production of middle-ear fluid (DeMaria et al., 1984a).

Interferon

Local production of interferon in the middle ear was suggested by findings of higher concentrations in specimens of middle-ear fluid when compared with levels in serum (Howie et al., 1982). The presence of interferon suggests a current or antecedent viral infection or possibly a bacterial infection. Salonen and colleagues recovered interferon in middle-ear fluids positive for RSV antigen and failed to detect interferon in antigen-negative specimens (Salonen et al., 1984). In contrast, Howie and colleagues demonstrated the presence of interferon in middle-ear fluids containing pathogenic bacteria in the absence of detectable viruses, suggesting bacterial induction of interferon (Howie et al., 1982). The role of interferon in middle-ear infection remains to be elucidated.

TABLE 21–12. Bacteriologic Results of 179 Chronic Middle-Ear Effusions in Children 1 to 16 Years of Age

TYPE OF ORGANISM	PERCENTAGE OF EARS WITH MIDDLE-EAR EFFUSION			
	Serous (48 ears)	Mucoid (112 ears)	Purulent (19 ears)	Total (179 ears)
S. pneumoniae	4	4	—	4
H. influenzae	8*	11	16	11
Streptococcus	—	—	5	0.6
B. catarrhalis	2	4	16	4
S. aureus	4	3	—	3
S. epidermidis	15	12	5	12
Others†	31	22	26	25
Percentage of ears with organism‡	52	43	68	48

*Includes one effusion with *H. influenzae* Type b; no ampicillin-resistant organisms were identified.

†Alpha- or nonhemolytic streptococci, microaerophilic streptococci, *Moraxella, Propionibacterium, Escherichia coli*, diphtheroids, *Candida albicans*.

‡This number is smaller than the sum of each percentage above because some ears contained more than one type of organism.

Modified from Riding, K. H., et al. 1978. Microbiology of recurrent and chronic otitis media with effusion. J. Pediatr. 93:739–743.

Neuraminidase

Neuraminidase identified at neutral pH was found in middle-ear fluids from patients with acute otitis media and otitis media with effusion. LaMarco and colleagues (1984) noted that almost all fluids that grew *S. pneumoniae* had neuraminidase activity, whereas only about one third of fluids that grew other bacteria or no bacteria had evidence of the enzyme. The plasma of patients lacked neuraminidase activity, indicating that the enzyme in the middle-ear fluid originated in the middle ear and was not a transudate from blood. Because mammalian neuraminidases have optimal activity near pH 4, these investigators concluded that the source of the neutral pH neuraminidase was microorganisms. The enzyme may be an important factor in the pathogenesis of disease caused by *S. pneumoniae*.

Chronic Otitis Media with Effusion

Chronic effusions have in the past been assumed to be sterile: several reports described unsuccessful attempts to culture bacteria (Harcourt and Brown, 1953; Robinson and Nicholas, 1951; Siirala and Vuori, 1956). Senturia and coworkers (1958), however, were able to identify bacteria by means of smears and cultures from 42 per cent of children with otitis media with effusion; since then other workers have reported similar results. The studies were performed by investigators in Columbus, Ohio (Liu et al., 1975), Boston (Healy and Teele, 1977), and Minneapolis (Giebink et al., 1979). The protocols were similar: most children were observed to have persistent effusion for at least 2 months; at the time of myringotomy or placement of tympanostomy tubes, fluid was obtained from the middle ear for culture of bacteria. In each study, 30 to 50 per cent of the children had bacteria in the middle-ear fluid. *S. pneumoniae, H. influenzae, B. catarrhalis*, or Group A streptococcus were isolated from 10 to 22 per cent of the fluids of these asymptomatic children.

These studies are cited because all included appropriate cleansing of the external canal prior to aspiration of the middle-ear fluid. Other studies are not included because of failure to cleanse the canal and thus may include bacteriologic results of middle-ear fluids contaminated by external canal flora. A special problem is presented by obtaining appropriate sampling for bacteria of the chronically draining ear. Cultures of fluid from draining ears require, first, removal of debris and fluid in the canal, which includes material from the middle ear mixed with external canal flora, and second, careful aspiration of fluid from the middle ear as it emerges through the tympanic membrane or by means of tympanocentesis. Without use of techniques of direct aspiration of fluid from the middle ear, microbiologic results must be considered of uncertain validity.

The bacteriologic results of chronic middle ear effusions of 179 Pittsburgh children aged 1 to 16 years are given in Table 21–12. Bacteria were cultured from 86 of 179 (48 per cent) chronic middle-ear effusions, and the organisms were present in serous, mucoid, and purulent effusions (Riding et al., 1978). The most common species were *H. influenzae, B. catarrhalis, S. pneumoniae*, and *S. aureus. S. epidermidis* was cultured from many middle ears when this organism was not cultured from the external canal of the same ear (a culture preceded sterilization and tympanocentesis). Bacteria were also cultured from 37 per cent of chronic middle-ear effusions found in Pittsburgh infants aged 1 to 12 months (Stanievich et al., 1981); *S. pneumoniae* and *H. influenzae* were present in 23 per cent of the ears. *S. pneumoniae* and *H. influenzae* were cultured from 50 per cent of 20 persistent middle-ear fluids of Pittsburgh infants with unrepaired cleft palates (Stanievich et al., 1981). More recent information from Pittsburgh contrasts the microbiologic results in acute otitis media with those in chronic otitis media with effusion (Fig. 21–62).

Anaerobic bacteria were isolated from the middle-ear fluids of few patients with chronic otitis media (Giebink et al., 1979; Sipilä et al., 1981; Teele et al., 1980a).

A higher incidence of bacterial pathogens was identified in fluids from persistent middle-ear infection in children 3 years of age or younger than in older children (Pelton et al., 1977).

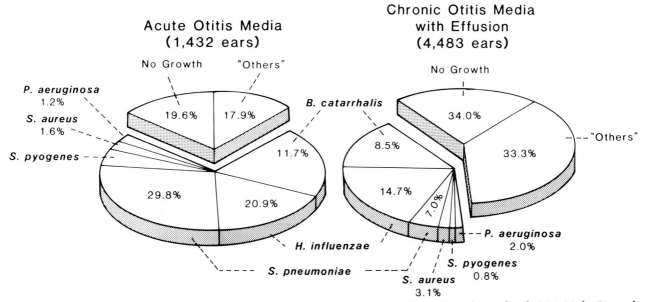

Figure 21–62. Microbiologic causes of acute otitis media and chronic otitis media with effusion (from the Pittsburgh Otitis Media Research Center, 1980 to 1985).

Herpes simplex virus was isolated from fluid of one child with persistent middle-ear effusion (Giebink et al., 1979), but use of an ELISA technique did not detect viral antigens in 96 such fluids (Sarkkinen et al., 1982).

Middle-ear fluid of asymptomatic children may harbor bacterial pathogens similar to those identified in acute otitis media, including *S. pneumoniae* and *H. influenzae*. The significance of this finding is at present uncertain. There were only minimal differences in the rates of isolation of bacteria from serous, mucoid, or purulent fluids. The bacteria may be present without provoking an inflammatory response, or they may produce a low-grade or subclinical infection, or the effusion may represent an immune response to the prolonged presence of the bacteria. Specific antibody to the bacteria isolated is present in the middle-ear fluid of children with persistent effusion (Bernstein et al., 1980; Lewis et al., 1979). This finding suggests that the bacteria are not passive in chronic middle-ear effusion but elicit an immunologic response and may be involved in the production and persistence of fluid.

Otitis Media in the Newborn

Bacteriologic data are available from aspiration of middle-ear fluids of 270 neonates with otitis media (see Table 21–10). *S. pneumoniae* and *H. influenzae* are the bacteria isolated most frequently in the very young, as is the case in older infants and children. However, organisms associated with local and systemic infection in the newborn infant, Group B streptococcus, *S. aureus*, and gram-negative enteric bacilli, are important pathogens in the newborn infant within 2 weeks after birth or in older infants who have remained in the nursery because of risk features (low birth weight

or prematurity) or disease (respiratory distress syndrome). When term infants who have had no problems with delivery or nursery experience develop otitis media 2 weeks or more after hospital discharge, the spectrum of bacterial pathogens is similar to that of older infants and most likely to be *S. pneumoniae* and *H. influenzae*.

External-Ear Canal

The microbial flora of the external canal is similar to the flora of skin elsewhere on the body. In various microbiologic studies there is a predominance of *S. epidermidis*, *S. aureus*, and diphtheroids and, to a lesser extent, anaerobic bacteria such as *P. acnes* and anaerobic cocci (Brook and Schwartz, 1981; Pelton et al., 1980; Riding et al., 1978). Pathogens, responsible for infection of the middle ear, *S. pneumoniae*, *H. influenzae*, or *B. catarrhalis*, are uncommonly found in cultures of the external auditory canal when the tympanic membrane is intact. Isolation of *S. epidermidis*, *S. aureus*, diphtheroids, or certain anaerobic bacteria from cultures of middle-ear fluids may represent contamination of the fluid by organisms present in the external canal. Adequate cleansing of the external canal is necessary before tympanocentesis is performed for the purpose of microbiologic diagnosis.

Diseases of the external canal are not considered here. The interested reader is referred to a monograph by Senturia and colleagues (1980*b*).

IMMUNOLOGY

The middle-ear mucosa has a secretory immune system similar to those of other areas of the respiratory tract (see Fig. 21–13). Immunologically active antigen interacts with immunocompetent cells in the lamina propria to produce a local immune response. The middle-ear effusion that results from acute or chronic infection contains the major classes of immunoglobulins, complement, cells, immune complexes of antigen and antibody, and various chemical mediators of inflammation (Table 21–13). The role of these substances in the course of otitis media with effusion is uncertain. The immune response to various antigens may prevent subsequent infection, assist in clearance of the middle-ear effusion, or contribute to the accumulation and persistence of fluid in the middle-ear cavity.

The immunologic effect of otitis media with effusion is a relatively new area of investigation. Almost all reports of important studies have been published since 1967.

Problems in Methodology

Immunologic studies of otitis media in the human are based on assays of serum, middle-ear effusion (obtained by needle aspiration through the tympanic membrane), and middle-ear mucosa (obtained by biopsy). Problems in methodology and limitations of data from human materials must be considered in evaluating results of these studies:

1. Effusion or mucosa is most readily obtained at operation. Therefore, most reports include patients with chronic disease who required an operative procedure. Only a few reports of materials obtained from patients with acute otitis media are available.

2. Without information gathered prospectively, the investigator cannot identify the stage of disease when material is obtained. In most reports the stage of otitis media is identified grossly as acute or chronic by the characteristic of the middle-ear effusion (serous, mucoid, purulent, or hemorrhagic). Few studies have results from more than one specimen or one observation. Thus, there is a paucity of information on the sequence of immune events.

3. Techniques for assay of the same function vary in sensitivity and specificity. Newer techniques may provide results at variance with those of previously used methods.

4. The quality and quantity of middle-ear fluid obtained by tympanocentesis is limited. The volume of most aspirates is 0.3 ml or less. Only a few studies can be performed with each sample. In addition, the liquid may be fibrinous or mucoid or filled with cellular debris, making homogenization difficult.

5. Materials are not usually available from "normal" patients, and controls are difficult to define.

6. The investigator may not be able to identify the origin of the substance in the effusion. Trauma may occur during the course of aspiration and contaminate the effusion with products of blood and tissue. The liquid represents the sum of substances derived from serum, inflamed middle-ear mucosa, degenerating white blood cells, or other cellular elements.

Experiments in animal models have provided important new information and stimulated new concepts. However, significant differences exist between species, and data derived from studies in animals must be viewed with caution. For the purposes of this discussion, only data derived from studies of humans is presented.

Immunology of Pharynx

Immunocompetent lymphoid tissue is present in the mucosa of the upper respiratory tract, the site of initial exposure for ingested and inhaled antigens. The lymphoid tissue of the pharynx includes the palatine tonsils and adenoids, lymphoid tissue at the base of the tongue (lingual tonsil), lymphoid tissue on the posterior wall of the pharynx (pharyngeal tonsil), and a circular ring of lymphoid tissue (Waldeyer ring). Plasma cells capable of producing all the major classes of immunoglobulins have been identified in the tonsils. The immunologic aspects of the tonsils have been reviewed by Wong and Ogra (1980).

The specific immunologic relationship of the tonsils and adenoids with the middle ear is unknown. The immunocompetent cells in the tonsils and adenoids are an important defense in excluding microbial and environmental antigens from the systemic lymphoid system, thus performing a "gatekeeper" function. Because microbial organisms responsible for infection of the middle ear proliferate first in the throat or nasopharynx, the tonsils may play a significant immunologic role in the host's defense against otitis media.

Humoral Factors

Immunoglobulin A and Secretory Immunoglobulin A

Immunoglobulin A (IgA) is secreted by plasma cells in lymphoid tissues lining the gastrointestinal, genitourinary, and respiratory tracts. Secretory component (SIgA) is a nonimmune glycoprotein, formed by local

TABLE 21–13. Substances Identified in Middle-Ear Effusion of Patients with Acute or Chronic Otitis Media with Effusion

Immunoglobulins	Oxidative Enzymes
G, A, M, E, D	Lactic dehydrogenase
Complement	Malic dehydrogenase
Rheumatoid factor	Succinic dehydrogenase
Prostaglandins E and F	Hydrolytic enzymes
Chemotactic substances	Lysozyme
Macrophage inhibitory factor	Acid phosphatase
Lactoferrin	Alkaline phosphatase
Histamine	Esterase
Granulocyte proteases	Leucine aminopeptidase
Protease inhibitors	Alanine aminopeptidase
Collagenase	

epithelial cells, that exists either in a bound state with IgA or in a free state in effusion fluids. Two IgA molecules combine with secretory component in the epithelium, and the complex (SIgA) is transported through the cell and into the lumen. The production of SIgA begins when antigen is presented to immunocompetent cells in the mucosa.

IgA is the predominant immunoglobulin in middle ear effusions. The ratio of IgA to IgG is higher in middle-ear effusion than in serum in most patients, and some patients have IgA in middle-ear fluid but not in serum. Fluorescent antibody staining of middle-ear mucosa demonstrates SIgA in the epithelium. Small amounts of free SIgA are present, but most secretory component in middle-ear effusions is bound to IgA (Mogi et al., 1973).

A specific IgA or SIgA response takes place in the middle-ear mucosa following exposure to antigen. IgA and SIgA specific for adenovirus, respiratory syncytial virus, and parainfluenza viruses have been identified in middle-ear fluids of children with otitis media with effusion (Meurman et al., 1980; Yamaguchi et al., 1984). The presence of specific IgA antibody for measles, mumps, rubella, and poliovirus in middle-ear fluid and its absence in some specimens of simultaneously obtained serum indicate that local antibody production takes place (Sloyer et al., 1977).

Specific IgA can interfere with adhesion of bacteria to mucous membrane and can neutralize viruses. In the intestine IgA prevents absorption of toxic proteins and antigens. Which, if any, of these functions applies to IgA and SIgA in the middle ear is unknown.

Immunoglobulin G

Immunoglobulin G (IgG) is present in the effusions of patients with both acute and chronic otitis media in concentrations suggesting that local development of IgG occurs in the middle ear. IgG is divided into subclasses IgG1, IgG2, IgG3, and IgG4 based on differences in structure of the gamma heavy polypeptide chain. Data presented by Freijd and coworkers (1985) suggest an association between plasma IgG2 concentrations and susceptibility to otitis media in children. Otitis-prone children (8 to 17 episodes by 30 months of age) had significantly lower plasma concentrations of IgG2 than did children who were not otitis prone (fewer than 2 episodes by 30 months of age) at ages 12 and 32 months. Concentrations of IgG1, IgG3, and IgG4 were similar in the two groups.

Immunoglobulin M

Immunoglobulin M (IgM) is produced in response to primary exposure to a microbial antigen; it is an effective mediator of complement fixation and regulates B-cell function. IgM is present in the middle-ear effusions of patients with both acute and chronic otitis media with effusion, but concentrations are lower than in serum, and studies of middle-ear mucosa obtained by biopsy in patients with chronic otitis media with effusion suggest that local synthesis of IgM does not occur.

Immunoglobulin D

Immunoglobulin D (IgD) has been identified in middle-ear effusions of patients with otitis media with effusion in excess of concentrations found in serum (Veltri and Sprinkle, 1973). IgD has no identifiable function (Lim and DeMaria, 1987).

Immunoglobulin E

Immunoglobulin E (IgE) is part of the external secretory system of antibody produced in the lymphoid tissue of the respiratory and gastrointestinal tracts. Increased concentration of IgE has been found in serum and secretions of patients with various atopic diseases. IgE antibody, when combined with appropriate antigen, causes release of histamine, slow-reacting substance, and chemotactic substance from mast cells and basophilic granulocytes.

IgE-producing plasma cells have been identified in biopsy of mucosa of the middle ear, and IgE has been found in the middle-ear effusions of patients with both acute and chronic otitis media. The source of IgE in the middle-ear fluid of patients with otitis media with effusion may be middle-ear mucosa in some patients (Bernstein, 1984a; Phillips et al., 1974a) and a transudate of serum in others (Lewis et al., 1978; Mogi et al., 1974).

Complement

The term complement represents a system that includes 11 discrete but interacting proteins and possesses a wide variety of activities, such as viral neutralization, phagocytosis, immune adherence, chemotaxis, anaphylatoxin activities on smooth muscle and blood vessels, and a cytotoxic effect that may serve a protective function, leading to destruction of foreign cells (Ward and McLean, 1978). Activation of complement occurs by the classic or alternate pathways. The classic pathway is usually activated by antigen-antibody complexes and proceeds in sequence from C1 to C9. The alternate pathways do not require immune complex for activation but utilize materials such as endotoxin or bacterial polysaccharide. The early factors of the classic pathway (C1, C2, C4) are not required, but properdin and C3 are involved in activation.

Evidence for activation of complement in the middle-ear effusions of patients with acute and chronic otitis media has been reviewed by Bernstein and colleagues (1978a) and Prellner and coworkers (1980). Studies of middle-ear effusion indicate that levels of C2, C3, C4, and C5 are all significantly depressed when compared with corresponding levels in serum and that the amounts of C3 breakdown products are significantly elevated in the middle-ear fluid of children with otitis media with effusion (Meri et al., 1984), indicating utilization of complement in the middle ear during the course of the disease. Meri and colleagues (1984) suggested that activation of complement in middle-ear fluid may play a significant role in the pathogenesis of otitis media with effusion either by decreasing local defenses against bacterial infection or by generating breakdown products that maintain and prolong the inflammatory process.

Rheumatoid Factor

Rheumatoid factor is an IgM that has the capacity to react with IgG *in vitro* and has been identified in the serum of patients with rheumatoid arthritis and other chronic inflammatory diseases. Rheumatoid factors may participate in the inflammatory process stimulated by immune complexes. DeMaria and colleagues (1984c) demonstrated rheumatoid factor in 85 per cent of 156 middle-ear fluids obtained from patients with otitis media with effusion; the factor was found in only 8 per cent of sera from the same patients. The investigators suggested that rheumatoid factor is produced in the middle ear and may participate in the pathogenesis of middle-ear effusion. These results were not corroborated by Bernstein (1984a); none of 21 middle-ear fluids tested showed positive results for rheumatoid factor.

Products of Immune and Inflammatory Reactions

A variety of other substances that take part in immune or inflammatory reactions have been identified in the middle-ear effusions of patients with chronic otitis media with effusion.

1. A chemotactic factor for neutrophils has been found (Bernstein, 1976). Chemotactic substances alter the pattern of movement of neutrophils so that cells, which otherwise would migrate randomly, are directed to the vicinity of the chemotactic substance.

2. Macrophage inhibition factor (MIF) inhibits the migration of macrophages *in vitro; in vivo* it serves to contain macrophages at the site of injury or inflammation (Bernstein, 1976). MIF augments the capacity of the macrophage to kill certain bacteria.

3. Lactoferrin inhibits growth of iron-dependent bacteria by competing for elemental iron. Bernstein and coworkers (1972) identified lactoferrin in mucoid but not serous effusions.

4. Prostaglandins have a wide range of biologic activities, including increasing capillary permeability, contraction of smooth muscles, and release of lysozymal enzymes. Bernstein and associates (1976) found prostaglandins E and F in middle-ear fluids; in some patients the concentration in the fluid was higher than it was in serum. The effect of prostaglandins on capillary permeability may play a role in development and persistence of middle-ear effusion.

5. Histamine was identified in 104 of 131 middle-ear fluids of patients with otitis media with effusion at time of placement of tympanostomy tubes. Berger and colleagues (1984) postulated that mast cells located in the middle-ear mucosa were triggered to degranulate and release histamine by a product derived from activation of the complement system.

6. Products derived from microorganisms that participate in immune or inflammatory responses (endotoxins, interferon, neuraminidase) are discussed under microbiology.

Cytology of Middle Ear and Middle-Ear Effusions

Neutrophils, macrophages, and lymphocytes are the predominant cell types in middle-ear effusions (Sipila and Karma, 1982; Yamanaka et al., 1982). The proportion of B and T lymphocytes varies widely in published reports. Bernstein and colleagues (1978b) found that mucoid middle-ear effusions contained many B cells but few T cells, whereas serous effusions contained mainly T cells but no B cells. Monocytes and phagocytes are present, but they occur in small numbers in most specimens. Occasionally, giant phagocytes with ingested cells, cell debris, and bacteria are seen. Eosinophils, mast cells, basophils, and plasma cells are rare. Epithelial cells include numerous flat endothelial cells and few ciliated and goblet cells.

After onset of acute otitis media, the middle-ear effusion contains large numbers of neutrophils and few lymphocytes, monocytes, and phagocytes. Initially, polymorphonuclear leukocytes may defend the middle ear from bacterial infection, as well as contribute to the middle-ear effusion by release of enzymes that stimulate an inflammatory response. After several weeks, the proportion of cells is reversed, and lymphocytes, monocytes, and phagocytes predominate (Qvarnberg et al., 1984).

Similar cell types are found in middle-ear mucosa obtained by biopsy of patients with otitis media with effusion. Inflammatory cells in the submucosa are predominantly of the mononuclear type. Plasma cells and small lymphocytes predominate. The presence of IgA and IgG was demonstrated by use of an immunofluorescent stain of mononuclear cells from middle-ear effusions; IgM and IgE were infrequently detected (Palva et al., 1976).

Immunology of Acute Otitis Media

Role of Serum Antibody

An immune response reflected in a rise in specific serum antibody occurs in some children after acute infection of the middle ear (Howie et al., 1973). The number of responders to pneumococcal infection is dependent on the age of the patient and the pneumococcal serotype: 18 per cent of Finnish children less than 1 year old, 48 per cent of 1-year-olds, and 39 per cent of children 2 to 7 years old had a significant increase in type-specific antibody following pneumococcal otitis media. Types 3 and 18 induced good antibody responses irrespective of age; Types 4, 7, 8, and 9 were intermediate; and Types 6, 19, and 23 were poor antigens, even in older children (Koskela et al., 1982). Similar results were found in Alabama children who had acute otitis media due to *Streptococcus pneumoniae*; only 12 per cent of children under 1 year of age had a significant rise in type-specific antibody in the convalescent serum, whereas 48 per cent of the children 2 years of age or older responded (Sloyer et al., 1974). The antibody responses to the type-specific pneumococcal infection were in general agreement with the responses to polysaccharide vaccine for children of similar ages.

A specific serum antibody response also occurs following acute otitis media due to nontypable *H. influenzae*. A majority of Alabama children 2 years of age or younger with *H. influenzae* infection had specific antibody in the convalescent serum (Sloyer et al., 1975). Shurin and coworkers (1980b) found similar immune responses in children 2 months to 12 years of age with acute otitis media due to nontypable strains of *H. influenzae*. Eleven per cent of the children had homotypic antibody in the acute serum, but 78 per cent had antibody in the convalescent specimen. Thus, an immune response to nontypable *H. influenzae* occurred in infants as well as older children.

Children with recurrent episodes of otitis media have new middle-ear infections due to the same spectrum of organisms that was responsible for the first episode. *S. pneumoniae* and nontypable *H. influenzae* are the most common bacteria in recurrent infections, but the new episodes are rarely due to the same serotype that infected the child in a prior episode. Austrian and colleagues (1977) found that approximately 1 per cent of isolates of *S. pneumoniae* in recurrent episodes of pneumococcal otitis media were due to the same serotype responsible for a prior episode. Recurrent episodes of otitis media due to nontypable *H. influenzae* are also associated with new types. Using outer membrane protein gel analysis and biotyping, Barenkamp and colleagues (1984) determined that episodes of early recurrence of otitis due to nontypable *H. influenzae* (less than 30 days after initial *H. influenzae* infection) had first and second isolates that were identical. In contrast, children with late recurrences of nontypable *H. influenzae* (more than 30 days after initial infection) had disease due to a different strain. These data suggest that infections due to *S. pneumoniae* or nontypable *H. influenzae* produce an immune response that protects the child against subsequent infection due to the same type. The specific protective mechanism, a serum or local antibody or other immune factor, is uncertain.

Role of Antibody in Clearance of Middle-Ear Effusion

Clearance of fluid from the middle ear in patients with acute otitis media due to *S. pneumoniae* and *H.*

influenzae was significantly associated with the presence and concentration of specific antibody to the infecting strain in the middle-ear fluid at the time of diagnosis (Sloyer et al., 1976). Clearing of the effusion by second visit (2 to 7 days following diagnosis) was associated with specific antibody in the middle-ear effusion obtained at first visit and was directly associated with the concentration of specific antibody. Infection due to *H. influenzae* was cleared rapidly in more children (45.3 per cent) than those with infection due to *S. pneumoniae* (13.6 per cent), whether or not antibody was present. The source for the antibody in the effusion at the time of presentation of acute otitis media is uncertain; antibody may have developed after a prior infection, may have developed rapidly after a current infection, or may indicate a delay of presentation until the time when the specimen of middle-ear fluid was obtained. If present from a prior infection, type-specific antibody did not protect the patient from a recurrent episode of acute otitis media but did reduce the duration of effusion. No other data are available to confirm or deny these findings.

Polymorphonuclear Leukocyte Response

Hill and coworkers (1977) identified defective chemotactic response in selected patients with recurrent episodes of otitis media and diarrhea. Ichimura (1982) identified defective neutrophil chemotaxis in 20 children who had had recurrent episodes of otitis media (four or more episodes during the preceding year) but were well at the time of examination. These data suggest that recurrent episodes of otitis media in some children may be due to or associated with depressed functions of polymorphonuclear leukocytes.

Immunology of Chronic Otitis Media with Effusion

Role of Antibody in Middle-Ear Fluid

All the major classes of immunoglobulins, IgA, IgG, IgM, IgD, and IgE, have been identified in the middle-ear fluids of patients with chronic otitis media with effusion. SIgA, IgA, and IgG are synthesized by the mucosa of the middle ear; synthesis of other immunoglobulins in the middle ear is less certain (Bernstein and Reisman, 1974). Both IgA and IgG are present in middle-ear effusions in concentrations higher than those found in simultaneously obtained serum, whereas IgM and IgE are present in equivalent or lower concentrations in effusion than are found in serum. The highest concentrations of each of the major classes of immunoglobulins are present in mucoid effusions; the lowest are found in serous effusions, and intermediate values occur in leukocytic middle-ear effusions.

Polymorphonuclear Leukocyte Response

Giebink and colleagues (1980) studied the polymorphonuclear leukocyte response in children with

chronic otitis media with effusion at the time of myringotomy or placement of ventilating tubes and, in a
few cases, 2 to 8 weeks later. In some children there
were transient abnormalities of polymorphonuclear
leukocyte motility (depressed chemotactic responsiveness), phagocytosis (depressed polymorphonuclear leukocyte bactericidal activity), or intracellular oxidation
(depressed polymorphonuclear leukocyte chemilumi-
nescence). Repeat studies performed after surgery
found these indexes to be normal in the majority of
children, suggesting that leukocyte dysfunction was
transient and probably associated with the inflammatory reaction that elicited the middle-ear fluid.

Immune Complexes

Some investigators suggest that chronic otitis media
with effusion may be an immune complex disease.
Antigen (microbial agents or allergens) may combine
with antibody (locally produced or derived from serum)
to form an immune complex, which activates the
complement sequence through the classic or alternate
pathways. Polymorphonuclear leukocytes and monocytes are attracted to the site. With the death of these
cells, intracellular enzymes are released, producing
local tissue damage and stimulating effusion. Maxim
and colleagues (1977) identified immune complexes in
middle-ear fluids by use of the fluorescent Raji cell
assay. Others have not been able to corroborate the
results (Bernstein et al, 1981). Yamanaka and associates
(1987) concluded, after a study of 245 patients with
otitis media with effusion, that immune complexes
formed in the middle ear might prolong the inflammatory process through complement activation following chemotaxis of neutrophils. If immune complexes
do occur in middle-ear fluid, they may represent
microbial antigen-antibody complexes as a part of the
normal process of elimination of infectious product
through phagocytosis.

Children with Defects of Immune System

Most children with recurrent episodes of otitis media
with effusion have no apparent systemic or local immune defect. These children have normal concentrations of immunoglobulin in serum, normal systemic
cell-mediated responses, and normal phagocytic and
bactericidal capacity of neutrophils in peripheral blood
(Giebink and Quie, 1978). Available data about the
immune system of the middle ear in children with
recurrent otitis media with effusion indicate that most
have the essential elements for immunologic resistance, including T- and B-cell responses that are fully
operative, macrophages that are available for engulfing
and ingesting antigenic material, and appropriate antibody response by middle-ear mucosa (Palva et al.,
1980).

Children with congenital or acquired immunodeficiency may have defects of phagocyte function or

humoral systems. Infections of the respiratory tract,
including otitis media, are associated with defects of
chemotaxis, phagocytosis (neutropenia or intrinsic cellular defects), or killing (chronic granulomatous disease); problems with the humoral system include
deficiency of circulating antibody (hypo- or agammaglobulinemia), mucosal antibody (IgA deficiency), or complement deficiency. Human immunodeficiency virus
(HIV), the organism responsible for AIDS, is highly
tropic for T lymphocytes. Children with AIDS have
abnormalities of T-cell, B-cell, and complement functions and phagocytosis. The children are susceptible
to local and systemic pyogenic infections, and otitis
media is only one of the many bacterial diseases that
may occur.

Multiple infections in the same system (respiratory
tract, urinary tract, or central nervous system) suggest
a local anatomic or physiologic defect. The vast majority of children with recurrent episodes of otitis media
as the sole form of recurrent infectious disease probably have an underlying defect that is not immunologically mediated (e.g., eustachian tube dysfunction). A
few children have recurrent respiratory tract infections, including recurrent otitis media and pyogenic
infections in other systems, as part of an immunodeficiency syndrome (Berdal et al., 1976; Johnston, 1984).
Occurrence of two or more serious pyogenic skin
infections (furunculosis, subcutaneous abscess, or cellulitis), accompanied by pneumonia or recurrent otitis
media, raises suspicion of neutropenia, defective chemotaxis, or problems with phagocytosis. A pattern of
subcutaneous abscesses of furunculosis, accompanied
by abscess formation in lymph nodes, liver, or lung,
and recurrent acute otitis media suggests chronic granulomatous disease. Meningitis, osteomyelitis, septic
arthritis with recurrent acute otitis media, or pneumonia raises concern for a deficiency of antibody or
C3. Protracted diarrhea, when accompanied by recurrent episodes of otitis media, sinusitis, or pneumonia,
suggests IgA deficiency (although many children with
deficiencies of IgA are otherwise normal without undue
susceptibility to infection). Children with selective
IgG2 or IgG3 subclass deficiency had recurrent sinopulmonary infections and otitis media (more than six
episodes per year) (Umetsu et al., 1985). However,
the significance of this finding of some IgG subclass
deficiencies remains unclear at present. Heiner (1987)
recommended that subjects with mild, relatively infrequent infections be given replacement therapy as
needed during periods of infection and patients with
chronic or repeated severe infections be given regular
doses of gamma globulin.

Patients with defects in splenic function are susceptible to overwhelming infection due to encapsulated
organisms such as *S. pneumoniae* or *H. influenzae*
Type b. Such patients, including those with congenital
or acquired asplenia and those with sickle cell disease,
have not been identified as groups with unusual susceptibility to infections at local sites, such as the skin
and soft tissues or middle ear.

Role of Allergy in Otitis Media

The role of allergy in etiology of otitis media with effusion is uncertain. The role of allergy in eustachian tube function is considered in discussion of physiology, pathophysiology, and pathogenesis above. Few critical studies of appropriate design are available to clarify the relationship of allergy and otitis media with effusion. Available studies are often biased (enrollees include children referred for allergy evaluation) and do not include appropriate control patients. However, the association of reaginic antibody with IgE provides a specific measure for precise definition of allergy and has already provided some significant information about the primary or secondary role of allergy in otitis media with effusion.

The evidence for a role for allergy in recurrent otitis media with effusion in some children was presented by Siegel (1979) and Bernstein (1980):

1. Many patients with recurrent otitis media with effusion have concomitant allergic respiratory disease.

2. A history of one or more major allergic illnesses in parents is usually present.

3. Nasal or peripheral eosinophils are often present in increased numbers.

4. Positive skin test reactions to allergens or positive results of radioallergosorbent tests (RAST) are present in many patients.

5. Elevated IgE levels in middle-ear effusions and in serum of some children have been identified.

6. Mast cells (some that are degranulating) are found frequently throughout the middle-ear mucosa.

Evidence against a major role for allergy in otitis media with effusion was summarized by Bernstein (1980).

1. In unselected series of cases of otitis media with effusion, fewer than one third of patients are atopic. Allergic airway disease was sought and found not to be a predisposing factor for Arizona Indian children with recurrent otitis media (Todd and Feldman, 1985). In these children other factors are likely responsible for the susceptibility to middle-ear infection.

2. The seasonal incidence of otitis media with effusion (winter to spring) is contrary to the season when grasses, trees, and pollens cause acute nasal allergy (late spring and early fall).

3. Most studies indicate an absence of eosinophils and absence of, or only small numbers of, IgE-producing cells in middle-ear fluids and middle-ear mucosa.

4. A failure to improve with aggressive allergic treatment, including hyposensitization and use of antihistamines, in spite of improvement in nasal symptoms, is seen in most patients.

Thus, many patients may be allergic and many children have recurrent otitis media, but there is no substantive evidence correlating the two conditions. However, it is likely that the allergic response plays a role in some children with otitis media with effusion or in some episodes of otitis media with effusion. The presence of specific IgE on mast cells in middle-ear mucosa could result in release of mediators of inflammation, with the mucosa functioning as a shock organ similar to respiratory mucosa in other areas. Alternately, the allergic reaction might be a predisposing factor producing congestion of the mucosa of the nose and eustachian tube, leading to obstruction of the tube with retention of fluid in the middle ear. Microbial and environmental antigens may act in a similar pattern of injury to middle-ear mucosa or elicit a similar response from cells with immune function in the mucosa.

Bacterial Vaccines and Immunoglobulins for Prevention of Otitis Media

If type-specific serum antibody is correlated with protection from homotypic infection, bacterial vaccines may be effective in preventing type-specific otitis media. Among bacterial vaccines currently under investigation, the meningococcal vaccines and the *H. influenzae* Type b vaccine are of limited interest because of the infrequency of acute otitis media caused by these organisms. A vaccine for nontypable *H. influenzae* is not available, but investigations have focused on use of outer membrane antigens for development of a vaccine (Gnehm et al., 1985). A multitype pneumococcal vaccine is available and is of major interest because of the importance of this organism as a cause of otitis media in all age groups. The clinical and microbiologic results of trials of pneumococcal vaccine to prevent recurrences of acute otitis media are presented in the discussion of immunoprophylaxis. Usage of immune globulins for prevention of acute otitis media is discussed below (p. 470).

PATHOLOGY

In the initial stages of classic acute otitis media the mucoperiosteum of the middle ear and mastoid air cells is hyperemic and edematous. This is followed by an exudation of polymorphonuclear leukocytes and serofibrinous fluid into the middle ear. The quantity of fluid increases until the middle ear is filled and pressure is exerted against the tympanic membrane (Fig. 21–63). If the disease progresses, the bulging tympanic membrane may rupture spontaneously. The resultant discharge is at first serosanguineous but then becomes mucopurulent. Throughout the middle ear and mastoid, the mucosa becomes markedly thickened by a mixture of inflammatory cells, new capillaries, and young fibrous tissue. This process may become associated with blockage of the aditus ad antrum, resulting in inadequate drainage of the mastoid air cells and a consequent mastoiditis. Extension beyond the mucoperiosteum may lead to intratemporal complications, such as facial paralysis, labyrinthitis, and petrositis, or intracranial complications, which may include lateral sinus thrombophlebitis, meningitis, oti-

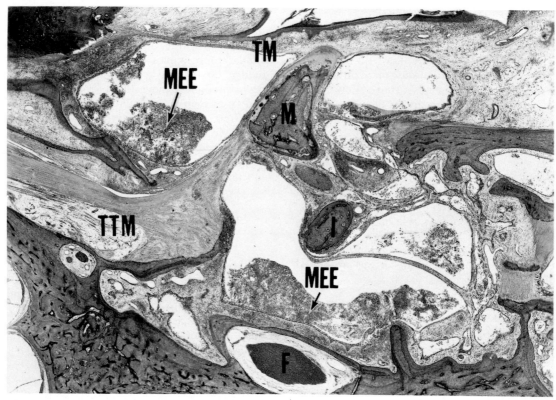

Figure 21–63. Acute otitis media (H & E, × 15). F, Facial nerve; I, incus; M, malleus; MEE, middle-ear effusion; TM, tympanic membrane; TTM, tensor tympani muscle. (Courtesy of H. F. Schuknecht, M.D.)

tic hydrocephalus, subdural abscess, epidural abscess, and brain abscess.

The pathologic findings associated with the serous (Fig. 21–64) or mucoid type of chronic middle-ear effusion are similar. There is an increase in the number of secretory cells, including glands and ciliated cells. The lamina propria or connective tissue layer becomes thickened by edema and infiltration of numerous inflammatory cells consisting of lymphocytes, plasma cells, macrophages, and polymorphonuclear leukocytes. These changes are more striking in the presence of a mucoid effusion than for a pure serous effusion in which tissue edema is the predominant finding, in addition to the presence of chronic inflammatory cells (Fig. 21–65). It is generally believed that mucoid effusions are mainly the result of secretion, whereas serous effusions are mostly transudates. Persistent atelectasis of the middle ear, chronic middle-ear effusions, or both are associated with a number of intratemporal complications and sequelae, including hearing loss, tympanosclerosis, adhesive otitis media, perforation with discharge, chronic mastoiditis, and cholesteatoma.

DIAGNOSIS

The methods of examination of a child with ear disease have been extensively described (including pneumatic otoscopy) in Chapter 8; however, the specific diagnostic features that characterize the various forms of otitis media and certain related conditions are presented below.

Clinical Description

For the clinician, the diagnosis of otitis media usually depends on a high index of suspicion and the presence of symptoms, but primarily on the pneumatic otoscopic findings.

Acute Otitis Media

The usual picture of acute otitis media is seen in a child who has an upper respiratory tract infection for several days and suddenly develops otalgia, fever, and hearing loss. Examination with the pneumatic otoscope reveals a hyperemic, opaque, bulging tympanic membrane that has poor mobility. Purulent otorrhea is usually also a reliable sign. In addition to fever, other systemic signs and symptoms may include irritability, lethargy, anorexia, vomiting, and diarrhea. However, all of these may be absent, and even earache and fever are unreliable guides and may frequently be absent (Schwartz et al., 1981d; Hayden and Schwartz, 1985). Likewise, otoscopic findings may consist only of a bulging or full, opaque, poorly mobile eardrum without evidence of erythema. Hearing loss will not be a complaint of the very young or even noted by the parents.

Tympanometry usually reveals an effusion pattern

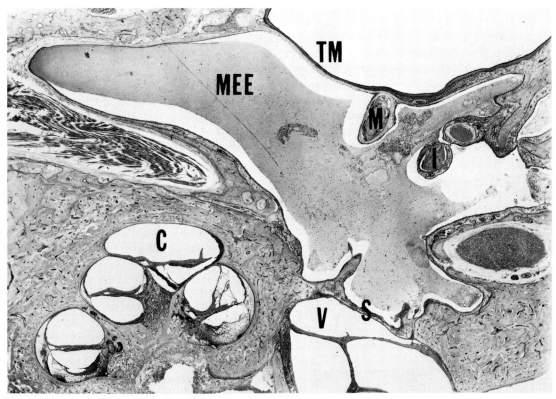

Figure 21–64. Otitis media with serous effusion (H & E, × 11). C, Cochlea; I, incus; M, malleus; MEE, middle-ear effusion; TM, tympanic membrane; S, stapes; V, vestibule. (Courtesy of H. F. Schuknecht, M.D.)

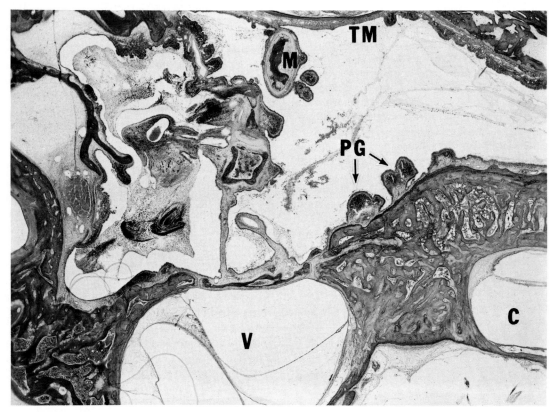

Figure 21–65. Chronic otitis media (H & E, × 15). C, Cochlea; M, malleus; PG, polypoid granulation tissue; TM, tympanic membrane; V, vestibule. (Courtesy of I. Sando, M.D.)

(flat) or a high positive-pressure pattern but may show a pattern that is not classically associated with an effusion.

When performed, tympanocentesis usually is productive of a purulent middle-ear aspirate, but in approximately 20 per cent a serous or mucoid effusion is present (Bluestone and Cantekin, 1979). Because of the variability of symptoms, infants and young children with diminished or absent mobility and opacification of the tympanic membrane should be suspected of having acute otitis media.

Otitis Media with Effusion

Most children with chronic middle-ear effusions are asymptomatic. Some may complain of hearing loss and, less commonly, tinnitus and vertigo. In children the attention of an alert parent or teacher may be drawn to a suspected hearing loss. Sometimes the child has a behavioral disorder due to the hearing deficit and consequent inability to communicate adequately. More often, the reason for referral is the detection of a hearing loss during a school hearing screening test or when acute otitis media fails to resolve completely. Occasionally, the first evidence of the disease is discovered during a routine examination or in evaluation of high-risk cases, such as children with a cleft palate.

Older children will describe a frank hearing loss or, more commonly, a "plugged" feeling or "popping" in their ears. The symptoms are usually bilateral. Unilateral signs and symptoms of chronic middle-ear effusion may result from a nasopharyngeal neoplasm such as an angiofibroma or even a malignancy.

Pneumatic otoscopy will frequently reveal either a retracted or full tympanic membrane that is usually opaque, but when it is translucent, an air-fluid level or air bubbles may be visualized, and a blue or amber color is noted. The mobility of the eardrum is almost always altered.

It is evident from the preceding clinical description of acute otitis media and chronic otitis media with effusion that there is considerable overlap; hence it is often difficult for the clinician to distinguish between acute and chronic forms unless the child has been observed over a period of time before the onset of disease or there are associated specific (otalgia) or systemic (fever) symptoms. It may not be possible to distinguish between the two even when the middle-ear effusion is aspirated (tympanocentesis), because in both acute and chronic otitis the effusion may be serous, mucoid, or purulent. In approximately half of chronic effusions, bacteria have been cultured that are frequently found in ears of children with classic signs and symptoms of acute otitis media (Riding et al., 1978a).

Atelectasis of the Tympanic Membrane–Middle Ear and High Negative Pressure

Atelectasis of the tympanic membrane may be acute or chronic, generalized or localized, and mild or se-

vere. The tympanic membrane may be retracted or collapsed. High negative pressure may be present or absent. When middle-ear effusion is also present the clinical picture is the same as described above when acute or chronic otitis media is present. In such cases, it is not unusual to visualize through the otoscope a severely retracted malleus in association with a tympanic membrane that is full or even bulging in the posterior portion. The malleus is retracted by concurrent high negative middle-ear pressure, chronic inflammation of the tensor tympani muscle or the malleolar ligaments, or both, whereas the hydrostatic pressure of the effusion (not completely filling the middle ear–mastoid air cell system) results in bulging of the most compliant (floppy) portion of the pars tensa, the posterosuperior and posteroinferior quadrants. Frequently an effusion is evident by the presence of an air-fluid level or bubbles behind a severely retracted tympanic membrane.

Just as when there is a middle-ear effusion present, there may be a lack of specific otologic symptoms when no effusion is present. The child may have a severely retracted translucent tympanic membrane with evidence of high negative pressure by pneumatic otoscopy (immobile to applied positive pressure and either decreased or absent mobility to applied negative pressure) or a high negative middle-ear pressure tracing on the tympanogram. The otoscopist can look through the tympanic membrane and see that there is no effusion present. Some children with such an otoscopic (and tympanometric) examination may not have any complaint, while others may have a feeling of fullness in the ear, otalgia, tinnitus, hearing loss, and even vertigo. The condition may be self-limited and in some it may be physiologic, owing to temporary eustachian tube obstruction. But in others, especially those with symptoms, the condition is pathologic and should be managed in a manner similar to that when an effusion is present.

When there is localized atelectasis or a retraction pocket, especially in the pars flaccida, or posterosuperior portion of the pars tensa of the tympanic membrane, then the condition may be more serious than when only generalized atelectasis is present. The child may be totally asymptomatic, but the retraction pocket may be associated with a significant conductive hearing loss, especially if there is erosion of one or more of the ossicles. Erosion of the long process of the incus may be present when a deep posterosuperior retraction pocket is visualized (Fig. 21–66). It is extremely important to visualize these areas of the tympanic membrane to determine if a retraction pocket is present, and, if so, whether there is destruction of one of the ossicles. It is important to distinguish between a retraction pocket and a cholesteatoma. If the otoscopic examination is not adequate to make this differential diagnosis, then the otomicroscope should be used; the clinician should not hesitate to perform otomicroscopic examination under general anesthesia when indicated. Cholesteatoma, like its precursor, the deep retraction pocket, may be without signs and symptoms (other

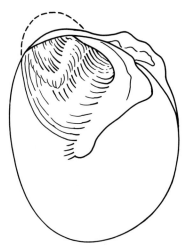

Figure 21–66. Illustration of an atelectatic right tympanic membrane that has a severe retraction pocket in the posterosuperior quadrant of the pars tensa.

than the otoscopic appearance) unless conductive hearing loss or otorrhea is present.

Eustachian Tube Dysfunction

Some children, especially older ones, will complain of a periodic popping or snapping sound in the ear, which may be preceded or accompanied by a feeling of fullness in the ear, hearing loss, tinnitus, or vertigo. Otoscopic examination may reveal a normal tympanic membrane or possibly slight retraction of the eardrum, but the middle-ear pressure is within normal limits. These children have obstruction of the eustachian tube that is not severe enough to cause atelectasis or a middle-ear effusion, but nevertheless may be quite disconcerting. When troublesome, the child should be managed in the same manner as children who have middle-ear effusion.

On occasion, older children may complain of autophony (hearing one's own voice in the ear) and hearing their own breathing. The eustachian tube is most likely patulous (abnormally patent), in which case the tympanic membrane will appear normal when visualized through the otoscope. Middle-ear pressure will be normal; however, if the child is asked to breathe forcefully through one nasal cavity, the opposite being

occluded with a finger, the posterosuperior portion of the tympanic membrane will be observed to move in and out with respiration, which will confirm the diagnosis. Tympanometry may also aid in diagnosis (see description of patulous tube test, p. 360).

Microbiologic Diagnosis

The correlation between bacterial cultures of the nasopharynx or the oropharynx and those of middle-ear fluids is poor. The poor correlation occurs because of the frequency of colonization of the upper respiratory tract with organisms of known pathogenicity for the middle ear and less commonly because of absence in cultures of the oropharynx or nasopharynx of the pathogen responsible for infection of the middle ear. Thus, cultures of the upper respiratory tract are of limited value in specific bacteriologic diagnosis of otitis media. Specific microbiologic diagnosis is achieved by culture of middle-ear fluid, obtained by needle aspiration through the intact tympanic membrane. If the patient has toxic signs or symptoms or has a localized infection elsewhere, culture of the blood or the focus of infection should be performed. Bacteremia is rarely associated with otitis media due to nontypable strains of *H. influenzae*, uncommonly associated with otitis media due to *S. pneumoniae*, but frequently associated with otitis media due to Type b strains of *H. influenzae* (Harding et al., 1973).

The consistent results of microbiologic studies of middle-ear fluid of children with acute otitis media provide an accurate guide to the most likely pathogens. Thus, initial therapy in the uncomplicated case does not require obtaining specimens for bacterial diagnosis. If the patient is critically ill when first seen, or has altered host defenses (as is the case with the newborn infant, the patient with malignancy, or the patient with immunologic disease), or fails to respond appropriately to initial therapy for acute otitis media and has toxic signs or symptoms, culture of the middle-ear fluid is indicated. In addition, culture of the blood is warranted for critically ill children and those with altered defenses.

Figure 21–67. Tympanocentesis is needle aspiration of a middle-ear effusion primarily for diagnosis of the presence or absence of an effusion and for microbiologic study. Myringotomy is an incision in the tympanic membrane primarily for therapeutic drainage.

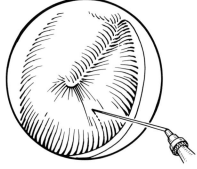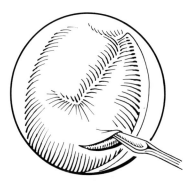

Tympanocentesis   Myringotomy

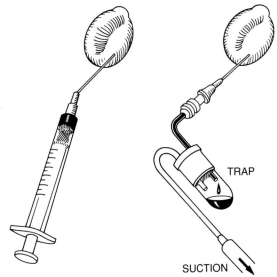

TRAP

SUCTION

Figure 21–68. Tympanocentesis can be performed by employing a needle attached to a tuberculin syringe (left) or by using an Alden-Senturia trap (Storz Instrument Co., St. Louis, MO) with a needle attached (right). (From Bluestone, C. D., and Klein, J. O. 1988. Otitis Media in Infants and Children. Philadelphia, W. B. Saunders Co.)

Diagnostic Aspiration of Middle Ear

When the diagnosis of acute otitis media is in doubt or when determination of the causative agent is desirable, aspiration of the middle ear should be performed (Fig. 21–67). Indications for tympanocentesis or myringotomy include the following:

1. Otitis media in patients who are seriously ill or have toxic signs or symptoms.
2. Unsatisfactory response to antimicrobial therapy.
3. Onset of otitis media in a patient who is receiving antimicrobial agents.
4. Presence of suppurative complications.
5. Otitis media in the newborn, the very young infant, or the immunologically deficient patient, in each of whom an unusual organism may be suspected.

Both of these procedures can usually be performed without general anesthesia. In certain instances, premedication with a combination of a short-acting barbiturate and either morphine or meperidine, or even a general anesthetic, is advisable. The procedures can be carried out with an otoscope with a surgical head or with the otomicroscope. Adequate immobilization of the patient is essential when a general anesthetic is not used.

Diagnostic aspiration may be performed through the inferior portion of the tympanic membrane employing an 18-gauge spinal needle attached to a syringe or collection trap (Fig. 21–68). Culture of the ear canal and cleansing of the canal with alcohol should precede the procedure (Fig. 21–69). The canal culture is helpful in determining whether organisms cultured are contaminants from the exterior canal or pathogens from the middle ear. When therapeutic drainage is required, a myringotomy knife should be employed and the incision should be large enough to allow for ade-

quate drainage and aeration of the middle ear (see discussion of myringotomy, p. 449).

Following tympanocentesis, the effusion caught in the syringe or collection trap is sent to the laboratory for culture. A gram-stained smear may provide immediate information about the bacterial pathogens.

The external ear swab and the fluid aspirated from the middle ear are inoculated onto appropriate solid media and into broth to isolate the likely organisms. Sensitivities of organisms isolated should be tested by the standard method described by Bauer and coworkers (1966).

Nasopharyngeal Culture

In an attempt to identify the causative organism in a child with acute otitis media, obtaining a nasopharyngeal specimen for culture would be less traumatic than a tympanocentesis or myringotomy. The concept is attractive because the bacteria found in middle-ear aspirates are the same type found in the nasopharynx of children with acute otitis media. However, the correlation between the organisms found in the middle ear and nasopharynx as reported in the past has not proved to be high enough to warrant the procedure. Schwartz and associates (1979) and Long and colleagues (1984) reported a technique that improved the correlation of organisms isolated by the nasopharyngeal culture with bacteria identified by culture of middle-ear fluid. The method used involved immediate plating of the nasopharyngeal swab on solid media and a semiquantitative estimation of colonies growing on culture plates.

Blood Culture

Bacteremia is rarely associated with otitis media due to nontypable strains of *H. influenzae*, uncommonly associated with otitis media due to *S. pneumoniae*, and frequently associated with otitis media due to Type b strains of *H. influenzae* (Harding et al., 1973).

Blood for culture was obtained from 600 consecutive children 1 to 24 months of age coming to a Boston hospital walk-in clinic with fever: 166 children had a diagnosis of otitis; only 2 (1.2 per cent) had concomitant bacteremia (Teele et al., 1975). Studies of young infants include information that is selected because those who had cultures of blood showed toxic symptoms or were hospitalized. In four series of infants 8 weeks of age or younger (Crain and Shelov, 1982; Greene et al., 1981; Roberts and Borzy, 1977; Shurin et al., 1978) and in two series of patients 3 months of age or younger (Schlesinger, 1982; Tetzlaff et al., 1977), 5 of 136 infants (3.7 per cent) with otitis media had positive blood cultures (two Group B streptococcus, one *S. pneumoniae*, one *P. aeruginosa*, and one enterococcus). The yield of cultures of blood is low in children with uncomplicated otitis media, but it is likely to be higher in children who have toxic symptoms, high fever, or concurrent infection at other foci (pneumonia, meningitis).

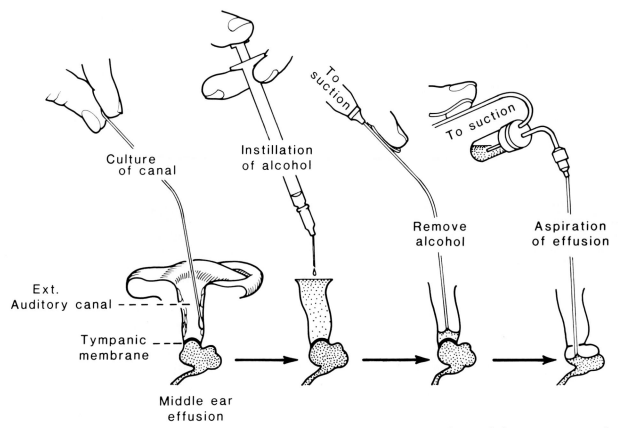

Figure 21–69. Method recommended for tympanocentesis and aspiration of a middle-ear effusion for microbiologic assessment. A culture of the external auditory canal is obtained with a Calgiswab (Falton, Oxnard, CA) that has been moistened with trypticase soy broth. The canal is then filled with 70 per cent ethyl alcohol for 1 minute, after which as much as possible of the alcohol is removed from the ear canal by aspiration. Tympanocentesis is performed in the inferior portion of the tympanic membrane with an Alden-Senturia trap (Storz Instrument Co., St. Louis, MO) with a needle attached. Care is taken not to close the suction hole in the trap before entering the middle ear.

White Blood Cell Count

Although white blood cell counts are too variable to be helpful in distinguishing the child with otitis media due to a bacterial pathogen from the child with otitis media and a sterile effusion, data suggest that the mean white blood cell count of children with bacterial otitis media is higher than that of children with sterile middle-ear effusion. Lahikainen (1953) noted that the mean white blood cell counts (per cubic millimeter) of children with otitis due to *S. pyogenes* was 13,400; due to *S. pneumoniae*, 10,500; and due to *H. influenzae*, 11,500, and of children with sterile middle-ear effusion, 8700. Mortimer and Watterson (1956) found similar results in children who had a bacterial pathogen in the middle-ear effusion, the mean white blood cell count (per mm³) being 10,300; the mean white blood cell count was 6700 in children with sterile effusions. Feingold and colleagues (1966) found an association of higher white blood cell counts with isolation of bacterial pathogen from the middle-ear effusion; of 35 children with white blood cell counts of 15,000 or more, 27 (77 per cent) had a bacterial pathogen grown from the middle-ear effusion, whereas of children with a white blood cell count of 9000 or less, 8 of 20 (40 per cent) had a bacterial pathogen grown from the middle-ear effusion.

C-Reactive Protein

Several investigators have shown that elevation of C-reactive proteins can be related to bacterial acute otitis media caused by *S. pneumoniae* and *H. influenzae*, but when *B. catarrhalis* was isolated from middle-ear aspirates, the serum C-reactive protein levels were comparable to those of patients with sterile effusions (Komoroski et al., 1987; Karma et al., 1987).

Sedimentation Rate

Lahikainen (1953) found increases in sedimentation rate in children with otitis media and differences among the bacterial pathogens isolated from the middle-ear effusion. The mean sedimentation rate for 104 children with otitis media due to *S. pyogenes* was 43.7; for 171 children with otitis media due to *S. pneumoniae*, 30.2; for 43 with otitis media due to *H. influenzae*, 17.3; and for 85 children with sterile effusion, 21.3.

Allergy Testing

Allergy testing is indicated in patients who have recurrent acute or chronic middle-ear effusions in association with signs and symptoms of allergy of the upper respiratory tract. Methods are discussed in Chapter 42.

Radiologic Imaging

For the uncomplicated case of acute otitis media with effusion, radiographs of the temporal bone are not indicated. However, when recurrent acute or chronic otitis media with effusion is present, roentgenographic evaluation of the paranasal sinuses may be helpful in identifying sinusitis that may be related causally to the otitis media. When there are signs and symptoms of sinusitis present (e.g., purulent nasal discharge, cough, and fetor oris), conventional radiographic examination of the paranasal sinuses is the simplest, least expensive, and most practical examination. The occipitomental (Waters), frontal (Caldwell), basal (submentovertical), and lateral erect views should be obtained. In addition, the lateral view is beneficial in assessing the adenoid size in relation to the nasopharynx. The submentovertical view is helpful in evaluation of ethmoid and sphenoid sinuses. Both lateral and submentovertical views can be diagnostic of a nasopharyngeal tumor, which can mechanically obstruct the eustachian tube and cause otitis media with effusion. Chronic nasal obstruction, with or without epistaxis or cervical lymphadenopathy, in association with otitis media should prompt the clinician to suspect a nasopharyngeal tumor. The A-mode ultrasound can also be useful in determining the presence of an effusion in the maxillary sinuses (Edell and Isaacson, 1978; Revonta, 1979). Computed tomography and nuclear magnetic resonance imaging are more definitive than either plain radiography or ultrasound (Chap. 30).

When certain complications or sequelae of otitis media are suspect or present, then radiologic evaluation of the temporal bone is indicated. Plain radiographs (Towne, Laws, Stenvers) may be helpful in the diagnosis of osteitis of the mastoid or a cholesteatoma, but CT scans are more precise and should be obtained if a suppurative intratemporal or intracranial complication is suspected (see Chaps. 22 and 23). In addition, CT can be an aid in visualizing the eustachian tube (Naito et al., 1987) (see Chap. 10).

Acoustic (Impedance) Immittance Measurement, Including Tympanometry

The function of the electroacoustic (impedance) immittance audiometer depends on the principles of sound in relation to the physiologic characteristics of the ear. (For a more complete description of acoustic immittance, see Chap. 9.) The most effective transfer of energy occurs when a force flows from one medium to another medium of similar impedance (i.e., with similar mechanical properties of stiffness, mass, and friction). The middle ear facilitates the transfer of

sound energy from an air medium with low impedance to a liquid medium with relatively high impedance (cochlea) (see Fig. 9–3A). The tympanic membrane and middle ear, therefore, act as an impedance matching transformer. Abnormalities that interfere with this function impair hearing. Three basic observations about acoustic impedance can be made with the electroacoustic impedance bridge: a tympanogram can be obtained, and middle-ear muscle reflex and static compliance can be measured. The instrument has become increasingly popular, and it is currently used in a wide variety of clinical settings for both diagnosis and screening. A tympanic membrane–middle ear system that has an increase in one or more of the components of impedance (stiffness, mass, or friction) will not transfer sound energy efficiently to the cochlear fluids. In such an instance, acoustic impedance is increased, or, stated reciprocally, acoustic compliance is reduced. Therefore, a greater amount of sound energy will be reflected from the tympanic membrane–middle ear region and a smaller amount of sound energy will be transmitted to the cochlea. An excellent example of this type is a middle ear that contains an effusion (see Fig. 9–3B). Conversely, the tympanic membrane and middle ear may have a decrease in impedance (or increase in compliance), such as may occur with disarticulation of the ossicular chain, in which case an increased amount of sound energy is received by the middle ear but is not transmitted to the cochlea (see Fig. 9–3C).

Electroacoustic Immittance Audiometer

Measurements made with the electroacoustic immittance audiometer (alternatively known as electroacoustic impedance bridge) provide an objective assessment of the mobility of the tympanic membrane and the dynamics of the ossicular chain, the intraaural muscles with their attachments, and the middle-ear air cushion. Its design permits the introduction of a signal through one of three small openings in the probe tip, which is hermetically sealed in the external auditory canal (Fig. 21–70). A certain amount of the signal is transmitted into and through the tympanic membrane and middle ear, whereas a certain amount is reflected back into the ear canal. The reflected sound is received by a microphone circuit, connected to a second opening in the probe tip in the ear canal, which has a certain amplitude and phase related to the mechanical properties of the tympanic membrane; the frequency of the signal is determined by the frequency of the probe tip, which is usually 220 Hz. The third aperture of the probe is connected to an air pump that varies the air pressure in the closed ear canal. With this arrangement, impedance can be monitored with a varying air pressure load on the tympanic membrane, or with a static air pressure load. The air pressure can be varied either manually or automatically with most bridges. The measurement of impedance changes at the tympanic membrane with a dynamic air pressure load is called tympanometry, and, when there is a

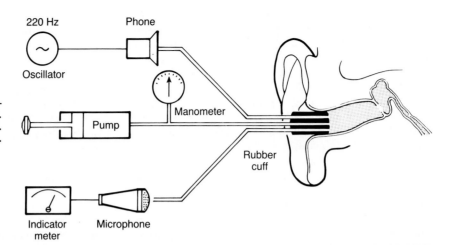

Figure 21–70. Schematic design of electro-acoustic immittance audiometer (see text). (From Bluestone, C. D., and Klein, J. O. 1988. Otitis Media in Infants and Children. Philadelphia, W. B. Saunders Co.)

static pressure load, static compliance can be measured.

IMMITTANCE INSTRUMENTATION

During the last 20 years, an increasing number of instrument companies have introduced electroacoustic immittance audiometers to the market. This has been primarily due to the widespread acceptance of this technique of assessment, which is related to the ever-growing number of studies that have shown that impedance testing improves the accuracy of diagnosing otitis media and related conditions. Tympanometry is a reliable, simple procedure that is easily carried out in a short time by nonprofessional personnel. For all of these reasons, the instruments have become enormously popular, and with this has come a technologic explosion in instrumentation that has resulted in confusion among professionals who wish to purchase new instruments and concern by those who find their relatively new instruments outdated in only a few years. In addition, most of the new or modified instruments are not field tested and validated prior to their introduction to the market; this presents a distinct hazard to the clinician who wishes to use a validated, reliable instrument. However, some of the instruments have been validated and are reliable, as demonstrated over many years of use by both clinicians and investigators.

The first commercially available instrument to measure acoustic impedance was developed in Denmark during the 1950's by Terkildsen and Nielson (1960), and in 1958 it was manufactured by Madsen Electronics as model ZO61. In 1963, Madsen introduced model ZO70, which rapidly became the prototype for all of the impedance bridges that followed and has provided the latest information on the invaluable diagnostic capabilities of electroacoustic impedance measurements. In 1971, Madsen introduced the ZO72, which incorporated an audiometer so that a contralateral acoustic reflex could be measured, and a later model added the ability to measure the ipsilateral acoustic reflex. In 1970, the Grason-Stadler Company introduced the otoadmittance meter, which measures the complex components of acoustic impedance. The measurement as described by the developers is termed acoustic admittance, which is divided into acoustic susceptance (compliance) and acoustic conductance (resistance) and is expressed in acoustic milliohms (Grason, 1972). Subsequent to the popularity of the Madsen model ZO70, many other companies have entered into manufacturing immittance audiometers. Some are designed for diagnostic use, others are purely for screening, and still others can be used for both diagnostic and screening purposes. The clinician should make a decision regarding which instrument to purchase based on need; however, availability of repair services should also be a consideration.

The only instruments that have been validated by comparing the patterns obtained with a bridge and the findings at myringotomy are (1) Madsen model ZO70 (Bluestone et al., 1973; Cantekin et al., 1977b; Paradise et al., 1976), (2) Grason-Stadler model 1720 (Beery et al., 1975a; Cantekin et al., 1977b; Shurin et al., 1977), and (3) Grason-Stadler model 1722 (Fria et al., 1980).

Tympanometry

Tympanometry employing most available instruments involves varying canal air pressure in a single sweep from 200 to -400 mm H_2O (or -600 mm H_2O), thereby altering the stiffness of the tympanic membrane. Changing the stiffness of the tympanic membrane results in an alteration of the relationship between the probe tone and the sound pressure level (SPL) in the canal; this changing relationship is recorded as tympanic membrane impedance, which can be calculated and displayed graphically as a tympanogram. The abscissa of the tympanogram records air pressure in millimeters of water, and the ordinate records compliance, an arbitrary unit (see Fig. 9–5). Because the tympanic membrane compliance is maximum when the air pressure on both sides of the drum is equal, the peak of the normal tympanogram tracing occurs at approximately 0 mm H_2O. If pressure within the middle ear is negative, the tympanometric peak will be in the negative-pressure zone of the tympanogram (see Fig. 9–6). Thus, the position of the peak of the trace along the horizontal axis usually is indicative of the middle-ear pressure. Also important is the height of the peak. Normally, the height of the peak is between half and full scale on the ordinate. Conditions that increase the impedance of the tympanic membrane–middle ear system (e.g., otitis media with effusion) can result in a tympanogram peak that is less than half scale, showing low compliance. Conversely, conditions that decrease the impedance of the system (e.g., a flaccid tympanic membrane) elevate the peak to exceed full-scale deflection. Therefore, the position of the peak along both the ordinate and the abscissa provides information regarding middle-ear pressure and the acoustic impedance of the system. In addition, the shape of the peak or, more specifically, the gradient (slope) is also important. A peak that has a gradual slope (rounded) rather than a steep one is usually associated with some degree of tympanic membrane–middle ear disorder.

VALIDATION OF TYMPANOMETRY

By assessing the pressure, compliance, and shape of the tympanometric trace, the normal tympanic membrane–middle ear system can be distinguished from the abnormal one with a reasonable degree of certainty. In addition, the types of abnormality may also be determined. To this end, the tympanometric patterns have been classified and related to various pathologic conditions involving the eardrum and middle ear. Bluestone and associates (1973) attempted to relate these patterns (with the Madsen instrument) to the presence or absence of effusion at myringotomy but found a high percentage of false-positive results (i.e., the tympanometric patterns indicated the presence of an effusion but none was found at myringotomy). Paradise and colleagues (1976) proposed a pattern classification with the same type of instrument for the identification of middle-ear effusion based on otoscopy and, in many instances, the myringotomy findings. The accuracy of the diagnosis of effusion was higher with Paradise and colleagues' (1976) classification than with the previously proposed patterns. The study also demonstrated that tympanometry in infants less than 7 months of age was not valid because of their highly compliant external auditory canals. A more recent study confirmed the diagnostic accuracy of this pattern classification (Gates et al., 1986). Beery and coworkers (1975a), employing the Grason-Stadler otoadmittance meter, also related myringotomy findings to the tympanometric patterns and proposed a pattern classification for the diagnosis of middle-ear effusion. The patterns were 93 per cent accurate. Shurin and associates (1977) also employed the Grason-Stadler instrument and proposed a pattern classification based on measurements with a planimeter. Cantekin and coworkers (1977a) compared the two instruments—the Madsen electroacoustic impedance bridge and the Grason-Stadler otoadmittance meter—as to their abilities to identify middle-ear effusions; the tympanometric findings were validated by myringotomy, and the same number of false-negative and false-positive patterns were recorded for both instruments.

TYMPANOMETRIC PATTERNS

From all of these studies, it appears that using the electroacoustic impedance bridge is an accurate way of identifying middle-ear effusions, but it is not perfect. The instrument can be an invaluable aid in diagnosis and, under certain conditions, in screening for middle-ear disease. Figure 21–71 shows the types of tympanograms and their common variants that relate to expected conditions of the eardrum and middle ear. This chart is currently employed by the authors, and much of this information is based on the myringotomy findings of a study of 425 ears of 238 subjects ranging in age from 7 months to 15 years, with a median age of 6 years (Bluestone and Cantekin, 1979). Tympanograms that are considered normal are those included in the first frame of the figure. Ears that yield tympanograms of Variant a will on occasion (2 per cent) be found to have an effusion, especially a scant, thin, serous effusion usually seen as an air-fluid level or bubbles behind a translucent eardrum. Variant b, even though it has a somewhat low compliance, is usually not obtained when an effusion is present. The tympanogram type that has an open end (peak off graph) at or near the normal pressure zone (Frame 2) is the result of high compliance and is most commonly associated with a flaccid tympanic membrane that is attributable to wide fluctuations in middle-ear pressure and loss of drum elasticity resulting from eustachian tube dysfunction. However, an effusion is not present. When this type of tympanogram is associated with a significant conductive hearing loss (usually between 40 and 60 dB), then an ossicular discontinuity should be suspected.

The negative-pressure type of tympanogram (Frame 3) has many variants, of which the four most common are shown. Unfortunately, at present there is no totally reliable way of predicting the presence or absence of effusion by the variant, as all may be associated with a middle-ear effusion. However, the probability that an ear yielding a tympanogram of Variant a has an effusion is less than the probability of effusion in ears giving the other three variants, and an ear from which a tympanogram of Variant d (with a rounded peak) is recorded has the highest probability of having an effusion present. When the tympanogram trace is open without a peak and is in the negative-pressure zone (Frame 4), the tympanic membrane is flaccid and only rarely will an effusion be present within the middle ear. The explanation for the floppy tympanic membrane is the same as that described for the type of tympanogram in Frame 2, but, in this type, negative pressure is evident at the time of testing. Again, as described above (Frame 2), if a significant air-bone audiometric gap is found, an ossicular chain discontinuity should be suspected. The tympanogram type that shows a high positive pressure (Frame 5) may be

TYMPANOGRAM TYPES AND VARIANTS RELATED TO CLINICAL FINDINGS

TYMPANOGRAM TYPES	COMMON VARIANTS	PRESUMPTIVE DIAGNOSIS OF TYMPANIC MEMBRANE MIDDLE EAR CONDITION
1. NORMAL	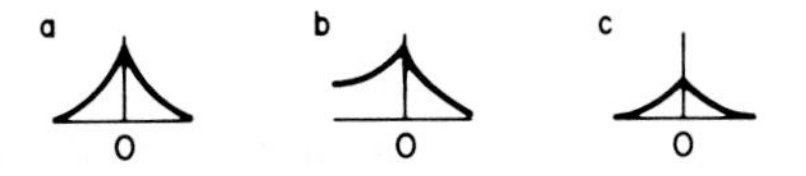	NORMAL
2. HIGH COMPLIANCE (NORMAL PRESSURE)	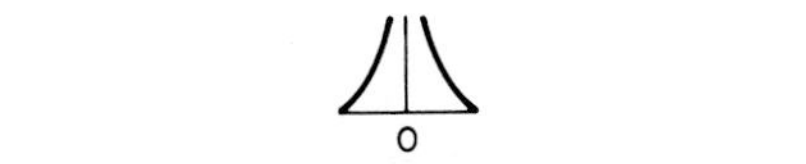	FLACCID TYMPANIC MEMBRANE OR OSSICULAR DISCONTINUITY
3. NEGATIVE PRESSURE (NORMAL COMPLIANCE)	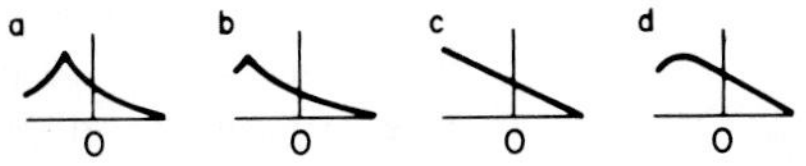	HIGH NEGATIVE PRESSURE WITH OR WITHOUT MIDDLE EAR EFFUSION
4. HIGH NEGATIVE PRESSURE AND HIGH COMPLIANCE	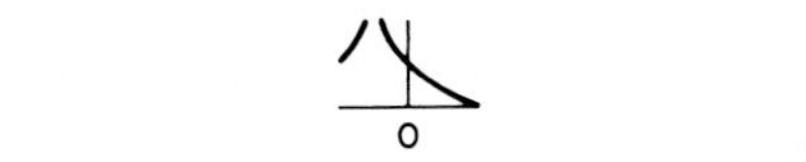	FLACCID TYMPANIC MEMBRANE AND HIGH NEGATIVE PRESSURE (OR OSSICULAR DISCONTINUITY AND HIGH NEGATIVE PRESSURE)
5. HIGH POSITIVE PRESSURE		HIGH POSITIVE PRESSURE WITH OR WITHOUT MIDDLE EAR EFFUSION
6. LOW COMPLIANCE	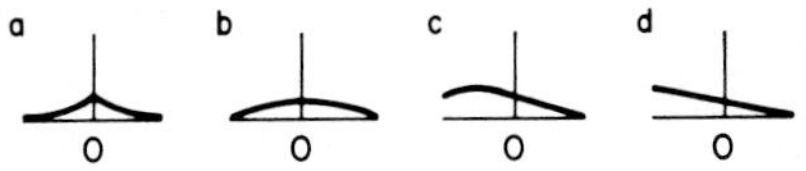	MIDDLE EAR EFFUSION, &/OR THICKENED TYMPANIC MEMBRANE, &/OR OSSICULAR FIXATION &/OR ADHESIVE OTITIS MEDIA

Figure 21–71. Tympanogram types related to presumptive conditions of the middle ear (see text). (From Bluestone, C. D., and Klein, J. O. 1988. Otitis Media in Infants and Children. Philadelphia, W. B. Saunders Co.)

associated with an effusion, usually an acute otitis media with effusion, particularly with Variant b. All of the variants shown for the types of tympanograms that have low compliance (Frame 6) are usually associated with a middle-ear effusion; ears from which tympanograms of Variants a and b are recorded may or may not have an effusion, whereas 90 per cent of ears with tympanograms of Variants c and d will have an effusion. Other pathologic conditions that can result in this type of pattern are those that increase the acoustic impedance of the system (e.g., thickening of the tympanic membrane, ossicular chain fixation, or adhesive otitis media).

The problem in attempting to diagnose either a fixation or a discontinuity of the ossicular chain by the tympanogram pattern is that other parts of the tympanic membrane–middle ear system may be abnormal and mask the condition. An example of this would be a middle ear in which one of the ossicles is fixed (e.g., stapes, with adhesive otitis media) but the tympanogram either is normal or reveals high compliance because the tympanic membrane is flaccid. Therefore, making a definitive diagnosis of an ossicular pathologic disorder usually must depend on the audiogram or, ultimately, an exploratory tympanotomy.

Acoustic Middle-Ear Muscle Reflex

Acoustic impedance instrumentation can also be used to detect the contraction of the middle-ear mus-

cles, the stapedius and tensor tympani, to intense sound stimulation. This contraction is called the acoustic middle-ear muscle reflex, or, simply, the acoustic reflex.

The anatomy of the acoustic reflex arc is depicted in Figure 21–72. The afferent portion of the arc, up to and including the superior olivary complex, is shared with the hearing mechanism. The efferent fibers of the acoustic reflex arc arise from neuronal connections in the brain stem between the olivary and the facial nerve nucleus for the stapedius muscle and the trigeminal nerve nucleus for the tensor tympani muscle.

The acoustic immittance audiometer indicates the status of the acoustic reflex in two ways: first, the reflex results in a stiffening of the ossicular chain and a concomitant increase in impedance; second, because the reflex is bilateral to a unilateral stimulus (the muscles of both sides contract when one ear is stimulated), an earphone can be placed on one ear to deliver an intense stimulus, and the probe tip of the immittance audiometer, inserted in the opposite ear, can detect the impedance change caused by the reflex.

When the immittance audiometer is used to detect an acoustic reflex elicited by stimulating the opposite ear, the response is commonly called the "contralateral" or "crossed" acoustic reflex. Many immittance audiometers marketed today have probe tips designed both to stimulate and to detect the acoustic reflex in the same ear; the reflex is elicited and its effect on impedance is detected in the same ear. Under these

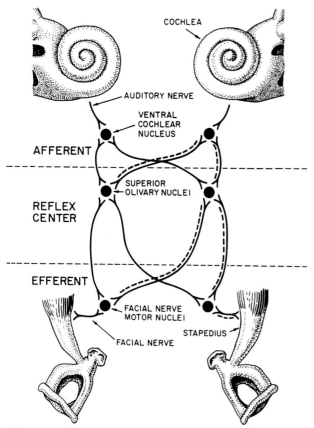

Figure 21–72. Diagrammatic representation of the acoustic reflex arc (see text). (From Bluestone, C. D., and Klein, J. O. 1988. Otitis Media in Infants and Children. Philadelphia, W. B. Saunders Co.)

conditions, the response is called the "ipsilateral" or "uncrossed" acoustic reflex.

The influence of a middle-ear effusion and attendant conductive hearing loss on the reflex is not simply a result of the mode of reflex stimulation. Ipsilateral acoustic reflex tests stimulate and detect the response in the same ear through the immittance audiometer probe tip. In the middle ear with an effusion, the impedance is already abnormally altered, and further changes in impedance, due to middle-ear muscle contraction, may not be observable; to be detectable, these changes may require elevated stimulus intensity levels.

It follows that ipsilateral acoustic reflex testing in a middle ear with an effusion will most probably yield no response; if the response is present, the threshold of the response will tend to be elevated.

The influence of a middle-ear effusion on the contralateral acoustic reflex may be somewhat harder to understand. The contralateral reflex will probably be absent if the middle ear having the probe tip has an effusion or if the effusion-filled middle ear having the stimulus earphone has a moderate to moderately severe conductive hearing loss. The reason for the first situation was described above. In the second situation, the conductive hearing loss necessitates reflex stimulus levels that may be beyond the instrument's output capabilities. For these reasons, the contralateral acous-

tic reflex is generally absent in cases of bilateral otitis media with effusion. When the effusion is unilateral, the contralateral reflex will probably be absent for both ears, if the impaired ear has a moderate to moderately severe conductive hearing loss (Chap. 9).

Static Compliance (Physical Volume Test)

Compliance, or the mobility of the tympanic membrane–middle ear system, can be measured by the amplitude of the tympanogram trace and can also be measured separately—it is usually expressed in absolute units of volume (cubic centimeters). However, the measurement has limited clinical value except for determining the volume of the system, which can be used to determine whether the tympanic membrane is intact or perforated or if a functioning tympanostomy tube is present. Clinically, a microscopic perforation can be detected with the measurement, even when the tympanic membrane appears to be mobile when positive or negative pressure is applied by the pneumatic otoscope (assuming that the perforation is small enough and the magnitude of the pressure exerted by the otoscope is sufficient to move the eardrum). A similar condition frequently exists when a tympanostomy tube is in the tympanic membrane but the patency of the tube is questionable. The volume measured by all of the currently available bridges is probably not accurate, but the technique is still useful for determination of an intact or nonintact tympanic membrane.

The volume of the middle ear is measured by applying 200 mm H_2O pressure to the external canal with the impedance bridge. If the tympanic membrane is intact, the measurement should be approximately 0.6 to 0.8 cc in a younger child and between 1.0 and 1.5 cc in the older child and adult. If the eardrum is not intact, then greater values are found: more than 2 cc in the child and 2.5 cc in the adult. However, some children have rather large ear canal volumes that may exceed 2 cc when the tympanic membrane is intact. Therefore, in such a case an additional method should be attempted to determine if a nonintact tympanic membrane is present. The external canal pressure should be raised to 400 mm H_2O, and, if the eardrum has an opening, the eustachian tube will be forced open in most children and rapid drops in pressure will be noted on the immittance audiometer's manometer. All infants and children from whom a tympanogram is obtained should have static compliance (volume) recorded also, as a flat or rounded tympanogram apparently indicating an effusion may be found in a child who actually has a nonintact eardrum.

Screening

SCREENING FOR EAR DISEASE WITH ACOUSTIC IMMITTANCE MEASUREMENTS

Emphasis has been placed on interpreting the three acoustic immittance measurements—tympanometry, static compliance, and the acoustic reflex—as a whole.

This approach provides the best opportunity for accurate diagnostic assessment. There have been numerous attempts, however, to separate certain impedance measurements as screening tools, particularly for the detection of middle-ear disease in children.

Several published investigations have evaluated the screening effectiveness of tympanometry, the acoustic reflex, or both (Brooks, 1973, 1976, 1977; Cooper et al., 1974; Ferrer, 1974; Harker and Van Wagoner, 1974; Lewis et al., 1974; McCandless and Thomas, 1974; McCurdy et al., 1976; Orchik and Herdman, 1974; Renvall et al., 1973; Roberts, 1976). Brooks (1978) supported the utility of the acoustic reflex alone as a screening tool for detection of middle-ear disease in children. These investigators commonly agree that impedance measurements are easy to perform, noninvasive, reliable, and highly sensitive to the presence of middle-ear disease. These factors would favor the use of tympanometry and the acoustic reflex as screening measurements for the detection of disease. However, definitive data supporting the validity of using impedance measurements for screening are still lacking. Although the measurements are sensitive to disease, when it is present, they are considerably less accurate in sorting out children without disease, and the percentage of false-positive errors obtained is uncomfortably high (Fria et al., 1978; Paradise and Smith, 1978; Wachtendorf et al., 1984). The resulting over-referral rate argues against the cost-effectiveness of *mass* screening for middle-ear disease with acoustic impedance measurements. A review of the state-of-the-art and suggested guidelines for impedance screening for middle-ear disease in children was presented by Bluestone and coworkers (1986).

TYMPANOMETRIC SCREENING FOR OTITIS MEDIA WITH EFFUSION

Screening for otitis media with effusion is a process that is intended to identify children who may have the disease but in whom it would otherwise go undetected. Otitis media is a disease that appears to be important to identify because it is highly prevalent, is associated with varying degrees of conductive hearing loss, and may lead to other, more serious complications and sequelae. Otoscopy performed by an expert is an excellent screening method and should be employed by professionals who care for children as a routine part of the examination. This is especially important in infants and young children. However, for mass screening, otoscopy is not feasible. Audiometry, employing the routine audiologic screening criteria, has been shown to identify only half of a group of children with middle-ear effusion (Bluestone et al., 1973). In addition, audiometry, employing standard methods, cannot be obtained on young infants in whom the prevalence of the disease is the highest. However, impedance screening employing tympanometry and possibly the acoustic reflex is a highly sensitive method to screen for otitis media with effusion. Impedance testing is acceptable to both the child and the health care provider because it is safe, noninvasive, and simply executed. Studies have shown impedance measurements to be reliable, but these studies have not involved subjects of all age groups or all instruments that are available, many of which have been designed specifically for screening purposes.

The validity of criteria for referral for specific diagnostic criteria based on impedance measurements (i.e., their association, singly or in combination, with the presence or absence of middle-ear effusion) has not been established completely, and further studies are required. In addition, neither the epidemiology nor the natural history of the disease has been adequately studied in the various age groups affected, which makes most of the methods of management currently employed difficult to evaluate. Otitis media with effusion in many instances spontaneously disappears. Because of these problems, the referral criteria for children who are identified with a middle-ear effusion remain controversial.

CURRENT RECOMMENDATIONS

A 1977 task force addressed the use of tympanometry for screening for ear disease and advised against mass screening on a routine basis for the detection of middle-ear disorders in children of any age group (Harford et al., 1978). Although not recommending mass screening, the task force did advise screening methods that employed impedance measurements in small, carefully controlled programs to determine the best method for larger screening programs. More recently, mass screening for otitis media was not advised (Bluestone et al., 1986).

The following is a summary of the 1977 task force's recommendations. Middle-ear effusion has its highest prevalence and incidence in the age group between 6 and 36 months. Following episodes of acute infection, asymptomatic otitis media with effusion continues for extended periods in a large number of infants, and there is concern about the possible effects of undetected effusions on a child's function and development. In children younger than 7 months of age, the relations between tympanometric findings and middle-ear disease are not well understood, although the limited data now available indicate that the sensitivity of tympanometry as usually performed is relatively low. There are also feasibility problems associated with impedance screening of infants. Logistically, it may be difficult to gather infants for testing after they leave their place of birth. Moreover, impedance testing in infants may sometimes be difficult and time consuming. However, if these difficulties can be overcome, impedance testing of infants should be attempted, if feasible.

Even though mass screening of preschool and school-age children by impedance measurements is not recommended at present, it should be carried out in a planned manner in a smaller program. The following procedures and criteria have been judged to be minimal:

TABLE 21–14. Schema for Tympanometric Screening

CLASSIFICATION	INITIAL SCREEN	RETEST	SUBJECT OUTCOME
I	Acoustic reflex present and	Not required	Cleared
	Tympanogram normal		
II	Acoustic reflex absent and/or	Acoustic reflex absent and/or	Referred
	Typanogram normal	Tympanogram normal	
III	Acoustic reflex absent and/or	Acoustic reflex present and	At risk—recheck at later date
	Tympanogram abnormal	Tympanogram normal	

1. A combination of tympanometry and acoustic reflex measurement should be used.

2. For eliciting the acoustic reflex, a signal of 105-dB hearing threshold level (HTL) should be used in the contralateral mode, or a signal of 105-dB sound pressure level (SPL) in the ipsilateral mode, or both.

3. Whether broad-band noise or pure tone is preferable as an eliciting stimulus for the acoustic reflex remains to be established. A pure tone between 1000 and 3000 Hz would be acceptable for this purpose. The stimulus should be specified, described, or both.

4. Acoustic reflex measurements can be obtained either with the ear canal air pressure that results in minimal acoustic impedance or with ear canal air pressure equal to ambient pressure. The condition used should be specified.

5. For tympanometry, a 220-Hz probe tone is preferred.

6. For tympanometry, an air pressure range of -400 to $+100$ mm H_2O is preferred. However, a range of -300 to $+100$ mm H_2O is acceptable. Automatic recording should be used whenever possible, and the rate of air pressure change should be specified.

7. Failure on the initial screening test is denoted by either an absent acoustic reflex or an abnormal tympanogram. An abnormal tympanogram is defined as one that either is flat or rounded (i.e., without a definite peak) or has a peak at, or more negative than, -200 mm H_2O. Flat or rounded tympanograms appear to be more highly correlated with middle-ear effusions than are tympanograms with peaks at negative-pressure readings.

8. Any child failing the initial screening should be retested in 4 to 6 weeks. Parents or guardians should be advised accordingly. Any child who has an acoustic reflex and a normal tympanogram result on the initial screening passes and is "cleared."

9. The schema on Table 21–14 is recommended for various screening findings. Classifications I and II should constitute the majority of children in a given population. Referral, when indicated after confirmatory retesting, should be made to an appropriate health care provider in the community. Classification III constitutes a group of children that require special monitoring by the agency responsible for the screening program. These "at risk" children should be retested periodically to determine the best possible need for future medical referral.

10. An optimal time and frequency for screening or referring particular populations could not be advised because of lack of adequate information. Future research is needed.

11. The agency responsible for a testing program must have facilities available for referral that include expert management. Prior to the initiation of a screening program, referral and management procedures must be defined.

12. Impedance testing should be supervised by professionals who are qualified by training and experience to perform and interpret impedance measurements.

13. Programs should be designed to gather information of value in defining the role of impedance measurement in screening children for middle ear disease.

The Committee on School Health of the Academy of Pediatrics (Zanga et al., 1987) recommends the following:

1. The impedance bridge should not be used in mass screening programs for the detection of hearing loss *or* middle-ear effusion.

2. The impedance bridge may be used in the school setting only as an aid in the diagnosis of individual children who are at high risk for, or who are suspected of having, otitis media with effusion.

3. Hearing screening by pure-tone audiometry be used as the primary method of detection of hearing loss in school children.

4. The impedance bridge should not be used as a replacement for audiometric screening, because it will not detect sensory neural hearing loss and may lead to overreferral of children with asymptomatic middle-ear effusion.

5. Any persistent abnormality detected by either the impedance bridge or pure-tone audiometry should result in a prompt referral to the child's pediatrician.

Acoustic Reflectometry

The acoustic otoscope, or reflectometer,* is a hand-held instrument that is placed next to the opening of the child's external ear canal (Fig. 21–73); it uses an

---

*Endeco Medical, Marion, MA.

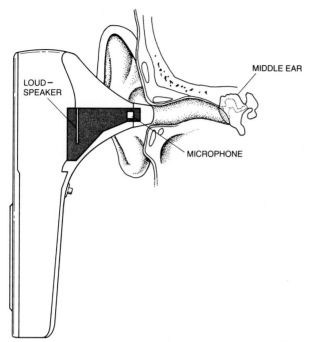

Figure 21–73. Cutaway view of probe assembly, showing relative position of microphone and loudspeaker. (From Bluestone, C. D., and Klein, J. O. 1988. Otitis Media in Infants and Children. Philadelphia, W. B. Saunders Co.)

80-dB sound source that varies from 2000 to 4500 Hz over a 100-msec period (Teele and Teele, 1984; Schwartz and Schwartz, 1987; Oyiborhiro et al., 1987). A microphone located in the probe tip measures the total level of transmitted and reflected sound (Fig. 21–74). Because no pressurization of the external canal is required, no seal with the canal is needed. Acoustic energy is reflected back toward the probe tip from the ear canal and eardrum. The operating principle is that a sound wave in a closed tube will be reflected when it strikes the end of the tube. Reflected sound waves from the middle ear cancel the transmitted sound one quarter of a wavelength from the eardrum, thus providing information related to the presence or absence of a middle-ear effusion, as will an estimate of ear canal length; the more sound reflected, the greater is the likelihood of an effusion being present. Sound reflectivity is measured in units ranging from zero through nine; a vertical scale indicates status of the middle ear by the sound reflected, and a horizontal score indicates canal length.

Assessment of Hearing

The assessment of hearing in infants and children is not an accurate method for identifying the presence of a middle-ear effusion but can be valuable in determining the effect of middle-ear disease on hearing function and is important in decision-making regarding management.

Hearing loss is by far the most prevalent complication and morbid outcome of otitis media, and it may be caused by one or more of the intraaural complications or sequelae. To a varying degree, fluctuating or persistent loss of hearing is almost always associated with otitis media. The audiogram usually reveals a mild to moderate conductive loss; when otitis media is present the average loss is 27 dB (Fria et al., 1985). However, there may be a sensorineural component, generally attributed to the effect of increased tension and stiffness of the round window membrane. This hearing loss is usually reversible with resolution of the effusion, but permanent conductive hearing loss can result from irreversible changes caused by recurrent acute or chronic inflammation (e.g., adhesive otitis, tympanosclerosis, or ossicular discontinuity). Irreparable sensorineural loss may also occur, presumably as the result of spread of infection through the round or oval window membrane (Paparella et al., 1972) or a labyrinthitis due to perilymphatic fistulas (Supance and Bluestone, 1983). Audiometry can be reliably per-

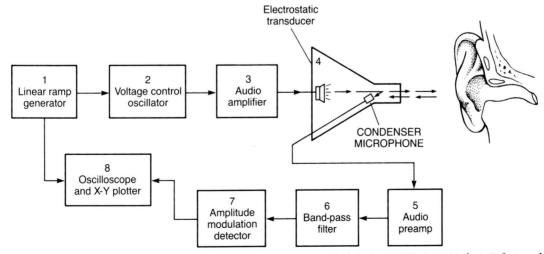

Figure 21–74. Block diagram of acoustic reflectometer. (From Bluestone, C. D., and Klein, J. O. 1988. Otitis Media in Infants and Children. Philadelphia, W. B. Saunders Co.)

formed in infants and children. Some infants and young children may require nonbehavioral tests of hearing.

All infants and children should have their hearing evaluated, if possible, when a chronic middle-ear effusion is present because the type (i.e., conductive, sensorineural, or both) and the degree of hearing loss will have a bearing on the selection and timing of the various management options available to the clinician. (For a more complete description of hearing evaluation, the reader is referred to Chapter 9.)

Methods

In general, there are two methods to evaluate hearing in children: behavioral and nonbehavioral. The age and the ability of the child to cooperate usually dictate the test selection (Northern and Downs, 1978).

BEHAVIORAL TESTS

The neonatal reactions to sudden, intense sound are predominantly reflexive and include the Moro reflex, the aural palpebral reflex, and the arousal and cessation responses.

The *Moro reflex* is a generalized motor response that is commonly known as the startle reflex. Classically, the neonate (also most infants) will thrust the head backward and suddenly move the arms and legs up and outward when a stimulus of 80- to 85-dB SPL is presented. The *aural palpebral reflex*, or "eyeblink" reflex, consists of a contraction of the orbicularis oculi muscles and, frequently, closing of the eyelids. A stimulus of 105- to 115-dB SPL will usually be required. The *arousal* and *cessation reflexes* involve clear contrasts in the neonate's pre- and poststimulus activity. A stimulus of 90-dB SPL should awaken or arouse the sleeping or drowsy neonate; in the cessation reflex, a decrease or inhibition of activity in the restless or crying baby is observed. However, these reactions are primarily reflexive, require rather intense stimuli, and are qualitative rather than quantitative.

Behavioral observation audiometry (BOA) is a technique used for neonates and young infants in which the examiner presents a stimulus sound and observes the child's associated behavioral response, which does not require conditioning. Simple noisemakers, such as rattles, squeak toys, and bells, are common stimulus devices used in the office setting, but calibrated stimuli are used in a test booth in audiology centers.

Visual reinforcement audiometry (VRA) also involves the preservation of a stimulus sound and the observation of the child's associated behavioral response (Fig. 21–75). The response, however, is rewarded with a visual reinforcement, such as a blinking light, an illuminated picture or toy, or an animated toy that is located above the loudspeaker through which the stimulus is presented. The test is most successful for assessing infants in the second year of life, but it may be used for younger infants.

Tangible reinforcement audiometry, or *tangible reinforcement operant conditioning audiometry*

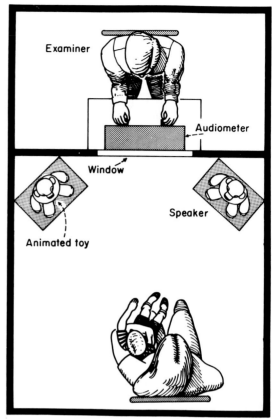

Figure 21–75. Visual reinforcement audiometry (VRA). Infant sits on mother's lap and is observed by examiner, who presents a sound stimulus through speaker to right or left of child. The infant's response, a head turn toward the sound stimulus, is rewarded by activation and illumination of the animated toy. (From Bluestone, C. D., and Klein, J. O. 1988. Otitis Media in Infants and Children. Philadelphia, W. B. Saunders Co.)

(TROCA), uses candy, cereal, or tangible rewards for pressing a bar when the sound stimulus is presented (Fig. 21–76). It is a test appropriate for assessment of difficult-to-test children, such as the mentally retarded, as well as infants.

Results of these tests will provide some indication of the degree of hearing loss present but not the type (conductive or sensorineural). However, in some children, the VRA and TROCA tests may be able to determine the hearing level in the individual ear. They are appropriate for children younger than 3 years of age.

Play audiometry is similar to conventional tests given to older children and adults and can be used to assess the hearing of children 2 years of age and older. Conventional audiometric techniques can be used, but they must be modified to be more interesting for the young child and usually take the form of "play." The assessment can provide information regarding both speech and pure-tone stimuli and can determine the degree of loss for the individual ear. In addition, play audiometry can provide threshold information on both air and bone conduction and, therefore, can determine whether a loss is conductive or sensorineural, or both.

Conventional audiometry is usually reserved for the

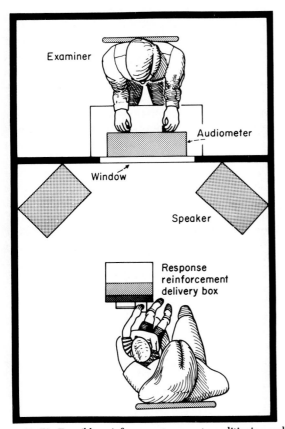

Figure 21–76. Tangible reinforcement operant conditioning audiometry (TROCA). Infant or young child sits on mother's lap and is observed by audiologist, who presents sound stimulus through speaker to right or left of child. The infant or child responds by pressing the bar on the TROCA device. Correct responses are rewarded by delivery of a tangible object, such as cereal, candy or small toys. (From Bluestone, C. D., and Klein, J. O. 1988. Otitis Media in Infants and Children. Philadelphia, W. B. Saunders Co.)

child 5 years of age and older but can be used for certain younger children, depending on the examiner and the cooperation of the child. The assessment should include pure-tone and speech audiometry to determine air and bone conduction thresholds on children with chronic otitis media with effusion to determine the type and degree of hearing loss for each ear.

NONBEHAVIORAL (PHYSIOLOGIC) TESTS

The nonbehavioral techniques to assess hearing include acoustic impedance measurements, auditory brain stem response recordings, cardiac audiometry, and respiratory audiometry. However, of all of these tests, the *auditory brain stem response* (ABR) is currently the best available and most widely used method. It is a test that is relatively independent of the child's behavioral response and is ordinarily used to evaluate infants and children for whom information on behavioral hearing tests is either unobtainable or unreliable. Three miniature electrodes placed on the scalp are used to record the responses. The ABR consists of five to seven vertex-positive waves labeled I to VII, occur-

ring in the first 10 msec following the onset of the stimulus (Fig. 21–77). Waves I through III presumably reflect activity of the eighth cranial nerve fibers (Wave I) and auditory centers in the pons (Waves II and III). Waves IV and V apparently reflect activity of the auditory centers in the mid to rostral pons and the caudal midbrain, respectively, whereas the neural generators for Waves VI and VII are less certain.

The electric configuration for the ABR includes the active electrode on the vertex of the skull, or midforehead at the hairline, and the reference and ground electrodes, respectively, on the ipsilateral and contralateral mastoid processes, or earlobes. The responses to 2000- to 4000-Hz clicks, filtered clicks, or brief, pure-tone bursts are typically averaged for each stimulus intensity employed. The stimuli are presented at a rapid rate (10 to 30/second) and a complete run, at a given stimulus intensity, requires 1.5 minutes; the entire procedure for both ears, in most cases, at several stimulus intensities, average less than an hour.

Because excessive muscle activity can interfere with the test, the child must be completely relaxed or, preferably, asleep. Natural sleep can be facilitated by feeding babies, up to about 6 months of age, immediately prior to the test. Children 7 years of age or older can lie quietly for the procedure; however, infants and children between these ages require sedation or even a general anesthesia.

The test can be sensitive in identifying a conductive hearing loss associated with a chronic middle-ear effusion, and it is especially valuable in the young infant. However, the technique does not assess the perceptual event called hearing. The ABR reflects auditory neural electric responses that are adequately correlated to behavioral hearing thresholds, but a normal result on the ABR only suggests that the auditory system up to midbrain level is responsive to the stimulus employed—it does not guarantee normal "hearing."

NORMAL ADULT

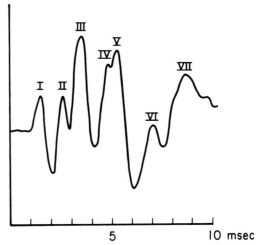

Figure 21–77. ABR to a 60-dB normal hearing level click stimulus in patient with normal hearing. Major wave components are labeled with Roman numerals I through VII. (From Bluestone, C. D., and Klein, J. O. 1988. Otitis Media in Infants and Children. Philadelphia, W. B. Saunders Co.)

In cases of middle-ear impairment, the entire series of ABR waves is delayed in time by an amount commensurate with the degree of attendant conductive hearing loss (Fria and Sabo, 1980). Latency of Wave I provides a better index of middle-ear impairment (Fig. 21–78). The consistent nature of the ABR in young infants makes it particularly useful in the evaluation of hearing when a chronic middle-ear effusion is present.

Indications for Hearing Assessment

Infants and children who have frequently recurrent otitis media or chronic otitis media with effusion, or both, should have their hearing assessed. It is important to know the degree of hearing loss and if that loss is conductive, sensorineural, or both. If the loss is only conductive and mild, management may consist of watchful waiting in hopes that the natural history of the effusion is in favor of spontaneous resolution. On the other hand, if there is significant bilateral conductive loss (e.g., greater than 30 dB), surgical intervention (e.g., insertion of tympanostomy tubes) may be an appropriate option, as the hearing loss may interfere with the child's development. The degree of conductive loss present in each ear would be more desirable information, because there may be a sequela or chronic middle-ear effusion present in one ear and not in the other. An ossicular chain disarticulation produced by rarefying osteitis, or ossicular fixation resulting from adhesive otitis media, may cause a maximal conductive hearing loss (i.e., 50 to 60 dB). In addition, a cholesteatoma may also be present even though there is no apparent defect in the tympanic membrane, and this may cause ossicular damage and a conductive loss. When the hearing loss (conductive) appears to be out of proportion to that expected with chronic otitis media with effusion, an examination employing the otomicroscope is necessary to exclude the possibility of a retraction pocket, cholesteatoma, or both in either the pars flaccida or the posterosuperior quadrant of the pars tensa. If the awake child cannot be examined

adequately, then general anesthesia will be required. At this time, a myringotomy and aspiration can be performed and a tympanostomy tube can be inserted. In addition, if the patient is too young for assessment of hearing with behavioral methods, difficult to assess, or not cooperative, then an ABR can be performed at the time of general anesthesia. The test should be performed after the aspiration of the effusion to determine if a residual conductive hearing loss is present that might be indicative of the presence of an ossicular abnormality.

When a conductive hearing loss is present in association with a middle-ear effusion and the effusion either spontaneously resolves in response to medical treatment or is removed by myringotomy, another audiogram should be obtained to verify that hearing has returned to normal limits. An audiogram should be obtained on every child approximately 2 weeks following the insertion of tympanostomy tubes (as long as there is no otorrhea present). A persistent, marked conductive hearing loss in the absence of an effusion would be presumptive evidence of an acquired ossicular defect or a concurrent congenital anomaly. The presence of both a chronic otitis media with effusion and a congenital ossicular deformity occurs quite frequently in the child with Down syndrome.

When a mixed hearing loss (conductive and sensorineural) is identified after the assessment, the clinician must suspect a middle-ear effusion that may be causing a serous ("toxic") labyrinthitis resulting from penetration of the round window or, possibly, a congenital or acquired defect in the oval or the round window, or both; in these cases the infection spreads directly into the labyrinth. Progressive or fluctuating sensorineural hearing loss with or without vertigo may be present, and, if documented, the patient should have further assessment (e.g., vestibular testing and CT of the temporal bone), and possible exploration (tympanotomy) of the middle ear in search for a perilymphatic fistula (Supance and Bluestone, 1983).

If the sensorineural hearing loss is not due to a

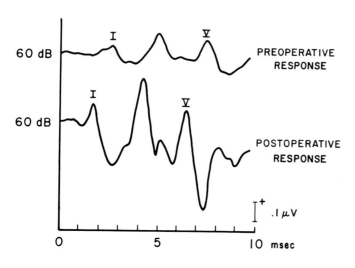

Figure 21–78. The ABR in a 6-month-old infant with otitis media with effusion, showing an example of latency delay. The top trace was recorded immediately prior to myringotomy and the bottom trace immediately after myringotomy. (With permission from Fria, T. J., and Sabo, D. L. 1980. Auditory brainstem responses in children with otitis media and effusion. Ann. Otol. Rhinol. Laryngol. 89[68]:200–206.)

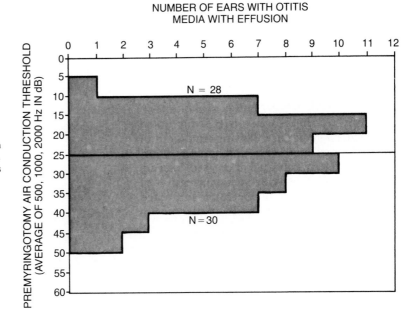

Figure 21–79. Audiometric findings in 58 ears with middle-ear effusion (see text). (From Bluestone, C. D., and Klein, J. O. 1988. Otitis Media in Infants and Children. Philadelphia, W. B. Saunders Co.)

condition that can be corrected, as described above, but to a known cause of sensorineural hearing loss in children (such as neonatal asphyxia or meningitis), then more aggressive management of chronic otitis media with effusion may be required than is needed for a child who does not have a sensorineural hearing loss. The added conductive hearing loss to a permanent sensorineural hearing loss may be quite handicapping for the child. This is especially true for the patient who has a moderate to severe sensorineural hearing loss and is mainstreamed in a regular school or is in a school for the deaf. Myringotomy and tympanostomy tubes are early treatment options for such children, rather than prolonged observation. Again, if a mixed hearing loss is suspected because the degree of loss appears to be greater than would be expected due to otitis media with effusion, then an accurate assessment of hearing is mandatory, regardless of the child's age. High-risk infants and children, in whom there is a family history of sensorineural hearing loss, would be of greatest concern. For such an infant, a procedure including an examination under anesthesia, a myringotomy, and insertion of tubes, followed by an ABR, is the best method to establish a definitive diagnosis as well as treat the chronic otitis media with effusion.

Screening for Hearing Loss

The identification of hearing loss is an important part of screening programs for preschool and school-age children, as identification of significant hearing problems must be followed by more definitive testing, evaluation, and, possibly, habilitation or rehabilitation of the child. However, audiometric screening to identify a middle-ear effusion does not have a high enough sensitivity and specificity to warrant its use. Bluestone and coworkers (1973) found that only half of a group of children (58 ears) with chronic middle-ear effusion

would have been identified by using an auditory screening test if 25 dB had been used as the criterion for failure (Fig. 21–79). However, audiometric screening is still necessary to identify those children with sensorineural hearing loss.

Vestibular Testing

Otitis media with effusion and eustachian tube dysfunction are the most common causes of dysequilibrium (e.g., vertigo, falling, and "clumsiness") in infants and children. The dysequilibrium almost invariably is resolved when the middle-ear effusion is absent or the child no longer has fluctuating middle-ear pressures. Frequently, the parents will report a dramatic disappearance of dysequilibrium immediately following insertion of tympanostomy tubes for recurrent acute or chronic otitis media with effusion or eustachian tube obstruction (fluctuating high negative pressure).

For most infants and children with otitis media and signs and symptoms of dysequilibrium, sophisticated vestibular testing is not indicated, as nonsurgical or surgical management of the eustachian tube–middle ear disorder will resolve the problem. In addition, the tests that are currently available are usually not feasible in children, especially infants. However, when the dysequilibrium persists despite the resolution of the middle-ear effusion and the presence of normal middle-ear pressures, then the child should be referred to an otolaryngologist for assessment of vestibular function to rule out the possibility of another cause of imbalance (see Chap. 15). Also, children who have frequent attacks of vertigo, with or without fluctuating or progressive sensorineural hearing loss, in association with otitis should be suspect of having a labyrinthine fistula.

The tests that can access vestibular function in

infants and children have been described in Chapter 11. Rotational tests and gross caloric testing can be performed in the infant and young child, and electronystagmography is feasible in the older child.

Endoscopy of the Nasopharynx

When infants or children have the possibility of nasal or nasopharyngeal pathologic state contributing to their middle-ear disease, transnasal endoscopy can be helpful, if other diagnostic methods are not definitive. Nasopharyngeal disease, such as choanal polyps, and neoplasms can obstruct the eustachian tube (Honjo et al., 1984).

HIGH–RISK POPULATIONS

Cleft Palate

In patients with cleft palate, ear disease and hearing loss have long been recognized as common problems. This association was first reported by Alt in 1878, who noted hearing improvement following treatment of otorrhea associated with cleft palate. Thorington (1892) reported increased hearing in a patient following artificial correction of a destroyed palate. In 1893, Gutzmann noted hearing loss in one half of his patients with cleft palate. Lannois (1901) reported the association of middle-ear disease and hearing loss in patients with cleft palate. In 1906, the need for otologic examination of patients with cleft palate was stressed by Brunck. Since these early descriptions, many reports have appeared in the literature related to the incidence, nature, and degree of hearing loss in patients with cleft palate.

Hearing Loss

The prevalence of hearing loss in the cleft palate population, as reported in the literature, varies considerably. Findings range from no hearing loss (Goetzinger et al., 1960) to 90 per cent prevalence (Sataloff and Fraser, 1952), but of all the studies, the average prevalence is approximately 50 per cent. Even though the criteria of hearing loss were not generally agreed on, it has been identified as conductive and usually bilateral. Halfond and Ballenger (1956) found that, of the 69 patients tested, 37 (54 per cent) had a hearing loss of 20 dB or greater. Miller (1956) reported that 19 (54 per cent) of 35 children with cleft palate had a hearing loss greater than 30 dB. That the prevalence may be even greater is suggested by Walton (1973), who studied 93 school-age children with cleft palate: one half of those who would have passed conventional audiometric screening at the 20-dB level were found to have air-bone gaps indicative of conductive hearing loss. This contention is supported by the study of

Bluestone and associates (1973), who found high-viscosity middle-ear effusions in children, including those with cleft palate, who would have passed a 25-dB screening audiogram. Even though a conductive hearing impairment would be expected, Bennett and colleagues (1968) reported that 30 per cent of 100 adults with cleft palate had either sensorineural or mixed hearing loss. This finding might be explained by the work of Paparella and coworkers (1972), who found sensorineural hearing loss in some patients with otitis media, and ascribed this to directly associated pathologic changes in the inner ear, presumably mediated via the round window. Unfortunately, no information is available in the literature concerning hearing in the infant with cleft palate.

Aural Pathology

INFANTS. Variot, in 1904, was the first to report ear disease in an infant with cleft palate. In 1936, Beatty described "acute tubotympanic congestion frequently found between the ages of three months and two years." Sataloff and Fraser (1952) reported that, in their experience, "examination of the ears of very young children with cleft palate reveals a high incidence of pathologic changes, despite the absence of subjective symptoms of otitis media." In 1958, Skolnick reported that only 6 per cent of cleft palate patients below the age of 1 year, and only 27 per cent of those between the ages of 1 and 4 years, had aural pathologic changes. Linthicum and coworkers (1959), however, discovered ear pathologic findings in 77 per cent of a group of 100 infants and children with cleft palate. In 1967, Stool and Randall reported that middle-ear effusion was present at myringotomy in 94 per cent of 25 cleft palate infants. Paradise and coworkers (1969), employing standard office otoscopy, diagnosed middle-ear disease in 49 of 50 infants with cleft palate. Most had full or bulging, opaque, immobile tympanic membranes, although spontaneous perforations and otorrhea were observed. Subsequent studies by the same team indicate that, throughout the first 2 years of life in infants with unrepaired cleft palate, otitis media is a virtually constant complication (Bluestone, 1971; Paradise and Bluestone, 1974). The otitis is usually characterized by an inflammatory effusion of variable viscosity; suppuration also occurs occasionally (Bluestone, 1971; Paradise, 1980).

OLDER CHILDREN AND ADULTS. Although the criteria of aural pathologic state in older children and adults with cleft palate vary considerably, its prevalence appears to be quite high. Meissner (1939) examined 213 such patients between the ages of 10 and 35 years and found that 83 per cent had abnormal tympanic membranes. Skolnick (1958) found that the prevalence of aural pathologic changes was 67 per cent in patients above the age of 5 years. Graham and Lierle (1962) found ear pathologic changes in 44 per cent of 29 patients with cleft palate and in 55 per cent of 146 with a cleft of both palate and lip. In a group of 82 patients, Aschan (1966) found that 78 per cent had aural abnormalities. In a retrospective, longitudinal study of 191 patients with cleft palate between 5 and 27 years of age, Severeid (1972) reported that 83 per cent had a middle-ear effusion confirmed by myringotomy. In Bennett's (1972) study of 100 adults with cleft palate, 30 per cent had aural pathologic findings consisting of signs of eustachian tube obstruction (13 per cent), chronic suppurative otitis media with or without mastoiditis (8 per cent), dry tympanic membrane perforation (6 per cent), and chronic adhesive otitis media (3 per cent).

Schools and Programs for the Deaf

Severely to profoundly deaf children (primarily those whose hearing loss is sensorineural), whether enrolled in a special class, in a regular school (mainstreamed), or in a residential school for the deaf, are of particular concern. Should a conductive hearing loss due to chronic or recurrent otitis media with effusion or high negative pressure, or both, be superimposed on the preexisting hearing loss, auditory input may be severely affected. This may critically interfere with the education of such children (Ruben and Math, 1978).

The incidence of middle-ear problems in deaf children has not been studied systematically, but the few studies that have been reported indicate the incidence to be equal to or possibly higher than that in nondeaf children. Porter (1974) found that 25 per cent of 79 deaf children aged 6 to 10 years had abnormal tympanograms. Brooks (1974) reported that 5-year-old children in a residential school for the deaf in England had a higher incidence of abnormal tympanograms than did nondeaf children. Mehta and Erlich (1978) found a high incidence of otitis media with effusion in children in a school for the deaf. Rubin (1978) reported the incidence of middle-ear effusion in children 3 to 6 years of age to be 30 per cent. Over a period of 1 year, Stool and coworkers (1980) conducted otoscopic, tympanometric, and audiometric evaluations on 446 students at a school for the deaf and reported that the incidence of middle-ear effusions was 8 per cent,

whereas that of high negative middle-ear pressure was 21 per cent. However, the incidence of otitis media with effusion in this study was 26 per cent in the 2- to 5-year age group. In addition, they found that 79 per cent of the students who initially were identified as having high negative middle-ear pressure consistently had abnormal negative pressures during the 1-year observation period.

From these few studies, it is apparent that continuous surveillance for middle-ear disease and early treatment should be part of every program or school for deaf children. This is especially critical for those children with some residual hearing who benefit from amplification because even the slightest conductive hearing loss may decrease or eliminate the efficacy of amplification. It is recommended that every school for deaf children be afforded appropriate health care professionals who are competent in otoscopy, tympanometry, audiometry, and treatment of otologic disorders to carry out this program. Most schools for the deaf do not have sufficient provisions for such care of the child.

Because the external canals of deaf children are frequently obstructed with cerumen, frequent examination and removal of the cerumen may be extremely beneficial, especially for those who wear a hearing aid (Riding et al., 1978b). This finding alone is reason enough for frequent periodic otologic examination; however, a schedule for screening for otitis media with effusion and high negative pressure should be established. Until a formal long-term study has been completed that will offer recommendations for a screening program in schools for the deaf, the following schedule of examinations of such children is proposed based on preliminary findings (Findlay et al., 1977; Riding et al., 1978b; Craig et al., 1979; Stool et al., 1980): all children should have an otoscopic, tympanometric, and audiometric examination on entering the school and periodically during the first school year (Table 21–15). Because infants and young children are at highest risk, they should be examined once a month by otoscopy (and tympanometry when indicated) during this first year. Older children and adolescents probably can be evaluated on entry and every 3 months during the first year, as the incidence of middle ear disease in

TABLE 21–15. Suggested Screening for Middle-Ear Disease in Programs and Schools for Deaf Children

	INFANTS AND YOUNG CHILDREN (ALSO MULTIPLY HANDICAPPED CHILDREN OF ALL AGES)		OLDER CHILDREN AND ADOLESCENTS		
First Year upon Entry					
Frequency of examination	Monthly*		Every 3 Months*		
Experience at the end of the first year	No disease or infrequent and of short duration	Frequently recurrent and/or chronic	No disease	Infrequent and of short duration	Frequently recurrent and/or chronic
Second Year					
And each succeeding year until experience changes	Every 2–3 months*	Monthly*	Yearly	Every 3 months*	Monthly*

*And with every upper respiratory tract infection and/or otologic signs and symptoms (e.g., otalgia, otorrhea).

this age group is less than in the younger age group. All students should be examined during periods of upper respiratory tract infection and whenever there are signs or symptoms related to the ear, such as otalgia or otorrhea. In addition, a child should be examined if the teacher or parent suspects a middle-ear problem owing to a noticeable lack of attention, sudden or gradual failure to benefit from amplification, or overt and progressive loss of hearing. After the first year of follow-up the children will usually separate into one of four groups, based on the occurrence of otitis media with effusion, high negative pressure, or both: (1) no disease; (2) infrequent disease and, when present, of short duration; (3) frequently recurrent disease; and (4) chronic disease. Infants and young children who fit into either of the first two categories based on examinations during the first year may be examined at less frequent intervals, such as every 2 to 3 months during the second year. Older children who have no evidence of disease during the first year probably can be examined once a year, either on entering in the fall or, more ideally, during the winter months. Older children with infrequent problems during the first year should probably be examined every 3 months during the second year. All infants and children who have frequently recurrent or chronic middle-ear disease during the first year must be examined every month and with each upper respiratory tract infection until they, too, have a year without significant problems. Screening during the succeeding years should be related to the middle-ear disease experience in the preceding year. Children who have multiple handicaps, in addition to deafness, are considered to be at high risk for middle-ear disease, which can significantly compound their handicap owing to the attendant conductive hearing loss. Therefore, screening for all such students during the first year should be the program recommended for infants and young children.

Ideally, every examination should be conducted by a physician who is expert in the diseases of the middle ear, but this is not always feasible. Therefore, a nurse should be trained to perform routine otoscopy, examination of the nose and throat, and removal of cerumen from the external canal when present. Tympanometry can be performed by the nurse, a technician, or, if available, an audiologist. Even though an otologist cannot examine every child with the frequency recommended, every school for the deaf must have a physician, preferably an otologist, assigned to the school for diagnosis and treatment of those children found to have middle-ear disease.

It is important that all children with severe or profound deafness be considered to be at risk for developing middle-ear disease. Therefore, they should have regular periodic examinations of the ear by competent health care professionals and appropriate early management instituted so that their educational handicap is not further compromised by a condition that is amenable to medical or surgical management.

Other Possible High-Risk Populations

Infants and children who have parents or siblings with otitis media with effusion appear to have a greater risk of developing otitis media with effusion than do those whose parents or siblings have no evidence of disease. Teele and associates (1980c) studied 2565 infants from birth to their third birthdays. They found that children who had single or recurrent episodes of otitis media were more likely to have parents or siblings with histories of significant middle-ear infections than were children who had no episodes of otitis media. Therefore, children whose siblings have had otitis media are at higher risk and should have more frequent otologic examinations than children whose siblings have not had the disease.

Upper respiratory tract allergy is thought to be involved in the etiology of otitis media and therefore requires close surveillance. Even though there is no proof that children who have an upper respiratory tract allergy have a higher incidence of otitis media than do children without such an allergy, they should be examined frequently for possible occurrence of otitis media.

Other possible risk factors, such as prematurity or some other reason for placing the infant in a neonatal intensive-care unit (Berman et al., 1978), first episode of otitis media during early infancy (Howie et al., 1975), malnutrition, and child abuse (Downs, 1980), are not proven but warrant consideration for close surveillance until these factors are disproved by further studies.

OVERVIEW OF MANAGEMENT

The different stages of otitis media and atelectasis are most frequently a continuum, and it is often difficult for the clinician to diagnose the precise stage of a patient's illness accurately. Before the detailed methods of management are presented, an initial overall management plan for each clinical type and the treatment options available (Table 21–16) will be described.

TABLE 21–16. Options for Managing Various Stages of Otitis Media

Antimicrobials
Decongestants
Antihistamines
Corticosteroids
Immunization
Hyposensitization (allergy control)
Inflation of eustachian tube and middle ear
Myringotomy with or without
   tympanostomy tube
Adenoidectomy with or without tonsillectomy
Tympanoplasty
Tympanomastoidectomy
Watchful waiting
Hearing aid

Acute Otitis Media

Figure 21–80 is a diagram of a recommended management plan for children with acute otitis media. Infants and children who have signs and symptoms of acute otitis media should receive antimicrobial therapy; however, several investigators have questioned the need for antimicrobial agents in all cases (Diamant and Diamant, 1974; Laxdal et al., 1970; Mygind et al., 1981; van Buchem et al., 1981). Because the rate of suppurative complications has decreased in the antibiotic era (Sorenson, 1977), antimicrobial therapy is still the treatment of choice (see p. 410).

Choice of Antimicrobial Agent

Amoxicillin or ampicillin is the currently preferred orally administered drug for initial empiric treatment of otitis media, as both are active both *in vitro* and *in vivo* against the two most common causative organisms, *Streptococcus pneumoniae* and *Haemophilus influenzae*. Other regimens that are satisfactory include amoxicillin-clavulanate, trimethoprim-sulfamethoxazole, cefaclor, cefuroxime axetil, cefixime, and combinations of a sulfonamide with benzathine penicillin G (administered by the intramuscular route as a single injection), oral penicillin G or V, or erythromycin. For the child who is allergic to penicillins, trimethoprim-sulfamethoxazole and erythromycin or clindamycin combined with a sulfonamide provide equivalent antimicrobial coverage. If the child has acute otitis media with otorrhea or tympanocentesis was initially performed, Gram stain, culture, and susceptibility studies of the causative organism will provide more precise data for selection of an antimicrobial agent (Table 21–17).

Dosage Schedules and Duration of Therapy

Dosage schedules have been determined on the basis of studies of clinical pharmacology and results of clinical trials. Physicians must rely on empirically derived schedules of therapy to plan drug regimens that lead to rapid and complete resolution of disease but minimal risk in terms of clinical or microbiologic failure or drug toxicity. The dosage schedules presented in Table 21–18 are appropriate for a 10-day course on the basis of currently available data. Methodologic problems, most importantly including ab-

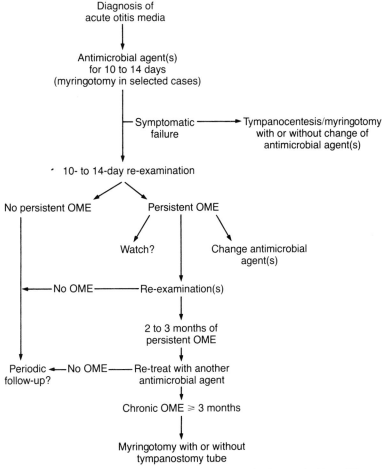

Figure 21–80. Recommended management plan for children with acute otitis media (see text). (From Bluestone, C. D., and Klein, J. O. 1988. Otitis Media in Infants and Children. Philadelphia, W. B. Saunders Co.)

TABLE 21–17. Efficacy of Selected Antimicrobial Agents for Common Pathogens in Acute Otitis Media

ANTIMICROBIAL AGENTS	S. PNEUMONIAE	H. INFLUENZAE Non–Beta-lactamase	H. INFLUENZAE Beta-lactamase	B. CATARRHALIS Non–Beta-lactamase	B. CATARRHALIS Beta-lactamase	S. PYOGENES
Ampicillin or amoxicillin	+	+	−	+	−	+
Amoxicillin-clavulanate	+	+	+	+	+	+
Penicillin V	+	−	−	+	−	+
Erythromycin	+	±	−	+	+	+
Sulfonamides	−	+	+	+	+	−
Erythromycin-sulfisoxazole	+	+	+	+	+	+
Trimethoprim-sulfamethoxazole	+	+	+	+	+	−
Cefaclor	+	+	+	+	±	+
Cefuroxime axetil	+	+	+	+	+	+
Cefixime	+	+	+	+	+	+

Based on available data from clinical trials and in vitro studies. +, Effective; −, not effective; ±, variable effectiveness.

sence of microbiologic diagnosis, limit the validity of the results.

Clinical Course

With appropriate antimicrobial therapy, most children with acute bacterial otitis media are significantly improved within 48 to 72 hours. The physician should be in contact with the patient to ascertain that improvement has occurred; children whose course has become worse after initial antimicrobial therapy has been given should be reexamined by the clinician, because a suppurative complication may have developed or a serious concurrent infection, such as meningitis, might be present. At this stage a tympanocentesis for micro-

biologic diagnosis and possibly myringotomy for drainage is an effective management option. Complications of otitis media are described in Chapters 22 and 23.

If there is persistence or recurrence of otalgia or fever, or both, then the child should also be reexamined before the completion of the antibiotic course. For children in whom severe signs and symptoms of acute infection are present, or for social considerations (e.g., poor home environment), it may be more advantageous to reexamine the child 48 to 72 hours after therapy is initiated. However, at this time the appearance of the tympanic membrane alone should not determine a change in the treatment. Almost all children will have a persistent middle-ear effusion, and even erythema and bulging of the tympanic membrane may still be present. If signs persist but the child shows no toxic symptoms and aspiration to culture the middle-ear effusion is not performed, the initial antimicrobial agent should be changed to a regimen to which beta-lactamase–producing *H. influenzae* or *B. catarrhalis* would be sensitive. If ampicillin or amoxicillin was initially given, then amoxicillin-clavulanate, cefaclor, cefuroxime axetil, cefixime, or a combination of erythromycin-sulfisoxazole or amoxicillin-clavulanate or trimethoprim-sulfamethoxazole should be administered. Trimethoprim-sulfamethoxazole is not effective when *S. pyogenes* is the causative organism and therefore should not be the drug of choice for initial treatment of otitis media. When *B. catarrhalis* is the causative organism, cefaclor would also not be the drug choice; cefixime is not indicated when *S. aureus* is the causative agent.

In patients with unusually severe earache or toxic symptoms, tympanocentesis and myringotomy may be performed initially to provide immediate relief. Tympanocentesis (and possibly myringotomy) should also be performed if the child develops acute otitis media while taking for another condition an antimicrobial agent that should have been effective against the common pathogens that cause otitis. When therapeutic drainage is required for the indications that will be outlined, a myringotomy knife should be used and the incision should be large enough to allow for adequate drainage of the middle ear.

Children may be reexamined at the end of the

TABLE 21–18. Daily Dosage Schedule for Antimicrobial Agents Useful in Otitis Media

AGENT	DOSAGE/24 HOURS
Penicillin G	50,000 U/kg in 4 doses*
Penicillin G (benzathine salt)†	600,000 U in 1 dose for ≤ 30-kg child
	1,200,000 U in 1 dose for > 30-kg child
Penicillin V	50 mg/kg in 4 doses
Amoxicillin	40 mg/kg in 3 doses
Ampicillin	50–100 mg/kg in 4 doses*
Amoxicillin-clavulanate	40 mg/kg in 3 doses
Bacampicillin	25–50 mg/kg in 2 doses
Cyclacillin	50–100 mg/kg in 3 doses
Oxacillin	50 mg/kg in 4 doses*
Cloxacillin	50 mg/kg in 4 doses*
Dicloxacillin	25 mg/kg in 4 doses*
Nafcillin	50 mg/kg in 4 doses*
Cephalexin	100 mg/kg in 4 doses*
Cefaclor	40 mg/kg in 3 doses
Cefuroxime axetil	125 mg 2 times per day below 2 years
	250 mg 2 times per day above 2 years
Cefixime	8 mg/kg in 1 dose
Erythromycin	40 mg/kg in 4 doses
Clindamycin	25 mg/kg in 4 doses
Sulfisoxazole	120 mg/kg in 4 doses
Trisulfapyrimidine	120 mg/kg in 4 doses
Trimethoprim-sulfamethoxazole (TMP-SMZ)	8 mg TMP and 40 mg SMZ in 2 doses

*Schedule at least 1 hour before or 2 hours after meals.
†Intramuscular route; all others are oral dosages.

course of antibiotic therapy, after 10 to 14 days. At this time, some children will have a persistent middle-ear effusion: Table 21–4 shows this proportion to be approximately half of those treated with antibiotics. Because persistence of middle-ear effusion after a 10-day trial of an antimicrobial agent is common, the presence of fluid in the middle ear is not sufficient grounds for continuing antibiotic therapy or performing surgery such as myringotomy and tympanostomy tube insertion. At 10 to 14 days, children who have continued minimal signs of persistent infection, either systemic (low-grade fever, failure to return to former level of activity) or otologic (continued inflammation of middle-ear mucosa) may benefit from an additional 10 days of antimicrobial therapy.

Although some children who fail clinically at the conclusion of a course of therapy do so because of a bacterial pathogen resistant to initial therapy (Schwartz et al., 1981b), many children have bacteria that are susceptible to the drug, and some have negative bacterial cultures and presumably have either a nonbacterial microorganism as the cause of otitis media or some other reason for the persistent fever.

Neonates and Immunocompromised Children

The method of management of acute otitis media may vary with the age of the patient. Acute otitis media during the first month of life may warrant more aggressive management than such a condition in an older child. Bland (1972) reported that otitis media in neonates was frequently caused by a more unusual organism than those that usually cause such problems in older infants and in children (i.e., gram-negative bacilli or S. aureus). Following this report, many authorities advocated treating these babies in the hospital according to protocols for neonatal sepsis, because the infection could be life threatening. However, other investigators (Schwartz et al., 1978; Shurin et al., 1976, 1978; Tetzlaff et al., 1977; Karma et al., 1987) have shown that the incidence of these unusual organisms is relatively low, especially in neonates who were apparently well when discharged from the hospital following birth and then developed an acute otitis media while at home. For these neonates, the acute otitis media should be treated as described above for older infants and children. However, if the neonate appears to be severely ill with toxic symptoms, hospitalization and a tympanocentesis and, possibly, myringotomy are indicated. If the baby is still hospitalized following delivery and develops otitis media, tympanocentesis and myringotomy provide microbiologic diagnosis. Culture of the middle-ear aspirate may reveal an unusual organism that would require treatment with an antimicrobial agent different from the antibiotics recommended for treatment of acute otitis media in older children.

The management of acute otitis media may be different in certain infants and children whose underlying condition is known to be caused by an unusual organism. Such children would be primarily those who are immunologically compromised. Tympanocentesis possibly followed by myringotomy would be indicated in an effort to identify the causative organisms and to promote drainage.

Adjunctive Therapies

Additional supportive therapy, including analgesics, antipyretics, and local heat, will usually be helpful. An oral decongestant, such as pseudoephedrine hydrochloride, may relieve nasal congestion, and antihistamines may help patients with known or suspected nasal allergy. However, the efficacy of antihistamines and decongestants in the treatment of acute otitis media has not been proved.

Complete clearing of the effusion may take 6 weeks or longer. Within 2 to 3 months the tympanic membrane should be entirely normal. If complete resolution has occurred and the episode represents the only known attack, the patient may be discharged. However, periodic follow-up is indicated for patients who have had recurrent episodes.

Persistent Middle-Ear Effusion

If the middle-ear fluid is persistent after the initial 10 to 14 days of antimicrobial therapy, one or more of the following treatment options have been advocated to hasten the resolution of the effusion during the next, subacute, phase:

1. Another 10- to 14-day course of the antimicrobial agent prescribed originally, because the ideal duration of therapy has yet to be established.
2. A course of an antimicrobial agent different from the initial one, based on the possibility that a resistant organism is present (Schwartz et al., 1981b).
3. A topical or systemic nasal decongestant or antihistamine, or a combination of these drugs.
4. Eustachian tube–middle ear inflation employing the method of Valsalva or Politzer.

Unfortunately, none of these commonly employed methods have been proved to be advantageous; they have not been shown to be effective in randomized, controlled trials of children with subacute otitis media with effusion, and the combination of systemic decongestant and antihistamine has been shown to be ineffective for this stage of otitis media (Cantekin et al., 1983). At present, the best treatment for children who have asymptomatic otitis media with effusion still present after 2 weeks is watchful waiting with reexamination of the ears 6 weeks later (i.e., 2 months after the initial visit). At this time, most patients should have a middle ear that is effusion free (see Table 21–4). However, another 10-day course of an antimicrobial agent such as amoxicillin might be helpful at this stage (Mandel et al., 1987; Corwin et al., 1986) or treatment with another antimicrobial that is effective against possible resistant bacteria is a reasonable alternative. If the child still has otitis media with effusion after

2 or 3 months, the effusion is chronic and should be treated as described below for management of otitis media with effusion (p. 413).

Recurrent Acute Otitis Media

It is not uncommon for an infant to have recurrent bouts of acute otitis media. Some children develop an acute episode with almost every respiratory tract infection, have more or less dramatic symptoms, respond well to therapy, and improve with advancing age. Others may have persistent middle-ear effusion and suffer recurrent episodes of acute otitis media superimposed on the chronic disorder. The child with recurrent acute otitis media that completely clears between episodes may be managed as outlined above. However, if the bouts are frequent and close together, prevention of further attacks is desirable, and the patient requires further evaluation. Several avenues of investigation are open: a search for respiratory allergy may prove fruitful; roentgenograms of the paranasal sinuses may reveal sinusitis; immunologic studies may be of value if other organs are involved (e.g., the lung). In addition, more thorough physical examination may reveal abnormalities, such as submucous cleft palate or a tumor of the nasopharynx, that require definitive management. If none of these conditions is present, then one or more of the popular methods of prevention may be attempted; however, the efficacy of these various modalities has yet to be proved in acceptable clinical trials. For infants and children who have frequent episodes (such as three or more episodes within the preceding 6 months) of acute otitis media without middle-ear effusion between the bouts, the most common nonsurgical and surgical methods currently employed for prevention are (1) chemoprophylaxis with one or more of the following—antibiotics, topical or systemic nasal decongestants, or antihistamines; (2) myringotomy with insertion of tympanostomy tubes; and (3) adenoidectomy with or without tonsillectomy. Pneumococcal vaccine is of limited efficacy in children less than 24 months of age and should be considered only for other children.

Chemoprophylaxis implies use of drugs in anticipation of infection, whereas treatment implies use of drugs after infection has taken place or signs of infectious disease are evident. Studies (Klein and Bluestone, 1982) suggest that chemoprophylaxis may be effective in children with recurrent episodes of acute otitis media, which is discussed in the section on the use of antimicrobial agents in this chapter (p. 442).

At present, there is no evidence that a topical or systemic nasal decongestant or antihistamine, either alone or in combination, administered daily or at the onset of an upper respiratory tract infection, prevents recurrent acute otitis media. Therefore, the use of such medications for prophylaxis is not recommended until their efficacy is proved.

Myringotomy as initial treatment for acute otitis media should only be considered in selected patients.

Myringotomy with insertion of tympanostomy tubes is commonly performed to prevent recurrent episodes of acute otitis media. The procedure is usually done after the signs and symptoms of the acute otitis media have resolved, but it may be performed during an acute episode if persistent otalgia or fever, or both, are present in a child who has had frequently recurrent episodes. A prospective randomized study by Gebhart (1981) was conducted in 95 children who had multiple episodes of acute otitis media. Comparison of infection rates was made between patients treated with conventional antibiotic therapy for each episode and patients who had tympanostomy tubes placed. Placement of tympanostomy tubes significantly decreased the number of episodes of acute purulent otitis media during a 6-month observation period. However, children with and without middle-ear effusions were admitted into the study.

Adenoidectomy with or without tonsillectomy is frequently advocated for the prevention of recurrent acute otitis media, but randomized, controlled studies reported in the past have not proved the efficacy of these procedures for prevention of recurrent acute otitis media (Bluestone, 1979). However, some children may be benefited by adenoidectomy (and possibly tonsillectomy), whereas others fail to show a reduction in the number of subsequent episodes following these procedures, and still others improve with advancing age without being subjected to these procedures. At present, adenoidectomy, or tonsillectomy, or both procedures, must remain of uncertain benefit for children who have recurrent acute otitis media, and recommendations for these procedures should be individualized. For example, children who frequently have recurrent pharyngotonsillitis or moderate to severe airway obstruction caused by tonsils or adenoids, would be more likely candidates than those who lack these conditions.

In summary, the parents of a child who has frequently recurrent episodes of acute otitis media in whom the effusion appears to clear between bouts should be offered the following management options: (1) antimicrobial treatment of each episode, (2) antimicrobial prophylaxis, (3) myringotomy and tympanostomy tube insertion, and (4) administration of pneumococcal vaccine if the patient is 2 years of age or older. The treatment option selected should involve the parents and possibly the child (if old enough) in the decision-making process. A few parents choose to watch and wait, usually if the episodes have been mild or relatively infrequent. At present, the decision should be between administering an antibiotic in a prophylactic dose or performing myringotomy and insertion of a tympanostomy tube. Because neither of these two procedures has been shown to be superior to the other, or even to watchful waiting, the decision should be based upon the parent's (and child's) willingness to have the child take daily medication as a preventive measure or to have surgery performed on the child's ear, which usually involves the administration of general anesthetic. The possibility of an adverse reaction occurring with either method should be discussed fully with the family. Usually a decision in favor of one of the treatment options is arrived at by this method, as some parents are unwilling to give a daily antibiotic or are concerned about the possible side effects of long-term antibiotic treatment, whereas other parents are concerned about the possible complications and sequelae of tympanostomy tube insertion or complications of a general anesthetic, or both. If the parents are undecided, then a trial of antimicrobial prophylaxis, such as amoxicillin or sulfisoxazole given in one dose before bedtime, can be offered with the option to perform a myringotomy and tympanostomy tube insertion if the chemoprophylaxis fails to prevent recurrent otitis media or if the signs or symptoms of eustachian tube dysfunction persist. Antimicrobial prophylaxis, if effective, is recommended during winter and spring, the seasons of highest risk, and then a period without prophylaxis can be tried to determine if indeed the child has improved.

For the rarely encountered child in whom tympanostomy tubes fail to prevent frequently recurrent acute otitis media (i.e., those who have otorrhea through the tube), the combination of antimicrobial prophylaxis and tympanostomy tubes is usually effective in preventing the recurrent episodes.

The above management options should be offered only to those children in whom chronic middle-ear effusion is not present between episodes (Fig. 21–81). If recurrent bouts of acute otitis media are superimposed on the chronic condition, the child should be treated as described below for management of chronic otitis media with effusion.

Otitis Media with Effusion

Infants and children who have otitis media with effusion ("secretory" otitis media) most likely have a condition that is an extension of an upper respiratory tract infection and that resolves spontaneously in most cases without active treatment. Treatment may be indicated in some children, as there are possible complications and sequelae associated with this condition. Because little information is currently available regarding the incidence of these complications and sequelae and the natural history of these effusions has not been studied formally, some thoughtful clinicians would take a watch-and-wait position and not actively treat such a child. However, hearing loss of some degree usually accompanies a middle-ear effusion. Although the significance of this hearing loss is still uncertain, such a loss may impair cognitive and language function and result in disturbances in psychosocial adjustment. With these uncertainties in mind, the clinician should decide whether or not to treat or to watch, and, if treatment is decided on, to choose one or more treatment options that appear to be most appropriate in eliminating the middle-ear effusion in the individual child. Many factors should be considered in this decision-making process. A child with a unilateral, asymptomatic otitis media with effusion of recent onset, in whom there is only a mild hearing loss and in whom there are no serious secondary changes in the tympanic membrane, may be a candidate for watchful waiting. Conversely, a child with bilateral chronic middle-ear effusions who has an associated marked hearing loss would be a more likely candidate for active treatment.

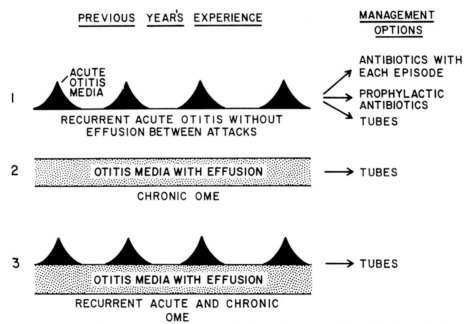

Figure 21–81. Three examples of children with recurrent acute or chronic otitis media, or both, related to available management options. (1) Patients with recurrent acute otitis media without middle-ear effusion between attacks can be treated with a prophylactic antimicrobial agent, tympanotomy tubes, or continuation of treatment of each episode. (2) Children with 3 months or more of chronic middle-ear effusion should be considered to be candidates for tympanostomy tubes. (3) When recurrent acute otitis media is superimposed on chronic otitis media with effusion, then tympanostomy tubes should be advised (see text). OME, Otitis media with effusion. (From Bluestone, C. D., and Klein, J. O. 1988. Otitis Media in Infants and Children. Philadelphia, W. B. Saunders Co.)

Important factors that should be considered in addition to hearing loss when the decision is made to treat or not to treat (and which treatment) would be one or more of the following: (1) occurrence in young infants, as they are unable to communicate about their symptoms and may have suppurative disease; (2) an associated acute purulent upper respiratory tract infection; (3) concurrent permanent conductive or sensorineural hearing loss; (4) vertigo; (5) alterations of the tympanic membrane, such as severe atelectasis, especially a deep retraction pocket in the posterosuperior quadrant or the pars flaccida, or both; (6) middle-ear changes, such as adhesive otitis or ossicular involvement; (7) effusion that persists for 3 months or longer; or (8) episodes that are frequently recurrent, resulting in an accumulation of an excessive duration of middle-ear effusion during a given period of time, such as 6 out of 12 months.

Before a nonsurgical or surgical method of management of chronic effusion is begun, a thorough search for an underlying origin (e.g., paranasal sinusitis, upper respiratory tract allergy, submucous cleft palate, or nasopharyngeal tumor) should be attempted.

Of the many methods of management that are available for otitis media with effusion, only a few have been shown to be effective in acceptable clinical trials. However, the clinician is forced to make a decision regarding all possible nonsurgical or surgical treatment options that are reasonable and most appropriate for the individual child. If treatment is chosen, the most rational approach initially should be a trial of one or more of the nonsurgical methods, and if the effusion is still persistent, then periodic observation or surgical intervention should be considered; the decision between these latter options should be based on the signs and symptoms present and should consider the potential complications and sequelae of both.

Probably the most popular method of management, a trial with an orally administered combination of a decongestant and antihistamine, has been shown to be ineffective in infants and children with acute, subacute, and chronic otitis media with effusion (Cantekin et al., 1983). The use of these agents for this disease in children is not recommended, but they may be effective in adolescents and adults or patients of all ages in whom there is evidence of upper respiratory tract allergy, because the study did not test the efficacy of this drug combination in these populations.

The efficacy of topical intranasal and systemic corticosteroid therapy has been tested, but convincing clinical trials showing benefit have not been reported; Maknin and Jones (1985) showed a lack of efficacy following treatment with systemically administered dexamethasone. In addition, some thoughtful clinicians consider that the risks of corticosteroid therapy for otitis media with effusion in children outweigh its possible benefits. Even though clinical trials have not tested the efficacy of immunotherapy and control of allergy in children with evidence of upper respiratory tract allergy, this method of management seems reasonable in children who have frequently recurrent or

chronic otitis media with effusion. Likewise, inflation of the eustachian tube–middle ear system by using the method of Politzer or employing the Valsalva maneuver has been advocated for over a century. Inflation that achieves a positive middle-ear pressure should enhance drainage of a thin (serous) middle-ear effusion down the eustachian tube and into the nasopharynx. Unfortunately, no randomized controlled trials have been reported to establish the efficacy of such procedures and, therefore, it is seldom recommended, especially in children with chronic otitis media with effusion.

Of all the medical treatments that have been advocated, a trial of an antimicrobial agent appears to be most appropriate in those children who have not received therapy recently. Because bacteria similar to those found in acute otitis media have been isolated from a significant proportion of middle-ear aspirates in children with chronic otitis media with effusion (Healy and Teele, 1977; Liu et al., 1976; Riding et al., 1978a; Senturia et al., 1958; Stanievich et al., 1981), the antibiotic chosen and duration of treatment should be the same as recommended for children who have acute otitis media. In a study recently reported by Mandel and associates (1987), amoxicillin (40 mg/kg/day in three divided doses) given for 14 days was twice as effective as placebo. Therefore, amoxicillin would be a reasonable agent, but if the effusion is chronic and unresponsive to amoxicillin therapy, a trial with an antimicrobial agent effective against ampicillin-resistant bacteria might be of benefit prior to consideration for surgery. Appropriate agents would be amoxicillin-clavulanate, erythromycin and sulfisoxazole, trimethoprim-sulfamethoxazole, cefaclor, cefuroxime axetil, or cefixime; however, clinical trials have not been reported that have shown these antimicrobials to be superior to amoxicillin for otitis media with effusion.

If nonsurgical methods of management fail, then surgical intervention should be considered. Myringotomy with aspiration of the middle-ear effusions would appear to be appropriate in those children in whom the procedure can be performed without the aid of a general anesthetic, because a second myringotomy with or without the insertion of a tympanostomy tube would be indicated if the effusion is present soon after the myringotomy incision heals (i.e., if the disease is persistent). It is desirable to avoid the risk of administering a second general anesthetic: if myringotomy is elected and general anesthesia is required, a tympanostomy tube should be inserted at the time of the initial myringotomy to preclude, if possible, the necessity of performing a second procedure under general anesthesia should a tube later be required (Mandel et al., 1984; Gates et al., 1987). This method of management appears at present to be the most reasonable. Following spontaneous extubation of the tympanostomy tube, reinsertion for recurrence of effusion would be indicated only after antimicrobial treatment has failed and the effusion has persisted for 3 months. Adenoidectomy with or without tonsillectomy either alone or in combination with myringotomy and with or without tympanostomy tube insertion may also be of benefit. Maw (1984), Paradise and coworkers (1987), and Gates and associates (1987) reported the efficacy of adenoidectomy in reducing the recurrence rate of otitis media with effusion. However, some children failed to improve following the procedure, whereas others improved without undergoing an adenoidectomy.

In some children myringotomy and placement of tympanostomy tubes must be repeated until the child grows older. For children who have had chronic otitis media with effusion that appears to be resistant to the methods of management described previously, mastoidectomy has been advocated (Proud and Duff, 1976), but this procedure is rarely indicated and should be reserved for those children in whom mastoid osteitis or a cholesteatoma is suspected, as almost all chronic effusions are at least temporarily eliminated after tympanostomy tube insertion.

Atelectasis of the Tympanic Membrane and High Negative Middle-Ear Pressure

Atelectasis of the tympanic membrane can be acute or chronic, localized or generalized, and mild or severe and may or may not be associated with abnormal negative pressure. Retraction of the tympanic membrane may be attributable to the presence of high negative pressure. However, a flaccid, atelectatic tympanic membrane may not be associated with high negative intratympanic pressure: the abnormal negative pressure may have been the original cause of such a condition of the membrane but may no longer be present. Localized atelectasis or a retraction pocket may be seen in the area of a healed perforation or at the site where a tympanostomy tube had been inserted ("atrophic scar" or dimeric membrane). A retraction pocket in the posterosuperior portion of the pars tensa or a pars flaccida retraction pocket is more frequently associated with the development of more serious sequelae (ossicular discontinuity or cholesteatoma) than is a retraction pocket in other areas of the tympanic membrane. These variations should be kept in mind when deciding how to manage atelectasis.

If a chronic middle-ear effusion is present concurrently with atelectasis, then the child should be treated as previously outlined for patients with otitis media with effusion. However, whether or not a middle-ear effusion is present, if a chronic severe retraction pocket of the posterosuperior area of the pars tensa or of the pars flaccida, or both, is present, myringotomy and insertion of a tympanostomy tube should be performed to prevent possible irreversible changes in the middle ear. After insertion of a tympanostomy tube, the tympanic membrane in the area of the retraction pocket should return to a more neutral position within several weeks or months, but if the retraction area remains adherent to the ossicles or middle ear, or both (Fig. 21–82), then adhesive otitis media is present, and tympanoplasty should be considered to prevent

further progression of the disease process (such as ossicular discontinuity or cholesteatoma formation, or both). Even though this method of management has not been tested in appropriately controlled clinical trials and the natural history of retraction pockets in these areas has not been studied adequately, this method of management would appear to be reasonable at present (Bluestone et al., 1977b).

For less severe cases in which the atelectasis of the tympanic membrane is apparently not associated with a middle-ear effusion and a retraction pocket is not present in the posterosuperior portion or pars flaccida, the management options become less obvious and more controversial. Generalized atelectasis, or even a localized area that is retracted for only a short time (acute retraction), is usually caused by transient high negative middle-ear pressure associated with an acute upper respiratory tract infection (and occasionally due to barotrauma). This condition is quite common in children and usually is self-limited. No specific treatment should be directed toward the middle ear unless the child complains of severe otalgia, hearing loss, tinnitus, or vertigo. The atelectasis (and high negative intratympanic pressure) and associated symptoms, if present, will usually subside when the acute upper respiratory tract infection disappears. Treatment at this time should be directed toward relief of the nasal symptoms. Topical or systemic nasal decongestants may provide relief of these symptoms and may also relieve congestion of the eustachian tube, although their effectiveness in this latter area has not yet been shown. If the symptoms become severe enough, myringotomy may be necessary to provide relief by returning middle-ear pressure to ambient levels. Inflation of the eustachian tube–middle ear system by employing the methods of Valsalva or Politzer has been advocated, but studies in animals indicate that these methods will not return the middle-ear pressure to normal for a sustained period when the eustachian tube is obstructed (Cantekin et al., 1980b). Controlled trials in children have not been reported to demonstrate the efficacy of these methods.

When the atelectasis is chronic and there is no evidence of a deep retraction pocket in the posterosuperior quadrant or pars flaccida, a thorough search should be made for an underlying origin, as described above for recurrent acute otitis media with effusion. If none is found, then the management options include only watchful waiting and active treatment. The decision for or against treatment should rest on the presence or absence of other, associated symptoms, and whether or not there is abnormal negative pressure within the middle ear. The presence of persistent or transient otalgia, hearing loss, vertigo, or tinnitus that is troublesome to the patient warrants active treatment. For chronic atelectasis in this case, a trial with a topical or systemic nasal decongestant with or without an antihistamine may be helpful; however, this type of treatment is often disappointing. Inflation of the eustachian tube and middle ear may provide temporary relief but usually must be repeated for permanent

Retraction Pocket–Atelectasis

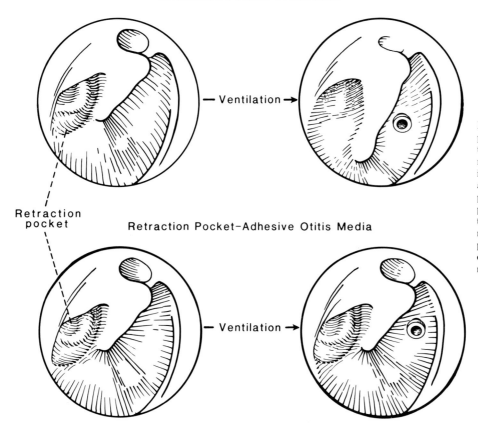

Retraction pocket

Retraction Pocket–Adhesive Otitis Media

Figure 21–82. When a retraction pocket is in the posterosuperior portion of the pars tensa of the tympanic membrane and adhesive otitis media is not present between the eardrum and ossicles, the insertion of a tympanostomy tube may return the tympanic membrane to the neutral position. However, if adhesive otitis media is present, the retraction pocket will persist in spite of the presence of a tympanostomy tube and middle-ear ventilation.

control of the symptoms and to maintain the tympanic membrane in a more normal position. For most children, myringotomy with insertion of a tympanostomy tube will usually be necessary to provide long-term relief. The procedure will prevent the sustained or transient high negative pressure due to eustachian tube obstruction that is responsible for the active retraction of the tympanic membrane. If the severely atelectatic tympanic membrane does not return to a more normal position after the insertion of the tympanostomy tube, or if the tube cannot be inserted owing to lack of a suitable aerated space within the middle ear, tympanoplasty should be considered.

When a flaccid tympanic membrane is passively collapsed on the ossicles and middle ear and high negative middle-ear pressure is not present, the nonsurgical and surgical management options described above may not be effective in restoring the tympanic membrane to a more normal position. Fortunately, symptoms of high negative middle-ear pressure and eustachian tube obstruction are frequently absent, so no treatment may be necessary. Even myringotomy and tympanostomy tube insertion may not be beneficial, as the tympanic membrane is no longer actively being retracted by high negative middle-ear pressure. In addition, at this stage, adhesive otitis media may also be present, and portions of the tympanic membrane may be adherent to the middle ear. The posterior or epitympanic (attic) portions of the middle ear

may become separated from the anterior portion by adhesions, and, subsequently, ventilation from the eustachian tube or a tympanostomy tube does not aerate the affected area. In such cases there are two management options: tympanoplasty or periodic (once or twice a year) observation.

Eustachian Tube Dysfunction

Otitis media with effusion and atelectasis with or without effusion are usually the result of dysfunction of the eustachian tube. However, abnormal function of the eustachian tube may cause otologic symptoms without an apparent effusion or severe atelectasis. The tympanic membrane may have a normal appearance, and mobility may be unimpaired when tested with a pneumatic otoscope or by tympanometry. Two types of eustachian tube dysfunction can be present: obstruction or abnormal patency. When the eustachian tube is obstructed but no effusion is present, the tube periodically opens to ventilate the middle-ear cavity but at less frequent intervals than normal; in this case high negative intratympanic pressure may be present for relatively long but transient periods. This type of intermittent middle-ear ventilation may cause periods of otalgia, a feeling of fullness or pressure, hearing loss, popping and snapping noises, tinnitus, and even vertigo. Management of this situation should be similar to that described for generalized atelectasis of the tympanic membrane. If the condition is present only during an acute upper respiratory tract infection, medical treatment should be directed toward relief of the nasal congestion. If the symptoms are of a chronic nature, a search for an underlying cause should be attempted, and, if found, appropriate management should be instituted. If no underlying cause is uncovered, then a trial with a decongestant or antihistamines, or both, may be helpful or eustachian tube–middle ear inflation may be tried, but if the nonsurgical methods are not successful, then myringotomy and insertion of a tympanostomy tube may be necessary.

At the other end of the spectrum of eustachian tube dysfunction is abnormal patency. In its extreme form, the hyperpatent eustachian tube is open even at rest (i.e., patulous). Lesser degrees of abnormal patency result in a semipatulous eustachian tube that is closed at rest but has low tubal resistance to airflow in comparison with the normal tube. A patulous eustachian tube may be caused by abnormal tube geometry or a decrease in extramural pressure, such as occurs as a result of weight loss or, possibly, mural or intraluminal changes. These last conditions may be seen when the extracellular fluid is altered by medical treatment of another unrelated condition. Interruption of the innervation of the tensor veli palatini muscle has also been shown to be a cause of a hyperpatent eustachian tube (Perlman, 1939).

Clinically, a patulous eustachian tube may be present in adolescents and adults but is less common in children. The patient frequently complains of hearing his or her own breathing in the ear or of autophony. Otoscopic examination reveals a tympanic membrane that moves medially on inspiration and laterally on expiration; the movement can be exaggerated with forced respiration. The condition is relieved when the patient is recumbent, as extramural pressure in the eustachian tube is increased by paratubal venous engorgement in this position. The patient should therefore be examined in the sitting position. The diagnosis can also be made by measuring the impedance of the middle ear (Bluestone, 1980). A tympanogram is obtained while the patient is breathing normally, and a second one is obtained while the patient holds his or her breath. Fluctuation in the tympanometric line should coincide with breathing. The fluctuation can be exaggerated by asking the patient to occlude one nostril and close the mouth during forced inspiration and expiration, or by performing the Toynbee or Valsalva maneuver.

Management of a patulous eustachian tube depends on first determining the cause of the problem. If the symptoms are of relatively short duration, the condition may subside without any active treatment. In children and teen-agers this condition is usually self-limited and probably related to changes in the structure and function of the eustachian tube and adjacent areas secondary to rapid growth and development. When a medication can be identified as the agent responsible, cessation of the medication usually alleviates the problem. However, in most instances the condition is idiopathic. When the symptoms are disturbing and the condition is chronic, active treatment is indicated. Myringotomy with insertion of a tympanostomy tube may be performed but usually does not alter the symptoms in most cases and occasionally results in increasing the patient's discomfort. Insufflation of powders into the eustachian tube and instillation of 2 per cent iodine or 5 per cent trichloroacetic acid solution have also been advocated (Mawson, 1974). Infusion of an absorbable gelatin sponge solution has also been suggested (Ogawa et al., 1976), as has injection of polytetrafluoroethylene (Teflon) into the paratubal area (Pulec, 1967), but all of these methods have major disadvantages. They are, for the most part, irreversible and may not improve the condition or may provide only temporary relief. Total obstruction of the eustachian tube can also be a complication. Stroud and associates (1974) have suggested the transposition of the tensor veli palatini through a palatal incision, but the procedure has not been shown to be safe and effective in a large number of patients by other investigators.

At present, the most logical choice for relief when the discomfort becomes severe is a procedure that would alleviate the symptoms simply, reversibly, and without untoward reactions. The technique described below has been found to fulfill these criteria and has been successful in relieving the symptoms of patulous eustachian tube (Bluestone and Cantekin, 1981). An anterior tympanotomy approach is used to insert an indwelling intravenous catheter with a flared tip (Medicut*) into the protympanic, or bony, portion of the eustachian tube (Fig. 21–83). The flared end of the catheter rests in the middle ear end of the eustachian tube. Prior to insertion, the lumen of the catheter is filled with methyl methacrylate to prevent the passage of air through the catheter; thus, the catheter occludes the eustachian tube. Following insertion of the catheter, a tympanostomy tube is inserted into the tympanic membrane to aerate the middle ear through the membrane. Even though spontaneous extrusion of the tympanostomy tube may occur, the middle ear may

*Argyle Medicut, Sherwood Medical Industries, St. Louis, MO 63013.

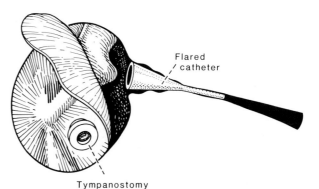

Flared catheter

Tympanostomy

Figure 21–83. Illustration of the placement of an indwelling catheter used to obstruct a patulous eustachian tube.

remain aerated with relief of symptoms and without development of high negative pressure, effusion, or both. The catheter most likely does not totally obstruct the eustachian tube, and adequate ventilation of the middle ear is provided around the catheter. Only a small number of patients have had the procedure, but the results have been gratifying. The indwelling eustachian tube catheter can be removed at any time, especially if and when the cause of this most perplexing otologic problem is uncovered and a nonsurgical or surgical method of management is shown to be more efficacious. In the meantime, this method to partially obstruct the eustachian tube appears to be effective in providing relief of symptoms of a patulous eustachian tube.

SPECIFIC MANAGEMENT OPTIONS

Antimicrobial Agents

An antimicrobial agent should be considered in any patient with a diagnosis of acute otitis media. Thus, use of antimicrobial agents for otitis media accounts for a large proportion of usage of these agents in infants and children. In 1986, 44.5 million antibiotics were prescribed for children under 10 years of age; 42 per cent of these prescriptions were for otitis media.

Decisions about optimal chemotherapy for otitis media are based on information about (1) the pathogens isolated from middle-ear fluids; (2) the *in vitro* activity of antimicrobial agents against these pathogens; (3) the clinical pharmacologic action of antimicrobial agents of value, including concentrations of drug achieved in middle-ear fluid; and (4) the results of clinical and microbiologic studies. These factors in choice of antimicrobial agents for treatment of children with otitis media with effusion are discussed below.

Microbiology of Otitis Media: Therapeutic Implications

The preferred antimicrobial agent for the patient with otitis media must be active against *S. pneumoniae*, *H. influenzae*, and *B. catarrhalis*, the three most important bacterial pathogens in all age groups. Group A streptococcus and *S. aureus* are less frequent causes of acute otitis media. Gram-negative enteric bacilli must be considered when otitis media occurs in the newborn infant, the immunocompromised host, and in those with suppurative complications or postoperative wound infections of the head and neck area. Anaerobic bacteria appear to have a limited role in chronic and a minimal role in acute otitis media. The bacterial pathogens are discussed above under microbiology of otitis media (p. 372).

STREPTOCOCCUS PNEUMONIAE

S. pneumoniae is markedly susceptible to penicillins, cephalosporins, erythromycin, clindamycin, and the

combination trimethoprim-sulfamethoxazole. Chloramphenicol and sulfonamides have moderate activity. Aminoglycosides are relatively ineffective.

Since the introduction of the penicillins more than 40 years ago, almost all strains of *S. pneumoniae* have been uniformly and markedly sensitive to penicillin G and other penicillins. However, moderate and high resistance to penicillin G and other antimicrobial agents has appeared and in some cases has been responsible for lack of clinical response and microbiologic failure. There are three facets to the problem: strains that are moderately resistant to penicillin G but susceptible to other antimicrobial agents, strains that are highly resistant to penicillin G and highly resistant to other antimicrobial agents, and strains that are sensitive to penicillin G but resistant to some other antimicrobial agents. The clinical and epidemiologic aspects of antibiotic-resistant pneumococci were reviewed by Ward (1981).

During the past 15 years, an increasing number of strains of *S. pneumoniae* have had decreased susceptibility to penicillins (Appelbaum, 1987). The susceptibility of most strains of *S. pneumoniae* is less than 0.05 μg/ml, whereas moderately resistant strains are 2 to 20 times less sensitive to penicillin G, requiring 0.1 to 1.0 μg/ml of penicillin G for inhibition (Table 21–19). Because usual dosage schedules of penicillin G or V achieve concentrations of 0.2 μg/ml to 4 μg/ml in middle-ear fluid, infection due to some moderately resistant strains may result in microbiologic and clinical failure (Howard et al., 1976; Kamme, 1970). Clinical and microbiologic failure in cases of pneumococcal meningitis due to moderately resistant strains treated with penicillin G has been reported (Mace et al., 1977; Paredes et al., 1976). Although the number of moderately resistant strains is now low (approximately 1 to 3 per cent of pneumococcal isolates tested in the authors' laboratory [Klein, 1987] and reported from laboratories in the United States and Western Europe), if the incidence of moderately resistant strains increases, physicians will have to reevaluate initial therapy or dosage schedules for treatment of otitis media.

Multiply-resistant strains of pneumococci were noted in 1977 by Appelbaum and colleagues. These strains were highly resistant to penicillin G, requiring more than 4 μg/ml for inhibition and were resistant to other drugs that serve as alternatives to penicillin G in pneumococcal disease, including other penicillins and cephalosporins, tetracyclines, chloramphenicol, erythromycin, clindamycin, sulfonamides, and rifampin. Some children with sepsis and meningitis due to a highly resistant pneumococcus died when treated with penicillin G alone. Since 1977, these strains have continued to appear in South Africa, mainly in Durban and Johannesburg, but have been reported rarely outside that country. Cases appearing elsewhere have usually been in immunosuppressed patients (Cates et al., 1978). The reason for the relative restriction of these strains to South Africa is unknown.

Strains of *S. pneumoniae* sensitive to penicillins but resistant to other antimicrobial agents are not uncom-

TABLE 21–19. In vitro Susceptibility of *Streptococcus pneumoniae* and *Haemophilus influenzae* Isolated from Middle-Ear Effusions of Children with Acute Otitis Media

| | MINIMAL INHIBITORY CONCENTRATION (MIC) (μg/ml), MEDIAN* | | | |
| | *S. pneumoniae* | | *H. influenzae* | |
ANTIMICROBIAL AGENT	Sensitive†	Resistant‡	Sensitive§	Resistant‖
Penicillin G	0.01	0.4	1.6	100
Penicillin V	0.01	0.4	12.5	100
Ampicillin	0.03	0.1	0.8	100
Nafcillin	0.01	0.8	25	50
Cephalexin	3.2	3.2	100	50
Cefaclor	0.4	1.6	12.5	25
Erythromycin	0.05	0.03	3.1	3.1
Clindamycin	0.05	0.05	3.1	6.3
Chloramphenicol	3.2	3.2	0.4	0.8
Tetracycline	0.2	25	0.4	0.4
Trimethoprim	1.6	3.2	0.8	1.6
Sulfamethoxazole	100	100	100	100
Timethoprim-sulfamethoxazole¶	0.3/6	0.3/6	0.2/3	0.2/3

*Inocula replicator method: 10^0 dilution for *S. pneumoniae;* 10^{-2} dilution for *H. influenzae.*
†Twenty-two strains with MIC for penicillin G, <0.1 μg/ml.
‡One strain with MIC for penicillin G, ≥ 0.1 μg/ml.
§Beta-lactamase–negative strains, including three Type b and 20 nontypable.
‖Beta-lactamase–positive strains, including three Type b and four nontypable.
¶Trimethoprim-sulfamethoxazole, 1 part trimethoprim/19 parts sulfamethoxazole.
From Teele, D. W., Norton, C. C., Mayer, J., Klein, J. O. 1976–1979. Unpublished data.

mon. Resistance has been noted in some strains to tetracycline, chloramphenicol, sulfonamides, erythromycin, and lincomycin. Susceptibility testing should be considered for strains of *S. pneumoniae* causing otitis media that do not respond to an appropriate course of a usually effective antimicrobial agent.

HAEMOPHILUS INFLUENZAE

Strains of *H. influenzae* responsible for otitis media may be subdivided on the basis of susceptibility to ampicillin. Ampicillin-sensitive strains are only slightly less susceptible to penicillin G than they are to ampicillin, but they are much less susceptible to penicillin V and the penicillinase-resistant penicillins. "Second-generation" cephalosporins—cefoxitin, cefamandole, cefuroxime, and cefaclor—and the "third-generation" cephalosporins—moxalactam, cefoperazone, cefotaxime, ceftizoxime, ceftriaxone, and cefixime—have significant activity against *H. influenzae* and are effective against ampicillin-sensitive and resistant strains. The third-generation cephalosporins are the most active antimicrobial agents *in vitro* against *H. influenzae* (Table 21–20). Chloramphenicol and tetracycline are effective against both ampicillin-sensitive and ampicillin-resistant strains, as are less active agents such as aminoglycosides, erythromycins, and clindamycin. Addition of a beta-lactamase inhibitor, clavulanic acid, to amoxicillin provides activity against *H. influenzae* without regard to production of the enzyme.

In recent years, ampicillin-resistant strains of both nontypable and Type b *H. influenzae* have been reported throughout the United States. The resistance appears to be a new phenomenon; few resistant strains were detected before 1972. Resistance to ampicillin is based on production of penicillinase, a beta-lactamase

that hydrolyzes the penicillin nucleus. Thus, all penicillins that are susceptible to beta-lactamase, including penicillin G, penicillin V, ampicillin, amoxicillin, carbenicillin, and ticarcillin, are likely to be ineffective against infections caused by these strains (see Table 21–19). In the United States, approximately 10 to 30 per cent of strains of nontypable (Schwartz, et al.,

TABLE 21–20. Cephalosporins, 1989

GENERIC NAME	TRADE NAME	ROUTE
First Generation		
Cephalothin	Keflin	IM, IV
Cefazolin	Ancef, Kefzol	IM, IV
Cephapirin	Cefadyl	IM, IV
Cephalexin	Keflex	PO
Cephradine	Velosef	PO, IM, IV
Cefadroxil	Ultracef, Duricef	PO
Second Generation		
Cefamandole	Mandol	IM, IV
Cefoxitin	Mefoxin	IM, IV
Cefaclor	Ceclor	PO
Cefuroxime	Zinacef	IM, IV
Cefuroxime axetil	Ceftin	PO
Ceforanide*	Precef	IM, IV
Cefonicid*	Monocid	IM, IV
Cefotetan*	Cefotan	IM, IV
Third Generation		
Moxalactam	Moxam	IM, IV
Cefoperazone*	Cefobid	IM, IV
Cefotaxime	Claforan	IM, IV
Ceftizoxime	Cefizox	IM, IV
Ceftriaxone	Rocephin	IM, IV
Ceftazidime	Fortaz, Tazidime	IM, IV
Cefixime	Suprax	PO

*Not approved for infants and/or children (8/89).

1982) and 5 to 20 per cent of Type b *H. influenzae* (Ward et al., 1978) isolated from children with disease are beta-lactamase–producing strains. Ampicillin-resistant strains of *H. influenzae* that do not produce beta-lactamase have been detected but are relatively uncommon. Children with suppurative life-threatening complications of otitis media (including sepsis or meningitis) in which *H. influenzae* may be the causative agent must receive a drug of uniform efficacy, such as chloramphenicol. Chloramphenicol-resistant strains of *H. influenzae* (most of which are susceptible to ampicillin) are uncommon, but meningitis due to such a strain has been reported (Kinmonth et al., 1978). Resistance is based on production of an acetyltransferase capable of inactivating chloramphenicol. Strains of *H. influenzae* resistant to both ampicillin and chloramphenicol are rare in the United States, but a high incidence has been noted in Barcelona (Campos et al., 1984).

Ampicillin or amoxicillin alone is still appropriate oral therapy for children with mild to moderately severe disease of the respiratory tract, including otitis media. But if the patient fails to respond favorably, the presence of a resistant strain must be considered and therapy changed to include a drug effective against beta-lactamase–producing *H. influenzae* (amoxicillin-clavulanate, a sulfonamide, trimethoprim-sulfamethoxazole, cefaclor, cefuroxime axetil, or cefixime).

Beta-lactamase–producing organisms (including *H. influenzae, S. aureus,* and *B. catarrhalis*) may inactivate drugs that would be effective for other susceptible organisms present at the same site. This effect is more likely to occur on a mucosal surface (the pharynx) than in a body fluid, but it is possible that such an effect would occur in a middle-ear fluid containing mixed cultures, including an ampicillin-resistant, beta-lactamase–producing strain *(H. influenzae)* and an ampicillin-sensitive strain *(S. pneumoniae)*, resulting in inactivation of the ampicillin and uninhibited growth of *S. pneumoniae* and *H. influenzae.*

BRANHAMELLA CATARRHALIS

Most, if not all, current strains of *B. catarrhalis* produce beta-lactamase and are not susceptible to penicillin G and ampicillin. These strains are resistant to ampicillin, amoxicillin, and other beta-lactamase–susceptible penicillins but are susceptible to the combination amoxicillin-clavulanate (ampicillin-sulbactam), various cephalosporins, erythromycin, chloramphenicol, and trimethoprim-sulfamethoxazole; about half of the beta-lactamase–producing strains are relatively resistant to cefaclor (Marchant et al., 1986). Methicillin and other penicillinase-resistant penicillins and clindamycin are ineffective. As is the case with *H. influenzae,* the isolation of beta-lactamase–producing strains of *B. catarrhalis* is a new phenomenon. In 1970, Kamme reported that all 108 strains of *B. catarrhalis* isolated in the Department of Clinical Bacteriology in Lund, Sweden, were highly susceptible to penicillin G and ampicillin. In 1980, Kamme

reported that 15 per cent of strains of *B. catarrhalis* isolated in the same laboratory produced beta-lactamase. His *in vitro* studies showed that trimethoprim-sulfamethoxazole and erythromycin were the preferred drugs for beta-lactamase–producing strains.

More recently, Marchant and coworkers (1984a) and Kovatch and associates (1984) from Cleveland and Pittsburgh, respectively, reported that over 20 per cent of isolates for acute middle-ear effusion had *B. catarrhalis,* and that three fourths of those isolates produced beta-lactamase. Several studies have shown that amoxicillin-clavulanate was effective against beta-lactamase–producing strains of *B. catarrhalis* (Bluestone, 1985; Odio et al., 1985; Kaleida et al., 1987).

GROUPS A AND B STREPTOCOCCI

There are no known strains of Group A and B streptococci that are resistant to the penicillins. These streptococci are markedly sensitive to the penicillins, cephalosporins, erythromycin, chloramphenicol, and clindamycin. They are relatively resistant to aminoglycosides and to sulfonamides. Trimethoprim-sulfamethoxazole in combination is more active than either component alone, but clinical efficacy is uncertain against Group A streptococci.

STAPHYLOCOCCUS AUREUS AND EPIDERMIDIS

Most strains of *S. aureus* that cause otitis media in hospitalized patients produce penicillinase and are resistant to penicillin G and ampicillin; the number of strains of resistant staphylococci in patients who have community-acquired disease is lower but significant. Thus, the penicillinase-resistant penicillins are the drugs of choice for initial management of the patient with suspected or documented staphylococcal otitis media. Most cephalosporins are also effective against penicillinase-producing strains; cefixime does not have effective activity against *S. aureus.* The efficacy of erythromycins, clindamycin, chloramphenicol, and the aminoglycosides is variable, and tests of susceptibility should be used to guide the choice for the patient who is suspected or known to have a staphylococcal infection and is allergic to penicillin. Amoxicillin-clavulanate would also be a choice if the organism produces beta-lactamase.

Disease due to methicillin-resistant staphylococci was reported shortly after the introduction of the drug. The strains are usually resistant to all penicillinase-resistant penicillins and to most cephalosporins. Bacterial resistance must be considered as a possible cause of therapeutic failure whenever a patient with staphylococcal disease who is on an adequate dosage schedule of a penicillinase-resistant penicillin does not respond favorably. Vancomycin is usually effective for these strains.

Most strains of *S. epidermidis* produce beta-lactamase that inactivates penicillin G, penicillin V, and ampicillin. *S. epidermidis* is also more resistant than *S. aureus* to the penicillinase-resistant penicillins, cephalosporins, erythromycin, and clindamycin. Vancomycin is usually effective against methicillin-resistant *S. epidermidis*.

GRAM-NEGATIVE ENTERIC BACILLI

The choice of antibiotics for infections due to gram-negative bacteria depends on the particular pattern of susceptibility in the hospital or community. These patterns vary in different hospitals or communities and from time to time within the same institution. In most areas, the most effective agents for *E. coli*, *Proteus* (indole-positive and -negative) species, *Klebsiella* and *Enterobacter* species, and *P. aeruginosa* are the aminoglycosides tobramycin, gentamicin, netilmicin, and amikacin. Some of the new cephalosporins (cefoxitin, moxalactam, cefoperazone, cefotaxime, ceftriaxone, and ceftazidime) have significant activity. Many gram-negative enteric bacilli are resistant to streptomycin, tetracycline, ampicillin, and the early cephalosporins such as cephalothin. Because the susceptibility of gram-negative enteric bacilli is variable and unpredictable, isolates should be tested to determine optimal choice of antimicrobial agents.

ANAEROBIC BACTERIA

Most anaerobic bacteria responsible for infection and disease in the upper respiratory tract, including anaerobic cocci, gram-positive nonsporulating anaerobic bacilli, and anaerobic gram-negative bacilli, are susceptible to penicillin G. Some strains of the gram-negative bacilli, such as *Bacteroides melaninogenicus*, are resistant to penicillin G. *Bacteroides fragilis* is an uncommon pathogen in the respiratory tract; most strains are resistant to penicillin G and susceptible only to clindamycin, chloramphenicol, or carbenicillin. Finegold (1981) has reviewed therapeutic implications for anaerobic infections in otolaryngology.

CHLAMYDIA TRACHOMATIS

C. trachomatis is susceptible to erythromycin, sulfonamides, tetracyclines, and chloramphenicol. Because this organism is likely to be associated with infection of the respiratory tract, including otitis media, in young infants, erythromycin or sulfisoxazole has been recommended for documented or suspected infection. Although controlled trials of efficacy of these drugs in young infants with respiratory tract infection have not been performed, results of uncontrolled studies suggest that either shortens the course of the illness. No data are available about efficacy of any antimicrobial drugs for otitis media due to *C. trachomatis*.

MYCOPLASMA PNEUMONIAE

Otitis media may accompany respiratory infection due to *M. pneumoniae*. The organisms are susceptible to erythromycin and tetracyclines. Controlled trials indicate that the duration of signs of lower respiratory tract infection such as cough, rales, and fever is less

in patients receiving one of these drugs, but there are no data about efficacy of the antibiotics for otitis media due to *M. pneumoniae*.

Clinical Pharmacology of Antimicrobial Agents of Value in Therapy of Otitis Media and Its Suppurative Complications

PENICILLINS (Table 21–21)

Penicillin G and Penicillin V

It is remarkable that in the more than 40 years that this drug has been in use, some organisms have remained exquisitely sensitive to penicillin G and no resistant strains have emerged. Thus, there are no penicillin G–resistant strains of Groups A or B streptococci. In contrast, the vast majority of strains of *S. aureus* and *S. epidermidis* are now resistant to penicillin G.

Oral preparations of buffered penicillin G and phenoxymethyl penicillin (penicillin V) are absorbed well from the gastrointestinal tract; the peak level of serum activity of penicillin V is approximately 40 per cent (4 to 8 µg/ml), and that of buffered penicillin G is approximately 20 per cent (1 to 4 µg/ml), of the level achieved by the same dose of aqueous penicillin G administered intramuscularly. Therefore, oral penicillins may be satisfactory for treatment of mild to mod-

TABLE 21–21. Penicillins, 1989

GENERIC NAME	TRADE NAME	ROUTE
Traditional		
Penicillin G	Many	PO
Aqueous	Many	IM, IV
Procaine	Many	IM
Benzathine	Bicillin, Permapen	IM
Penicillin V	Many	PO
Penicillinase Resistant		
Methicillin	Staphcillin, Celbenin	IM, IV
Oxacillin	Prostaphlin, Bactocill	PO, IM, IV
Nafcillin	Unipen, Nafcil	PO, IM, IV
Cloxacillin	Tegopen, Cloxapen	PO
Dicloxacillin	Dynapen, Pathocil, Veracillin	PO
Broad Spectrum		
Ampicillin	Many	PO, IM, IV
Amoxicillin	Many	PO
Amoxicillin-clavulanate	Augmentin	PO
Bacampicillin	Spectrobid	PO
Cyclacillin	Cyclapen	PO
Extended Spectrum		
Carbenicillin	Geopen, Pyopen	IM, IV
	Geocillin	PO
Ticarcillin	Ticar	IM, IV
Ticarcillin-clavulanate*	Timentin	IM, IV
Azlocillin	Azlin	IM, IV
Mezlocillin	Mezlin	IM, IV
Piperacillin*	Pipracil	IM, IV
Carbapenem		
Imipenem*	Primaxin	IM, IV

*Not available for infants and/or children under 12 years of age (8/89).

erately severe infections due to sensitive organisms. Penicillin V and penicillin G are of approximately equivalent efficacy *in vitro* against gram-positive cocci, but penicillin V is much less effective than penicillin G against *H. influenzae*. The efficacy of penicillin G against *H. influenzae in vitro* is only two times less than that of ampicillin (see Table 21–19).

Parenteral preparations include the salts potassium or sodium aqueous, and procaine and benzathine penicillin G, which modify absorption and thereby produce different patterns of peak and duration of antibacterial activity in serum and tissues. Aqueous penicillin G produces high peak levels of antibacterial activity in serum within 30 minutes after intramuscular administration but is rapidly excreted; thus, the concentration in serum is low within 2 to 4 hours after administration. If aqueous penicillin G is given by the intravenous route, the peak is higher and earlier, and the duration of antibacterial activity in serum is shorter (approximately 2 hours). Aqueous penicillin G, given intramuscularly or intravenously, is used for severe disease, including suspected sepsis and meningitis due to organisms known to be, or suspected to be, highly susceptible. In such cases the drug should be given at frequent intervals, usually every 4 hours, until the infection has been brought under control.

Procaine penicillin G given intramuscularly produces lower levels of serum antibacterial activity (approximately 10 to 30 per cent of the peak level achieved by the same dose of the aqueous form), but activity persists in serum for as long as 12 hours. Intramuscular administration of procaine penicillin G should be reserved for the patient with mild to moderate disease who cannot tolerate oral penicillins (those who are vomiting or have diarrhea or the comatose patient) or the patient who requires the reliability of parenteral administration, although the disease is not severe enough to warrant frequent intramuscular or intravenous doses of aqueous penicillin G.

Benzathine penicillin G given intramuscularly is a repository preparation providing low levels of serum activity (approximately 1 to 2 per cent of the peak level achieved by the same dose of the aqueous form). After administration of this drug, low concentrations of penicillin activity are measurable in serum for 14 days or more and in urine for several months. Significant pain at the site of injection is the major deterrent to widespread usage of this unique antibiotic. Combination of the benzathine and procaine salts (900,000 and 300,000 units, respectively) is less painful and comparable in efficacy to benzathine alone (1,200,000 units) for treatment of streptococcal pharyngitis (Bass et al., 1976). Benzathine penicillin G is appropriate only for highly sensitive organisms present in tissues that are well vascularized, so that the drug can diffuse readily to the site of infection. Thus, benzathine penicillin G is suitable for treatment of children with otitis media due to *S. pneumoniae* but not *H. influenzae*, and it should not be used for otitis media alone unless the pathogen is known and is susceptible. The place of intramuscular benzathine penicillin G in treatment

and prevention of infections in infants and children was reviewed (Klein, 1985).

Penicillinase-Resistant Penicillins

Methicillin was the first penicillinase-resistant penicillin to be introduced and is available in parenteral form only. Oxacillin and nafcillin are available in both parenteral and oral preparations and have greater *in vitro* activity against gram-positive cocci. Cloxacillin and dicloxacillin are available in oral forms only and are absorbed more efficiently from the gastrointestinal tract than are the other oral drugs. Differences among these five penicillins include degree of binding to proteins, degree of degradation by beta-lactamases, and *in vitro* level of susceptibility; however, all are effective for treatment of staphylococcal disease, and clinical studies have shown them to be comparable when used according to appropriate dosage schedules. In addition, all but methicillin have proved to be effective against infections due to *S. pneumoniae* and beta-hemolytic streptococci. The penicillinase-resistant penicillins can be used for initial therapy when the otitis is suspected to be due to *S. aureus*.

Broad-Spectrum Penicillins

Ampicillin and Amoxicillin. Ampicillin and amoxicillin are effective *in vitro* against a wide spectrum of bacteria, including gram-positive cocci (*S. pneumoniae*, beta-hemolytic streptococci, nonpenicillinase-producing strains of *S. aureus*, and oropharyngeal strains of anaerobic bacteria), gram-negative cocci, gram-negative coccobacilli (nonpenicillinase-producing strains of *H. influenzae*), and some gram-negative enteric bacilli (*E. coli* and *Proteus mirabilis*). The broad spectrum of activity of ampicillin and amoxicillin provides the basis for their use as a single agent for treatment of otitis media.

Both drugs are available for oral administration; ampicillin alone is available in a parenteral form. Amoxicillin provides levels of activity in serum that are higher and more prolonged than those achieved with equivalent doses of ampicillin; thus, amoxicillin can be given in lower doses and three times a day rather than four times, as required for ampicillin. An additional advantage of amoxicillin is that absorption is not altered when the antibiotic is administered with food, whereas absorption of ampicillin is decreased significantly when it is given with food.

Cyclacillin and Bacampicillin. These two preparations are chemically and pharmacologically similar to ampicillin. Cyclacillin is an oral penicillin with a spectrum of activity similar to that of ampicillin. *In vitro* activity of cyclacillin against gram-positive and gram-negative microorganisms, however, is 25 to 50 per cent below that of ampicillin. Cyclacillin is inactivated by the beta-lactamase of *H. influenzae* and *S. aureus*. Peak serum concentrations of cyclacillin are three to four times greater than equivalent doses of ampicillin. Patients who received cyclacillin had fewer side effects, including diarrhea and rash, than did patients who received ampicillin in a double-blind clinical trial involving 2581 patients (McLinn et al., 1982).

Bacampicillin is a semisynthetic ester of ampicillin. After absorption, bacampicillin is completely hydrolyzed to yield ampicillin. The antibacterial activity of bacampicillin is similar to that of ampicillin. The drug is rapidly and completely absorbed after oral administration and achieves peak serum levels that are more than twice as high as those of ampicillin and approximately 30 per cent greater than those of amoxicillin. Ingestion with food does not decrease or delay absorption. The peak serum level is achieved earlier than is the case with ampicillin, and the duration of activity is more prolonged. As a result of the more prolonged activity, dosage schedules require only two doses per day. The clinical usage and adverse effects are similar to those of ampicillin. Early clinical experience with bacampicillin was summarized by Craig and Kirby (1981).

Amoxicillin-Clavulanate. Amoxicillin in combination with clavulanate potassium (Augmentin) was introduced in 1984 for oral administration. Clavulanate potassium is the salt of clavulanic acid, a beta-lactam antibiotic with poor *in vitro* activity against pathogenic bacteria but potent activity as an inhibitor of beta-lactamase enzymes. The combination drug is equivalent to amoxicillin alone in activity against amoxicillin-susceptible organisms. The addition of clavulanic acid extends the *in vitro* activity of amoxicillin to include beta-lactamase–producing strains of *S. aureus* (but not methicillin-resistant strains), *H. influenzae*, *B. catarrhalis*, *Neisseria gonorrhoeae*, *E. coli*, *Proteus* species, and anaerobic bacteria, including *B. fragilis*. The pharmacokinetics of the two drugs are similar; both are rapidly absorbed and are not affected when taken with meals. Initial studies indicate that diarrhea, abdominal pain, and nausea are more frequent with the combination than with amoxicillin alone.

The combination of amoxicillin and clavulanate potassium may be considered if a beta-lactamase–producing organism is known or suspected to be the cause of otitis media. The combination may be of importance if the proportion of beta-lactamase–producing strains of *H. influenzae* increases or if these strains or those of *B. catarrhalis* (the majority of which are beta-lactamase producers), or both, are identified more frequently as pathogens in otitis media, sinusitis, and other respiratory tract infections.

Carbenicillin and Ticarcillin. These two agents are effective against gram-positive cocci; anaerobic bacteria, including *Bacteroides* species; and gram-negative enteric bacilli, including *Enterobacter* species, indole-positive *Proteus* species, and *P. aeruginosa*. High concentrations of these drugs are required to inhibit the gram-negative organisms, but this advantage is overcome in part by the low toxicity of the drugs, even when they are given in large intravenous doses. Combination of these penicillins with an aminoglycoside such as gentamicin or tobramycin produces synergistic activity against many gram-negative enteric bacilli. These combinations have been used effectively in

initial therapy of sepsis of unknown origin or sepsis suspected to be due to gram-negative enteric bacilli in patients with malignancy or immunosuppressive disease (Kirby, 1970). An oral form of carbenicillin produces low concentrations of drug in serum and should be restricted to therapy of infections of the urinary tract and not used for otitis media or its complications.

Ticarcillin is similar to carbenicillin, but it is more active against some strains of *P. aeruginosa* and less active against gram-positive cocci. Because of the increased activity, smaller dosages of ticarcillin than of carbenicillin may be used for treatment of disease due to gram-negative organisms (Fuchs et al., 1977). Ticarcillin in combination with potassium clavulanate was introduced in 1985. This combination drug extends the antibacterial activity of ticarcillin to include beta-lactamase–producing strains of *S. aureus*, *Klebsiella pneumoniae*, and *B. fragilis*. At present, the combination drug is not approved for children under 12 years of age.

Although ticarcillin and carbenicillin have no dose-related toxicity, both drugs are disodium salts; the large amounts in which they are given include significant quantities of sodium: 1 gm of carbenicillin contains 4.7 mEq, or 108 mg, of sodium per gram of drug; 1 gm of ticarcillin contains 5.2 mEq, or 120 mg, of sodium per gram of drug. The amount of sodium administered may be of concern in the treatment of certain patients with renal or cardiac disease.

For otitis media, the primary roles of carbenicillin, ticarcillin, or ticarcillin-clavulanate are in cases of chronic suppurative otitis media with perforation and discharge due to *P. aeruginosa* or *Proteus* species that are unresponsive to other forms of medical treatment, such as ototopical drops.

Piperacillin, Mezlocillin, and Azlocillin. These parenteral penicillins have a spectrum of activity similar to that of carbenicillin and ticarcillin but show greater activity *in vitro* against some gram-negative bacilli and anaerobic bacteria. Piperacillin and azlocillin are more active than carbenicillin, ticarcillin, or mezlocillin against *P. aeruginosa*. Piperacillin and mezlocillin are more active *in vitro* than carbenicillin or ticarcillin against susceptible strains of *E. coli* and *Klebsiella*, *Enterobacter*, and *Serratia* species. Each of these penicillins is inactivated by beta-lactamases. Combination with an aminoglycoside results in synergy against some gram-negative enteric bacilli.

Use of one of these penicillins (usually in combination with an aminoglycoside) in adults has included intraabdominal, gynecologic, and urinary tract infections and sepsis in patients with altered host defenses. The clinical experience with these drugs in infants and children is limited. The available data from children and adults indicate that each penicillin is effective against susceptible organisms, but the evidence is inadequate to demonstrate a significant advantage of any single drug (carbenicillin, ticarcillin, piperacillin, mezlocillin, or azlocillin). The last three drugs have half the sodium content per gram of carbenicillin or ticarcillin, a factor of some importance in patients who require large amounts of the penicillin and have cardiac or renal disease.

Bluestone and colleagues (Kenna et al., 1986) used azlocillin and other antipseudomonal agents for treatment of chronic suppurative otitis media due to *P. aeruginosa*. A significant proportion of children were cured and did not require surgery. The results of this study suggest that use of a broad-spectrum penicillin may be effective alone for children with chronic suppurative middle-ear infections.

Imipenem. Imipenem was introduced in 1985 as the first carbapenem antibiotic. Carbapenems have the same ring structure of the penicillins with the substitution of carbon for sulphur and presence of unsaturation in the five-member ring. The parent compound is thienamycin. Imipenem, the active thienamycin, is combined with cilastatin, which inhibits inactivation of imipenem. Imipenem has the broadest antimicrobial spectrum available among beta-lactam antibiotics, including gram-positive cocci, gram-negative cocci, gram-negative bacilli, and anaerobic bacteria. The uses include single-drug therapy for the immunocompromised patient with suspected sepsis, as an alternative to combination therapy for serious intraabdominal infections, and for serious, hospital-acquired infections. The drug is not approved for use in children less than 12 years old. The role of the drug in infections of the head and neck is unclear.

Toxicity and Sensitization

The penicillins are unique among antimicrobial agents in having low dose-related toxicity. Seizures may occur under circumstances that result in high concentrations of penicillin in nervous tissues: rapid intravenous infusion of single large doses, large dosage schedules for prolonged periods in patients with impaired renal function, high concentrations given by an intrathecal route, or direct application of penicillin to brain tissue (as might occur inadvertently during a neurosurgical procedure). Nephritis has followed administration of some penicillins, most frequently after use of methicillin. The mechanism of the nephrotoxicity is uncertain, but data suggest that the renal injury is probably an immunologic reaction and not a direct toxic effect (Barza, 1978). Thrombocytopenia with purpura due to drug-induced platelet aggregation has been noted after use of carbenicillin and penicillin G. These reports indicate a low incidence of toxicity, so low as to preclude any change in the choice of therapy for the patient with an infection due to susceptible bacteria. However, when patients with impaired renal function are receiving prolonged parenteral courses of penicillin therapy (more than 1 week), the concentration of drug in serum should be determined to make certain that serum levels of the drug are not excessive.

If toxicity is not a significant concern with the penicillins, sensitization is a most important factor. Four types of reactions may occur after administration of a penicillin (or any drug or antigen).

1. Immediate or anaphylactic reactions occur within 30 minutes after administration and are life-threatening events. Clinical signs include hypotension or shock, urticaria, laryngeal edema, and bronchospasm. Acute anaphylaxis is rare after administration of penicillin (approximately one case per 20,000 courses of treatment in adults), but a significant number of fatalities occur each year because of the extensive use of these drugs. Children are believed to have fewer systemic reactions than adults, presumably because of less previous exposure to penicillin antigens. Oral preparations are less likely to result in an immediate reaction than are parenteral forms, perhaps because antigens are altered in the gastrointestinal tract or because of slower absorption.

2. Accelerated reactions occur from 1 to 72 hours after administration. The signs are similar to those of the immediate reaction but occur in a less severe form.

3. Late allergic reactions usually occur after 3 days. The major sign is skin rash. This is the most perplexing reaction to penicillin because it is nonspecific, and the rash may also be due to other drugs given at the same time or may be a sign of the infectious disease. Skin rash is associated with approximately 4 per cent of courses of penicillins (up to 7 per cent in the case of ampicillin).

4. Immune-complex reactions include serum sickness, hemolytic anemia, and drug fever. Penicillin-induced hemolytic anemia is associated with high and sustained levels of penicillin in blood. Circulating red blood cells are coated with a penicillin hapten, the patient makes antibody to the penicillin antigen, the antibody binds to the altered red blood cell surface, and the cell undergoes lysis or sequestration (Petz and Fudenberg, 1966).

Identification of the patient who will have a significant reaction if penicillin is administered is still difficult. Serologic assays for detection of antibodies to penicillin have been considered; however, such assays lack specificity. Because the immediate reaction is largely mediated by IgE reagin or skin-sensitizing antibody, the patient who may subsequently respond with a life-threatening reaction could be identified by use of intradermal tests with appropriate antigens. Selection of the antigens to be used for skin testing, however, is an uncertain procedure because many different antigens play roles in the allergic reaction: at least 10 metabolic breakdown products of the penicillin nucleus have been identified, macromolecular impurities are present in solutions of the drug and high-molecular-weight penicillin polymers can be found in poorly buffered penicillin solutions standing for prolonged periods, side chains of the various penicillins may be responsible for reactions, and, finally, bacterial enzymes (amidases) used to prepare semisynthetic penicillins may cause an allergic reaction (Parker, 1972). Thus, investigators have had difficulty in choosing sensitive and specific antigens to use for skin-testing purposes.

The most promising studies of skin-test antigens have come from the laboratories of Levine (1966) and of Parker (1972). Levine identified two materials for use in skin testing, penicilloyl polylysine* and "a minor determinant mixture," a preparation of a dilute solution of aqueous crystalline penicillin G that includes metabolic breakdown products. In contrast, Parker used four skin-test antigens associated with penicillin and its products. A positive result is indicated by a wheal-and-flare reaction in 10 to 15 minutes and suggests a significant chance of reaction on subsequent administration of a penicillin; a negative result suggests that a significant allergic reaction will not take place. Although much effort has gone into clinical tests of these antigens, their prognostic value in children is still uncertain (Green et al., 1977; Levine et al., 1966).

At present, the physician must rely on the patient's history of an adverse reaction after administration of a penicillin to identify the patient who is likely to be allergic. If the reaction appears to be related to the administration of penicillin, the drug should be avoided for minor infections. If a life-threatening infection should occur and penicillin is clearly the drug of choice, as in the case of overwhelming disease due to *S. pneumoniae*, the physician may choose to administer the drug under carefully controlled conditions. A small dose may be injected initially in an extremity and may be followed by increasingly larger doses given every 30 minutes. Epinephrine, a tourniquet, and equipment for tracheotomy should be available in the event of a severe reaction during the testing period. All penicillins are cross-reactive in regard to sensitization, and allergy to any one implies sensitization to all.

ANTIMICROBIAL AGENTS USED AS ALTERNATIVES TO PENICILLIN

Cephalosporins (See Table 21–20)

The cephalosporins have a broad range of activity that includes gram-positive cocci, gram-negative enteric bacilli, and anaerobic bacteria. Most cephalosporins are relatively resistant to hydrolysis by beta-lactamases produced by *S. aureus*. At present, 20 cephalosporins are available in the United States, and many more are undergoing clinical trials. Some of the cephalosporins are of importance in therapy of otitis media and its complications. Many new products are introduced before clinical data on infants and children are available; physicians should read the package insert for current restrictions on usage in the pediatric age groups.

For simplicity, the cephalosporins have been categorized as first, second, and third generations (see Table 21–20), based on time of introduction and, to some extent, similar *in vitro* activity. Most of the parenteral drugs can be administered by the intravenous or intramuscular routes, although for some, intramuscular injection is painful and intravenous administration is preferred. The oral products are absorbed well from the gastrointetinal tract, and the presence of food does not alter absorption.

The cephalosporins, like the penicillins, are safe for children and have almost no dose-related toxicity. Physicians should be alert for the uncommon reactions, including kidney problems, alcohol intolerance, serum sickness–like reactions, and bleeding. Nephrotoxicity has been reported in adults who received cephalothin in combination with gentamicin (Barza, 1978). A response similar to that induced by disulfuram (Antabuse) occurred in patients taking alcoholic beverages following administration of cefamandole, moxalactam, and cefoperazone. Bleeding problems due to hypoprothrombinemia, thrombocytopenia, or platelet dysfunction have been associated with several cephalosporins but, in particular, moxalactam. If due to hypoprothrombinemia, bleeding was reversed by administration of vitamin K.

The cephalosporins may produce allergic reactions similar to those caused by the penicillins. There is cross-sensitization among the cephalosporins, and allergy to one implies (as is the case with the penicillins) allergy to all. Various degrees of immunologic cross-reaction of penicillins and cephalosporins have been demonstrated *in vitro* and in animal models (Petz, 1978). Patients with a history of penicillin allergy have shown increased reactivity to cephalosporins. However, some patients who are allergic to penicillin have increased incidence of hypersensitivity to unrelated drugs, and it is still uncertain whether or not the penicillin-allergic patient reacts to a cephalosporin because of cross-allergenicity. Most patients who are believed to be allergic to penicillin may be given cephalosporins without an adverse reaction. Although a cephalosporin may be used with caution as an alternative to penicillin in children who have an ambiguous history of skin rash, these cephalosporins should be avoided for the patient with a known immediate or accelerated reaction to a penicillin.

An unusual serum sickness–like reaction has been reported in children who received cefaclor (Murray et al., 1980). The children developed a generalized pruritic rash, similar to erythema multiforme; in some cases it was accompanied by purpura and arthritis with pain and swelling in knees and ankles. The signs appeared 5 to 19 days after the start of therapy with cefaclor and generally disappeared within 4 to 5 days after the drug was discontinued. The children had no prior history of allergy to a penicillin or a cephalosporin. Three hundred and eleven cases, including 289 children, were reported to the manufacturer by the winter of 1982 (Getty, 1982). Approximately 3 million courses had been administered, suggesting a minimal (considering the likelihood of underreporting) incidence of one reaction per 10,000 courses.

First-Generation Cephalosporins. The first-generation cephalosporins are effective against gram-positive cocci, including beta-lactamase–producing *S. aureus* and have variable activity against gram-negative enteric bacilli. Six first-generation cephalosporins are currently available for use in infants and children: the parenteral drugs cephalothin, cefazolin, and cephapirin; the oral products cephalexin and cefadroxil; and

---

*Pre-pen, Kremers-Urban Co., Milwaukee, Wis.

cephradine, which is available in both oral and parenteral forms. Cephalothin and cephapirin are painful on intramuscular injection, and the intravenous route is preferred. Cefazolin produces higher concentrations in blood than the other parenteral first-generation drugs. The three oral preparations have comparable *in vitro* activity (Moellering and Swartz, 1976).

These drugs are alternatives to penicillin for disease caused by *S. aureus*, *S. pyogenes*, *S. pneumoniae*, and susceptible gram-negative enteric bacilli that are resistant to other drugs. Activity against *H. influenzae* is limited. First-generation cephalosporins are not the drug of choice for any pediatric infection but are of value for children with disease due to susceptible organisms who are known or suspected to be allergic to penicillin. Because of the uncertain aspects of cross-reactivity, cephalosporins should not be used if the patient has had an immediate or accelerated reaction to penicillin.

Second-Generation Cephalosporins. The second-generation cephalosporins consist of six parenteral drugs—cefamandole, cefoxitin, cefuroxime, ceforanide, cefonicid, cefotetan—and one oral preparation, cefaclor. Ceforanide, cefotetan, and cefonicid are not approved for use in infants and children.

Cefoxitin has excellent activity against anaerobic organisms, particularly *B. fragilis*, and selective activity against gram-negative enteric bacilli. Cefoxitin has been effective for therapy of intraabdominal, gynecologic, and respiratory tract infections due to mixed bacterial pathogens, including anaerobic bacteria. Cefotetan was introduced in 1986 with an *in vitro* spectrum of activity and clinical usage similar to that of cefoxitin. Its safety and effectiveness have not been established in children.

Cefamandole is active against gram-positive cocci, including *S. aureus*, and was the first cephalosporin to be effective for infections due to *H. influenzae* (including beta-lactamase–producing strains). Reports of clinical and microbiologic failure in a small number of cases of meningitis due to *H. influenzae* (presumably due to inadequate concentrations of drug in cerebrospinal fluid) indicate limited use of cefamandole for disease in which sepsis is not a concern.

Cefuroxime has an *in vitro* spectrum of activity similar to that of cefamandole but has been effective in meningitis due to *H. influenzae*. Cefuroxime is of value in the treatment of diseases in which gram-positive cocci, particularly *S. aureus* as well as *H. influenzae*, are the likely pathogens, as in septic arthritis, orbital cellulitis, and severe pneumonias. Cefuroxime offers the advantage of single-drug therapy of these diseases, whereas, previously, a combination of a penicillinase-resistant penicillin plus chloramphenicol was required.

The oral form cefuroxime axetil has recently been made available and is effective against the common bacteria that cause acute otitis media, including beta-lactamase–producing strains of *H. influenzae*, *B. catarrhalis*, and *S. aureus*. However, at present, there is no liquid formulation available of cefuroxime axetil.

Ceforanide possesses an antibacterial spectrum that is similar to that of cefamandole and cefuroxime; however, its *in vitro* activity is less. Experience in children is limited, and safety and effectiveness have not been established for children under 1 year of age. The main use in adults is perioperative prophylaxis.

Cefaclor is the only oral cephalosporin with activity that includes gram-positive cocci and *H. influenzae*. Clinical trials suggest efficacy in therapy of otitis media, sinusitis, and mild to moderate cases of pneumonia. Cefaclor is a suitable alternative to amoxicillin for treatment of the child with diseases due to susceptible bacteria and suspected allergy to penicillin or when a beta-lactamase–producing strain of *H. influenzae* is known or suspected to be a cause of disease. However, serum sickness and Stevens-Johnson syndrome have been reported following repeated courses of cefaclor (Levine, 1985).

Cefonicid has a spectrum of activity similar to that of cefamandole. The serum half-life is approximately 5 hours, and efficacy has been demonstrated for a single daily dose schedule. The drug is not approved for infants and children.

Third-Generation Cephalosporins. Cefoperazone, cefotaxime, moxalactam, ceftriaxone, and ceftazidine are effective *in vitro* against gram-negative enteric bacilli and *H. influenzae* and have variable efficacy for gram-positive organisms. Cefoperazone has not been approved for use in children under 12 years of age. The *in vitro* activity of moxalactam and cefotaxime against *E. coli* and *S. pneumoniae* is greater than that from any other antibiotic now available. Moxalactam is not effective against Group B streptococcus or *S. aureus*, and neither moxalactam nor cefotaxime is effective against *Enterococcus* species or *Listeria monocytogenes*. Moxalactam was equivalent to ampicillin or chloramphenicol for treatment of meningitis in children due to *H. influenzae* (Kaplan et al., 1984) and equivalent (when each was used in combination with ampicillin) to amikacin for treatment of meningitis in neonates that was caused by gram-negative enteric bacilli (McCracken et al., 1984). Moxalactam alone was successful in curing cases of chronic suppurative otitis media and malignant external otitis due to *P. aeruginosa* (Haverkos et al., 1982).

Ceftriaxone is effective against gram-positive cocci, including *S. aureus*, *S. pyogenes*, *S. pneumoniae*, and *H. influenzae*, and selected gram-negative enteric bacilli. The most unusual quality of ceftriaxone is the long duration of effective concentrations of drug in blood and tissues. The half-life in children is between 4.5 and 6.5 hours. Although meningitis due to *S. pneumoniae* and *H. influenzae* has been cured with regimens of ceftriaxone administered once per day, the recommended dosage schedule for treatment of serious disease is administration every 12 hours. For diseases requiring prolonged therapy, ceftriaxone may be of value for use outside the hospital. After the acute signs of disease have diminished and the child remains in the hospital only for parenteral therapy, discharge and daily administration of ceftriaxone in the home or clinic may be considered (Higham et al., 1985).

Ceftizoxime has a spectrum of activity similar to that of cefotaxime and moxalactam. Clinical experience with the drug in children is limited. Although ceftizoxime has been approved for treatment of meningitis due to *H. influenzae* and *S. pneumoniae*, its role in pediatric infectious diseases is uncertain.

Ceftazidime was introduced for clinical use in the United States in 1985. The drug is highly resistant to inactivation by a broad spectrum of beta-lactamases and has excellent activity *in vitro* against *P. aeruginosa*, including strains resistant to antipseudomonal penicillins. On a weight basis, ceftazidime is the most effective of all antimicrobial agents against *P. aeruginosa*. Its use in middle-ear infections in children is likely to focus on chronic suppurative otitis media or other infections in which *P. aeruginosa* plays an important role.

Cefixime is the only third-generation cephalosporin available for oral administration. This recently approved drug is effective *in vitro* against the common organisms causing acute otitis media, with the notable exception of *S. aureus*, and has been found to be effective and safe for treatment of acute otitis media in infants and children (Kenna et al., 1987).

Use of the Cephalosporins in Infants and Children. Although many cephalosporins are available, there are relatively few infectious diseases in children for which one of these drugs offers a unique advantage over previously available antimicrobial agents. Some of the cephalosporins are appropriate alternatives when a previously available drug cannot be used (e.g., penicillin allergy), and some have potential advantages that have not been adequately studied in children. For treatment of otitis media and its complications, cephalosporins may be considered in the following circumstances:

1. Disease caused by *S. aureus*, *S. pyogenes*, and *S. pneumoniae* in children with known or suspected allergy to penicillin—oral or parenteral first-generation cephalosporin.
2. Otitis media, sinusitis, and mild lower respiratory tract infections—cefaclor, cefuroxime axetil, and cefixime.
3. Mixed infections, including anaerobic bacteria—cefoxitin.
4. Orbital cellulitis—cefuroxime or ceftriaxone.
5. Severe complications due to gram-negative enteric bacilli—cefotaxime or moxalactam.
6. Ambulatory therapy for patients requiring prolonged courses of therapy for disease—ceftriaxone.
7. Infections due to or suspected to be due to *P. aeruginosa*—ceftazidime.

Aztreonam

Aztreonam is the first monocyclic beta-lactam drug (monobactam). It has excellent activity against aerobic gram-negative bacilli including *H. influenzae*, *E. coli*, *K. pneumoniae*, and *Proteus* species. *Serratia* and *Enterobacter* species are somewhat less susceptible. Aztreonam in combination acts synergistically with aminoglycosides against *P. aeruginosa* and many gram-negative enteric bacilli. The drug is unaffected by gram-negative beta-lactamases. Activity against gram-positive organisms is limited. As a beta-lactam antibiotic, the drug is well tolerated, with no dose-related toxicity. Although clinical data in children are still limited (and it is not approved for usage in infants 3 months of age and younger), the drug alone or in combination with aminoglycosides may have a role in therapy of chronic suppurative otitis media.

Erythromycin

For otitis media, erythromycin is effective *in vitro* against the gram-positive cocci, *S. pneumoniae*, *S. pyogenes*, and penicillinase- and non–penicillinase-producing strains of *S. aureus* but possesses only moderate activity against *H. influenzae*. Erythromycin is effective for infection due to chlamydia, a cause of otitis in young infants, and for infection due to *M. pneumoniae*, a possible cause of otitis in school-age children, adolescents, and young adults who have other respiratory manifestations of disease due to this organism.

Several preparations are available for oral administration. Because the erythromycin base is unstable in the acidic environment of the stomach, better-absorbed products were prepared by adding a protective enteric coating or by altering the chemical structure through formation of salts and esters. The derivatives of erythromycin are absorbed more efficiently from the gastrointestinal tract than is the base form; these derivations include the ethylsuccinate or propionate (esters), the stearate (a salt), and the estolate (salt of an ester). The estolate provides the highest concentration of antimicrobial activity in serum, but there is still controversy about which of the preparations provides the most biologically active drug at the site of infection. Because the base is the active component, all the erythromycin preparations must be hydrolyzed to the base after absorption.

Two erythromycin preparations are available for intravenous administration, the glucoheptonate (gluceptate) and the lactobionate forms. Intramuscular administration of these forms is painful and should be avoided. Phlebitis frequently occurs during intravenous administration and may limit the duration of use of these drugs.

The erythromycins administered by mouth are well tolerated, and all but the estolate are nontoxic. The estolate may give rise to a cholestatic jaundice that is believed to be due to a hypersensitivity reaction. Because this syndrome has been observed less frequently with other forms of erythromycin, the ester is thought to be responsible for the hepatotoxicity. The jaundice has been reported to occur almost exclusively in adults who receive the estolate for more than 14 days and to resolve usually when administration of the drug is stopped. Few cases of jaundice in children have been reported. At present, potential hepatotoxicity is not considered a contraindication to the use of the estolate in children. Nevertheless, physicians prescribing this preparation should limit duration of therapy to 10 days and should be alert for signs of liver toxicity (Braun, 1969).

Erythromycin may be considered for treatment of otitis media due to *S. pneumoniae*, *S. pyogenes*, and *S. aureus* (mild to moderate disease) in patients who are known or suspected to be allergic to penicillins. Serious disease due to *S. aureus* should be treated with a combination of erythromycin and another effective agent such as chloramphenicol because of the rapid development of resistance to erythromycin when prolonged use is required. Erythromycin has variable activity against *H. influenzae* and thus should not be relied on as the single antibiotic in treatment of otitis media (see Table 21–19). *C. trachomatis* may be an important cause of otitis media in young infants (2 weeks to 6 months of age); this disease appears to respond to therapy with either sulfonamides or erythromycin.

A fixed combination of erythromycin ethylsuccinate and sulfisoxazole is now available. Each 5 ml contains 200 mg of erythromycin activity and the equivalent of 600 mg of the sulfonamide. The combination provides activity against the pneumococcus and ampicillin-sensitive and -resistant strains of *H. influenzae*. The combination drug is of value for children who are allergic to penicillin or who fail to respond initially when treated with ampicillin or amoxicillin and may have infection due to an ampicillin-resistant strain of *H. influenzae*.

Clindamycin and Lincomycin

These agents are effective *in vitro* against gram-positive cocci, including *S. pneumoniae*. Clindamycin is also active against a wide range of anaerobic bacteria, including penicillin-resistant *Bacteroides* species. Clindamycin provides higher levels of activity in serum than does lincomycin, and, in contrast to the case with lincomycin, oral absorption is not decreased when the drug is taken with food.

Diarrhea and pseudomembranous enterocolitis may occur after use of clindamycin. Antibiotic-associated colitis has been reported in as many as 10 per cent of patients after treatment with clindamycin. The epithelium of the colon undergoes necrosis, the mucous glands dilate and an inflammatory plaque forms and adheres loosely to the underlying epithelium. This disease has been associated with other antibiotics that alter intestinal flora, including ampicillin (Auritt et al., 1978), tetracycline, chloramphenicol, and lincomycin. Overgrowth of toxin-producing strains of *Clostridium difficile* is responsible for most cases of antibiotic-associated colitis. The antibiotic suppresses the normal flora in the colon, and the *C. difficile* organisms proliferate and produce an enterotoxin that is responsible for the disease. Most of these reactions have occurred in elderly patients, those with severe illness, or those receiving multiple antimicrobial agents (Gorbach and Bartlett, 1977). Clindamycin has been well tolerated by children. Diarrhea is a common side effect, but enterocolitis occurs rarely in this age group.

Clindamycin may be considered an alternative to penicillin for the patient who is believed to be allergic and has disease due to Group A beta-hemolytic streptococci, *S. pneumoniae*, or *S. aureus*. Clindamycin should also be considered when infection is due to anaerobic bacteria, particularly *Bacteroides* species. Because of its limited activity against *H. influenzae*, clindamycin can be used as initial therapy for otitis only when combined with an agent, such as a sulfonamide, that is active against this organism.

Sulfonamides and Trimethoprim-Sulfamethoxazole

The first sulfonamide (and the first drug of the modern antimicrobial era), Prontosil, was reported in 1935 by Domagk to be effective against infections due to beta-hemolytic streptococci. Sulfapyridine was introduced in 1938 and was the first antimicrobial agent effective against pneumococcal pneumonia. Soon after the introduction of these drugs, however, both streptococci and pneumococci developed resistance to the sulfonamides. Today, sulfonamides are used in the treatment of a wide variety of infections in children, including otitis media due to nontypable strains of *H. influenzae*, usually in combination with a penicillin or erythromycin to provide coverage for *S. pneumoniae*. Sulfisoxazole was used by Perrin and colleagues (1974) for prophylaxis in children with recurrent episodes of acute otitis media.

Trimethoprim-sulfamethoxazole is an antimicrobial combination with significant activity against a broad spectrum of gram-positive cocci and gram-negative enteric pathogens. Trimethoprim is more active than the sulfonamide, but the mixture is significantly more effective than either drug alone (see Table 21–19). The drugs act in synergy by blocking the sequence of steps by which folic acid is metabolized: the sulfonamide competes with and displaces para-aminobenzoic acid in the synthesis of dihydrofolate; trimethoprim binds dihydrofolate reductase, inhibiting conversion of dihydrofolate to tetrahydrofolate. The effect of sulfonamide in bacteria is circumvented in the mammal, which obtains folates from food sources. The reaction inhibited by trimethoprim is similar in bacteria and mammals but differs quantitatively in the extent of binding of the drug to the enzyme. Mammalian dihydrofolate reductase is 60,000 times less sensitive to trimethoprim than is the enzyme from *E. coli*.

Sulfamethoxazole was chosen as the sulfonamide to use in combination with trimethoprim because the drugs have similar patterns of absorption and excretion. Both are well absorbed from the gastrointestinal tract, and food does not affect absorption. A parenteral preparation is available. Rapid absorption and peak serum activity occur between 1 and 4 hours after oral administration; serum activity persists for more than 12 hours, but there is no significant accumulation after repeated doses given at 12-hour intervals.

Adverse reactions to the combination include rashes similar to those previously associated with sulfonamides (maculopapular or urticarial rashes, purpura, photosensitivity reactions, and erythema multiforme bullosum) and gastrointestinal symptoms, primarily nausea and vomiting. Hematologic indexes have been carefully evaluated because of the antifolate activity of trimethoprim. Leukopenia, thrombocytopenia, agranulocytosis, and aplastic anemia have been associated with administration of trimethoprim-sulfamethoxazole; the incidence of these adverse reactions is low, but deaths have resulted from this drug combination following administration for otitis media in children (Salter, 1982). Hemolysis may occur in patients with erythrocyte deficiency of glucose-6-phosphate dehydrogenase.

The combination of trimethoprim and sulfamethoxazole in children has been effective in the treatment of acute otitis media due to S. pneumoniae or H. influenzae (including beta-lactamase–producing strains). However, the drug is not effective when S. pyogenes or S. aureus is the causative organism of acute otitis media. It also is not recommended for pharyngitis due to S. pyogenes. The combination has been used with success for children who are allergic to penicillins or who fail after an initial course of ampicillin due to beta-lactamase–producing strains of H. influenzae (Schwartz and Schwartz, 1980; Teele et al., 1981b).

Vancomycin

Vancomycin is a parenterally administered antimicrobial agent with a spectrum of activity limited to gram-positive organisms. It is usually administered by the intravenous route because intramuscular injection causes pain and tissue necrosis. Ototoxicity and nephrotoxicity resulted from high concentrations in serum of early preparations, but improvements in the manufacturing process have resulted in a product that is believed to have lower toxicity. The principal uses in children are treatment of serious staphylococcal disease caused by strains resistant to the penicillinase-resistant penicillins and of sepsis caused by enterococci in the patient who has a significant history of allergy to penicillin. Vancomycin is one of the few drugs (rifampin, fusidic acid, and bacitracin are others) effective in vitro against the highly resistant strains of S. pneumoniae isolated recently in South Africa; it may become an important therapeutic agent if this strain becomes more widespread (Jacobs et al., 1978).

Tetracyclines

Tetracyclines are effective against a broad range of microorganisms, including gram-positive cocci and some gram-negative enteric bacilli. Tetracycline should not be considered to be a substitute for penicillin for patients with otitis media due to or suspected to be due to gram-positive cocci, because a significant proportion of Group A streptococci and some strains of S. pneumoniae are resistant.

Seven tetracycline compounds are available for oral administration in the United States: tetracycline, chlortetracycline, oxytetracycline, declomycin (demethyl-chlortetracycline), methacycline, doxycycline, and minocycline. Tetracycline, chlortetracycline, doxycycline, and minocycline are also available for intravenous administration. With few exceptions, there are only minor differences in the in vitro activity of the different preparations. However, minocycline may be effective against some strains of S. aureus, and doxycycline may inhibit strains of B. fragilis resistant to the other tetracyclines (Neu, 1978).

Tetracyclines are deposited in teeth during the early stages of calcification and cause dental staining. A relationship between the total dose and the degree of visible staining has been established. Tetracyclines cross the placenta, and discoloration of teeth has been seen in babies of mothers who received tetracycline or its analogues after the sixth month of pregnancy. The permanent teeth are stained if the drug is administered after 6 months and before 6 years of age. Other adverse effects include phototoxicity (particularly with declomycin), nephrotoxicity (with tetracycline hydrochloride, oxytetracycline, and declomycin), and vestibular toxicity (with minocycline).

There are few indications for administering a tetracycline to a young child; other effective drugs are available for almost all infections for which tetracycline might be considered. There is little reason to consider a tetracycline in the treatment of otitis media in children.

DRUGS EFFECTIVE AGAINST GRAM-NEGATIVE ENTERIC BACILLI

Aminoglycosides

Aminoglycosides are drugs of value because they provide broad coverage against gram-negative enteric bacilli and some gram-positive organisms (such as S. aureus), are rapidly bactericidal, and are readily absorbed after administration. The major concerns in their use are nephrotoxicity, ototoxicity, and poor diffusion across biologic membranes, including passage into cerebrospinal fluid. The aminoglycosides of current importance include streptomycin, kanamycin, gentamicin, tobramycin, netilmicin, and amikacin.

The in vitro activity of these antibiotics against gram-negative enteric bacilli varies and must be defined for each institution on the basis of current sensitivity tests. Streptomycin is not included in routine disc sensitivity tests nowadays because results for many years indicated that it is ineffective against a significant proportion of gram-negative enteric bacilli. The other aminoglycosides are active against most isolates of E. coli and Enterobacter, Klebsiella, and Proteus species. At present, gentamicin, tobramycin, netilmicin, and amikacin are the most active of the aminoglycosides against these organisms and against P. aeruginosa. The spectrums of activity of gentamicin, netilmicin, and tobramycin are similar, and strains resistant to one are usually resistant to the other. The major advantage of tobramycin is its activity against some strains of P. aeruginosa that are resistant to gentamicin. The spectrum of activity of amikacin is similar to that of gentamicin, netilmicin, and tobramycin, but there is little cross-resistance, and some gram-negative organisms resistant to these aminoglycosides are sensitive to amikacin.

The aminoglycosides have significant *in vitro* activity against *S. aureus* but are less effective for Groups A and B beta-hemolytic streptococci and *S. pneumoniae*. A combination of a penicillin and an aminoglycoside results in more rapid killing and lower concentration of drug required to inhibit selected strains of gram-negative enteric bacilli and enterococci.

After parenteral administration, the aminoglycosides distribute rapidly in extracellular body water, with slow accumulation in tissues. Peak levels occur in serum between 1 and 2 hours after administration, and significant activity persists for 6 to 8 hours. Penetration across biologic membranes is variable, and diffusion into cerebrospinal fluid is limited (the concentration in cerebrospinal fluid is approximately 10 per cent of the peak serum concentration).

All aminoglycosides may produce renal injury and ototoxicity. In general, gentamicin and tobramycin are more likely to affect vestibular function, and amikacin and kanamycin are more likely to damage the cochlear apparatus, but both functions may be affected by each drug. The cochlear effect may occur as a high-frequency hearing loss or tinnitus; vestibular disturbances include vertigo, nystagmus, and ataxia. Some of the effects may be reversible, but permanent damage is frequent. Nephrotoxicity may be noted as albuminuria, the presence of white and red blood cells and casts in the urine sediment, or elevation of blood urea nitrogen or serum creatinine levels. Toxicity appears to be dose related, although eighth nerve damage has followed the use of relatively small doses in patients with renal failure. Toxicity has not been a significant problem in children with normal kidney function who were treated with aminoglycosides according to currently recommended dosage schedules. Toxicity has usually been associated with administration of high doses for a long time, previous therapy with other aminoglycosides, administration of drugs to patients with impaired kidney function, or concurrent administration of other agents that are potentially nephrotoxic (e.g., the diuretics furosemide and ethacrynic acid).

Animal studies suggest that netilmicin has less ototoxicity and less nephrotoxicity than gentamicin. Comparable safety data in children are limited. The clinical role of netilmicin is probably similar to that of gentamicin, but its assets over those of previously available aminoglycosides are yet to be demonstrated.

Concentrations of aminoglycosides in serum are variable and unpredictable. Patients who receive a prolonged course of aminoglycosides or who have impaired renal function require careful monitoring to determine safety as well as efficacy of the aminoglycoside. Blood should be obtained to determine drug concentration at the expected peak (1 to 2 hours after parenteral administration) or trough (prior to the next dose, that is, 8 or 12 hours after last administration). Specimens of blood should be obtained early in the

course of therapy (within the first 3 days) to be certain that effective levels in serum are achieved and at subsequent intervals (every 3 to 4 days) to determine that the concentration of aminoglycoside in serum is below the level of toxicity (Evans et al., 1978). The desired peaks for the aminoglycosides are as follows: gentamicin and tobramycin, 5 to 10 µg/ml; kanamycin and amikacin, 15 to 25 µg/ml. The trough should not exceed 2 µg/ml for gentamicin and tobramycin and 10 µg/ml for kanamycin and amikacin. The toxic ranges are considered to be 14 µg/ml for gentamicin and tobramycin and 40 µg/ml for kanamycin and amikacin. Dosage schedules should be modified if concentrations in serum are either too low, and therefore inadequate for optimal therapy, or too high and potentially toxic.

The major use of aminoglycosides for otitis media in children is for serious disease that is due to, or suspected to be due to, gram-negative enteric bacilli; these include infections of the neonate and suppurative complications of acute otitis media in the child with malignancy or immunologic defect. Aminoglycosides may be of value alone or in combination with a broad-spectrum penicillin for chronic suppurative otitis media due to *P. aeruginosa*. The aminoglycosides may be administered by the intramuscular or intravenous (by slow drip over 1 to 2 hours) route. Oral preparations are not absorbed.

Published proceedings of symposia should be consulted for more specific information about the pharmacologic actions and clinical uses of gentamicin (Finland and Hewitt, 1971), tobramycin (Finland and Neu, 1976), and amikacin (Finland et al., 1976).

Chloramphenicol

Chloramphenicol is active against many gram-positive and gram-negative bacteria and chlamydiae. Oral preparations are well absorbed. The intravenous route is preferred for parenteral administration, because lower levels of serum activity follow intramuscular use. The drug diffuses well across biologic membranes, even in the absence of inflammatory reaction. Approximately 70 per cent of the concentration of chloramphenicol in serum is present in cerebrospinal fluid of patients with meningitis.

The major limiting factor in the use of chloramphenicol is its toxic effect on bone marrow. A dose-related anemia occurs in most patients receiving high dosages for more than a few days. The anemia is concurrent with therapy, ceases when the drug is discontinued, and is characterized by decreased reticulocyte count, increased concentration of serum iron, and cytoplasmic vacuolization of early erythroid and myeloid precursors in bone marrow (Scott et al., 1965).

Aplastic anemia is a rare (approximately one case per 20,000 to 40,000 courses of treatment) idiosyncratic reaction that is usually fatal. Most cases of aplastic anemia follow use of the oral preparation of chloramphenicol; few reports have been published of aplastic anemia that followed parenteral administration alone (Domart et al., 1961; Grilliat et al., 1966; Restrepo and Zambrano, 1968; Wallerstein et al., 1969). In some of these cases other drugs or the patient's disease could have been responsible for the aplastic anemia. Because few patients receive chloramphenicol by the parenteral route only, as compared with the extensive worldwide oral usage of chloramphenicol (particularly in many countries of Central and South America and Africa, where the oral drug is available without a prescription), and because the incidence of aplastic anemia is so low, one cannot be certain that aplastic anemia occurring almost exclusively after oral usage, rather than after parenteral administration, is a true event or one of statistical chance. Because cases of aplastic anemia following parenteral administration are extraordinarily rare, clinicians should not avoid use of intravenous chloramphenicol when it is indicated.

Because of the significant proportion of ampicillin-resistant strains of *H. influenzae*, chloramphenicol should be used in the initial treatment of severe and life-threatening complications of otitis media that are due to, or suspected to be due to, *H. influenzae* Type b (such as meningitis). The initial regimen should be reevaluated when results of cultures and susceptibility tests are available. Chloramphenicol may be an effective drug in the treatment of some cases of otitis media due to gram-negative enteric bacilli.

Wide variability occurs in concentrations of chloramphenicol in serum of infants and children. Peak serum concentrations should be 15 to 25 μg/ml to be safe and effective (Friedman et al., 1979).

Polymyxins

Polymyxin and colistin are highly effective *in vitro* against a broad spectrum of gram-negative enteric bacilli, including *P. aeruginosa*. These drugs do not diffuse well across biologic membranes, however, and are usually effective only when they are applied topically.

ANTIVIRAL AGENTS

Although three agents that have activity against respiratory viruses are available or under active investigation, no data are available about their efficacy in prevention or treatment of acute otitis media. Undoubtedly, this will change during the next few years.

Amantadine (Symmetrel), 1-adamantanamine hydrochloride, is active against influenza A and has been used extensively for prevention of illness. It has only modest therapeutic effect. The drug has little or no activity against influenza B, and higher concentrations than can be safely achieved in humans are required to inhibit rubella, parainfluenza, and respiratory syncytial viruses. Although the precise mode of action is unknown, antiviral activity appears to be due to interference with virus uncoating, rather than direct inactivation of infectious virus.

Ribavirin is a synthetic nucleoside that inhibits a wide variety of DNA and RNA viruses. Infants with bronchiolitis or pneumonia due to RSV substantially improved with aerosolized ribavirin (Hall et al., 1983). The drug (Virazole) was introduced in the United States in 1986. Ribavirin is rapidly transported into cells, where it is converted by cellular enzymes to monophosphate, diphosphate, and triphosphate derivates that then inhibit viral or virally induced enzymes involved in viral nucleic acid synthesis.

Interferons are proteins that are released by cells in response to infection or other stimuli and induce a temporary antiviral state in uninfected cells. Until recently, only limited supplies of interferon were available; the drug was prepared by exposure of peripheral blood lymphocytes to a paramyxovirus. The interferon genes have been cloned into bacterial and yeast plasmids, and large quantities of interferon will be available now for investigational purposes. Alpha$_2$-interferon has been administered as an intranasal spray against infection due to rhinoviruses and coronaviruses, causes of the common cold. Recently published studies identify the efficacy of alpha-interferon admin-

TABLE 21–22. Concentrations of Antimicrobial Agents in Serum and Middle-Ear Fluids of Children with Acute Otitis Media

AGENT	DOSAGE (mg/kg)	CONCENTRATION (μg/ml)*			REFERENCE
		S	MEF	MEF/S	
Penicillin V	13 PO	8.1	1.8	0.22	Kamme et al., 1969
	26 PO	15.5	6.3	0.41	
Ampicillin	10 PO	4.3	1.2	0.28	Lahikainen et al., 1977
Amoxicillin	10 PO	4.8	2.2	0.46	Howard et al., 1976
Bacampicillin	800 IM†	7.7	2.4	0.31	Virtanen and Lahikainen, 1979
Cefaclor	10 PO	7.0	1.3	0.19	Ginsburg et al., 1981
Cefotaxime	25 IM/IV	5.8	2.1	0.36	Danon, 1980
Erythromycin					Ginsburg et al., 1981
Estolate	15 PO	3.6	1.7	0.49	
Ethylsuccinate	15 PO	1.2	0.5	0.42	
Sulfonamide (trisulfapyrimidine)	30 PO	13.4	8.3	0.62	Howard et al., 1976

*Concentration achieved 0.5 to 2.5 hours after administration.
†Single dose administered to adults.
S, Serum; MEF, middle-ear fluids.

TABLE 21–23. Concentrations of Antibiotics in Serum and Middle-Ear Fluids of Children with Chronic Serous Otitis Media

ANTIBIOTIC (DOSE)*	SAMPLE	CONCENTRATION (μg/ml) Sample Time (minutes)					
		0–30	30–60	60–90	90–120	120–180	180–240
Amoxicillin (15 mg/kg)	S	6.8	6.5	13.6	9.4	5.8	3.1
	MEF	0.17	2.2	2.0	2.3	5.6	2.7
	MEF/S	0.03	0.34	0.15	0.24	0.97	0.87
Cefaclor (15 mg/kg)	S	12.8	16.8	11.2	6.9	—	—
	MEF	3.8	2.8	2.3	1.3	—	—
	MEF/S	0.30	0.17	0.21	0.19	—	—

*Specimens obtained after single dose.
S, Serum; MEF, middle-ear fluids.
With permission from Krause, P. J., et al. 1982. Penetration of amoxicillin, cefaclor, erythromycin-sulfisoxazole, and trimethoprim-sulfamethoxazole into the middle ear fluid of patients with serous otitis media. J. Infect. Dis. 145:815–821.

istered as a nasal spray for short-term prophylaxis against the common cold in the household. Almost all the effect was against rhinovirus infections, with no preventive benefit for colds due to other agents (Douglas et al., 1986; Hayden et al., 1986).

Diffusion of Antimicrobial Agents into Middle-Ear Fluids

Although studies of concentrations of various drugs in serum and middle-ear fluid cited in Tables 21–22 through 21–24 differ in dosage schedules, time of collection, and methods of assay, the results indicate that most antimicrobial agents of value for treatment of acute otitis media achieve significant concentrations in middle-ear fluid. Because the middle ear is embryologically, morphologically, and physiologically part of the respiratory tract, penetration of systemically administered antibiotics into middle-ear mucosa and middle-ear fluid provides a model for dynamics of diffusion of antibiotics in other areas of the respiratory tract.

Data about diffusion of the listed antimicrobial agent into middle-ear fluid of patients with acute or chronic middle-ear infection are available: penicillin G (Lahikainen, 1970; Silverstein et al., 1966); penicillin V (Howard et al., 1976; Kamme et al., 1969; Lundgren et al., 1979; Nelson et al., 1981); ampicillin (Coffey,

1968; Klimek et al., 1977; Lahikainen et al., 1977); amoxicillin (Klimek et al., 1977; Nelson et al., 1981); erythromycin estolate, ethyl succinate (Bass et al., 1971; Ginsburg et al., 1981; Nelson et al., 1981; Sundberg et al., 1979); trimethoprim-sulfamethoxazole (Klimek et al., 1980; Kohonen et al., 1983; Nelson et al., 1981); cefaclor (Ginsburg et al., 1981; Lildholdt et al., 1981; Nelson et al., 1981); bacampicillin (Virtanen and Lahikainen, 1979); cefotaxime (Danon, 1980); oxytetracycline (Silverstein et al., 1966); and metronidazole (Jokipii et al., 1978). These studies of penetration of systemically administered antibiotics have significant flaws in design:

1. Most include specimens obtained after a single dose, whereas Sundberg and coworkers (1979) showed that concentrations of erythromycin increased in middle-ear fluids when specimens were obtained after multiple doses.

2. Standard curves of antibiotic concentrations are prepared in buffered solutions, which may not represent an adequate control for middle-ear fluid.

3. Results of assays of materials obtained at various intervals after administration of drug give different concentrations in middle-ear fluids and different ratios of middle-ear fluid to simultaneously obtained serum concentrations. Peak values occur at different times for different drugs. Therefore, values taken at one

TABLE 21–24. Concentrations of Orally Administered Antimicrobial Agents in Serum and Middle-Ear Fluids of Children with Chronic Otitis Media with Effusion

AGENT	DOSAGE	CONCENTRATION (μg/ml)*			REFERENCE
		S	MEF	MEF/S	
Penicillin V	10 mg/kg	—	0.2	—	Nelson et al., 1981
Ampicillin	1 gm	22.4	1.5	0.07	Klimek et al., 1977
Amoxicillin	1 gm	15.3	6.2	0.41	Klimek et al., 1977
Trimethoprim	4 mg/kg	1.9	1.4	0.76	
Sulfamethoxazole	20 mg/kg	40.4	8.2	0.20	
Cefaclor	15 mg/kg	8.0	0.5	0.06	Lildholdt et al., 1981
Erythromycin	10 mg/kg				Nelson et al., 1981
Estolate		—	2.0	—	
Ethylsuccinate		—	0.3	—	

*Concentration achieved 0.5 to 2.5 hours after administration.
†Administered as the combination but assayed separately.
S, Serum; MEF, middle-ear fluid.

sample time may not provide adequate indication of penetration into middle-ear fluid.

4. Homogenization of mucoid or purulent middle-ear fluid is difficult.

5. Specimens containing blood are not always excluded.

6. The condition of the mucosa is not accurately portrayed. Differences in penetration may vary, depending on the degree of inflammation of the mucosa, and this may not be identified or known by the investigator.

In spite of these significant limitations, data from assays of concentrations of drug in middle-ear fluid provide useful information, which along with *in vitro* susceptibility data guide the choice of antimicrobial agents for otitis media.

Significant concentrations of each of the drugs tested appeared promptly in middle-ear fluid. The concentrations of drug in the middle-ear fluid were, in general, parallel though lower than those in serum. The peak activity in middle-ear fluid was delayed when compared with peak activity achieved in serum, but duration of activity was similar in both serum and middle-ear fluid. Concentrations of penicillin V and ampicillin in middle-ear fluid of patients with chronic otitis media were lower than concentrations in fluid of patients with acute disease, but concentrations of amoxicillin, erythromycins, and cefaclor were similar in acute and chronic effusions.

In children with chronic otitis media, concentrations of drug in purulent fluids were higher than those in mucoid or serous fluids, and concentrations were similar to those found in purulent fluids of children with acute otitis media (Nelson et al., 1981).

Penicillin V, ampicillin, bacampicillin, and cefaclor achieved concentrations in middle-ear fluid that were approximately one fifth to one third of the levels in serum. Approximately 50 per cent of serum concentrations were achieved in middle-ear fluid after administration of amoxicillin, erythromycins, and sulfonamides. Thus, usual dosage schedules of ampicillin, amoxicillin, bacampicillin, cefaclor, and trimethoprim-sulfamethoxazole produced concentrations of antimicrobial activity in middle-ear fluid that were sufficient to inhibit *S. pneumoniae* and most strains of *H. influenzae* (excluding beta-lactamase–producing strains in the case of ampicillin, amoxicillin, and bacampicillin). The concentrations achieved in middle-ear fluid after administration of penicillin V and erythromycins were sufficient to inhibit *S. pneumoniae* but were not adequate to inhibit most strains of *H. influenzae*.

Selected Aspects of Administration of Antimicrobial Agents

DOSAGE SCHEDULES FOR INFANTS AND CHILDREN

Dosage schedules of antimicrobial agents useful in otitis media for infants (beyond the newborn period) and children are listed in Table 21–18. Oral regimens are used for otitis media due to susceptible organisms

in the absence of suppurative complications. Parenteral administration should be considered for severe infections due to less susceptible organisms and when sepsis or suppurative complications are present or imminent (Table 21–25).

DOSAGE SCHEDULES FOR NEWBORN INFANTS

The clinical pharmacologic action of antimicrobial agents administered to the newborn infant is unique and cannot be extrapolated from the results of studies done in older children or adults. Physiologic and metabolic processes that affect the distribution, metabolism, and excretion of drugs undergo rapid changes during the first few weeks of life. The increased efficiency of kidney function after the first 7 days of life requires a decrease in the interval between doses of penicillins and aminoglycosides to maintain high concentrations of drug in blood and tissues. Thus, different dosage schedules are provided for the first week of life and for subsequent weeks of the neonatal period (Table 21–26). McCracken and Nelson (1983) provided detailed information about the clinical phar-

TABLE 21–25. Daily Dosage Schedules for Parenteral Antimicrobial Agents of Value in Infants (Other than Neonates) and Children with Sepsis or Suppurative Complications of Otitis Media

DRUG	ROUTE	DOSAGE/kg/24 HOURS*
Penicillin G	IV, IM	100,000–400,000 U in 4–6 doses
Methicillin	IV, IM	200 mg in 4–6 doses
Oxacillin	IV, IM	200 mg in 4–6 doses
Nafcillin	IV, IM	200 mg in 4–6 doses
Ampicillin	IV, IM	200–300 mg in 4–6 doses
Carbenicillin	IV, IM	400–600 mg in 4–6 doses
Ticarcillin	IV, IM	200–300 mg in 4–6 doses
Mezlocillin	IV	200–300 mg in 4–6 doses
Azlocillin	IV	200–300 mg in 4–6 doses
Cephalothin	IV, IM	100–150 mg in 4–6 doses
Cefazolin	IV, IM	50–150 mg in 4 doses†
Cefoxitin	IV, IM	80–160 mg in 3 doses
Ceftizoxime	IV, IM	150–200 mg in 3–4 doses
Cefuroxime	IV, IM	175–240 mg in 4–6 doses
Moxalactam	IV	150–200 mg in 3–4 doses
Cefotaxime	IV, IM	150–200 mg in 4 doses
Ceftriaxone	IV, IM	50–75 mg in 2 doses
Ceftazidime	IV	125–150 mg in 3 doses
Erythromycin	IV	50 mg in 4 doses†
Clindamycin	IM, IV	40 mg in 3–4 doses
Vancomycin	IV	40–60 mg in 4 doses
Chloramphenicol	IV	50–100 mg in 4 doses
Kanamycin	IV, IM	15 mg in 2–3 doses†
Gentamicin	IV, IM	5–7.5 mg in 3 doses†
Tobramycin	IV, IM	5 mg in 3 doses†
Amikacin	IV, IM	15 mg in 2 doses†
Sulfisoxazole	IV	120 mg in 4 doses
Trimethoprim-sulfamethoxazole	IV	8 mg TMP/40 mg SMZ in 2 doses

*Use high-dosage schedule if meningitis is diagnosed or suspected.

†Administer in continuous drip or by slow infusion in 30 to 60 minutes or more.

TABLE 21–26. Daily Dosage Schedule for Parenteral Antibacterial Agents for Newborn Infants with Sepsis or Suppurative Complications of Otitis Media

DRUG	ROUTE	DOSAGE/kg/24 HOURS*	
		7 Days of Age	7–28 Days of Age
Penicillin G, Crystalline	IV, IM	50,000–75,000 U in 2–3 doses	75,000–100,000 U in 3–4 doses
Penicillinase-Resistant Penicillins			
Methicillin	IV, IM	50–75 mg in 2 doses	75–100 mg in 3 doses
Oxacillin	IV, IM	50–75 mg in 2 doses	75–100 mg in 3 doses
Nafcillin	IM	50–75 mg in 2 doses	75–100 mg in 3 doses
Broad-Spectrum Penicillins			
Ampicillin	IV, IM	50–75 mg in 2 doses	75–100 mg in 3–4 doses
Carbenicillin	IV, IM	200–300 mg in 2–3 doses	300–400 mg in 3–4 doses
Ticarcillin	IV, IM	150–225 mg in 2–3 doses	225–300 mg in 3–4 doses
Cephalosporin			
Moxalactam	IV	100 mg in 2 doses	150 mg in 3 doses
Cefotaxime	IV, IM	100 mg in 2 doses	150 mg in 3 doses
Ceftazidime	IV, IM	60 mg in 2 doses	90 mg in 3 doses
Aminoglycosides†			
Kanamycin	IV,‡ IM	15 mg in 2 doses	15 mg in 3 doses
Gentamicin	IV,‡ IM	5 mg in 2 doses	7.5 mg in 3 doses
Tobramycin	IV,‡ IM	4 mg in 2 doses	6 mg in 3 doses
Amikacin	IV,‡ IM	15 mg in 2 doses	15 mg in 3 doses
Chloramphenicol†	IV	Premature—25 mg in 1 dose Term—25 mg in 1 dose	Premature—25 mg in 2 doses Term—50 mg in 2 doses
Vancomycin	IV§	20 mg in 2 doses	30 mg in 3 doses

*The higher dose is recommended in the treatment of meningitis.
†Serum concentrations should be assayed to determine the optimal dose.
‡Intravenous administration given in a 20- to 30-minute interval.
§Intravenous administration given in a 30- to 60-minute interval.

macologic activity of antimicrobial agents in the newborn infant.

FOOD INTERFERENCE WITH ABSORPTION

The absorption of some oral antimicrobial agents is significantly decreased when the drug is taken with food or near mealtime. These drugs include unbuffered penicillin G, penicillinase-resistant penicillins (nafcillin, oxacillin, cloxacillin, and dicloxacillin), ampicillin, and lincomycin. Milk, milk products, and other foods or medications containing calcium or magnesium salts interfere with absorption of the tetracyclines. Absorption of penicillin V, buffered penicillin G, amoxicillin, cephalexin, cefaclor, chloramphenicol, erythromycin, and clindamycin is only slightly affected by food. Antibiotics whose absorption is affected by concurrent administration of food should be taken one or more hours before or 2 or more hours after meals. A four-times-per-day dosage schedule should call for the drug to be given on arising, one hour before lunch, one hour before supper, and at bedtime.

INTRAVENOUS AND INTRAMUSCULAR ADMINISTRATION

After intravenous administration of most antimicrobial agents, there is a period when the concentration

of drug in serum is higher than that following intramuscular administration. However, no therapeutic advantage of intravenous as opposed to intramuscular administration has been demonstrated. Intravenous administration should be used if the patient is in shock or has a bleeding diathesis. If prolonged parenteral therapy is anticipated, the pain on injection and the small muscle mass of the young child preclude the intramuscular route and make intravenous therapy preferable.

Antibacterial concentrations in blood are similar after oral and intravenous administration of chloramphenicol and trimethoprim-sulfamethoxazole. Parenteral administration may be preferred because of hypothesized lesser bone marrow toxicity of chloramphenicol and ease of administration for the patient unable to take oral trimethoprim-sulfamethoxazole.

Chloramphenicol, the tetracyclines, and erythromycin should be administered parenterally by the intravenous, rather than the intramuscular, route. Chloramphenicol has variable absorption from intramuscular sites. The intramuscular injection of parenteral tetracyclines and erythromycin causes local irritation and pain.

The physician must be alert for thrombophlebitis that may result from prolonged intravenous administration and sterile abscesses that may follow intramuscular administration. The technique and complications of intramuscular injections were reviewed by Bergeson and colleagues (1982). In general, the site of injection in young infants is the upper lateral thigh; in children over 2 years of age, the gluteal area; and for older children, the deltoid muscle. After selection of the proper site and insertion of the needle into the muscle, negative pressure is applied by pulling back on the plunger to be certain that the needle is not in a blood vessel.

USE OF DRUGS FOR CHILDREN IN SCHOOL OR GROUP DAY-CARE CENTERS

Infants and children may return to the school or day-care center during a course of antimicrobial therapy. Because of the problems with administration of drugs outside the home, physicians should use medications that are given infrequently and need only simple directions. Drugs that are administered twice or three times a day are preferred. Use of chewable tablets, when available, may be of value in reducing the need for the school nurse or day-care provider to measure specific amounts of liquid suspension. Single-dosage regimens, such as intramuscular benzathine penicillin G for Group A streptococcal infections, may be advantageous. Guidelines for administration of medications in school have been published (Zanga et al., 1984) and may also serve as a model for the physician who is prescribing drugs to be administered in day-care settings. Administration of medications in day-care situations has been addressed (Smith and Aaronson, 1986).

PATIENT COMPLIANCE

The most frequent drug-related factor in failure of antibiotic therapy is inadequate compliance. Physicians overestimate the degree of compliance of their patients. Unacceptable taste or odor of drugs may result in poor compliance. Penicillin V, amoxicillin, and ampicillin are somewhat bitter, but acceptance is usually not a problem. Erythromycin preparations, alone or in fixed combination with sulfonamide, and cefaclor are well accepted. Trimethoprim-sulfamethoxazole and the oral penicillinase-resistant penicillins have a bitter aftertaste, and compliance problems should be anticipated in instructions to parents (Nelson and McCracken, 1980; Schwartz and Schwartz, 1980). Diarrhea leads to discontinuance of courses more frequently with ampicillin than with amoxicillin or trimethoprim-sulfamethoxazole (Feder, 1982) and is a particular problem with amoxicillin-clavulanate.

Mattar and colleagues (1975) evaluated treatment given at home for children with otitis media. Full compliance with prescribed medications occurred in only 5 of 100 patients. Factors limiting compliance included incorrect dosage schedules (36 per cent), early termination (37 per cent), inadequate dispensing of medication at drugstores (15 per cent), spilled medicine (7 per cent), and a series of other errors by physician, pharmacist, and parent (Table 21–27). Com-

pliance improved to more than half when hospital pharmacy personnel gave patients and parents verbal and written instructions for administration of medications that were dispensed with a calibrated measuring device and a calendar to record doses taken.

Other drug-related factors include inappropriate dosage schedule and inadequate duration of therapy. Some antimicrobial agents deteriorate on prolonged storage. Adherence to expiration dates recommended by the manufacturer safeguards against inadequate potency of the drug.

PHARMACOLOGIC INTERACTIONS

Concurrent administration of an antimicrobial agent and a second drug may result in altered pharmacokinetics of either drug.

The tubular secretion of penicillins and most cephalosporins is blocked by probenecid. This effect can be exploited by coadministration of probenecid (in a dose of 10 mg/kg four times a day in children to a maximum dose of 500 mg/kg four times a day) to produce a higher peak and more sustained level of antimicrobial activity.

Administration of chloramphenicol succinate with the anticonvulsant drugs phenobarbital and phenytoin leads to significant changes in concentrations of the antibiotic in serum: lower serum concentrations of chloramphenicol resulted when phenobarbital was coadministered, whereas higher serum concentrations of chloramphenicol were detected when phenytoin was coadministered. Phenobarbital may have induced the activity of hepatic endoplasmic reticulum, thereby increasing the metabolism of chloramphenicol, resulting in decreased concentrations of active antibiotic in

TABLE 21–27. Factors in Failure of Patients to Comply with Prescribed Medication

Physician Errors
Action of drugs and possible side effects not explained to parent
Dosage schedule ambiguous or incorrect
Instructions absent or incomplete
Multiple drugs prescribed, resulting in confusion
Cost of expensive trade brand used exceeds Medicaid reimbursement rate

Pharmacist Errors
Misleading or incorrect labels
Underfilling of prescriptions

Community Factors
Drugstores not open at time of day when parents seek medication

Parent and Home Factors
Difficulty in giving medication—two people often necessary to administer drug
Use of household teaspoon unsatisfactory
Bottles broken or spilled
Schedule of administration unrealistic for parent—baby sitter inadequate to dispense medication

Data from Mattar, M. E., et al., 1975. Pharmaceutic factors affecting pediatric compliance. Pediatrics 55:101–108.

serum and tissues. Phenytoin may cause induction of hepatic microsomal enzymes and compete with chloramphenicol for binding sites, resulting in elevated serum concentration of one or both drugs, possibly to toxic levels. Patients who receive chloramphenicol and anticonvulsant therapy require monitoring of serum concentrations to be certain of the safety and efficacy of the antibiotic (Krasinski et al., 1982).

Erythromycin interferes with the hepatic metabolization of theophylline, resulting in increased serum concentrations of theophylline that may produce nausea, vomiting, and other signs of toxicity. Coadministration of the two drugs is frequent in children with asthma. An alternative antibiotic should be considered, and if a suitable alternative is not optimal therapy, the dosage schedule of theophylline should be reduced and serum levels monitored (Prince et al., 1981).

OTOTOPICAL USE OF ANTIMICROBIAL AGENTS

Ototopical antimicrobial agents are used for otitis media when a perforation of the tympanic membrane (or tympanostomy tube) and a discharge are present. Neomycin, polymyxin B, chloramphenicol, and gentamicin are the most commonly used drugs. All of the agents are potentially ototoxic and should be used only when absolutely necessary. Sensitization does not appear to be an important problem with topical antibiotics, although some patients with chronic dermatoses may react to certain agents, such as neomycin.

Results of Clinical Trials of Antimicrobial Agents for Otitis Media

ASSESSMENT OF EFFICACY OF ANTIMICROBIAL AGENTS

The efficacy of antimicrobial agents for otitis media may be assessed in terms of clinical, microbiologic, and immunologic testing results (Table 21–28). Clinically, effective drugs are expected to produce a significant decrease in signs and symptoms of disease in 48 to 72 hours, to limit the duration of time of middle-ear effusion, and to prevent complications of disease that occur by extension to adjacent tissues. Studies by Mandel and colleagues (1982) and McLinn (1980) indicate that more children who received cefaclor were free of effusion at 14 days after onset of therapy than children who received amoxicillin. The basis for this effect is unknown, but the data suggest that time to

---

TABLE 21–28. Efficacy of Antimicrobial Agents for Treatment of Otitis Media

Clinical Efficacy
Resolution of acute signs
Decrease in duration of middle-ear effusion
Prevention of complications

Microbiologic Efficacy
Sterilization of infection
Elimination of microbial antigens

Immunologic Efficacy
Development of local and systemic immunity

---

resolution of middle-ear effusion should be included in assessment of antimicrobial agents evaluated for use in otitis media.

The major microbiologic criterion for efficacy of antimicrobial drugs is sterilization of the middle-ear infection. Studies by Howie and Ploussard (1969) attest to the value of the information provided by this *"in vivo* susceptibility test." Recent studies indicate that bacterial antigens persist in middle-ear fluid, although the antibiotic may have rid the ear of viable organisms. Pneumococcal polysaccharide has been identified in the vast majority of fluids in which the organism is isolated and in many specimens that have no bacterial growth (Karma et al., 1985; Palva and Lehtinen, 1987). The role of these bacterial products in diseases and the effect of antibacterial drugs in processing and eliminating the antigens are unknown but may be important in dealing with the problem of effusion that persists after acute infection.

The immunologic process of otitis media is incompletely understood, and little information is available about the effect of antimicrobial agents on the development of local and systemic immunity after acute or chronic otitis media. Do antibiotics limit the immune response to infection in the middle ear? Do antibiotics differ in their effect on local or systemic immunity of the middle ear? How will these features of the immune response affect the duration of fluid in the middle ear? How will these features affect type-specific protection against the same bacteria? Antimicrobial agents undoubtedly play a role in modulating the immune response of the mucosa of the middle ear, but little is known about that role.

HISTORY OF CLINICAL TRIALS

The design of clinical trials for evaluation of efficacy of antimicrobial agents in children with acute otitis media has undergone significant changes in the past 35 years. Prior to 1960, most American studies were performed without tympanocentesis and, thus, without a specific microbiologic diagnosis. Often large numbers of children were enrolled to evaluate two or more drugs, the definition of otitis media was broadly stated and included such signs as inflammation of the tympanic membrane (which most experts now do not accept as a suitable sole criterion for otitis media with effusion), the drugs were assigned by some random method, and results of therapy were presented in general terms such as "good response" or "therapeutic failure." The results were usually ambiguous and demonstrated only minimal differences between the drugs studied (Stickler and McBean, 1964). A review of such articles today would yield little information of value in assessment of use of various antimicrobial agents available for management of acute otitis media.

Tympanocentesis to define the causative agent in the middle-ear fluid of children with otitis media with effusion had been common to clinical trials by Scandinavian investigators, but it became customary in American studies only in the 1960's. About this time, more investigators, both in the private practice of pediatrics and in academic centers, became interested in various aspects of infection of the middle ear, including evaluation of antimicrobial agents. The study designs were more precise: many studies were double blind, sterilization was defined in some studies by reaspiration of persisting middle-ear fluid, compliance was evaluated by assessment of use of the drug (weighing of returned bottles of medication or assay of urine for antimicrobial activity), the clinical course was followed with precise end points, and side effects and toxicity of the antimicrobial agents were carefully assessed by clinical evaluation and laboratory tests.

ARE ANTIMICROBIAL AGENTS INDICATED FOR ACUTE OTITIS MEDIA?

Prior to the introduction of sulfonamides in 1936, management of acute otitis media included watchful waiting or, when the suppurative process produced severe clinical signs or complications, use of myringotomy to drain the middle-ear abscess. Spread of infection to the mastoid, meninges, or other intracranial foci was a feared complication of otitis media.

After the advent of sulfonamides and later of penicillin and other antibiotics, the frequency of complications of otitis media showed a dramatic decline. In 1938, the frequency of mastoidectomy associated with acute otitis media was 20 per cent; by 1948 it was 2.5 per cent (Sorensen, 1977). In some studies it dropped to zero (Herberts et al., 1971). Mortality from acute otitis media was a concern prior to the advent of use of antimicrobial agents (Sorensen, 1977).

Most experts agree that acute otitis media should be treated with antimicrobial agents. This consensus is based on the facts that susceptible organisms, predominantly bacterial pathogens, are isolated from the majority of middle-ear effusions of children who have acute otitis media and that there has been a significant decline in the incidence of suppurative intratemporal and intracranial complications of otitis media since the advent of use of antimicrobial agents. On the other hand, some physicians believe that antimicrobial therapy is used too frequently and should not be instituted for episodes of otitis media with minimal symptoms, that instead, it should be reserved for severe cases, for otitis media associated with suppurative complications, for effusions that become chronic, or for otitis media in certain high-risk children (Diamant and Diamant, 1974; van Buchem et al., 1981, 1985). Bluestone and associates (1984) concluded that "there may be some merit in withholding antimicrobial therapy in selected patients who have acute otitis media, but the criteria for identifying patients for whom this type of management will be safe have not been defined." They recommended appropriate clinical trials to answer the question but concluded that an antimicrobial agent was indicated for treatment of acute otitis media (Bluestone et al., 1984).

RESULTS OF THERAPEUTIC TRIALS INCLUDING CHILDREN WHO RECEIVE A PLACEBO

Many children with acute otitis media improve without use of antimicrobial agents. The use of a placebo group in a comparative trial with one or more antimicrobial agents has been studied by many investigators in the past 35 years. Some of these studies yield important information on the course of infection of the middle ear unmodified by an antimicrobial agent (at least, at onset).* Results from representative studies provide important insights into the value of antimicrobial agents and use of myringotomy alone or in combination with a drug. Only studies that used a method of aspiration of middle-ear fluid to define the microbiologic agents are cited.

1. Rudberg (1954) evaluated 1365 patients with acute, uncomplicated otitis media treated as inpatients or outpatients between January 1951 and May 1952. All patients were confined to bed and had their ears drained by syringe daily, as long as discharge was present. If spontaneous perforation did not occur, myringotomy was performed. Four regimens of antimicrobial agents were used: penicillin G tablets or a triple-sulfonamide preparation alone or in combination, or an intramuscular injection of a combination of benzathine and procaine penicillin G. A fifth group received none of the drug regimens. The criteria for efficacy included the duration of discharge and incidence of complications. Between 236 and 333 cases were included in each group. The results were as follows:

Duration of ear discharge was significantly shortened in infections due to the pneumococcus and *H. influenzae* in patients who received penicillin or sulfonamide preparations, when compared with those who received placebo. Infections due to *S. aureus* and beta-hemolytic streptococcus were favorably altered by use of penicillin, but the results in the sulfonamide group were not significantly different from those for the placebo group. Complications, including exacerbation of clinical signs, mastoiditis, and failure of the infection to subside, occurred significantly more often in the placebo group than in the groups receiving penicillin, but the complications in patients receiving a sulfonamide were not significantly different from those of the placebo group. Mastoiditis occurred in 44 of 254 (17 per cent) of patients receiving placebo, in 4 of 267 patients treated with sulfonamides, and in none of 844 patients managed with one of the penicillin regimens. The highest incidence of complications occurred in patients with disease due to beta-hemolytic streptococcus and *H. influenzae*.

2. In 1953 Lahikainen reported a study of children who were managed by use of myringotomy alone or in combination with penicillin G. The duration of discharge was significantly decreased in the group who received the antibiotic. No complications occurred in the penicillin-treated group, but 9 of 153 patients who had myringotomy alone developed complications, including 7 cases of mastoiditis, 1 case of meningitis, and 1 case of sinus thrombosis and brain abscess.

---

*These studies should not be considered to describe the natural course of otitis media, as all include a procedure that drains variable amounts of fluid: tympanocentesis (aspiration) or myringotomy (incision and drainage). In some cases, the procedure was repeated at frequent intervals.

3. Van Dishoeck and associates (1959) reported that 50 per cent of 400 children treated with eardrops alone recovered in 7 to 17 days, but 13 children developed mastoiditis requiring operation.

4. Halstead and colleagues (1968) identified clinical improvement in a majority of untreated patients with suppurative otitis (almost all had cultures that were positive for *S. pneumoniae* or *H. influenzae*), but one third of the children (13 of 19) continued to be ill.

5. Howie and Ploussard (1972) evaluated various antimicrobial agents and included a group without antimicrobial therapy. Clinical resolution and microbiologic eradication occurred without use of antibiotics in a small number of patients with otitis media due to *S. pneumoniae* (9 of 45, 20 per cent) and in a larger number of those with disease due to *H. influenzae* (9 of 21, 43 per cent).

6. Lorentzen and Haugsten (1977) evaluated 505 children, and, from these, three treatment groups were defined: myringotomy, penicillin V, and penicillin V in combination with myringotomy. Significantly more failures occurred in the myringotomy group (15 per cent) than in the penicillin group (4 per cent) or the penicillin plus myringotomy group (5 per cent). Thus, penicillin V was more efficacious than myringotomy alone, but myringotomy did not add to the effectiveness of the drug.

7. Van Buchem and coworkers (1981) reported that antimicrobial therapy had no effect on the outcome of children with acute otitis media. The investigators treated 171 children in a double-blind study of four regimens: amoxicillin alone, amoxicillin plus myringotomy, myringotomy alone, and neither drug nor surgery. Children aged 2 to 12 years were enrolled by 12 general practitioners in or near Tilburg, the Netherlands. The results suggested that the clinical course (pain, temperature, otoscopic appearances, and recurrence rate) was not different in any of the groups, although ears had discharge for a longer time and eardrums took longer to heal (neither difference significant) in the children treated without antibiotics. The authors concluded that "symptomatic therapy with nosedrops and analgesics seems a reasonable initial approach to acute otitis media in children" (van Buchem et al., 1981).

The study has been discussed extensively and criticized (Saah et al., 1982). The critics of the study identify flaws in the study design and analysis of results and question the validity of the conclusions. In general, the criticisms focus on the age of the patients (excluding infants, who have the highest age-specific incidence of disease), the small number of patients in each treatment group, the methods of statistical analysis, the absence of microbiologic data, the absence of definition of disease, the failure to assess observer reliability for the many participating physicians, and the failure to consider important variables of disease in randomization for therapy.

Van Buchem and colleagues (1985) performed a second trial in which 4860 children 2 years of age or older with acute otitis media were treated with nose drops and analgesics alone for the first 3 to 4 days. Children whose condition took "an unsatisfactory course" (high temperature, otalgia, or persistent discharge) were treated with antimicrobial drug alone or in combination with myringotomy. More than 90 per cent of the children recovered within a few days using this regimen, but two developed mastoiditis. Group A streptococci was cultured from ear fluids of 39 per cent of the children with the "unsatisfactory course" who underwent myringotomy; *S. pneumoniae* was cultured from 17 per cent, but *H. influenzae* was cultured from only one child (1.4 per cent).

8. Mygind and associates (1981) compared penicillin with placebo for acute otitis media in Danish children and concluded that antibiotic therapy was more effective.

These studies suggest that many cases of infection of the middle ear resolve spontaneously or with the assistance of surgical drainage. The reasons for resolution are listed in Table 21–29. Many cases improve because the contents of the middle-ear infection are discharged through the eustachian tube or after spontaneous perforation of the tympanic membrane. In addition, many children have acute otitis media due to viruses or other microorganisms that are not susceptible to currently used antimicrobial drugs. The major advantages of antimicrobial agents as compared with placebo (the latter usually including some drainage procedure) are (1) the duration of drainage and other signs of clinical disease are decreased, and (2) the incidence of complications, though low, is significantly decreased, almost to zero (Sorenson, 1977).

In a recently reported study by Puczynski and coworkers (1987), a single dose of amoxicillin was compared with the standard 10-day course. The trial was prematurely halted after only 17 patients had been entered owing to the occurrence of three treatment failures in the single-dose group, whereas in the group treated for 10 days, no treatment failures occurred.

RESULTS OF RECENT CLINICAL TRIALS

A summary of results of selected clinical trials of various antimicrobial agents in children with acute otitis media is given in Table 21–30. The reports were published between 1969 and 1987, and the list includes only studies that identified the bacterial cause by aspiration of middle-ear fluid. The clinical results were consistent with the results that would be expected based on *in vitro* studies of the activity of antimicrobial agents (see Table 21–19) and data about concentrations of drug achieved in middle-ear fluid (see Tables 21–22 through 21–24).

TABLE 21–29. Reasons for Resolution of Otitis Media with Effusion without Use of Antimicrobial Agents

Effusion is due to nonbacterial organism
Effusion is due to a noninfectious cause
Effusion persists from a prior episode of otitis media
Effusion is cleared by
    Drainage through eustachian tube
    Drainage through spontaneous perforation of tympanic
      membrane
    Absorption by middle-ear mucosa

TABLE 21–30. Selected Trials of Antimicrobial Agents for Acute Otitis Media

| INVESTIGATOR | DRUGS | CLINICAL EFFICACY* | | |
		S. pneumoniae	H. influenzae	B. catarrhalis
Nilson et al., 1969	Penicillin V	+	−	N/A
	Penicillin V and trisulfapyrimidines	+	+	
	Ampicillin	+	+	
Howie and Ploussard, 1972	Placebo	−	−	N/A
	Ampicillin	+	+	
	Erythromycin estolate (E)	+	−	
	Trisulfapyrimidines (S)	−	+	
	E&S	+	+	
Feigin et al., 1973a	Ampicillin	+	+	N/A
	Clindamycin	+	−	
Howie et al., 1974	Ampicillin	+	+	N/A
	Amoxicillin	+	+	
Howard et al., 1976	Amoxicillin	+	+	N/A
	Penicillin V	+	−	
	Erythromycin estolate	+	−	
	E&S	+	+	
Stechenberg et al., 1976	Ampicillin	+	+	N/A
	Cephalexin	+	−	
Shurin et al., 1980a	Ampicillin	+	+	N/A
	Trimethoprim-sulfamethoxazole	+	+	
Mandel et al., 1982	Amoxicillin	+	+	+
	Cefaclor	+	+	+
Berman and Laver, 1983	Cefaclor	+	+	+
	Amoxicillin	+	+	+
Blumer et al., 1984	Trimethoprim-sulfamethoxazole	+	+	+
	Cefaclor	+	+	+
Marchant et al., 1984a	Trimethoprim-sulfamethoxazole	+	+	+
	Cefaclor	+	−	−
Odio et al., 1985	Amoxicillin-clavulanate	+	+	+
	Cefaclor	+	+	+
Howie et al., 1985	Trimethoprim-sulfamethoxazole	−	−	N/A
	Cefaclor	−	−	N/A
Rodriguez et al., 1985	Erythromycin-sulfamethoxazole	+	+	+
	Amoxicillin	+	+	+
Marchant et al., 1986	Amoxicillin-clavulanate	+	+	+
	Cefaclor	−	−	−
Bergeron et al., 1987	Erythromycin-sulfisoxazole	+	+	+
	Cefaclor	+	+	+
Kaleida et al., 1987	Amoxicillin-clavulanate	+	+	+
	Cefaclor	+	+	+
Kenna et al., 1987	Cefixime	+	+	+
	Cefaclor	+	+	+

*Clinical results are defined as satisfactory (+) or unsatisfactory (−); N/A, not reported.

Because of the marked susceptibility of the pneumococcus for all drugs tested (with the sole exception of sulfonamides), clinical results of drugs for otitis media due to S. pneumoniae were satisfactory. The efficacy of the drugs for infections due to H. influenzae was variable. Ampicillin, amoxicillin, cyclacillin, amoxicillin-clavulanate, sulfonamides, and trimethoprim-sulfamethoxazole were effective in some but not all cases. Penicillin V, erythromycins, and clindamycin were ineffective. Prior to 1980, B. catarrhalis was not thought to be a pathogen in acute otitis media, however, since then studies have evaluated drug efficacy when this organism was present in the initial isolate. Erythromycin-sulfamethaoxale, trimethaprim-sulfisoxazole, and amoxicillin-clavulanate appeared to be effective.

RELAPSE AND RECURRENCE

The reasons for antimicrobial failure have been addressed in several studies. Children whose clinical signs did not resolve after initial therapy with a 10-day course of ampicillin, amoxicillin, or erythromycin-sulfonamide mixture were evaluated (Schwartz et al., 1981b). Middle-ear fluid was aspirated and cultured for bacteria: ampicillin-resistant H. influenzae was found in about one third (31 per cent), ampicillin-susceptible strains of S. pneumoniae or H. influenzae were identified in about one half (51 per cent), and no bacterial growth was found in the other fluids. Boston children who failed to respond to therapy were studied in a similar fashion with the following results: 19 per cent had organisms resistant to initial therapy, and 57 per cent had no bacteria isolated from the middle-ear fluids (Teele et al., 1981*b*). Some children who fail clinically do so because of a bacterial pathogen resistant to initial therapy, but many children have bacteria that are susceptible to the drug, and some have negative bacterial cultures and presumably have a nonbacterial microorganism as the cause of otitis media or some other reason for the persistent fever. The child who fails to respond to therapy in 48 to 72 hours, or later relapses, should receive a new antimicrobial regimen that provides effective activity against organisms that might be resistant to the initial therapy (i.e., beta-lactamase–producing organisms that would inactivate ampicillin). Harrison and coworkers (1985) found that, when children treated with amoxicillin initially had an early recurrence, a resistant organism was frequently found on aspiration of the middle ear; recurrences that appeared later in time did not show this difference in bacterial etiology.

The bacteriologic features of middle-ear infection in children who have recurrent episodes of acute otitis media are, in general, similar to those found in first episodes: the predominant pathogens are *S. pneumoniae* (though of different serotypes) and nontypable strains of *H. influenzae*. Thus, the child with recurrent episodes of otitis media may be treated initially with the same antimicrobial regimens as the child with a first episode of middle-ear infection.

STERILIZATION OF MIDDLE-EAR FLUIDS BY ANTIMICROBIAL AGENTS

Howie and Ploussard have contributed significant information about the epidemiology, diagnosis, and management of otitis media. The *in vivo* sensitivity test is one of their most valuable studies (1969). The middle-ear fluid of children with acute otitis media was aspirated and cultured prior to the start of therapy with various antimicrobial agents. All drugs were prescribed in usual dosage schedules, and patients were advised to return in 2 to 5 days. If fluid was still present at the second visit, a culture of the fluid was obtained by needle aspiration. The results of these cultures are listed in Table 21–31. Their studies are consistent with expected results based on *in vitro* data (see Table 21–19) and achievable concentrations of drug in middle-ear fluid (see Tables 21–22 through 21–24). Penicillins G and V, intramuscular benzathine penicillin G, and erythromycin were successful in eradicating *S. pneumoniae* from middle-ear fluid. Sulfonamides and tetracyclines did not eradicate *S. pneu-*

TABLE 21–31. Results of Antimicrobial Therapy in Otitis Media—*In Vivo* Sensitivity Test

DRUG	NUMBER OF PATIENTS FROM WHOM ORGANISM WAS RECOVERED DURING THERAPY*/NUMBER WITH BACTERIAL OTITIS MEDIA		
	S. pneumoniae	*H. influenzae*	*B. catarrhalis*
Data from Howie and Ploussard, 1969			
Phenoxymethyl penicillin	0/2	7/7	N/A
Phenoxymethyl penicillin with sulfonamides	0/17	2/6	N/A
Ampicillin	1/20	0/17	N/A
Benzathine, procaine, aqueous penicillin	1/9	7/7	N/A
Erythromycin ethylsuccinate	1/15	17/20	N/A
Erythromycin ethylsuccinate plus triple sulfonamide suspension	3/8	2/7	N/A
Triple sulfonamide suspension	8/18	3/8	N/A
Data from Howie et al., 1985†			
Trimethoprim-sulfamethoxazole	10/23	11/26	N/A
Amoxicillin	6/42	4/17	N/A
Cefaclor	10/17	16/30	N/A
Data from McLinn, 1980‡; McLinn and Serlin, 1983§; Marchant et al., 1984a, 1986‖			
Amoxicillin‡	4/37	3/14	0/6
Amoxicillin§	0/35	0/23	0/4
Cyclacillin‡	0/40	0/18	1/5
Trimethoprim-sulfamethoxazole‖	0/19	1/14	0/9
Cefaclor,‖ three times daily	1/37	3/20	0/2
Cefaclor,‖ twice daily	4/20	8/18	0/8
Amoxicillin-clavulanate‖	0/21	1/15	0/4
Cefaclor, 3 times daily‖	2/14	4/14	2/7

*Two to 10 days after beginning therapy.
†Studied from 1976 to 1980.
‡Reaspiration of middle-ear fluid 2 days after therapy.
§Reaspiration of middle-ear fluid 2 to 3 days after therapy.
‖Reaspiration of middle-ear fluid 3 to 6 days after therapy.
N/A, not reported.

moniae. H. influenzae was eradicated by ampicillin but not by penicillin V, intramuscular benzathine penicillin G, and erythromycin. The high minimal inhibitory concentration of penicillin V for *H. influenzae* and the relatively low concentrations of benzathine penicillin G achieved in serum (and by extrapolation in middle-ear fluid) are the probable reasons for failure of these two penicillins to sterilize *H. influenzae* from the middle-ear fluid. An oral form of penicillin G was not studied.

Studies using the methods of the *in vivo* sensitivity test add information about additional antimicrobial agents (McLinn, 1980; McLinn and Serlin, 1983; Marchant et al., 1984a, 1986; Chonmaitree et al., 1986). Amoxicillin, cyclacillin, trimethoprim-sulfamethoxazole, and amoxicillin-clavulanate were effective in sterilizing middle-ear fluids 2 to 6 days after identification of otitis media due to *S. pneumoniae, H. influenzae,* and *B. catarrhalis.* When clinical outcome was evaluated, the efficacy of cefaclor was satisfactory for the common pathogens. However, in the *in vivo* studies reported by Howie and associates (1985) and Marchant and colleagues (1986), cefaclor failed to eradicate the causative organisms in several cases when reaspiration was performed 3 to 5 days after initiation of therapy; when amoxicillin-clavulanate was tested, all but 1 of 36 subjects had eradication of the initial isolate (Marchant et al., 1986). Even though the *in vivo* method of testing efficacy is only one measure of outcome, these findings are important.

EFFECT OF ANTIMICROBIAL AGENTS
ON DURATION OF EFFUSION

The primary role of antimicrobial agents is to eradicate the local infection and to prevent spread to contiguous and distant tissues. Studies demonstrating the persistence of middle-ear effusions after acute infection suggest a need to consider duration of fluid in the middle ear among the criteria for efficacy of an antimicrobial agent. Few investigations have been designed to answer this question. Mandel and colleagues (1982) compared the results obtained by cefaclor and amoxicillin in children with acute otitis media. Fourteen days after onset of therapy, more children who received cefaclor had aeration of the middle ear (59 of 106, 55.7 per cent) than did children who received amoxicillin (40 of 97, 41.2 per cent; p = 0.05). On day 42, the proportion of children with normal aerated ears was the same, 68.9 per cent for cefaclor and 67.5 per cent for amoxicillin. McLinn (1980) demonstrated similar findings in a study of ampicillin and cefaclor. It is possible that the differences on day 14 were related to differing effects of the antimicrobial drugs on the inflammatory response in the middle ear, whereas, by day 42, host factors were dominant and little difference would be expected, irrespective of the antibiotic used.

EFFECT OF ANTIMICROBIAL AGENTS
ON CHRONIC OTITIS MEDIA WITH EFFUSION

Bacterial pathogens are identified in about one third of children with chronic otitis media with effusion (see

discussion of microbiology). The role of the bacteria in persistence of fluid in the middle ear is uncertain. One hypothesis is that the bacteria or their products are a factor in the continued production of fluid. Would a course of an appropriate antimicrobial agent assist in ridding the ear of fluid? Healy (1984) administered trimethoprim-sulfamethoxazole (8 mg of trimethoprim and 40 mg of sulfamethoxazole per kilogram per day in two doses) for 4 weeks to 200 children 2 to 5 years of age with middle-ear effusion present for longer than 12 weeks. The proportion of children who were free of effusion at the 4-week observation was significantly higher for the antibiotic group (58 per cent), as compared with an observation group (6 per cent).

Mandel and coworkers (1987) demonstrated that amoxicillin was more effective than placebo for otitis media with effusion, but almost 70 per cent of the patients had persistent effusion at the end of the treatment period and there was a 50 per cent recurrence rate over the succeeding 3 months, irrespective of the treatment received initially. A similar benefit of cefaclor for treatment of otitis media with effusion was identified by Ernstson and Anari (1985).

These data suggest that viable bacteria play a role in persistent middle-ear effusion and that eradication of the bacteria by antimicrobial agents results in resolution of fluid in some children. These data are sufficiently compelling to warrant consideration of a 10-day course of an appropriate antimicrobial agent immediately prior to placement of ventilating tubes.

Strategy for Management of Acute Otitis Media

CHOICE OF ANTIMICROBIAL AGENTS

At present, antimicrobial agents should be administered to children who have acute otitis media (see Fig. 21–80). Because the same bacteria found in acute middle-ear effusions have been isolated from ears of children who lack the classic signs and symptoms of acute otitis media and also from ears of children with chronic effusions, all children who have otitis media, regardless of the stage, should be considered candidates for a course of an antimicrobial agent if one has not been given during the recent past. However, in asymptomatic children who have otitis media with effusion of recent onset, spontaneous resolution can occur 90 per cent of the time (Casselbrant et al., 1985).

Amoxicillin or ampicillin is the currently preferred drug for initial treatment of acute otitis media, as they are active both *in vitro* and *in vivo* against *S. pneumoniae* and *H. influenzae.* The current incidence of strains of ampicillin-resistant *H. influenzae* is low (only 4 to 9 per cent of all cases of acute otitis media), and occurrence of ampicillin-resistant *B. catarrhalis* is variable from community to community; these resistance patterns do not require a change in recommendations for initial therapy. Other regimens that are satisfactory include trimethoprim-sulfamethoxazole, cefaclor, cefuroxime axetil, cefixime, amoxicillin-clavulanate, and combinations of a sulfonamide with benzathine penicillin G (administered by the intramuscular route as a single injection), oral penicillin G or V, clindamycin, or erythromycin. For the child who is allergic to penicillins, trimethoprim-sulfamethoxazole, cefaclor, or erythromycin or clindamycin combined with a sulfonamide provide equivalent antimicrobial coverage.

Intramuscular benzathine penicillin G is an alternative choice if the child is vomiting, if there is difficulty in oral administration, or if there is doubt concerning patient compliance with the prescribed regimen. This agent is effective against S. pneumoniae and S. pyogenes but must be combined with a sulfonamide for coverage of H. influenzae.

For neonates, immunosuppressed children, or those in whom an unusual organism has been isolated by culture of the middle-ear fluid, the appropriate antimicrobial agent should be selected according to the results of sensitivity testing.

DOSAGE SCHEDULES

Dosage schedules have been determined on the basis of studies of clinical pharmacology and results of clinical trials (see Table 21–22). Oral ampicillin, 50 to 100 mg/kg/24 hours, in four divided doses for 10 days, is recommended. Amoxicillin, 40 mg/kg/24 hours, is equally effective, can be given in three divided doses, and has fewer side effects, such as diarrhea. Ten days of treatment is recommended. If the child is allergic to the penicillins, then a combination of oral erythromycin, 40 mg/kg/24 hours, and sulfisoxazole, 120 mg/kg/24 hours, or trimethoprim-sulfamethoxazole 8 mg of trimethoprim and 40 mg of sulfamethoxazole per kilogram per 24 hours, is a suitable alternative. The availability of a fixed combination of erythromycin and sulfisoxazole antimicrobial agents (Pediazole) makes the combination an attractive choice, as patient compliance is improved when only one medication need be given instead of two. If beta-lactamase–producing H. influenzae or B. catarrhalis is suspected or documented by tympanocentesis, then appropriate choices would be amoxicillin-clavulanate (dosage based on amoxicillin content), erythromycin and sulfisoxazole, trimethoprim-sulfamethoxazole (8 mg of trimethoprim and 40 mg of sulfamethoxazole per kilogram per 24 hours) or cefaclor (40 mg/kg/24 hours in three divided doses).

FAILURE TO RESPOND TO INITIAL THERAPY

With appropriate antimicrobial therapy, most children with acute bacterial otitis media are significantly improved within 48 to 72 hours. The physician should be in contact with the parent to ascertain that improvement has occurred. If the patient does not respond to initial therapy with ampicillin or amoxicillin, infection with a resistant strain of H. influenzae should be considered. If signs persist but the child has no toxic signs or symptoms and aspiration to culture the middle-ear effusion is not performed, the initial antimicrobial agent should be changed to a regimen to which most uncommon organisms, such as a beta-lactamase–

producing H. influenzae or S. aureus, would be sensitive. Toxicity with persistent or recurrent fever or otalgia, or both, should prompt the clinician to recommend tympanocentesis or myringotomy, or both, to identify the causative organism; a specific antimicrobial agent may then be chosen on the basis of the results of culture of the middle-ear effusion and sensitivity testing. If ampicillin or amoxicillin was initially given, then the combinations of erythromycin-sulfisoxazole or amoxicillin-clavulanate or cefaclor should be administered. Trimethoprim-sulfamethoxazole (8 mg of trimethoprim and 40 mg of sulfamethoxazole per kilogram per 24 hours in three divided doses) appears to be effective when ampicillin-resistant H. influenzae is present or suspected to be present. However, trimethoprim-sulfamethoxazole is usually not effective when S. pyogenes is the causative organism. The newer oral cefalosporins, cefuroxime axetil and cefixime, would also be suitable choices; however, cefixime is not effective when S. aureus is the causative agent.

DURATION OF THERAPY

Physicians must rely on empirically derived schedules of therapy to plan drug regimens that lead to rapid and complete resolution of disease but are of minimal risk in terms of clinical or microbiologic failure or drug toxicity. For treatment of otitis media, opinions vary and the data are not easy to interpret. The dosage schedules presented in Table 21–18 appear appropriate for a 10-day course on the basis of currently available data.

Other dosage schedules (longer or shorter) than the traditional 10- to 14-day course may be as good, if not better. Studies compared the results of 3- and 10-day courses of amoxicillin (Chaput de Saintonge et al., 1982), treatment with penicillin V for 2 and 7 days (Meistrup-Larsen et al., 1983), and penicillin V administered for 5 or 10 days (Ingvarsson and Lundgren, 1982). In each study, the shorter course was similar in clinical results to the longer course. Methodologic problems, including absence of microbiologic diagnosis, limit the validity of the results. Nevertheless, there is reason to believe that for most children shorter courses may be as appropriate as 10 to 14 days, but the efficacy of longer courses, as yet not tested, may be superior to that of shorter courses.

Chemoprophylaxis for Recurrent Acute Otitis Media

Chemoprophylaxis implies use of drugs in anticipation of infection, whereas treatment implies use of drugs after infection has taken place or signs of infectious disease are evident. Although indiscriminate use of antimicrobial agents for prophylaxis is to be avoided, many forms of chemoprophylaxis have been extensively tested and are of proven value. Studies suggest that chemoprophylaxis may be effective in children with recurrent episodes of acute otitis media.

CRITERIA FOR USE OF CHEMOPROPHYLAXIS

Because prolonged courses of any drug may have harmful effects, the physician must be assured that the benefits of freedom from infection outweigh the risk of a prolonged course of a modified dosage schedule of drug. For any form of chemoprophylaxis, the following criteria should be considered:

1. The patient is at risk if infection occurs.
2. The microorganisms are known and are consistent causes of disease.
3. The microorganisms are unlikely to develop resistance to the drug used for a prolonged course.
4. The drug is well tolerated and can be administered in a convenient dosage and form.
5. The drug has limited side effects or toxicity.

Otitis media is a disease of sufficient importance to warrant chemoprophylaxis. The bacteriologic aspects of otitis media are well documented, and S. pneumoniae and nontypable strains of H. influenzae are the major bacterial pathogens in all studies. Resistance has not occurred during prolonged use of sulfonamides or ampicillin. The experience with penicillins and sulfonamides for prevention of streptococcal infections in patients with rheumatic heart disease may provide some support for the concept that resistance of the upper respiratory tract flora is unlikely to occur. The sulfonamides and penicillins are available in a variety of convenient forms that are well tolerated in infants and older children. Drug toxicity is not a problem, although allergic reactions are to be expected in a small number of children. Parents must be made alert for signs indicative of known side effects or toxicity.

Children are at risk for recurrent episodes of acute otitis media during a relatively short period of life: most episodes occur between 6 and 24 months of age. If the child who is susceptible to recurrent otitis media could be protected from infection during this period, the morbidity of middle-ear disease might be avoided. Thus, the concept of prophylaxis is a worthy one and deserves careful study, and it may be helpful when used appropriately by physicians who care for children.

PUBLISHED REPORTS

Nine controlled trials suggest the value of chemoprophylaxis in children with recurrent episodes of acute otitis media.

Maynard and associates (1972) studied Alaskan Eskimo children. Ampicillin or a placebo was administered for 1 year to children under 7 years of age living in Alaskan Eskimo villages. The children received a daily dose of oral ampicillin—125 mg for those up to 2.5 years of age and 250 mg for older children. Otitis media was defined as a new episode of otorrhea by history or observation of a research nurse who made monthly visits to the villages. The incidence of otorrhea was reduced by approximately 50 per cent in the 173 children receiving ampicillin, compared with the incidence in 191 children who received a placebo.

Perrin and coworkers (1974) administered sulfisoxazole or a placebo to 54 children, who were 11 months to 8 years of age and had histories of recurrent episodes of acute otitis media (three or more episodes in the previous 18 months, or a total of more than five episodes). Children received a placebo or 500 mg of sulfisoxazole twice a day for 3 months. They were then switched to the alternate regimen for another 3-month period. No specific criteria for otitis media were used by the participating pediatricians. A significant decrease in new episodes of acute otitis media occurred in the group of children receiving the antimicrobial agent. The older children, 6 to 8 years of age, showed minimal or insignificant decrease in incidence of otitis media when on the prophylactic regimen. The results of the study are given in Table 21–32.

Biedel (1978) evaluated the effectiveness of sulfonamides (sulfisoxazole or trisulfapyrimidine in a dosage of 100 to 130 mg/kg/24 hours, or sulfamethoxazole in a dosage of 55 mg/kg/24 hours) used at the onset of signs of infection of the upper respiratory tract. Children were enrolled in the program after recovery from a recent acute episode of otitis media. They were placed alternately into treatment (sulfonamide) or control (decongestant) groups when parents called the physician and reported any sign of a new upper respiratory tract infection. Treatment was prescribed for a minimum of 6 days, and any new episodes of otitis media that occurred during the 8 weeks following recovery from the original episode were recorded. Otitis media was found to recur with a new upper respiratory tract infection more frequently in children receiving decongestants than in children receiving sulfonamide.

Six other studies of prophylaxis for recurrent acute otitis media (Schwartz et al., 1982; Liston et al., 1983; Schuller, 1983; Varsano et al., 1985; Persico et al., 1985; Lampe and Weir, 1986) corroborated the results in the initial studies. Of the nine studies, six used a sulfonamide (sulfisoxazole in five and sulfamethoxazole in one), two used a penicillin (ampicillin or penicillin V), and erythromycin was used in one.

Reduction in number of episodes of acute infection in children in the prophylactic group, when compared with results for the controls, varied from 47 per cent (Maynard et al., 1972) to 90 per cent (Schuller, 1983).

TABLE 21–32. Effects of Chemoprophylaxis on Recurrence of Otitis Media

DRUG	NUMBER OF CHILDREN (n = 54)	NUMBER OF EPISODES	
		None	One or More
First Trial (12/72 to 2/73)			
Sulfisoxazole	28	25	3
Placebo	26	14	12
Second Trial (3/73 to 5/73)			
Sulfisoxazole	26	25	1
Placebo	28	19	9

With permission from Perrin, J. M., et al. 1974. Sulfisoxazole as chemoprophylaxis for recurrent otitis media: A double-blind cross-over study in pediatric practice. N. Engl. J. Med. 291:664–667.

These additional features were noted in one or more of the studies:

1. Age was an important factor—infants under 2 years of age were most likely to be benefited by chemoprophylaxis.

2. Compliance was critical to success of the program.

3. A carry-over effect was noted in some of the studies (Liston et al., 1983; Schwartz et al., 1982). Children had less disease in the months after conclusion of the prophylactic regimen.

4. No increase in drug resistance of organisms in the upper respiratory tract occurred. The data about bacterial resistance are limited and must be evaluated from studies in progress.

5. No significant incidence of side effects occurred when sulfonamides or ampicillin was used. Allergic reactions in children on prolonged modified courses for prophylaxis occurred at a rate similar to those expected from usage of the drugs for therapy of acute disease.

6. Duration of middle-ear effusion was not significantly different in treated and control children.

PLAN FOR PROPHYLAXIS

Although the available studies do not provide conclusive evidence of the validity of chemoprophylaxis, the data are persuasive that children who are prone to recurrent episodes of acute infection of the middle ear are benefited. While definitive studies of chemoprophylaxis are awaited, it is reasonable to consider the following program:

Who? Children who have had three documented episodes of acute otitis media in 6 months or four episodes in 12 months should be considered for the program.

Which Drugs? Sulfisoxazole and ampicillin (amoxicillin is preferable) were the agents used in published studies and provide the advantages of demonstrated efficacy, safety, and low cost.

What Dosage? Half the therapeutic dose should be administered once a day (usually at bedtime offers maximal compliance, but any single time during the day would be satisfactory). Dosage is amoxicillin, 20 mg/kg, or sulfisoxazole, 50 mg/kg.

How Long? During the winter and spring period, when respiratory tract infections are most frequent, treatment should be given for a period up to 6 months.

What Type of Follow-up? Children should be examined at 4- to 6-week intervals when free of acute signs to determine if middle-ear effusion is present. Management of prolonged middle-ear effusion should be considered separately from prevention of recurrences of acute infection (see Fig. 21–81).

How Should Acute Infections Be Treated? Acute infections should be treated with an alternative regimen. Amoxicillin-clavulanate would be a suitable alternative irrespective of the drug used for prophylaxis. If a sulfonamide was used for prophylaxis, ampicillin or cefaclor would also be appropriate choices for treat-

ment. If ampicillin or amoxicillin was used for prophylaxis, erythromycin-sulfisoxazole, trimethoprim-sulfamethoxazole, or cefaclor would be adequate to treat the acute infection.

Other Medical Therapies

Decongestants and Antihistamines

Nasal and oral decongestants, administered either alone or in combination with an antihistamine, are currently among the most popular medications for the treatment of otitis media with effusion. The common concept is that these drugs reduce congestion of the mucosa of the eustachian tube; however, the efficacy of this mode of therapy for otitis media with effusion has not been demonstrated.

A number of investigators have evaluated decongestants with or without antihistamines, but the quality of design of the programs has varied and therefore the results are difficult to interpret.

1. Collipp (1961) evaluated the use of phenylephrine hydrochloride nose drops in treating acute purulent otitis media with effusion in 180 children aged 2 to 14 years. Half of the children were treated with nasal spray by their parents four times per day; the other half received no decongestant. All subjects were given an initial injection of procaine penicillin G and a 10-day course of sulfisoxazole, chlorpheniramine maleate, and phenylephrine hydrochloride. No statistical differences were noted in the otologic status of the children who received the nasal spray and those who did not.

2. Rubenstein and coworkers (1965) treated 462 episodes of otitis media with effusion using several antimicrobial agents and the decongestant pseudoephedrine. Although some improvement was noted to be the result of treatment with the antimicrobial agents, the addition of pseudoephedrine to the medication regimen did not appear to improve treatment results significantly.

3. Miller (1970) evaluated the effect of a decongestant mixture containing carbinoxamine maleate and pseudoephedrine hydrochloride on 13 children with tympanostomy tubes that had been inserted to treat recurrent otitis media with effusion. The study used drug or placebo in a limited double-blind cross-over design. The success of the placebo or drug was determined by the results of eustachian tube function tests that measured the ability to equilibrate applied negative middle-ear pressures. An almost equal number of patients demonstrated "suggestive" positive response or no response to the drug, whereas none of the children showed any response to the placebo.

4. Stickler and colleagues (1967), in a follow-up to Rubenstein's (1965) study, evaluated the effects of penicillin and antihistamine (chlorpheniramine maleate), of penicillin alone, and of penicillin with sulfonamides on otitis media with effusion. Although sulfonamides did not improve the effects of the penicillin,

the addition of the antihistaminic agent to penicillin did produce better results.

5. Olson and coworkers (1978) evaluated the efficacy of pseudoephedrine hydrochloride by studying the response to treatment of 96 children who had had acute otitis media with effusion that had not responded to treatment for 2 weeks. Following a double-blind protocol that compared the effects of the drug with those of the placebo, the children were treated for up to 4 weeks or more and were reexamined by pneumatic otoscopy and tympanometry. No significant differences between the treatment groups were found. Although the findings were not statistically significant, these researchers did note that males and children with an allergic history did worse with the decongestant regimen.

6. Holmquist (1977) reported the effect of a combination of ephedrine and antihistamine compared with that of a placebo in a double-blind study on eustachian tube function in 58 patients (62 ears). The eustachian tube function was evaluated by means of air pressure equalization and tympanometry. In the 28 ears of patients who received the drug, a "positive effect" was noted in 16 (57 per cent), whereas of the 34 ears of subjects who received the placebo, a "positive effect" was reported in only 6 (18 per cent); the difference was statistically significant at the 95 per cent confidence level.

7. Fraser and associates (1977) compared ephedrine nose drops; a combination of brompheniramine maleate, phenylephrine hydrochloride, and phenylpropanolamine hydrochloride; autoinflation; and no treatment in children with otitis media with effusion and found no difference in tympanic membrane compliance, middle-ear pressure, or audiometric findings among the treatment groups. In addition to problems associated with documentation of otitis media with effusion, the investigators had eight treatment regimens with only 10 or 11 subjects in each group, which leads one to question the design and statistical analysis of the study.

8. In a double-blind study, Roth and coworkers (1977) showed that pseudoephedrine hydrochloride decreased nasal resistance in adults who had an upper respiratory tract infection.

Past studies, employing a modified inflation-deflation manometric technique to assess eustachian tube function in children who had had recurrent or chronic otitis media with effusion, showed that the obstruction of the eustachian tube was functional rather than mechanical (Bluestone et al., 1974; Cantekin et al., 1976). However, further studies during periods of upper respiratory tract infection showed that eustachian tube function was decreased from the baseline measurements at these times (Bluestone et al., 1977a). This decrease was attributed to intrinsic mechanical obstruction superimposed on the functional obstruction.

9. In an attempt to determine the effect of an oral decongestant with or without an antihistamine on the ventilatory function of the eustachian tube, two separate studies were conducted in 50 children who had had chronic or recurrent otitis media with effusion and in whom tympanostomy tubes had been inserted previously (Cantekin et al., 1980a). The first was a double-blind study that compared the effect of an oral decongestant, pseudoephedrine hydrochloride, with that of a placebo in 22 children who developed an upper respiratory tract infection during an observation period. Certain measures of eustachian tube function were significantly elevated above baseline values during the upper respiratory tract infection, which was attributed to intrinsic mechanical obstruction of the eustachian tube. It was found that oral decongestants tended to alter these measures of eustachian tube function in the direction of the baseline (before upper respiratory tract infection) values. Even though the effect was statistically significant, the favorable changes in measurements of tubal function were only partial and were more prominent on the second day of the trial, after the subjects had received four doses of the decongestant. However, the administration of a nasal spray of 1 per cent ephedrine had no effect on eustachian tube function in these children.

The second study was a double-blind cross-over design. In this study of 28 children who did not have an upper respiratory tract infection, the effect of a decongestant-antihistamine combination (pseudoephedrine hydrochloride and chlorpheniramine maleate) was compared with that of a placebo. When the subjects were given the decongestant-antihistamine medication, there were favorable changes in certain eustachian tube function measures that were not observed when the children received the placebo. Again, the response differences between the two groups were statistically significant. Even though these two studies indicated that an oral decongestant appeared to affect favorably the eustachian tube function of children who had an upper respiratory tract infection and that the combination of an oral decongestant and antihistamine had a similar effect on tubal function in children without an upper respiratory tract infection, an evaluation of the efficacy of these commonly employed medications must await the results of controlled clinical trials in children with otitis media with effusion.

10. Lildholdt and coworkers (1982) evaluated the effect of a topical nasal decongestant spray on eustachian tube function in 40 children with tympanostomy tubes. Five tubal function variables were assessed, employing a modified-inflation test and forced-response test before and after spraying the nose with either oxymetazoline hydrochloride or placebo, according to a double-blind study design. The results showed no significant differences between the two treatment groups of the study children who had severe functional tubal dysfunction, as documented by the constrictions of eustachian tube lumen during swallowing.

11. Cantekin and coworkers (1983), in a double-blind, placebo-controlled, randomized clinical trial of an oral decongestant and antihistamine combination in 553 infants and children with otitis media with effusion, showed *no* efficacy of these drugs. In addition, side

effects such as irritability and sleepiness were more common in children in the drug group than in subjects who received placebo.

12. Mandel and associates (1987) reported that amoxicillin was effective when compared with placebo, in the treatment of otitis media with effusion. However, the addition of a combination of an oral decongestant and antihistamine to amoxicillin provided no additional benefit over amoxicillin alone; more side effects were noted in children who received the decongestant and antihistamine combination.

The conclusion from these studies is that topical or systemic decongestants and antihistamines for otitis media with effusion are not warranted but may be effective for less severe conditions such as eustachian tube obstruction (Cantekin et al., 1980a). In children receiving these agents, however, side effects are common, and some, such as visual hallucinations, are quite disturbing.

Corticosteroids

The administration of adrenocorticosteroids in the form of either a topical nasal spray or a systemic preparation has been advocated for treatment of otitis media with effusion for the past 2 decades. Heisse (1963) reported excellent results with depomethylprednisone in 30 allergic patients who had otitis media with effusion. Oppenheimer (1968, 1975) recommended a short-term trial of corticosteroids in children. Shea (1971) also reported success in treating allergic children who had middle-ear effusions with a 4-day course of prednisone. Persico and colleagues (1978) treated one group of 160 children with prednisone and ampicillin and another group of 116 children with ampicillin only. They reported 53 per cent in the group that received the steroid and ampicillin treatment resolved their effusion compared with 13 per cent in the group that was treated only with the antibiotic. However, none of these studies was a randomized, controlled trial.

Schwartz and colleagues (1980) reported 70 per cent success in treating 41 children with a 7-day course of prednisone in a double-blind, placebo-controlled, cross-over study. The steroid appeared to be equally effective in those children who did and in those who did not have a history of allergy. Berman and associates (1987) also found benefit but the study was limited, owing to the small number of subjects studied. However, Macknin and Jones (1985) conducted a controlled trial in children with either otitis media with effusion or persistent middle-ear effusion after acute otitis media who were randomly assigned to enter a course of dexamethasone or placebo. The study was stopped before the trial was completed, because the investigators found no benefit in giving the drug.

Studies have evaluated the effects of administering a topical corticosteroid nasal spray. However, Schwartz and coworkers (1980) noted that when beclomethasone dipropionate spray was given to ten children with otitis media with effusion, it was only effective in three.

Lildholdt and associates (1982), in a double-blind study employing beclomethasone nasal spray in children with otitis media with effusion, failed to show efficacy.

If, indeed, adrenocorticosteroid therapy is effective in the treatment of otitis media with effusion, the mode of action remains only speculative at this time but may be related to the antiinflammatory action of the drug. Persico and coworkers (1978) postulated that the drug altered surface tension forces within the lumen of the eustachian tube. Schwartz and colleagues (1980) suggested that steroids may shrink the lymphoid tissue around the eustachian tube, acting on mucoproteins to decrease the viscosity of the middle-ear effusion by reducing tubal edema or reversing metaplasia of the middle-ear mucosa.

From these few studies it appears that a short course of systemic adrenocorticosteroid therapy is of uncertain efficacy in alleviating the problems of otitis media with effusion in children. At this time, the potential adverse side effects associated with the administration of a systemic adrenocorticosteroid (Shapiro et al., 1982) does not appear to justify its use in infants and children for otitis media.

Immunotherapy and Allergy Control

Because the precise role of allergy in the development of otitis media with effusion has not been documented, and because at times it is difficult to establish or confirm the diagnosis of allergy with certainty, it is not possible at present to quantify the relative efficacy of allergic management of otitis media with effusion in children. This topic is discussed further in the section on allergy and eustachian tube function (see p. 366). In spite of this dilemma, owing to a lack of information, there are clinicians who advocate allergy management for infants and children who have recurrent or chronic otitis media with effusion. Other physicians doubt that allergy plays any part in the origin of otitis media with effusion and rarely, if ever, consider directing their treatment of a patient with this problem to a possible underlying allergy. For example, Bluestone and Shurin (1974) and Paradise (1980), in extensive reviews of otitis media in infants and children, did not include control of allergy as a management option. On the other hand, there are those who include allergy in the differential diagnosis if there are one or more of the following: (1) past or present atopy in the child, (2) family history of allergy, or (3) signs of upper respiratory tract allergy present at the time of the clinical examination. These investigators have employed various regimens in their management of allergies, but all have reported obtaining good results from such treatment (Draper, 1967, 1974; Fernandez and McGovern, 1965; Kjellman et al., 1976; Phillips et al., 1974; Rapp and Fahey, 1973; Whitcomb, 1965).

Clemis (1976) considers inhalant allergy easiest to identify and treat and therefore advocates searching for inhalant sensitivities before looking for allergies to foods and chemicals. In his experience, house dust is the most frequent inhalant allergen identified. When house dust is identified as the problem, he advises "dust-proofing" the child's environment (especially the child's bedroom) and using electrostatic air filters. If environmental control measures are not successful in reducing symptoms, then hyposensitization to house dust may be considered. Mold spores are the second most common aeroallergen responsible for nonpollen allergy, for which he advocates environmental control, and if unsuccessful, hyposensitization. The treatment of choice when an adverse food reactivity is suspected is total dietary elimination of that food. In Clemis's experience, pollinosis plays a much less dominant role than that of dusts, molds, and foods in causing otitis media, but when pollinosis is present, he recommends hyposensitization. Pets may also be a source of allergy, but in this case, hyposensitization is not as successful as exclusion of the offending pet from the house. In Clemis's (1976) view, antihistamines are not of benefit in treating otitis media caused by allergy, and he advises against the use of cortisone, in either the systemic or topical intranasal forms, for therapy. Waickman (1979) agrees with Clemis that house dust is the most common allergic offender in patients who have otitis media with effusion that persists for 2 weeks or longer and has been unresponsive to adequate therapy for infection. Other inhalant antigens are considered to be less common offenders than dust, but for all inhalants the Rinkel (1962, 1963) method of immunotherapy is advocated.

In a double-blind, cross-over study by Friedman and coworkers (1983) that involved adult volunteers without otitis media, eustachian tubes became obstructed when the subjects were challenged intranasally with the antigen to which they were sensitive but not when they were challenged with a placebo (i.e., an antigen to which they were not sensitive).

Unfortunately, none of these studies was based on randomized, controlled trials in children with otitis media. Nevertheless, there does appear to be some evidence that chronic and recurrent otitis media with effusion may be associated with upper respiratory tract allergy. Therefore, until knowledge of the origin, method of diagnosis, and management of allergy in relation to otitis media with effusion increases, when a child has recurrent or chronic middle-ear disease and evidence of upper respiratory tract allergy, management of the allergy should be considered as a treatment option. A history of itching of the eyes, nose, or throat; of paroxysms of sneezing; and of chronic or frequently recurrent watery rhinorrhea in the presence or absence of the classic signs of nasal allergy should prompt the clinician to evaluate further the possibility that the child has an upper respiratory tract allergy. However, because no convincing clinical trials of the treatment options have been reported, no single method of treatment can be recommended. It does not seem favorable at present to treat for allergy those children who have recurrent or chronic middle-ear effusion, or both types, and who lack the signs and symptoms of upper respiratory tract allergy. This could change, however, if convincing data were presented to establish that the middle ear is a shock organ.

Inflation of the Eustachian Tube

Procedures that force air through the eustachian tube and into the middle ear and mastoid cavities have been employed for over 100 years in an effort to normalize negative intratympanic pressure and eliminate middle-ear effusion. The methods of Valsalva (1949) and Politzer (1909) are the most commonly used in children. Catheterization of the eustachian tube has also been utilized but is of limited usefulness in children, because the procedure can be frightening and is technically difficult to perform in young patients. All three of these methods are also crude tests of eustachian tube patency and have been described under physiology, pathophysiology, and pathogenesis (p. 341).

From a physiologic standpoint, inflation of the eustachian tube, middle ear, and mastoid has merit. Figure 21–84 shows the flask model of the nasopharynx–eustachian tube–middle ear system: liquid is shown in the body and narrow neck of an inverted flask. Relative negative pressure inside the body of the flask prevents the flow of the liquid out of the flask. This is analogous to an effusion in a middle ear that has abnormally high negative pressure. If air is insufflated up into the liquid, through the neck and into the body of the flask, the negative pressure is converted to ambient or positive pressure and the liquid will flow out of the flask. However, if the liquid is of high viscosity, the likelihood of air's being forced through the liquid into the body of the flask is remote, especially if the thick liquid completely fills the cham-

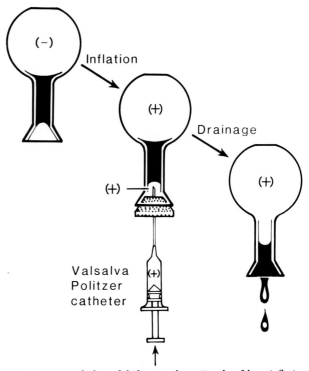

Figure 21–84. Flask model showing the rationale of how inflation of the middle ear promotes drainage down the eustachian tube. The eustachian tube–middle ear–mastoid air cell system can be likened to an inverted flask with a long, narrow neck (see text).

ber. Therefore, in the human system a thin, or serous, effusion would be more likely to flow out of the middle ear and down the eustachian tube than would a thick, mucoid effusion that fills the middle ear and mastoid cavities. The method probably is not effective in maintaining normal middle-ear pressure in children who have atelectasis caused by eustachian tube obstruction (i.e., high negative pressure), as experiments in animals have shown inflation of the middle ear not to be effective (Cantekin et al., 1980b).

Theoretically, then, inflation of the eustachian tube and middle ear should be an effective treatment option for children with certain types of otitis media with effusion or atelectasis, or both; however, in reality, there are several problems with this method of management. The self-inflation method of Valsalva is somewhat difficult for children to learn, because it is a technique involving forced nasal expiration with the nose and lips closed (Fig. 21–85). Cantekin and colleagues (1976) tested 66 children between the ages of 2 and 6 years who had had chronic or recurrent otitis media with effusion and who had functioning tympanostomy tubes in place. They asked each subject to try to blow his or her nose with the glottis closed. None of these children could passively open their eustachian tubes and force air into the middle ear by the Valsalva method, even though they developed a maximum nasopharyngeal pressure of 538.8 ± 237.0 mm H_2O. It was concluded that the Valsalva method of opening the eustachian tube in this age group was not successful owing to possible tubal compliance problems. Unfortunately, children in this age group have a high incidence of otitis media; for infants, who have the highest incidence of otitis media, the procedure cannot be used at all.

Politzer's method of opening the eustachian tube involves inserting the tip of a rubber air bulb into one nostril while the other nostril is compressed by finger pressure (Fig. 21–86) and then asking the child to swallow while the rubber bulb is compressed. Some children complain of a sudden "pop" in the ear as the positive pressure is forced up the eustachian tube and have discomfort with the procedure. However, this method is also extremely difficult to perform in infants.

The major difficulty with both methods is determining whether the middle ear is actually inflated by the

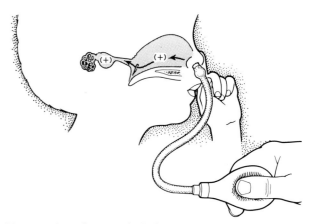

Figure 21–86. Politzer method of inflation of the eustachian tube–middle ear.

procedure. If a child hears a "pop" or has a pressure sensation in the ear, there is only presumptive evidence of passage of air into the middle ear. Auscultation of the ear (listening for the sound of air entering the middle ear during the procedure) is helpful in determining whether or not the procedure is successful, but a sound may be heard even when air does not enter the middle ear. Objective otoscopic evidence that the middle ear is actually inflated would be constituted by the presence of bubbles or a fluid level behind the tympanic membrane when these findings were not present prior to inflation. Another excellent method for determining objectively if the inflation is successful is to obtain a tympanogram before and after the procedure: the compliance peak should shift toward or be in the positive-pressure zone after inflation (Fig. 21–87). If none of the results of these presumptive or objective methods of determining the success of inflation is definitive, then the clinician cannot be certain that the procedure has been therapeutic. Failure to achieve a successful result may be related to (1) inability of the patient to learn the method; (2) insufficient nasopharyngeal overpressure to open the eustachian tube passively; (3) eustachian tube abnormality; or (4) a middle ear filled with a thick, mucoid effusion.

Unfortunately, the beneficial effect of the Valsalva and Politzer methods of inflation for treatment of otitis media with effusion or atelectasis has not been subjected to any acceptable randomized, controlled trials. Most of the evidence has been anecdotal. Gottschalk (1966, 1980) described remarkable success with a modification of the Politzer method in over 12,000 patients; the average course of treatment was a minimum of 12 inflations in the office on 3 separate days. Schwartz and coworkers (1978) have shown that it is possible to inflate the middle ears of children at home by the Politzer method; they documented the results of the method by tympanometry but did not test its efficacy. The only controlled trial of this method was reported by Fraser and colleagues (1977), and they were not able to demonstrate that it was efficacious.

Until well-controlled clinical trials are reported, it would appear reasonable to use the Politzer method

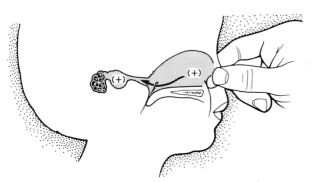

Figure 21–85. Self-inflation of the eustachian tube–middle ear employing the method of Valsalva.

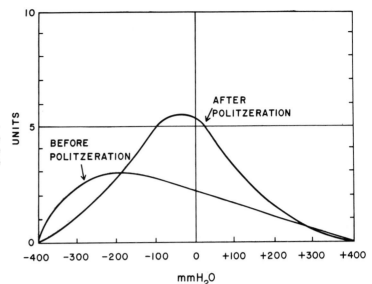

Figure 21–87. Tympanogram demonstrating objective evidence that inflation of the middle ear is successful. Before inflation, the compliance peak is in the negative-pressure zone (an effusion pattern), whereas after inflation, the peak is shifted toward the positive-pressure zone.

of inflating the middle ear for the following conditions: Barotrauma (following flying or swimming) should respond ideally to the Politzer procedure if atelectasis with high negative pressure or otitis media with effusion, or both, are present. Inflation of the middle ear should be helpful under these circumstances, because this condition is usually not due to chronic eustachian tube dysfunction, and inflation may resolve the acute, subacute, or chronic disorder rapidly. When a middle-ear effusion not due to barotrauma is found in a patient who only occasionally has a problem and in whom frequently recurrent or chronic disease is not suspected, then the procedure may also be successful, especially if a small amount of serous effusion is visible behind a translucent tympanic membrane. However, it is unlikely that a mucoid or purulent effusion could be evacuated by this technique; if it could be, it would probably recur immediately after the procedure. Atelectasis of the tympanic membrane and middle ear, with or without high negative pressure, can also be treated by repeated autoinflation (Valsalva) or the Politzer method, but even if the middle ear is successfully inflated, the benefit is usually only of short duration and the procedure must be repeated frequently. Therefore, it is unlikely that inflation will be successful in alleviating for any length of time frequently recurrent or chronic eustachian tube dysfunction. There is also a remote possibility that bacteria can be forced into the middle ear from the nasopharynx during this procedure.

In conclusion, these procedures may be worthwhile for children with barotitis and for children who have an occasional episode of otitis media with effusion or atelectasis, but they are probably not helpful in children who have chronic or frequently recurrent middle-ear effusion or atelectasis, or both.

Surgical Management

Myringotomy and Tympanocentesis

Myringotomy, or the incision of the tympanic membrane for acute otitis media, was first described by Sir

Ashley Cooper in 1802 (Alberti, 1974). This procedure became increasingly popular until the 1940's, when antimicrobial agents came into wide use. Nowadays myringotomy is reserved only for selected cases and performed primarily by otolaryngologists and a handful of primary care physicians; the indications are usually limited to those children who have severe otalgia, suppurative complications, or both. However, facing an apparent recent increase in the prevalence and incidence of acute and chronic otitis media with effusion, there has been considerably more effort to study the efficacy of myringotomy in the management of this disease. The potential benefit from more liberal use of the procedure in cases of acute otitis media might be relief of otalgia and a decrease in persistence and recurrence rates. When chronic otitis media with effusion is present, myringotomy may be as effective in eliminating the middle-ear effusion as the insertion of a tympanostomy tube, with its attendant complications and sequelae (assuming a surgical procedure is indicated at all).

The results of studies conducted in the past to determine the efficacy of myringotomy for acute otitis media are shown in Table 21–33. In the study by Roddey and coworkers (1966), all 181 children received an antimicrobial agent, and, in approximately half of the subjects, myringotomy was performed as well. The only significant difference between the two groups—judged by otoscopy at 2, 10, 30 and 60 days and by audiometry at 3 to 6 months—was more rapid pain relief among a small group who had severe otalgia initially. Fewer children who had the myringotomy and antimicrobial therapy had middle-ear effusion at the end of 6 weeks than did those who received antimicrobial agents alone, but the difference was not statistically significant. However, if a larger number of children had been involved in the study, the difference might have achieved statistical significance. Herberts and colleagues (1971) found no difference in the percentages of children with persistent effusion 10 days after either myringotomy and antimicrobial therapy or

TABLE 21–33. Percentage of Patients with Persistent Middle-Ear Effusion Following Initial Myringotomy and Antimicrobial Therapy Compared with Those Receiving Antimicrobial Therapy Alone for Acute Otitis Media

INVESTIGATOR	PROCEDURE*	NUMBER OF SUBJECTS	PERCENTAGE WITH PERSISTENT EFFUSION AFTER			STATISTICAL SIGNIFICANCE ACHIEVED
			10–14 Days	4 Weeks	6 Weeks	
Roddey et al., 1966	AB	121	35	7	2	No
	AB&M	94	24	9	1	
Herberts et al., 1971	AB	81	10	—	—	No
	AB&M	91	18	—	—	
Lorentzen and Haugsten, 1977	AB	190	16	6		No
	AB&M	164	20†	6		
Puhakka et al. 1979	AB	90	78	29	—	Yes
	AB&M	68	29	10	—	
Qvarnberg and Palva, 1980	AB	151	50	—	—	Yes
	AB&M	97	28	—	—	
Schwartz and Schwartz, 1980	AB	361	47	—	—	No
	AB&M	415	51	—	—	

*AB, Antibiotic; AB&M, antibiotic and myringotomy.
†Estimated.

antimicrobial therapy alone. Lorentzen and Haugsten (1977) found the "myringotomy only" group to have the same recovery rate (88 per cent) as both the group treated with penicillin V alone and the group treated with penicillin V and myringotomy. Puhakka and coworkers (1979) repeated the same study with 158 children and found that 4 weeks after the onset of acute otitis media, 71 per cent of the children who did not undergo myringotomy but were treated with penicillin V were cured, whereas 90 per cent of the group that had myringotomy and penicillin V treatment had the same outcome, indicating that "myringotomy clearly accelerates the recovery rate from acute otitis media." Qvarnberg and Palva (1980) reported results of their study of 248 children, in which they compared the efficacy of penicillin V and myringotomy, penicillin V alone, and amoxicillin, and concluded that if the first attack of acute otitis media is treated with myringotomy and antibiotics (penicillin V or amoxicillin), cure is the rule, but that if antibiotics alone (either one) are used, 10 per cent of the patients will run a prolonged course. Schwartz and associates (1981c) treated 776 children with a variety of antimicrobial agents, half of whom also had myringotomy (without aspiration), and found no difference in the relief of pain or in the percentage with persistent effusion 10 days after myringotomy therapy.

Unfortunately, all of these studies had design and methodologic flaws that make interpreting their results and determining the value of myringotomy for acute otitis media difficult. For example, in the study conducted by Puhakka and coworkers (1979), myringotomy was performed along with aspiration of the middle-ear effusion, but it was a nonrandomized trial. However, children who received a myringotomy had a significantly shorter course of their disease than those who did not have a myringotomy. On the other hand, Schwartz and associates (1981c) failed to find a difference between those children who did and those who did not receive a myringotomy. There was no attempt to aspirate the middle-ear effusion, and the children

were not randomly assigned into the two treatment groups.

INDICATIONS

In spite of the lack of convincing evidence to support the routine use of myringotomy for *all* children with acute otitis media, there are certain indications for which there is consensus at present:

SUPPURATIVE COMPLICATIONS. Whenever a child has acute mastoiditis, labyrinthitis, facial paralysis, or one or more of the intracranial suppurative complications such as meningitis, myringotomy and aspiration should be performed as an emergency procedure. Tympanocentesis should precede myringotomy to identify the causative organism. In addition, in such cases the insertion of a tympanostomy tube should be attempted to provide prolonged drainage.

SEVERE OTALGIA REQUIRING IMMEDIATE RELIEF. Even though some studies have failed to show that myringotomy alleviated earache (Schwartz et al., 1981c), Roddey and colleagues (1966) did show that acute pain was relieved in those children who received myringotomy. Culture of the effusion is reasonable, because the middle ear is being opened, but it is not absolutely necessary if there is no reason to suspect the presence of an unusual organism.

TYMPANOCENTESIS AND MYRINGOTOMY. Although not as compelling as the above indications, whenever diagnostic tympanocentesis is indicated, myringotomy for drainage may follow the needle aspiration, especially when a copious amount of middle-ear effusion is identified by the tympanocentesis. Myringotomy may then reasonably follow tympanocentesis when acute otitis media is present and (1) when the child is critically ill; (2) when there is persistent or recurrent otalgia or fever, or both, in spite of adequate and appropriate antimicrobial therapy; (3) when acute otitis media occurs during the course of antimicrobial therapy given for another infection, and when the agent should be effective against the most common organisms causing otitis (for example, amoxicillin or ampicillin); (4) when otitis media occurs in the neonatal period; and (5) when it occurs in the immunologically compromised host. The specific indications and techniques for tympanocentesis have also been described above (p. 392).

The benefit of performing myringotomy on all infants and children with acute otitis media is uncertain at present but it is a reasonable procedure, especially if otalgia is present. If a middle-ear effusion persists after 10 to 14 days of antimicrobial therapy, myringotomy may also be appropriate if the child is still symptomatic, but if the child is relatively asymptomatic, the indications for the procedure would be less valid, as most effusions at this stage would be expected to clear spontaneously during the subsequent several weeks. If the middle-ear effusion persists for longer than 3 months, surgical drainage would appear to be a reasonable choice. If the procedure can be performed without a general anesthetic, myringotomy alone would seem appropriate, with the physician reserving the insertion of a tympanostomy tube in case the effusion recurs soon after the myringotomy incision heals. However, if a general anesthetic is required to perform the surgical drainage of chronic otitis media with effusion, myringotomy and tympanostomy tube insertion would seem a valid option at present. This recommendation is appropriate because Mandel and coworkers (1984) showed that myringotomy with insertion of a tympanostomy tube was more effective than myringotomy alone in a control group. The study was conducted in over 100 children who had chronic otitis media with effusion, which was unresponsive to amoxicillin treatment. Gates and associates (1987) also demonstrated superiority of myringotomy with tube insertion over myringotomy alone in children with chronic otitis media with effusion that was unresponsive to antimicrobial therapy.

TECHNIQUE OF MYRINGOTOMY

Tympanocentesis is a needle aspiration of the middle-ear contents for diagnostic purposes, but myringotomy is a procedure in which an incision of the tympanic membrane by a myringotomy knife is made to provide adequate drainage (Fig. 21–88). To accomplish this goal, the incision should be large enough to provide not only adequate and prolonged drainage into the external auditory canal but also aeration of the middle ear to enhance drainage down the eustachian tube. When acute otitis media is present in the infant or young child, adequate restraint employing a sheet or board especially designed for restraining children may be all that is needed; sedation is not necessary. However, for older children, sedation or even general anesthesia may be required. Iontophoresis does not effectively provide anesthesia of the tympanic membrane when acute otitis media is present. However, when myringotomy is to be performed for a middle-ear effusion when acute disease is not present, iontophoresis may be a satisfactory method. The use of a topical solution of phenol gently applied to the exact

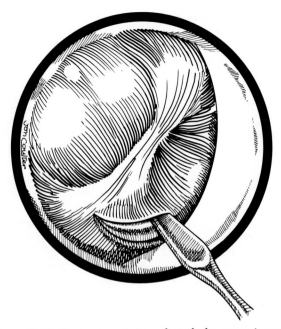

Figure 21–88. Myringotomy incision through the tympanic membrane for drainage of the middle ear. (From Bluestone, C. D., and Klein, J. O. 1988. Otitis Media in Infants and Children. Philadelphia, W. B. Saunders Co.)

spot on the tympanic membrane to be opened may be all that is necessary in older children and teen-agers. The myringotomy incision should be a wide circumferential incision encompassing both inferior quadrants of the tympanic membrane to provide adequate drainage, and an attempt should be made to aspirate as much of the middle-ear effusion as possible. Frequently, insertion of the suction tip through the incision on the tympanic membrane will enhance removal of the effusion and provide a larger opening which, it is hoped, will remain open longer than just an incision alone.

The procedure can be performed through an otoscope with a surgical head attached, or, for better magnification and binocular vision, the otomicroscope is desirable. For the routine case, the otoscope is quite adequate and makes the procedure readily available to the clinician in settings other than an operating room or otologic outpatient area, where an otomicroscope would be available. By becoming proficient with the otoscope in performing myringotomy, the physician can perform the procedure in emergency rooms, inpatient pediatric floors, the child's home, or any other setting in which a child is examined and is in need of myringotomy.

In almost all conditions in which myringotomy is performed, diagnostic tympanocentesis may precede it. In such instances, the procedure should be performed as described above.

The complications of a properly performed myringotomy are few. The persistent otorrhea that follows the procedure and is the most common finding after myringotomy can hardly be considered a complication, as it is the desired outcome; however, the discharge may become profuse and cause an eczematoid external otitis. If this occurs, meticulous cleaning of the external auditory canal with a cotton-tipped applicator; instillation of otic drops containing hydrocortisone, neomycin, and polymyxin; and insertion of a small piece of cotton (which should be changed frequently) in the outer canal will usually eliminate the problem. Dislocation of the incudostapedial joint, severing the facial nerve, and puncturing an exposed jugular bulb are dreaded complications but are so rare in experienced hands that they should not deter the trained practitioner from employing the procedure when indicated. The most common sequelae of the procedure are persistent perforation, atrophic scar, and tympanocentesis at the site of the incision. Even though the incidence of these conditions has not been systematically studied in a prospective manner, the risk of any or all occurring should not outweigh the benefits of myringotomy when indicated. The incidence of these sequelae would rise in children who require repeated myringotomy, and, in these patients, a tympanostomy tube should be considered, even though this is not without complications and sequelae.

Tympanostomy Tube Insertion

Myringotomy with insertion of tympanostomy tubes is currently the most common surgical procedure performed in children that requires general anesthesia. The use of tympanostomy tubes was first suggested by Politzer over 100 years ago, but they did not become readily available until they were reintroduced by Armstrong in 1954. Since then they have become increasingly popular. It has been estimated that in 1976 2 million tubes were manufactured and, presumably, inserted through the tympanic membranes of probably more than 1 million patients (Paradise, 1977).

CLINICAL TRIALS

Several studies have addressed the question of the efficacy of myringotomy and the insertion of tympanostomy tubes for the treatment of otitis media with effusion.

1. Shah (1971) performed a myringotomy and aspiration in one ear and a myringotomy and aspiration with tympanostomy tube insertion on the opposite ear of children with bilateral mucoid otitis media with effusion. Adenoidectomies were performed on all of these children at the time of ear surgery. Shah found that the hearing in the ears into which the tympanostomy tubes had been inserted was better than the hearing in the other ears 6 to 12 months after the procedures.

2. Kilby and colleagues (1972) also performed bilateral myringotomies (and inserted a tympanostomy tube into only one ear) in a series of children but did not perform an adenoidectomy at the same time. These investigators found no difference in the hearing in the two ears of these children 2 years after surgery, when all the tubes had been extruded.

3. Kokko (1974) compared findings in the ears of children who had undergone adenoidectomy, myringotomy, and tympanostomy tube insertion with the findings in the ears of those who had undergone adenoidectomy and myringotomy without insertion of tubes. He found, 4.5 years after the procedures, no differences in the pathologic conditions of the tympanic membranes or in the degree of hearing loss in the two groups.

4. Yagi (1977) compared 100 children who underwent an adenoidectomy, myringotomy, and tympanostomy tube insertion with 100 children who underwent only adenoidectomy. There were no significant differences between the two groups in (1) the number of children whose hearing problems were "cured" without further surgery, (2) the number of those requiring insertion of tubes due to recurrence of problems after initial treatment, (3) the number of patients having abnormal tympanic membranes, and (4) the number of patients with more than a 20-dB hearing loss 18 months after treatment.

5. Mawson and Fagan (1972) performed adenoidectomy, myringotomy, and tympanostomy tube insertion on a number of children and found that the degree of hearing loss and the number of tympanic membrane abnormalities (such as tympanosclerosis) noted increased the longer the children were followed. They reported that 76 per cent of the children in their study required insertion of another tympanostomy tube within 4 years of initial treatment.

6. Tos and Poulsen (1976) performed adenoidectomy, myringotomy, and tympanostomy tube insertion on 108 children. During a 5- to 8-year follow-up period, they reported that only 2.5 per cent of the children into whose ears tympanostomy tubes had been placed had hearing losses, but that scarring was a frequently observed abnormality.

7. Marshak and Neriah (1981) did a retrospective study on 58 children, half of whom had undergone adenoidectomy and myringotomy for chronic otitis media with effusion and the other half of whom had only had tympanostomy tubes inserted. Only 20.7 per cent of the adenoidectomized children had normal hearing and aerated middle ears during a 2-year follow-up, whereas 59 per cent of the children who had had tympanostomy tubes inserted had normal hearing and aerated middle ears at the same period.

8. Mandel and coworkers (1984) conducted a study in 102 children who had chronic otitis media with effusion that had been unresponsive to antimicrobial therapy and randomly assigned subjects to receive (1) myringotomy, (2) myringotomy and tube insertion, or (3) no surgery (control). During the first year of the trial, subjects who had tympanostomy tubes inserted had less frequent middle-ear disease and better hearing than either children who had only myringotomy perforation or those subjects in whom no surgery had been performed. In addition, half of the subjects in the myringotomy group had to have tympanostomy tubes inserted during the year, owing to an excessive number of myringotomies to control their disease. Likewise, half of the subjects in the control group

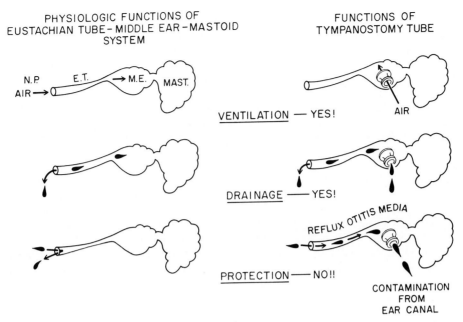

Figure 21–89. Physiologic functions of the eustachian tube that are related to the middle ear (see text). N.P., Nasopharynx; E.T., eustachian tube; M.E., middle ear; MAST., mastoid. (From Bluestone, C. D., and Klein, J. O. 1988. Otitis Media in Infants and Children, Philadelphia, W. B. Saunders Co.)

required tympanostomy tube insertion during the course of the year because of development of "significant" hearing loss associated with their chronic middle-ear effusion, even though none of the children had this degree of hearing loss when they entered the trial. Gates and associates (1987) showed similar results (see discussion of tonsillectomy and adenoidectomy, p. 457).

RATIONALE FOR USE OF TYMPANOSTOMY TUBES

Even though the completed controlled clinical trials have not been reported, tympanostomy tube insertion would appear to be beneficial, because hearing is restored and permanent structural changes within the middle ear may be prevented. The rationale for the procedure may be found in certain physiologic and pathophysiologic aspects of the nasopharynx, eustachian tube, middle ear, and mastoid air cell system that are related to the pathogenesis of otitis media. The eustachian tube has three important physiologic functions in relation to the middle ear (Fig. 21–89): (1) middle-ear pressure regulation, (2) drainage of secretions down the eustachian tube, and (3) protection of the middle ear from the entrance of unwanted nasopharyngeal secretions (Bluestone and Beery, 1976).

A functioning tympanostomy tube would maintain ambient pressure within the middle ear and mastoid and provide adequate drainage both down the eustachian tube and through the tympanostomy tube. Therefore, two physiologic functions of the eustachian tube are fulfilled by the tympanostomy tube. However, the protective function of the eustachian tube may be impaired by tympanostomy tube insertion, because all of the conventional tympanostomy tubes used leave an opening in the tympanic membrane, and the physiologic middle-ear air cushion is not present if the tympanic membrane is open. Therefore, reflux of nasopharyngeal secretions into the middle ear may be enhanced when a tympanostomy tube eliminates the middle-ear air cushion, a situation that can result in "reflux otitis media" and otorrhea.

The ideal eustachian tube prosthesis would be a transtympanic tube that fulfilled all three of the important physiologic functions of the eustachian tube: pressure regulation, drainage, *and* protection.

RECOMMENDED INDICATIONS

Even though the efficacy of tympanostomy tubes has not been established, current indications for their use seem reasonable in selected cases until such controlled studies are reported.

CHRONIC OTITIS MEDIA WITH EFFUSION. Patients who have had otitis media with effusion that has been unresponsive to a course of antimicrobial therapy for at least 3 months are reasonable candidates for the insertion of tympanostomy tubes. The use of antimicrobial agents is based on results of several studies that have demonstrated the presence of bacteria in chronic middle-ear effusions (Healy and Teele, 1977; Liu et al., 1975; Riding et al., 1978a; Senturia et al., 1958). If antimicrobial therapy is unsuccessful, then removal of the middle-ear effusion through a myringotomy incision is warranted. Persistence of otitis media with effusion immediately following myringotomy and aspiration of the effusion would be a compelling indication for the use of a tympanostomy tube. It would seem reasonable to attempt a myringotomy and aspiration of the middle ear effusion prior to insertion of a tympanostomy tube in both children and adults who do *not* require general anesthesia. However, if general anesthesia is necessary to perform a myringotomy, insertion of a tympanostomy tube at the same time would appear to be reasonable.

Removal of a middle-ear effusion that is asymptomatic, especially when significant hearing loss is not present, is questionable. If air is visualized behind a translucent tympanic membrane (i.e., bubbles or a fluid level are visible), the condition would appear to be less severe. However, all such children have some degree of conductive hearing loss, and the short- or long-term effects of even modest degrees of hearing loss on the development of a child have not been measured adequately (Hanson and Ulvestad, 1979). In addition, it is not known what chronic irreversible changes such as adhesive otitis media, tympanosclerosis, ossicular discontinuity, or cholesteatoma might occur in the middle-ear space if such an effusion is not treated. Therefore, the ultimate decision for use of tympanostomy tubes for chronic otitis media with effusion must be based on many factors, most of which remain arbitrary. At present, however, it seems to be reasonable to insert tympanostomy tubes to restore hearing and prevent possible complications and sequelae of recurrent and chronic otitis media with effusion.

RECURRENT ACUTE OTITIS MEDIA. Many children, especially infants, have recurrent episodes of acute otitis media that respond to medical therapy or resolve spontaneously, and in these children the middle-ear effusion does not become chronic. However, it would still be desirable to prevent these episodes when they occur frequently over a relatively short period of time, because hearing is affected when the middle-ear effusion is present and the child may be uncomfortable because of accompanying otalgia and fever. At present, there are three popular treatments for such episodes: (1) antimicrobial prophylaxis (Biedel, 1978; Ensign et al., 1960; Maynard et al., 1972; Perrin et al., 1974), (2) adenoidectomy with or without tonsillectomy (Bluestone et al., 1972c, 1975a), and (3) myringotomy with insertion of tympanostomy tubes (Gebhart, 1981).

In spite of the relative lack of proof of their efficacy, tympanostomy tubes may reasonably be assumed to prevent acute otitis media. Presumably, the tube could prevent aspiration of infected nasopharyngeal secretions into the middle ear, because ambient, rather than negative, middle-ear pressure would be present. Absence of negative middle-ear pressure could also prevent accumulation of a noninfected middle-ear effusion. In addition, a nonintact tympanic membrane would allow for excellent drainage down the eustachian tube of any secretions entering the middle ear. However, in children with semipatulous eustachian tubes, reflux of nasopharyngeal secretions could be enhanced when the tympanic membrane is not intact, resulting in otorrhea secondary to reflux otitis media. Studies of appropriate design to test these hypotheses are lacking. Although data are not available, myringotomy with insertion of a tympanostomy tube appears to the authors to be helpful for children who have frequent,

recurrent attacks of acute otitis media. Three or more episodes during the preceding 6 months, or at least four episodes during the preceding year (with the last episode occurring during the preceding 6 months), would be indications for performing this procedure. However, for such children a trial of antimicrobial prophylaxis would be an acceptable alternative management option, and myringotomy with insertion of tympanostomy tubes should be reserved for those children in whom chemoprophylaxis has failed. Antimicrobial prophylaxis should be considered only in those children who have *no* evidence of a middle-ear effusion between the acute attacks. For those children who have recurrent acute episodes superimposed on a chronic otitis media with effusion, tympanostomy tubes should be inserted.

EUSTACHIAN TUBE DYSFUNCTION AND ATELECTASIS OF THE TYMPANIC MEMBRANE. Tympanostomy tubes may restore normal middle-ear pressure in patients who have eustachian tube dysfunction but who do *not* have a middle-ear effusion when one or more of the following conditions is present: (1) otalgia, (2) significant and symptomatic conductive hearing loss, (3) vertigo, or (4) tinnitus. If these signs and symptoms are believed to be due to eustachian tube obstruction and not related to a condition that can be improved by medical treatment (e.g., sinusitis), then tympanostomy tubes often provide relief. This is not usually the case in patients with a patulous or semipatulous eustachian tube. When an abnormally patent eustachian tube is suspected, a trial with just myringotomy should first be attempted. If the patient is symptom free when the tympanic membrane is not intact, a tympanostomy tube can then be inserted. However, if the symptoms are not eliminated or become worse, a tympanostomy tube should not be inserted. While the tympanic membrane is open, a test of eustachian tube function should be performed in an effort to determine the specific type of dysfunction present. If the function of the eustachian tube is normal, another cause of the symptoms (e.g., inner-ear disease) should be sought.

Atelectasis of the middle ear may be the result either of passive collapse of the tympanic membrane, due to lack of stiffness of the drum, or of active retraction of the tympanic membrane resulting from high negative middle-ear pressure. Atelectasis may be generalized or localized, or both, and may be accompanied by a retraction pocket in the pars flaccida or posterosuperior portion of the tympanic membrane. These two portions of the tympanic membrane are the most compliant areas of the drum (Khanna and Tonndorf, 1972). A severe retraction pocket in the posterosuperior portion of the tympanic membrane may cause irreversible destruction of the incus, with resultant conductive hearing loss. Progression of such a retraction pocket may also result in a cholesteatoma. This sequence of events has been shown to be associated with eustachian tube dysfunction (Bluestone et al., 1977b) and may be reversed by insertion of a tympanostomy tube. However, if the retraction pocket is associated with adhesive otitis media in which the

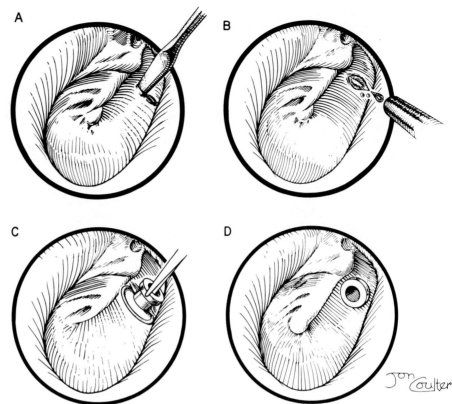

Figure 21–90. Method of insertion of a tympanostomy tube. *A,* Radial incision in the tympanic membrane. *B,* Middle-ear effusion aspirated. *C,* Short, biflanged tympanostomy tube (Armstrong type) inserted using alligator forceps. *D,* Tube position in anterosuperior portion of tympanic membrane.

tympanic membrane is adherent to the incudostapedial joint and the surrounding area, restoration of normal intratympanic pressure with a tympanostomy tube may not be successful in returning the tympanic membrane to its neutral position. Following tympanostomy tube insertion, persistence of such a retraction pocket in the attic or in the posterosuperior quadrant, or in both, may require a tympanoplastic procedure in an effort to prevent progressive disease. However, when tympanoplasty is performed in such ears and eustachian tube function is abnormal, insertion of a tympanostomy tube should be considered postoperatively to maintain normal middle-ear regulation of pressure, which should prevent recurrence of the retraction pocket and possibly development of a cholesteatoma (Bluestone et al., 1978, 1979*a*).

SURGICAL TECHNIQUE AND TYPE OF TUBE EMPLOYED

Insertion of a tympanostomy tube into the posterosuperior quadrant of the tympanic membrane is not advised, as this is the most compliant part of the pars tensa and may result in a permanent perforation or an atrophic scar with subsequent retraction pocket. A retraction pocket could lead to necrosis of the incus or formation of a cholesteatoma, or both. Insertion of a tympanostomy tube under the annulus also may result in a cholesteatoma. It seems more appropriate to insert the tube into the anterior portion of the pars tensa. In fact, when there is severe generalized atelectasis, the

anterosuperior portion may be the only area into which a tympanostomy tube can be inserted (Fig. 21–90).

The type of tube employed varies with the surgeon. The short, double-flanged tubes appear to provide adequate middle-ear aeration without a high incidence of obstruction of the lumen by mucus or cerumen, but water can more readily enter the ear through a short tube. However, when the longer type of tube is used, there is a greater chance of obstruction of the lumen. The size of the lumen of the tube is quite variable, but, again, if the lumen is too small, obstruction is a problem, and if the lumen is too large, removal or spontaneous extrusion of the tube could result in a persistent perforation. Tubes are made of various materials, but no data are available to show the superiority of one type of biocompatible material over another.

Much controversy exists concerning the indications for insertion of tympanostomy tubes that are more or less "permanent." Insertion of such tubes may be warranted in selected patients: those in whom tympanostomy tubes have frequently been tried and in whom eustachian tube dysfunction appears to be not only chronic but also not likely to improve in the near future. "Permanent" tubes may also be used in adults with long-standing chronic otitis media with effusion or severe atelectasis. However, these tubes should not be used in children, because the incidence of otitis media with effusion and atelectasis of the tympanic membrane progressively decreases with advancing age during childhood. This is true even for children with cleft palates who have had repeated myringotomies.

On the infrequent occasions when permanent tympanostomy tubes are used in children, the function of the eustachian tube should be tested periodically to determine when or if there is evidence of improvement so that the tube may be removed.

Even though many ways to assess eustachian tube function have been tried, there is currently no known method that surpasses observation of the middle ear when the tympanic membrane is intact. Therefore, the best way to determine if a patient needs another tympanostomy tube after the tube extrudes spontaneously is to examine the ears frequently.

WHEN SHOULD TYMPANOSTOMY TUBES BE REMOVED?

In general, after tubes have been inserted, they should be permitted to extrude spontaneously into the external auditory canal and not be removed surgically. The rationale for such management is based on experience rather than on any controlled clinical trials: in children with tympanostomy tubes in place, eustachian tube function has not been shown to change significantly, even after several years (Beery et al., 1979).

There are, however, some exceptions to this generalization. Serial eustachian tube function tests should be carried out, and if significant improvement does occur, then the tympanostomy tube may be removed.

Most tympanostomy tubes remain in the tympanic membrane for 6 to 12 months, although some have been known to have remained in place for years. In children in whom tympanostomy tubes have been inserted bilaterally and in whom one tube subsequently extrudes but the other remains in place for a prolonged period, the remaining tube can usually be removed if the opposite middle ear remains free of high negative middle-ear pressure or middle-ear effusion, or both, for at least 1 year after the spontaneous extrusion of the opposite tube. This method of management is based on the observation that eustachian tube function is usually about the same in both ears in children. If high negative middle-ear pressure or otitis media with effusion, or both, occur during the observation period, the tube in the opposite ear should not be removed. Unfortunately, this method of management cannot be employed in adults, as eustachian tube function may not be symmetric.

COMPLICATIONS AND SEQUELAE

Complications of insertion of tympanostomy tubes include scarring of the tympanic membrane (tympanosclerosis) and localized or diffuse membrane atrophy, with or without retraction pockets, or atelectasis, or both (Kokko, 1974; Mawson and Fagan, 1972; Muenker, 1980). Much less commonly, a perforation may remain at the insertion site following extrusion of the tube, or a cholesteatoma may develop. Other complications include secondary infection accompanied by otorrhea through the tube and dislocation of the tube into the middle-ear cavity.

The most common complication of tympanostomy

tube insertion is otorrhea through the lumen of the tube. This is usually the result of reflux of nasopharyngeal secretions into the middle ear. Otorrhea occurs in two thirds of infants with unrepaired cleft palates who have had tympanostomy tubes inserted to treat chronic otitis media with effusion and who are followed during the first 2 years of life (Paradise and Bluestone, 1974). However, otorrhea may also occur in children without cleft palates in whom tubes have been inserted. When this occurs, a culture should be obtained from the middle ear by obtaining an aspirate through the tympanostomy tube. A preliminary culture of the ear canal and meticulous cleaning of the ear canal should precede the aspiration of the middle ear. Oral systemic antimicrobial therapy should be guided by middle-ear culture and sensitivity studies. Topical antimicrobials and irrigation of the middle ear with a variety of agents has been advocated, but the ototoxic effect of these medications must be considered (see discussion of chronic suppurative otitis media in Chap. 22).

When frequently recurrent episodes of acute otitis media occur despite the presence of a functioning tympanostomy tube, antimicrobial prophylaxis should be given to prevent the recurrent middle-ear infection and otorrhea. The selection of antibiotic and dose would be the same as recommended for antimicrobial prophylaxis alone (see discussion of prevention, p. 442).

PROTECTION OF EAR WHEN TUBES ARE IN PLACE

Water from bathing or swimming should not be allowed to enter the middle ear through the tympanostomy tube, as contamination usually results in otitis media and discharge. During bathing or hair washing, a wad of either lamb's wool or cotton covered with petroleum jelly should be inserted into the external auditory meatus. Ear defenders* are usually effective in protecting the middle ear and may be used to permit the patient to swim; surface swimming only is recommended, as diving or swimming deeply under water may lead to contamination of the middle ear.

CONCLUSIONS

It is extremely important to continue to determine the efficacy of insertion of tympanostomy tubes in patients with recurrent acute or chronic otitis media with effusion, as well as with certain related conditions such as atelectasis of the tympanic membrane and middle ear. However, the apparent beneficial results obtained by this technique warrant its continued use. It does not seem that the use of tympanostomy tubes is a modern fad that will become obsolete in the near future. Recurrent acute otitis media and chronic otitis media with effusion are extremely prevalent in infants and young children but are conditions that are highly age related. Because hearing loss attributable to otitis

---

*Mine Safety Appliance Co., Pittsburgh, PA.

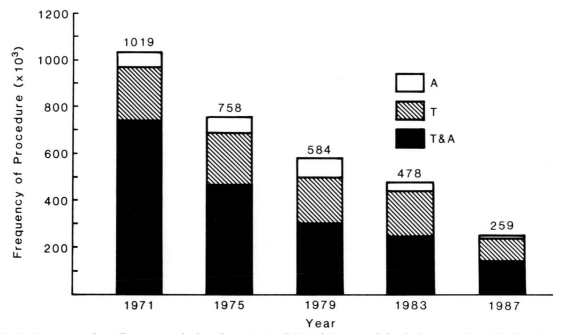

Figure 21–91. Frequency of tonsillectomies and adenoidectomies in all United States nonfederal, short-term hospitals (based on National Center for Health Statistics, National Hospital Discharge Survey, from non-federal, short-stay hospitals, 1986). Frequency (in 1000's) tonsillectomy (T), adenoidectomy (A), and T & A, 1971–1987.

media during infancy and early childhood may impair language or cognitive development, and because insertion of tympanostomy tubes permits hearing preservation and probably prevents many of the complications and sequelae of otitis media while the tubes are in place, their use is advocated even though otitis media usually improves with increasing age. Tympanostomy tubes are indicated in the following types of cases: (1) chronic otitis media with effusion that has been present for at least 3 months and is unresponsive to or not improving progressively with antimicrobial therapy and whose duration is either documented or evident from the history; (2) at least three episodes of recurrent acute otitis media within the preceding 6 months, the frequency documented or evident from the history, especially when antimicrobial prophylaxis has failed or is not deemed feasible or desirable; (3) eustachian tube dysfunction resulting in one or more of the following: significant and symptomatic hearing loss, otalgia, vertigo, tinnitus, or severe atelectasis, especially in those ears in which a deep retraction pocket is present in the posterosuperior quadrant or pars flaccida, or both; (4) following tympanoplasty, when eustachian tube function is known to be poor; and (5) when a suppurative complication is present, such as facial paralysis, as tympanostomy tubes can provide drainage of the middle ear.

Tonsillectomy and Adenoidectomy

Adenoidectomy performed either separately or in combination with tonsillectomy is the most common major surgical procedure employed to prevent otitis media; myringotomy with tympanostomy tube inser-

tion is the most common minor surgical procedure for otitis media (Paradise, 1977).

Tonsil and adenoid surgery are the most common major operations performed in the United States; approximately one fourth of all children undergo tonsillectomy and adenoidectomy during childhood. Such operations account for about one half of all major surgical operations performed on children, one fourth of all hospital admissions of children, and 10 per cent of hospital bed-days utilized by children. In 1985, about 400,000 procedures on the tonsils and adenoids were performed in the United States, which, as shown in Figure 21–91, represents a significant reduction from the over 1 million such operations performed 10 years earlier.

However, this decrease in the total number of tonsil and adenoid operations may be related to a demographic change, as the total reduction during the same period in the number of children in the age group concerned was approximately 20 per cent. Although the number of adenoidectomies without tonsillectomy remained relatively small in comparison with the number of tonsillectomies performed either separately or in combination with adenoidectomy, there was more than a twofold increase in the performance of adenoidectomy without tonsillectomy. Also, there appears to be a wide variation in the rate of performance of these operations by region of the country; the rates for adenoidectomy vary the most widely (National Center for Health Statistics, 1974). However, there are no data available related to the indications for which these operations were performed. Certainly, for many of these surgical procedures, otitis media was one of the indications, and in many instances the only indication, for adenoidectomy either with or without tonsillectomy.

CLINICAL TRIALS

The following is a summary of the results of the clinical trials that have been conducted as they relate to the efficacy of adenoidectomy and tonsillectomy for prevention of otitis media. In 1930, Kaiser reported the results of following 4400 children, on one half of whom tonsillectomy and adenoidectomy were performed (the indications for surgery were not reported). Table 21–34 shows the results of his retrospective analysis of the prevalence of purulent otorrhea 10 years after surgery. Even though there was no difference in incidence of purulent otorrhea in the children who had been operated on and those who had not, the study cannot be considered to indicate conclusively the lack of efficacy of tonsillectomy and adenoidectomy in preventing otitis media because (1) the two groups may not have been similar at the outset, (2) they were not randomized, (3) the analysis was retrospective, and (4) only purulent otorrhea was considered as a measurement of the effectiveness of tonsillectomy and adenoidectomy.

The first truly prospective clinical trial of tonsillectomy and adenoidectomy was reported by McKee (1963a). The criterion for entry into the study was a history of at least three episodes of "throat infection" or of acute upper respiratory tract infection with cervical adenitis during the preceding year. Table 21–35 shows the mean incidence of otitis media 1 and 2 years following treatment, in those (randomly chosen) children who underwent tonsillectomy and adenoidectomy compared with those who did not.

The mean incidence of otitis media among control subjects was twice as high as among children having the tonsillectomy and adenoidectomy during the first year of the trial, but during the second year there was no difference in incidence of otitis media in the group that had been operated on and the control group. However, this study was based on the occurrence of sore throats and not on the presence of middle-ear disease in the year preceding the study. In fact, subjects were initially excluded from the study if they had "marked deafness, or recurrent or chronic otitis media." In addition, the follow-up evaluation was based solely on interview data, with no objective examinations being made, and no attempt was made

TABLE 21–34. Prevalence of Purulent Otorrhea in 2200 Children Who Received Tonsillectomy with Adenoidectomy and 2200 "Comparable" Children Who Did Not

	T&A (%)	NO T&A (%)
Before operation	15	12
10 years after operation	5	6

T&A, Tonsillectomy and adenoidectomy.
With permission from Kaiser, A. D. 1930. Results of tonsillectomy: A comparative study of 2,200 tonsillectomized children with an equal number of controls three and ten years after operation. JAMA 95:837–842. Copyright 1930, American Medical Association.

TABLE 21–35. Mean Incidence of Otitis Media in Children Aged 2 to 15 Years Receiving Tonsillectomy with Adenoidectomy Compared with Control Group

	CONTROL (NUMBER)	T&A (NUMBER)	t
First year	0.33 (154)	0.17 (222)	2.52*
Second year	0.17 (139)	0.14 (213)	0.54

*Significant change p < 0.01.
T&A, Tonsillectomy and adenoidectomy.
With permission from McKee, W. J. 1963. A controlled study of the effects of tonsillectomy and adenoidectomy in children. Br. J. Prev. Soc. Med. 17:46–49.

to detect asymptomatic otitis media with effusion or impairment of hearing.

In a second study, McKee (1963b) attempted to distinguish the effects of tonsillectomy from those of adenoidectomy. The criterion for entry into the study was the same as in the first study and, again, children with deafness and otitis media were excluded. Two hundred children were randomly assigned to undergo either tonsillectomy and adenoidectomy or adenoidectomy only. The mean incidence of otitis media in each of the two surgical groups was approximately the same.

Therefore, McKee concluded from the two studies that otitis media was infrequent after adenoidectomy or tonsillectomy and adenoidectomy and that the combined operation did not offer any particular advantages in the prevention of the disease. Even though the studies did not select children with a high morbidity of otitis media, McKee stated that it was reasonable to infer that adenoidectomy without tonsillectomy was indicated for the prevention of otitis media with effusion.

Mawson and associates (1967) reported a prospective study of tonsillectomy and adenoidectomy. The design of their experiment was similar to that of the first McKee study in that an unspecified number of children who were severely affected were excluded and operated on. Minimal criteria for entry were not described. Table 21–36 shows the relative incidence of earache and otitis media before and 1 and 2 years after randomization of 404 children into either the tonsillectomy and adenoidectomy or control group.

There was no apparent difference at any age between the two groups. However, over one half of the children did not have otitis media prior to entry (Table 21–36), and the occurrence of asymptomatic otitis media with effusion or the incidence of hearing loss was not reported.

A study from New Zealand used an experimental design similar to McKee's (Roydhouse, 1970). In addition to the group of children who were referred for tonsillectomy and adenoidectomy and who were randomized into surgical and no-surgery groups, a third matched group of children who were presumably normal were followed during the trial. Table 21–37 shows the mean incidence of otitis media in the three groups:

TABLE 21–36. Relative Frequency of Earache and Otitis Media in 404 Children Receiving Tonsillectomy and Adenoidectomy Compared with Control Group

NUMBER OF EPISODES	YEAR PRIOR TO TRIAL (%)		FIRST YEAR OF TRIAL (%)		SECOND YEAR OF TRIAL (%)	
	T&A	Control	T&A	Control	T&A	Control
0	63	65	59	57	58.5	57.5
1	5	4.5	7.5	15	7	9.5
2–3	19	22.5	15.5	18	9	11
4–6	6	3	3.5	2	1	1.5
>7	5	4		2.5		1

T&A, Tonsillectomy and adenoidectomy.

With permission from Mawson, S. R., Adlington, R., and Evans, M. 1967. A controlled study evaluation of adeno-tonsillectomy in children. J. Laryngol. Otol. 81:777–790.

tonsillectomy and adenoidectomy, tonsillectomy and adenoidectomy withheld, and controls. The results were similar to those reported by McKee, in that there was a reduction in the incidence of otitis media in the first year after tonsillectomy and adenoidectomy, but this difference was not maintained into the second year. However, in the second year of the trial, the total duration of episodes of otitis media in the tonsillectomy and adenoidectomy group was less than 60 per cent of the duration of those that occurred before surgery. Roydhouse (1970) concluded that the operation not only reduced the incidence of otitis media quickly in the first year but also reduced the severity in both the first and second years after surgery. However, as in the previous studies, patients whose main symptoms were aural were excluded, and there was no attempt to detect asymptomatic otitis media with effusion or impairment in hearing.

In a second clinical trial, Roydhouse (1980) randomly divided 100 children with persistent otitis media into two groups, adenoidectomy with tympanostomy tube insertion and tympanostomy tube insertion alone. All had failed to respond to a nonsurgical treatment regimen. He compared these two groups with a third group of 69 other children who had had otitis media but had all been found to be free of middle-ear effusion following nonsurgical management and received no surgical treatment.

The cure rate was similar in each of the operative groups, with a greater relapse rate in the nonadenoidectomy group, who required 9 per cent more tympanostomy tube insertions. An estimation from radiographs of the size of the adenoids showed that the group cured without surgery had somewhat smaller adenoids. The relapse rate in the group who received tympanostomy tubes only was independent of the size

of the adenoids. The study failed to show a favorable outcome following adenoidectomy.

In a study of children with bilateral chronic otitis media with effusion, Maw (1984) randomly assigned subjects into (1) adenoidectomy, (2) adenoidectomy and tonsillectomy, and (3) nonsurgical control. Tympanostomy tubes were inserted into only one ear of each child; the contralateral ear was not operated on and was observed for 1 year. One third of the children in the nonsurgical control group had resolution of their middle-ear effusion during the year, and one third of the two surgical groups had persistent or recurrent disease following adenoidectomy with or without tonsillectomy (Fig. 21–92). Maw concluded that adenoidectomy conferred benefit in about one third of the subjects, but those children likely to benefit by the operation could not be identified prior to surgery. In addition, he reported that the addition of tonsillectomy to the adenoidectomy had no more beneficial effect than adenoidectomy alone.

Unfortunately, all of these prospective controlled studies had one or more of the following limitations in experimental design: (1) entry into the study was based on the occurrence of a sore throat and not on the presence of otitis media; (2) objective evidence of otitis media was not documented by tympanometry or audiometry; (3) other surgical procedures that may have been performed (myringotomy or tympanostomy tube insertions, for example) were not reported; (4) the technique of adenoidectomy (e.g., "midline sweep" or thorough removal of adenoid tissue from the fossa of Rosenmüller) was not described, nor was evidence of complete removal of the adenoids documented; and (5) nasal and eustachian tube function were not assessed objectively.

In a recent study by Gates and associates (1987),

TABLE 21–37. Mean Incidence per Year of Otitis Media in Children Receiving Tonsillectomy and Adenoidectomy Compared with Two Control Groups

	T&A		T&A WITHHELD		CONTROL	
	Mean Incidence	Number of Children	Mean Incidence	Number of Children	Mean Incidence	Number of Children
First year of trial	0.19	251	0.29	175	0.12	173
Second year of trial	0.09	204	0.07	122	0.08	173

T&A, Tonsillectomy and adenoidectomy.

Data extracted from Roydhouse, N. 1970. A controlled study of adenotonsillectomy. Arch. Otolaryngol. 92:611–616.

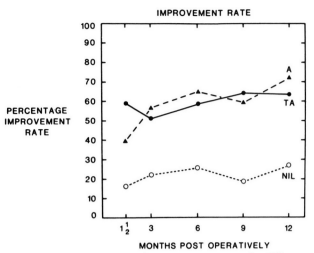

Figure 21–92. Percentage of improvement rate of middle-ear effusion following adenoidectomy (A), tonsillectomy and adenoidectomy (TA), and no surgery (NIL). (From Maw, A. R. 1984. Chronic otitis media with effusion and adenotonsillectomy: A prospective randomized controlled study. *In* Lim, D. J., Bluestone, C. D., Klein, J. O., and Nelson, J. D. [eds.]: Recent Advances in Otitis Media with Effusion. Toronto, B. C. Decker, p. 301.)

578 4- to 8-year-old children with chronic otitis media with effusion, which was unresponsive to a course of antimicrobial therapy, were randomized to receive (1) myringotomy, (2) myringotomy and tympanostomy tube insertion, (3) adenoidectomy and myringotomy, and (4) adenoidectomy, myringotomy, and tympanostomy tube insertion. Table 21–38 shows a summary of the outcome of this trial. The myringotomy group had a greater percentage of time with middle-ear effusion, greater percentage of time with hearing loss, the shortest time to first recurrence, and more repeat surgical procedures, over the 2-year follow-up period, than did the other three groups. Adenoidectomy and myringotomy, with and without tympanostomy tube insertion, was more effective than myringotomy and tube insertion; however, the mean time to first recurrence was longer in both groups that included tympanostomy tube insertion. Gates and associates (1987) concluded that adenoidectomy, irrespective of adenoid size, should be considered when surgical therapy is indicated in children (of the age group studied) who are severely affected by chronic otitis media with effusion; their recommendation is for adenoidectomy and myringotomy, without tympanostomy tube insertion, because purulent otorrhea through the tube was a problem in their study.

Children's Hospital of Pittsburgh Studies

At the Children's Hospital of Pittsburgh randomized, controlled trials are currently in progress to determine the efficacy of tonsillectomy and adenoidectomy (see Chap. 53; see also Paradise et al., 1988; Mandel et al., 1988). The effect of adenoidectomy on otitis media is one of the primary research questions, and an attempt is being made to document and control those factors cited as lacking in the previous studies cited above. The criterion for entry into the study (to deal with the problem of performing adenoidectomies for otitis media with effusion) is documented episodes of recurrent acute otitis media or chronic otitis media with effusion in a child who has had a myringotomy and insertion of a tympanostomy tube at least once previously. Applying stringent surgical indications, of course, requires careful evaluation. After initial examination, each patient is examined every 6 weeks and at the time of any respiratory illness. Pneumatic otoscopy is always performed at every visit. A trained interviewer telephones each home every 2 weeks to determine whether there has been apparent or suspected illness, to make sure that any ill child is brought in promptly for examination, and to obtain routine information on school attendance, medication usage, and a number of minor symptoms.

Allergy screening is part of every child's work-up. A nasal smear is examined for eosinophils, and a battery of skin tests using common inhalant allergens is applied. Other regularly performed studies include lateral soft tissue radiography of the nasopharynx, to assess adenoid size; sinus radiography, when sinusitis is suspected; and audiometry and tympanometry, to evaluate hearing and middle-ear status and tympanic membrane compliance.

The degree of middle-ear disease developing in the adenoidectomy and nonadenoidectomy groups, respectively, is measured on the basis of three main variables: (1) number of episodes per year of otitis media with effusion, (2) months of middle-ear effusion, and (3) frequency with which myringotomy is carried out subsequent to the child's entering the clinical trial.

TABLE 21–38. Effectiveness of Various Treatments in 578 Children with Chronic Otitis Media with Effusion

OUTCOME*	MYRINGOTOMY	MYRINGOTOMY AND TUBE INSERTION	ADENOIDECTOMY AND MYRINGOTOMY	ADENOIDECTOMY, MYRINGOTOMY, AND TUBE INSERTION
Percentage of time with effusion	49.1%	34.9%	30.2%	25.8%
Percentage of time with hearing loss†	37.5%	30.4%	22.0%	22.4%
Median time to first recurrence	54 days	222 days	92 days	240 days
No surgical retreatments	66	36	17	17

*During 2-year follow-up.
†Hearing loss equal to or greater than 20 dB.
Adapted with permission from Gates, G. A., et al. 1987. Effectiveness of adenoidectomy and tympanostomy tubes in treatment of chronic otitis media with effusion. N. Engl. J. Med. 317:1444.

Data concerning subjects assigned randomly either to receive adenoidectomy or to enter the nonadenoidectomy control group are maintained separately from data concerning subjects whose parents decline randomization and opt for or against adenoidectomy.

Preliminary analyses of data currently available may be summarized by stating that, in study subjects (1) adenoidectomy by no means eliminates the problem of recurrent otitis media in some children, whereas (2) adenoidectomy does somewhat reduce the rate, severity, or duration of recurrent episodes of middle-ear effusion in others; the rate of recurrent acute otitis media was not significantly reduced and children with nasal allergy had no demonstrable reduction in otitis media after adenoidectomy (Paradise et al., 1987). The following variables are being examined as potentially important in affecting the outcome of adenoidectomy for otitis media with effusion and in identifying which children might or might not benefit from surgery: age, sex, race, allergy, adenoid size, and eustachian tube function.

This study does not address the question of whether tonsillectomy and adenoidectomy is more effective in the prevention of otitis media with effusion than adenoidectomy alone, nor will it answer the question of the relative value of adenoidectomy with or without tonsillectomy for children who have not received myringotomy and insertion of tympanostomy tubes in the past. These questions are being addressed in a randomized clinical trial currently being conducted at the same institution.

EFFECT OF ADENOIDECTOMY ON EUSTACHIAN TUBE FUNCTION

In an attempt to improve criteria for the preoperative selection of patients for adenoidectomy, radiographic studies of the nasopharynx and eustachian tube prior to surgery and after adenoidectomy were reported (Bluestone et al., 1972c). Of 27 patients who had preoperative obstruction of the nasopharyngeal end of the eustachian tube, adenoidectomy appeared to be helpful in 19 (70 per cent). Results appeared to be quite poor in children with nasal allergy: only two of ten had good results. Furthermore, children who preoperatively showed reflux of contrast medium from the nasopharynx into the middle ear did not benefit from adenoidectomy. In this study, 20 of 33 (60 per cent) children seemed to have a favorable response to adenoidectomy, but 8 had more severe middle-ear disease after the operation than before. For example, a few of the children who had asymptomatic otitis media with effusion prior to adenoidectomy developed recurrent acute symptomatic otitis media with effusion following the procedure.

Figure 21–93 shows a lateral roentgenographic study of a child with chronic secretory otitis media who received an adenoidectomy. Before surgery the adenoids were adjudged to be of only moderate size. Eight weeks following the adenoidectomy the adenoid size appeared only somewhat smaller. However, when the pre- and postadenoidectomy submentovertex views were compared in the same child, the function of the eustachian tube at the nasopharyngeal end appeared obstructed before the operation and normal following the operation (Fig. 21–94). This example demonstrates that lateral roentgenographic views alone may not be sufficient to assess the effect of the adenoids on the nasopharyngeal end of the eustachian tube.

The ventilatory function of the eustachian tube has been studied using the inflation-deflation manometric technique both before and after adenoidectomy in a group of children with otitis media with effusion in whom a tympanostomy tube had been inserted (Bluestone et al., 1975a). Inflation-deflation studies of the eustachian tube were obtained in ears that remained intubated, aerated, and dry both before and 8 weeks after adenoidectomy. Nasal pressures during swallowing were also determined in some. The results of this study indicated that, following adenoidectomy, eustachian tube ventilatory function improved in some, remained the same in others, and appeared to have been made worse in a few children. Improvement was related to a reduction of extrinsic mechanical obstruction of the eustachian tube (Fig. 21–95) or to nasal obstruction by the adenoids (Fig. 21–96), whereas in those in whom the function was adjudged worse, the tube was considered to be more pliant after the adenoidectomy than before. This increase in compliance was attributed to loss of adenoid support of the eustachian tube in the fossa of Rosenmüller (Fig. 21–97). A comparable situation was described in the radiographic study in which several of the children demonstrated reflux of radiopaque liquid medium from the nasopharynx into the middle ear after the adenoidectomy but not before (Fig. 21–98).

However, neither of these studies (Bluestone et al., 1972, 1975) included control subjects. In one of the current investigations of adenoidectomy conducted at the Children's Hospital of Pittsburgh (Mandel et al., 1988), eustachian tube ventilatory function studies employing the inflation-deflation manometric technique are performed prior to and after randomized selection of children for the study and at any time an upper respiratory tract infection supervenes; the degree of nasal obstruction is also being assessed. Because eustachian tube ventilatory function has been shown to be affected adversely by an upper respiratory tract infection (Bluestone et al., 1977a), it is important to assess this function when an upper respiratory tract infection is present as well as when infection is absent in children both before and after randomization into either the adenoidectomy or the control group. The goal of this study is to determine if adenoidectomy is efficacious in preventing otitis media with effusion in children, and if so, whether or not a simple eustachian tube function test may be helpful in determining who may be helped by the procedure. An additional question would be which type of adenoidectomy ("midline sweep" or also removing the adenoids from the fossa of Rosenmüller) is indicated for the individual child. It is hoped that some or all of these questions will be answered by studies under way.

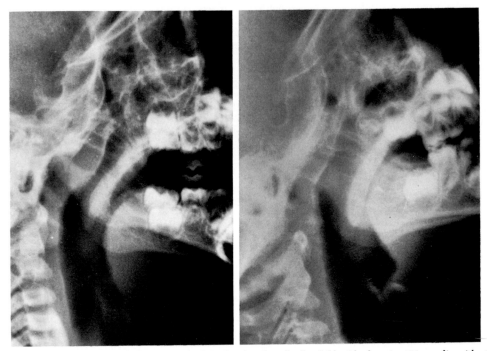

Figure 21–93. Lateral roentgenograms of the soft tissues of the head and neck of a child with chronic otitis media with effusion. Prior to adenoidectomy, the adenoids were considered to be of only moderate size (left). On the postadenoidectomy roentgenogram, they appeared slightly smaller (right).

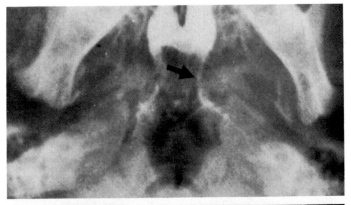

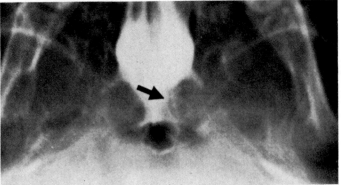

Figure 21–94. Preadenoidectomy submentovertex roentgenogram (top) demonstrating extrinsic compression of the nasopharyngeal end of the eustachian tube (arrow) in the same child described in Figure 21–93. Following adenoidectomy (bottom), contrast material entered the mouth of the eustachian tube, and the torus tubarius (arrow) was not obstructed by the adenoids.

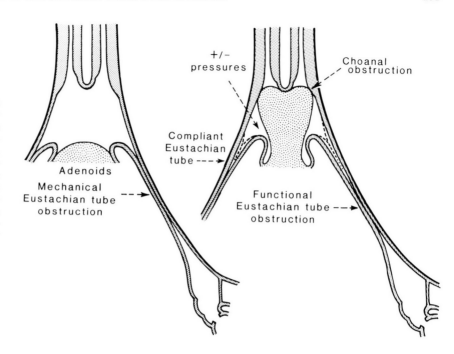

Figure 21–95. Two proposed mechanisms by which obstructive adenoids could alter eustachian tube function. The adenoids can cause extrinsic mechanical compression of the eustachian tube in the fossa of Rosenmüller (left). Obstruction of the posterior nasal choanae may result in abnormal nasopharyngeal pressures that develop during swallowing (Toynbee phenomenon); it may cause insufflation into the middle ear of nasopharyngeal secretions, prevent the tube from opening, or both (right).

CONCLUSIONS

Prospective studies conducted prior to the 1980's to determine the efficacy of tonsillectomy and adenoidectomy or adenoidectomy alone for otitis media showed a modest reduction in the incidence of ear disease following surgery in some studies (McKee, 1963a and b; Roydhouse, 1970) but no reduction in others (Kaiser, 1930; Mawson et al., 1967; Roydhouse, 1980). However, all of these studies had shortcomings in design and method. Three recently reported randomized clinical trials (Maw, 1983; Paradise et al., 1987; Gates et al., 1987), in which most of the problems of the earlier studies were eliminated, have shown a modest, but significant reduction in the morbidity of

chronic otitis media with effusion following adenoidectomy, which appeared to be independent of adenoid size. However, only in the Paradise and associates' (1987) trial was the question of efficacy of adenoidectomy for prevention of recurrent acute otitis media addressed, and the results did demonstrate benefit following the operation. In addition, all three studies showed that some subjects who received adenoidectomy had recurrent otitis media despite the surgery, whereas others who did not have an adenoidectomy were relatively free of the disease.

The ongoing studies of tonsillectomy and adenoidectomy being conducted at the Children's Hospital of Pittsburgh (Paradise et al., 1988; Mandel et al., 1988)

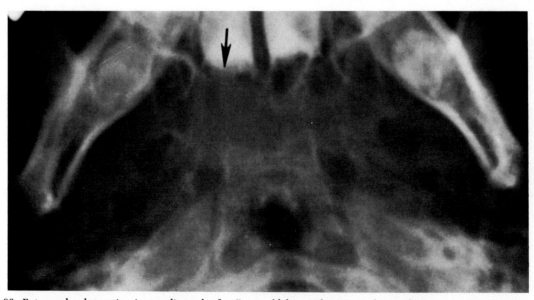

Figure 21–96. Retrograde obstruction in a radiograph of a 5-year-old boy with otitis media. Radiopaque medium failed to enter the nasopharyngeal portion of the eustachian tube during both open-nose and closed-nose swallowing. Note enlarged adenoids (arrow). (From Bluestone, C. D., and Klein, J. O. 1988. Otitis Media in Infants and Children. Philadelphia, W. B. Saunders Co.)

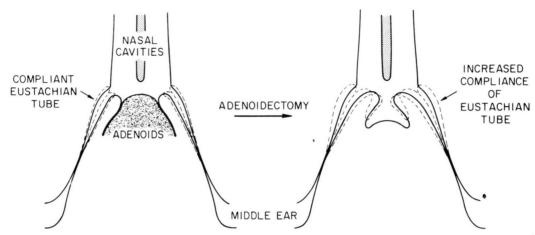

Figure 21–97. Proposed mechanism by which removal of adenoids can result in a more pliant eustachian tube after surgery than before. The increase in compliance following the surgery may be due to decrease in tubal support as a result of the adenoids being removed from the fossa of Rosenmüller.

are attempting to determine whether adenoidectomy, with or without tonsillectomy, is helpful in decreasing the morbidity of otitis media, so that children who stand to benefit can be helped, whereas those who may not can be spared the cost, discomfort, and risks of surgery. At present, the clinician who is faced with a child who has recurrent or chronic otitis media must decide if the potential benefits of these operative procedures outweigh the costs and potential risks following assessment of each child individually. That assessment should include, among others (1) type of otitis media (i.e., recurrent or chronic otitis media with effusion or recurrent acute otitis media, or both); (2) frequency, duration, and severity of the middle-ear disease; (3) age of the child; (4) presence of other, coexisting conditions that would make adenoidectomy or tonsillectomy more compelling, such as frequently recurrent pharyngotonsillitis (Paradise et al., 1984) or upper airway obstruction caused by obstructive adenoids or tonsils (Chap. 53); (5) presence or absence of upper respiratory tract allergy or infection, or both; and (6) thoughtful consideration to other management options, such as watchful waiting, antimicrobial prophylaxis, or myringotomy and insertion of tympanos-

tomy tubes. Decisions for or against these options should include the child (if old enough to comprehend) and the parents.

Tympanoplasty for Atelectasis of Tympanic Membrane

In selected cases in which severe atelectasis is present, a tympanoplastic procedure may be indicated. The most compelling indication for such a procedure would be the presence of a deep retraction pocket in the posterosuperior portion of the pars tensa that is unresponsive to nonsurgical and other surgical methods of management previously described for this defect. For example, if a tympanostomy tube had been inserted previously but the retraction pocket did not return to the neutral position after several months of equalization of the intratympanic pressure, tympanoplasty should be considered, as adhesive otitis media is most likely binding the drum to the ossicles and surrounding structures within the middle ear. Even though the natural history of such deep retraction pockets has not been formally studied, the risk of erosion necrosis of the incus or formation of a choles-

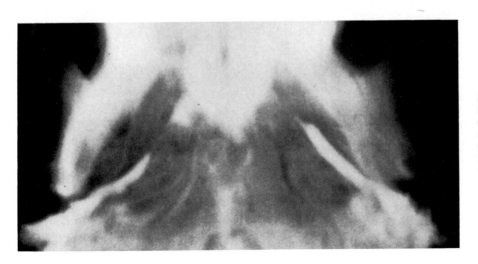

Figure 21–98. Postadenoidectomy roentgenogram of a child who demonstrated reflux of radiopaque media from the nasopharynx into the middle ear. This did not occur during the preadenoidectomy roentgenographic study.

teatoma, or both, appears to be quite high. It is frequently difficult to determine if there is only a retraction pocket present or if a cholesteatoma has already developed; therefore, a thorough examination of the entire external canal and tympanic membrane should be performed with the otomicroscope. An examination under general anesthesia will be required for all infants and children in whom the examination is unsatisfactory without general anesthesia. With the patient anesthetized, a thorough examination of the retraction pocket, employing a curved, blunt probe, should be performed to determine the extent of the pocket. In addition, the continuity of the incus and stapes should be assessed, because erosion of the long process of the incus may require surgical correction. Frequently, when nitrous oxide is employed as one of the anesthetic agents, the retraction pocket can be seen to balloon laterally, as visualized through the otomicroscope. When this occurs, insertion of the tympanostomy tube will usually be sufficient to prevent recurrence of the retraction pocket. However, reinsertion of the tube may be needed if a retraction pocket recurs after spontaneous extubation.

There are many techniques advocated for repair of a severely atelectatic tympanic membrane, many of which have been shown to be quite successful (Goodhill, 1979; Sheehy, 1977). However, the surgeon should be cautioned that even though the graft "takes," the child will most likely have persistent eustachian tube dysfunction with sustained fluctuating or negative intratympanic pressure after the procedure, which could result in recurrence of the retraction pocket months or years later. Therefore, a tympanostomy tube should be inserted at the time of the tympanoplastic surgery and reinserted if atelectasis begins to recur after the tympanostomy tube is spontaneously extruded. Some surgeons prefer using tragal cartilage attached to its perichondrium to cover the area of the retraction pocket so that recurrence of an attic or posterosuperior retraction pocket can be prevented (Heermann et al., 1970).

All children who require tympanoplasty for severe atelectasis must be followed at relatively frequent intervals for the first year after the procedure and at appropriate intervals for several succeeding years, since recurrence of the atelectasis should always be anticipated.

Mastoidectomy and Middle-Ear Surgery for Chronic Otitis Media with Effusion

On rare occasions a child will require mastoidectomy and middle-ear surgery to eliminate chronic otitis media with effusion when *all* other nonsurgical and surgical methods of management have failed. The operation, which has been advocated by Proctor (1971) and Paparella (1973) and described in detail by Proud and Duff (1976), should be reserved for children in whom a thorough search for an underlying origin of the chronic middle-ear effusion has failed to uncover a cause, or, if a cause was found, appropriate management (e.g., cleft palate repair) has failed to alleviate the problem. In addition, all attempts should have been made to maintain an aerated middle-ear space by means of myringotomy and insertion of a tympanostomy tube, even though the procedure may have to be repeated many times for years. If, however, the myringotomy and thorough aspiration of the middle-ear fluid is unsuccessful in eliminating the effusion and the insertion of a tympanostomy tube fails to provide an aerated middle-ear space, the child may be considered a candidate for a mastoidectomy. Examination of the mastoid and middle-ear space at the time of surgery may reveal a previously unsuspected mastoid osteitis, cholesterol granuloma, or cholesteatoma (Chap. 22). However, even when these conditions are not present, the usual findings will be a cellular mastoid containing edematous, hyperplastic mucosa, with granulomatous tissue, polypoid tissue, and a thick mucoid effusion. The condition is usually reversible with mastoid–middle ear surgery, but an aerated middle ear–mastoid air cell system should be maintained by the insertion of a tympanostomy tube at the time of the mastoid surgery; the tube should be reinserted if otitis media with effusion or atelectasis, or both, recurs.

It should be stressed that mastoidectomy and middle ear surgery is *rarely* indicated and should be performed only in those few children for whom other appropriate methods have been unsuccessful.

Hearing Aids

A management option recommended by some clinicians as an alternative to surgical intervention is fitting a hearing aid on a child who has conductive hearing loss due to chronic otitis media with effusion or chronic atelectasis of the tympanic membrane, or both. The rationale is that the hearing loss may interfere with normal development of speech, language, and learning and that the middle-ear condition is self-limited and should improve as the child grows older. The fallacy in this argument is that the natural history of chronic middle-ear effusions and atelectasis is not known. In some cases, these conditions can lead to middle-ear damage. An excellent example is the population of children who have cleft palate, in whom cholesteatoma formation is a frequent sequela in spite of what apparently is aggressive medical, and even surgical, management of their ever-present chronic middle-ear effusions and atelectasis. Therefore, the fitting of a hearing aid on such individuals could obscure the pathologic complications and sequelae of otitis media in an effort to promote adequate hearing.

On the other hand, fitting a hearing aid on selected children should be considered and attempted when the hearing loss is interfering with the child's development and the middle-ear disease cannot be reversed by medical or surgical methods. Insertion of tympanostomy tubes usually restores hearing to adequate levels when chronic otitis media with effusion is present. In some ears, especially those with severe atelectasis of the tympanic membrane, a tympanostomy tube either is difficult to insert or only remains in place for a short period. Fluctuating hearing loss in children so affected could be detrimental, and amplification of the hearing may be beneficial. Likewise, a child who already has damage to the ossicular chain and must wait to grow older before reconstructive middle-ear surgery is performed may also be a good candidate for a hearing aid.

Therefore, the fitting of hearing aids should be considered in selected children, but close medical monitoring of such children is mandatory so that the possible development of complications and sequelae of otitis media and atelectasis are not masked.

Management of Special Populations

There are certain types of children who are known to be at high risk for developing otitis media and in whom continuing surveillance and more attentive management is necessary to prevent the complications and sequelae of the disease. In addition, children who have handicaps otherwise unrelated to middle-ear disease may deserve special attention, as the occurrence of otitis media with its attendant conductive hearing loss may further compromise the preexisting handicap and possibly interfere with the educational and social development of the child.

Infants and Children with Cleft Palate

Because otitis media with effusion is a universal finding in infants with an unrepaired cleft palate (Paradise et al., 1969; Stool and Randall, 1967), it seems reasonable to attempt to maintain the middle ears of these children free of effusion and with normal pressures. Because there is always a conductive hearing loss and usually discomfort associated with a middle-ear effusion, elimination of otitis media as early in life as possible should be the goal of management. Medical treatment, such as a trial of antimicrobial therapy in young infants with an unrepaired cleft palate, has not been systematically tested; however, in older infants and children, the nonsurgical methods of management have usually been unsuccessful in eliminating middle-ear effusion and restoring hearing. Therefore, the most reasonable method of management for young infants with an unrepaired cleft palate would be the insertion of a tympanostomy tube as early in life as feasible, because these infants have functional obstruction of the eustachian tube (Bluestone, 1971; Paradise and Bluestone, 1974; Doyle, 1985). If a repair of a cleft lip is performed at 2 or 3 months of age, the tympanostomy tubes can be inserted at this time. In any event, a tympanostomy tube should probably be inserted sometime during the first 6 months of life. The overall reduction in middle-ear disease that follows palate repair would appear to constitute a basis for consideration of earlier repair than might otherwise be undertaken (Paradise and Bluestone, 1974). Paradise and

colleagues (1969) pointed out that the middle-ear damage and hearing loss prevalent during later life in patients who had cleft palates probably originated with chronic middle-ear effusion in infancy; they further suggest that the possible restrictions in language skill (McWilliams, 1966) and speech articulation that also seem to be prevalent in these patients later in life may have the same origin, because the persistent middle-ear effusion of infants with cleft palates is probably accompanied by variable degrees of hearing loss. When spontaneous extubation occurs in these children, the tubes should be reinserted if otitis media with effusion recurs.

Patients with a cleft palate and otitis media should be considered uncertain candidates for adenoidectomy; there is a distinct possibility that the operation may worsen velopharyngeal function. In a retrospective study by Severeid (1972), adenoidectomy was not found to be effective in relieving otitis media in children with cleft palates.

Other Craniofacial Malformations

All children with craniofacial malformations who have an associated cleft palate will have a high incidence of otitis media early in life. Otitis media in these children should be managed as previously outlined for children with only cleft palates. Children in this category include those with Pierre Robin syndrome (glossoptosis, micrognathia, and cleft of the soft palate) and those with trisomy 21 (Down syndrome). The latter have an extremely high incidence of otitis media with effusion owing to eustachian tube dysfunction (White et al., 1984). Balkany and coworkers (1978, 1979) have reported that over 50 per cent of such children will have a middle-ear effusion and that more than three fourths have a conductive hearing loss. Antimicrobial therapy is usually not successful in eliminating the effusion, and most will require myringotomy and tympanostomy tube insertion to restore the hearing to normal. If a conductive hearing loss persists after successful placement of a tympanostomy tube (the middle ear appears to be aerated), then an ossicular malformation should be suspected, because this congenital anomaly is commonly found in association with these syndromes.

Even though the incidence of otitis media with effusion in many of the infants and children with craniofacial malformations has not been formally studied, children with some of the following malformations are considered to be at high risk for developing middle-ear effusions: mandibulofacial dysostosis (Treacher Collins syndrome), craniofacial dysostosis (Crouzon disease), gonadal dysgenesis (Turner syndrome), and mucopolysaccharidosis (Hunter-Hurler syndrome) (Table 21–39). However, any child with a congenital craniofacial malformation should be followed to detect the development of otitis media with effusion; a child acquiring this problem might most reasonably be managed by myringotomy with insertion of a tympanostomy tube.

TABLE 21–39. Craniofacial Malformations and Syndromes Associated with High Incidence of Otitis Media with Effusion

Cleft palate, micrognathia, glossoptosis (Pierre Robin anomalad)
Trisomy 21 (Down syndrome)
Trisomy 13–15 (Patau syndrome)
Mandibulofacial dysostosis (Treacher Collins syndrome)
Oculoauriculovertebral dysplasia (Goldenhar syndrome)
Acrocephalosyndactyly (Apert syndrome)
Gonadal dysgenesis (Turner syndrome)
Craniometaphyseal dysplasia (Pyle disease)
Osteopetrosis (Albers-Schönberg disease)
Achondroplasia (Parrot disease)
Mucopolysaccharidosis (Hunter-Hurler syndrome)
Orofacial-digital syndrome (Mohr syndrome)
Craniofacial dysostosis (Crouzon disease)

Racial Groups

Certain racial groups are believed to have a high incidence of otitis media with effusion: American natives (Indians and Eskimos), the Maori of New Zealand, natives of Guam, Greenland Eskimos, Australian aborigines, and Laplanders. Early in life the children of these populations appear to develop recurrent acute otitis media, perforation of the tympanic membrane, otorrhea, and a propensity for chronic otitis media with discharge as a later sequela. When infants in these racial groups contract upper respiratory tract infections, which are so frequently associated with the ear disease, they should be aggressively treated by medical means, and antimicrobial therapy should be instituted for otitis media as early as possible. A perforation appears to be part of the natural history of ear disease in these children, and if it occurs, meticulous cleansing of the purulent material from the canal (aural toilet) should be performed frequently. In addition, an appropriate topical aural antibiotic, selected on the basis of culture, should be instilled. Antimicrobial prophylaxis is a reasonable treatment option for such children. Ensign and associates (1960) demonstrated a decreased incidence of otitis media in American Indians when prophylactic doses of a sulfonamide were administered. In a later study, Maynard and coworkers (1972) were able to decrease the incidence of otorrhea in about 50 per cent of Alaskan Eskimos who were given a prophylactic daily dose of ampicillin over a 1-year period. For those children in whom compliance was considered best, there was a two thirds reduction in the incidence of ear discharge.

The insertion of tympanostomy tubes into the ears of such children has not been as successful in alleviating the recurrent otitis media as it has in children with cleft palates. This may be due to the basic differences in the origin and pathogenesis of the disease in these two groups of children: children with cleft palates usually have otitis media with effusion, whereas American natives more commonly have recurrent otitis media, followed by perforation and discharge.

If a perforation persists in infants and children who have a racial predilection for developing otitis media

and tympanoplasty is not performed, a hearing aid should be fitted to help restore the child's hearing.

Immunocompromised Host

Infants and children who have congenital, acquired, or drug-induced compromise of their immune systems require special consideration when otitis media is present (Table 21–40). Children with congenital conditions that compromise their defense systems are more susceptible to infections in general and may be more susceptible to otitis media in particular. When otitis media is present in patients with immune deficiency, the possibility of an unusual organism should be considered (Table 21–41). Medications such as corticosteroids, antibiotics, and cytotoxic drugs may compromise the immune system. Lymphoproliferative disease states such as lymphoma or leukemia may also compromise the host's defenses.

For such children, the occurrence of acute signs and symptoms of otitis media warrants identification of the causative organism employing tympanocentesis and possibly drainage (i.e., myringotomy). Culture and sensitivity testing of the middle-ear aspirate will be helpful in selecting the appropriate antimicrobial agent effective against the causative organism. In certain children who are immunocompromised, frequently recurrent and chronic otitis media are potentially life threatening, and more permanent drainage may be required. Myringotomy and insertion of a tympanostomy tube should be considered to eliminate the middle-ear effusion and prevent recurrence of suppurative disease, so as to prevent intracranial and intratemporal complications such as labyrinthitis and meningitis.

Immotile Cilia Syndrome

Infants and children with chronic otitis media with effusion, paranasal sinusitis, and bronchitis (and bronchiectasis) should be suspected of having a chronic respiratory tract infection produced by abnormal cilia, which will significantly interfere with the mucociliary transport system (Eliasson et al., 1977). It is now appreciated that Kartagener syndrome (dextrocardia with situs inversus, bronchiectasis, sinusitis, or agenesis of the frontal sinuses) is associated with the immotile cilia syndrome. Patients with this condition should undergo bilateral myringotomy and tympanostomy tube insertion to eliminate the middle-ear effusion, restore the hearing, and prevent the complications and sequelae of otitis media with effusion. Nonsurgical methods of management, such as antimicrobial prophylaxis, may be effective, but when a persistent effusion is present, myringotomy with insertion of a tympanostomy tube is indicated.

Concurrent Permanent Hearing Loss

Infants and children with preexisting hearing losses who subsequently develop otitis media with effusion

TABLE 21–40. Classification of Conditions That Resulted in Increased Susceptibility to Infections, Including Otitis Media in Which Unusual Organism Should Be Suspected

CONGENITAL	ACQUIRED	DRUG-INDUCED
B-cell Deficiency	Neoplasms	Antiinflammatory
Hypogammaglobulinemia	Acute and chronic leukemia	Aspirin
X-linked agammaglobulinemia	Hodgkin disease	Corticosteroid
IgA deficiency	Non-Hodgkin lymphoma	Indomethacin
Common variable deficiency	Sarcoma	Phenylbutazone
T-cell deficiency	Carcinoma	Gold salts
DiGeorge syndrome	Weber-Christian disease	Antiparasitics
Nucleoside phosphorylase deficiency	Inflammatory	Levamisole
Thymic dysplasia	Acute infection	Niridazole
Chronic mucocutaneous candidiasis	Neonatal infections	Suramin
T- and B-cell deficiencies	Lepromatous leprosy	Cytotoxic
Cartilage-hair hypoplasia	Felty syndrome	Cyclophosphamide
Ataxia telangiectasia	Rheumatoid arthritis	Azathioprine
Wiskott-Aldrich syndrome	Metabolic	Methotrexate
Reticular dysgenesis	Diabetes mellitus	6-Mercaptopurine
Nezelof syndrome	Renal disease	5-Fluorouracil
Phagocyte defects	Hepatic cirrhosis	Phenothiazines
Neutropenia	Hyperosmolar states	Chlorpromazine
Chronic granulomatous disease	Protein-calorie malnutrition	Mepazine
Chediak-Higashi syndrome	Storage diseases	Diuretics
Lazy leukocyte syndrome	Anemias	Thiazides
Myeloperoxidase deficiency	Neutropenia	Ethacrynic acid
Hyper IgE syndrome	Chronic hemolytic anemia	Mercurial diuretics
Others	Sickle cell disease	Antithyroid
Down syndrome	Others	Thiouracil derivatives
Complement deficiencies	Alcoholism	Methimazole
Glucose-6-phosphate dehydrogenase deficiency	Malakoplakia	Antiarrhythmics
Hyper IgE syndrome (with normal phagocytes)	Burn	Quinidine
	Systemic lupus erythematosus	Procainamide
		Propranolol
		Anticonvulsants
		Phenytoin
		Phenobarbital
		Other
		Anesthesia

or abnormal negative middle-ear pressure (atelectasis), or both, are at higher risk for impairment of language acquisition and learning than are those children whose hearing loss is due to the middle-ear effusion and negative pressure alone. Therefore, the former children should be observed at more frequent intervals than children without a concurrent permanent hearing loss and may require more aggressive management for the superimposed conductive hearing loss, because it is amenable to treatment. The preexisting hearing loss may be conductive, sensorineural, or mixed. The child with a congenital malformation of the middle-ear ossicles who has a conductive hearing loss may develop persistent or recurrent otitis media with effusion or high negative pressure, which would increase his or her hearing handicap. Likewise, children who have a preexisting sensorineural hearing loss of some degree are often severely handicapped socially and educationally if they then acquire a middle-ear effusion. These children should be managed in the same way as those without a concurrent hearing loss from another cause, but it is even more important to eliminate the middle-ear effusion in these children rapidly and to prevent the development of any further hearing loss, if possi-

ble. If medical treatment does not eliminate the superimposed conductive hearing loss within a relatively short time, myringotomy and insertion of a tympanostomy tube should be considered at an earlier time than for children without a concurrent hearing loss. Middle-ear effusion is common in all children but appears to have an even higher incidence in some children with a congenital middle-ear malformation (e.g., in Down syndrome) and those who have a sensorineural loss. For this reason, surgical intervention should be considered earlier in children who have recurrent middle-ear effusion and persistent or fluctuating conductive hearing loss to prevent further impairment of hearing and, consequently, of development.

Today many children with moderate to severe permanent hearing losses attend regular schools (mainstreaming), and some may not even require a hearing aid. Regardless of their functional level of hearing, however, any child who has such a hearing loss should be evaluated more frequently for possible occurrence of otitis media with effusion than should the child without a permanent hearing loss. Children of all ages are at high risk, but infants, preschoolers, and young school-age children are at particular risk, because the

TABLE 21–41. Unusual Microbial Agents That May Be Found in Otitis Media of Compromised Host

BACTERIA

Aerobic and/or Facultative Anaerobic

Gram-negative bacilli	Gram-positive cocci
Pseudomonas species	*Streptococcus* species
Proteus species	*Staphylococcus* species
Klebsiella species	*Enterococcus* species
Escherichia coli	Non-*Enterococcus* species
Enterobacter species	Gram-positive bacilli
Serratia species	*Bacillus* species
Gram-negative cocci or	*Corynebacterium* species
coccobacilli	*Listeria monocytogenes*
Moraxella lacunata	

Anaerobic	**Higher Bacteria**
Peptococcus	*Actinomyces israelii*
Bacteroides species	*Mycobacterium* species
	Nocardia species

FUNGI

Candida species
Aspergillus species

incidence of otitis media is higher in these age groups. Examination of such infants and children twice a year would appear to be a reasonable goal if the child had no past history or evidence of the disease, but more frequent evaluation (three or four times per year) is desirable for those children who have had recurrent middle-ear effusions. Because all infants and young children are at high risk for developing otitis media with effusion and high negative pressure, all infants identified as having a sensorineural hearing loss early in life should be more frequently examined for possible recurrence of otitis media. Even if such children show no objective evidence of middle-ear effusion by otoscopy, tympanometry, or both, if there is a history of fluctuating hearing loss the child should be actively treated, as even the presence of transient high negative pressure may lead to a compounding of the educational handicap.

Schools or Programs for Deaf

Children with severe to profound deafness who are enrolled in schools for the deaf or in special programs in regular schools who are mainstreamed are at high risk for compounding their handicaps if they develop an added conductive hearing loss due to otitis media with effusion, high negative pressure, or both. The incidence of intercurrent middle-ear problems appears to be high in such children; thus, early identification employing a formal screening program such as the one proposed above is mandatory. Some children develop troublesome cerumen that obstructs the ear canal and may interfere with the function of a hearing aid. Such children should be examined frequently, and cerumen should be periodically removed. As suggested above, otitis media with effusion, high negative pressure, or both should be suspected during periods of upper

respiratory tract infection, or when the children have signs and symptoms of otologic disease such as otorrhea and otalgia, or when there has been a noticeable loss of hearing reported by the parents or teachers. Regular periodic screening employing otoscopy, tympanometry, or both will identify those children with middle-ear problems who might otherwise be overlooked because obvious signs and symptoms associated with hearing loss may be absent.

Treatment of such children would depend on the type, severity, frequency, and duration of the middle-ear problem. However, more aggressive treatment is indicated for this special population. Myringotomy and tympanostomy tube insertion should be considered earlier in such children when otitis media with effusion is frequently recurrent or chronic. Because sustained or transient high negative middle-ear pressure without a middle-ear effusion can cause a persistent or fluctuating conductive hearing loss, the insertion of tympanostomy tubes should also be considered at an earlier time than in nondeaf children. The presence of a hearing aid will not interfere with the function of tympanostomy tubes, as a small hole can be bored in the ear mold to provide ventilation. It is important when tympanostomy tubes are inserted in such children that a short tube be used so that the ear mold may be inserted.

Early identification and appropriate management of middle-ear disease in a child with severe to profound deafness, especially those who utilize their residual hearing, are imperative so that maximum rehabilitation may be accomplished.

Immunoprophylaxis

S. pneumoniae is the most frequent bacterial organism isolated from middle-ear fluids of children with acute otitis media (Klein, 1981). Relatively few serotypes are responsible for most infections; more than 90 per cent of isolates of *S. pneumoniae* from middle-ear fluids are among the 23 types present in the available pneumococcal vaccines (Klein, 1981). A 14-type pneumococcal polysaccharide vaccine was licensed for use in the United States in 1978. A 23-valent vaccine was licensed in 1983 and replaces the 14-type product. The vaccine contains purified polysaccharide antigens of types associated with otitis media in children. These include Danish Types 1, 2, 3, 4, 5, 6B, 7F, 8, 9N, 9V, 10A, 11A, 12F, 14, 15B, 17F, 18C, 19A, 19F, 20, 22F, 23F, and 33F. Each polysaccharide is extracted, separated, and combined into the final vaccine. A 0.5-ml dose contains 25 µg of each polysaccharide type dissolved in isotonic saline solution containing 0.25 per cent phenol as a preservative; it is administered subcutaneously or intramuscularly. The vaccine is well tolerated. Children who receive the vaccine have some pain, erythema, and induration at the site of injection, and a small number have a minimal elevation in temperature. No significant reactions have been noted in children.

Each antigen produces an independent antibody

response. In older children (older than 2 years of age) and adults, antibody develops in about 2 weeks. Studies in children indicate that, as with polysaccharide vaccines prepared from capsular materials of *H. influenzae* Type b and *N. meningitidis* Group C, children less than 2 years of age exhibit unsatisfactory serologic responses to a single dose regimen. However, *N. meningitidis* Group A (Gold et al., 1978) and *S. pneumoniae* Type 3 (Makela et al., 1980) evoke significant antibody responses in infants as young as 6 months, suggesting that some polysaccharides are adequate immunogens in young infants.

CLINICAL TRIALS

RESULTS OF THE PNEUMOCOCCAL VACCINE TRIALS. Because of the frequency and morbidity of otitis media in young children, the importance of the pneumococcus as an etiologic agent, and the limited number of serotypes responsible for most disease, investigations of 8- or 14-type pneumococcal vaccines for prevention of recurrent episodes of acute otitis media were initiated (Karma et al., 1980; Makela et al., 1980, 1981; Sloyer et al., 1981; Teele et al., 1981*a*). Results were evaluated by number of clinical episodes of acute otitis media and by bacteriologic features of the infection, identified by aspiration of middle-ear fluids.

Types of *S. pneumoniae* present in the vaccine were isolated less frequently from middle-ear fluids of children in the vaccine group with acute episodes of otitis media following immunization than from children in the control group in each of the studies. If the estimates of relative risk for the studies are combined, the overall risk indicates a significant protective effect in children who received the vaccine.

The number of episodes of otitis media due to types not present in the vaccine and due to other pathogens (predominantly *H. influenzae*) was similar in the vaccine and control groups. Finnish children 2 to 7 years of age who received pneumococcal vaccines had 50 per cent fewer episodes of otitis media caused by types present in the vaccine. Acute otitis media was also reduced in a Swedish study of children between 2 and 5 years of age: Rosen and colleagues (1983) performed a double-blind trial of the 14-type vaccine; in contrast with the other vaccine studies, results were identified only by clinical evaluation.

In spite of the decrease in middle-ear infections due to pneumococcal types present in the vaccine, the clinical experience of children under 2 years of age in the vaccine groups was similar to that of children in the control groups. In general, the number of children who had one or more episodes of otitis media and the mean number of episodes of acute otitis media after immunization were similar in the vaccine and control groups. There were differences in some subsets; Huntsville, Alabama, children, 6 to 12 months of age, in the vaccine group had fewer episodes of otitis media than did children in the control group (Sloyer et al., 1981). The pneumococcal vaccine was effective in prevention of new clinical episodes of otitis media in black children 6 to 11 months of age in Huntsville, but the vaccine was ineffective in preventing otitis media in white infants of the same age (Howie et al., 1984). These data suggest racial differences in terms of preventing disease; prior studies had suggested genetic difference in response to polysaccharide vaccines (Ambrosino et al., 1986; Granoff et al., 1983). The duration of middle-ear effusion following an episode of pneumococcal otitis media was similar for the vaccine and the control groups (analyzed only by the Boston group [Teele et al., 1981*a*]).

CONCLUSIONS OF THE VACCINE TRIALS. There are both promise and disappointment in the results of the pneumococcal vaccine trials for prevention of new episodes of acute otitis media. The vaccine *was* effective. Children who received either the 8- or 14-type vaccine had significantly fewer episodes of acute otitis media due to types of *S. pneumoniae* present in the vaccine. The disappointment occurred because the clinical experience with otitis media was not significantly altered; the reduction in pneumococcal type-specific infection in vaccinated children was of insufficient magnitude to affect the number of episodes of otitis media after immunization.

From the results of these studies, pneumococcal vaccine is not indicated for prevention of otitis media in children under 2 years of age but may be of value for children older than 2 years who still experience recurrent episodes of acute otitis media.

FUTURE VACCINES

New conjugate vaccines combining the polysaccharides of the pneumococcus or *H. influenzae* Type b with a protein carrier such as diphtheria or tetanus toxoids, a nontoxic mutant of diphtheria toxin, or an outer membrane protein of group B meningococcus are now in development and in clinical trial (Bluestone et al., 1989). These products are immunogenic in infants as young as 3 months of age (Eskola et al., 1985). It is conceivable that within a few years polysaccharide conjugate vaccines including four or more pneumococcal types, *H. influenzae* Type b, and one or more meningococcal groups will be administered with diphtheria and tetanus toxoid and pertussis vaccine to children as young as 2 months of age.

Because nontypable *H. influenzae* lacks capsular materials, different techniques will be necessary to develop a vaccine. Recent investigations focused on use of outer membrane proteins as candidate antigens for development of a vaccine (Gnehm et al., 1985).

PROTECTIVE EFFECT OF IMMUNOGLOBULINS

Specific serum antibody is correlated with protection from homotypic infection, and prevention of disease may be achieved (albeit for limited duration) by administration of immunoglobulins. Since infants who have recurrent episodes of acute otitis media usually improve with age, it is possible that a program of passive immunization might be effective.

Diamont and colleagues (1961) suggested that patients with recurrent episodes of acute otitis media associated with hypo- or agammaglobulinemia are benefited by frequent administration of gamma globulin. In their investigation children aged 1 to 7 years were enrolled after the first visit. Children born on an odd date were given gamma globulin at their first visit and then once a month for 6 months. Children born on an even date received no gamma globulin. Of the 113 children treated, 10 had one or more episodes of acute otitis media during the months of administration of the gamma globulin; of 118 untreated children, 25 had one or more episodes of the disease during the same period of time. The protective effect of the gamma globulin persisted during the 8 months following cessation of administration; 25 episodes occurred in the treated group and 53 in the untreated group. In the untreated group, some patients had up to five episodes, whereas no patient in the treated group had more than two bouts of acute otitis media (Diamont et al., 1961). Investigations are now under way to evaluate the protective effect of hyperimmune globulins among American Indian children, who are highly susceptible to recurrent episodes of acute otitis media (Shurin, unpublished data).

Acknowledgment: *The authors want to thank Ms. Mary Scheetz for her patient, diligent, and painstaking work during the preparation of this chapter and Chapters 22 and 23. They would also like to thank Mr. Jon Coulter for design and preparation of the artwork; William J. Doyle for assistance in preparation of the section on anatomy of the nasopharynx–eustachian tube–middle ear system; and Thomas Fria and Robert Nozza for their assistance in preparation of the section "Immittance and Assessment of Hearing" in this chapter.*

SELECTED REFERENCES

Sade, J. (ed.) 1986. Acute and Secretory Otitis Media. Amsterdam, Kugler Publications.

This book is a collection of the papers presented at the International Conference on Acute and Secretory Otitis Media held in Jerusalem, November 1985.

Bluestone, C. D., and Doyle, W. J. 1985. Eustachian tube function: Physiology and role in otitis media. Ann. Otol. Rhinol. Laryngol. 94.

The supplement is an excellent state of knowledge of the anatomy, pathology, physiology, and pathophysiology of the eustachian tube.

Lim, D. J., Bluestone, C. D., Klein, J. O., and Nelson, J. D. (eds.) 1988. Recent Advances in Otitis Media with Effusion. Toronto, B. C. Decker.

This book is the Proceedings of the Fourth International Symposium on Otitis Media held in 1987. It contains 155 extended abstracts on most aspects of the disease.

Kumazawa, T., and Kawamoto, K. (eds.) Proceedings Extraordinary International Symposium on Recent Advances in Otitis Media with Effusion 1985. Auris Nasus Larynx 12 (Suppl. 1).

This supplement contains many excellent extended abstracts on the basic science aspects and management of otitis media of presentations from an international meeting held in Kyoto, Japan, in 1985.

Schuknecht, H. F. 1974. Pathology of the Ear. Cambridge, MA, Harvard University Press, pp. 23–40, 97–105, 215–224.

This text has the best description of the pathologic changes in otitis media and certain related conditions.

REFERENCES

Ackerman, M. N., Friedman, R. A., Doyle, W. J., et al. 1984. Antigen-induced eustachian tube obstruction: An intranasal provocative challenge test. J. Allergy Clin. Immunol. 73:604.

Alberti, P. W. 1974. Myringotomy and ventilating tubes in the 19th century. Laryngoscope 84:805.

Alberti, P. W., and Kristensen, R. 1970. The clinical application of impedance audiometry: A preliminary appraisal of an electroacoustic impedance bridge. Laryngoscope 80:735.

Albiin, N., Hellström, S., and Stenfors, L-E. 1983. Clearance of effusion material from the attic space—an experimental study in the rat. Int. J. Pediatr. Otorhinolaryngol. 5:1.

Alt, A. 1878, 1879. Heilunger taubstummheit erzielte durch beseitigung einer otorrhoe und einer angebornen gaumenspalate. Arch. Augen Ohrenh 7:211, and Schmidt's Jahrbuecher 183:277.

Ambrosino, D. M., Barrus, V. A., DeLange, G. G., and Siber, G. R. 1986. Correlation of the Km(l) immunoglobulin allotypes with human anti-polysaccharide antibody concentrations. J. Clin. Invest. 78:361.

Ambrosino, D. M., Schiffman, G., Gotschlisch, E. C., et al. 1985. Correlation between G2m(n) immunoglobin allotype and human antibody response and susceptibility to polysaccharide encapsulated bacteria. J. Clin. Invest. 75:1935.

Ament, R. P. 1980. Hospital Record Study, Professional Activity Study. Ann Arbor, MI, Commission on Professional and Hospital Activities.

American Academy of Pediatrics. 1977. Otitis Media. Evanston, IL, Committee on Infectious Diseases, pp. 160–163.

Ammann, A. J., and Shannon, K. 1985. Recognition of acquired immunodeficiency syndrome (AIDS) in children. Ped. Rev. 7:101.

Andersson, B., Eriksson, B., Falsen, E., et al. 1981. Adhesion of *Streptococcus pneumoniae* to human pharyngeal epithelial cells in vitro: Differences in adhesive capacity among strains isolated from subjects with otitis media, septicemia, or meningitis or from healthy carriers. Infect. Immun. 32:311.

Anson, B. (ed.). 1967. Morris' Human Anatomy. New York, McGraw-Hill Book Co., pp. 1195–1196.

Anson, B., and Donaldson, J. 1967. The Surgical Anatomy of the Temporal Bone and Ear. Philadelphia, W. B. Saunders Co., pp. 29–30.

Appelbaum, P. C. 1987. World-wide development of antibiotic resistance in pneumococci. Eur. J. Clin. Microbiol. 6:367.

Appelbaum, P. C., Bhamjee, A., Scragg, J. N., et al. 1977. *Streptococcus pneumoniae* resistant to penicillin and chloramphenicol. Lancet 2:995.

Armstrong, B. W. 1954. A new treatment for chronic secretory otitis media. Arch. Otolaryngol. 59:653.

Aschan, G. K. 1952. Observations on the eustachian tube. Acta Soc. Med. Upsalien 57:1.

Aschan, G. 1954. The eustachian tube. Acta Otolaryngol. (Stockh.) 44:295.

Aschan, G. K. 1955. The anatomy of the eustachian tube with regard to its function. Acta Soc. Med. Upsalien 60:131.

Aschan, G. K. 1966. Hearing and nasal function correlated to postoperative speech in cleft palate patients with velopharyngoplasty. Acta Otolaryngol. (Stockh.) 61:371.

Auritt, W. A., Hervada, A. R., and Fendrick, G. 1978. Fatal pseudomembranous enterocolitis following oral ampicillin therapy. J. Pediatr. 93:882.

Austrian, R., Howie, V. M., and Ploussard, J. H. 1977. The bacteriology of pneumococcal otitis media. Johns Hopkins Med. J. 141:104.

Baba, S. 1985. Recent aspects of clinical bacteriology in otitis media. Presented at Presymposium on Management of Otitis Media, Kyoto, Japan, January 12, 1985.

Bacher, J. A. 1912. The applied anatomy of the eustachian tube. Laryngoscope 22:21.

Bakwin, H., and Jacobinzer, H. 1939. Prevention of purulent otitis media in infants. J. Pediatr. 14:730.

Balkany, T. J., Berman, S. A., Simmons, M. A., and Jafek, B. W. 1978. Middle ear effusions in neonates. Laryngoscope 88:398.

Balkany, T. J., Downs, M. P., Jafek, B. W., and Krajicek, M. J.

1979. Hearing loss in Down's syndrome. A treatable handicap more common than generally recognized. Clin. Pediatr. 18:116.

Barenkamp, S. J., Shurin, P. A., Marchant, C. D., et al. 1984. Do children with recurrent *Hemophilus influenzae* otitis media become infected with a new organism or reacquire the original strain? J. Pediatr. 105:533.

Barza, M. 1978. The nephrotoxicity of cephalosporins: An overview. J. Infect. Dis. 137:S60.

Bass, J. W., Craft, F. W., Knowles, C. R., et al. 1976. Streptococcal pharyngitis in children. A comparison of four treatment schedules with intramuscular penicillin G benzothine. J.A.M.A. 235:1112.

Bass, J. W., Steele, R. W., Wiebe, R. A., and Dierdorff, E. P. 1971. Erythromycin concentrations in middle ear exudates. Pediatrics 48:417.

Bauer, A. W., Kirby, W. M., Sherris, J. C., and Turck, M. 1966. Antibiotic susceptibility testing by a standardized single disk method. Am. J. Clin. Pathol. 45:493.

Bauer, F. 1975. Tubal function in the glue ear: Urea for glue ears. J. Laryngol. Otol. 89:63.

Beatty, H. G. 1936. The care of cleft palate patients. Laryngoscope 46:203.

Beery, Q. C., Bluestone, C. D., Andrus, W. S., and Cantekin, E. I. 1975a. Tympanometric pattern classification in relation to middle ear effusions. Ann. Otol. Rhinol. Laryngol. 84:56.

Beery, Q. C., Bluestone, C. D., and Cantekin, E. I. 1975b. Otologic history, audiometry and tympanometry as a case finding procedure for school screening. Laryngoscope 85:1976.

Beery, Q. C., Doyle, W. J., Cantekin, E. I., and Bluestone, C. D. 1979. Longitudinal assessment of eustachian tube function in children. Laryngoscope 89:1446.

Beery, Q. C., Doyle, W. J., Cantekin, E. I., et al. 1980. Eustachian tube function in an American Indian population. Ann. Otol. Rhinol. Laryngol. 89:28.

Bennett, M. 1972. The older cleft palate patient: A clinical otologic-audiologic study. Laryngoscope 82:1217.

Bennett, M., Ward, R. H., and Tait, C. A. 1968. Otologic-audiologic study of cleft palate children. Laryngoscope 78:1011.

Berdal, P., Brandtzaeg, P., Froland, S., et al. 1976. Immunodeficiency syndromes with otorhinolaryngological manifestations. Acta Otolaryngol. (Stockh.) 82:185.

Berger, G., Hawke, M., Proops, D. W., et al. 1984. Histamine levels in middle ear effusions. Acta Otolaryngol. (Stockh.) 98:385.

Bergeron, M. G., Ahronheim, G., Richard, J. E., et al. 1987. Comparative efficacy of erythromycin-sulfisoxazole and cefaclor in acute otitis media: A double blind randomized trial. Pediatr. Infect. Dis. 6:654.

Bergeson, P. S., Singer, S. A., and Kaplan, A. M. 1982. Intramuscular injections in children. Pediatrics 70:944.

Bergman, A. B., and Haggerty, R. J. 1962. The emergency clinic: A study of its role in a teaching hospital. Am. J. Dis. Child. 104:36.

Bergstrom, L. 1978. Congenital and acquired deafness in clefting and craniofacial syndromes. Cleft Palate J. 15:254.

Berman, S. A., Balkany, T. J., and Simmons, M. A. 1978. Otitis media in the neonatal intensive care unit. Pediatrics 62:198.

Berman, S., Grose, K., and Zerbe, G. O. 1987. Medical management of chronic middle ear effusion: Results of a clinical trial of prednisone combined with sulfamethoxazole and trimethoprim. Am. J. Dis. Child. 141:690.

Berman, S., and Laver, B. A. 1983. A controlled trial of cefaclor versus amoxicillin for treatment of acute otitis media in early infancy. Pediatr. Infect. Dis. 2:30.

Bernstein, J. M. 1976. Biological mediators of inflammation in middle ear effusions. Ann. Otol. Rhinol. Laryngol. 85:90.

Bernstein, J. M. 1980. Immunological reactivity in otitis media with effusion. In Oehling, A., Mathov, E., Glazer, I., and Arbesman, C. (eds.): Advances in Allergology and Immunology. Oxford, Pergamon Press, pp. 139–146.

Bernstein, J. M. 1984a. Observations on immune mechanisms in otitis media with effusion. Int. J. Pediatr. Otorhinolaryngol. 8:125.

Bernstein, J. M. 1984b. Immunologic reactivity in otitis media with effusion. Clin. Rev. Allergy 2:303.

Bernstein, J. M., Brentjens, J., and Vladutziu, A. 1981. Immune complex determination in otitis media with effusion. Presented at the ARO Midwinter Meeting, St. Petersburg, FL, January 1981.

Bernstein, J. M., Dryja, D., and Neter, E. 1984. The clinical significance of coagulase negative staphylococci in otitis media with effusion. In Lim, D. J., Bluestone, C. D., Klein, J. O., and Nelson, J. D. (eds.): Recent Advances in Otitis Media with Effusion. Toronto, B. C. Decker Inc., pp. 114–116.

Bernstein, J. M., Hayes, E. R., Ishikawa, T., et al. 1972. Secretory otitis media: A histopathologic and immunochemical report. TAAOO 76:1305.

Bernstein, J. M., Myers, D., Kosinski, D., et al. 1980. Antibody coated bacteria in otitis media with effusions. Ann. Otol. Rhinol. Laryngol. 89:104.

Bernstein, J. M., and Ogra, P. L. 1980. Mucosal immune system: Implications in otitis media with effusion. Ann. Otol. Rhinol. Laryngol. 89:326.

Bernstein, J. M., Okazaki, T., and Reisman, R. E. 1976. Prostaglandins in middle ear effusions. Arch. Otolaryngol. 102:257.

Bernstein, J. M., and Reisman, R. 1974. The role of acute hypersensitivity in secretory otitis media. TAAOO 78:ORL 120.

Bernstein, J. M., Schenkein, H. A., Genco, R. J., and Bartholomew, W. 1978a. Complement activity in middle ear effusions. Clin. Exp. Immunol. 33:340.

Bernstein, J. M., Szymanski, C., Albini, B., et al. 1978b. Lymphocyte subpopulations in otitis media with effusion. Pediatr. Res. 12:786.

Berry, M. F., and Eisenson, J. 1956. Speech Disorders: Principles and Practices of Therapy. New York, Appleton-Century-Crofts.

Bess, F. H., Lewis, H. D., and Cieliczka, B. T. 1975. Acoustic impedance measurements in cleft palate children. J. Speech Hear. Res. 40:13.

Biedel, C. W. 1978. Modification of recurrent otitis media by short-term sulfonamide therapy. Am. J. Dis. Child. 132:681.

Birch, L., and Elbrønd, O. 1985. Daily impedance audiometric screening of children in a day-care institution: Changes through one month. Scand. Audiol. 14:5.

Birkin, E. A., and Brookler, K. H. 1972. Surface tension lowering substance of the canine eustachian tube. Ann. Otol. Rhinol. Laryngol. 81:268.

Bjuggren, G., and Tunevall, G. 1952. Otitis in childhood: A clinical and serobacteriological study with special reference to the significance of *Haemophilus influenzae* in relapses. Acta Otolaryngol. 42:311.

Bland, R. D. 1972. Otitis media in the first six weeks of life: Diagnosis, bacteriology, and management. Pediatrics 49:187.

Bluestone, C. D. 1971. Eustachian tube obstruction in the infant with cleft palate. Ann. Otol. Rhinol. Laryngol. 80:1.

Bluestone, C. D. 1975. Assessment of eustachian tube function. In Jerger, J. (ed.): Handbook of Clinical Impedance Audiometry. New York, American Electromedics Corp., pp. 127–148.

Bluestone, C. D. 1978. Eustachian tube function and allergy in otitis media. Pediatrics 61:753.

Bluestone, C. D. 1979. Eustachian tube dysfunction. In Wiet, R. J., and Coulthard, S. W. (eds.): Proceedings of the Second National Conference on Otitis Media. Columbus, OH, Ross Laboratories, pp. 50–58.

Bluestone, C. D. 1980. Assessment of eustachian tube function. In Jerger, J., and Northern, J. (eds.): Clinical Impedance Audiometry. Acton, MA, American Electromedics Corp., pp. 83–108.

Bluestone, C. D. 1984. State of the art: Definitions and classifications. In Lim, D. J., Bluestone, C. D., Klein, J. O., and Nelson, J. D. Recent Advances in Otitis Media with Effusion. Toronto, B. C. Decker, pp. 1–4.

Bluestone, C. D. 1985. Current concepts in eustachian tube function related to otitis media. Auris Nasus Larynx 12:1.

Bluestone, C. D. 1987. Otitis media and sinusitis: Management and when to refer to the otolaryngologist. Pediatr. Infect. Dis. J. 6:100.

Bluestone, C. D. 1988. Management of otitis media in infants and children: Current role of old and new antimicrobial agents. Pediatr. Infect. Dis. J. 7:S129.

Bluestone, C. D., and Beery, Q. C. 1976. Concepts on the pathogenesis of middle ear effusions. Ann. Otol. Rhinol. Laryngol. 85:182.

Bluestone, C. D., Beery, Q. C., and Andrus, W. S. 1974. Mechanics of the eustachian tube as it influences susceptibility to and persistence of middle ear effusions in children. Ann. Otol. Rhinol. Laryngol. 83:27.

Bluestone, C. D., Beery, Q. C., and Paradise, J. L. 1973. Audiometry and tympanometry in relation to middle ear effusions in children. Laryngoscope 83:594.

Bluestone, C. D., and Cantekin, E. I. 1979. Design factors in the characterization and identification of otitis media and certain related conditions. Ann. Otol. Rhinol. Laryngol. 88:13.

Bluestone, C. D., and Cantekin, E. I. 1981. Management of the patulous eustachian tube. Laryngoscope 91:149.

Bluestone, C. D., Cantekin, E. I., and Beery, Q. C. 1975a. Certain effects of adenoidectomy on eustachian tube ventilatory function. Laryngoscope 85:113.

Bluestone, C. D., Cantekin, E. I., and Beery, Q. C. 1977a. Effect of inflammation on the ventilatory function of the eustachian tube. Laryngoscope 87:493.

Bluestone, C. D., Cantekin, E. I., Beery, Q. C., et al. 1977b. Functional eustachian tube obstruction in acquired cholesteatoma and related conditions. In McCabe, B. F., Sade, J., and Abramson, M. (eds.): Cholesteatoma: First International Congress. Birmingham, Aesculapius Pub. Co., pp. 325–335.

Bluestone, C. D., Cantekin, E. I., Beery, Q. C., et al. 1975b. Eustachian tube ventilatory function in relation to cleft palate. Ann. Otol. Rhinol. Laryngol. 84:333.

Bluestone, C. D., Cantekin, E. I., Beery, Q. C., et al. 1978. Function of the eustachian tube related to surgical management of acquired aural cholesteatoma in children. Laryngoscope 88:1155.

Bluestone, C. D., Cantekin, E. I., and Douglas, G. S. 1979a. Eustachian tube function related to the results of tympanoplasty in children. Laryngoscope 89:450.

Bluestone, C. D., Casselbrant, M. L., and Cantekin, E. I. 1981. Functional Obstruction of the Eustachian Tube in the Pathogenesis of Acquired Cholesteatoma in Children. Amsterdam, Kugler Publications, pp. 211–224.

Bluestone, C. D., and Doyle, W. J. (eds.). 1985. Eustachian tube function: Physiology and role in otitis media: Workshop report. Ann. Otol. Rhinol. Laryngol. 94 (Suppl. 120):1.

Bluestone, C. D., Fria, T. J., Arjona, S. K., et al. 1986. Controversies in screening for middle ear disease and hearing loss in children. Pediatrics 77:57.

Bluestone, C. D., Gellis, S. S., Rundkrantz, H., et al. 1984. Panel Discussion: Controversies in antimicrobial therapy for otitis media. In Lim, D. J., Bluestone, C. D., Klein, J. O., and Nelson, J. D. (eds.): Recent Advances in Otitis Media with Effusion. Toronto, B. C. Decker, pp. 290–292.

Bluestone, C. D., Michaels, R. H., Stool, S. E., et al. 1979b. Cefaclor compared with amoxicillin in acute otitis media with effusion: A preliminary report. Postgrad. Med. J. 55:42.

Bluestone, C. D., Nelson, J. D., and Sheetz, M. D. (eds.) 1989. Proceedings of a workshop on vaccines for otitis media. Pediatr. Infect. Dis. J. 8 (Suppl. 1):8.

Bluestone, C. D., Paradise, J. L., and Beery, Q. C. 1972a. Physiology of the eustachian tube in the pathogenesis and management of middle ear effusions. Laryngoscope 82:1654.

Bluestone, C. D., Paradise, J. L., Beery, Q. C., et al. 1972b. Certain effects of cleft palate repair on eustachian tube function. Cleft Palate J. 9:183.

Bluestone, C. D., and Shurin, P. A. 1974. Middle ear diseases in children: Pathogenesis, diagnosis, and management. Pediatr. Clin. North Am. 21:379.

Bluestone, C. D., Wittel, R. A., Paradise, J. L., et al. 1972c. Eustachian tube function as related to adenoidectomy for otitis media. TAAOO 76:1325.

Bluestone, C. D., Wittel, R. A., and Paradise, J. L. 1972d. Roentgenographic evaluation of eustachian tube function in infants with cleft and normal palates. Cleft Palate J. 9:93.

Blumer, J. L., Bertino, J. S., and Husak, M. P. 1984. Comparison of cefaclor and trimethoprim-sulfamethoxazole in the treatment of acute otitis media. Pediatr. Infect. Dis. 3:25.

Bodor, F. F. 1982. Conjunctivitis-otitis syndrome. Pediatrics 69:695.

Bodor, F. F., Marchant, C. D., Shurin, P. A., and Barenkamp, S. J. 1985. Bacterial etiology of conjunctivitis-otitis media syndrome. Pediatrics 76:26.

Bordley, J. E., and Kapur, Y. P. 1972. The histopathological changes in the temporal bone resulting from acute smallpox and chickenpox infection. Laryngoscope 82:1477.

Brash, J. (ed.). Cunningham's Textbook of Anatomy, 9th ed. London, Oxford Press, 1951.

Braun, P. 1969. Hepatotoxicity of erythromycin. J. Infect. Dis. 119:300.

Brook, I. 1979. Bacteriology and treatment of chronic otitis media. Laryngoscope 89:1129.

Brook, I. 1987. The role of anaerobic bacteria in otitis media: Microbiology, pathogenesis, and implications on therapy. Am. J. Otolaryngol. 8:109.

Brook, I., Anthony, B. F., and Finegold, S. M. 1978. Aerobic and anaerobic bacteriology of acute otitis media in children. J. Pediatr. 92:13.

Brook, I., and Schwartz, R. 1981. Anaerobic bacteria in acute otitis media. Acta Otolaryngol. 91:111.

Brooks, D. N. 1968. An objective method of detecting fluid in the middle ear. Int. Audiol. 7:280.

Brooks, D. N. 1969. The use of the electroacoustic impedance bridge in the assessment of middle ear function. Int. Audiol. 8:563.

Brooks, D. N. 1971. Electroacoustic impedance bridge studies on normal ears of children. J. Speech Hear. Res. 14:247.

Brooks, D. N. 1973. A comparative study of an impedance method and pure tone screening. Scand. Audiol. 2:67.

Brooks, D. N. 1974. Impedance bridge studies on normal and hearing impaired children. Acta Otorhinolaryngol. Belg. 28:140.

Brooks, D. N. 1976. School screening for middle ear effusions. Ann. Otol. Rhinol. Laryngol. 25:223.

Brooks, D. N. 1977. Mass screening with acoustic impedance. In Proceedings of the Third International Symposium on Impedance Audiometry. New York, American Electromedics Co.

Brooks, D. N. 1978. Impedance screening for school children—state of the art. In Harford, E. R., Bess, F. H., Bluestone, C. D., and Klein, J. O. (eds.): Impedance Screening for Middle Ear Disease in Children. New York, Grune & Stratton, pp. 173–180.

Brunck, W. 1906. Die Systematische Untersuchung des Sprachorganes bei Angeborenen Gaumendefekte in Ihrer Beziehung zur Prognose und Therapie. Leipzig, B. Angestein.

Bryant, W. S. 1907. The eustachian tube: Its anatomy and its movement: With a description of the cartilages, muscles, fasciae, and the fossa of Rosenmuller. Med. Rec. 71:931.

Bush, P. J., and Rabin, D. L. 1980. Racial differences in encounter rates for otitis media. Pediatr. Res. 14:1115.

Bylander, A. 1980. Comparison of eustachian tube function in children and adults with normal ears. Ann. Otol. Rhinol. Laryngol. 89:20.

Bylander, A., and Tjernstrom, O. 1983. Changes in eustachian tube function with age in children with normal ears. A longitudinal study. Acta Otolaryngol. (Stockh.) 96:467.

Bylander, A., Tjernstrom, O., and Ivarsson, A. 1983. Pressure opening and closing functions of the eustachian tube by inflation and deflation in children and adults with normal ears. Acta Otolaryngol. (Stockh.) 96:255.

Cambon, K., Galbraith, J. D., and Kong, G. 1965. Middle ear diseases in Indians of the Mount Currie reservation, British Columbia. Can. Med. Assoc. J. 93:1301.

Campos, J., Garcia-Tornel, S., and Sanfeliu, I. 1984. Susceptibility studies of multiply resistant Haemophilus influenzae isolated from pediatric patients and contacts. Antimicrob. Agents Chemother. 25:706.

Cantekin, E. I. 1984. State of the art: Physiology and pathophysiology of the eustachian tube. In Lim, D. J., Bluestone, C. D., Klein, J. O., and Nelson, J. (eds.): Recent Advances in Otitis Media with Effusion. Toronto, B. C. Decker, pp. 45–49.

Cantekin, E. I., Beery, Q. C., and Bluestone, C. D. 1977b. Tympanometric patterns found in middle ear effusions. Ann. Otol. Rhinol. Laryngol. 86:16.

Cantekin, E. I., and Bluestone, C. D. 1976. A membrane ventilating tube for the middle ear. Ann. Otol. Rhinol. Laryngol. 85:270.

Cantekin, E. I., Bluestone, C. D., and Parkin, L. P. 1976. Eustachian tube ventilatory function in children. Ann. Otol. Rhinol. Laryngol. 85:171.

Cantekin, E. I., Bluestone, C. D., Rockette, H. E., et al. 1980a. Effect of decongestant with or without antihistamine on eustachian tube function. Ann. Otol. Rhinol. Laryngol. 89:290.

Cantekin, E. I., Bluestone, C. D., Saez, C. A., et al. 1977a. Normal and abnormal middle ear ventilation. Ann. Otol. Rhinol. Laryngol. 86:1.

Cantekin, E. I., Doyle, W. J., and Bluestone, C. D. 1983a. Effect of levator veli palatini muscle excision on eustachian tube function. Arch. Otolaryngol. 109:281.

Cantekin, E. I., Doyle, W. J., Phillips, C. D., et al. 1980b. Gas absorption in the middle ear. Ann. Otol. Rhinol. Laryngol. 89:71.

Cantekin, E. I., Doyle, W. J., Reichert, T. J., et al. 1979a. Dilation of the eustachian tube by electrical stimulation of the mandibular nerve. Ann. Otol. Rhinol. Laryngol. 88:40.

Cantekin, E. I., Mandel, E. M., Bluestone, C. D., et al. 1983b. Lack of efficacy of a decongestant-antihistamine combination for otitis media with effusion ("secretory" otitis media) in children. N. Engl. J. Med. 308:297.

Cantekin, E. I., Phillips, C. D., Doyle, W. J., et al. 1980c. Effect of surgical alterations of the tensor veli palatini muscle on eustachian tube function. Ann. Otol. Rhinol. Laryngol. 89:47.

Cantekin, E. I., Saez, C. A., Bluestone, C. D., et al. 1979b. Airflow through the eustachian tube. Ann. Otol. Rhinol. Laryngol. 88:603.

Carlin, S. A., Marchant, C. D., Shurin, P. A., et al. 1987. Early recurrences of otitis media: Reinfection or relapse? J. Pediatr. 110:20.

Carlsson, B., Lundberg, C., and Ohlsson, K. 1983. Granulocyte protease inhibition in acute and chronic middle ear effusion. Acta Otolaryngol. (Stockh.) 95:341.

Carson, J. L., Collier, A. M., and Hu, S. S. 1985. Acquired ciliary defects in nasal epithelium of children with acute viral upper respiratory infections. N. Engl. J. Med. 312:463.

Casselbrant, M. L., Brostoff, L. B., Cantekin, E. I., et al. 1986. Otitis media in children in the United States. In Sade, J. Acute and Secretory Otitis Media. Amsterdam, Kugler Publications.

Casselbrant, M. L., Brostoff, L. M., Cantekin, E. I., et al. 1985. Otitis media with effusion in preschool children. Laryngoscope 95:428.

Casselbrant, M. L., Okeowo, P. A., Flaherty, M. R., et al. 1984. Prevalence and incidence of otitis media in a group of preschool children in the United States. In Lim, D. J., Bluestone, C. D., Klein, J. O., and Nelson, J. D. (eds.): Recent Advances in Otitis Media with Effusion. Toronto, B. C. Decker, pp. 16–19.

Cates, K. L., Gerrard, J. M., Giebink, G. S., et al. 1978. A penicillin-resistant pneumococcus. J. Pediatr. 93:624.

Chandra, R. K. 1979. Prospective studies of the effect of breast feeding on incidence of infection and allergy. Acta Paediatr. Scand. 68:691.

Chang, M. J., Rodriguez, W. J., and Mohla, C. 1982. Chlamydia trachomatis in otitis media in children. Pediatr. Infect. Dis. J. 1:95.

Chaput de Saintonge, D. M., Levine, D. F., Templae Savage, I., et al. 1982. Trial of three-day and ten-day courses of amoxycillin in otitis media. Br. Med. J. 284:1078.

Chaudhuri, P. K., and Bowen-Jones, E. 1978. An otorhinolaryngological study of children with cleft palates. J. Laryngol. Otol. 92:29.

Chonmaitree, T., Howie, V. M., and Truant, A. L. 1986. Presence of respiratory viruses in middle ear fluids and nasal wash specimens from children with acute otitis media. Pediatrics 77:698.

Clarke, T. A. 1962. Deafness in children: Otitis media and other causes; a selective survey of prevention and treatment and of educational problems. Proc. R. Soc. Med. 55:61.

Clements, D. A. 1968. Otitis media and hearing loss in a small aboriginal community. Med. J. Aust. 1:665.

Clemis, J. D. 1976. Allergic factors in management of middle ear effusions. Ann. Otol. Rhinol. Laryngol. 85:259.

Coffey, J. D., Jr. 1966. Otitis media in the practice of pediatrics: Bacteriological and clinical observations. Pediatrics 38:25.

Coffey, J. D., Jr. 1968. Concentration of ampicillin in exudate from acute otitis media. J. Pediatr. 72:693.

Coffey, J. D., Jr., Martin, A. D., and Booth, H. N. 1967. Neisseria catarrhalis in exudative otitis media. Arch. Otolaryngol. 86:403.

Cohn, A. M., Schwaber, M. K., Anthony, L. S., and Jerger, J. F. 1979. Eustachian tube function and tympanoplasty. Ann. Otol. Rhinol. Laryngol. 88:339.

Collipp, P. J. 1961. Evaluation of nose drops for otitis media in children. Northwest Med. 60:999.

Committee on School Health. 1987. Impedance bridge (tympanometer) as a screening device in schools. Pediatrics 79:472.

Compere, W. E., Jr. 1960. The radiologic evaluation of eustachian tube function. Arch. Otolaryngol. 71:386.

Compere, W. E., Jr. 1970. Radiologic evaluation of the eustachian tube. Otolaryngol. Clin. North Am. 3:45.

Cooper, J. C., Gates, G., Owen, J., and Dickson, H. 1974. An abbreviated impedance bridge technique for school screening. J. Speech Hear. Dis. 40:260.

Corwin, M. J., Weiner, L. B., and Daniels, D. 1986. Efficacy of oral antibiotics for treatment of persistent otitis media with effusion. Int. J. Pediatr. Otorhinolaryngol. 11:109.

Craig, H. B., Stool, S. E., and Laird, M. A. 1979. Project "Ears": Otologic maintenance in a school for the deaf. Am. Ann. Deaf 124:458.

Craig, W. A., and Kirby, W. M. M. (eds.) 1981. Pulse dosing of antimicrobial drugs with special reference to bacampicillin. Rev. Infect. Dis. 3:1.

Crain, E. F., and Shelov, S. P. 1982. Febrile infants: Predictors of bacteremia. J. Pediatr. 101:686.

Crysdale, W. S. 1976. Rational management of middle ear effusions in cleft palate patients. J. Otolaryngol. 5:463.

Cunningham, A. S. 1977. Morbidity in breast-fed and artificially fed infants. J. Pediatr. 90:726.

Danon, J. 1980. Cefotaxime concentrations in otitis media effusion. J. Antimicrob. Chemother. 6 (Suppl. A):131.

Dawson, C., Wood, T. R., Rose, L., and Hanna, L. 1967. Experimental inclusion conjunctivitis in man. Keratitis and other complications. Arch. Ophthalmol. 78:341.

Deinard, A. S., Dassenko, D., Kloster, B., et al. 1980. Otogenous tetanus. J.A.M.A. 243:2156.

DeMaria, T. F., Briggs, B. R., Okazaki, N., and Lim, D. J. 1984a. Experimental otitis media with effusion following middle ear inoculation of nonviable H. influenzae. Ann. Otol. Rhinol. Laryngol. 93:52.

DeMaria, T. F., Lim, D. J., Barnishan, J., et al. 1984b. Biotypes of serologically nontypable Hemophilus influenzae isolated from the middle ears and nasopharynges of patients with otitis media with effusion. J. Clin. Microbiol. 20:1102.

DeMaria, T. F., McGhee, R. B., Jr., and Lim, D. J. 1984c. Rheumatoid factor in otitis media with effusion. Arch. Otolaryngol. 110:279.

DeMaria, T. F., Prior, R. B., Briggs, B. R., et al. 1984d. Endotoxin in middle ear effusions from patients with chronic otitis media with effusion. In Lim, D. J., Bluestone, C. D., Klein, J. O., and Nelson, J. D. (eds.): Recent Advances in Otitis Media with Effusion. Toronto, B. C. Decker, pp. 123–124.

Dever, G. J., Stewart, J. L., and David, A. 1985. Prevalence of otitis media in selected populations on Pohnpei; a preliminary study. Int. J. Pediatr. Otorhinolaryngol. 10:143.

Diamant, M., and Diamant, B. 1974. Abuse and timing of use of antibiotics in acute otitis media. Arch. Otolaryngol. 100:226.

Diamant, M., Ek, S., Kallos, P., et al. 1961. Gammaglobulin treatment and protection against infections. Acta Otolaryngol. (Stockh.) 53:317.

Doege, T. C., Heath, C. W., Jr., and Sherman, I. L., 1962. Diphtheria in the United States 1959–1960. Pediatrics 30:194.

Domagk, G. 1935. Ein beitrag zur Chemotherapie der bakteriellen Infektionen. Dtsch. Med. Wochenschr. 61:250.

Domart, A., Hazard, J., and Husson, R. 1961. Fatal bone marrow aplasia after intramuscular chloramphenicol administration in two adults. Sem. Hop. Paris 37:2256.

Douglas, R. M., Moore, B. W., Miles, H. B., et al. 1986. Prophylactic efficacy of intranasal alpha 2-interferon against rhinovirus infections in the family setting. N. Engl. J. Med. 314:65.

Downes, J. J. 1959. Primary diphtheritic otitis media. Arch. Otolaryngol. 70:27.

Downham, M. A., Scott, R., Sims, D. G., et al. 1976. Breast-feeding protects against respiratory syncytial virus infections. Br. Med. J. 2:274.

Downs, M. P. 1980. Identification of children at risk for middle ear effusion problems. Ann. Otol. Rhinol. Laryngol. 89:168.

Doyle, W. J. 1977. A functiono-anatomic description of eustachian tube vector relations in four ethnic populations—an osteologic study. Ph.D. dissertation.

Doyle, W. J. 1979. Boston genetic study. Personal communication.

Doyle, W. J. 1985. Eustachian tube function in special populations: Cleft palate children. Ann. Otol. Rhinol. Laryngol. 94:39.

Doyle, W. J., Cantekin, E. I., and Bluestone, C. D. 1980a. Eustachian tube function in cleft palate children. Ann. Otol. Rhinol. Laryngol. 89:34.

Doyle, W. J., Cantekin, E. I., Bluestone, C. D., et al. 1980b. Nonhuman primate model of cleft palate and its implications for middle ear pathology. Ann. Otol. Rhinol. Laryngol. 89:41.

Doyle, W. J., Friedman, R., Fireman, P., et al. 1984a. Eustachian tube obstruction after provocative nasal antigen challenge. Arch. Otolaryngol. 110:508.

Doyle, W. J., Ingraham, A. S., Saad, M., et al. 1984b. A primate model of cleft palate and middle ear disease: Results of a one-year postcleft follow-up. In Lim, D. J., Bluestone, C. D., Klein, J. O., and Nelson, J. D. (eds.): Recent Advances in Otitis Media with Effusion. Toronto, B. C. Decker, pp. 215–218.

Draper, W. L. 1967. Secretory otitis media in children: A study of 540 children. Laryngoscope 77:636.

Draper, W. L. 1974. Allergy in relationship to the eustachian tube and middle ear. Otolaryngol. Clin. North Am. 7:749.

Drettner, B. 1960. The nasal airway and hearing in patients with cleft palate. Acta Otolaryngol. (Stockh.) 52:131.

Drury, D. W. 1925. Diphtheria of the ear. Arch. Otolaryngol. 1:221.

Dugdale, A. E., Canty, A., Lewis, A. N., et al. 1978. The natural history of chronic middle ear disease in Australian aboriginals: A cross-sectional study. Med. J. Aust. Spec. Suppl. 1:6.

Dugdale, A. E., Lewis, A. N., and Canty, A. A. 1982. The natural history of chronic otitis media. N. Engl. J. Med. 307:1459.

Edell, S. L., and Isaacson, S. 1978. A-mode ultrasound evaluation of the maxillary sinus. Otolaryngol. Clin. North Am. 11:531.

Eden, A., and Gannon, P. I. 1987. Neural control of middle ear aeration. Arch. Otol. Head Neck Surg. 113:133.

Eguchi, S. 1975. A new acoustical measurement of tubal opening. Otologia (Fukuoka) 21:154.

Ekvall, L. 1970. Eustachian tube function in tympanoplasty. Acta Otolaryngol. (Stockh.) Suppl. 263:33.

Eliasson, R., Mossberg, B., Camner, P., et al. 1977. The immotile cilia syndrome: A congenital ciliary abnormality as an etiologic factor in chronic airway infections and male sterility. N. Engl. J. Med. 297:1.

Elbrønd, O., and Larsen, E. 1976. Mucociliary function of the eustachian tube. Arch. Otolaryngol. 102:539.

Elner, A. 1972. Indirect determination of gas absorption from the middle ear. Acta Otolaryngol. (Stockh.) 74:191.

Elner, A. 1977. Quantitative studies of gas absorption from the normal middle ear. Acta Otolaryngol. (Stockh.) 83:25.

Elner, A., Ingelstedt, S., and Ivarsson, A. 1971a. A method for studies of middle ear mechanics. Acta Otolaryngol. (Stockh.) 72:191.

Elner, A., Ingelstedt, S., and Ivarsson, A. 1971b. Indirect determination of the middle ear pressure. Acta Otolaryngol. (Stockh.) 72:255.

Elner, A., Ingelstedt, S., and Ivarrson, A. 1971c. The elastic properties of the tympanic membrane system. Acta Otolaryngol. (Stockh.) 72:397.

Elner, A., Ingelstedt, S., and Ivarsson, A. 1971d. The normal function of the eustachian tube: A study of 102 cases. Acta Otolaryngol. (Stockh.) 72:320.

Elpern, B. S., Naunton, R. F., and Perlman, H. B. 1964. Objective measurement of middle ear function: The eustachian tube. Laryngoscope 74:359.

Ensign, P. R., Ubanich, E. M., and Moran, M. 1960. Prophylaxis for otitis media in an Indian population. Am. J. Public Health 50:195.

Ernston, S., and Anari, M. 1985. Cefaclor in the treatment of otitis media with effusion. Acta Otolaryngol. (Stockh.) Suppl. 100:17.

Eskola, J., Käyhty, H., and Peltola, H. 1985. Antibody levels achieved in infants by course of Haemophilus influenzae type b polysaccharide/diphtheria toxoid conjugate vaccine. Lancet 1:1184.

Evans, W. E., Feldman, S., Barker, L. F., et al. 1978. Use of gentamicin serum levels to individualize therapy in children. J. Pediatr. 93:133.

Falk, B., and Magnuson, B. 1984. Eustachian tube closing failure in children with persistent middle ear effusion. Int. J. Pediatr. Otorhinolaryngol. 7:97.

Feder, H. M., Jr. 1982. Comparative tolerability of ampicillin,

amoxicillin, and trimethoprim-sulfamethoxazole suspension in children with otitis media. Antimicrob. Agents Chemother. 121:426.

Feigin, R. D., Kenney, R. E., Nusrala, J., et al. 1973a. Efficacy of clindamycin therapy for otitis media. Arch. Otolaryngol. 98:27.

Feigin, R. D., Shackelford, P. G., Campbell, J., et al. 1973b. Assessment of the role of Staphylococcus epidermidis as a cause of otitis media. Pediatrics 52:569.

Feingold, M., Klein, J. O., Haslam, G. E., et al. 1966. Acute otitis media in children: Bacteriological findings in middle ear fluid obtained by needle aspiration. Am. J. Dis. Child. 111:361.

Ferber, A., and Holmquist, J. 1973. Roentgenographic demonstration of the eustachian tube in chronic otitis media. Acta Radiol. (Diagn.) (Stockh.) 14:667.

Fernandez, A. A., and McGovern, J. P. 1965. Secretory otitis media in allergic infants and children. South. Med. J. 58:581.

Ferrer, H. 1974. Use of impedance audiometry in school screening. Public Health 88:153.

Fiellau-Nikolajsen, M. 1979. Tympanometry in three-year-old children. II. Seasonal influence on tympanometric results in nonselected groups of three-year-old children. Scand. Audiol. 8:181.

Fiellau-Nikolajsen, M., Lous, J., Vang Pedersen, S., et al. 1977. Tympanometry in three-year-old children. I. A regional prevalence study on the distribution of tympanometric results in a nonselected population of three-year-old children. Scand. Audiol. 6:99.

Findlay, R. C., Stool, S. E., and Svitko, C. A. 1977. Tympanometric and otoscopic evaluations of a school-age deaf population: A longitudinal study. Am. Ann. Deaf 122:407.

Finegold, S. M. 1981. Anaerobic infections in otolaryngology. Ann. Otol. Rhinol. Laryngol. 90:13.

Finland, M., Brumfitt, W., and Kass, E. H. (eds.). 1976. Advances in aminoglycoside therapy: Amikacin. J. Infect. Dis. 134:S235.

Finland, M., and Hewitt, W. L. (eds.). 1971. Second international symposium on gentamicin, an aminoglycoside antibiotic. J. Infect. Dis. 124:S1.

Finland, M., and Neu, H. C. (eds.). 1976. Tobramycin. Symposium of the ninth international congress of chemotherapy in London, England. J. Infect. Dis. 134:S1.

Fischer, G. W., Sunakorn, P., and Duangman, C. 1977. Otogenous tetanus: A sequela of chronic ear infections. Am. J. Dis. Child. 131:445.

Fischer, J. J., McAdams, J. A., Entis, G. N., et al. 1978. Middle ear ciliary defect in Kartagener's syndrome. Pediatrics 62:443.

Fisher, R., McManus, J., Entis, G., et al. 1978. Middle ear ciliary defect in Kartagener's syndrome. Pediatrics 62:443.

Flisberg, K. 1966. Ventilatory studies on the eustachian tube: A clinical investigation of cases with perforated eardrums. Acta Otolaryngol. (Stockh.) Suppl. 219.

Fraser, J. G., Mehta, M., and Fraser, P. M. 1977. The medical treatment of secretory otitis media: A clinical trial of three commonly used regimens. J. Laryngol. Otol. 91:757.

Freijd, A., Oxelius, V.-A., and Rynnel-Dagoo, B. 1985. A prospective study demonstrating an association between plasma IgG2 concentrations and susceptibility to otitis media in children. Scand. J. Infect. Dis. 17:115.

Fria, T. J., Cantekin, E. I., and Eichler, J. A. 1985. Hearing acuity of children with otitis media with effusion. Arch. Otolaryngol. 111:10.

Fria, T. J., Cantekin, E. I., and Probst, G. 1980. Validation of an automatic otoadmittance middle ear analyzer. Ann. Otol. Rhinol. Laryngol. 89:253.

Fria, T. J., and Sabo, D. L. 1980. Auditory brainstem responses in children with otitis media with effusion. Ann. Otol. Rhinol. Laryngol. 89:200.

Fria, T. J., Sabo, D., and Beery, Q. C. 1978. The acoustic reflex in the identification of otitis media with effusion. Presented at the American Speech and Hearing Association National Convention, 1978.

Friedman, C. A., Lovejoy, F. C., and Smith, A. L. 1979. Chloramphenicol disposition in infants and children. J. Pediatr. 95:1071.

Friedman, R. A., Doyle, W. J., Casselbrant, M. L., et al. 1983. Immunologic-mediated eustachian tube obstruction: A double-blind crossover study. J. Allergy Clin. Immunol. 71:442.

Fuchs, P. C., Gavan, T. L., Gerlach, E. H., et al. 1977. Ticarcillin:

A collaborative *in vitro* comparison with carbenicillin against over 9,000 clinical bacterial isolates. Am. J. Med. Sci. 274:255.

Ganstrom, G., Holmquist, J., Jarlstedt, J., et al. 1985. Collagenase activity in middle ear effusion. Acta Otolaryngol. (Stockh.) 100:405.

Gates, G. A., Avery, C., Cooper, J. C., et al. 1986. Predictive value of tympanometry in middle ear effusion. Ann. Otol. Rhinol. Laryngol. 95:46.

Gates, G. A., Avery, C. S., Phihooa, T. J., et al. 1987. Effectiveness of adenoidectomy and tympanostomy tubes in the treatment of chronic otitis media with effusion. N. Engl. J. Med. 317:1444.

Gebhart, D. E. 1981. Tympanostomy tubes in the otitis media–prone child. Laryngoscope 91:849.

Gerrity, T. R., Cotromanes, E., Garrard, C. S., et al. 1983. The effect of aspirin on lung mucociliary clearance. N. Engl. J. Med. 308:139.

Gershel, J., Kruger, B., Giraudi-Perry, D., et al. 1985. Accuracy of the Welch Allyn audioscope and traditional hearing screening for children with known hearing loss. J. Pediatr. 106:15.

Getty, J. (Marketing Plans Manager, Eli Lilly) 1982. *In* Nelson, J. D., and McCraken, G. H., Jr. (eds.): Pediatric Infectious Disease Newsletter, Vol. 8, No. 3.

Giebink, G. S., Berzins, I. K., Cates, K. L., et al. 1980. Polymorphonuclear leukocyte function during otitis media. Ann. Otol. Rhinol. Laryngol. 89:138.

Giebink, G. S., Mills, E. L., Huff, J. S., et al. 1979. The microbiology of serous and mucoid otitis media. Pediatrics 63:915.

Giebink, G. S., and Quie, P. G. 1978. Otitis media: The spectrum of middle ear inflammation. Ann. Rev. Med. 29:285.

Ginsburg, C. M., McCracken, G. H., and Nelson, J. D. 1981. Pharmacology of oral antibiotics used for treatment of otitis media and tonsillopharyngitis in infants and children. Ann. Otol. Rhinol. Laryngol. 90:37.

Glew, R. H., Diven, W. F., and Bluestone, C. D. 1981. Lysosomal hydrolases in middle ear effusions. Ann. Otol. Rhinol. Laryngol. 90:148.

Gnehm, H. E., Pelton, S. I., Gulati, S., et al. 1985. Characterization of antigens from nontypable *Haemophilus influenzae* recognized by human bactericidal antibodies. J. Clin. Invest. 75:1645.

Goetzinger, C. P., Embrey, J. E., Brooks, R., et al. 1960. Auditory assessment of cleft palate adults. Acta Otolaryngol. (Stockh.) 52:551.

Gold, J. A., Hegarty, C. P., Deitch, M. W., et al. 1979. Double-blind clinical trials of oral cyclacillin and ampicillin. Antimicrob. Agents Chemother. 15:55.

Gold, R., Lepow, M. L., Goldschneider, I., et al. 1978. Antibody responses of human infants to three doses of Group A *Neisseria meningitidis* polysaccharide vaccine administered at two, four, and six months of age. J. Infect. Dis. 138:731.

Goodhill, V. 1979. Ear Diseases, Deafness, and Dizziness. Hagerstown, MD, Harper & Row, pp. 356–379.

Gorbach, S. L., and Bartlett, J. G. 1977. Pseudomembranous enterocolitis: A review of its diverse forms. J. Infect. Dis. 135:S89.

Goss, C. (ed.). 1967. Gray's Anatomy of the Human Body. Philadelphia, Lea & Febiger, p. 1087.

Gottschalk, G. H. 1966. Further experience with controlled middle ear inflation in treatment of serous otitis. EENT Monthly 45:49.

Gottschalk, G. H. 1980. Nonsurgical management of otitis media with effusion. Ann. Otol. Rhinol. Laryngol. 89:301.

Grace, A., Kwok, P., and Hawke, M. 1987. Surfactant in middle ear effusions. Otol. Head Neck Surg. 96:335.

Graham, M. D. 1963. A longitudinal study of ear disease and hearing loss in patients with cleft lips and palates. TAAOO 67:213.

Graham, M. D., and Lierle, D. M. 1962. Posterior pharyngeal flap palatoplasty and its relation to ear disease and hearing loss: A preliminary report. Laryngoscope 72:1750.

Granoff, D. M., Squires, J. E., Munson, R. S., Jr., et al. 1983. Siblings of patients with *Haemophilus* meningitis have impaired anticapsular antibody responses to *Haemophilus* vaccine. J. Pediatr. 103:185.

Granstrom, E., Holmquist, J., Jarlstedt, J., et al. 1985. Collagenase activity in middle ear effusion. Acta Otolaryngol. (Stockh.) 100:405.

Grason, R. L. 1972. Otoadmittance meters. *In* Proceedings of Impedance Symposium. Rochester, MN.

Graves, G. O., and Edwards, L. F. 1944. The eustachian tube: Review of its descriptive, microscopic, topographic, and clinical anatomy. Arch. Otolaryngol. 39:359.

Gray, B. M., Converse, G. M., and Dillon, H. C., Jr. 1979. Serotypes of *Streptococcus pneumoniae* causing disease. J. Infect. Dis. 140:979.

Green, G. R., Rosenblum, A. H., and Sweet, L. C. 1977. Evaluation of penicillin hypersensitivity: Value of clinical history and skin testing with penicilloylpolysine and penicillin G. A cooperative prospective study of the penicillin study group of the American Academy of Allergy. J. Allergy Clin. Immunol. 60:339.

Greene, J. W., Hara, C., O'Connor, S., et al. 1981. Management of febrile outpatient neonates. Clin. Pediatr. 20:375.

Grilliat, J. P., Streiff, F., and Hua, G. 1966. Fatal cytopenia after chloramphenicol hemisuccinate therapy. Ann. Med. (Nancy) 5:754.

Gronroos, J. A., Kortekangas, A. E., Ojala, L., et al. 1964. The aetiology of acute middle ear infection. Acta Otolaryngol. (Stockh.) 58:149.

Guillerm, R., Riu, R., Badre, R., et al. 1966. Une nouvelle technique d'exploration fonctionelle de la trompe d'Eustache: La sonomanometrie tubaire. Ann. Otolaryngol. Chir. Cervicofac. 83:523.

Gutzmann, H. 1893. Zur Prognose und Behandlung der angeborenen Gaumendefekte. Mschr. Sprachheilk.

Gyergyay, A. 1932. Neue Wege zur Erkennung der Physiologie und Pathologie der Ohrtrompete. Monatsschr. Ohrenheilkd. Laryngorhinol. 66:769.

Hagen, W. E. 1977. Surface tension lowering substance in eustachian tube function. Laryngoscope 87:1033.

Hagerman, R. J., Altshul-Stark, D., and McBogg, P. 1987. Recurrent otitis media in the fragile X syndrome. Am. J. Dis. Child. 141:184.

Halfond, M. M., and Ballenger, J. J. 1956. An audiologic and otorhinologic study of cleft lip and cleft palate cases. Arch. Otolaryngol. 64:58.

Hall, C. B., McBride, J. T., Walsh, E. E., et al. 1983. Aerosolized ribavirin treatment of infants with respiratory syncytial viral infection. A randomized double-blind study. N. Engl. J. Med. 308:1443.

Halstead, C., Lepow, M. L., Balassanian, N., et al. 1968. Otitis media: Clinical observations, microbiology and evaluation of therapy. Am. J. Dis. Child. 115:542.

Hammerschlag, M. R., Hammerschlag, P. E., and Alexander, E. R. 1980. The role of *Chlamydia trachomatis* in middle ear effusion in children. Pediatrics 66:615.

Hanson, D. G., and Ulvestad, R. F. (eds.). 1979. Otitis media and child development: Speech, language, and education. Ann. Otol. Rhinol. Laryngol. 88:1.

Hanson, L. A., Andersson, B., Carlsson, B., et al. 1985. Defense of mucous membranes by antibodies, receptor analogues and nonspecific host factors. Infection 13:S166.

Harcourt, F. L., and Brown, A. K. 1953. Hydrotympanum (secretory otitis media). Arch. Otolaryngol. 57:12.

Harding, A. L., Anderson, P., Howie, V. M., et al. 1973. *Haemophilus influenzae* isolated from children with otitis media. *In* Sell, S. H. W., and Kargon, D. T. (eds.): *Haemophilus influenzae*. Nashville, Vanderbilt University Press, pp. 21–28.

Harford, E. R., Bess, F. H., Bluestone, C. D., et al. (eds.) 1978. Impedance Screening for Middle Ear Disease in Children. New York, Grune & Stratton.

Harker, L. A., and Van Wagoner, R. 1974. Application of impedance audiometry as a screening instrument. Acta Otolaryngol. (Stockh.) 77:198.

Harrison, C. J., Marks, M. I., and Welch, D. F. 1985. Microbiology of recently treated acute otitis media compared with previously untreated acute otitis media. Pediatr. Infect. Dis. 4:641.

Harrison, R. J., and Phillips, B. J. 1971. Observations on hearing losses of preschool cleft palate children. J. Speech Hear. Disord. 36:252.

Haverkos, H. W., Caparosa, R., Ya, V. L., et al. 1982. Moxalactam therapy. Its use in chronic suppurative otitis media and malignant external otitis. Arch. Otolaryngol. 108:329.

Hayden, F. G., Albrecht, J. K., Kaiser, D. L., et al. 1986. Prevention of natural colds by contact prophylaxis with intranasal alpha 2-interferon. N. Engl. J. Med. 314:71.

Hayden, G. F., and Schwartz, R. H. 1985. Characteristics of earache among children with acute otitis media. Am. J. Dis. Child. 139:721.

Healy, G. B. 1984. Antimicrobial therapy of chronic otitis media with effusion. Int. J. Pediatr. Otorhinolaryngol. 8:13.

Healy, G. B., and Teele, D. W. 1977. The microbiology of chronic middle ear effusions in young children. Laryngoscope 87:1472.

Heermann, J., Jr., Heermann, H., and Kopstein, E. 1970. Fascia and cartilage palisade tympanoplasty: Nine years experience. Arch. Otolaryngol. 91:228.

Heiner, D. C. 1987. Recognition and management of IgG subclass deficiencies. Pediatr. Infect. Dis. 6:235.

Heisse, J. W., Jr. 1963. Secretory otitis media: Treatment with depomethylprednisone. Laryngoscope 73:54.

Heller, J. C., Hochberg, L., and Milano, G. 1970. Audiologic and otologic evaluation of cleft palate children. Cleft Palate J. 7:774.

Henderson, F. W., Collier, A. M., Clyde, W. A., Jr., et al. 1977. The epidemiology of acute otitis media in childhood. Abstract, Interscience Conference on Antimicrobial Agents and Chemotherapeutics.

Henderson, F. W., Collier, A. M., Sanyal, M. A., et al. 1982. A longitudinal study of respiratory viruses and bacteria in the etiology of acute otitis media with effusion. N. Engl. J. Med. 306:1377.

Herberts, G., Jeppson, P. H., Nylen, O., et al. 1971. Acute otitis media: Etiological and therapeutical aspects of acute otitis media. Prac. Otol. Rhinol. Laryngol. 33:191.

Herva, E., Haiva, V.-M., Koskela, M., et al. 1984. Pneumococci and their capsular polysaccharide antigens in middle ear effusion in acute otitis media. In Lim, D. J., Bluestone, C. D., Klein, J. O., and Nelson, J. D. (eds.): Recent Advances in Otitis Media with Effusion. Toronto, B. C. Decker, pp. 120–122.

Hewitt, W. L., and McHenry, M. C. 1978. Blood level determinations of antimicrobial drugs. Some clinical considerations. Med. Clin. North Am. 62:1119.

Higham, M., Cunningham, F. M., and Teele, D. W. 1985. Ceftriaxone administered once or twice a day for treatment of bacterial infections of childhood. Pediatr. Infect. Dis. 4:22.

Hill, H. R., Book, L. S., Hemming, V. G., et al. 1977. Defective neutrophil chemotactic responses in patients with recurrent episodes of otitis media and chronic diarrhea. Am. J. Dis. Child. 131:433.

Hills, B. A. 1984a. Analysis of eustachian surfactant and its function as a release agent. Arch. Otolaryngol. 110:3.

Hills, B. A. 1984b. Hydrophobic lining of the eustachian tube imparted by surfactant. Arch. Otolaryngol. 110:779.

Hoekelman, R. A. 1977. Infectious illness during the first year of life. Pediatrics 59:119.

Holborow, C. 1970. Eustachian tube function: Changes in anatomy and function with age and the relationship of these changes with aural pathology. Arch. Otolaryngol. 92:624.

Holborow, C. 1975. Eustachian tube function: Changes throughout childhood and neuro-muscular control. J. Laryngol. Otol. 89:47.

Holmes, E. M., and Reed, G. F. 1955. Hearing and deafness in cleft palate patients. Arch. Otolaryngol. 62:620.

Holmquist, J. 1968. The role of the eustachian tube in myringoplasty. Acta Otolaryngol. (Stockh.) 66:289.

Holmquist, J. 1969a. Eustachian tube function in patients with eardrum perforations following chronic otitis media. Acta Otolaryngol. (Stockh.) 68:391.

Holmquist, J. 1969b. Eustachian tube function assessed with tympanometry. Acta Otolaryngol. (Stockh.) 68:501.

Holmquist, J. 1970. Middle ear ventilation in chronic otitis media. Arch. Otolaryngol. 92:617.

Holmquist, J. 1972. Tympanometry in testing auditory tubal function. Audiology 11:209.

Holmquist, J. 1977. Medical treatment in ears with eustachian tube dysfunction. Presented at the Symposium on Physiology and Pathophysiology of the Eustachian Tube and Middle Ear, Freiburg, West Germany.

Honjo, I. 1981. Experimental study of the pumping function of the eustachian tube. Acta Otolaryngol. 91:85.

Honjo, I. 1987. Localization of motor neurons innervating the eustachian tube muscles in cats. Acta Otolaryngol. (Stockh.) 104:108.

Honjo, I., Hayashi, M., Ito, S., et al. 1985. Pumping and clearance function of the eustachian tube. Am. J. Otolaryngol. 6:241.

Honjo, I., Okazaki, N., and Kumazawa, T. 1979. Experimental study of the eustachian tube function with regard to its related muscles. Acta Otolaryngol. (Stockh.) 87:84.

Honjo, I., Ushiro, K., Hajo, T., et al. 1983. Role of tensor tympani muscle in eustachian tube function. Acta Otolaryngol. (Stockh.) 95:329.

Honjo, I., Ushiro, K., Mitoma, T., et al. 1984. Eustachian function of children with secretory otitis media. Pract. Otol. (Kyoto) 77:1111.

Honjo, I., Ushiro, K., Okazaki, N., et al. 1981. Evaluation of eustachian tube function by contrast roentgenography. Arch. Otolaryngol. 107:350.

Howard, J. E., Nelson, J. D., Clashen, J., et al. 1976. Otitis media of infancy and early childhood: A double-blind study of four treatment regimens. Am. J. Dis. Child. 130:965.

Howie, V. M. 1975. Natural history of otitis media. Ann. Otol. Rhinol. Laryngol. 84 (Suppl. 19):67.

Howie, V. M., Dillaro, R., and Lawrence, B., 1985. In vivo sensitivity in otitis media: Efficacy of antibiotics. Pediatrics 75:8.

Howie, V. M., and Ploussard, J. H. 1969. The "in vivo sensitivity test": Bacteriology of middle ear exudate during antimicrobial therapy in otitis media. Pediatrics 44:940.

Howie, V. M., and Ploussard, J. H. 1972. Efficacy of fixed combination antibiotics versus separate components in otitis media. Clin. Pediatr. (Phila.) 11:205.

Howie, V. M., Ploussard, J. H., and Lester, R. L. 1970. Otitis media: A clinical and bacteriological correlation. Pediatrics 45:29.

Howie, V. M., Ploussard, J. H., and Sloyer, J. 1974. Comparison of ampicillin and amoxicillin in the treatment of otitis media in children. J. Infect. Dis. 129:S181.

Howie, V. M., Ploussard, J. H., and Sloyer, J. 1975. The "otitis prone" condition. Am. J. Dis. Child. 129:676.

Howie, V. M., Ploussard, J. H., Sloyer, J. L., et al. 1984. Use of pneumococcal polysaccharide vaccine in preventing otitis media in infants: Different results between racial groups. Pediatrics 73:79.

Howie, V. M., Ploussard, J. H., Sloyer, J. L., et al. 1973. Immunoglobulins of the middle ear fluid in acute otitis media: Relationship to serum immunoglobulin concentrations and bacterial cultures. Infect. Immun. 7:589.

Howie, V. M., Pollard, R. B., Kleyn, K., et al. 1982. Presence of interferon during bacterial otitis media. J. Infect. Dis. 145:811.

Hubbaro, T. W., Paradise, T. L., McWilliams, B. J., et al. 1985. Consequences of unremitting middle-ear disease in early life. N. Engl. J. Med. 312:1529.

Ichimura, K. 1982. Neutrophil chemotaxis in children with recurrent otitis media. Int. J. Pediatr. Otorhinolaryngol. 4:47.

Ingelstedt, S., and Bylander, A. 1978. A comparison of the eustachian tube function in fifty children and fifty adults with normal ears. Presented at the Association for Research in Otolaryngology Meeting, St. Petersburg, FL.

Ingelstedt, S., Ivarsson, A., and Jonson, B. 1967a. Mechanics of the human middle ear; pressure regulation in aviation and diving: A nontraumatic method. Acta Otolaryngol. (Stockh.) Suppl. 228.

Ingelstedt, S., Ivarsson, A., and Jonson, B. 1967b. Quantitative determination of tubal ventilation during changes in ambient pressure as during ascent and descent in aviation. Acta Otolaryngol. (Stockh.) Suppl. 228:31.

Ingelstedt, S., and Ortegren, U. 1963. Qualitative testing of the eustachian tube function. Acta Otolaryngol. (Stockh.) Suppl. 182:7.

Ingvarsson, L. 1982. Acute otalgia in children—findings and diagnosis. Acta Pediatr. Scand. 71:705.

Ingvarsson, L., and Lundgren, K. 1982. The duration of penicillin treatment of acute otitis media children. Acta Otolaryngol. (Stockh.) Suppl. 386:112.

Ito, J., Oyagi, S., and Honjo, I. 1987. Localization of motoneurons innervating the eustachian tube muscles in cat. Acta Otolaryngol. (Stockh.) 104:108.

Jacobs, M. R., Koornhof, H. J., Robins-Browne, R. M., et al. 1978. Emergence of multiply resistant pneumococci. N. Engl. J. Med. 299:735.

Jaffe, B. F., Hurtado, F., and Hurtado, E. 1970. Tympanic membrane mobility in the newborn with seven months follow-up. Laryngoscope 80:36.

Jaumann, M. P., Steiner, W., and Berg, M. 1980. Endoscopy of the pharyngeal eustachian tube. Ann. Otol. Rhinol. Laryngol. 89 (Suppl. 68):54.

Jensen, K. J., Senterfit, L. B., Scully, W. E., et al. 1967. *Mycoplasma pneumoniae* infections in children. An epidemiologic appraisal in families treated with oxytetracycline. Am. J. Epidemiol. 86:419.

Jerger, J. 1970. Clinical experience with impedance audiometry. Arch. Otolaryngol. 92:311.

Johnston, R. B., Jr. 1984. Recurrent bacterial infections in children. N. Engl. J. Med. 310:1237.

Jokipii, L., Karma, P., and Jokipii, A. M. 1978. Access of metronidazole into the chronically inflamed middle ear with reference to anaerobic bacterial infection. Arch. Otolaryngol. 220:167.

Jonson, B., and Rundcrantz, H. 1969. Posture and pressure within the internal jugular vein. Acta Otolaryngol. (Stockh.) 68:271.

Jorgensen, F., Andersson, B., Larsson, S. H., et al. 1984. Children with frequent attacks of acute otitis media: A re-examination after eight years concerning middle ear changes, hearing, tubal function, and bacterial adhesion to pharyngeal epithelial cells. *In* Lim, D. J., Bluestone, C. D., Klein, J. O., and Nelson, J. D. (eds.): Recent Advances in Otitis Media with Effusion. Toronto, B. C. Decker, pp. 141–144.

Jorgensen, F., and Holmquist, J. 1984. Toynbee phenomenon and middle ear disease. Am. J. Otolaryngol. 4:291.

Juhn, S. K., and Huff, J. S. 1976. Biochemical characteristics of middle ear effusions. Ann. Otol. Rhinol. Laryngol. 85:110.

Kaiser, A. D. 1930. Results of tonsillectomy: A comparative study of 2,200 tonsillectomized children with an equal number of controls three and ten years after operation. J.A.M.A. 95:837.

Kaleida, P. H., Bluestone, C. D., Blatter, M. M., et al. 1986. Sultamicillin (ampicillin-sulbactam) in the treatment of acute otitis media in children. Pediatr. Infect. Dis. 5:33.

Kaleida, P. H., Bluestone, C. D., Rockette, H. E., et al. 1987. Amoxicillin-clavulanate potassium compared with cefaclor for acute otitis media in infants and children. Pediatr. Infect. Dis. 6:265.

Kamme, C. 1970. Evaluation of the *in vitro* sensitivity of *Neisseria catarrhalis* to antibiotics with respect to acute otitis media. Scand. J. Infect. Dis. 2:117.

Kamme, C. 1980. Penicillin-resistant *Branhamella catarrhalis*. Lakartidningen 77:4858.

Kamme, C., Ageberg, M., and Lundgren, K. 1970. Distribution of *Diplococcus pneumoniae* types in acute otitis media in children and influence of the types on the clinical course in penicillin V therapy. Scand. J. Infect. Dis. 2:183.

Kamme, C., Lundgren, K., and Rundcrantz, H. 1969. The concentration of penicillin V in serum and middle ear exudate in acute otitis media in children. Scand. J. Infect. Dis. 1:77.

Kaplan, G. J., Fleshman, J. K., Bender, T. R., et al. 1973. Long-term effects of otitis media: A ten-year cohort study of Alaskan Eskimo children. Pediatrics 52:577.

Kaplan, S. L., Mason, E. O., Jr., Mason, S. K., et al. 1984. Prospective comparative trial of moxalactam versus ampicillin or chloramphenicol for treatment of *Haemophilus influenzae* type b meningitis in children. J. Pediatr. 104:447.

Karma, P., Luotonen, J., Timonen, M., et al. 1980. Efficacy of pneumococcal vaccination against recurrent otitis media. Preliminary results of a field trial in Finland. Ann. Otol. Rhinol. Laryngol. 89:357.

Karma, P., Palva, A., and Kokko, E. 1976. Immunological defects in children with chronic otitis media. Acta Otolaryngol. (Stockh.) 82:193.

Karma, P., Pukander, J., Sipilä, M., et al. 1987. Middle ear fluid bacteriology or acute otitis media in neonates and very young infants. Int. J. Pediatr. Otorhinolaryngol. 14:141.

Karma, P., Sipilä, P., Virtanen, T., et al. 1985. Pneumococcal bacteriology after pneumococcal otitis media with special reference to pneumococcal antigens. Int. J. Pediatr. Otorhinolaryngol. 10:181.

Kass, E. H., and Evans, D. A. (eds.). 1979. Future prospects and past problems in antimicrobial therapy: The role of cefoxitin. Rev. Infect. Dis. 1:1.

Kaufman, R. S. 1970. Hearing loss in children with cleft palates. N.Y. State J. Med. 70:2555.

Kenna, M. A., Bluestone, C. D., Fall, P., et al. 1987. Cefixime vs. cefaclor in the treatment of acute otitis media in infants and children. Pediatr. Infect. Dis. 6:992.

Kenna, M. A., Bluestone, C. D., Reilly, J. S., et al. 1986. Medical management of chronic suppurative otitis media without cholesteatoma in children. Laryngoscope 96:146.

Kero, P., and Piekkala, P. 1987. Factors affecting the occurrence of acute otitis media during the first year of life. Acta Pediatr. Scand. 76:618.

Kessner, D. M., Snow, C. K., and Singer, J. 1974. Assessment of Medical Care for Children, Vol. 3. Washington, DC, Institute of Medicine, National Academy of Sciences.

Khanna, S. M., and Tonndorf, J. 1972. Tympanic membrane vibrations in cats studied by time-averaged holography. J. Acoust. Soc. Am. 51:1904.

Kilby, D., Richards, S. H., and Hart, G. 1972. Grommets and glue ears. Two year results. J. Laryngol. Otol. 86:881.

Kinmonth, A. L., Storrs, C. N., and Mitchell, R. G. 1978. Meningitis due to chloramphenicol-resistant *Haemophilus influenzae* type b. Br. Med. J. 1:694.

Kirby, W. M. M. (Chrmn.) 1970. Symposium on carbenicillin. A clinical profile. J. Infect. Dis. 122:S1.

Kitajiri, M., Sando, I., Hashida, Y., and Doyle, W. 1984. Histopathology of otitis media in infants with cleft and high arched palates. *In* Lim, D. J., Bluestone, C. D., Klein, J. O., and Nelson, J. D. (eds.): Recent Advances in Otitis Media with Effusion. Toronto, B. C. Decker, pp. 195–198.

Kitajiri, M., Sando, I., and Takahara, T. 1987. Postnatal development of the eustachian tube and its surrounding structures. Ann. Otol. Laryngol. 96:191.

Kjellman, N. I., Synnerstad, B., and Hansson, L. O. 1976. Atopic allergy and immunoglobulins in children with adenoids and recurrent otitis media. Acta Paediatr. Scand. 65:593.

Klein, B. S., Dollete, F. R., and Yolken, R. H. 1982. The role of respiratory syncytial virus and other viral pathogens in acute otitis media. J. Pediatr. 101:16.

Klein, J. O. 1976. Otitis media in the newborn infant. *In* Remington, J. S., and Klein, J. O. (eds.): Infectious Diseases of the Fetus and Newborn Infant. Philadelphia, W. B. Saunders Co., p. 807.

Klein, J. O. 1981. Epidemiology of pneumococcal disorders in infants and children. Rev. Infect. Dis. 3:246.

Klein, J. O. (ed.). 1985. Symposium on long-acting penicillins. Pediatr. Infect. Dis. 4:569.

Klein, J. O., and Bluestone, C. D. 1982. Acute otitis media. Pediatr. Infect. Dis. 1:66.

Klein, J. O., and Bratton, L. 1973. Unpublished data.

Klein, J. O., and Marcy, S. M. 1983. Bacterial sepsis and meningitis. *In* Remington, J. S., and Klein, J. O. (eds.): Infectious Diseases of the Fetus and Newborn Infant, 2nd ed. Philadelphia, W. B. Saunders Co., pp. 679–735.

Klein, J. O., and Teele, D. W. 1976. Isolation of viruses and mycoplasmas from middle ear effusions: A review. Ann. Otol. Rhinol. Laryngol. 85 (Suppl. 25):140.

Klimek, J. J., Bates, T. R., Nightingale, C., et al. 1980. Penetration characteristics of trimethoprim-sulfamethoxazole in middle ear fluid of patients with chronic serous otitis media. J. Pediatr. 96:1087.

Klimek, J. J., Nightingale, C., Lehmann, W. B., et al. 1977. Comparison of concentrations of amoxicillin and ampicillin in serum and middle ear fluid of children with chronic otitis media. J. Infect. Dis. 135:999.

Koch, H., and Dennison, N. J. 1974. Office visits to pediatricians. Hyattsville, MD, National Ambulatory Medical Care Service, National Center for Health Statistics.

Kokko, E. 1974. Chronic secretory otitis media in children: A clinical study. Acta Otolaryngol. (Stockh.) Suppl. 327:7.

Korsan-Bengstein, M., and Nylen, O. 1974. A follow-up study of cleft children treated with primary bone grafting. Scand. J. Plast. Reconstr. Surg. 8:161.

Koskela, M., Leinonen, M., and Luotonen, J. 1982. Serum antibody response to pneumococcal otitis media. Pediatr. Infect. Dis. 1:245.

Kovatch, A. L., Wald, E. R., and Michaels, R. H. 1983. β-Lactamase–producing *Branhamella catarrhalis* causing otitis media in children. J. Pediatr. 102:261.

Kraemer, R. J., Richardson, M. A., Weiss, N. S., et al. 1983. Risk factors for persistent middle-ear effusions. J.A.M.A. 249:1022.

Krasinski, K., Kusmeisz, H., and Nelson, J. D. 1982. Pharmacologic interactions among chloramphenicol, phenytoin and phenobarbital. Pediatr. Infect. Dis. 1:232.

Krause, P. J., Owens, N. G., Nightingale, C. H., et al. 1982. Penetration of amoxicillin, cefaclor, erythromycin-sulfisoxazole, and trimethoprim-sulfamethoxazole into the middle ear fluid of patients with chronic serous otitis media. J. Infect. Dis. 145:815.

Kunin, C. M. 1972. Antibiotic usage in patients with renal impairment. Hosp. Pract. 7:141.

LaFaye, M., Gaillard de Collogny, L., Jourde, H., et al. 1974. Étude de la permeabilité de la trompe d'Eustache par les radio-isotopes. Ann. Otolaryngol. Chir. Cervicofac. 91:665.

Lahikainen, E. A. 1953. Clinico-bacteriologic studies on acute otitis media: Aspiration of tympanum as diagnostic and therapeutic method. Acta Otolaryngol. (Stockh.) Suppl. 107:1.

Lahikainen, E. A. 1970. Penicillin concentration in middle ear secretion in otitis. Acta Otolaryngol. (Stockh.) 70:358.

Lahikainen, E. A., Vuori, M., and Virtanen, S. 1977. Azidocillin and ampicillin concentrations in middle ear effusion. Acta Otolaryngol. (Stockh.) 84:227.

LaMarco, K. L., Diven, W. F., Glew, R. H., et al. 1984. Neuraminidase activity in middle ear effusion. Ann. Otol. Rhinol. Laryngol. 93:76.

Lampe, R. M., and Weir, M. R. 1986. Erythromycin prophylaxis for recurrent otitis media. Clin. Pediatr. 25:510.

Lampe, R. M., Weir, M. R., Spier, J., et al. 1985. Acoustic reflectometry in the detection of middle ear effusion. Pediatrics 76:75.

Lang, R. W., Liu, Y. S., Lim, D. J., et al. 1976. Antimicrobial factors and bacterial correlation in chronic otitis media with effusion. Ann. Otol. Rhinol. Laryngol. 85:145.

Lannois, M. 1901. De l'état de l'oreille moyenne dans les fissures congenitales du palais. Rev. Hebd. Laryngol. 21:177.

Laxdal, O. E., Merida, J., and Trefor Jones, R. H. 1970. Treatment of acute otitis media: A controlled study of 142 children. Can. Med. Assoc. J. 102:263.

Lee, K., and Schuknecht, H. F. 1971. Results of tympanoplasty and mastoidectomy at the Massachusetts Eye and Ear Infirmary. Laryngoscope 81:529.

Leinonen M., Luotonen, J., Herva, E., et al. 1981. Preliminary serologic evidence for a pathogenic role of Branhamella catarrhalis. J. Infect. Dis. 144:570.

Levine, B. B. 1966. Immunologic mechanisms of penicillin allergy. A haptenic model system for the study of allergic diseases of man. N. Engl. J. Med. 275:1115.

Levine, B. B., Redmond, A. P., Fellner, M. J., et al. 1966. Penicillin allergy and the heterogeneous immune responses of man to benzylpenicillin. J. Clin. Invest. 45:1895.

Levine, L. R. 1985. Quantitative comparison of adverse reactions to cefaclor vs. amoxicillin in a surveillance study. Pediatr. Infect. Dis. 4:358.

Lewis, A. N., Barry, M., and Stuart, J. 1974. Screening procedures for the identification of hearing and ear disorders in Australian aboriginal children. J. Laryngol. Otol. 88:335.

Lewis, D. M., Schram, J. L., Birck, H. G., et al. 1979. Antibody activity in otitis media with effusion. Ann. Otol. Rhinol. Laryngol. 88:392.

Lewis, D. M., Schram, J. L., Lim, D. J., et al. 1978. Immunoglobulin E in chronic middle ear effusions: Comparison of RIST, PRIST, and RIA techniques. Ann. Otol. Rhinol. Laryngol. 87:197.

Lildholdt, T., Cantekin, E. I., Bluestone, C. D., et al. 1982. Effect of nasal decongestant on eustachian tube function in children with tympanostomy tubes. Acta Otolaryngol. (Stockh.) 94:93.

Lildholdt, T., Cantekin, E. I., Marshak, G., et al. 1981. Pharmacokinetics of cefaclor in chronic middle ear effusions. Ann. Otol. Rhinol. Laryngol. 90:44.

Lim, D. J., and DeMaria, T. F. 1987. Immunobarriers of the tubotympanum. Acta Otolaryngol. (Stockh.) 103:355.

Lindsay, W. K., LeMeusurier, A. B., and Farmer, A. W. 1962. A study of the speech results of a large series of cleft palate patients. Plast. Reconstr. Surg. 29:273.

Ling, D., McCoy, R. H., and Levinson, E. D. 1969. The incidence of middle ear disease and its educational implications among Baffin Island Eskimo children. Can. J. Public Health 60:385.

Linthicum, F. H., Body, H., and Keaster, J. 1959. Incidence of middle ear disease in children with cleft palate. Cleft Palate Bull. 9:23.

Liston, T. E., Foshee, W. S., and Pierson, W. D. 1983. Sulfisoxazole chemoprophylaxis for frequent otitis media. Pediatrics 71:524.

Liu, Y. S., Lim, D. J., Lang, R. W., et al. 1975. Chronic middle ear effusions: Immunochemical and bacteriological investigations. Arch. Otolaryngol. 101:278.

Liu, Y. S., Lim, D. J., Lang, R., et al. 1976. Micro-organisms in chronic otitis media with effusion. Ann. Otol. Rhinol. Laryngol. 85:245.

Loda, F. A., Glezen, W. P., and Clyde, W. A. 1972. Respiratory disease in group day care. Pediatrics 49:428.

Loeb, M. R., and Smith, D. H. 1980. Outer membrane protein composition in disease isolates of Haemophilus influenzae: Pathogenic and epidemiological implications. Infect. Immun. 30:710.

Loeb, W. J. 1964. Speech, hearing and the cleft palate. Arch. Otolaryngol. 79:1.

Long, S. S., Henretig, F. M., Teter, M. J., et al. 1984. Nasopharyngeal flora and acute otitis media. Infect. Immun. 41:987.

Lorentzen, P., and Haugsten, P. 1977. Treatment of acute suppurative otitis media. J. Laryngol. Otol. 91:331.

Lous, J., and Fiellau-Nikolajsen, M. 1981. Epidemiology of middle ear effusion and tubal dysfunction: A one year prospective study comprising monthly tympanometry in 387 nonselected seven year old children. Int. J. Pediatr. Otorhinolaryngol. 3:303.

Lundgren, K., Ingvarsson, L., and Olofsson, B. 1984. Epidemiologic aspects in children with recurrent otitis media. In Lim, D. J., Bluestone, C. D., Klein, J. O., and Nelson, J. D. (eds.): Recent Advances in Otitis Media with Effusion. Toronto, B. C. Decker, pp. 22–25.

Lundgren, K., Ingvarsson, L., and Rundcrantz, H. 1979. The concentration of penicillin V in middle ear exudate. Int. J. Pediatr. Otorhinolaryngol. 1:93.

Luotonen, J., Herva, E., Karma, P., et al. 1981. The bacteriology of acute otitis media in children with special reference to Streptococcus pneumoniae as studied by bacteriological and antigen detection methods. Scand. J. Infect. Dis. 13:177.

Luotonen, J., Jokipii, A. M. M., Vayrynen, J., et al. 1982. Aerobic and anaerobic bacteria in the middle ear and ear canal in acute otitis media. Acta Otolaryngol. (Stockh.) 386:100.

Lupin, A. J. 1969. The relationship of the tensor tympani and tensor palati muscles. Ann. Otol. Rhinol. Laryngol. 78:792.

Lynn, G. E., and Benitez, J. T. 1974. Temporal bone preservation in a 2600 year old Egyptian mummy. Science 183:200.

MacAdam, A. M., and Rubio, T. 1977. Tuberculous otomastoiditis in children. Am. J. Dis. Child. 131:152.

Macbeth, R. 1960. Some thoughts on the eustachian tube. Proc. R. Soc. Med. 53:151.

Mace, J. W., Janik, D. S., Sauer, R. L., et al. 1977. Penicillin-resistant pneumococcal meningitis in an immunocompromised infant. J. Pediatr. 91:506.

Mach, E., and Kessel, J. 1872. Die Function der Trommelhohle und der Tuber Eustachii sitzungsber. Weiner Akad. Math. Natur. Wiss. 66:329.

Magnus, A. 1864. Werhalten des Gehor-organs in konprimirter Luft. Arch. Ohren. 1:269.

Makela, P. H., Leinonen, M., Tukander, J., et al. 1981. A study of the polyvaccine in prevention of clinically acute attacks of recurrent otitis media. Rev. Infect. Dis. 3:S124.

Makela, P. H., Sibakov, M., Herva, E., et al. 1980. Pneumococcal vaccine and otitis media. Lancet 2:547.

Maknin, M. L., and Jones, P. K. 1985. Oral dexamethasone for treatment of persistent middle ear effusion. Pediatrics 75:329.

Mandel, E. M., Bluestone, C. D., Cantekin, E. I., et al. 1981. Comparison of cefaclor and amoxicillin for acute otitis media with effusion. Ann. Otol. Rhinol. Laryngol. 90:48.

Mandel, E. M., Bluestone, C. D., Paradise, J. L., et al. 1984. Efficacy of myringotomy with and without tympanostomy tube insertion in the treatment of chronic otitis media with effusion in infants and children: Results for the first year of a randomized clinical trial. In Lim, D. J., Bluestone, C. D., Klein, J. O., and Nelson, J. D. (eds.): Recent Advances in Otitis Media with Effusion. Toronto, B. C. Decker, pp. 308–311.

Mandel, E. M., Bluestone, C. D., Rockette, H. E., et al. 1982.

Duration of effusion after antibiotic treatment for acute otitis media: Comparison of cefaclor and amoxicillin. Pediatr. Infect. Dis. 1:310.

Mandel, E. M., Casselbrant, M. L., Bluestone, C. D., et al. 1988. Adenoidectomy, eustachian tube function, and otitis media. Ann. Otol. Rhinol. Laryngol. 97(Suppl. 133):52.

Mandel, E. M., Rockette, H. E., Bluestone, C. D., et al. 1987. Efficacy of amoxicillin with and without decongestant-antihistamine for otitis media with effusion in children: Results of a double-blind, randomized trial. N. Engl. J. Med. 316:432.

Marchant, C. D., Shurin, P. A., Johnson, C. E., et al. 1986. A randomized controlled trial of amoxicillin plus clavulanate compared with cefaclor for treatment of acute otitis media. J. Pediatr. 109:891.

Marchant, C. D., Shurin, P. A., Turcyzk, V. A., et al. 1984a. A randomized controlled trial of cefaclor compared with trimethoprim-sulfamethoxazole for treatment of acute otitis media. J. Pediatr. 105:633.

Marchant, C. D., Shurin, P. A., Turcyzk, V. A., et al. 1984b. Course and outcome of otitis media in early infancy: A prospective study. J. Pediatr. 104:826.

Marshak, G., and Neriah, Z. B. 1981. Adenoidectomy versus tympanostomy in chronic secretory otitis media. Ann. Otol. Rhinol. Laryngol. 89:316.

Masters, F. W., Bingham, H. G., and Robinson, D. W. 1960. The prevention and treatment of hearing loss in the cleft palate child. Plast. Reconstr. Surg. 25:503.

Mattar, M. E., Markello, J., and Yaffe, S. J. 1975. Pharmaceutic factors affecting pediatric compliance. Pediatrics 55:101.

Maw, A. R. 1983. Chronic otitis media with effusion and adenotonsillectomy—a prospective randomized controlled study. Int. J. Pediatr. Otorhinolaryngol. 6:239.

Maw, A. R. 1984. Chronic otitis media with effusion and adenotonsillectomy: A prospective randomized controlled study. In Lim, D. J., Bluestone, C. D., Klein, J. O., and Nelson, J. D. (eds.): Recent Advances in Otitis Media with Effusion. Toronto, B. C. Decker, pp. 299–302.

Mawson, S. R. 1974. The eustachian tube. In Mawson, S. R.: Diseases of the Ear. Baltimore, Williams & Wilkins Co.

Mawson, S. R., Adlington, R., and Evans, M. 1967. A controlled study evaluation of adeno-tonsillectomy in children. J. Laryngol. Otol. 81:77.

Mawson, S. R., and Fagan, P. 1972. Tympanic effusions in children: Long-term results of treatment by myringotomy, aspiration, and indwelling tubes (grommets). J. Laryngol. Otol. 86:105.

Maxim, P. E., Veltri, R. W., Sprinkle, P. M., et al. 1977. Chronic serous otitis media: An immune complex disease. TAAOO 84:234.

Maynard, J. E., Fleshman, J. K., and Tschopp, C. F. 1972. Otitis media in Alaskan Eskimo children: Prospective evaluation of chemoprophylaxis. J.A.M.A. 219:597.

McCandless, G. A., and Thomas, G. K. 1974. Impedance audiometry as a screening procedure for middle ear disease. TAAOO 78:98.

McCracken, G. H., Jr., and Nelson, J. D. 1983. Antimicrobial Therapy for Newborns, 2nd ed. New York, Grune & Stratton.

McCracken, G. H., Jr., Threlkeld, N., Mize, S., et al. 1984. Moxalactam therapy for neonatal meningitis due to gram-negative enteric bacilli. A prospective controlled evaluation. J.A.M.A. 252:1427.

McCurdy, J. A., Goldstein, J. L., and Gorski, D. 1976. Auditory screening of preschool children with impedance audiometry—a comparison with pure tone audiometry. Clin. Pediatr. 15:436.

McKee, W. J. 1963a. A controlled study of the effects of tonsillectomy and adenoidectomy in children. Br. J. Prev. Soc. Med. 17:46.

McKee, W. J. 1963b. The part played by adenoidectomy in the combined operation of tonsillectomy with adenoidectomy: Second part of a controlled study in children. Br. J. Prev. Soc. Med. 17:133.

McLinn, S. E. 1976. Letter: Cephalosporins in otitis media. Can. Med. Assoc. J. 114:13.

McLinn, S. E. 1980. Cefaclor in treatment of otitis media and pharyngitis in children. Am. J. Dis. Child. 134:560.

McLinn, S. E., Goldberg, F., Kramer, R., et al. 1982. Double-blind multicenter comparison of cyclacillin and amoxicillin for the treatment of acute otitis media. J. Pediatr. 101:607.

McLinn, S. E., and Serlin, S. 1983. Cyclacillin versus amoxicillin as treatment for acute otitis media. Pediatrics 71:196.

McMyn, J. K. 1940. The anatomy of the salpingopharyngeus muscle. J. Laryngol. Otol. 55:1.

McNicoll, W. D. 1982. Remediable eustachian tube dysfunction in diving recruits: Assessment, investigation, and management. Undersea Biomed. Res. 9:37.

McNicoll, W. D., and Scanlon, S. G. 1979. Submucous resection: The treatment of choice in the nose-ear distress syndrome. J. Laryngol. Otol. 93:357.

McWilliams, B. J. 1966. Speech and hearing problems in children with cleft palate. J. Am. Med. Wom. Assoc. 21:1005.

Means, B. J., and Irwin, J. V. 1954. An analysis of certain measures of intelligence and hearing loss in a sample of Wisconsin cleft palate population. Cleft Palate Bull. 4:4.

Mehta, D., and Erlich, M. 1978. Serous otitis media in school for the deaf. Volta Rev. 80:75.

Meissner, K. 1939. Ohrenerkrankungen bei Gaumen-spalten. Hals-Nasen-und Ohrenarzt 30:6.

Meistrup-Larsen, K.-I., Sorensen, H., Johnson, N.-J., et al. 1983. Two versus seven days penicillin treatment for acute otitis media. A placebo controlled trial in children. Acta Otolaryngol. (Stockh.) 96:99.

Meri, S., Lehtinen, T., and Palva, T. 1984. Complement in chronic secretory otitis media: C3 breakdown and C3 splitting activity. Arch. Otolaryngol. 110:774.

Metz, O. 1946. The acoustic impedance measured in normal and pathological ears. Acta Otolaryngol. (Stockh.) Suppl. 63.

Meurman, O. H., Sarkkinen, H. K., Puhakka, H. J., et al. 1980. Local IgA-class antibodies against respiratory viruses in middle ear and nasopharyngeal secretions of children with secretory otitis media. Laryngoscope 90:304.

Miller, G. F., Jr. 1965. Eustachian tube function in normal and diseased ears. Arch. Otolaryngol. 81:41.

Miller, G. F. 1970. Influence of an oral decongestant on eustachian tube function in children. J. Allergy 45:187.

Miller, G. F., and Bilodeau, R. 1967. Preoperative evaluation of eustachian tubal function in tympanoplasty. South. Med. J. 60:868.

Miller, M. H. 1956. Hearing losses in cleft palate cases: The incidence, type, and significance. Laryngoscope 66:1492.

Miller, S. A., Omene, J. A., Bluestone, C. D., et al. 1983. A point prevalence of otitis media in a Nigerian village. Int. J. Pediatr. Otolaryngol. 5:19.

Mitchell, G. A. C. 1954. The autonomic nerve supply of the throat, nose and ear. J. Laryngol. Otol. 68:495.

Moellering, R. C., Jr. (ed.). 1978. Symposium on cefamandole. J. Infect. Dis. 137 (Suppl.):S1.

Moellering, R. C., Jr., and Swartz, M. N. 1976. Drug therapy. The newer cephalosporins. N. Engl. J. Med. 294:24.

Mogi, G., Honjo, S., Maeda, S., et al. 1974. Immunoglobulin E (IgE) in middle ear effusions. Ann. Otol. Rhinol. Laryngol. 83:393.

Mogi, G., Maeda, S., Yoshida, T., et al. 1976. Immunochemistry of otitis media with effusion. J. Infect. Dis. 133:126.

Mogi, G., Yoshida, T., Honjo, S., et al. 1973. Middle ear effusions: Quantitative analysis of immunoglobulins. Ann. Otol. Rhinol. Laryngol. 82:196.

Mortimer, E. A., Jr., and Watterson, R. L., Jr. 1956. A bacteriologic investigation of otitis media in infancy. Pediatrics 17:359.

Muenker, G. 1980. Results after treatment of otitis media with effusion. Ann. Otol. Rhinol. Laryngol. 89:308.

Mumtaz, M. A., Schwartz, R. H., Grundfast, K. M., et al. 1983. Tuberculosis of the middle ear and mastoid. Pediatr. Infect. Dis. 2:234.

Murphy, T. F., and Apicella, M. A. 1985. Antigenic heterogenicity of outer membrane proteins of nontypable Haemophilus influenzae as a basis for serotyping system. Infect. Immun. 50:15.

Murphy, T. F., Bernstein, J. M., Dryja, D. M., et al. 1987. Outer membrane protein and lipooligosaccharide analysis of paired nasopharyngeal and middle ear isolates in otitis media due to nontypable Haemophilus influenzae: Pathogenic and epidemiological observations. J. Infect. Dis. 156:723.

Murrary, D. L., Singer, D. A., and Singer, A. B. 1980. Cefaclor: A cluster of adverse reactions. N. Engl. J. Med. 303:1003.

Murti, K. G., Stern, R. M., Cantekin, E. I., et al. 1980. Sonometric evaluation of eustachian tube function using broadband stimuli. Ann. Otol. Rhinol. Laryngol. 89:178.

Myers, E. N., Beery, Q. C., Bluestone, C. D., et al. 1984. Effect of certain head and neck tumors and their management on the ventilatory function of the eustachian tube. Ann. Otol. Rhinol. Laryngol. 93 (Suppl. 114):3.

Mygind, N., Meistrup-Larsen, K. I., Thomsen, J., et al. 1981. Penicillin in acute otitis media: A double-blind placebo-controlled trial. Clin. Otolaryngol. 6:5.

Mygind, N., and Pedersen, M. 1983. Nose, sinus and ear symptoms in 27 patients with primary ciliary dyskinesia. Eur. J. Respir. Dis. 64 (Suppl. 127):96.

Naiditch, M. J., and Bower, A. G. 1954. Diphtheria: A study of 1,433 cases observed during a ten-year period at Los Angeles County Hospital. Am. J. Med. 17:229.

Naito, Y., Hrono, Y., Honjo, I., et al. 1987. Magnetic resonance imaging of the eustachian tube. Arch. Otolaryngol. Head Neck Surg. 113:1281.

Nathanson, S. E., and Jackson, R. T. 1976. Vidian nerve and the eustachian tube. Ann. Otol. Rhinol. Laryngol. 85:83.

National Center for Health Statistics. 1974. Surgical Operations in Short-Stay Hospitals: United States—1971. DHEW Publication No. HRA-75-1769. Rockville, MD, United States Department of Health, Education and Welfare.

Naunton, R. F., and Galluser, J. 1967. Measurements of eustachian tube function. Ann. Otol. Rhinol. Laryngol. 76:455.

NDTI Review. 1970. Leading diagnoses and reasons for patient visits. 1:18.

Nelson, J. D. 1978. Oral antibiotic therapy for serious infections in hospitalized patients. J. Pediatr. 92:175.

Nelson, J. D., Howard, J. B., and Shelton, S. 1978. Oral antibiotic therapy for skeletal infections of children. J. Pediatr. 92:131.

Nelson, J. D., Ginsburg, C. M., McLeland, O., et al. 1981. Concentrations of antimicrobial agents in middle ear fluid, saliva and tears. Int. J. Pediatr. Otorhinolaryngol. 3:327.

Nelson, J. D., and McCracken, G. H. 1980. The drug of choice for otitis media? J. Pediatr. Infect. Dis. 6:5.

Nelson, W. L., Kuritsky, J. N., Kennedy, D. L., et al. 1987. Outpatient pediatric antibiotic use in the US: Trends and therapy for otitis media, 1977–1986. In Program and Abstracts of the 27th Interscience Conference on Antimicrobial Agents and Chemotherapy. Washington, DC, American Society for Microbiology.

Neu, H. C. 1978. A symposium on the tetracyclines: A major appraisal. Introduction. Bull. N.Y. Acad. Med. 54:141.

Nilson, B. W., Poland, R. L., Thompson, R. S., et al. 1969. Acute otitis media: Treatment results in relation to bacterial etiology. Pediatrics 43:351.

Noone, R. B., Randall, P., Stool, S. E., et al. 1973. The effect on middle ear disease of fracture of the pterygoid hamulus during palatoplasty. Cleft Palate J. 10:23.

Northern, J. L., and Downs, M. P. (eds.). 1978. Hearing in Children, 2nd ed. Baltimore, Williams & Wilkins Co.

Nozoe, T., Okazaki, N., Koda, Y., et al. 1984. Fluid clearance of the eustachian tube. In Lim, D. J., Bluestone, C. D., Klein, J. O., and Nelson, J. D. (eds.): Recent Advances in Otitis Media with Effusion. Toronto, B. C. Decker, pp. 66–68.

Odio, C. M., Kusmiesz, H., Shelton, S., et al. 1985. Comparative treatment trial of augmentin versus cefaclor for acute otitis media with effusion. Pediatrics 75:819.

Odio, H., Proud, G. O., and Toledo, P. S. 1971. Effects of pterygoid hamulotomy upon eustachian tube function. Laryngoscope 81:1242.

Ogawa, S., Satoh, I., and Tanaka, H. 1976. Patulous eustachian tube. A new treatment with infusion of absorbable gelatin sponge solution. Arch. Otolaryngol. 102:276.

Ohashi, Y., Nakai, Y., and Kihara, S. 1985. Ciliary activity of the middle ear in guinea pigs. Ann. Otol. Rhinol. Laryngol. 94:419.

Ohashi, Y., Nakai, Y., Koshimo, H., et al. 1986. Ciliary activity in the in vitro tubotympanum. Arch. Otorhinolaryngol. 243:317.

Olson, A. L., Klein, S. W., Charney, E., et al. 1978. Prevention and therapy of serous otitis media by oral decongestant: A double-blind study in pediatric practice. Pediatrics 61:679.

Oppenheimer, P. 1968. Short-term steroid therapy—treatment of serous otitis media in children. Arch. Otolaryngol. 88:138.

Oppenheimer, R. P. 1975. Serous otitis: Review of 992 patients. EENT Monthly 54:316.

Orchik, D. J., and Herdman, S. 1974. Impedance audiometry as a screening device with school-age children. J. Aud. Res. 14:283.

Ostfeld, E., and Altmann, G. L. 1980. Evaluation of countercurrent immunoelectrophoresis as a diagnostic tool in bacterial otitis media. Ann. Otol. Rhinol. Laryngol. 89:110.

Ostfeld, E., and Rubinstein, E. 1980. Acute gram-negative bacillary infections of middle ear and mastoid. Ann. Otol. Rhinol. Laryngol. 89:33.

Oyagi, S., Ito, J., and Honjo, I. 1987. The origin of autonomic nerves of the middle ear as studied by horseradish peroxidase tracer method. Acta Otolaryngol. (Stockh.) 104:463.

Oyiborhoro, J. M. A., Olaniyan, S. O., Newman, C. W., et al. 1987. Efficacy of acoustic otoscopy in detecting middle ear effusion in children. Laryngoscope 97:495.

Page, J. R. 1935. Report of acute infections of middle ear and mastoid process at Manhattan Eye, Ear, and Throat Hospital during 1934: Their prevalence and virulence. Laryngoscope 45:839.

Palva, T., Hayry, P., and Ylikoski, J. 1980. Lymphocyte morphology in middle ear effusions. Ann. Otol. Rhinol. Laryngol. 89:143.

Palva, T., Holopainen, E., and Karma, P. 1976. Protein and cellular protein of glue ear secretions. Ann. Otol. Rhinol. Laryngol. 85:103.

Palva, T., and Lehtinen, T. 1987. Pneumococcal antigens and endotoxin in effusions from patients with secretory otitis media. Int. J. Pediatr. Otolaryngol. 14:123.

Pannbacker, M. 1969. Hearing loss and cleft palate. Cleft Palate J. 6:50.

Paparella, M. M. 1980. The middle ear effusions. In Paparella, M. M., and Shumrick, D. A. (eds.): Otolaryngology, Vol. II. Philadelphia, W. B. Saunders Co., pp. 1422–1443.

Paparella, M. M., and Dickson, R. I. 1969. The recurrent middle ear effusions. Otolaryngol. Clin. North Am. 2:53.

Paparella, M. M., Hiraide, F., Juhn, S. K., et al. 1970. Cellular events involved in middle ear fluid production. Ann. Otol. Rhinol. Laryngol. 79:766.

Paparella, M. M., Oda, M., Hiraide, F., et al. 1972. Pathology of sensorineural hearing loss in otitis media. Ann. Otol. Rhinol. Laryngol. 81:632.

Paradise, J. L. 1977. On tympanostomy tubes: Rationale, results, reservations, and recommendations. Pediatrics 60:86.

Paradise, J. L. 1980. Otitis media in infants and children. Pediatrics 65:917.

Paradise, J. L. 1987. On classifying otitis media as suppurative or nonsuppurative with a suggested clinical schema. J. Pediatr. 111:948.

Paradise, J. L., and Bluestone, C. D. 1974. Early treatment of the universal otitis media of infants with cleft palate. Pediatrics 53:48.

Paradise, J. L., Bluestone, C. D., Bachman, R. Z., et al. 1984. Efficacy of tonsillectomy for recurrent throat infection in severely affected children: Results of parallel randomized and nonrandomized clinical trials. N. Engl. J. Med. 310:674.

Paradise, J. L., Bluestone, C. D., and Felder, H. 1969. The universality of otitis media in fifty infants with cleft palate. Pediatrics 44:35.

Paradise, J. L., Bluestone, C. D., Rogers, K. D., et al. 1980. Efficacy of adenoidectomy in recurrent otitis media: Historical overview and preliminary results from a randomized, controlled trial. Ann. Otol. Rhinol. Laryngol. 89:319.

Paradise, J. L., Bluestone, C. D., Rogers, K. D., et al. 1987. Efficacy of adenoidectomy for recurrent otitis media: Results from parallel random and nonrandom trials. Pediatr. Res. 21:286A.

Paradise, J. L., Bluestone, C. D., Rogers, K. D., et al. 1988. Adenoidectomy with and without tonsillectomy for otitis media. Ann. Otol. Rhinol. Laryngol. 97 (Suppl. 133):52.

Paradise, J. L., and Elster, B. A. 1984. Breast milk protects against otitis media with effusion. Pediatr. Res. 18:283A.

Paradise, J. L., and Smith, C. G. 1978. Impedance screening for preschool children—state of the art. In Harford, E. R., Bess, F. H., Bluestone, C. D., and Klein, J. O. (eds.): Impedance Screening for Middle Ear Disease in Children. New York, Grune & Stratton, pp. 113–124.

Paradise, J. L., Smith, C. G., and Bluestone, C. D. 1976. Tympanometric detection of middle ear effusion in infants and young children. Pediatrics 58:198.

Paredes, A., Taber, L. H., Yow, M. D., et al. 1976. Prolonged pneumococcal meningitis due to an organism with increased resistance to penicillin. Pediatrics 58:378.

Parisier, S. C., and Khilnani, M. T. 1970. The roentgenographic evaluation of eustachian tubal function. Laryngoscope 80:1201.

Parker, C. W. 1972. Allergic drug responses—mechanisms and unsolved problems. CRC Crit. Rev. Toxicol. 1:261.

Pederson, C. B., and Zachau-Christiansen, B. 1986. Otitis media in Greenland children: Acute, chronic and secretory otitis media in three to eight year olds. J. Otolaryngol. 15:332.

Pelton, S. I., Shurin, P. A., and Klein, J. O. 1977. Persistence of middle ear effusion after otitis media. Pediatr. Res. 11:504.

Pelton, S. I., Teele, D. W., Shurin, P. A., et al. 1980. Disparate cultures of middle ear fluids. Am. J. Dis. Child. 134:951.

Perlman, H. B. 1939. The eustachian tube: Abnormal patency and normal physiologic state. Arch. Otolaryngol. 30:212.

Perlman, H. B. 1951. Observations on the eustachian tube. Arch. Otolaryngol. 53:370.

Perrin, J. M., Charney, E., MacWhinney, J. B., Jr., et al. 1974. Sulfisoxazole as chemoprophylaxis for recurrent otitis media: A double-blind crossover study in pediatric practice. N. Engl. J. Med. 291:664.

Persico, M., Barker, G. A., and Mitchell, D. P. 1985. Purulent otitis media—a "silent" source of sepsis in the pediatric intensive care unit. Otolaryngol. Head Neck Surg. 93:330.

Persico, M., Podoshin, L., and Fradis, M. 1978. Otitis media with effusion: A steroid and antibiotic therapeutic trial before surgery. Ann. Otol. Rhinol. Laryngol. 87:191.

Pestalozza, G. 1984. Otitis media in newborn infants. Int. J. Pediatr. Otorhinolaryngol. 8:109.

Petz, L. D. 1978. Immunologic cross-reactivity between penicillins and cephalosporins: A review. J. Infect. Dis. 137:S74.

Petz, L. D., and Fudenberg, H. H. 1966. Coombs-positive hemolytic anemia caused by penicillin administration. N. Engl. J. Med. 274:171.

Pfisterer, H. 1958. Recent knowledge concerning impairment of hearing in patients with palatal fissure. HNO (Berl.) 6:307.

Phillips, M. J., Knight, N. J., Manning, H., et al. 1974a. IgE and secretory otitis media. Lancet 2:1176.

Phillips, M. J., Manning, H., Knight, N. J., et al. 1974b. Secretory otitis media. Lancet 2:1176.

Pieraggi, J. 1974. Interet de la sonomanometrie dans le prognostic de la microchirurgie auriculaire. Rev. Laryngol. Otol. Rhinol. (Bord.) 95:319.

Pisacane, A., and Ruas, I. 1982. Bacteriology of otitis media in Mozambique. Lancet 1:1305.

Ploussard, J. H. 1984. Evaluation of 5 days of cefaclor vs. ten days of amoxicillin therapy in acute otitis media. Curr. Ther. Res. 36:641.

Politzer, A. 1862. Ueber die willkurlichen bewegungen des trommelfells. Weiner Med. Halle. Nr. 18:103.

Politzer, A. 1865, 1869. Lehrbuch der Ohrenheilkunde. 5. Auflage Vol. I. Stuttgart, F. Enke.

Politzer, A. 1883. Diseases of the Ear. Cassells, J. P. (trans.-ed.) Philadelphia, Henry C. Lea's Son and Co., pp. 375–377.

Politzer, A. 1909. Diseases of the Ear. Philadelphia, Lea & Febiger.

Porter, T. A. 1974. Otoadmittance measurements in a residential deaf population. Am. Ann. Deaf 119:47.

Potsic, W. P., Cohen, M., Randall, P., et al. 1979. A retrospective study of hearing impairment in three groups of cleft palate patients. Cleft Palate J. 16:56.

Poulson, G., and Tos, M. 1978. Screening tympanometry in newborn infants and during the first six months of life. Scand. Audiol. 7:159.

Prellner, K., Hallberg, T., Kalm, O., and Mansson, B. 1985. Recurrent otitis media: Genetic immunoglobulin markers in children and their parents. Int. J. Pediatr. Otorhinolaryngol. 9:219.

Prellner, K., Nilsson, N. I., Johnson, U., et al. 1980. Complement and C1q binding substances in otitis media. Ann. Otol. Rhinol. Laryngol. 89:129.

Prince, R. A., Wing, D. S., Weinberger, M. M., et al. 1981. Effect of erythromycin on theophylline kinetics. J. Allergy Clin. Immunol. 68:427.

Proctor, B. 1967. Embryology and anatomy of the eustachian tube. Arch. Otolaryngol. 86:503.

Proctor, B. 1971. Attic-aditus block and the tympanic diaphragm. Ann. Otol. Rhinol. Laryngol. 80:371.

Proud, G. O., and Duff, W. E. 1976. Mastoidectomy and epitympanotomy. Ann. Otol. Rhinol. Laryngol. 85:289.

Puczynski, M. S., Stankienwicz, J. A., and O'Keefe, J. P. 1987. Single dose amoxicillin treatment of acute otitis media. Laryngoscope 97:16.

Puhakka, H., Virolainen, E., Aantaa, E., et al. 1979. Myringotomy in the treatment of acute otitis media in children. Acta Otolaryngol. (Stockh.) 88:122.

Pukander, J. 1982. Occurrence of acute otitis media. Academic dissertation. Acta Universitatis Tamperensis Ser. A Vol. 135.

Pukander, J., Luotonen, J., Sipilä, M., et al. 1982. Incidence of acute otitis media. Acta Otolaryngol. (Stockh.) 93:447.

Pukander, J., Luotonen, J., Timonen, M., et al. 1985. Risk factors affecting the occurrence of acute otitis media among 2-3-year-old urban children. Acta Otolaryngol. (Stockh.) 100:260.

Pukander, J., Sipilä, M., and Karma, P. 1984. Occurrence of and risk factors in acute otitis media. In Lim, D. J., Bluestone, C. D., Klein, J. O., and Nelson, J. D. (eds.): Recent Advances in Otitis Media with Effusion. Toronto, B. C. Decker, pp. 9–13.

Pulec, J. L. 1967. Abnormally patent eustachian tubes: Treatment with injection of polytetrafluoroethylene (Teflon) paste. Laryngoscope 77:1543.

Qvarnberg, Y., Holopainen, E., and Palva, T. 1984. Aspiration cytology in acute otitis media. Acta Otolaryngol. (Stockh.) 97:443.

Qvarnberg, Y., and Palva, T. 1980. Active and conservative treatment of acute otitis media: Prospective studies. Ann. Otol. Rhinol. Laryngol. 89:269.

Raikundalia, K. B. 1975. Analysis of suppurative otitis media in children: Aetiology of non-suppurative otitis media. Med. J. Aust. 1:749.

Rapp, D. J., and Fahey, D. 1973. Review of chronic secretory otitis and allergy. J. Asthma Res. 10:193.

Rapport, P. N., Lim, D. J., and Weiss, H. J. 1975. Surface active agent in eustachian tube function. Arch. Otolaryngol. 101:305.

Rathbun, T. A., and Mallin, R. 1977. Middle ear disease in a prehistoric Iranian population. Bull. N.Y. Acad. Med. 53:901.

Reed, D., Struve, S., and Maynard, J. E. 1967. Otitis media and hearing deficiency among Eskimo children: A cohort study. Am. J. Public Health 57:1657.

Rees-Jones, G. F., and McGibbon, J. E. 1941. Radiological visualization of the eustachian tube. Lancet 2:660.

Renvall, U., Liden, G., Jungert, S., et al. 1973. Impedance audiometry as a screening method in schoolchildren. Scand. Audiol. 2:133.

Restrepo, M. A., and Zambrano, F. 1968. II. Late onset aplastic anemia secondary to chloramphenicol. Report of ten cases. Antioquia Medica 18:593.

Revonta, M. 1979. A-mode ultrasound of maxillary sinusitis in children (letter). Lancet 1:320.

Rich, A. R. 1920a. The innervation of the tensor veli palatini and levator veli palatini muscles. Bull. Johns Hopkins Hosp. 31:305.

Rich, A. R. 1920b. A physiological study of the eustachian tube and its related muscles. Bull. Johns Hopkins Hosp. 31:206.

Richman, D. D., Cleveland, P. H., Redfield, D. C., et al. 1984. Rapid viral diagnosis. Rev. Infect. Dis. 149:298.

Riding, K. H., Bluestone, C. D., Michaels, R. H., et al. 1978a. Microbiology of recurrent and chronic otitis media with effusion. J. Pediatr. 93:739.

Riding, K. H., Reichert, T. J., Findlay, R. C., et al. 1978b. Tympanometric and otologic evaluation of students in a school for the deaf. In Harford, E. R., Bess, F. H., Bluestone, C. D., and Klein, J. O. (eds.): Impedance Screening for Middle Ear Disease in Children. New York, Grune & Stratton, pp. 279–291.

Rifkind, D. R., Chanock, R. M., Kravetz, H., et al. 1962. Ear involvement (myringitis) and primary atypical pneumonia following inoculation of volunteers with Eaton agent. Am. Rev. Respir. Dis. 85:479.

Rinkel, H. J. 1962, 1963. The management of clinical allergy. Arch. Otolaryngol. Part I—76:491, 1962: Part II—77:42, 1963; Part III—77:205, 1963; Part IV—77:302, 1963.

Riu, R., Flottes, L., Bouche, J., et al. 1966. La Physiologie de la Trompe d'Eustache. Paris, Librairie Anette.

Roberts, D. B. 1980. The etiology of bullous myringitis and the role of mycoplasmas in ear disease: A review. Pediatrics 65:761.

Roberts, K. B., and Borzy, M. S. 1977. Fever in the first eight weeks of life. Johns Hopkins Med. J. 11:9.

Roberts, M. E. 1976. Comparative study of pure tone, impedance, and otoscopic hearing screening methods. Arch. Otolaryngol. 102:690.

Robinson, J. M., and Nicholas, H. O. 1951. Catarrhal otitis media with effusion—a disease of a retropharyngeal and lymphatic system. South. Med. J. 44:777.

Roddey, O. F., Jr., Earle, R., Jr., and Haggerty, R. 1966. Myringotomy in acute otitis media: A controlled study. J.A.M.A. 197:849.

Rodriguez, W. J., Schwartz, R. H., Sait, T., et al. 1985. Erythromycin-sulfisoxazole vs amoxicillin in treatment of acute otitis media in children. Am. J. Dis. Child. 139:766.

Rogers, R. L., Kirchner, F. R., and Proud, G. O. 1962. The evaluation of eustachian tubal function by fluorescent dye studies. Laryngoscope 72:456.

Rood, S. R. 1973. Morphology of m. tensor veli palatini in the five-month human fetus. Am. J. Anat. 138:191.

Rood, S. R., and Doyle, W. J. 1978. Morphology of tensor veli palatini, tensor tympani, and dilatator tubae muscles. Ann. Otol. Rhinol. Laryngol. 87:202.

Rood, S. R., and Doyle, W. J. 1982. The nasopharyngeal orifice of the auditory tube: Implications for tubal dynamics anatomy. Cleft Palate J. 19:119.

Rosen, C., Christensen, P., Hovelius, B., et al. 1983. Effect of pneumococcal vaccination on upper respiratory tract infections in children. Design of a follow-up study. Scand. J. Infect. Dis. (Suppl.) 39:39.

Rosen, L. M. 1970. The morphology of the salpingopharyngeus muscle. Unpublished master's thesis, University of Pittsburgh.

Ross, M. 1971. Functional anatomy of the tensor palati—its relevance in cleft palate surgery. Arch. Otolaryngol. 93:1.

Roth, R. P., Cantekin, E. I., Bluestone, C. D., et al. 1977. Nasal decongestant activity of pseudoephedrine. Ann. Otol. Rhinol. Laryngol. 86:235.

Roydhouse, N. 1970. A controlled study of adenotonsillectomy. Arch. Otolaryngol. 92:611.

Roydhouse, N. 1980. Adenoidectomy for otitis media with mucoid effusion. Ann. Otol. Rhinol. Laryngol. 89:312.

Ruben, R. J., and Math, R. 1978. Serous otitis media associated with sensorineural hearing loss in children. Laryngoscope 88:1139.

Rubenstein, M. M., McBean, J. B., Hedgecock, L. D., et al. 1965. The treatment of acute otitis media in children: A third clinical trial. Am. J. Dis. Child. 109:308.

Rubin, M. 1978. Serous otitis media in severely to profoundly hearing impaired children, ages 0 to 6. Volta Rev. 80:81.

Rudberg, R. D. 1954. Acute otitis media: Comparative therapeutic results of sulfonamide and penicillin administered in various forms. Acta Otolaryngol. 113:1.

Rudin, R., Welin, L., Svardsudd, K., et al. 1985. Middle ear disease in samples from the general population. II. History of otitis and otorrhea in relation to tympanic membrane pathology, the study of men born in 1913 and 1923. Acta Otolaryngol. (Stockh.) 99:53.

Saah, A. J., Blackwelder, W. C., and Kaslow, R. A. 1982. Commentary: Treatment of acute otitis media. J.A.M.A. 248:1071.

Saarinen, U. M. 1982. Prolonged breast feeding as prophylaxis for recurrent otitis media. Acta Pediatr. Scand. 71:567.

Sade, J. 1966. Pathology and pathogenesis of serous otitis media. Arch. Otolaryngol. 84:297.

Sade, J., and Afula, F. 1967. Ciliary activity and middle ear clearance. Arch. Otolaryngol. 86:128.

Sade, J., and Eliezer, N. 1970. Secretory otitis media and the nature of the mucociliary system. Acta Otolaryngol. 70:351.

Salonen, R., Sarkkinen, H., and Ruuskanen, O. 1984. Presence of interferon in middle ear fluid during acute otitis media. J. Infect. Dis. 19:480.

Salter, A. J. 1982. Trimethoprim-sulfamethoxazole: An assessment of more than 12 years of use. Rev. Infect. Dis. 4:196.

Sanyal, M. A., Henderson, F. W., Stempel, E. C., et al. 1980. Effect of upper respiratory tract infection on eustachian tube ventilatory function in the preschool child. J. Pediatr. 97:11.

Sarkkinen, H., Meurman, O., Puhakka, H., et al. 1982. Failure to detect viral antigens in the middle ear secretions of patients with secretory otitis media. Acta Otolaryngol. (Stockh.) 386:106.

Sarkkinen, H., Ruuskanen, O., Meurman, O., et al. 1985. Identification of respiratory virus antigens in middle ear fluids of children with acute otitis media. J. Infect. Dis. 151:444.

Sataloff, J., and Fraser, M. 1952. Hearing loss in children with cleft palates. Arch. Otolaryngol. 55:61.

Satoh, I., Watanabe, I., and Saindo, T. 1970. Measurement of eustachian tube function. Arch. Otolaryngol. 92:329.

Savic, D., and Djeric, D. 1985. Anatomical variations and relations in the medial wall of the bony portion of the eustachian tube. Acta Otolaryngol. (Stockh.) 99:551.

Schachter, J., Grossman, M., Holt, J., et al. 1979. Prospective study of chlamydial infection in neonates. Lancet 2:377.

Schaefer, O. 1971. Otitis media and bottle-feeding. An epidemiological study of infant feeding habits and incidence of recurrent and chronic middle ear disease in Canadian Eskimos. Can. J. Public Health 62:478.

Schlesinger, P. C. 1982. The significance of fever in infants less than three months old: A retrospective review of one year's experience at Boston City Hospital's pediatric walk-in clinic. Thesis submitted to the Yale University School of Medicine.

Schuller, D. E. 1983. Prophylaxis of otitis media in asthmatic children. Pediatr. Infect. Dis. 2:280.

Schwartz, D. M., and Schwartz, R. H. 1978. Acoustic impedance and otoscopic findings in young children with Down's syndrome. Arch. Otolaryngol. 104:652.

Schwartz, D. M., and Schwartz, R. H. 1987. Validity of acoustic reflectometry in detecting middle ear effusion. Pediatrics 79:739.

Schwartz, D. M., Schwartz, R. H., and Redfield, N. P. 1978. Treatment of negative middle ear pressure and serous otitis media with Politzer's technique: An old procedure revised. Arch. Otolaryngol. 104:487.

Schwartz, R. H. 1981. Bacteriology of otitis media: A review. Otolaryngol. Head Neck Surg. 89:444.

Schwartz, R. H., Barsanti, R. G., and Rodriguez, W. J. 1978. Private practice view of otitis media. Pediatrics 61:937.

Schwartz, R. H., Puglese, J., and Rodriguez, W. J. 1982. Sulfamethoxazole prophylaxis in the otitis-prone child. Arch. Dis. Child. 57:590.

Schwartz, R. H., Puglese, J., and Schwartz, D. M. 1980. Use of a short course of prednisone for treating middle ear effusion: A double-blind crossover study. Ann. Otol. Rhinol. Laryngol. 89:296.

Schwartz, R. H., and Rodriguez, W. J. 1981. Acute otitis media in children eight years old and older: A reappraisal of the role of *Haemophilus influenzae*. Am. J. Otolaryngol. 2:19.

Schwartz, R. H., Rodriguez, W. J., Brook, I., et al. 1981a. The febrile response in acute otitis media. J.A.M.A. 245:2057.

Schwartz, R. H., Rodriguez, W. J., and Khan, W. N. 1981b. Persistent purulent otitis media. Clin. Pediatr. 20:445.

Schwartz, R. H., Rodriguez, W. J., Khan, W. N., et al. 1977. Acute purulent otitis media in children older than five years: Incidence of *Haemophilus* as a causative organism. J.A.M.A. 238:1032.

Schwartz, R., Rodriguez, W. J., Mann, R., et al. 1979. The nasopharyngeal culture in acute otitis media: A reappraisal of its usefulness. J.A.M.A. 241:2170.

Schwartz, R. H., Rodriguez, W. J., and Schwartz, D. M. 1981c. Office myringotomy for acute otitis media: Its value in preventing middle ear effusion. Laryngoscope 91:616.

Schwartz, R. H., and Schwartz, D. M. 1980. Acute otitis media: Diagnosis and drug therapy. Drugs 19:107.

Schwartz, R. N., Stool, S. E., Rodriguez, W. J., et al. 1981d. Acute otitis media: Toward a more precise diagnosis. Clin. Pediatr. 20:549.

Scott, J. L., Finegold, S. M., Belkin, G. A., et al. 1965. A controlled double-blind study of the hematologic toxicity of chloramphenicol. N. Engl. J. Med. 272:1137.

Sellars, S. L., and Seid, A. B. 1973. Aural tuberculosis in childhood. S. Afr. Med. J. 47:216.

Senturia, B. H., Bluestone, C. D., Klein, J. O., et al. 1980a. Report of the ad hoc committee on definition and classification of otitis media with effusion. Ann. Otol. Rhinol. Laryngol. 89:3.

Senturia, B. H., Gessert, C. F., Carr, C. D., et al. 1958. Studies concerned with tubotympanitis. Ann. Otol. Rhinol. Laryngol. 67:440.

Senturia, B. H., Marcus, M. D., and Lucente, F. E. 1980b.

Diseases of the External Ear: An Otologic-Dermatologic Manual, 2nd ed. New York, Grune & Stratton.

Severeid, L. R. 1972. A longitudinal study of the efficacy of adenoidectomy in children with cleft palate and secondary otitis media. TAAOO 76:1319.

Shah, K. N., and Desai, M. P. 1969. *Ascaris lumbricoides* from the right ear. Indian Pediatr. 6:92.

Shah, N. 1971. Use of grommets in "glue" ears. J. Laryngol. Otol. 85:283.

Shapiro, G. G., Biermon, C. W., Furukawa, C. T., et al. 1982. Treatment of persistent eustachian tube dysfunction in children with aerosolized nasal dexamethasone phosphate versus placebo. Ann. Allergy 49:81.

Shaw, J. R., Todd, N. W., Goodwin, M. H., et al. 1979. Observations on otitis media among four Indian populations in Arizona. *In* Wiet, R. J., and Coulthard, S. (eds.): Proceedings of the Second National Conference on Otitis Media. Columbus, OH, Ross Laboratories.

Shea, J. J. 1971. Autoinflation treatment of serous otitis media in children. J. Laryngol. Otol. 85:1254.

Sheehy, J. L. 1977. Surgery of chronic otitis media. *In* English, G. (ed.): Otolaryngology, Vol. I. Hagerstown, MD, Harper & Row.

Shurin, P. A., Howie, V. M., Pelton, S. I., et al. 1978. Bacterial etiology of otitis media during the first six weeks of life. J. Pediatr. 92:893.

Shurin, P. A., Marchant, C. D., Kim, C. H., et al. 1983. Emergence of beta-lactamase–producing strains of *Branhamella catarrhalis* as important agents of acute otitis media. Pediatr. Infect. Dis. 2:34.

Shurin, P. A., Pelton, S. I., Donner, A., et al. 1980a. Trimethoprim-sulfamethoxazole compared with ampicillin in the treatment of acute otitis media. J. Pediatr. 96:1081.

Shurin, P. A., Pelton, S. I., and Finkelstein, B. A. 1977. Tympanometry in the diagnosis of middle ear effusions. N. Engl. J. Med. 296:412.

Shurin, P. A., Pelton, S. I., and Klein, J. O. 1976. Otitis media in the newborn infant. Ann. Otol. Rhinol. Laryngol. 85:216.

Shurin, P. A., Pelton, S. I., Tager, I. B., et al. 1980b. Bactericidal antibody and susceptibility to otitis media caused by non-typable strains of *Haemophilus influenzae*. J. Pediatr. 97:364.

Siber, G. R., Smith, A. L., and Levin, M. J. 1979. Predictability of peak serum gentamicin concentration with dosage based on body surface area. J. Pediatr. 94:135.

Siedentop, K. H. 1972. Eustachian tube dynamics, size of the mastoid air cell system, and results with tympanoplasty. Otolaryngol. Clin. North Am. 5:33.

Siedentop, K. H., Loewy, A., Corrigan, R. A., et al. 1978. Eustachian tube function assessed with tympanometry. Ann. Otol. Rhinol. Laryngol. 87:163.

Siegel, S. C. 1979. Allergy as it relates to otitis media. *In* Wiet, R. J., and Coulthard, S. W. (eds.): Proceedings of the Second National Conference on Otitis Media. Columbus, OH, Ross Laboratories, pp. 25–29.

Siirala, U., and Lahikainen, E. A. 1952. Some observations on the bacteriostatic effect of the exudate in otitis media. Acta Otolaryngol. (Stockh.) Suppl. 100:20.

Siirala, U., Tarpila, S., and Halonen, P. 1961. Inhibitory effect of sterile otitis media exudates on the cytopathogenicity of herpes simplex, poliomyelitis, and adenoviruses in HeLa cells. Acta Otolaryngol. (Stockh.) 53:230.

Siirala, U., and Vuori, M. 1956. The problem of sterile otitis media. Prac. Otorhinolaryngol. 19:159.

Silverstein, H., Bernstein, J. M., and Lerner, P. I. 1966. Antibiotic concentrations in middle ear effusion. Pediatrics 38:33.

Simkins, C. 1943. Functional anatomy of the eustachian tube. Arch. Otolaryngol. 38:476.

Sipilä, M., Pukander, J., and Karma, P. 1987. Incidence of acute otitis media up to the age of 1 1/2 years in urban infants. Acta Otolaryngol. (Stockh.) 104:138.

Sipilä, P., Jokipii, A. M. M., Jokipii, L., et al. 1981. Bacteria in the middle ear and ear canal of patients with secretory otitis media and with noninflamed ears. Acta Otolaryngol. (Stockh.) 92:123.

Sipilä, P., and Karma, P. 1982. Inflammatory cells in mucoid effusion of secretory otitis media. Acta Otolaryngol. (Stockh.) 94:467.

Skolnick, E. M. 1958. Otologic evaluation in cleft palate patients. Laryngoscope 68:1908.

Skolnik, P. R., Nadol, J. B., Jr., and Baker, A. S. 1986. Tuberculosis of the middle ear: Review of the literature with an instructive case report. Rev. Infect. Dis. 8:403.

Sloyer, J. L., Jr., Cate, C. C., Howie, V. M. 1975. The immune response to acute otitis media in children. II. Serum and middle ear antibody in otitis media due to *Haemophilus influenzae*. J. Infect. Dis. 132:685.

Sloyer, J. L., Jr., Howie, V. M., Ploussard, J. H., et al. 1974. Immune response to acute otitis media in children. I. Serotypes isolated in serum and middle ear fluid antibody in pneumococcal otitis media. Infect. Immun. 9:1028.

Sloyer, J. L., Jr., Howie, V. M., Ploussard, J. H., et al. 1977. Immune response to acute otitis media in children. II. Implications of viral antibody in middle ear fluid. J. Immunol. 118:248.

Sloyer, J. L., Jr., Howie, V. M., Ploussard, J. H., et al. 1976. Immune response to acute otitis media: Association between middle ear antibody and the clearing of clinical infection. J. Clin. Microbiol. 4:306.

Sloyer, J. L., Jr., Ploussard, J. H., and Howie, V. M. 1981. Efficacy of polysaccharide vaccine in preventing acute otitis media in infants in Huntsville, Alabama. Rev. Infect. Dis. 3:S119.

Sly, R. M., Zambie, M. F., Fernandes, D. A., et al. 1980. Tympanometry in kindergarten children. Ann. Allergy. 44:1.

Smith, H., and Aronson, S. S. 1986. Organizational approach to medication administration in day care. Rev. Infect. Dis. 8:657.

Sobeslavsky, O., Syrucek, L., Bruckoya, M., et al. 1965. The etiological role of *Mycoplasma pneumoniae* in otitis media in children. Pediatrics 35:652.

Solomon, N. E., and Harris, L. J. 1976. Otitis Media in Children. Assessing the Quality of Medical Care Using Short-Term Outcome Measures: Eight Disease-Specific Applications. Santa Monica, CA, Rand Corp.

Sorensen, H. 1977. Antibiotics in suppurative otitis media. Otolaryngol. Clin. North Am. 10:45.

Speilberg, W. 1927. Visualization of the eustachian tube by roentgen ray. Arch. Otolaryngol. 5:334.

Spivey, G. H., and Hirschhorn, N. 1977. A migrant study of adopted Apache children. Johns Hopkins Med. J. 140:43.

Spriesterbach, D. C., Lierle, D. M., Moll, K. L., et al. 1962. Hearing loss in children with cleft palates. Plast. Reconstr. Surg. 30:336.

Stangerup, S.-E., and Tos, M. 1986. Epidemiology of acute suppurative otitis media. Am. J. Otolaryngol. 7:47.

Stanievich, J. F., Bluestone, C. D., Lima, J. A., et al. 1981. Microbiology of chronic and recurrent otitis media with effusion in young infants. Int. J. Pediatr. Otorhinolaryngol. 3:137.

Stechenberg, B. W., Anderson, D., Chang, M. J., et al. 1976. Cephalexin compared to ampicillin treatment of otitis media. Pediatrics 58:532.

Steinberg, E. A., Overturf, G. D., Wilkins, J., et al. 1978. Failure of cefamandole in treatment of meningitis due to *Haemophilus influenzae* type b. J. Infect. Dis. 137:S180.

Stenfors, L. E., Hellstrom, S., and Albiin, N. 1985. Middle ear clearance in eustachian tube function: Physiology and role in otitis media. Ann. Otol. Rhinol. Laryngol. 94:30.

Stickler, G. B., and McBean, J. B. 1964. The treatment of acute otitis media in children: A second clinical trial. J.A.M.A. 187:85.

Stickler, G. B., Rubenstein, M. M., McBean, J. B., et al. 1967. Treatment of acute otitis media in children: A fourth clinical trial. Am. J. Dis. Child. 114:123.

Stool, S. E., Craig, H. B., and Laird, M. A. 1980. Screening for middle ear disease in a school for the deaf. Ann. Otol. Rhinol. Laryngol. 89:172.

Stool, S. E., and Randall, P. 1967. Unexpected ear disease in infants with cleft palate. Cleft Palate J. 4:99.

Strangert, K. 1977. Otitis media in young children in different types of day-care. Scand. J. Infect. Dis. 9:119.

Stroud, M. H., Spector, G. J., and Maisel, R. H. 1974. Patulous eustachian tube syndrome: Preliminary report of the use of the tensor veli palatini transposition procedure. Arch. Otolaryngol. 99:419.

Suehs, O. W. 1952. Secretory otitis media. Laryngoscope 62:998.

Sugita, R., Kawamura, S., Ichikawa, G., et al. 1983. Bacteriology of acute otitis media in Japan and chemotherapy, with special reference to *Haemophilus influenzae*. Int. J. Pediatr. Otorhinolaryngol. 6:135.

Sumaya, C. V., and Ench, Y. 1985. Epstein-Barr virus infectious mononucleosis in children. I. Clinical and general laboratory findings. Pediatrics 75:1003.

Sundberg, L., Eden, T., Ernstson, S., et al. 1979. Penetration of erythromycin through respiratory mucosa. Acta Otolaryngol. (Stockh.) Suppl. 365:1.

Supance, J. S., and Bluestone, C. D. 1983. Perilymph fistulas in infants and children. Otolaryngol. Head Neck Surg. 91:663.

Swarts, J. D., Rood, S. R., and Doyle, W. J. 1986. Fetal development of the auditory tube and paratubal musculature. Cleft Palate J. 23:289.

Tager, I. B., Weiss, S. T., Munoz, A., et al. 1983. Longitudinal study of the effects of maternal smoking on pulmonary function in children. N. Engl. J. Med. 309:699.

Takahara, T., Sando, I., Bluestone, C. D., et al. 1986. Lymphoma invading the anterior eustachian tube: Temporal bone histopathology of functional tubal obstruction. Ann. Otol. Rhinol. Laryngol. 95:101.

Takahashi, H., Masahiko, M., and Honjo, I. 1987. Compliance of the eustachian tube in patients with otitis media with effusion. Am. J. Otolaryngol. 3:154.

Taylor, G. D. 1972. The bifid uvula. Laryngoscope 82:771.

Teele, D. W., Healy, G. B., and Tally, F. P. 1980a. Persistent effusions of the middle ear: Cultures for anaerobic bacteria. Ann. Otol. Rhinol. Laryngol. 89:102.

Teele, D. W., Klein, J. O., and the Greater Boston Collaborative Otitis Media Program. 1980b. Beneficial effects of breastfeeding on the duration of middle ear effusion after the first episode of acute otitis media. Pediatr. Res. 14:494.

Teele, D. W., Klein, J. O., and the Greater Boston Collaborative Otitis Media Study Group. 1981a. Use of polyvaccine for prevention of recurrent acute otitis media in infants in Boston. Rev. Infect. Dis. 3:S113.

Teele, D. W., Klein, J. O., and Rosner, B. A. 1980c. Epidemiology of otitis media in children. Ann. Otol. Rhinol. Laryngol. 89:5.

Teele, D. W., Klein, J. O., and Rosner, B. 1984. Otitis media with effusion during the first three years of life and development of speech and language. Pediatrics 74:282.

Teele, D. W., Klein, J. O., Rosner, B., et al. 1983. Burden and the practice of pediatrics: Middle ear disease during the first five years of life. J.A.M.A. 249:1026.

Teele, D. W., Klein, J. O., Rosner, B., and the Greater Boston Otitis Media Study Group. 1989. Epidemiology of otitis media during the first seven years of life in children in greater Boston: A prospective, cohort study. J. Infect. Dis. (in press).

Teele, D. W., Pelton, S. I., Grant, M. J. A., et al. 1975. Bacteremia in febrile children under 2 years of age: Results of cultures of blood of 600 consecutive febrile children seen in a walk-in clinic. J. Pediatr. 87:227.

Teele, D. W., Pelton, S. I., and Klein, J. O. 1981b. Bacteriology of acute otitis media unresponsive to initial antimicrobial therapy. J. Pediatr. 98:537.

Teele, D. W., and Teele, J. 1984. Detection of middle ear effusion by acoustic reflectometry. J. Pediatr. 104:832.

Terkildsen, K., and Nielsen, S. S. 1960. An electroacoustic impedance measuring bridge for clinical use. Arch. Otolaryngol. 72:339.

Terracol, A., Corone, A., and Guerrier, G. 1949. La Trompe D'Eustache. Paris, Masson.

Tetzlaff, T. R., Ashworth, C., and Nelson, J. D. 1977. Otitis media in children less than 12 weeks of age. Pediatrics 59:827.

Tetzlaff, T. R., McCracken, G. H., Jr., and Nelson, J. D. 1978. Oral antibiotic therapy for skeletal infections of children. II. Therapy of osteomyelitis and suppurative arthritis. J. Pediatr. 92:485.

Thomsen, J., Meistrup-Larson, K. I., Sorensen, H., et al. 1980. Penicillin and acute otitis: Short and long term results. Ann. Otol. Rhinol. Laryngol. 89:271.

Thomsen, J., and Tos, M. 1981. Spontaneous improvement of secretory otitis. A long-term study. Acta Otolaryngol. (Stockh.) 92:493.

Thomsen, K. A. 1957. Studies on the function of the eustachian tube in a series of normal individuals. Acta Otolaryngol. (Stockh.) 48:516.

Thomsen, K. A. 1958a. Investigations on the tubal function and measurement of the middle ear pressure in pressure chamber. Acta Otolaryngol. (Stockh.) Suppl. 140:269.

Thomsen, K. A. 1958b. Investigations on Toynbee's experiment in normal individuals. Acta Otolaryngol. (Stockh.) Suppl. 140:263.

Thorington, J. 1892. Almost total destruction of the velum palati corrected by an artificial soft palate, producing not only greatly improved speech, but an immediate increase of audition. Med. News 61:269, and Ann. Mal l'Oreille Larynx, p. 694.

Timmermans, F. J., and Gerson, S. 1980. Chronic granulomatous otitis media in bottle-fed Inuit children. Can. Med. Assoc. J. 122:545.

Tipple, M. A., Beem, M. O., and Saxon, E. M. 1979. Clinical characteristics of the afebrile pneumonia associated with Chlamydia trachomatis infection in infants less than six months of age. Pediatrics 63:192.

Todd, N. W., and Bowman, C. A. 1985. Otitis media at Canyon Day, Ariz. 1985. A 16-year follow-up in Apache Indians. Arch. Otolaryngol. 111:606.

Todd, N. W., and Feldman, C. M. 1985. Allergic airway disease and otitis media in children. Int. J. Pediatr. Otorhinolaryngol. 10:27.

Todhunter, J. S., Siegel, M. I., and Doyle, W. J. 1984. Computer-generated eustachian tube shape analysis. In Lim, D. J., Bluestone, C. D., Klein, J. O., and Nelson, J. D. (eds.): Recent Advances in Otitis Media with Effusion. Toronto, B. C. Decker, pp. 101–104.

Tos, M. 1980. Spontaneous improvement of secretory otitis and impedance screening. Arch. Otolaryngol. 106:345.

Tos, M. 1984. Anatomy and histology of the middle ear. Clin. Rev. Allergy 2:267.

Tos, M., Holm-Jensen, S., Hjort Sorensen, C., et al. 1982. Spontaneous course and frequency of secretory otitis in four-year-old children. Arch. Otolaryngol. 108:4.

Tos, M., and Poulsen, G. 1976. Secretory otitis media: Late results of treatment with grommets. Arch. Otolaryngol. 102:672.

Tos, M., and Poulsen, G. 1979. Tympanometry in two-year-old children. Seasonal influence on frequency of secretory otitis and tubal function. ORL 41:1.

Tos, M., Poulsen, G., and Borch, J. 1978. Tympanometry in two-year-old children. ORL 40:77.

Tos, M., Poulsen, G., and Hancke, A. B. 1979. Screening tympanometry during the first year of life. Acta Otolaryngol. (Stockh.) 88:388.

Trujillo, H., Callejas, R., Mejia de R, G. I. 1981. Otitis media aguda. Medicina U.P.B. 1:31.

Turner, A. L., and Fraser, J. S. 1915. Tuberculosis of the middle ear cleft in children: A clinical and pathological study. J. Laryngol. Rhinol. Otol. 30:209.

Umetsu, D. T., Ambrosino, D. M., Quinti, I., et al. 1985. Recurrent sinopulmonary infection and impaired antibody response to bacterial capsular polysaccharide antigen in children with selective IgG-subclass deficiency. N. Engl. J. Med. 313:1247.

Valsalva, A. 1949. Trachus de aure humana. In Stevenson, R. S., and Guthrie, D. (eds.): A History of Otolaryngology. Edinburgh, E. and S. Livingstone.

van Buchem, F. L., Dunk, J. H. M., and van't Hof, M. A. 1981. Therapy of acute otitis media: Myringotomy, antibiotics, or neither? A double-blind study in children. Lancet 2:883.

van Buchem, F. L., Peeters, M. F., and van't Hof, M. A. 1985. Acute otitis media: A new treatment strategy. Par. Med. J. (Clin. Res.) 290:1033.

Van Dishoeck, H. A. E. 1947. Resistance measuring of the eustachian tube and the ostium and isthmus valve mechanisms. Acta Otolaryngol. (Stockh.) 35:317.

Van Dishoeck, H. A. E., Derks, A. C. W., and Voorhorst, R. 1959. Bacteriology and treatment of acute otitis media in children. Acta Otolaryngol. (Stockh.) 50:250.

Variot, G. 1904. Écoulement de lait par l'oreille d'un mourisson atteint de division congenitale du voile du palais. Bull. Soc. Pediatr. Paris 6:387.

Varsano, I., Volvitz, B., and Mimouni, F. 1985. Sulfisoxazole prophylaxis of middle ear with effusion and recurrent acute otitis media. Am. J. Dis. Child. 139:632.

Veltri, R. W., and Sprinkle, P. M. 1973. Serous otitis media: Immunoglobulin and lysozyme levels in middle ear fluids and serum. Ann. Otol. Rhinol. Laryngol. 82:297.

Venker, H. 1973. Sonomanometric investigation of the eustachian tube function and tympanoplasty. ORL 35:233.

Vinther, B., Elbrønd, O., and Pedersen, C. 1979. A population study of otitis media in childhood. Acta Otolaryngol. (Stockh.) 360:135.

Vinther, B., Elbrønd, O., and Pedersen, C. B. 1982. Otitis media in childhood, socio-medical aspects with special reference to daycare and housing conditions. Acta Otolaryngol. (Stockh.) 386:121.

Virolainen, E., Puhakka, H., Aantaa, E., et al. 1980. Prevalence of secretory otitis media in seven to eight year old school children. Ann. Otol. Rhinol. Laryngol. 89:7.

Virtanen, H. 1977. Eustachian tube sound conduction—sonotubometry, an acoustical method for objective measurement of auditory tubal opening. Thesis, Department of Otolaryngology, University of Helsinki, Finland.

Virtanen, H. 1978. Sonotubometry: An acoustical method for objective measurement of auditory tubal opening. Acta Otolaryngol. (Stockh.) 86:93.

Virtanen, H., Palva, T., and Jauhiainen, T. 1980. The prognostic value of eustachian tube function measurements in tympanoplastic surgery. Acta Otolaryngol. (Stockh.) 90:317.

Virtanen, S., and Lahikainen, E. A. 1979. Ampicillin concentrations in middle ear effusions in acute otitis media after administration of bacampicillin. Infection 7:472.

Wachtendorf, C. A., Lopez, L. L., Cooper, J. C., et al. 1984. The efficacy of school screening for otitis media. In Lim, D. J., Bluestone, C. D., Klein, J. O., and Nelson, J. D. (eds.): Recent Advances in Otitis Media. Toronto, B. C. Decker, pp. 242–246.

Waickman, F. G. 1979. Allergic management of otitis media. Transactions of the Second National Conference on Otitis Media. Columbus, OH, Ross Laboratories, pp. 109–114.

Wald, E. R., Dashefsky, B., Byers, C., et al. 1988. Frequency and severity of infections in day care. J. Pediatr. 112:540.

Wallerstein, R. O., Condit, P. K., Kasper, C. K., et al. 1969. Statewide study of chloramphenicol therapy and fatal aplastic anemia. J.A.M.A. 208:2045.

Walton, W. K. 1973. Audiometrically "normal" conductive hearing losses among the cleft palate. Cleft Palate J. 10:99.

Ward, J. 1981. Antibiotic-resistant Streptococus pneumoniae: Clinical and epidemiological aspects. Rev. Infect. Dis. 3:254.

Ward, J. I., Tsai, T. F., Filice, G. A., and Fraser, D. W. 1978. Prevalence of ampicillin- and chloramphenicol-resistant strains of Haemophilus influenzae causing meningitis and bacteremia: National survey of hospital laboratories. J. Infect. Dis. 138:421.

Ward, P. A., and McClean, R. 1978. Complement activity. In Bellanti, J. A. (ed.): Immunology II. Philadelphia, W. B. Saunders Co. pp. 138–150.

Warren, W. S., and Stool, S. E. 1971. Otitis media in low-birth-weight infants. J. Pediatr. 79:740.

Webster, J. C. 1980. Middle ear function in the cleft palate patient. J. Laryngol. Otol. 94:31.

Welin, S. 1947. On the radiologic examination of the eustachian tube in cases of chronic otitis. Acta Radiol. (Stockh.) 28:95.

Whaley, J. B. 1957. Otolaryngologist's role in the care of cleft palate patients. J. Can. Dent. Assoc. 23:574.

Whitcomb, N. J. 1965. Allergy therapy in serous otitis media associated with allergic rhinitis. Clin. Allergy 23:232.

White, B. L., Doyle, W. J., and Bluestone, C. D. 1984. Eustachian tube function in infants and children with Down's syndrome. In Lim, D. J., Bluestone, C. D., Klein, J. O., et al. (eds.): Recent Advances in Otitis Media with Effusion. Toronto, B. C. Decker, pp. 62–66.

Willis, R. 1985. Otitis media and the Australian aboriginal. Am. J. Otol. 6:316.

Wittenborg, M. H., and Neuhauser, E. B. 1963. Simple roentgenographic demonstration of eustachian tubes and abnormalities. Am. J. Roentgenol. Rad. Ther. Nucl. Med. 89:1194.

Wolff, D: 1931. Microscopic observation of the eustachian tube. Oto-Rhino-Laryngol. 40B:1055.

Wolff, D. 1934. The microscopic anatomy of the eustachian tube. Ann. Otol. Rhinol. Laryngol. 43:483.

Wong, D. T., and Ogra, P. L. 1980. Immunology of tonsils and adenoids—an update. Int. J. Pediatr. Otorhinolaryngol. 2:181.

Wright, P. F., McConnell, K. B., Thompson, J. M., et al. 1985. A longitudinal study of the detection of otitis media in the first two years of life. Int. J. Pediatr. Otorhinolaryngol. 10:245.

Yaffe, S. J. 1975. Requiem for tetracyclines. Pediatrics 55:142.

Yagi, H. A. 1977. The surgical treatment of secretory otitis media in children. J. Laryngol. Otol. 91:267.

Yamaguchi, T., Urasawa, T., and Kataura, A. 1984. Secretory immunoglobulin A antibodies to respiratory viruses in middle ear effusion of chronic otitis media with effusion. Ann. Otol. Rhinol. Laryngol. 93:73.

Yamanaka, N., Somekawa, Y., Suzuki, T., et al. 1987. Immunologic and cytologic studies in otitis media with effusion. Acta Otolaryngol. (Stockh.) 104:481.

Yamanaka, T., Bernstein, J. B., Cumella, J., et al. 1982. Immunologic aspects of otitis media with effusion: Characteristics of lymphocyte and macrophage reactivity. J. Infect. Dis. 145:804.

Yamashita, K. 1983. Pneumatic endoscopy of the eustachian tube. Endoscopy 15:257.

Yules, R. B. 1970. Hearing in cleft palate patients. Arch. Otolaryngol. 91:319.

Zanga, J., Donland, M. A., Newton, J., et al. 1984. Administration of medication in school. Pediatrics 74:433.

Zollner, R. 1942. Anatomie, Physiologie und Klinik der Ohrtrompete. Berlin, Springer-Verlag.

Zonis, R. D. 1968. Chronic otitis media in the Southwestern American Indian. Arch. Otolaryngol. 88:360.

Chapter 22

INTRATEMPORAL COMPLICATIONS AND SEQUELAE OF OTITIS MEDIA

Charles D. Bluestone, M.D.   Jerome O. Klein, M.D.

Intracranial suppurative complications of otitis media, including meningitis, brain abscess, and lateral sinus thrombosis, are relatively uncommon today. Intratemporal complications, those that occur within the aural cavity and adjacent structures of the temporal bone, are more common. These include acute and chronic perforation of the tympanic membrane, chronic suppurative otitis media, mastoiditis, petrositis, cholesteatoma and retraction pocket, adhesive otitis media, tympanosclerosis, ossicular discontinuity and fixation, infectious eczematoid dermatitis, and cholesterol granuloma (Fig. 22–1). The most frequent complication or sequela of otitis media is hearing loss that accompanies most episodes of otitis media (Bluestone et al., 1983). Recent studies indicate that children who had recurrent episodes of otitis media or persistent middle-ear effusion perform less well on tests of speech and language than do their disease-free peers. These data suggest that delay or impairment of development may be an important sequela of otitis media. In this chapter, the authors discuss the epidemiology, pathogenesis, microbiology, and management of intratemporal complications and sequelae of otitis

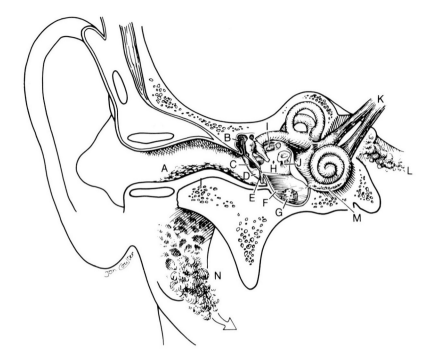

Figure 22–1. Intratemporal complications and sequelae of otitis media include (A) infectious eczematoid dermatitis, (B) cholesteatoma, (C) retraction pocket of the tympanic membrane, (D) tympanosclerosis, (E) perforation of the tympanic membrane, (F) chronic suppurative otitis media, (G) cholesterol granuloma, (H) ossicular discontinuity, (I) facial paralysis, (J) adhesive otitis media with fixation of the ossicles, (K) hearing loss, (L) petrositis, (M) labyrinthitis, (N) mastoiditis with extension into the neck (Bezold abscess).

media. In the next chapter, similar information is presented for intracranial complications and sequelae.

For many of the aural and intratemporal complications and sequelae of otitis media, surgery is indicated, but the emphasis in this chapter is on concepts of surgical management as they relate to infants and children, rather than on explicit descriptions of surgical techniques. For details of the surgical techniques, the reader is referred to current texts and atlases.

HEARING LOSS

Fluctuating or persisting loss of hearing is present in most children who have middle-ear effusion; impairment of hearing is the most prevalent complication of otitis media.

Conductive Hearing Loss

Audiograms of children with middle-ear effusion usually reveal a mild to moderate conductive loss in the range of 15 to 40 dB. With such deficits, the softer speech sounds and voiceless consonants may be missed. The average audiogram of a child with otitis media with effusion is presented in Figure 22–2. The hearing loss is influenced by the quantity of fluid in the middle ear; ears with thin fluids are impaired to the same degree as those with fluids of gluelike consistency (Brown et al., 1983; Weiderhold et al., 1980). Ears that are partially filled with fluid (identified otoscopically by the presence of bubbles or an air-fluid level) have lesser hearing impairment than ears that are completely filled with fluid (Fria et al., 1985). The hearing impairment is usually reversed with resolution

of the effusion. On occasion, permanent conductive hearing loss occurs owing to irreversible changes resulting from recurrent acute or chronic inflammation (e.g., adhesive otitis media or ossicular discontinuity). High negative pressure in the ear, or atelectasis, in the absence of effusion is another cause of conductive hearing loss.

Sensorineural Hearing Loss

Sensorineural hearing loss may also result from acute otitis media or otitis media with effusion. A reversible hearing impairment is generally attributed to the effect of increased tension and stiffness of the round window membrane. A permanent sensorineural loss may occur, presumably as a result of spread of infection or products of inflammation through the round window membrane (Morizono et al., 1985; Paparella et al., 1972, 1984; Vartiainen and Karjalainen, 1987; Walby et al., 1983), occurrence of a perilymphatic fistula in the oval or round window in association with otitis media (Grundfast and Bluestone, 1978; Supance and Bluestone, 1983), or a suppurative complication such as labyrinthitis.

Studies of Hearing Loss with Acute Otitis Media

Few studies of hearing have been performed during acute episodes of otitis media. Olmstead and coworkers (1964) studied children 2½ to 12 years of age with a diagnosis of acute otitis media who were seen in the Outpatient Department of St. Christopher's Hospital in Philadelphia. Of 82 children enrolled in the study,

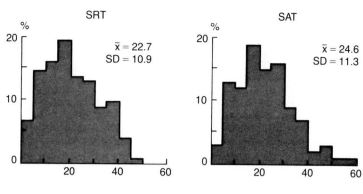

Figure 22–2. Frequency distribution of thresholds for speech stimuli associated with otitis media with effusion. *Left,* Speech reception threshold (SRT) of 540 children; *right,* speech awareness threshold (SAT) of 222 infants. HL indicates hearing level. (From Fria T. J., Cantekin, E. I., and Eichler, J. A. 1985. Hearing acuity of children with otitis media with effusion. Arch. Otolaryngol. 111:10–16. Copyright 1985, American Medical Association.)

33 per cent had no loss of hearing on the initial audiometric test following acute infection; 40 per cent had loss of hearing (up to 15 dB) initially, which disappeared in one to six months; 12 per cent had loss of hearing throughout the six-month period of observation; and 15 per cent had loss of hearing initially but were lost to the study between one and four months after the acute episode of otitis media. The children had no prior history of hearing difficulty or chronic ear infection. Otoscopic examinations were not performed after initial diagnosis, and data were not presented concerning duration of fluid in the middle ear. These data indicate that after a single episode of acute otitis media, many children have prolonged impairment of hearing.

Hearing loss has also been identified in children who have apparently recovered from acute otitis media. A longitudinal study of Alaskan Eskimo children showed a statistically significant association between the frequency of episodes of otitis media and hearing loss of greater than 26 dB. Of children who had one or more attacks of otitis media per year, 49 per cent had hearing loss; hearing loss was evident in 15 per cent of children with no diagnosed episodes of otitis media (Reed et al., 1967). Other studies with differing criteria have found the incidence of hearing loss associated with acute otitis media to vary between 6 and 30 per cent (Lowe et al., 1963; Neil et al., 1966).

Studies of Hearing Loss with Otitis Media with Effusion

Hearing loss is a frequent accompaniment of persistent middle-ear effusion (documented at the time of surgery) (Bluestone et al., 1973; Kokko, 1974). Fria and colleagues (1985) evaluated hearing in 222 infants (aged 7 to 24 months) and 540 older children (aged 2 to 12 years). Both the younger and the older children had, on average, thresholds for speech reception and speech awareness of 24.6 and 22.7 dB, respectively (Fig. 22–2). Not all children with middle-ear effusion have apparent hearing impairment. About one third of the children had air-conduction thresholds of 15 dB, but approximately 25 per cent of children with middle-ear effusion had thresholds of up to 30 dB. The

cumulative frequency curves were similar for children of various ages and for duration of effusion. This large study provides a very complete picture of the number of children affected and the extent of the hearing loss when middle-ear effusion is present.

Audiometric techniques for children of various ages are discussed in Chapter 9.

EFFECTS OF OTITIS MEDIA ON DEVELOPMENT OF THE CHILD

Do children who have had acute otitis media or persistent effusions of the middle ear suffer long-term sequelae because of impairment of hearing? Much has been written about the handicap imposed on the severely hearing-impaired child, but less is known about the effects on the young child of the mild and fluctuating hearing loss associated with otitis media (Menyuk, 1980, 1986; Feagans, 1986).

Sensorineural hearing loss has been associated with impairment in the cognitive, language, and emotional development of children. Children with sensorineural hearing impairment, when compared with peers who have normal hearing, are significantly retarded in development of vocabulary (Young and McConnell, 1957), are placed below their grade level in school (Kodman, 1963), have poorer articulation and auditory discriminatory abilities (Goetzinger et al., 1964), and have a high rate of maladjusted behavior patterns (Fisher, 1966) and disturbances in psychosocial adjustment (Peckham et al., 1972).

The first months of life are important in language acquisition. The infant is capable of speech sound discrimination as early as 1 month of age. By 6 weeks of age, the infant is attracted to human voices more than to environmental sounds and to female more than to male voices. At 5 to 6 months, the infant enters the babble phase and plays with sound-making. The child is putting words together in sentences by 18 months of age, and by 4 years the child produces all the basic syntactic structures that he or she will ever use (Menyuk, 1977).

Since so much progress in language acquisition is made during infancy, any problems in receiving or interpreting sound signals might have a significant

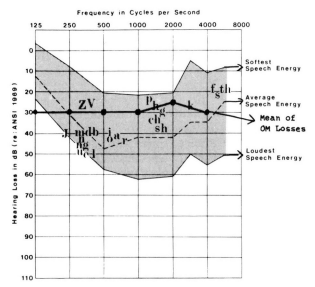

Figure 22–3. Range of speech energy related to standard audiogram. Shaded area shows range of sound energy present in normal speech, and dashed line indicates average of speech energy (adapted from Skinner, 1978). Line connected by solid circles shows mean of hearing losses from otitis media. It can be seen that softer speech sounds may not be heard when otitis media is present. (From Bluestone, C. D., and Klein, J. O. 1988. Otitis Media in Infants and Children. Philadelphia, W. B. Saunders Co.)

effect on development of speech and language. Softer speech sounds and voiceless consonants, in particular, may be missed or confused when effusion is present in the middle ear (Fig. 22–3) (Downs, 1983). Important differences have been identified in the early patterns of vocalization of the hearing-impaired infant when compared with hearing infants. How these data about differences in infant babble relate to ultimate development of speech and language when the hearing impairment is mild and fluctuating is unknown.

The current hypothesis for the effects of otitis media on development of the child is presented in Figure 22–4. Children with severe or recurrent otitis media have prolonged time spent with middle-ear effusion. Hearing impairment (average loss approximately 25 dB) accompanies the effusion in most children, and if the hearing impairment occurs at a time of rapid intellectual growth, the result may be impaired development of speech, language, and cognitive abilities.

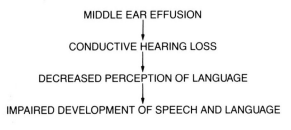

Figure 22–4. Long-term sequelae of middle-ear effusion. (From Bluestone, C. D., and Klein, J. O. 1988. Otitis Media in Infants and Children. Philadelphia, W. B. Saunders Co.)

Studies

The results of more than a dozen studies suggest that children with histories of recurrent episodes of acute otitis media score lower in tests of speech and language than do disease-free peers. A brief resume of the results of selected studies follows:

1. One of the earliest and most widely cited studies is that of Holm and Kunze of Seattle (1969). Children aged 5 to 9 years who had a history of chronic otitis media with onset before 2 years of age were compared with children in a control group matched for age, sex, and socioeconomic background. Children with a history of ear disease were delayed in all language skills requiring the receiving or processing of auditory stimuli, but the groups were similar in tests measuring visual and motor skills (Fig. 22–5). Diagnosis of otitis media was made on the basis of history. Otoscopic and audiometric examinations were not performed, and the sample size was small (16 children in each group).

2. Eskimo children were observed prospectively during the first four years of life and had tests of hearing, intelligence, and assessment of school performance at age 10 years (Kaplan et al., 1973). Children with recurrent episodes of otitis media (defined as the presence of a draining ear) during the first two years of life and with loss of hearing of 26 dB or more had lower scores in tests of reading, mathematics, and language than did children who had little or no disease in infancy. Otorrhea was the sole criterion for otitis media; data were not available about the presence or

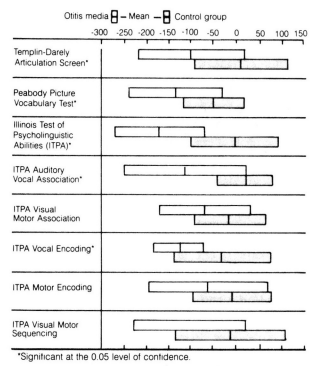

Figure 22–5. Results of language tests in children with and without otitis media (standard score mean and standard deviation). (From Holm, V. A., and Kunze, L. H. 1969. Effects of chronic otitis media on language and speech development. Reproduced by permission of Pediatrics, vol. 43, page 833, copyright 1969.)

duration of middle-ear effusions or episodes of acute otitis media that did not result in otorrhea.

3. Aboriginal children from Brisbane, Australia, were studied by Lewis (1976). Children aged 7 to 9 years who "failed otoscopic examinations" and had hearing deficits measured by audiometry or tympanometry over a four-year period were compared with age-matched control children who had consistently passed the audiometric tests and were assumed to be disease-free. Children with ear disease had mean scores for speech and language development that were significantly lower than those of the children without ear disease. The sample size was small—14 children with disease and 18 control subjects.

4. Needleman (1977) evaluated 20 children 3 to 8 years of age with a history of recurrent otitis media and first episode before age 18 months. Twenty control subjects who had no history of hearing problems or recurrent ear infections were matched with the patients for age, grade, and socioeconomic status. The children were evaluated for their ability to use speech sounds expressively and receptively. Children with a history of ear disease had poorer phonologic abilities than did matched control children. Diagnosis of ear disease was based on history alone.

5. Sak and Ruben (1982) used a sibling control for children with histories of otitis media. Children received tests of speech and language between 8 and 11 years of age. One sibling of each pair had had a documented history of persistent otitis media beginning before 5 years of age, whereas the other sibling had had no middle-ear problem. The children who had had otitis media showed a lower verbal IQ, poorer auditory reception, and lower spelling achievement than their matched sibling controls.

More of the siblings with otitis were boys than were the control siblings, and more minor abnormalities of the middle ear identified by audiometry or tympanometry were prevalent among the otitis media siblings than among the control siblings, suggesting the possibility that deficits were associated with recent, rather than earlier, disease of the middle ear.

6. Friel-Patti and coworkers (1982) examined the association of otitis media early in life with language development at 12, 18, and 24 months. The infants had been selected from intensive care units of low-birth-weight nurseries and were predominantly from low socioeconomic groups. Frequent episodes of otitis media were correlated with a higher prevalence of language delay, but no correlation was found between hearing impairment measured by auditory brain stem response testing and language delay.

7. To determine the association between time spent with middle-ear effusion and development of speech, language, and cognitive abilities, Teele and colleagues (1984) studied 190 white children of varying socioeconomic strata from Greater Boston. The children were selected from a cohort of children in five health centers who were followed from birth with regular examinations of the middle ear at each visit to office or clinic, whether for illness or for routine care. The study was prospective, used uniform criteria for diagnosis of acute otitis media and middle-ear effusion, and tested children from all socioeconomic strata (Teele et al., 1984).

Tests of speech and language administered at the third birthday included the Peabody Picture Vocabulary Test (a test of both early receptive and expressive language), the Fisher-Logemann and Goldman-Fristoe Tests of Articulation (tests of production of speech sound), and other measurements of complexity of language structure and estimates of intelligibility.

Children who had spent fewer than 30 days with middle-ear effusion during the first three years of life were compared with those who had spent 30 to 129 days with middle-ear effusion during the first three years of life and with those who had spent 130 or more days with middle-ear effusion from birth to age 3 years. In summary, the results identified (1) lower scores on tests for the total number of children tested, but significant differences were present only in the scores of children from the high socioeconomic group. No significant differences were found for children from low socioeconomic groups (Table 22–1). The basis for the difference in results for children in lower and upper socioeconomic strata is unclear but might be accounted for by the lower scores of children in the low socioeconomic group. The tests used may have been insensitive to differences in performance by these children at 3 years of age. (2) Increased time with middle-ear effusion during the first year of life was most significantly associated with lower scores in children tested at 3 years of age. Confounding variables such as race and birth order were either controlled for or excluded.

From the cohort of Greater Boston children followed from birth, 196 children were selected for testing within three months of their seventh birthday. Time spent with middle-ear effusion during the first three

TABLE 22–1. Otitis Media with Effusion and Scores of Tests of Speech and Language at Age Three Years, Peabody Picture Vocabulary Test*

TIME WITH MIDDLE-EAR EFFUSION	ALL CHILDREN	HIGH SOCIOECONOMIC STATUS	LOW SOCIOECONOMIC STATUS
Less than 30 days	101.4	104.8	96.6
More than 130 days	96.4	99.6	92.5
	p = 0.002	p = 0.0001	p = nonsignificant

*Total sample, 190 children: 106, high socioeconomic status; 84, low socioeconomic status.
From Bluestone, C. D., and Klein, J. O. 1988. Otitis Media in Infants and Children. Philadelphia, W. B. Saunders Co.

years of life and especially during the first year was associated with significantly lower scores in many aspects of cognitive ability, speech, and language at age 7 years. Time spent with middle-ear effusion during the first three years of life was also associated with significantly lower scores in mathematics and in reading (Klein et al., 1987).

8. Hubbard and colleagues in Pittsburgh (Hubbard et al., 1985) evaluated two matched pairs of children with repaired palatal clefts. The treatment of the children had been equivalent, with the exception that one group had undergone early myringotomy with placement of tympanostomy tubes (mean age, 3 months), and the other group had undergone initial myringotomy later (mean age, 30.8 months) or not at all. Hearing acuity and consonant articulation were significantly less impaired in the group undergoing early myringotomy. Mean verbal performance and full scale IQs and scores on psychosocial indices were normal in both groups and did not differ significantly between the groups.

9. Watanabe and colleagues (1985) studied total speaking time in infants and children with and without middle-ear effusion. To support the premise that improvements in the child's performance occurred when hearing improved with resolution of middle-ear effusion, the authors developed a technique to identify time of vibration of the vocal cords. Duration of speaking time was measured in children with otitis media with effusion before and after placement of tympanostomy tubes. Preoperative speaking time was found to be eight minutes and two seconds per measured hour when middle-ear effusion was present and 10 minutes per hour when the effusion cleared following placement of tympanostomy tubes. The implications of this innovative study are uncertain but suggest that hearing improvement increases speaking time and causes the child's ordinary behavior to be more animate.

Other studies of otitis media and language performance include a study of Montreal children, aged 3 to 5 years, that identified significant differences among the children with histories of otitis media and matched controls (Schlieper et al., 1985), a study of Danish children 3 to 9 years of age that did not show an effect of otitis media with effusion early in life on reading achievement (Lous and Fiellau-Nikolajsen, 1984), and evaluation of Apache Indian children 6 to 8 years of age who had contrasting histories of otitis media but no significant difference in language performance (Fischler et al., 1985).

Roberts and coworkers (1986) examined 61 socioeconomically disadvantaged children during the first years of life and administered standardized tests of intelligence and academic performance when they were 3½ to 6 years of age. These investigators found no relationship between number of days with otitis media and later performance on verbal components of the intelligence tests or later academic achievement.

These reports are disturbing but most have one or more flaws in design: (1) reliance on retrospective history of acute otitis media, (2) uncertain validity of diagnosis of otitis media, (3) lack of information about middle-ear effusion, (4) presence of significant hearing impairment in subjects at time of tests of speech and language, (5) small numbers of subjects, (6) special populations tested (e.g., Australian aborigines or Alaskan Eskimos, or children with cleft palate), and (7) inadequate criteria for selection of children without disease used for comparison. Hignett summarized the study design issues and evaluated the effectiveness of 10 early studies of otitis media and speech, language, and behavior (Hignett, 1983). The studies of Teele and coworkers (1984) and Hubbard and associates (1985) represent significant advances in study design when compared with prior investigations. But each of these studies has been subject to criticism (Leviton and Bellinger, 1985; Paradise and Rogers, 1986) because of perceived limitations and deficiencies. These inadequacies of study design prevent general application of these results to planning care for young children, but they do not prevent concern that many children may suffer from the sequelae of otitis media with persistent middle-ear effusion in infancy.

Factors of Importance in Analysis of Studies of Otitis Media and Development of Speech, Language, and Cognitive Abilities

QUALITY OF PARENTING. Language development is an interactive process in which the quality of parent-child interaction is an important factor. The quality of parenting is difficult to measure but undoubtedly plays a significant role in the development of language for the child.

FAMILY STRESS. The parents and siblings of a child with recurrent otitis media must contend with earaches in the middle of the night, irritability and inattentiveness of the child, and the expense and inconvenience of frequent visits to the physician. Although some families can accept and cope with the stress of a child's recurrent illnesses, other families cannot. A constellation of disturbances in psychosocial development may result.

RECURRENT AND PERSISTENT OTITIS MEDIA AS A CHRONIC DISEASE. The systemic effects of illness, including irritability, malaise, lethargy, and local or generalized pain, may be sufficiently distracting to affect development. These effects of a chronic illness must be distinguished from the specific effects of otitis media (i.e., hearing loss) in the interpretation of the sequelae of the disease. Is the child treated differently by the parents, siblings, peers, or teachers because of the recurrent illnesses? Is the child vulnerable to effects unassociated with the specific morbidity of the disease (kept indoors, away from peers, or out of exercise and athletic programs)?

CRITICAL AGES FOR EFFECTS OF OTITIS MEDIA. Otitis media of similar duration may affect children differently at different ages. There may be critical periods of perception of language when the child is most vulnerable to mild, fluctuating, or persistent hearing loss. The results of the Boston study suggested that the children were most affected by middle-ear effusion when disease occurred during the first year of life (Teele et al., 1984). During early stages of language development, the child learns the sounds of the language; different or changing auditory signals resulting from persistent or fluctuating hearing deficits may impede the child's abilities to form linguistic categories (Berko-Gleason, 1983).

AUDITORY DEPRIVATION. Studies in birds and rodents indicate that deprivation of sound early in life leads to identifiable changes in auditory sectors of the brain. A decrease in the size and the number of neurons in the auditory nuclei of mice occurred when the animals were deprived of auditory stimuli during early development (Webster, 1983). In normal postnatal development of the mouse, the neurons of the auditory brain stem reach adult size by age 12 days, the time of onset of hearing. Mice that underwent auditory deprivation by experimentally produced conductive hearing loss from 4 to 45 days after birth had auditory brain stem neurons that were significantly smaller than normal. If the mice who underwent induced hearing loss early in life were returned to normal hearing after 45 days, the smaller-than-normal neurons were retained. The size of the neurons was not altered in mice raised in a normal sound environment until 45 days and then deprived of sound until 90 days of age.

These data demonstrate that a period exists in the development of mice during which adequate sound stimulation is needed to establish the normal size of neuronal cells in the auditory brain stem. These experimental data in animals raise concerns about irreparable damage from temporary conductive hearing loss in infants. However, Webster points out that the factors in the experimental model differ from the mild to moderate hearing losses of otitis media with effusion in humans; in the experimental model the conductive loss is approximately 50 dB, greater than the loss in most cases of otitis media with effusion. The loss is persistent rather than fluctuating, and the impairment starts at the inception of hearing in the mouse, whereas inception of sound occurs prenatally in the human. The author concludes that although the restrictions of the animal model must be kept in mind, "the fact that early auditory restriction has a profound effect on the central nervous system in one mammal must arouse concern about possible related effects in humans."

UNILATERAL HEARING LOSS. Unilateral hearing loss has not been considered a handicap for children. However, data indicate that children with unilateral hearing impairment score less well on auditory, linguistic, and behavioral tests than do children without hearing impairment (Bess and Tharpe, 1984). Although the children studied had sensorineural hearing deficits, the data suggest that we should no longer accept as benign a unilateral hearing loss. Children with unilateral conductive loss may also suffer during critical periods of language perception by confused speech signals.

EFFECTS OF GROUP DAY CARE. Respiratory infections are readily spread among children in day care, and children in day care are likely to have more episodes of otitis media than will children in home care. In relation to development of language, the quantity and quality of the speech sounds around the infants in group care differ from those presented to the child in home care. The factors of increased number of infections and differences in the speech environment in group day care will need to be considered in future studies.

PSYCHOSOCIAL EFFECTS OF OTITIS MEDIA. Does otitis media with mild and fluctuating hearing loss affect the child's motivation and perception of others? Gray (1983) suggested that inconsistencies in the child's ability to hear may have a lasting effect on the child's motivation to achieve and may cause strain in relationships with teachers and parents.

OTHER PRIMARY VARIABLES THAT MAY RELATE TO EARLY CHILDHOOD LANGUAGE DEVELOPMENT. Future study designs must also consider these additional factors: visual status, physical and motor development, social and emotional development, nutritional status and history of medications, dialect exposure, birth order, and number of siblings.

TEST RESULTS AND FUNCTIONAL SIGNIFICANCE. Do a few percentage points of one or more standard tests of speech, language, or cognitive abilities affect the child's capability to function in the school, play, and home settings? Some investigators question whether these are statistical differences of limited importance to child development. But there are reasons for concern. Since the data are expressed here in terms of mean differences, the scores of some children will be close to or better than the norm, but others will have scores that are much lower. Otitis media is so common in early childhood that even if a small percentage of children are adversely affected in terms of development, the number of children who suffer is large. Of the 3.7 million children born in the United States each year, more than one third will have recurrent episodes of otitis media (three or more) by 3 years of age. If only 10 per cent of the children with recurrent episodes are affected adversely, the national impact is greater: More than 100,000 of each year's newborn infants would be involved.

Since the tests measure the child's potential for achievement, it is possible that the loss suffered by the child with frequent and recurrent episodes of otitis media accompanied by hearing loss in early infancy is never perceived by the parents, teachers, or physicians. The child is not obviously slow or behind his peers. The failure of the child to reach his or her potential is a loss for the child and the family, and because the number of children is large each year, it must be considered a national concern.

Summary: Role of Otitis Media in Infant Development

The accumulated results of the various studies of otitis media and development of speech, language, and cognitive abilities suggest that children do suffer long-term effects from otitis media early in life. However, the scientific evidence remains incomplete. Some experts are skeptical about available data (Paradise, 1983; Ventry, 1983). Ventry concluded that no causal link had been established (by 1982) between early recurrent middle-ear effusion and language delay or learning problems. Rapin (1979) noted that no studies published by 1977 "met the standards of rigor needed to provide a definitive answer to this question, although the burden of the evidence is that a persistent and mild hearing loss, especially if present since infancy, probably has a measurably deleterious effect on the language of most, but not all, children." The authors believe that Dr. Rapin's statement is as applicable today as it was in 1977.

The difficulties in study design needed to resolve the issues and to account for many of the variables are formidable. The optimal design will need to include frequent otoscopic observations beginning soon after birth to develop a chronology of time spent with middle-ear effusion. Assessments of hearing will need to be performed in infants when they have effusion and are free of effusion to measure the duration and severity of hearing deficits. All this will need to be done in the first years of life, when hearing assessments are more difficult and less precise than in the older child. The study will need to be cross-sectional and prospective from birth and should be performed by validated otoscopists. Tests of speech, language, and cognitive abilities will need to be selected that are accurate and standardized for the populations to be tested. The tests should be performed at least annually to define the time of onset or the effect of otitis media on development. The previous section identified the other variables that will need to be considered, including the quality of parenting, the effect of siblings, and the time spent in group day care.

Concern about the association of disease of the middle ear and development of speech and language was expressed in a recent policy statement of the American Academy of Pediatrics. Although recognizing the validity of criticism of published studies, the Committee on Early Childhood, Adoption, and Dependent Care concluded that "there is growing evidence demonstrating a correlation between middle-ear disease with hearing impairment and delays in the development of speech, language, and cognitive skills. . . . When a child has frequently recurring acute otitis media and/or middle-ear effusion persisting for longer than three months, hearing should be assessed and the development of communicative skills must be monitored" (American Academy of Pediatrics, 1984). Until definitive answers are available from studies of appropriate design to evaluate the sequelae of otitis media in early infancy, the physician must decide, for each child in his or her care, the optimal management of persistent middle-ear effusion. Chapter 21, on management, provides guidelines for such care.

Pertinent to these issues of speech, language, and otitis media, the words of the Chilean poet Gabriela

Mistral seem appropriate, "Many of the things we need can wait. The child cannot. Right now is the time his bones are being formed, his blood is being made, and his senses are being developed. To him we cannot answer tomorrow. His name is today."

PERFORATION OF THE TYMPANIC MEMBRANE

A perforation of the tympanic membrane that is secondary to otitis media (and certain related conditions, such as atelectasis of the tympanic membrane) can be classified according to its duration, the area of the eardrum involved, its size, and the presence or absence of associated conditions, such as otitis media or cholesteatoma. In addition, the perforation may not be spontaneous (a result of a middle-ear infection) but may be a complication of a surgical procedure to manage otitis media, such as a myringotomy and tympanostomy tube insertion. An acute perforation is most frequently secondary to an episode of acute otitis media, whereas if it persists for two or three months, it is considered chronic. These perforations occur in the pars tensa and involve one or more of the following quadrants: anterosuperior, anteroinferior, posterosuperior, or posteroinferior. The defect may involve almost the entire pars tensa or may be so small as to be detectable only when visualized with the otomicroscope or when the electroacoustic impedance bridge measures a volume larger than the expected ear canal volume. Otitis media (with or without discharge) may be present or absent; when chronic otitis media with discharge is present, the condition is called chronic suppurative otitis media, which is described in detail in the next section. Likewise, a perforation may be associated with some of the other complications and sequelae described in this chapter.

In the past, perforations have been classified into "central" and "marginal" types. Regardless of size, if there is a rim of tympanic membrane remaining at all borders, the perforation has been classified as being of the "central" type, whereas when any part of the perforation extends to the annulus, it has been termed a "marginal perforation." Similarly, a defect in the pars flaccida has been commonly called an "attic perforation." However, the so-called "marginal perforation" of the pars tensa, which usually occurs in the posterosuperior portion, and the "attic perforation" are in reality either a deep retraction pocket or a cholesteatoma (Fig. 22–6). There is usually no continuity between the *defect* in the membrane and the middle ear until late in the disease process, when infection destroys the membrane of the pocket or the matrix of the cholesteatoma. Therefore, the terms "marginal perforation" and "attic perforation" are misnomers; they were applied on the basis of observations made prior to the availability of the otomicroscope, modern surgery of the middle ear, advances in temporal bone histopathology, the use of the electroacoustic impedance bridge, and a better understanding of the patho-

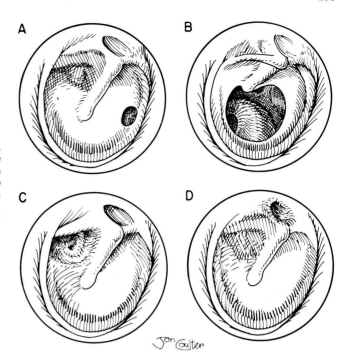

Figure 22–6. Examples of defects in the tympanic membrane. *A*, A small "central" perforation in the anteroinferior portion of the pars tensa of the tympanic membrane. *B*, A "central" perforation that involves approximately half of the pars tensa. *C*, A deep retraction pocket in the posterosuperior portion of the pars tensa that has been incorrectly called a "marginal perforation." *D*, A deep retraction pocket in the pars flaccida that has been inappropriately called an "attic perforation."

genesis of a retraction pocket and cholesteatoma (both of which are described in a separate section in this chapter). In this section, only acute and chronic perforations (with and without acute otitis media) will be discussed.

Acute Perforation

Etiology

An acute perforation (not due to trauma) is usually secondary to acute otitis media but may also occur during the course of chronic otitis media with effusion. Since a spontaneous perforation commonly accompanies an episode of acute middle-ear infection, it may be part of the natural history of the disease process rather than a complication. Because such a perforation allows pus to drain into the external canal and enhances drainage of pus down the eustachian tube (see Chap. 21), a perforation of the eardrum that adequately drains the middle ear may prevent further spread of infection within the temporal bone or, more important, into the intracranial cavity. Infants and children of certain racial groups, such as Alaskan natives (Eskimos) and American Indians, have a high incidence of spontaneous perforation with discharge; the eardrum is perforated spontaneously with almost every episode of acute otitis media. The disease runs a similar course in certain other children not belonging to these high-risk populations.

Pathogenesis

The perforation may occur in high-risk populations because of the presence of a semipatulous eustachian tube (Beery et al., 1980): A eustachian tube with low resistance would permit a larger bolus of bacteria-laden purulent material from the nasopharynx to enter the middle ear, causing a more fulminating infection than would occur if the eustachian tube had either normal or high resistance. An alternative explanation of why some children seem to suffer a perforated eardrum with each episode of acute otitis media, while others do not, could be that there are differences in the virulence of the bacteria or decreased resistance of the host.

Microbiology

The organisms that are most frequently cultured from an aural discharge when acute otitis media is present are the same as those that have been cultured from acute middle-ear effusions when a tympanocentesis has been performed (e.g., *Streptococcus pneumoniae* and *Haemophilus influenzae*). *Streptococcus pyogenes*, when present and untreated, has been associated with acute perforation of the tympanic membrane.

Management

Antimicrobial therapy for children with perforated eardrums should be the same as that recommended for those with acute otitis media when a perforation is not present (see Chap. 21). However, when an aural discharge is present, it may be desirable to culture the drainage in all cases, if feasible. Indications for obtaining a culture in selected patients would be similar to those for performing a tympanocentesis when acute otitis media (without a perforation) is present: (1) the child is critically ill or toxic; (2) there is an unsatisfactory clinical response to antimicrobial therapy, such as persistence or recurrence of fever or otalgia, or both;

(3) a suppurative complication, such as acute mastoiditis with periosteitis, is present or impending; (4) a discharge is occurring in the neonate, the very young infant, or the immunologically deficient patient, in each of whom an unusual organism may be present; and (5) the purulent otorrhea persists in spite of a full course of antimicrobial therapy. The antimicrobial agent(s) can then be adjusted according to the results of the Gram stain culture and susceptibility testing. The most effective method to obtain a sample of the discharge is to remove as much as possible of the purulent material from the external canal by suction or cotton-tipped applicator and then to aspirate pus directly at or through the perforation, using a spinal needle attached to a tuberculin syringe or an Alden-Senturia trap (Storz Instrument Co., St. Louis) and suction.

Even though some experts would argue against the use of ototopical medication when a perforation is present because of the potential danger of ototoxicity, some children should have otic drops instilled into the external canal. In particular, ototopical medication will usually be beneficial when infectious eczematoid external otitis complicates the picture (see section on infectious eczematoid dermatitis, p. 531). The application of an antibiotic-cortisone otic medication whenever a discharge is present has been advocated by many clinicians despite the possibility of ototoxicity, since the topical medication may prevent an external canal infection from occurring and hasten the resolution of the middle-ear infection.

In any event, the discharge, especially when profuse, should be prevented from draining onto the pinna and adjacent areas, since this usually results in dermatitis. The parent should be instructed to keep cotton in the external auditory meatus and change it as often as necessary to keep the canal as dry as possible. Cotton-tipped applicators should not be used by the child or the parent.

Healing of the tympanic membrane frequently follows cessation of the suppurative process. The defect usually closes within a week of the onset of the infection; however, when persistent discharge lasts longer than the initial ten-day course of antibiotic treatment, the child requires more intensive evaluation and aggressive management. In addition to obtaining a culture of the purulent material from the middle ear and adjusting the antimicrobial agent(s), frequent cleaning of the canal followed by instillation of ototopical drops may also be required. The presence of acute mastoiditis with periosteitis or acute mastoid osteitis should be suspected if the child has persistent otalgia, tenderness of the ear to touch, erythema, and swelling in the postauricular area. Roentgenograms of the mastoids may be helpful, but even computed tomograms are not always diagnostic of mastoid osteitis (see section on mastoiditis, p. 523). Spread of the infection outside the middle ear and mastoid may be diagnosed on computed tomograms. Even if an intratemporal (or intracranial) complication is not readily apparent, if the aural discharge persists for two or

three weeks after the onset of the acute otitis media, the child should be hospitalized if appropriately administered oral antibiotics (selected on the basis of the culture results) have failed to resolve the infection. The child should also be evaluated again thoroughly to search for an underlying illness that would interfere with the resolution of the infection. The otologic assessment should include an examination of the entire external canal and tympanic membrane, using the otomicroscope to determine if another otologic condition is present, such as a cholesteatoma or neoplasm. If an adequate examination cannot be performed with the child awake, it should be carried out with the patient under general anesthesia, at which time a culture directly from the middle ear (or biopsy) can be obtained. If no other condition besides the perforation and subacute otitis media is found, parenteral antimicrobial agents should be administered, and appropriate ototopical drops should be directly instilled once or twice a day (using a needle attached to a syringe) into the middle ear through the perforation, with the aid of the otomicroscope. The selection of both the systemic and topical antimicrobial agents should be based on the results of the culture (see Tables 21–17 and 22–2). Frequently, a gram-negative organism (e.g., *Pseudomonas aeruginosa*) is present at this stage, and management is essentially as recommended under Chronic Suppurative Otitis Media.

With this method of management, the infection will usually subside; however, if the discharge persists, an exploratory tympanotomy and complete simple mastoidectomy are indicated, even if there are no signs and symptoms of mastoid osteitis present and if the roentgenograms fail to show osteitis, that is, "coalescence." During the surgery on the middle ear and mastoid, a thorough search for another cause of the persistent infection must be made. On occasion, a cholesteatoma or neoplasm that could not be visualized through the otomicroscope will be found. Resolution of the infection in the middle ear and mastoid will invariably follow the surgery, since mastoid osteitis is the usual cause of this complication of acute otitis media.

Fortunately, nowadays, the occurrence of such cases is uncommon, and the perforation usually heals rap-

TABLE 22–2. Ototopical Agents Available for Treating Otitis Media with Perforation, Discharge, and Secondary Eczematoid External Otitis*

GENERIC NAME	TRADE NAME
Chloramphenicol	Chloromycetin Otic
Colistin sulfate; neomycin sulfate; thonzonium bromide; hydrocortisone acetate	Coly-Mycin S Otic
Polymyxin B; neomycin sulfate; gramicidin; hydrocortisone	Cortisporin Cream and Cortisporin Ointment
Polymyxin B; neomycin sulfate; hydrocortisone	Cortisporin Otic Suspension
Polymyxin B; hydrocortisone	Pyocidin-Otic Solution

*These drugs should be used with care in cases of nonintact eardrum because of the possibility of ototoxicity.

idly; however, not infrequently, the defect will remain open without evidence of otitis media (with or without discharge). If the perforation remains free of infection, it will frequently close in a few months. At this stage, no attempt at surgical closure of an uncomplicated perforation, even though there are no signs of otitis media, is indicated. If there is no sign of progressive healing after three or more months, management should be as described next for a chronic perforation of the tympanic membrane.

Chronic Perforation

A perforation of the tympanic membrane may remain open after an episode of acute otitis media or following spontaneous extrusion (or removal) of a tympanostomy tube. When the perforation is present with no signs of healing and there are no signs of otitis media for several months, the perforation is considered to be chronic and possibly "permanent." If chronic suppurative otitis media is present, the perforation may close spontaneously following appropriate treatment. The healing of the perforation is most probably being prevented by the presence of squamous epithelium at the edges of the perforation. The effect on hearing of a small chronic perforation, regardless of its location, and in the absence of other abnormalities of the middle ear, is not significant. However, a large perforation can be associated with an appreciable conductive hearing loss (e.g., 20 to 30 dB).

The incidence of chronic perforation in the pediatric population has not been formally studied, but chronic perforation is a frequent reason for referral to an otolaryngologist. The incidence of tympanoplasties performed in children would not accurately reflect the true incidence of chronic perforation, since many physicians elect to withhold surgery until later in the child's life. However, next to myringotomy, with or without tympanostomy tube insertion, tympanoplasty is the most common ear operation performed in children (Avery et al., 1976).

Chronic perforations, as complications of otitis media, are more prevalent in racial groups that also have a high prevalence and incidence of perforations associated with acute infection of the middle ear. In 1970, new cases of chronic perforation (with or without chronic suppurative otitis media), were reported in 8 per cent of the native population of Alaska, although this rate appears to be dropping (Wiet et al., 1980). Similar rates have been reported in American Indian populations. Zonis (1970) reported that of 207 Apache Indian children examined in Canyon Day, Arizona, 17 (8 per cent) had chronic perforations as their only sign of otitis media, whereas 16 years later, Todd and Bowman (1985) returned to the same village in 1983, examined 145 Indian children living there at the time, and found only one child who had a perforation of the tympanic membrane but 12 (8 per cent) children who had other evidence of otitis media. Of 1062 ears of children who received tympanostomy tubes in one

study reported from West Germany, 26 ears (2.5 per cent) had a persistent perforation (Muenker, 1980). However, this figure is dependent on the site of the tube placement and the type of tube used (see section on tympanostomy tubes, p. 453).

Management

The management of so-called "dry" chronic perforations in children is both difficult and controversial. On the one hand, the perforation provides ventilation and drainage of the middle ear, but on the other hand, the physiologic protective function of the eustachian tube–middle ear system is impaired. The middle ear and mastoid air cells no longer have an air cushion to prevent nasopharyngeal secretions from entering the ear, which can result in "reflux otitis media" (Figs. 22–7 and 22–8). In addition, the open tympanic membrane can permit contaminated water to enter the middle ear during bathing and swimming. Therefore, the dilemma of when to close such a perforation is comparable to that regarding the most appropriate time to remove a tympanostomy tube; a small, uncomplicated chronic perforation and a tympanostomy tube have similar benefits and risks. Like a tympanostomy tube, a perforation may be beneficial for a child who had had recurrent or chronic otitis media with effusion prior to the development of the perforation, but recurrent acute "reflux otitis media" with discharge may become a problem, making closure of the eardrum defect a consideration. However, recurrent acute otitis media that results in otorrhea through a chronic perforation can be effectively treated and even prevented without repair of the tympanic membrane.

When the episodes are infrequent, the treatment of each bout should be the same as recommended for an acute perforation that is associated with acute otitis media. However, if the episodes of acute infection are frequent and the interval between bouts short, then a prolonged course of a prophylactic antimicrobial agent (e.g., amoxicillin, 20 mg/kg given before bedtime) will usually prevent the recurrent middle-ear infection and discharge. The selection of the agent should be based

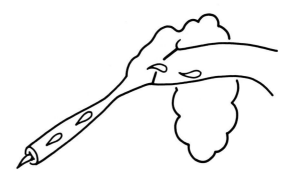

Figure 22–7. The presence of a perforation of the tympanic membrane may promote the reflux of secretions into the middle ear from the nasopharynx, since the middle-ear air cushion is not present (see also Fig. 22–8). (From Bluestone, C. D., and Klein, J. O. 1988. Otitis Media in Infants and Children. Philadelphia, W. B. Saunders Co.)

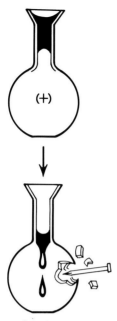

Figure 22–8. Flask model showing how a perforation of the tympanic membrane may result in reflux of nasopharyngeal secretions into the middle ear. The nasopharynx–eustachian tube–middle ear–mastoid air cell system is likened to a flask with a narrow neck. When the system is intact, liquid is prevented from entering the body of the flask, but when the body of the flask is not intact (i.e., when a perforation is present), liquid can readily flow through the system.

on the results of the cultures obtained from the previous episodes of discharge. Dosage and duration of the treatment should be the same as recommended for children who have had frequently recurrent acute otitis media without a perforation (see Chap. 21, section on antimicrobial agents for prophylaxis). Children in whom an attack of acute middle-ear infection and discharge persists despite adequate medical treatment and in whom the infection is thought to be chronic should be evaluated and managed as described in the section Chronic Suppurative Otitis Media. Fortunately, most children who have a defect in the eardrum that is thought to be preventing otitis media can be watched until the risk of recurrence of infection is low enough to consider surgical closure of the perforation. Since the perforation, like a tympanostomy tube, may be preventing the development of a retraction pocket and, subsequently, of a cholesteatoma if the function of the eustachian tube is poor, it is desirable to delay such surgery as long as possible in order to prevent such complications. On the other hand, surgery for a chronic perforation should not necessarily be withheld in children because of recurrent episodes of otitis media and discharge, since the perforation may be causing the middle-ear infection (owing to reflux from the nasopharynx), rather than preventing disease.

INDICATIONS FOR REPAIR OF THE PERFORATION. Indications for repair of a chronic perforation in adults have been defined by many surgeons, but there remains no agreement on the indications for tympanoplasty in children. Some surgeons have reported that

pediatric tympanoplasty is as successful as that in adults (Lee and Schuknecht, 1971; Buchwacd and Birck, 1980; Friedberg and Gillis, 1980; Raine and Singh, 1983; Bergen et al., 1983; Adkins and White, 1984; Hildmann et al., 1985; Lau and Tos, 1986), but others have had the opposite experience (Armstrong, 1965; Goodey and Smyth, 1972; Mawson and Ludman, 1979). When criteria for a successful tympanoplasty include other outcome measures than just healing of the graft, the success rate is frequently lower in children as compared to adults. Even though Lau and Tos (1986) reported that 92 per cent of the grafts healed, the success of the procedure over time fell to 64 per cent. During the follow-up period, 14 per cent required tympanostomy tube insertion, 5 per cent had persistent middle-ear effusion, and 9 per cent had postoperative atelectasis. Similar outcomes were reported by Manning and colleagues (1987) in a study of 56 children (63 ears). Even though 78 per cent of the grafts healed, only 52 per cent of the children had a healed graft and adequate middle-ear function during the postoperative follow-up period. Some surgeons attribute these differences between adult and pediatric tympanoplasty to the higher incidence of upper respiratory tract infection leading to otitis media in children and the unpredictability of their eustachian tube function. Optimal ages at which to perform tympanoplastic surgery have variously been stated to be from 3 years to puberty (Mawson and Ludman, 1979; Bailey, 1976; Glasscock, 1976; Storrs, 1976). Paparella (1977) states that tympanoplasty can be performed in children of almost any age. However, Sheehy and Anderson (1980) do not recommend elective tympanic membrane grafting in children who are younger than 7 years of age because of the possibility of postoperative otitis media. This observation is confirmed by recent epidemiologic studies of otitis media in children (see Chap. 21, section on epidemiology) and is consistent with the maturation of the structure and function of the eustachian tube (see Chap. 21, section on physiology and pathophysiology). However, on occasion, the surgeon must operate on an infant or a young child, such as when cholesteatoma is present.

Studying eustachian tube function before the patient with a chronic perforation of the tympanic membrane is operated on may be helpful in determining the potential results of tympanoplasty surgery. Holmquist (1968) studied eustachian tube function in adults before and after tympanoplasty and reported that the operation had a high rate of success in patients with good eustachian tube function (i.e., those who could equilibrate applied negative pressure) but that in patients without good tubal function, surgery frequently failed to close the perforation. Miller and Bilodeau (1967) and Siedentop (1968) reported similar findings, but Ekvall (1970), Lee and Schuknecht (1971), Andreasson and Harris (1979), Cohn and colleagues (1979), and Virtanen and associates (1980) found no correlation between the results of the inflation-deflation tests and success or failure of tympanoplasty. Most of these studies failed to define the criteria for "success," and the postoperative follow-up period was too short. Bluestone and coworkers (1979) assessed children prior to tympanoplasty and found that of 51 ears of 45 children, 8 ears could equilibrate an applied negative pressure (-200 mm H_2O) to some degree, and in 7 of these ears the graft healed, no middle-ear effusion occurred, and no other perforation developed during a follow-up period of between one and two years. However, as was found in studies in adults, failure to equilibrate an applied negative pressure did not predict failure of the tympanoplasty.

More recently from the same institution, Manning and colleagues (1987) reported that good eustachian tube function was shown to be predictive of a good outcome, but poor tubal function was not helpful in predicting a poor outcome. In this study, an additional test of eustachian tube function was performed in conjunction with the inflation-deflation test that was used in the first study, the forced-response test. Using this latter test, there was a significant association between outcome and preoperative tubal function as determined by combining active and passive function parameters. In addition, these investigators reported that other factors, such as graft placement (medial or lateral), contralateral middle-ear status, and age of the child, were not associated with outcome (see Chap. 21, section on tests of ventilatory function).

The conclusion to be drawn from these studies is that if the child has good tubal function, regardless of age, the success of tympanoplasty is probable, but if poor function is present, these tests will not help the clinician in deciding not to operate. However, the value of testing a patient's tubal function lies in the possibility of determining from the test results if a young child is a candidate for tympanoplasty when one might decide on the basis of other findings alone to withhold surgery until the child is older. These tests are also of value in the diagnosis of severe or total mechanical obstruction, conditions that contraindicate the performance of a simple myringoplasty rather than a tympanoplasty; further evaluation and medical or surgical management of such patients may be indicated, depending upon the condition of the ear. The child should be examined for the possible presence of a nasopharyngeal tumor, and if none is found, the cause of obstruction could be mucosal swelling of the middle-ear end of the eustachian tube, which may respond to a medical treatment, such as ototopical medication. If the obstruction persists despite medical treatment and if a repair of the perforation is to be performed, an exploration of the middle ear and bony (protympanic) portion of the eustachian tube should be part of the examination. It is possible that an unsuspected cholesteatoma will be found to be the cause of the obstruction.

Even though not substantiated by the study by Manning and colleagues (1987), otoscopic and tympanometric assessment of the contralateral ear, if the tympanic membrane is intact, is thought by some surgeons (Bluestone et al., 1979; Ophir et al., 1987) to be helpful in predicting the success of tympanoplasty.

Since the best indication of eustachian tube function is obtained by observing the status of the middle ear over a period of at least one year (i.e., four seasons) and since eustachian tube function is usually the same bilaterally in children, the status of the contralateral ear with an intact tympanic membrane may be a good indicator of the expected functioning of the middle ear with a perforated eardrum following repair of the eardrum. If recurrent or persistent high negative pressure, effusion, or both are present within the middle ear or if there is a retraction pocket in the posterosuperior quadrant of the pars tensa or in the pars flaccida, or a cholesteatoma, tympanoplasty is usually unsuccessful. Figure 22–9 shows an example of test results of an ideal case for tympanoplasty, whereas Figure 22–10 is an example of results that would indicate that the child is an uncertain candidate for surgical repair of the tympanic membrane.

If a child has a unilateral perforation and if insertion of a tympanostomy tube is indicated in the opposite, intact side to prevent recurrent otitis media with effusion, or to eliminate a chronic middle-ear effusion, or to ventilate a severely atelectatic tympanic membrane (with or without a retraction pocket), tympanoplasty for an uncomplicated chronic perforation would be contraindicated until these conditions are absent and a tympanostomy tube is no longer required. Again, an observation period of at least one year will be required. If the child must have middle-ear surgery, and tubal function is known or suspected (because of age, usually less than age 6 years) to be poor, such as would be the case when the child has a perforation and a cholesteatoma, then either repair of the tympanic membrane can be delayed or the more preferred method of management can be employed, proceeding with a tympanoplasty, followed by insertion of a tympanostomy tube.

There is no available evidence to support the belief that removal of the adenoids (and tonsils) improves the success rate of tympanoplasty, and until such studies are available, surgical removal of these structures for the ear condition alone should be considered of uncertain benefit. Three retrospective studies in children failed to show that adenoidectomy had any effect on the outcome of tympanoplasty (Bluestone et al., 1979; Buchwach and Birck, 1980; Ophir et al., 1987). Most surgeons agree that there should be no signs of otitis media in the ear prior to a tympanoplasty; that is, the ear should be "dry," since the presence of discharge is associated with failure of the tympanoplasty (Armstrong, 1965). When an acquired cholesteatoma is found in the operated ear, tympanoplasty will most probably be less than optimally successful (Bluestone et al., 1979). When a tympanoplasty is withheld in a child who has significant hearing loss, a hearing aid should be considered until such time as the procedure is performed and hearing improvement is achieved.

In children who have bilateral perforations and in whom eustachian tube function tests show no active function when negative pressure is applied, it is uncertain whether or not tympanoplasty would be suc-

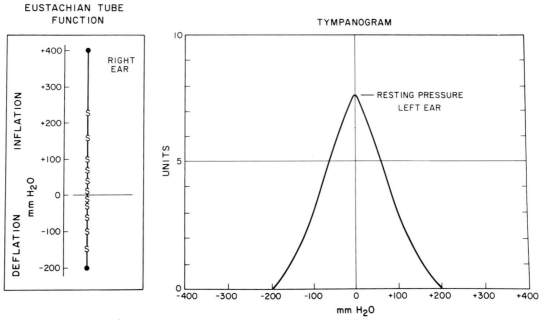

Figure 22–9. Pretympanoplasty evaluation of a child who had normal results on the inflation-deflation eustachian tube function test in the perforated ear and normal resting pressure in the contralateral ear with an intact tympanic membrane. S, swallow.

cessful. A better test of tubal function must be devised and the results correlated with the results of the surgery before it will be possible to determine the probable degree of success to be expected from tympanoplasty in these cases. When a tympanoplasty must be performed and the function of the eustachian tube is thought to be poor, a tympanostomy tube should be inserted.

SURGICAL TECHNIQUES. Once the decision is made to close a chronic perforation of the tympanic membrane of a "dry" ear surgically, a technique should be chosen that will have the greatest chance of success with the least risk to the child. To perform most surgical procedures to repair a perforation in children, a general anesthetic will be required, whereas in adults, especially when the perforation is small, local

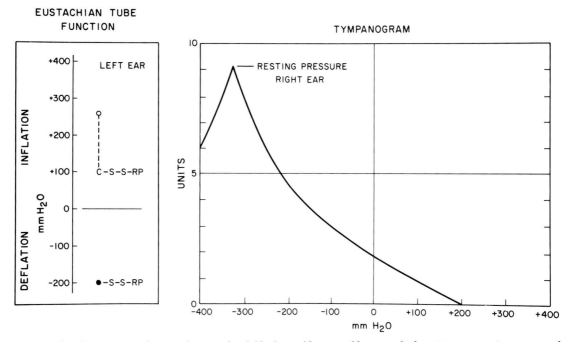

Figure 22–10. Results of pretympanoplasty evaluation of a child who could not equilibrate applied positive or negative pressure during the inflation-deflation eustachian tube test in the ear with the perforation. A tympanogram of the contralateral ear with an intact tympanic membrane revealed high negative pressure. O, opening pressure; C, closing pressure; S, swallow; RP, residual pressure.

anesthesia is adequate. Therefore, the benefits of surgery in a child must outweigh the risks of general anesthesia.

When no other abnormalities of the middle ear are present, a small perforation may heal if the epithelium is removed from its edges and if the circumference of the perforation is cauterized with trichloroacetic acid. A rayon, silk, or plastic wrap (e.g., Saran Wrap) patch can then be placed over the defect. This simple technique can be done as an outpatient procedure, with local anesthesia in older children and adolescents, but general anesthesia may be necessary in young children. The procedure should be performed only if the hearing is normal or only slightly impaired and if the remaining portion of the tympanic membrane is translucent; these two criteria must be met in order to avoid the possibility that the ossicles may be involved or that a tympanic membrane–middle ear cholesteatoma, that is, migration of squamous epithelium through the perforation into the middle ear, may be present. These same criteria also apply to the next, somewhat more involved, type of repair, a myringoplasty. This procedure is similar to the simple closure, except that cautery is usually not used, a larger defect can be repaired, and a fresh autograft should be employed, such as temporalis fascia, tragal perichondrium, or earlobe fat. However, neither procedure involves exploration of the middle ear; therefore, in most children, the middle ear (including the medial side of the tympanic membrane remnant) must be inspected during tympanoplasty to rule out the possible presence of another pathologic condition that may require more extensive surgery. In one large study reported by Sheehy and Anderson (1980), the 472 myringoplasties performed during the years 1967 to

1977 represented only 10 per cent of all the primary operations performed at their center, and of these, 88 per cent were performed in patients 16 years of age or older.

Of all the techniques of tympanoplasty that are currently advocated (see Selected References), none is specifically designed for children. In general, the surgical techniques are the same for children as for adults; however, certain considerations should be kept in mind when performing a tympanoplasty in a child. Since the external canal is frequently smaller in children than in adults, a postauricular (or endaural) approach may be required to achieve adequate visualization of the tympanic membrane and the middle ear. A transcanal approach should be reserved for only those children whose ear canals are large enough to provide proper exposure of the entire operative field. Autografts are preferred over homografts and heterografts, since we have inadequate information at present to determine the long-term effects of using the latter grafts. For the same reason, when an ossicular chain abnormality is present, a Type II or III tympanoplasty (Fig. 22–11), or an autograft ossicle, should be used for the ossiculoplasty rather than inert material (see Ossicular Discontinuity and Fixation). A Type IV tympanoplasty is invariably unsuccessful in children. The preference for a technique that involves placing the graft lateral to the tympanic membrane has some merit, since laterally placed grafts have been shown to have a higher initial "take rate" in children (Bluestone et al., 1979). The failure of medially placed grafts may be related to the fluctuating negative pressure that is so commonly present in the middle ears of children and that could conceivably enhance the take of a lateral graft but tend to pull a medial graft away from the

Figure 22–11. Tympanoplasty surgical procedures. Type I, ossicular chain intact; Type II, graft lies on incus; Type III, graft is on stapes superstructure; Type IV, graft is on stapes footplate.

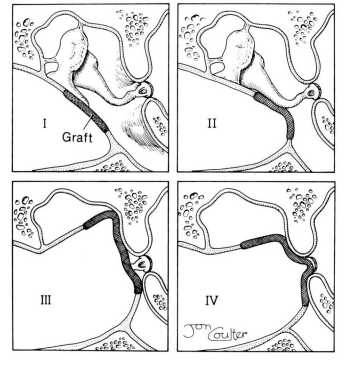

tympanic membrane. For smaller perforations, a medial graft may be satisfactory, but for a large perforation, the laterally placed fascia graft appears to give better results and, when performed properly, should not lead to the postoperative complication of "blunting" in the anterior sulcus or lateral healing of the graft (Sheehy and Anderson, 1980).

The routine addition of an extensive simple mastoidectomy to a tympanoplasty procedure in children who show no evidence of disease in the mastoid is not justified. The risk of prolonging the general anesthesia does not outweigh the remote possibility of finding occult disease, nor is the risk justified by increasing the middle ear–mastoid air volume, which has been purported to enhance the success rate of tympanoplasty. In addition, obtaining routine preoperative roentgenograms of the mastoid without any evidence of disease in the area also does not appear to be justified owing to the potential hazards of radiation.

The problems associated with postoperative care of the patient are greater when the patient is a child than an adult, especially if the patient is a young child. These problems must be considered before deciding to perform elective tympanic grafting.

Outcome

Unfortunately, regardless of the technique and despite adequate follow-up, tympanoplasty is not as successful in children as it is in adults, which is probably the reason that many surgeons wait until a child grows older to do the procedure. In children, the criteria that must be met for a tympanoplasty done to repair an uncomplicated perforation to be successful are take of the initial graft (the tympanic membrane remains intact) and absence of high negative middle-ear pressure, atelectasis, retraction pocket, otitis media with effusion, or cholesteatoma for a follow-up period of at least two years. Improvement in hearing is also an important goal. In two studies of children in which the preceding criteria were used to evaluate the outcome of tympanoplasty, about half of the tympanoplasties followed for one to two years were successful (Bluestone et al., 1979; Manning et al., 1987). However, some of these cases initially had cholesteatoma.

Conclusions

Children are uncertain candidates for tympanoplastic surgery (especially children below the age of 6 years), since as a group their eustachian tube function is not as good as that of adults. However, in selected cases, the procedure may be successful. For some children, tympanoplasty appears to be contraindicated, whereas in others, the outcome of the operation is less certain. The problem for the clinician is deciding which child should have the perforation repaired. The development of an improved method of testing the eustachian tube, a method that is more indicative of the actual function available for clinical use, could possibly help in this decision-making process. A controlled study of the indications for tympanoplasty and the most effective technique of repair (e.g., medial vs. lateral graft) in a large group of children is needed.

CHRONIC SUPPURATIVE OTITIS MEDIA

(Chronic Suppurative Otitis Media and Mastoiditis, Chronic Otitis Media with Perforation and Discharge, Chronic Otitis Media)

Chronic suppurative otitis media is a stage of ear disease in which there is chronic inflammation of the middle ear and mastoid and in which a nonintact tympanic membrane (perforation or tympanostomy tube) and discharge (otorrhea) are present. Mastoiditis is invariably a part of the pathologic process. The condition has been called simply chronic otitis media, but this term can be confused with chronic otitis media with effusion, in which no perforation is present. It is also called chronic suppurative otitis media and mastoiditis, chronic purulent otitis media, and chronic otomastoiditis. The most descriptive term is chronic otitis media with perforation, discharge, and mastoiditis (Senturia et al., 1980a), but this is not common usage. When a cholesteatoma is also present, the term chronic suppurative otitis media with cholesteatoma is used; however, because an acquired aural cholesteatoma does not have to be associated with chronic suppurative otitis media, cholesteatoma is not part of the pathology of the type of ear disease described in this section but is presented as a separate entity in the following section.

Epidemiology

Most studies that have reported the prevalence of chronic suppurative otitis media in children include children who also have cholesteatoma, so that accurate data on the incidence of chronic suppurative otitis media alone are not available. In a study conducted by the School Health Service in Great Britain, the number of children found to have chronic otitis media at the periodic medical inspections was about 9 in 1000 (Mawson and Ludman, 1979).

This type of chronic ear disease has a high prevalence in children of certain racial groups. The studies of American Indians (Cambon et al., 1965; Zonis, 1970; DeBlanc, 1975; Wiet et al., 1980), Canadian and Alaskan (Eskimo) natives (Maynard, 1969; Baxter and Ling, 1974; Baxter, 1982), Greenland natives (Innuits) (Pedersen and Zachau-Christiansen, 1986), Australian aboriginal children (McCafferty et al., 1977; Willis, 1985) and others, such as the Maoris of New Zealand, have shown an extremely high prevalence and incidence of chronic suppurtive otitis media among these populations. In addition, the prevalence of chronic suppurative otitis media is higher in children in these racial groups than in the white population living in the same area (Ratnesar, 1977). More recently, Todd and Bowman (1985) reported a sharp decline in the incidence of chronic draining ears in Apache Indian children living in the southwestern United States.

Cholesteatoma is not commonly associated with chronic ear disease found in these populations. In a study of 4193 Alaskan native school children (Tschopp, 1977), 1274 (30 per cent) had perforated tympanic membranes, but in only 144 (3 per cent) was cholesteatoma also diagnosed. Ratnesar (1977) reported similar findings in a study of Canadian Eskimos and Indians but also found a higher incidence of cholesteatoma in the whites living in the same area. Similarly, McCafferty and coworkers (1977) studied 3663 Australian aboriginal children and found that 70 per cent of their ears were abnormal; 12 per cent had chronic otitis media, but less than 1 per cent had cholesteatoma. Ear disease has an early onset in these children; Maynard (1969) reported that most Eskimo children had chronic otitis media before the age of 2 years.

These epidemiologic studies appear to be describing the etiology and pathogenesis of chronic suppurative otitis media that is *not* associated with cholesteatoma. By studying the natural history of the ear disease in these population groups, the pathogenesis of this type of ear disease can be better understood.

In addition to perforations that occur as part of the natural history of otitis media, an extremely large number of temporary perforations (tympanostomy tubes) are created by the surgical treatment of otitis media. It has been estimated that over one million tympanostomy tubes are inserted annually for recurrent acute otitis media and otitis media with effusion (Paradise, 1977). Herzon (1980) reported that of 140 patients, 21 per cent developed otorrhea one or more times with tubes in place, whereas McLelland (1980) reported that chronic drainage developed in 3.6 per cent of his patients with tympanostomy tubes.

Pathogenesis

The pathogenesis of chronic suppurative otitis media is not completely known, but it is considered to be the chronic stage that follows an attack of acute otitis media in which a perforation has developed, followed by continuous discharge. The sequence of events does not have to progress directly from the acute to the chronic form. A perforation secondary to acute otitis media can become chronic without evidence of middle-ear inflammation (i.e., "dry" perforation). Some authors consider this stage to be an "inactive" stage of chronic otitis media, since middle ear (and mastoid) infection with discharge through the perforation may occur at any time. However, some children have a perforation that rarely, if ever, has a discharge after the initial acute episode in which the perforation developed, and the middle-ear mucous membrane remains normal. Therefore, only a chronic perforation that is associated with chronic inflammation of the

middle ear–mastoid system should be considered to be chronic suppurative otitis media (see section on perforation of the tympanic membrane). However, the pathogenesis may be the same for acute or chronic perforations with or without otitis media. Most probably, the pathogenesis of chronic infection in the middle ear when a tympanostomy tube is in place is similar to that proposed earlier when a perforation is present (Fig. 22–12).

Anatomic differences in bony segment of the eustachian tube were identified in studies of the bony craniofacial structures of Eskimo, American Indian, white, and black individuals (Doyle, 1977). Beery and coworkers (1980) studied 25 White Mountain Apache Indians ranging in age from 3 to 36 years and found that their eustachian tubes were semipatulous (of low resistance) in comparison with those of a group of whites. In this study, the function of the eustachian tube was assessed directly through chronic perforations of the eardrum, employing the inflation-deflation and forced-response tests. These studies would appear to indicate that these racial groups and the segment of the white population that have chronic suppurative otitis media have eustachian tubes that permit reflux of nasopharyngeal secretions into the middle ear; reflux acute otitis media develops and the tympanic membrane perforates. In some individuals, the reflux of nasopharyngeal secretions continues after the initial episode, whereas in others, the process recurs with each upper respiratory tract infection. The perforation enhances the reflux of the secretions from the nasopharynx, since the middle ear–mastoid air cushion is abolished (see Chap. 21).

Individuals with a patulous eustachian tube rarely have a cholesteatoma in the posterosuperior quadrant of the pars tensa or in the pars flaccida, and if a cholesteatoma is present, it is usually due to migration of epithelium through the "central" perforation, an uncommon condition. An even more rare and unproven pathogenesis of cholesteatoma is that which is secondary to metaplasia of the middle-ear mucous membrane. Most cholesteatomas are the final step in a sequence of events that begins with negative middle-ear pressure, progresses to atelectasis, and then leads to a retraction pocket. Therefore, the development of

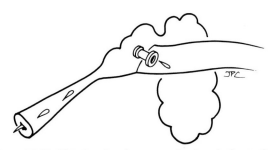

Figure 22–12. This drawing shows a mechanism similar to the one described when a perforation is present (see Fig. 22–7). A patent tympanostomy tube may promote reflux of secretions from the nasopharynx into the middle ear. (From Bluestone, C. D., and Klein, J. O. 1988. Otitis Media in Infants and Children. Philadelphia, W. B. Saunders Co.)

a cholesteatoma should be rare when a "central" perforation is present, since the middle-ear pressure is ambient. Thus, even though children who have chronic suppurative otitis media have a morbid process, they appear to be protected from developing an attic or posterosuperior type of cholesteatoma. It is important to keep these facts in mind when considering the surgical management of the perforation after elimination of the chronic middle-ear and mastoid infection.

Microbiology

Chronic suppurative otitis media develops from a chronic bacterial infection. However, the bacteria that caused the initial episode of acute otitis media with perforation are usually not those that are isolated from the chronic discharge when there is chronic infection in the middle ear and mastoid. Thus, the antimicrobial therapy recommended for acute otitis media will not be effective for most cases of chronic suppurative otitis media. Kenna, Bluestone, and Reilly (1986) reported that the most common organisms are *P. aeruginosa* and *Staphylococcus aureus* (Table 22–3). Anaerobic bacteria were isolated infrequently in this study. These organisms are most probably secondary invaders that gain entrance to the middle ear and mastoid from the external auditory canal during an episode of acute otitis

TABLE 22–3. Microbiological Findings in Middle-Ear Aspirates from 36 Infants and Children (51 Ears) with Chronic Suppurative Otitis Media

SPECIES	NUMBER OF ISOLATES
Pseudomonas aeruginosa	34
Staphylococcus aureus (7 beta-lactamase–positive strain)	10
Diphtheroids	10
Staphylococcus epidermidis	6
Streptococcus, alpha	4
Streptococcus pneumoniae	3
Escherichia coli	2
Candida albicans	2
Haemophilus influenzae, nontypable	2
Candida parapsilosis	2
Enterococcus	2
Pseudomonas maltophilia	2
Proteus mirabilis	2
Streptococcus pyogenes	1
Pseudomonas cepacia	1
Eikenella corrodens	1
Moraxella	1
Alcaligenes odorans	1
Haemophilus influenzae, type b	1
Branhamella catarrhalis	1
Acinetobacter calcoaceticus	1
Citrobacter freundii	1
Streptococcus, nonhemolytic	1
No growth	2
Total	93

From Kenna, M., Bluestone, C. D., and Reilly, J. 1986. Medical management of chronic suppurative otitis media without cholesteatoma in children. Laryngoscope 96:146–151.

media and otorrhea. In contrast, Brook (1985) isolated *Bacteroides melaninogenicus* in 40 per cent and *Peptococcus* species in 35 per cent of middle-ear exudates; collection of exudate was performed through the perforation in the tympanic membrane, using an 18-gauge needle covered by a plastic cannula. Although uncommon today, *Mycobacterium tuberculosis* is also a causative organism in suppurative otitis media (Munzel, 1978; Jeang and Fletcher, 1983).

Pathology

It is important to understand the pathologic process of chronic otitis media, since the decision for or against surgical intervention may depend on the pathologic changes in the middle ear and mastoid. These include edema, submucosal fibrosis, and infiltration with chronic inflammatory cells, which together cause thickening of the mucous membrane (Schuknecht, 1974). Polyps may result from excessive mucosal edema; in the more advanced stage, not only polypoid tissue and granulation tissue but also osteitis of the mastoid bone, ossicles, and labyrinth may be present. Adhesive otitis media and sclerosis of bone may occur with healing. Tympanosclerosis may also be present and is commonly associated with this disease in Alaskan (Eskimo) natives (Wiet et al., 1980). If intensive medical treatment is instituted early, these pathologic changes may be reversible without surgery. However, when longstanding chronic disease has led to irreversible changes, middle-ear and mastoid surgery is usually indicated to eradicate the infection.

Diagnosis

A purulent, mucoid, or serous discharge coming through a "central" perforation of the tympanic membrane for at least two or three months is evidence of chronic suppurative otitis media. Frequently, a polyp will be seen coming through the perforation (Fig. 22–13). The size of the perforation has no relation to the duration or severity of the disease, but frequently the defect involves most of the pars tensa. There is no otalgia, tenderness to touch in the mastoid area or pinna, vertigo, or fever. When any of these signs or symptoms is present, the examiner should look for a possible suppurative intratemporal or intracranial complication. A search for the underlying cause of the infection may reveal the presence of paranasal sinusitis, which must be actively treated, since the ear infection may not respond to medical treatment until the sinusitis resolves. An upper respiratory tract allergy or a nasopharyngeal tumor may also be contributing to the pathogenesis of chronic otitis media and will need to be managed appropriately (see Chap. 21).

The diagnostic evaluation must include a gram-stained smear, culture, and susceptibility testing of the discharge. This should be done as described in the

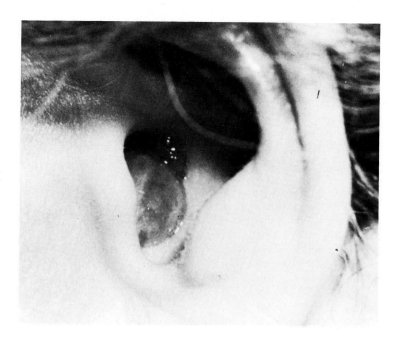

Figure 22–13. Aural polyp in external auditory meatus. The polyp came through a large perforation of an ear with chronic suppurative otitis media.

section on perforation of the tympanic membrane in this chapter.

However, one of the most important parts of the evaluation is a complete examination, with the aid of the otomicroscope, of the ear canal, tympanic membrane, and, if the perforation is large enough, the middle ear. If a satisfactory examination cannot be performed with the child awake, then an examination under general anesthesia will be necessary. At this time, the discharge can be aspirated, and a Gram stain and culture from the middle ear can be obtained; in addition, a search for a polyp or unsuspected cholesteatoma or neoplasm should be conducted.

A conductive hearing loss usually accompanies chronic otitis media. If greater than a 20 to 30 dB hearing loss is found, the ossicles may be involved; however, the patient may also have a sensorineural component, which is most probably due to a serous labyrinthitis (Paparella et al., 1972). Impedance testing may be helpful if purulent material in the ear canal prevents visualization of the eardrum adequate to identify a possible perforation. If a perforation is present, the measured volume of the external canal will be larger than expected; however, the tympanometric pattern may be flat despite the presence of a perforation if the volume of air in the middle ear and mastoid is small. When this is suspected, the pressure on the pump-manometer of the impedance bridge can be increased in an attempt to force open the eustachian tube; if the tube can be opened with positive air pressure from the pump-manometer, a perforation must be present.

If a defect in the bone due to osteitis is present, the area will appear on the roentgenogram. However, it is often difficult to distinguish between reversible (i.e., surgical) mastoiditis even when computed tomograms are obtained; magnetic resonance imaging does not provide as much diagnostic information as computed tomograms. Discontinuity of the ossicular chain, if present, may be visualized if tomography is used.

Unusual causes of a chronic draining ear include neoplasm, eosinophilic granuloma, and an unusual bacterial infection. These must be considered in the differential diagnosis of chronic suppurative otitis media.

Management

Medical management of chronic otitis media is directed toward eliminating the infection from the middle ear and mastoid. Since the bacteria most frequently cultured are gram-negative, antimicrobial agents should be selected to be effective against these organisms. Both a suspension containing polymyxin B, neomycin, and hydrocortisone (Cortisporin) and one that has neomycin, polymyxin E, and hydrocortisone (Coly-Mycin) have been advocated, but owing to the concern over the potential ototoxicity of these agents, caution is advised (Brummett et al., 1976; Meyerhoff et al., 1983) (see Table 22–2). Orally administered antibiotics are usually not effective unless the organisms are highly susceptible.

If topical antibiotic medication is elected, the child should return to the outpatient facility daily to have the discharge thoroughly aspirated (i.e., aural toilet) and to have ototopical medication directly instilled into the middle ear through the perforation or tympanostomy tube, employing the otomicroscope. Frequently, the discharge will rapidly improve with this type of treatment within a week, after which the ear drops may be administered at home until there is complete resolution of the middle ear–mastoid inflammation.

Because of concern over toxicity of the ototopical

agents, parents should be informed of this potential danger if such medications are used. As an alternative, the authors hospitalize patients and administer a parenteral beta-lactam antipseudomonal drug such as ticarcillin, azlocillin, piperacillin, and ceftazidime. The regimen can be altered when results of culture and susceptibility tests are available. The middle ear is aspirated daily. In almost all children, the middle ear will be free of discharge and the signs of otitis media will be greatly improved or absent within several days. If resolution does occur, the child should be discharged and followed on an ambulatory basis at periodic intervals to watch for signs of spontaneous closure of the perforation, which frequently happens after the middle ear and mastoid are no longer infected. If the perforation (or tympanostomy tube) and middle ear are not infected, and it is desirable to maintain middle-ear ventilation through a nonintact eardrum, recurrent episodes of otorrhea can usually be prevented with antimicrobial prophylaxis. The agent selected should be effective against the usual organisms that cause acute otitis media (e.g., pneumococci, *Haemophilus influenzae*) such as amoxicillin, 20 mg/kg given once daily before bedtime (see Chapter 21). If a tympanostomy tube is present and the middle ear is now dry, its removal may restore middle ear–eustachian tube physiology. However, removal of tympanostomy tubes may not be desirable, especially in infants and young children, and in these cases, antimicrobial prophylaxis should also be considered until the tubes spontaneously extrude.

If the perforation persists or another abnormality requiring surgery is present, such as an ossicular chain disarticulation, tympanoplastic surgery should be considered. When a chronic ("dry") perforation is present, the indications for repair of the tympanic membrane would be similar to those outlined in the previous section. Frequent episodes of acute and chronic infection would be a possible indication to explore the middle ear (and possibly the mastoid) and perform tympanoplasty. Routine mastoidectomy is not necessary if the perforation is not associated with another abnormality that would warrant an exploration of the mastoid. In most children who have had complete resolution of the infection in the middle ear and mastoid but who have a persistent, chronic ("dry") perforation and in whom a tympanoplasty is performed, the addition of a mastoidectomy is of limited value for either diagnosis or management. In such cases, the mastoid is likely to be converted to a more normal state if the discharge is absent for several months.

When the discharge fails to respond to intensive medical therapy within several days, surgery on the middle ear and mastoid is indicated. Kenna, Bluestone, and Reilly (1986) conducted a study in 36 pediatric patients with chronic suppurative otitis media who all received parenteral antimicrobial therapy and daily aural toilet. Thirty-two patients (89 per cent) had resolution of their infection with medical therapy alone; four children required tympanomastoidectomy.

For most children, a complete simple mastoidectomy combined with a transcanal tympanotomy with removal of the infected mucous membrane, granulation tissue, and bone will usually result in resolution of the chronic suppurative middle-ear infection and chronic irreversible mastoid osteitis. On occasion, a child may require a modified radical mastoidectomy if the surgeon is not convinced that there is adequate communication between the middle ear and the mastoid cavity. Failure to take down the canal wall in such a case can result in persistence and recurrence of the disease process. Some surgeons repair the tympanic membrane defect and, if required, reconstruct the ossicular chain at this time, whereas others prefer to withhold tympanoplasty and ossiculoplasty for a second stage. The decision for or against these procedures should be individualized, since there are many variables involved (e.g., age of the child, status of eustachian tube function, and severity of the disease). Most young children are prone to developing recurrence of otitis, which would make reconstructive surgery at the initial procedure less desirable than a planned second-stage procedure later in life, depending on the status of the ear during the postoperative period. Some young children may require a nonintact tympanic membrane (persistent perforation or tympanostomy tube insertion) or even prophylactic antimicrobial therapy until they grow older. On the other hand, an older child or adolescent may benefit by having an intact tympanic membrane to prevent reflux of nasopharyngeal secretions.

A child who has a chronic suppurative aural discharge and who develops one or more of the intratemporal suppurative complications, such as acute mastoid osteitis, labyrinthitis, facial paralysis, and an intracranial suppurative complication, will require immediate surgical intervention.

It is not uncommon that a cholesteatoma is present when an ear with chronic suppurative otitis media fails to respond to intensive medical treatment, even though no preoperative evidence for the presence of cholesteatoma was identified by otomicroscopy or computed tomography. The cholesteatoma usually is found in the middle ear (and mastoid) following migration of the squamous epithelium through the perforation in the tympanic membrane. When a cholesteatoma is found, surgical removal as outlined in the next section is indicated. With the possible exception of finding a cholesteatoma, there is seldom a reason to perform a radical mastoidectomy for chronic suppurative otitis media.

If the patient continues to have otorrhea despite mastoid surgery for chronic suppurative otitis media and mastoiditis, then a prolonged course of antimicrobial therapy with frequent débridement may be indicated, as is the case with osteomyelitis of the long bones. An alternative method of management for the rare child who fails to respond to mastoid surgery and prolonged antimicrobial therapy is to surgically obliterate the eustachian tube.

Conclusions

Most children who have chronic suppurative otitis media that is refractory to ototopical medication and orally administered antimicrobial agents will require (1) a thorough examination of the external canal and tympanic membrane with the otomicroscope (under general anesthesia, if necessary); (2) a gram-stained culture obtained directly from the middle ear; (3) thorough aspiration of the ear canal and, if possible, the middle ear (i.e., "aural toilet") and, ideally, direct instillation of the appropriate ototopical medication into the middle ear daily, using the otomicroscope to visualize the middle ear; and, (4) if the suppurative process is severe, hospitalization and the parenteral administration of an antimicrobial agent. The ototopical medication and the systemic antimicrobial therapy should be selected following microbiologic assessment of the discharge. If the infection can be eliminated using the methods previously described, prevention of recurrence can be achieved by the following options: (1) early and appropriate antimicrobial therapy for acute otitis media, in an attempt to prevent bacteria from the external canal from entering the middle ear; (2) prophylactic antimicrobial therapy; (3) removal of the tympanostomy tube; or (4) surgical repair of the tympanic membrane defect. The choice of these options will be dependent on the age of the child and the status of the function of the eustachian tube. Middle-ear and mastoid surgery should be reserved for the children who fail to respond to intensive medical therapy.

CHOLESTEATOMA AND RETRACTION POCKET

Keratinizing stratified squamous epithelium and an accumulation of desquamating epithelium of keratin within the middle ear or other pneumatized portions of the temporal bone is called a keratoma or, more commonly, a cholesteatoma. Aural cholesteatomas can be classified into two types: "congenital" and acquired. A "congenital" cholesteatoma has been defined as a congenital rest of epithelial tissue and appears as a white, cystlike structure within the middle ear (intratympanic) or temporal bone. The tympanic membrane is intact, and it is apparently not a sequela of otitis media or eustachian tube dysfunction (Cawthorne and Griffith, 1961; Derlacki and Clemis, 1965) (see Chap. 18). Acquired cholesteatoma may be secondary to implantation or may be a sequela of otitis media or a retraction pocket or both. Implantation cholesteatoma may develop either from epithelium that has migrated through a traumatic perforation of the tympanic membrane or from epithelium that has been inadvertently overlooked in the middle ear or mastoid during surgery of the ear (iatrogenic) (Brandow, 1977).

However, the most common cholesteatoma is the acquired type, which is secondary to middle-ear disease. In a study of 1024 patients (adults as well as

children), a cholesteatoma was found in the attic in 42 per cent, in the posterosuperior quadrant in 31 per cent, in 18 per cent when there was a "total" perforation, in 6 per cent when there was a "central" perforation, and in 3 per cent when there was no perforation (Sheehy et al., 1977). However, it is possible that the patients in whom the cholesteatoma was associated with a "total" perforation originally had involvement of the posterosuperior portion of the pars tensa. In children, the most common defect in the tympanic membrane begins developing in the posterosuperior quadrant of the pars tensa or, somewhat less commonly, in the pars flaccida. The term "marginal perforation" has been used to describe the defect in the posterosuperior quadrant, and the defect in the pars flaccida has been called an "attic perforation," but in reality, these are not perforations but are either retraction pockets or cholesteatomas that appear otoscopically to be perforations (Fig. 22–6). No continuity between the defect and the middle ear occurs until later in the disease process (see section on perforation of the tympanic membrane, p. 495). Retraction pockets of the tympanic membrane are also described in Chapter 21.

Epidemiology, Natural History, and Complications

Harker and Koontz (1977), in a study of the general population in Iowa, reported the overall incidence of cholesteatoma to be 6 per 100,000; in children up to 9 years of age, the incidence was 4.7 per 100,000, while in children 10 to 19 years old, the incidence of 9.2 per 100,000 was the highest for all age groups. Cholesteatoma is a common sequela in children with cleft palate. Severeid (1977) reviewed the records of 160 children and young adults with cleft palates (70 per cent were 10 to 16 years of age), all of whom had had a history of ear disease, and found the incidence of cholesteatoma to be 7.1 per cent; the posterosuperior portion of the pars tensa was the most common site; a later report from the same institution reported almost 10 per cent of children with cleft palate developed cholesteatoma (Harker and Severeid, 1982). In contrast to this high incidence of cholesteatoma in the cleft palate population is the rare occurrence of cholesteatoma in Alaskan (Eskimo) natives, American Indians (Hinchcliffe, 1977), and Australian aboriginal children (McCafferty et al., 1977), in whom other middle-ear disease is very common. This remarkable difference in the incidence of cholesteatoma in children with cleft palates and in certain racial groups, both of which have a high prevalence and incidence of otitis media, is most probably related to differences in the pathogenesis and natural history of the respective middle-ear disease processes.

Cholesteatoma in children is considered to be a more aggressive disease than that occurring in adults (Baron, 1969; Derlacki, 1973; Schuknecht, 1974) for two reasons: (1) Very extensive disease is found at the time of surgery more frequently in children than in adults, and (2) higher rates of residual (persistent) and recurrent cholesteatoma following surgery have been found in children compared to the rates in adults (Abramson et al., 1977). Palva and colleagues (1977) compared 65 children with cholesteatomas with 65 adults with the same disease and found that whereas 22 per cent of the children had extensive disease that filled the middle ear and mastoid, only 6 per cent of adults had such extensive disease. However, despite the finding that cholesteatomas in children tend to be more extensive than those occurring in adults, childhood cholesteatoma may still be confined to the mesotympanum or epitympanum.

Ritter (1977) compared an epidemiologic study in Michigan of 152 cases of cholesteatoma identified during the period from 1965 to 1970 to a similar study from Massachusetts of 303 cases that were identified during a period prior to the use of antimicrobial agents (1925 to 1936). He found in both series that about 45 per cent of cases of cholesteatoma were operated on before the patient was 20 years of age, that in approximately 65 per cent of the patients, the aural discharge had begun by 11 years of age, and that the distribution of sites on the tympanic membrane where the defect was located were about the same. He concluded that antimicrobial agents have not altered the incidence and natural history of cholesteatoma during the 40 years between the two studies.

However, prior to the advent of the widespread use of antimicrobial agents and modern otologic surgery, complications of cholesteatoma were common, and for many children when infection involved the intracranial cavity, the result was death. Nowadays, serious complications of cholesteatoma in children are uncommon. In a study of 181 children who had cholesteatoma, 8 (4.4 per cent) developed a labyrinthine fistula, and one suffered facial paralysis, but none had intracranial complications (Sheehy et al., 1977). However, in the same study, which also included 843 adults, the incidence of both intratemporal and intracranial complications increased the longer the cholesteatoma was present. Because most of the adults could date the onset of their disease to childhood and because diagnosis and surgery for cholesteatoma is the best way of preventing serious complications, physicians dealing with ear problems in children should treat suspected cholesteatoma early and aggressively.

The incidence of retraction pockets has not been formally studied, but a retraction pocket is a common sequela of atelectasis of the tympanic membrane with or without otitis medial with effusion (Sade et al., 1982). The incidence in individuals with cleft palates must be greater than that of cholesteatoma in this population (7.1 per cent), since a retraction pocket precedes the development of a cholesteatoma in children with cleft palate (Bluestone et al., 1982).

Pathogenesis

Many hypotheses regarding the pathogenesis of cholesteatoma have been proposed; the following are the most popular: (1) metaplasia of the middle ear and attic due to infection (Wendt, 1873; Tumarkin, 1938); (2) invasive hyperplasia of the basal layers of the meatal skin adjoining the upper margin of the tympanic membrane (Nager, 1925; Hellman, 1925; Lange, 1932; Ojala and Saxen, 1952; Ruedi, 1958); (3) invasive hyperkeratosis of the deep external auditory canal (McGuckin, 1961); and (4) retraction or collapse of the tympanic membrane with invagination secondary to eustachian tube dysfunction (Habermann, 1888; Bezold, 1889; Wittmaack, 1933). In addition, there are those who consider the condition not to be acquired at all but to be an embryonic epidermal rest occurring in the attic (McKenzie, 1931; Teed, 1936; Diamant, 1952).

Bluestone and associates (1977) reported preliminary findings of varying degrees of functional rather than mechanical (anatomic) obstruction of the eustachian tube in 13 children and adults who had a retraction pocket or an acquired cholesteatoma. Subsequently, the findings in 12 children with acquired cholesteatoma, all of whom had functional obstruction of the eustachian tube, were also reported by the same group (Bluestone et al., 1978). Children were specifically studied, since the development of an acquired cholesteatoma with its attendant irreversible changes was thought to occur early in life and since the function of the eustachian tube might improve with growth and development. In these children, the function of the eustachian tube was assessed by the modified inflation-deflation technique (after Ingelstedt et al., 1963). Another study was undertaken by Bluestone and coworkers (1982) to clarify further the cause of this functional obstruction by employing a new test of eustachian tube function, the forced-response test (Cantekin et al., 1979), and to evaluate a larger group of children who had either a cholesteatoma or a retraction pocket. In addition, children with an apparently "congenital" cholesteatoma were also studied, and the results obtained in both groups were then compared to the results of testing children who had traumatic perforation of the tympanic membrane but who otherwise were considered to be otologically "normal." Another goal of the study was to determine whether there were any differences in eustachian tube function among ears that had a posterosuperior or pars flaccida retraction pocket or cholesteatoma, a central perforation and a cholesteatoma, and ears with "congenital" cholesteatoma.

More recently, Lindeman and Holmquist (1987) showed similar findings in adults with acquired cholesteatoma. Compared to adults with traumatic perforations (i.e., control subjects), 20 adults with cholesteatoma had poor eustachian tube test results and smaller mastoid air cell areas as measured on roentgenograms.

From these studies, it appears that the basic problem in children with acquired cholesteatoma is functional obstruction of the eustachian tube due to constriction rather than dilatation of the tube during swallowing. (This type of functional obstruction of the eustachian tube was present in subjects with a retraction pocket or cholesteatoma regardless of the site.) Abnormal functioning of the tube then results in impaired ventilation of the middle ear–mastoid air cell system, which in turn results in fluctuating or sustained high negative middle-ear pressure. Periodic, rather than regular, ventilation could result in wide variations in middle-ear pressures that would produce greater than normal excursions of the tympanic membrane. The membrane would then lose elasticity and would become flaccid and, eventually, atelectatic. The most flaccid parts of the tympanic membrane are the posterosuperior and pars flaccida areas (Khanna and Tonndorf, 1972). When the atelectasis becomes severe and localized in these sites, a retraction pocket forms. Inflammation between the medial portion of the retracted or collapsed tympanic membrane could then result in adhesive changes and could fix the pocket to the ossicles or surrounding structures, or both. The next stage in this series of events would be discontinuity of the ossicles or cholesteatoma formation, or both. Figures 22–14 and 22–15 show the progression from the stage of a retraction pocket with atelectasis to adhesive otitis and, finally, to cholesteatoma.

The distinction between a deep retraction pocket and a cholesteatoma in either the posterosuperior quadrant of the pars tensa or the pars flaccida can be difficult even with the aid of the otomicroscope. The transition between the two conditions usually follows a progressive change from a retraction pocket to cholesteatoma; however, the factors involved in this transition remain obscure at present, although infection within the retraction pocket–sac appears to be important in the process.

Children who have a central perforation and cholesteatoma are of particular interest. The cholesteatoma in these cases most probably develops as a result of migration of epithelium from the tympanic membrane through the perforation and into the middle ear. However, it must be stressed that, in children, this type of acquired cholesteatoma is less common compared to the posterosuperior or attic type.

It is uncertain that "congenital" cholesteatomas are truly congenital in origin. Children who have an intratympanic cholesteatoma may have had otitis media with effusion. It could be argued, on the one hand, that intratympanic cholesteatoma is the result of metaplasia secondary to middle ear inflammation and that it is not "congenital" (Sade, 1977); on the other hand, otitis media with effusion, when present, may be unrelated to a congenital rest. The fact that children who have "congenital" cholesteatomas tend to be younger than those who present with a retraction pocket or acquired cholesteatoma would support the origin of a cholesteatoma medial to an intact tympanic membrane as being congenital. In any event, most acquired cholesteatomas not due to implantation are secondary to otitis media or a retraction pocket, or both, and some children who have an apparently "congenital" cholesteatoma may have developed the disease in the same way (Sobol et al., 1980). Levenson and colleagues (1986) believe that the pathogenesis of

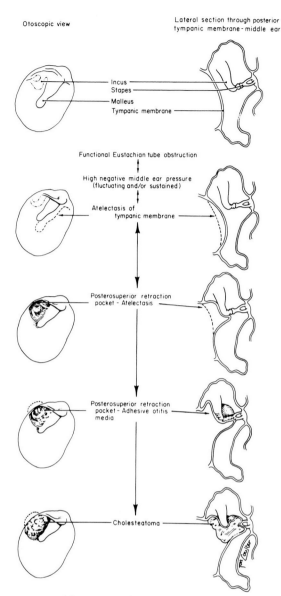

Figure 22–14. Chain of events in the pathogenesis of acquired aural cholesteatoma in the posterosuperior portion of the pars tensa or the tympanic membrane.

congenital cholesteatoma is an epithelial rest, which is stimulated to grow by otitis media.

Cholesteatoma is a common sequela of middle-ear disease in patients with cleft palate (Severeid, 1977; Harker and Severeid, 1982). It has been shown that all infants with an unrepaired cleft palate have otitis media with effusion (Stool and Randall, 1967; Paradise et al., 1969) and that they have functional obstruction of the eustachian tube due to impairment of the tubal opening mechanism (Bluestone, 1971; Bluestone et al., 1972, 1975). Studies of infants, children, and adolescents with cleft palate demonstrate constriction of the eustachian tube during the forced-response test (Doyle et al., 1980). Cholesteatoma is a common sequela of middle-ear disease in patients with cleft palate (Severeid, 1977). Therefore, the child with cleft

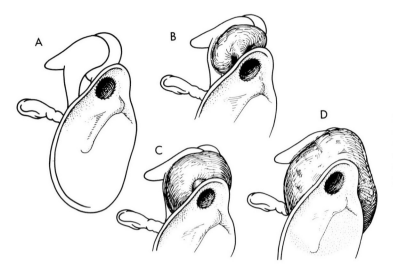

Figure 22–15. Evolution of acquired attic cholesteatoma. *A*, Attic retraction pocket (i.e., defect) that appears on otoscopic examination to be a "perforation." *B*, A narrow neck sac developing. *C*, Enlargement of the sac with erosion of the ossicles. *D*, A large cholesteatoma sac, a portion of which can be seen through the eardrum.

palate represents an *in vivo* model of the type of functional eustachian tube obstruction that can result in an acquired cholesteatoma. Because this type of dysfunction also occurs commonly in whites who have otitis media or atelectasis but who do not have cleft palate (Cantekin et al., 1979), they are also at risk for developing cholesteatoma.

On the other hand, cholesteatoma has rarely been identified in American Indian populations (Wiet et al., 1980). Jaffe (1969) reported that attic "perforations" are rarely found in Navajo children; in over 200 tympanoplasties performed to repair central perforations, no cholesteatoma was found. Wiet (1979), in a study of 600 White Mountain Apache Indians, also reported a low incidence of cholesteatoma; the few cases he found were mostly of the attic type. In a subsequent study by Beery and associates (1980), otoscopic examination of 25 Apache Indians revealed no cholesteatomas. The eustachian tube function was tested in these Indians employing the inflation-deflation and forced-response tests, which revealed the presence of a eustachian tube that had low resistance to airflow (was semipatulous) but had active muscle function. This type of tube would probably preclude the development of high negative middle-ear pressure, a retraction pocket, or cholesteatoma. The Apache Indian appears to have a eustachian tube that allows for easier passage of gas and liquid than does the white with or without cleft palate. The middle ear of the Apache individual is very easily ventilated and, consequently, is not protected from unwanted secretions from the nasopharynx. It appears that the structure of the eustachian tube of the Apache Indian of the White Mountain Reservation is conducive to the development of "reflux" otitis media, perforation, and discharge.

Therefore, some American Indian tribes would appear to be *in vivo* models of the semipatulous eustachian tube that actively dilates during swallowing. Cholesteatoma formation is rarely seen in such ears, since the middle ear is aerated either by the eustachian tube or by a central perforation, or both. By studying these *in vivo* models, we can gain a clearer perspective of the whole spectrum of eustachian tube dysfunction (see Chapter 21).

Microbiology

When a cholesteatoma is infected, the organisms cultured from the discharge are similar to those identified from ears with chronic suppurative otitis media: *Pseudomonas aeruginosa* and *Proteus* are the most commonly identified aerobic bacteria, and *Bacteroides* and *Peptococcus-Peptostreptococcus* are the most commonly seen anaerobic organisms. Multiple bacteria were cultured from the discharges of over half of 30 patients with cholesteatomas studied by Harker and Koontz (1977; Table 22–4). Karma and coworkers (1978) reported that when they cultured 18 infected cholesteatomas, in half of the cultures, both aerobic and anaerobic bacteria were found. From the results of the preceding studies, it seems that the most appropriate ototopical medication and systemic antimicrobial therapy for patients who have an infected cholesteatoma would be agents that are effective against gram-negative organisms and anaerobic bacteria; however, the results of culturing the discharge will aid in selecting the proper antimicrobial therapy. These considerations may be life-saving when an intratemporal or intracranial complication of cholesteatoma is present. In addition, preoperative and postoperative antimicrobial therapy for patients with profuse otorrhea may also be necessary to prevent development of a postoperative infection.

Pathology

The pathology of a cholesteatoma is characterized by the presence of keratinizing stratified squamous epithelium, with accumulation of desquamating epithelium or keratin within the middle-ear cleft or other pneumatized portions of the temporal bone. Usually, a cystlike structure is produced by the keratinizing

TABLE 22–4. Bacteriology of Infected Cholesteatomas in 30 Children and Adults

ORGANISM	NO. CASES PRESENT
Aerobes	
Pseudomonas aeruginosa	11
Pseudomonas fluorescens	2
Proteus	4
Escherichia coli	4
Klebsiella-Enterobacter-Serratia	4
Streptococcus	8
Alcaligenes-Achromobacter	3
Staphylococcus aureus	1
Staphylococcus epidermidis	2
CBC Group F	2
Anaerobes	
Bacteroides	13
Peptococcus-Peptostreptococcus	11
Propionibacterium acnes	8
Fusobacterium	4
Bifidobacterium	3
Clostridium	3
Eubacterium	2

Adapted from Harker, L. A., and Koontz, F. P. 1977. The bacteriology of cholesteatoma. *In* McCabe, B. F., Sade, J., and Abramson, M. (eds.): Cholesteatoma: First International Conference. New York, Aesculapius Pub., pp. 264–267.

squamous epithelium. Laminated keratin from its inverted surface accumulates within the cavity, which may also contain necrotic tissue and purulent material (Fig. 22–16). If the pocket is dry, the rate of exfoliation may be slow (Schuknecht, 1974). A cholesteatoma may or may not be infected or associated with chronic suppurative otitis media. Sheehy and coworkers (1977) reported that of 1024 children and adults with cholesteatoma, 26 per cent had no history of aural discharge in the past, in 53 per cent it had been intermittent, and in only 21 per cent of the patients was discharge reported as being continuous. When these patients had surgery, almost half had no evidence of discharge.

The cholesteatoma usually causes bone resorption, which is thought to be secondary to pressure erosion as the mass enlarges or possibly due to the activity of collagenase (Abramson, 1969). Erosion of bone can occur anywhere in the temporal bone, although the ossicles are commonly involved. Ossicular erosion can result in discontinuity (usually erosion of the long process of the incus) and a conductive hearing loss or fistulization of the labyrinth. (The lateral semicircular canal is a common site of erosion.)

Alternatively, the epidermis may invade the aerated space of the temporal bone and form an incomplete surface lining into which the desquamated keratin debris overflows. This process may give the impression that the mucous membrane is converted by metaplasia to keratinizing squamous epithelium (Sade, 1977); however, there apparently is no histopathologic support for this hypothesis (Schuknecht, 1974).

Cholesteatoma in children, in contrast to adults, will frequently extend into the cell tracts of the temporal bone, since pneumatization is usually more extensive in children than in adults (Schuknecht, 1974). This finding may explain the commonly held belief that cholesteatoma in children is more invasive than in adults and, therefore, that it is more difficult to cure surgically in younger patients.

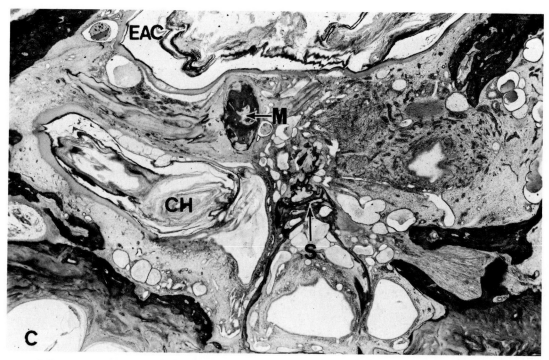

Figure 22–16. Cholesteatoma (H & E, × 16). CH, Cholesteatoma; EAC, external auditory canal; M, malleus; S, stapes; C, cochlea. (Courtesy of I. Sando, M.D.)

Diagnosis

The signs and symptoms of cholesteatoma are such that the disease may go undetected for many years in all age groups, but in children this is an even greater problem. Most adults have a history of hearing loss, which is usually progressive and associated with recurrent ear discharge. However, children rarely complain of hearing loss, especially if the disease is unilateral. Frequently, there is no discharge, and otalgia may be absent in most children and adults. In addition, children are usually unaware of the more subtle symptoms associated with the disease, such as fullness in the ear, tinnitus, mild vertigo, and the foul smell of the discharge, when present. Fever is not a sign of cholesteatoma; when it accompanies this disease, and especially when otalgia is also present, a search for an intratemporal or intracranial complication must be made. Other signs and symptoms, such as facial paralysis, severe vertigo, vomiting, and headache, should also alert the physician to the presence of a suppurative complication. In children, the attic type of cholesteatoma appears to be less symptomatic than a cholesteatoma in the posterosuperior quadrant, since the latter type is frequently preceded by symptomatic recurrent or chronic otitis media with effusion and an early onset of ossicular discontinuity with a significant hearing loss. However, in both types, the preceding atelectasis and retraction pocket may not be associated with significant symptoms in children. The intratympanic "congenital" cholesteatoma, which may be secondary to otitis media, is even more obscure, since hearing loss may be a late sequela and discharge is not present.

Examination of the ear with an otoscope or, more accurately, with the otomicroscope, is the most effective way of diagnosing cholesteatoma. Usually white, shiny, greasy flakes of debris, which may or may not be associated with a foul-smelling discharge, will be seen in a defect in the posterosuperior portion of the pars tensa or the attic or through a large perforation. A polyp may be seen coming through the defect, which, like a crust, can prevent adequate visualization of the tympanic membrane. A crust overlying the area of the posterosuperior quadrant or the pars flaccida must be removed, since a retraction pocket or cholesteatoma may be present. The size of the defect in the tympanic membrane may not be indicative of the extent of the cholesteatoma, since a small defect, especially in the attic, may be associated with extensive cholesteatoma. On the other hand, the cholesteatoma may be confined only to the attic or middle ear despite the presence of a large defect. If an adequate examination of the child's ear is not possible with the child awake, then an examination with the patient under anesthesia is indicated. Every child who must be given a general anesthetic for myringotomy (with or without the insertion of a typanostomy tube) should have an examination of the entire tympanic membrane in order to identify a possible cholesteatoma or its precursor, a retraction pocket. In addition, an intratympanic cholesteatoma may be visualized through the tympanic membrane or through the incision following a myringotomy.

It is not always possible to determine whether the defect is a retraction pocket or a "dry" cholesteatoma; however, even though this distinction cannot be made, the management of the defect will usually be the same.

There is no tympanometric pattern that is diagnostic of a cholesteatoma. An abnormal tympanogram should alert the clinician to the presence of middle-ear disease, but the tympanogram may be normal even when a cholesteatoma is present. Impedance testing may reveal a perforation of the tympanic membrane, but in children this occurs less commonly than in adults. Likewise, audiometric testing may reveal a conductive hearing impairment or possibly a mixed conductive and sensorineural deficit, but a cholesteatoma may be present without the presence of a loss of hearing. A sensorineural hearing loss is presumably due to serous labyrinthitis (Paparella et al., 1972) or possibly to a labyrinthine fistula.

Computed tomograms of the temporal bone should be obtained when a cholesteatoma is suspected. The computed tomograms should be studied carefully to identify the extent of the cholesteatoma, possible ossicular involvement, and any complication that might be present, such as a labyrinthine fistula. The scans should be restudied preoperatively when planning the surgical procedure; decisions concerning the surgical approach and the extent of surgery can be aided by obtaining computed tomograms.

When aural discharge accompanying cholesteatoma is profuse, microbiologic assessment of the discharge is indicated so the infection can be controlled preoperatively by administering the most appropriate antimicrobial agent(s) (see Table 21–26).

Prevention and Management

Rational management of children with cholesteatoma and conditions that may be causally related to this disease should be based on an understanding of its pathogenesis. The presence of a deep retraction pocket in the posterosuperior or pars flaccida area of the tympanic membrane, if persistent, must be managed promptly by insertion of a tympanostomy tube in an effort to return the tympanic membrane to the neutral position and to prevent formation of adhesions between the tympanic membrane and the middle-ear structures (Fig. 22–17, upper panel) (Buckingham and Ferrer, 1966). In children, the retraction pocket may be seen to distend during inhalation anesthesia (while looking through the otomicroscope); this is a good sign that the tympanic membrane will return to the normal position following the insertion of a tympanostomy tube. On the other hand, if the retraction pocket does not distend during anesthesia, then the surgeon should carefully examine the depth and extent of the pocket, probing gently with a blunt right-angled hook. Mirrors may also help to visualize the extent of the pocket, or the 90-degree needle telescope (Olympus Co.) may be

RETRACTION POCKET—ATELECTASIS

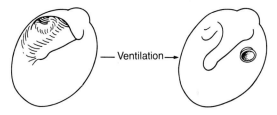

— Ventilation →

RETRACTION POCKET—ADHESIVE OTITIS

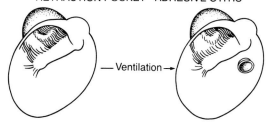

— Ventilation →

Figure 22–17. When a retraction pocket is in the posterosuperior portion of the pars tensa of the tympanic membrane and adhesive otitis media is not present between the eardrum and ossicles, the insertion of a tympanostomy tube may return the tympanic membrane to the neutral position. However, if adhesive otitis media is present, the retraction pocket will persist in spite of the presence of a tympanostomy tube and middle-ear ventilation. (From Bluestone, C. D., and Klein, J. O. 1988. Otitis Media in Infants and Children. Philadelphia, W. B. Saunders Co.)

used to determine the exact borders of the pocket (Fig. 22–18) (Gonzalez and Bluestone, 1986). A retraction pocket can extend into any area of the middle ear, but most frequently it is found extending into the epitympanum and sinus tympani. If the retraction pocket persists after the middle ear has been ventilated by a tympanostomy tube that has been in place for several weeks or months (Fig. 22–17, *lower panel*), then the surgeon should consider performing a tympanoplasty procedure to prevent ossicular discontinuity or the development of a cholesteatoma, or both. Heermann and coworkers (1970) advocate the use of cartilage to support the tympanic membrane graft to prevent recurrence of the retraction pocket. Especially in children, a tympanostomy tube should probably be inserted into the tympanic membrane remnant, since eustachian tube function will most probably remain poor postoperatively.

If a cholesteatoma is found in the posterosuperior or attic area during the examination of a child, an attempt should be made to remove the cholesteatoma debris. If most or all of this material can be removed and if the extent of the sac can be visualized adequately, then a tympanostomy tube should be inserted. A few children have been found to have normal tympanic membranes within one month following such "débridement" and tympanostomy tube insertion (Bluestone et al., 1982; Buckingham, 1982). However, when this uncommon event occurs, long-term follow-up of these children must include reinsertion of a tympanostomy tube if the retraction pocket recurs.

Surgical Procedures

When a cholesteatoma is present, surgical intervention is indicated. The only exceptions to this form of management would be unusual cases (just described) in which simple "débridement" and insertion of a tympanostomy tube are successful, or the presence of a concomitant disease that would make surgery under general anesthesia a hazard to the child's health. The surgical procedures that are currently employed to eradicate a cholesteatoma are briefly described next. These procedures may also be performed for other conditions described in this chapter, but for detailed descriptions of the surgical techniques, the reader is referred to the Selected References at the end of this chapter.

The procedures can be divided into those that provide exposure and removal of disease from the middle ear and mastoid and those that are designed to reconstruct the middle ear to preserve or restore hearing. A *tympanotomy* is a surgical procedure that opens the middle-ear space. In an *exploratory tympanotomy*, a tympanomeatal flap is elevated so that the middle ear and its structures can be viewed directly. Exploratory tympanotomy is indicated when it is suspected that there is an abnormality, such as intratympanic cholesteatoma or ossicular chain abnormality, or as a planned second-stage procedure after a tympanoplasty with or without a mastoidectomy has been performed to manage cholesteatoma.

A *myringoplasty* is the surgical repair of a defect in the tympanic membrane with no attempt made to explore the middle ear. A perforation (or retraction

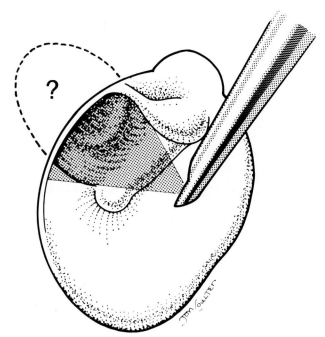

Figure 22–18. Visualization of the extent of retraction pocket can best be achieved utilizing the 90-degree needle telescope (Olympus Co., Japan). The retraction pocket in this artist's drawing is illustrated to be in the posterosuperior quadrant of a right tympanic membrane.

pocket) is commonly repaired by utilizing autogenous connective tissue graft (temporalis fascia or compressed adipose tissue from the earlobe) as a lattice onto which epithelial cells can migrate from the edges of the existing perforation. The procedure is employed to manage a simple uncomplicated tympanic membrane perforation without cholesteatoma. *Tympanoplasty* is the surgical reconstruction of the tympanic membrane–ossicle transformer mechanism. If a perforation is present, it is repaired with a connective tissue graft, but unlike a myringoplasty, the middle ear is explored. Ossicles can be repositioned (ossiculoplasty) to restore ossicular chain continuity. Traditionally, tympanoplasty operations are characterized according to the degree to which the reconstructed ossicular chain approximates the anatomic juxtaposition of ossicles in the normal middle ear (see sections on perforation of the tympanic membrane, p. 495, and ossicular chain discontinuity and fixation, p. 519).

Mastoidectomy involves the surgical exposure and removal of mastoid air cells. There are several types of mastoidectomy (Fig. 22–19). In a *complete simple "cortical" mastoidectomy* (Fig. 22–19A), the mastoid air cell system is exenterated, including the epitympanum, but the canal wall is left intact. The operation is performed when acute or chronic mastoid osteitis is present and is frequently part of the surgical procedure advocated by some surgeons for cholesteatoma. A *posterior tympanotomy* or *facial recess tympanotomy* (Fig. 22–19B) involves exenteration of mastoid air cells followed by formation of an opening between the mastoid and middle ear created in the posterior wall of the middle ear lateral to the facial nerve and medial to the chorda tympani. This procedure is an extension of the complete simple mastoidectomy that allows better visualization of the facial recess without removing the canal wall and is primarily advocated for ears in which a cholesteatoma is present. A *modified radical mastoidectomy* (Fig. 22–19C) is an operation in which a portion of the posterior ear canal wall is removed and a permanent mastoidectomy cavity is created, but the tympanic membrane and some or all of the ossicles are left. The procedure is usually performed when a cholesteatoma cannot be removed without removing the canal wall; some function may be preserved. *Radical mastoidectomy* (Fig. 22–19D) involves exenteration of all mastoid air cells, opening of the epitympanum, and removal of the posterior ear canal wall along with the tympanic membrane, the malleus, and the incus. Only the stapes, or the footplate of the stapes, remains. No attempt is made to preserve or improve function. By removing the posterior ear canal wall, the exenterated mastoid cellular area, middle ear, and external auditory canal communicate, forming a common single cavity. The procedure is indicated when there is extensive cholesteatoma present in the middle ear and mastoid that cannot be removed by a less radical procedure. In addition, the operation may be indicated when a suppurative complication of otitis media is present.

When a tympanoplasty operation is done in conjunction with mastoidectomy, the combined procedure is termed mastoidectomy-tympanoplasty. Mastoidectomy operations that leave the posterior ear canal wall intact are termed "closed cavity," "canal wall up," or "intact canal wall" procedures, whereas those in which the posterior canal is partially removed are called "open cavity" or "canal wall down" procedures.

Type of Surgical Procedure Related to Outcome

There has been a great deal of controversy concerning the best surgical methods to eradicate cholestea-

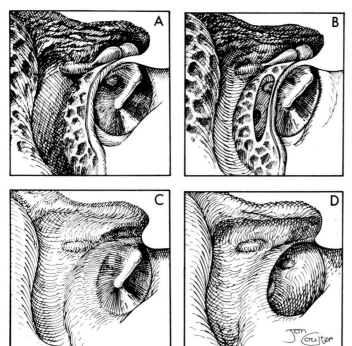

Figure 22–19. Examples of four types of mastoid surgery. *A,* Complete simple ("cortical") mastoidectomy in which the canal wall has been left intact. However, the exposure of the epitympanum is an important part of the surgical procedure. *B,* A posterior tympanotomy–facial recess access to the middle ear has been added to the complete simple mastoidectomy. *C,* Modified radical mastoidectomy. *D,* Radical mastoidectomy.

toma from the middle ear and mastoid in all age groups. Some surgeons prefer to perform mastoidectomy and surgery of the middle ear, or "canal wall up" procedures, in which the cholesteatoma is removed without leaving a mastoid cavity and in which function is preserved or restored by performing a tympanoplasty (with or without an ossiculoplasty) (Jansen, 1963; Sheehy and Patterson, 1967; Sheehy, 1985; Smyth, 1972; Austin, 1976; Glasscock, 1977; Glasscock et al., 1981; Smyth and Hassard, 1980; Sanna et al., 1987). Most of the surgeons who advocate the "intact canal wall" procedure perform a "planned second-stage" exploratory tympanotomy, at which time cholesteatoma can be removed that had been left either purposefully in a critical area, such as over a labyrinthine fistula, or inadvertently. However, opponents to this approach prefer to perform either a modified radical mastoidectomy or, when the cholesteatoma is extensive, a radical mastoidectomy, since they consider the rate of persistence (residual) or recurrence, or both, of cholesteatoma following the "intact canal wall" procedures to be unacceptably high (Abramson et al., 1977; Abramson, 1985). The advocates of the "canal wall down" approach would rather sacrifice the potential preservation or restoration of function (in some procedures leaving the patient with a "mastoid bowl") for a better chance at total removal of the cholesteatoma, that is, a low rate of residual and recurrent disease. Palva and colleagues (1977) advocate performing a modified radical mastoidectomy in which the mastoidectomy cavity is obliterated with subcutaneous tissue, that is, a Palva flap, to eliminate the "mastoid bowl," and an attempt is made to improve or preserve the hearing. However, when he compared 65 children and 65 adults who underwent the procedure to remove cholesteatoma, the three patients in whom a postoperative residual cholesteatoma occurred were children. Tos (1983) advocates fitting the procedure to the pathologic condition found at surgery.

Unfortunately, at present there have been no randomized controlled trials of these two approaches to determine the best method. Therefore, both are currently acceptable in adults, but when a cholesteatoma is present in the ear of a child, the evidence currently available would appear to direct the surgeon toward the "canal wall down" procedures. This approach in children is based on several factors, of which two have already been described: The first is that cholesteatoma is more invasive in children compared to adults, and the second is that several studies have shown that there is a higher rate of residual and recurrent cholesteatoma following intact canal wall mastoidectomy-tympanoplasty procedures in children than in adults (Smyth, 1977). Sheehy (1978) reported that residual cholesteatoma was either purposely left or found at the second-stage procedure in 51 per cent of children, compared to only 30 per cent of adults. Sanna and associates (1987) compared the results of treatment of 102 children who had acquired cholesteatoma. They reported that children had a 43.8 per cent incidence of recurrent cholesteatoma after intact canal wall tym-

panoplasty, which were much higher rates than they found in adults, 18.4 per cent and 3.9 per cent, respectively.

Abramson and coworkers (1977) found that children younger than the age of 9 years had a significantly greater rate of postoperative cholesteatoma than adults, following either an "intact canal wall" or a "canal wall down" procedure but that the rate in children who had "intact canal wall" mastoidectomy was more than twice as high as that in children who underwent modified radical mastoidectomy ("canal wall down").

Another factor that influences the type of procedure selected for children is that almost all children with cholesteatoma have poor eustachian tube function, which would make them at risk for developing recurrent or chronic middle-ear effusion following tympanoplasty (with or without mastoidectomy). Still another, more important factor is that the same sequence of events that led to development of the initial cholesteatoma can recur, particularly in the posterosuperior or pars flaccida area.

Current Recommendations

At either end of the spectrum of the disease, the decision as to the most appropriate surgical management of cholesteatoma is relatively straightforward. For children who have a small cystlike cholesteatoma that is localized to the mesotympanum or epitympanum and that can be removed easily, a tympanoplasty can be successful. Performance of a second-stage exploratory tympanotomy should be considered six months after the initial procedure to uncover residual or recurrent disease. This time interval is somewhat shorter than that advocated for adults, but residual cholesteatoma grows more rapidly in children than in adults. However, this may not be necessary if the tympanic membrane is translucent without evidence of progressive disease medial to the drum and if the hearing is stable during the postoperative follow-up period (and no second-stage ossiculoplasty is planned). In these cases, the child may be observed. However, a "second look" should be performed if the tympanic membrane is opaque or if a progressive loss of hearing develops. If residual cholesteatoma is found during this second procedure and if it is extensive, a "canal wall down" procedure should be performed, that is, a modified radical mastoidectomy or radical mastoidectomy. The use of the needle telescope can be very helpful in determining whether cholesteatoma is in the sinus tympani and facial recess during the initial operative procedure and at the time of the "second look" exploratory tympanotomy (Fig. 22–20). On rare occasions, only a small remnant of the original cholesteatoma will be found to be present at this second exploration (with no other apparent spread of cholesteatoma); this remnant should be removed, and a third-stage procedure should be planned. On the other hand, if no cholesteatoma is found at the planned second-stage procedure, the child is most probably

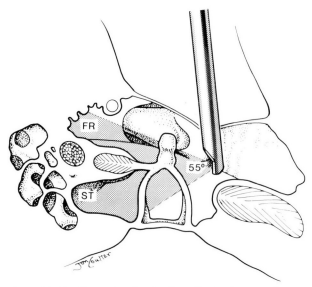

Figure 22–20. Illustration showing how during the operative procedure, the needle telescope can visualize the sinus tympani (**ST**) and facial recess (**FR**) areas to determine whether residual cholesteatoma is present.

free of the original cholesteatoma. These children must nevertheless be followed by periodic examination for years: If severe atelectasis or a retraction pocket develops, prompt myringotomy and insertion of a tympanostomy tube are indicated. An alternative approach for a small attic cholesteatoma would be *atticotomy*, that is, exteriorization, especially when a second-stage procedure is not feasible.

At the other end of the spectrum is the extensive cholesteatoma that involves all or most of the middle ear and mastoid, in which the disease has left only remnants of the ossicles. For this condition, a radical mastoidectomy would be indicated. However, the problem for the surgeon is deciding how to manage the majority of cholesteatomas in children that are neither small and easily removed nor so extensive that only radical surgery is indicated. The recommendation at this time is to select the operative procedure that most probably will give the best outcome for that individual child.

A modified mastoidectomy and, when possible, a tympanoplasty would appear to be the most appropriate procedures. All children do not have to have a "routine" planned second-stage exploratory operation, but if extensive disease was found at the initial procedure, an exploratory tympanotomy six months after the original surgery should be seriously considered, since there has been a high rate of residual cholesteatoma found in children, even after a "canal wall down" procedure. As advocated by Shambaugh (Shambaugh and Glasscock, 1980), a Bondy modified radical mastoidectomy using the endaural approach is still an excellent choice when an attic cholesteatoma is present. This procedure is especially appropriate for children in whom the cholesteatoma is lateral to the ossicles in the epitympanum and has spread into the mastoid but does not involve the mesotympanum.

When a modified radical or radical mastoidectomy has been performed, the open mastoid cavity should probably not be obliterated with a connective tissue flap, bone pate, or plastic material, since residual cholesteatoma may occur in the mastoid cavity and since the long-term outcome of these procedures in large groups of children has yet to be reported.

When tympanoplasty is performed in children at the same time that mastoidectomy is performed to eradicate a cholesteatoma, the results of the tympanoplasty may have a poor outcome (Bluestone et al., 1979). Failure of the tympanoplasty is associated with one or more of the following conditions: sloughing of the graft, recurrence of high negative middle-ear pressure and a retraction pocket, recurrent or chronic otitis media with effusion, or recurrence of cholesteatoma. Another study of a large number of adults and children who underwent tympanoplasties at the time of surgery to remove cholesteatoma also showed that tympanoplasties in such patients are not successful (Cody, 1977), while other studies have reported more favorable outcomes (Glasscock et al., 1981; Sheehy, 1985; Sanna et al., 1987). When chronic suppurative otitis media is present in addition to the cholesteatoma, a tympanoplasty should be withheld or performed as a second-stage procedure (see section on chronic suppurative otitis media, p. 502). In addition, when a cholesteatoma is infected, with or without the presence of chronic suppurative otitis media (and mastoiditis), preoperative control of the infection with antimicrobial agents is desirable, since the presence of infection may affect the outcome of the tympanoplasty as well as increase the risk of developing a postoperative wound infection. When a tympanoplasty for cholesteatoma is performed, then artificial ventilation of the middle ear must also be provided by a tympanostomy tube. However, in older children, eustachian tube function may be adequate to ventilate the middle ear, and tympanoplasty can be performed without tympanostomy tube insertion. When tympanoplasty is performed in children who have a defect in the posterosuperior quadrant of the pars tensa, or the pars flaccida, or both, cartilage should be placed to support the grafted tympanic membrane and thus prevent recurrence of cholesteatoma (Heerman et al., 1970).

When the cholesteatoma is extensive and a radical mastoidectomy is necessary to control the disease, then the middle-ear end of the poorly functioning eustachian tube should be closed surgically, since the middle ear–mastoidectomy cavity is then an open system (Bluestone et al., 1978). Otherwise, nasopharyngeal secretions could reflux into the middle ear–mastoidectomy cavity, resulting in inflammation and otorrhea (Fig. 22–21). The most effective way to obliterate the bony portion of the eustachian tube is with bone pate. Closure of the eustachian tube at the time of radical mastoidectomy, although not universally performed by modern otologic surgeons, is not a new addition to the procedure but has been advocated for many years. Closure of the middle-ear portion of the tube is also indicated for patients who have had a

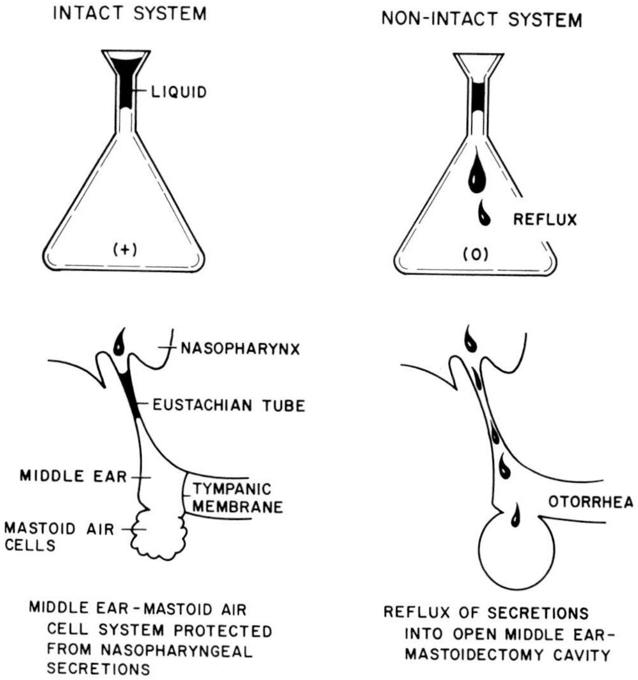

Figure 22–21. Liquid flow through a flask is compared with the nasopharynx–eustachian tube–middle ear–mastoid air cell system. When the system is intact, liquid is prevented from flowing into the body of the flask (middle ear–mastoid air cells). By contrast, the nonintact system permits liquid to reflux into the flask. This condition is analogous to a perforation of the tympanic membrane in which reflux of nasopharyngeal secretions could occur, since the middle ear–mastoid air cushion is lost. Similarly, following a radical mastoidectomy, the presence of a patent eustachian tube could cause troublesome otorrhea (see text).

radical mastoidectomy performed in the past and who have intermittent or persistent postoperative aural discharge. Eustachian tube function tests should be performed. If the tube is found to be patent, revision middle ear–mastoid surgery should be performed, and surgical closure of the eustachian tube should be done if a tympanoplasty is not going to be performed at the time of the revision surgery or planned in the future.

Conclusions

In children with a retraction pocket or acquired cholesteatoma in the posterosuperior or pars flaccida portion of the tympanic membrane, active function of the eustachian tube is abnormal; constriction, rather than dilatation, of the eustachian tube occurs during swallowing. Acquired cholesteatoma not secondary to implantation is a sequela of otitis media or a retraction pocket, or both. The type of surgery chosen to manage these conditions in children should be selected on the basis not only of the site and extent of the cholesteatoma but also of other factors, such as patient age, presence or absence of otitis media, eustachian tube function, and availability of health care. The operation must be tailored for each child. Prevention of the pathologic conditions that predispose to this type of cholesteatoma is the most effective method of management.

ADHESIVE OTITIS MEDIA

Adhesive otitis media is a result of healing following chronic inflammation of the middle ear and mastoid. The mucous membrane is thickened by proliferation of fibrous tissue, which frequently impairs the move-

ment of the ossicles, resulting in a conductive hearing loss. Schuknecht (1974) has described the pathologic condition as a proliferation of fibrous tissue within the middle ear and mastoid and has termed the condition fibrous sclerosis. When there are cystic spaces present, it is called fibrocystic sclerosis, and when there is new bone growth in the mastoid, he has classified it as fibroosseous sclerosis.

There are no data available on the prevalence of adhesive otitis media in children, but the condition is common in those who have had recurrent acute or chronic otitis media with effusion or atelectasis of the tympanic membrane–middle ear, or both. Unfortunately, we have no data from which to establish the probability with which a child who has a middle-ear effusion or atelectasis might develop adhesive otitis media. However, the possibility of adhesive changes occurring when inflammation is present in the middle ear and mastoid must be seriously considered when selecting the most appropriate medical or surgical treatment of children who have recurrent acute and chronic otitis media with effusion or atelectasis. In addition to fixation of the ossicles, adhesive otitis media may result in ossicular discontinuity and conductive hearing loss due to rarefying osteitis, especially of the long process of the incus. When there is severe localized atelectasis (a retraction pocket) in the posterosuperior portion of the pars tensa of the tympanic membrane, adhesive changes may bind the eardrum to the incus, stapes, and other surrounding middle-ear structures and cause resorption of the ossicles. Once adhesive changes bind the tympanic membrane in this area, the development of a cholesteatoma is also possible (Fig. 22–22). Timely ventilation of the middle ear and mastoid prior to the adhesive changes may return the tympanic membrane to the normal position, thus preventing ossicular damage. If medical

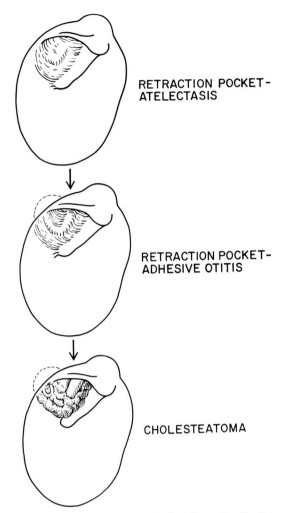

RETRACTION POCKET-
ATELECTASIS

RETRACTION POCKET-
ADHESIVE OTITIS

CHOLESTEATOMA

Figure 22–22. Sequence of events leading from a localized area of atelectasis (retraction pocket) in the posterosuperior portion of the pars tensa of the tympanic membrane to a cholesteatoma and ossicular discontinuity. Adhesive otitis media in this area is shown as the stage between atelectasis and the development of a cholesteatoma.

treatment fails, then a myringotomy should be performed, and a tympanostomy tube should be inserted in an attempt to reverse the potentially progressive pathologic condition. However, if the tympanic membrane is still attached to the ossicles in spite of tympanostomy tube insertion, then adhesive otitis media is present. In children, tympanoplasty should be considered to prevent further structural damage, since the process may progress owing to persistent eustachian tube obstruction.

When ossicular discontinuity or fixation has occurred, an ossiculoplasty may be performed to restore function but is not always successful. When the middle ear and mastoid are bound by adhesive otitis media, the results of ossiculoplasty frequently are not permanent owing to recurrence of the adhesive process. However, surgery should be considered (Shambaugh and Glasscock, 1980). The best method to manage adhesive otitis media is prevention, which involves the treating of its precursors, acute and chronic otitis media with effusion and atelectasis (see Chap. 21).

TYMPANOSCLEROSIS

Tympanosclerosis may be a sequela of chronic middle-ear inflammation or the result of trauma. It is characterized by the presence of whitish plaques in the tympanic membrane and nodular deposits in the submucosal layers of the middle ear (Igarashi et al., 1970). The pathologic condition in the tympanic membrane occurs in the lamina propria, while within the middle ear, the pathologic condition is in the basement membrane; in both sites, there is hyalinization followed by deposition of calcium and phosphate crystals. Conductive hearing loss may occur if the ossicles become imbedded in the deposits.

The condition was first described by von Troltsch (1869), who called it "sclerosis," but it was Zollner (1956) who called the disorder tympanosclerosis and differentiated it from otosclerosis. Schuknecht (1974) prefers the term "hyalinization" rather than tympanosclerosis, since the histopathologic condition is that of hyalin degeneration, which is the result of a healing reaction characterized by fibroblastic invasion of the submucosa, followed by thickening and fusion of collagenous fibers into a homogeneous mass. He also described the hyalinized collagen around the ossicles.

Even though no reliable data are available, tympanosclerosis of the tympanic membrane is a very common sequela in children who have or have had recurrent or chronic otitis media with effusion and also is common at the site of a healed, spontaneous perforation or following myringotomy, especially if a tympanostomy tube had been inserted. It would appear that the chalky patch seen in the tympanic membrane of children may be due to inflammation or trauma, or both. However, in the pediatric age group as a whole, the condition is not common in the middle ear, especially in infants and young children. In particular, ossicular involvement is rare in very young children. Of 311 cases of tympanosclerosis studied by Kinney (1978), only 20 per cent occurred in individuals 30 years of age or younger. This would imply that the condition in the middle ear may take many years to develop. However, Schiff and colleagues (1980) propose the hypothesis that tympanosclerosis has an immune component that occurs in the middle ear following an insult or mucosal disruption and that there is also a genetic component, which would explain the low incidence of the condition in children who have such a high prevalence and incidence of middle-ear inflammation.

The preceding hypothesis may be the explanation for the relatively high rate of tympanosclerosis among children who are Alaskan natives (Eskimos) and American Indians (Wiet, 1979; Jaffe, 1969; DeBlanc, 1975).

However, other factors may predispose these children to the disease, such as differences in eustachian tube function. Weider (Wiet et al., 1980) reported that tympanosclerosis affected a higher percentage of Alaskan native children than children of a similar age in his New Hampshire private practice; tympanosclerosis of the tympanic membrane or the ossicles or both was found in 78 (68 per cent) of 114 Alaskan native children who had tympanoplasty surgery, whereas only seven such cases were diagnosed in 377 consecutive tympanoplasties performed on children in his practice. In addition, he also found that far advanced tympanosclerosis that resulted in fixation of the ossicular chain occurred at an early age in the Alaskan native children but not in children in his practice.

No surgical correction, such as tympanoplasty, is indicated when tympanosclerosis of the tympanic membrane, even though extensive, is the only abnormality of the middle ear. If a middle-ear effusion is present and a myringotomy, with or without a tympanostomy tube insertion, is indicated, the incision should be placed, if possible, in an area without involvement, leaving the affected area untouched. Removal of large tympanosclerotic plaques may result in a permanent perforation of the tympanic membrane. When an incision must be made in an area of tympanosclerosis, then only the amount necessary to perform the procedure should be removed. When a tympanoplasty is being performed to repair a perforation of the tympanic membrane and tympanosclerosis is present in the drum remnant, removal of the plaque is optional: the plaque may remain if the area of tympanosclerosis does not interfere with the surgical procedure and is not impeding function. When tympanosclerosis is the cause of ossicular fixation and a tympanoplasty procedure is elected, the methods of removal of the plaques and ossiculoplasty described by Shambaugh and Glasscock (1980) are appropriate for the rare child with this advanced stage of tympanosclerosis. However, refixation of the ossicles is not uncommon even after apparently adequate surgical removal of the plaques and ossiculoplasty. If surgery is not performed or is not successful in restoring the hearing loss, then a hearing aid should be considered.

Even though the pathogenesis of tympanosclerosis is not understood, it seems most probable that appropriate management of recurrent and chronic middle-ear inflammation in infants and children is the best method of prevention. Since it also occurs following trauma to the tympanic membrane, myringotomy with tympanostomy tube placement should be performed with tympanosclerosis as one of the potential complications and sequelae in mind. However, in general, tympanosclerosis involving the tympanic membrane does not appreciably affect function, although when the ossicles are involved, the patient may have a significant conductive hearing loss. Thus, tympanostomy tubes may, on the one hand, increase the incidence of tympanosclerosis of the tympanic membrane, but on the other hand, their placement may decrease the frequency of ossicular fixation due to this disease later in life.

OSSICULAR DISCONTINUITY AND FIXATION

Ossicular interruption is the result of rarefying osteitis secondary to chronic inflammation of the middle ear. A retraction pocket or cholesteatoma may also cause resorption of the ossicles. The long process of the incus is most commonly involved, which results in incudostapedial disarticulation. The commonly accepted reason given for this portion of the incus being eroded is its poor blood supply; however, since the tympanic membrane frequently becomes attached to this part of the incus when a posterosuperior retraction pocket is present, adhesive otitis media may be the cause of the osteitis and subsequent erosion. Also, cholesteatoma is commonly found in the same area (Bluestone et al., 1977). The stapes, or more specifically its crural arches, is the second most commonly involved ossicle. The etiology of stapes fixation is more likely to be associated with presence of a retraction pocket or cholesteatoma rather than with decreased vascular supply. Less commonly, the body of the incus and the manubrium of the malleus may also be eroded. The ossicles may become fixed by fibrous tissue secondary to adhesive otitis media or, more rarely in children, secondary to tympanosclerosis. Neither the incidence of ossicular discontinuity and fixation nor the natural history of the pathologic conditions that precede these abnormalities has been formally studied in children. However, ossicular discontinuity is commonly associated with a deep retraction pocket or cholesteatoma in the posterosuperior portion of the tympanic membrane. Disarticulation or fixation of the ossicles may also occur when there is a central perforation of the tympanic membrane with or without the presence of chronic suppurative otitis media and, more rarely, when the tympanic membrane is intact.

The hearing loss is conductive when the ossicular chain is affected, and the degree is dependent on the site and the degree of involvement of the ossicle(s) as well as on the presence or absence of associated conditions such as a perforation of the tympanic membrane. When there is a discontinuity of the incudostapedial joint and the tympanic membrane is intact, a maximal conductive hearing loss may be present, that is, 50 to 60 dB. However, when the same ossicular pathologic condition is present and a perforation is also present, the hearing loss may be less severe. Erosion of the manubrium of the malleus is usually associated with a perforation of the tympanic membrane but does not contribute to the hearing loss.

Diagnosis

The diagnosis of the ossicular chain abnormalities that are secondary to otitis media and its related conditions can frequently be made by visualization of the defect through the otoscope or, more accurately, with the otomicroscope. Erosion of the long process of the incus can usually be seen when a deep posterosuperior retraction pocket is present. The presence of a significant conductive hearing loss, for example, greater than 30 dB, when a perforation of the tympanic membrane is present would be presumptive evidence of ossicular involvement. However, when the tympanic membrane is normal, a significant conductive loss may be due to inflammatory ossicular involvement that has occurred in the past, but congenital ossicular abnormalities and otosclerosis must be part of the differential diagnosis. In addition to the history, otoscopic examination, and conventional audiometric testing, impedance audiometry may aid in the diagnosis. A tympanogram showing high compliance would be presumptive evidence of ossicular chain discontinuity when there is a significant conductive hearing loss present. If the compliance is low, ossicular fixation would be more probable. However, the accuracy with which tympanometry can differentiate between ossicular discontinuity and fixation is not high, since several other parameters in the middle ear, such as mobility of the tympanic membrane, affect the shape of the tympanogram. Polytomography may also aid in identifying ossicular discontinuity but usually is of diagnostic benefit only when a large defect is present. The most accurate way of diagnosing these defects is exploration of the middle ear, either during exploratory tympanotomy, when the tympanic membrane is intact, or by inspection of the entire ossicular chain when surgery of the middle ear and mastoid, such as tympanoplasty, is indicated.

Management

Management of ossicular deformities in children is similar to that described for adults, with some notable exceptions. Most adults who have ossicular discontinuity or fixation no longer are at risk of developing otitis media with effusion or high negative pressure within the middle ear due to eustachian tube dysfunction, but many children still have or will have these conditions, which could interfere with the success of reconstructive middle-ear surgery generally and ossiculoplasty specifically. Therefore, the indications for timing and the type of middle ear surgery may be different for children. When an ossicular deformity is suspected and the tympanic membrane is intact without evidence of otitis media or any of its other complications or sequelae, such as retraction pocket or cholesteatoma, then the decision to perform an exploratory tympanotomy to diagnose and possibly repair the ossicular deformity would depend on several considerations. First, and most important, is the child still at risk of developing a middle-ear effusion or atelectasis (retraction pocket), or both? As a general rule, if neither condition has occurred in either ear for a year or longer, the risk is low; however, the younger the child, the higher the risk. If further middle-ear disease may still occur, the operation should be delayed. The second consideration is the degree of hearing loss and whether or not the defect is unilateral or bilateral. A child who has a maximum conductive hearing loss in both ears would be a very probable candidate for surgical intervention, while the child who only has a unilateral mild conductive loss should not be operated on. Another important consideration is the need for

general anesthesia to perform the surgery in all children. The benefit of surgery must be weighed against the risk of general anesthesia. For the child who has a bilateral maximum conductive hearing loss, the benefit of hearing improvement may outweigh the risk of general anesthesia, whereas the risk of anesthesia may not override the potential chance of improving the hearing in a child with only a unilateral loss of hearing. Withholding the reconstructive surgery until the child is able to tolerate a local anesthetic (adolescence) is a preferred option when the hearing loss is unilateral and especially when it is only mild to moderate in degree. Whenever the decision to operate is delayed until the child is older, a hearing aid should be considered, even when the hearing loss is unilateral.

When surgery of the middle ear is indicated owing to the presence of a perforation of the tympanic membrane with or without chronic suppurative otitis media, a cholesteatoma, or a retraction pocket, the very fact that the patient is a child still affects the decision as to whether or not to perform an ossiculoplasty. This is because children are at increased risk of suffering future episodes of otitis media and of developing atelectasis or adhesive otitis media. When these conditions are a possibility, the surgeon should consider staging the surgery and performing the ossiculoplasty when the child is older.

The various ways in which ossicles that are either eroded or fixed may be reconstructed have been adequately described elsewhere. However, it is important to reiterate that the type of ossiculoplasty chosen for a child may be different than that performed in an adult. We feel, and most experts agree, that in general, middle-ear ossicular implants should not be used in children unless absolutely necessary, as neither the safety nor the efficacy of these prostheses has been proved over a long enough period of time to warrant insertion in the middle ear of a child. However, some surgeons advocate the use of homograft ossicles in children. Whenever possible, only the child's own tissue should be used to reconstruct the ossicular chain. For the most common discontinuity encountered, that of the incudostapedial joint, an incus transposition or insertion of a fitted incus is the ideal procedure (Fig. 22–23). When the stapes crura are missing, the shaped incus can usually be inserted between the mobile footplate of the stapes and the malleus handle. For all age groups, whenever the stapes is fixed, a stapedectomy should not be performed unless the tympanic membrane is intact, and in children who have had otitis media, stapedectomy should rarely, if ever, be performed, even when the tympanic membrane is intact, since a recurrence of otitis media with suppurative labyrinthitis as a complication would be an ever-present risk. Freeing of other fixed ossicles can be attempted in children, but refixation often occurs, since adhesive otitis media, which is the most frequent cause of fixation, commonly leads to further fibrosis.

The most effective method of managing ossicular discontinuity and fixation is prevention of the diseases

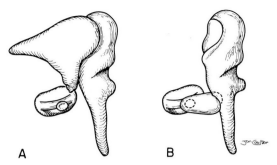

Figure 22–23. The most common ossicular discontinuity present in children is at the incudostapedial joint and is due to erosion of the long process of the incus (A). An autograft fitted incus is the recommended procedure for children (B).

that cause these ossicular abnormalities. Of special note is the early diagnosis and management, usually by insertion of a tympanostomy tube, of a postero-superior retraction pocket in which the tympanic membrane is lying on the incus and stapes (see Chap. 21, section on atelectasis of the tympanic membrane–middle ear and high negative middle-ear pressure).

MASTOIDITIS

The proximity of the mastoid to the middle-ear cleft suggests that most cases of suppurative otitis media are associated with inflammation of the mastoid air cells. However, the incidence of clinically significant mastoiditis is low since the introduction of antimicrobial agents. Nevertheless, acute and chronic disease still occurs and may be responsible for significant morbidity and life-threatening disease.

At birth, the mastoid consists of a single cell, the antrum, connected to the middle ear by a small channel, the aditus ad antrum (Fig. 22–24). Pneumatization of the mastoid bone takes place soon after birth and is usually extensive by 2 years of age. The process may continue throughout life. The clinical importance of the mastoid is related to contiguous structures, including the posterior cranial fossa, the middle cranial fossa, the sigmoid and lateral sinuses, the canal of the facial nerve, the semicircular canals, and the petrous tip of the temporal bone. The mastoid air cells are lined with modified respiratory mucosa, and all are interconnected with the antrum.

Infection in the mastoid proceeds after middle-ear infection through the following stages: (1) hyperemia and edema of the mucosal lining of the pneumatized cells, (2) accumulation of serous and then purulent exudates in the cells, (3) demineralization of the cellular walls and necrosis of bone due to pressure of the purulent exudate on the thin bony septa and ischemia of the septa caused by decrease in blood flow, (4) formation of abscess cavities due to the coalescence of adjacent cells following destruction of the cell walls, and (5) escape of pus into contiguous areas.

This process may halt at any stage, with subsequent resolution. However, when infection persists for more than a week or ten days, inflammatory granulation tissue forms in the pneumatic cavity. A hypertrophic osteitis develops, which results in thickening and sclerosis of the cellular walls and reduction in the size of the cellular space. There may be repeated cycles of absorption and deposition of bone. If the infection remains chronic but low-grade, there is thickening of the mucosa caused by a fibrinous exudate, which may

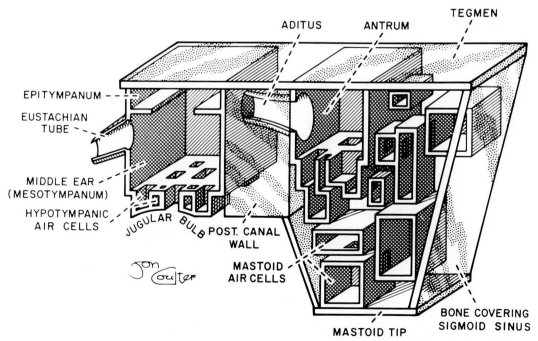

Figure 22–24. Diagrammatic representation of the anatomy of the middle ear and mastoid air cell system, showing the narrow connection (aditus ad antrum) between the two, which is sometimes referred to as the "bottleneck" when acute infection cannot drain from the mastoid into the middle ear.

become organized and may lead to permanent adhesions. Columnar metaplasia with new gland formation may lead to extensive production of mucus in the former cells.

Mastoiditis can be classified into acute and chronic. Acute mastoiditis is further subdivided according to the pathologic stage present, which has clinical significance, since management is dependent on the stage of the disease. Unfortunately, because of failure to appreciate the natural history and pathologic process of acute mastoiditis, there is a great deal of confusion in the minds of clinicians, as well as in the current literature, regarding the most appropriate management of each stage.

Acute Mastoiditis

In almost every child who has acute otitis media, the mastoid air cells are also inflamed; thus, acute mastoiditis is a natural extension and part of the pathologic process of the acute middle-ear infection. No specific signs or symptoms of the mastoid infection are present in this most common stage of mastoiditis. The hearing loss, otalgia, and fever are due primarily to the acute infection within the middle ear. Computed tomograms of the mastoid area are usually read as "cloudy mastoids," which is, in reality, indicative of inflammation. No mastoid osteitis is evident on the computed tomograms (Fig. 22–25). The process is usually reversible, as the middle ear–mastoid effusion resolves, either as a natural process or as a result of treatment of the acute infection. If resolution of the infection does not occur at this stage, one or more of the following conditions can develop: (1) acute mas-

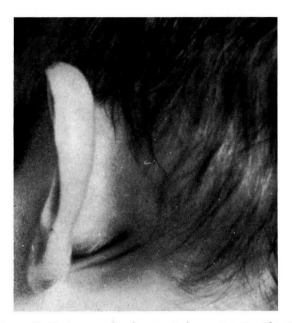

Figure 22–26. An example of postauricular periosteitis. This 2-year-old boy had acute otitis media and mastoiditis. In addition to fever and otalgia, there was postauricular swelling, erythema, tenderness to touch, and loss of the postauricular crease but no evidence of a subperiosteal abscess or roentgenographic evidence of mastoid osteitis. Management consisted of tympanocentesis-myringotomy (and tympanostomy tube insertion) and parenteral antimicrobial therapy, which resulted in complete resolution of the postauricular involvement 24 hours after the beginning of treatment.

toiditis with periosteitis, (2) acute mastoid osteitis (with or without a subperiosteal abscess), or (3) chronic mastoiditis.

A condition called "masked mastoiditis" has been described for which a complete simple mastoidectomy has been advocated (Mawson and Ludman, 1979). The disease appears to be a subacute stage of otitis media and mastoiditis (without osteitis) that is characterized by the same signs and symptoms as acute otitis media, except that they are persistent and less severe. The progression to this stage is attributed to failure of the initial antimicrobial agent to resolve the middle ear infection within a short period. Persistent otalgia and fever in a patient who is receiving an antimicrobial agent are indications for a tympanocentesis-myringotomy to identify the causative organism and to promote drainage. In selected children, especially for those patients who have had frequently recurrent episodes of acute otitis in the past, the insertion of a tympanostomy tube (in addition to the appropriate antimicrobial therapy) will resolve the problem. No mastoid surgery is indicated unless mastoid osteitis is present. However, infants and children may have a suppurative process in the mastoid, which may even result in an intratemporal or intracranial complication, in which the middle ear may not appear to be diseased and the patient lacks the classic signs and symptoms of otitis media and mastoiditis. This condition can be called "masked mastoiditis"; the diagnosis is usually made by computed tomographic imaging.

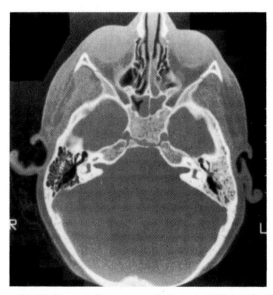

Figure 22–25. Computed tomogram of the temporal bone of a child with acute otitis media in which the mastoid air cells show signs of inflammation without osteitis. The diagnosis was acute mastoiditis, which is usually present during episodes of acute middle-ear infection and is most frequently self-limited. (From Bluestone, C. D., and Klein, J. O. 1988. Otitis Media in Infants and Children. Philadelphia, W. B. Saunders Co.)

Acute Mastoiditis with Periosteitis

At this stage, the infection within the mastoid air cells spreads to the periosteum covering the mastoid process, causing periosteitis (Fig. 22–26). The route of infection from the mastoid cells to the periosteum is by venous channels, usually the mastoid emissary vein. The condition should not be confused with the presence of a subperiosteal abscess, since the management of the latter condition requires incision and drainage of the abscess and a complete simple (cortical) mastoidectomy, while the former usually responds to immediate but less aggressive surgical intervention.

When acute mastoiditis with periosteitis occurs in the absence of roentgenographic evidence of osteitis of the mastoid, management should consist of hospitalization, immediate tympanocentesis (for aspiration and microbiologic assessment of the middle ear–mastoid effusion), and myringotomy for drainage of the system. The insertion of a tympanostomy tube is desirable and will enhance drainage over a longer period of time than myringotomy alone. Parenteral antimicrobial agents should be administered as described in the section on acute mastoid osteitis.

Resolution of the periosteal involvement should occur within 24 to 48 hours after the tympanic membrane has been opened for drainage and adequate and appropriate antimicrobial therapy has begun. Surgical drainage of the mastoid, that is, complete simple mastoidectomy, should be performed if the symptoms of the acute infection, such as fever and otalgia, persist, if the postauricular involvement does not progressively improve, or if a subperiosteal abscess develops.

Failure to institute immediate treatment at this stage may result in the development of acute mastoid osteitis with or without a subperiosteal abscess or, more dangerous to the child, a suppurative intratemporal or intracranial complication such as lateral sinus thrombosis, extradural abscess, or meningitis.

Acute Mastoid Osteitis (Acute "Coalescent" Mastoiditis, Acute Surgical Mastoiditis)

If the infection within the mastoid progresses, rarefying osteitis can cause destruction of the bony trabeculae that separate the mastoid cells, resulting in a "coalescence" of the cells. At this stage, a mastoid empyema is present. The pus may spread in one or more of the following directions: (1) anterior to the middle ear through the aditus ad antrum, in which case spontaneous resolution usually occurs; (2) lateral to the surface of the mastoid process, resulting in a subperiosteal abscess (Fig. 22–27); (3) anteriorly, burrowing beneath the skin to form a soft tissue abscess below the pinna or behind the attachment of the sternocleidomastoid muscle in the neck, which is known as a Bezold abscess (Fig. 22–28); (4) medial to the petrous air cells, resulting in petrositis; or (5) posterior to the occipital bone, which can result in osteomyelitis of the calvarium or a Citelli abscess.

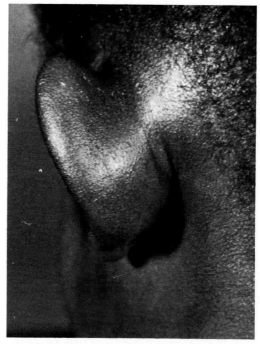

Figure 22–27. An example of a subperiosteal abscess in a child who had acute mastoid osteitis. Note that the pinna is displaced inferiorly and anteriorly, with obliteration of the postauricular crease resulting from the abscess.

Infection may also spread to the labyrinth and facial nerve or into the intracranial cavity, causing one or more suppurative complications, such as an extradural abscess or meningitis.

Clinically, the major signs of mastoid osteitis are a reflection of the underlying inflammatory process and include swelling, redness, and tenderness to touch over the mastoid bone. The pinna is displaced outward and downward (Fig. 22–29), and swelling or sagging of the posterosuperior canal wall may also be present. A purulent discharge may issue through a perforation in the tympanic membrane. Ear drainage may be persistent, and the ear canal is filled with pus and debris. Alternatively, there may be a nipplelike protrusion at the site of the perforation of the tympanic membrane. A fluctuant subperiosteal abscess may be present or even a draining fistula from the mastoid to the postauricular area (Fig. 22–30). The patient may be toxic and febrile with systemic signs of acute illness. In the subacute disease, fever may be prolonged and low-grade with occasional temperature spikes.

Conversely, the tympanic membrane and middle ear may appear almost normal when mastoid osteitis is present. In such cases, the acute middle-ear effusion drains through the eustachian tube, in which case there is resolution of the otitis media, but if an obstruction between the middle ear and mastoid is present, then infection in the mastoid becomes trapped and can cause osteitis. The obstruction is usually due to the presence of mucosal swelling or granulation

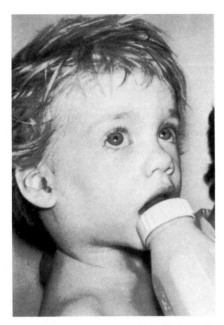

Figure 22–28. An abscess in the neck (Bezold abscess) can be seen in this child who has a draining ear owing to acute otitis media. The pus has extended from acute mastoid osteitis and empyema into the neck. (From Bluestone, C. D., and Klein, J. O. 1988. Otitis Media in Infants and Children. Philadelphia, W. B. Saunders Co.)

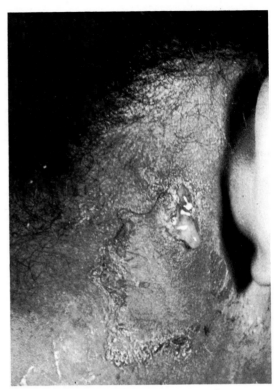

Figure 22–30. An example of a postauricular fistula with purulent discharge in a child who had acute mastoid osteitis.

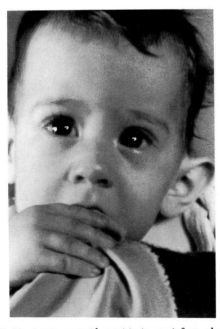

Figure 22–29. Acute mastoid osteitis in an infant, showing the outward displacement of the pinna. (From Bluestone, C. D., and Klein, J. O. 1988. Otitis Media in Infants and Children. Philadelphia, W. B. Saunders Co.)

tissue at the aditus ad antrum, or the "bottleneck" of the middle ear–mastoid system. In these cases, the condition of the tympanic membrane and middle ear may not be a reliable indication of mastoid infection. When no external stigmas of extension of pus from the mastoid, such as a subperiosteal abscess, are evident, roentgenograms of the mastoids must be obtained to rule out the presence of an acute mastoid osteitis when otitis media is not obvious. Any child with a fever of unknown origin should have, as part of the search for the cause of the fever, roentgenograms of the mastoids to rule out the possibility that the fever is caused by acute mastoid osteitis (without otitis media).

Epidemiology

Before antimicrobial agents were widely used, acute mastoid osteitis was the most common suppurative complication of acute otitis media and frequently resulted in death. The frequency of mastoidectomy for this condition in 1938 was 20 per cent, whereas it was 2.8 per cent in 1948, with an almost 90 per cent reduction in the mortality rate during that period (Sorensen, 1977). A more recent study from Finland found that 29 cases of acute mastoiditis were reported during the period from 1956 to 1971 (Juselius and Kaltiokallio, 1972). It would appear that the frequency of this complication has significantly dropped, but it is still present, even in this, the age of antibiotics.

Microbiology

Acute mastoiditis may be caused by the same organisms responsible for acute otitis media, *Streptococcus pneumoniae* and *Haemophilus influenzae.* In subacute or chronic cases, *Staphylococcus aureus* and gram-negative enteric bacilli, including *Escherichia coli, Proteus,* and *Pseudomonas aeruginosa,* may be present and are responsible for a persistent and indolent discharge. In a recent study from South Africa by Maharaj and colleagues (1987), 90 per cent of 32 patients with acute mastoiditis had bacteria isolated, and of these, the most frequently isolated were *S. aureus, Proteus mirabilis, Bacteroides melaninogenicus,* and *B. fragilis.*

Diagnosis

The diagnosis should be suspected on the basis of clinical signs. Computed tomograms of the mastoid area may show one or more of the following signs: (1) haziness, distortion, or destruction of the mastoid outline; (2) loss of sharpness of the shadows of cellular walls due to demineralization, atrophy, and ischemia of the bony septa (Fig. 22–31); (3) decrease in the density and cloudiness of the areas of pneumatization due to inflammatory swelling of the air cells; and (4) in long-standing cases, there is a chronic osteoblastic inflammatory reaction that may obliterate the cellular structure. Small abscess cavities in sclerotic bone may be confused with pneumatic cells. Computed tomograms may also be helpful in ruling out the coexistence of other suppurative intratemporal or intracranial complications of otitis media.

Cultures for bacteria from ear drainage must be taken with care and concern for discriminating fresh drainage from the debris in the external canal. The canal must be initially cleaned, and if fresh pus is exuding through a perforation in the tympanic membrane, the discharge is cultured at the point of exit from the tympanic membrane with a cotton-tipped wire swab or, preferably, a needle and syringe under direct view. A Gram stain of the pus provides immediate information about the responsible organisms.

Management

Antimicrobial agents are the mainstay of treatment of acute disease. If the case is otherwise uncomplicated (i.e., there was no prior infection), it is probable that *S. pneumoniae* or *H. influenzae* is responsible, and ampicillin in a dosage schedule for severe disease is suitable (see Table 21–25). If the disease has persisted for weeks or longer, coverage for *S. aureus* and gram-negative organisms must be provided. It is of the utmost importance to obtain cultures from the site of infection to guide therapy, but initial treatment may begin with a penicillinase-resistant penicillin (nafcillin, oxacillin, or methicillin) and an aminoglycoside (gentamicin or tobramycin) or monotherapy using a cephalosporin, such as cefuroxime. This regimen may be altered by the findings from a Gram stain of purulent material or by the results of cultures and sensitivity tests.

A complete simple ("cortical") mastoidectomy must be performed when there is evidence of acute mastoid osteitis, especially when the mastoid empyema has extended outside the mastoid bone. The procedure should be considered an emergency, but the timing of the operation must be dependent on the status of the child. Ideally, sepsis should be under control, and the patient must be able to tolerate a general anesthetic. The procedure is described in detail in current texts (Shambaugh and Glasscock, 1980) (see Fig. 22–19A), but in general, the goal is to clean out the mastoid infection and drain the mastoid air cell system into the middle ear by eliminating any obstruction that is caused by edema or granulation tissue in the aditus ad antrum and to provide external drainage. Drains should be inserted into the mastoid cavity and into any abscess that has developed adjacent to the mastoid cavity. To drain and ventilate the middle ear, a tympanostomy tube should be inserted, if it is not already in place. If a suppurative intratemporal or intracranial complication is also present, surgical intervention for these conditions may also be required (see Chap. 23).

Failure to control the infection in the acute stage of mastoid osteitis may lead to a chronic infection within the mastoid bone or to one of the suppurative complications.

Chronic Mastoiditis

Chronic mastoiditis is invariably associated with chronic suppurative otitis media. The mastoid may be poorly pneumatized or sclerotic. The chronic infection at this stage may be brought under control by medical treatment, but when there are extensive granulation tissue and osteitis in the mastoid, mastoidectomy is usually necessary to eliminate the chronic mastoid

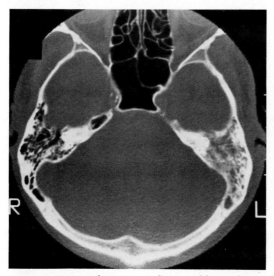

Figure 22–31. Computed tomogram of temporal bones showing left acute osteitis with loss of septa between the mastoid air cells, which has been termed acute "coalescent" mastoiditis; right mastoid is normal. Mastoid surgery was performed on this patient. (From Bluestone, C. D., and Klein, J. O. 1988. Otitis Media in Infants and Children. Philadelphia, W. B. Saunders Co.)

osteitis, especially if a cholesteatoma is present (see section on chronic suppurative otitis media, p. 502, and cholesteatoma and retraction pocket, p. 507).

PETROSITIS

Petrositis is a rare suppurative complication that is secondary to an extension of infection from the middle ear and mastoid into the petrous portion of the temporal bone. All the inflammatory and cellular changes described as occurring in the mastoid can also occur in the pneumatized petrous pyramid. Only about 30 per cent of the individuals have well-pneumatized petrous bones (Ranier, 1938). However, in these individuals, infection of the temporal petrosa may be more frequent than appreciated by clinical and roentgenographic signs, since there is communication of the petrosal air cells with the mastoid and middle ear. Pneumatization usually does not occur before 3 years of age.

Petrositis may be either acute or chronic. In the acute form, there is extension of acute otitis media and mastoiditis into the pneumatized petrous air cells. The condition, like acute mastoiditis, usually is self-limited with resolution of the acute middle ear and mastoid infection. However, on occasion the infection in the petrous portion of the temporal bone does not drain owing to mucosal swelling or because granulation is obstructing the passage from the petrous air cells to the mastoid and middle ear, which results in acute petrous osteomyelitis. Nowadays, the widespread use of antimicrobial agents has made this an extremely rare complication. However, chronic petrous osteomyelitis can be a complication of chronic suppurative otitis media or cholesteatoma, or both, and is much more common than the acute type. Pneumatization of the petrous portion of the temporal bone does not have to be present, since the infection can invade the area by thrombophlebitis, osteitis, or along fascial planes (Allam and Schuknecht, 1968). The infection may persist for months or years, with mild and intermittent signs and symptoms, or may spread to the intracranial cavity and result in one or more of the suppurative complications of ear disease, such as an extradural abscess or meningitis.

Microbiology

The organisms that cause acute petrositis are the same as those that cause acute mastoid osteitis: *S. pneumoniae* and *H. influenzae*. However, chronic petrous osteomyelitis may be caused by the bacteria found in association with chronic suppurative otitis media and cholesteatoma, such as *P. aeruginosa* or *Proteus*.

Diagnosis

The disease is characterized by pain behind the eye, deep ear pain, persistent ear discharge, and sixth nerve

palsy. Eye pain is due to irritation of the ophthalmic branch of the fifth cranial nerve. On occasion, the maxillary and mandibular divisions of the fifth nerve will be involved, and pain will occur in the teeth and jaw. A discharge from the ear is common with acute petrositis but may not be present with chronic disease. Paralysis of the sixth cranial nerve leading to diplopia is a late complication (Glasscock, 1972). Acute petrous osteomyelitis should be suspected when persistent purulent discharge follows a complete simple mastoidectomy for mastoid osteitis. The triad of pain behind the eye, aural discharge, and sixth nerve palsy is known as Gradenigo syndrome.

The diagnosis of acute petrous osteomyelitis is suggested by its unique clinical signs. Standard roentgenograms of the temporal bones may show clouding with loss of trabeculation of the petrous bone. The visualization is uncertain, however, because of normal variation in pneumatization (including asymmetry) and the obscuring of the petrous pyramids by superimposed shadows of other portions of the skull. However, polytomograms of the temporal bones can be diagnostic, and computed tomography should always be performed to rule out the possibility of an extension of the infection into the cranial cavity.

Management

Management of acute petrositis is similar to that described for acute mastoiditis, since at this stage it can be considered as further spread of infection within the pneumatized petrous portion of the temporal bone. However, when acute petrous osteomyelitis and acute mastoid osteitis are present together, a more aggressive surgical approach to management will be required than when only the mastoid is involved. As described for patients with acute mastoid osteitis, tympanocentesis-myringotomy (for smear and culture and for drainage) should be performed immediately, and adequate doses of antimicrobial agents should be administered. A complete simple mastoidectomy must also be performed to remove the irreversible mucosal and bone infection, but when the petrous part of the temporal bone is involved, wide exploration of the cell tracts from the mastoid to the petrous portion of the temporal bone should also be part of the surgical procedure to provide adequate drainage. A tympanostomy tube should be inserted into the tympanic membrane if one is not already present. When a large perforation of the tympanic membrane is present, no attempt at reconstruction should be made, since, like the tympanostomy tube, drainage of the middle ear is an important part of management. This approach will usually be adequate for resolution of the petrous infection; however, if drainage of the middle ear, mastoid, and petrosa cannot be achieved by performing a complete simple mastoidectomy, then a modified radical mastoidectomy or, more appropriately, a radical mastoidectomy, may be necessary. However, in children in whom an "extensive" complete simple mastoidectomy (or radical mastoidectomy) fails to resolve the persistent profuse discharge from the mastoid wound and middle ear and for most cases of chronic petrous osteomyelitis, more extensive temporal bone surgery is indicated. The various surgical approaches to the deep petrosal cells have been adequately described by Shambaugh and Glasscock (1980), including the approach through the middle cranial fossa, which usually can preserve the labyrinth, carotid artery, and facial nerve (Glasscock, 1969).

LABYRINTHITIS

This complication of otitis media occurs when infection spreads into the cochlear and vestibular apparatus. The usual portals of entry are the round window and, less commonly, the oval window, but invasion may take place from an infectious focus in an adjacent area, such as the mastoid antrum, the petrous bone, and the meninges, or as a result of bacteremia. Schuknecht (1974) has classified labyrinthitis into four types: (1) acute serous (toxic) labyrinthitis, in which there may be bacterial toxins or biochemical involvement, but no bacteria are present; (2) acute suppurative (purulent) labyrinthitis, in which bacteria have invaded the otic capsule; (3) chronic labyrinthitis, which is secondary to soft tissue invasions, usually by cholesteatoma and granulation tissue or fibrous tissue; and (4) labyrinthine sclerosis, in which there is replacement of the normal labyrinthine structures by fibrous tissue and bone. Labyrinthitis has also been classified into localized (circumscribed) and generalized types.

Acute Serous (Toxic) Labyrinthitis (with or without Perilymphatic Fistula)

The acute serous type of labyrinthitis is considered to be one of the most common suppurative complications of otitis media. Paparella and associates (1972) described the histopathologic evidence of serous labyrinthitis in most of the temporal bone specimens from patients who had otitis media. Bacterial toxins from the infection in the middle ear may enter the inner ear, primarily through an intact round window or through a congenital defect. The portal of entry may also be through an acquired defect of the labyrinth, such as from head trauma or previous middle ear or mastoid surgery. Biochemical changes within the labyrinth have also been found. The cochlea is usually more severely involved than the vestibular system. Paparella and coworkers (1980) reviewed the audiograms of 232 patients who had surgery for chronic otitis media and found a significant degree of bone-conduction loss in the younger age groups. In addition, there was a marked difference in the presence and degree of sensorineural hearing loss in the affected ear, as compared to the normal ear, in patients of all age groups who had unilateral disease. They postulated that the high-frequency sensorineural hearing loss that

frequently accompanies this disease is due to a pathologic insult to the basal turn of the cochlea. Fluctuating sensorineural hearing loss has been described in patients with otitis media and has been thought to be due to either endolymphatic hydrops (Paparella et al., 1979) or to a perilymphatic fistula (Grundfast and Bluestone, 1978; Supance and Bluestone, 1983).

The signs and symptoms of serous labyrinthitis (especially when a perilymphatic fistula is present) are a sudden, progressive, or fluctuating sensorineural hearing loss or vertigo, or both, in association with otitis media or one or more of its complications or sequelae, such as mastoid osteitis. The loss of hearing is usually mixed, that is, there are both conductive and sensorineural components, when serous labyrinthitis is a complication of otitis media. However, in some children who have recurrent middle-ear infection, the hearing may be normal between episodes, while in other children, a mild or moderate sensorineural hearing loss only will be present at all times. The presence of vertigo may not be obvious in children, especially infants. Older children may describe a feeling of spinning or turning, while younger children may not be able to verbalize concerning the symptoms but manifest the dysequilibrium by falling, stumbling, or "clumsiness." The vertigo may be mild and momentary, and it may tend to recur over months or years. Spontaneous nystagmus may also be present, but the signs and symptoms of acute suppurative labyrinthitis, such as nausea, vomiting, and deep-seated pain, are usually absent. Fever, if present, is usually due to a concurrent upper respiratory tract infection or acute otitis media.

The presence of a labyrinthine fistula may be identified by performing a fistula test employing a Siegle pneumatic otoscope or by applying positive and negative external canal pressure using the pump-manometer system of an impedance bridge. The fistula test is considered positive if nystagmus or vertigo is produced by the application of the pressures. Electronystagmography is an objective way of documenting the presence or absence of the nystagmus, but the findings of the fistula test may be misleading, since there can be false-positive and false-negative results. The test can be done in the presence of a perforation of the tympanic membrane or tympanostomy tube. Fistulas are frequently associated with congenital or acquired defects in the temporal bone, such as the Mondini malformation (Fig. 22–32). Computed tomograms may be helpful in identifying such defects (Fig. 22–33).

When otitis media with effusion is present, a tympanocentesis and myringotomy should be performed for microbiologic assessment of the middle-ear effusion and drainage. If possible, a tympanostomy tube should also be inserted for more prolonged drainage and in an attempt to ventilate the middle ear. Antimicrobial agents with efficacy against *S. pneumoniae*, *H. influenzae*, and *Branhamella catarrhalis*, such as amoxicillin, should be administered. Following resolution of the otitis media with effusion, the signs and symptoms of the labyrinthitis should rapidly disappear; however, sensorineural hearing loss may persist. If the diagnostic

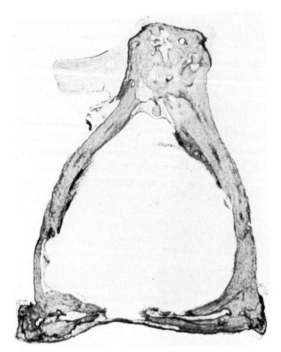

Figure 22–32. Congenital defect in the footplate of the stapes removed from an infant who had a Mondini malformation.

assessment is indicative of a possible congenital or acquired defect of the labyrinth, an exploratory tympanotomy should be performed as soon as the middle ear is free of infection. If a perilymphatic fistula is found, it should be repaired employing either adipose tissue from the earlobe, temporalis fascia, or tragal

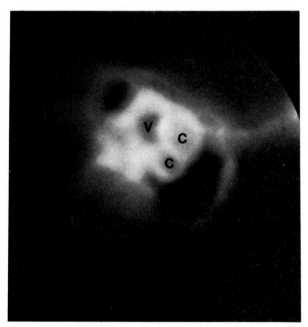

Figure 22–33. Polytomogram of the temporal bone of a 9-month-old girl, showing a dilated vestibule (V) and cochlea (C). The child had a fluctuating sensorineural hearing loss, ascertained by auditory brain stem response audiometry, when otitis media with effusion was present. Bilateral tympanotomy revealed a congenital defect of the oval window, with a perilymphatic fistula. Following repair of the oval window defect, the hearing remained normal.

perichondrium (Fig. 22–34). Even when no defect of the oval or round window is identified, but a fistula is still suspected, the stapes footplate and round window should be covered with connective tissue, since a leak may not be present at the time of the tympanotomy but may recur (Grundfast and Bluestone, 1978; Supance and Bluestone, 1983). A tympanostomy tube should be reinserted if recurrent otitis media persists.

When acute mastoid osteitis, chronic suppurative otitis media, or cholesteatoma is present, definitive medical and surgical management of these conditions is essential in eliminating the labyrinthine involvement. A careful search for a labyrinthine fistula must be performed when mastoid surgery is indicated. However, a labyrinthectomy is not indicated for serous labyrinthitis.

Any child with sensorineural hearing loss (with or without vertigo) who also has recurrent acute or chronic otitis media with effusion should be carefully evaluated for the possible existence of serous labyrinthitis, which can be secondary to a perilymphatic fistula. This combination appears to be quite common, and failure to identify this complication can result in irreversible severe to profound hearing loss, making early diagnosis and prevention imperative. Since prevention of sensorineural hearing loss due to other causes (such as congenital or viral causes) is not yet possible, our goal should be to prevent this loss of function in those children in whom it can be prevented. In addition, serous labyrinthitis may develop into acute suppurative labyrinthitis.

Acute Suppurative Labyrinthitis

Suppurative (purulent) labyrinthitis may develop as a complication of otitis media or may be one of its complications and sequelae when bacteria migrate from the middle ear into the perilymphatic fluid through the oval or round window, a preexisting temporal bone fracture, an area where bone has been eroded by cholesteatoma or chronic infection, or

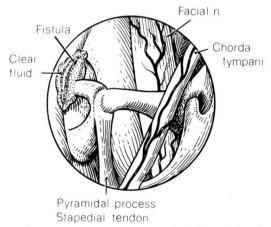

Figure 22–34. Abnormal stapes seen in the left ear. The anterior crus is straight rather than curved, and it joins the central portion rather than the anterior edge of the footplate.

through a congenital defect. (The most common way that bacteria enter the labyrinth is from the meninges, but migration by this route is usually not a complication of otitis media.)

The incidence of suppurative labyrinthitis as a complication of otitis media is unknown, but it is rare since the widespread use of antibiotics. In a series of 96 cases of suppurative intratemporal and intracranial complications of acute and chronic otitis media that were treated during the period from 1956 to 1971, there were only five cases of suppurative labyrinthitis, all of which were secondary to cholesteatoma that had caused a labyrinthine fistula (Juselius and Kaltiokallio, 1972).

The sudden onset of vertigo, dysequilibrium, deep-seated pain, nausea and vomiting, and sensorineural hearing loss during an episode of acute otitis media or an exacerbation of chronic suppurative otitis media indicates that labyrinthitis had developed. The hearing loss is severe, and there is loss of the child's ability to repeat words shouted in the affected ear, with masking of sound in the opposite ear. Often, spontaneous nystagmus and past pointing can be observed. Initially, the quick component of the nystagmus is toward the involved ear, and there is a tendency to fall toward the opposite side. However, when there is complete loss of vestibular function, the quick component will be toward the normal ear. Laboratory and radiographic studies are not of much diagnostic value. In the absence of associated meningitis, the cerebrospinal fluid pressure and cell count are normal.

Frequently, the onset of suppurative labyrinthitis may be followed by facial paralysis, meningitis, or both. In later stages, cerebellar abscess can develop. Thus, suppurative labyrinthitis is a serious complication of otitis media. The development of purulent labyrinthitis means that infection has spread to the fluid of the inner ear, and infection can then spread to the subarachnoid space through the cochlear aqueduct, the vestibular aqueduct, or the internal auditory canal.

The treatment of suppurative labyrinthitis in the absence of meningitis consists of otologic surgery combined with intensive antimicrobial therapy. If this complication is due to acute otitis media, immediate tympanocentesis and myringotomy with tympanostomy tube insertion are indicated, as described when serous labyrinthitis is present. If acute mastoid osteitis is present, a complete simple mastoidectomy should be performed; however, because this complication is usually secondary to cholesteatoma, a radical mastoidectomy or modified radical mastoidectomy is required. A radical or modified radical mastoidectomy is also appropriate when chronic suppurative otitis media is present without cholesteatoma. If meningitis has also occurred in association with suppurative labyrinthitis, then otologic surgery other than a diagnostic and therapeutic tympanocentesis-myringotomy should be delayed until the meningitis is under control. A labyrinthectomy should be performed only if there is complete loss of labyrinthine function or if the infection

spreads to the meninges in spite of adequate antimicrobial therapy. Initially, parenteral antimicrobial agents appropriate to manage the primary middle ear and mastoid disease present should be administered, but since cholesteatoma and chronic suppurative otitis media are the most frequent causes of suppurative labyrinthitis, antimicrobials effective for the gram-negative organisms (*Pseudomonas aeruginosa* and *Proteus*) are frequently required (see Table 21–26). However, the results of culturing the middle-ear effusion, purulent discharge, or the cerebrospinal fluid may alter the selection of the antibiotics.

Chronic Labyrinthitis

The most common cause of chronic labyrinthitis as a complication of middle-ear disease is a cholesteatoma that has eroded the labyrinth, resulting in a fistula. Osteitis may also cause bone erosion of the otic capsule. The fistula most commonly occurs in the lateral semicircular canal and is filled by squamous epithelium of a cholesteatoma, granulation tissue, or fibrous tissue entering the labyrinth. The middle ear and mastoid are usually separated at the site of the fistula from the inner ear by the soft tissue, but when there is continuity, acute suppurative labyrinthitis may develop.

The signs and symptoms of chronic labyrinthitis are similar to those of the acute forms of the disease (e.g., sensorineural hearing loss and vertigo) except that their onset is more subtle rather than more sudden. The disease is characterized by slowly progressive loss of cochlear and vestibular function over a prolonged period of time. The fistula test may be helpful in making the diagnosis of a labyrinthine fistula, and polytomography may reveal a defect. When there is complete loss of function, no signs or symptoms of labyrinthine dysfunction may be present.

Since a cholesteatoma is the most common cause of this type of labyrinthitis, middle ear and mastoid surgery must be performed. For children with a labyrinthine fistula due to a cholesteatoma, a modified radical or radical mastoidectomy is the procedure of choice. When labyrinthine function is still present, the cholesteatoma matrix overlying the fistula should be left undisturbed, since removal can result in total loss of function. Even though there are advocates of performing an intact canal wall procedure and also surgeons who prefer to remove the cholesteatoma matrix, either at the time of the initial surgery or in a second-stage procedure, the most conservative approach is recommended when a cholesteatoma has caused a labyrinthine fistula in a child.

Failure to make the diagnosis of this complication and to perform the surgery as soon as possible may result in complete loss of cochlear and vestibular function with possible development of labyrinthine sclerosis or an acute suppurative labyrinthitis, which can cause a life-threatening intracranial complication, such as meningitis.

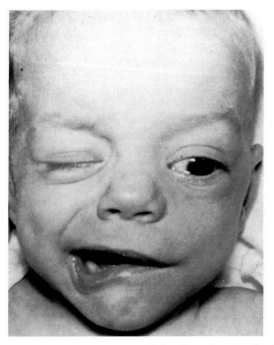

Figure 22–35. An infant in whom left facial paralysis developed a day after the onset of acute otitis media.

Labyrinthine Sclerosis

Labyrinthine sclerosis is caused by fibrous replacement or new bone formation (labyrinthitis ossificans) in part or all of the labyrinth, with resulting loss of labyrinthine function. Because this condition is the end stage of healing after acute or chronic labyrinthitis, prevention of disease of the middle ear is the most effective way to prevent labyrinthine sclerosis.

FACIAL PARALYSIS

Facial paralysis may occur during an episode of acute otitis media because of exposure of the facial nerve from a congenital bony dehiscence within the middle ear (Figs. 22–35 and 22–36). Facial paralysis is a relatively frequent complication of acute otitis media in infants and children, and when it occurs as an isolated complication, tympanocentesis and a myringotomy should be performed, and parenteral antibiotics should be administered. The paralysis will usually improve rapidly without requiring further surgery (facial nerve decompression). Mastoidectomy is not indicated unless acute mastoid osteitis (acute "coalescent" mastoiditis) is present. However, if there is complete loss of facial function and if electrophysiologic testing indicates the presence of degeneration or progressive deterioration of the nerve, then facial nerve decompression may be necessary to achieve complete return of function.

During the period from 1960 to 1980, there were 35 cases of facial paralysis associated with acute otitis media at the Children's Hospital of Pittsburgh and The Eye and Ear Hospital of Pittsburgh. The paralysis was partial in 22 (63 per cent) and complete in 13 (37 per cent). In most instances, initial treatment consisted of antimicrobial therapy and myringotomy. However, of these 35 individuals, seven (20 per cent) had further surgery; five underwent facial nerve decompression, and two had simple mastoidectomies (all seven of these children had complete facial paralysis; unpublished data).

When a facial paralysis develops in a child who has chronic suppurative otitis media with or without cholesteatoma, immediate surgical intervention is indicated (see Chap. 17).

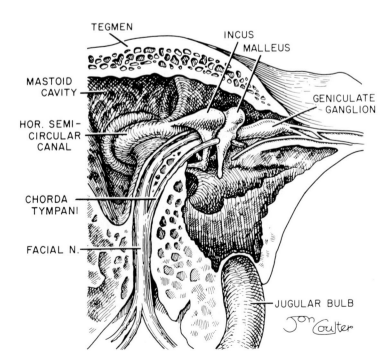

Figure 22–36. The course of the facial nerve shown in the middle ear and mastoid. The nerve can be affected by infection in these areas, which can result in facial paralysis.

CHOLESTEROL GRANULOMA

Cholesterol granuloma is a sequela of chronic otitis media with effusion. It has been described as "idiopathic hemotympanum," since clinically the tympanic membrane appears to be dark blue, a so-called "blue eardrum." However, this term is a misnomer, since there is no evidence that bleeding within the middle ear is related to the etiology of this disease, nor is the presence of fresh blood or microscopic amounts of old blood (Sade et al., 1980). The condition is rare in all age groups but does occur in children and is most likely due to long-standing changes associated with chronic otitis media with effusion (Paparella and Lim, 1967; Sheehy et al., 1969). The blue color of the tympanic membrane as visualized through the otoscope is probably due to the reflection of light from the thick liquid (granuloma) within the middle ear. The condition must be differentiated from an uncovered high jugular bulb and a glomus tumor, either tympanicus or jugulare (Valvassori and Buckingham, 1974) and, more commonly, chronic otitis media with effusion or barotitis.

The tissue has been described as being composed of chronic granulations, with foreign body giant cells and foam cells within the middle ear or mastoid, or both. Cholesterol crystals are usually present. The condition is similar to a chronic middle-ear effusion except that a soft brownish material that contains shining golden-yellow specks is present. The pathologic process present with cholesterol granuloma should not be confused with that of a cholesteatoma (Schuknecht, 1974). Similar granulomas have been described in other parts of the body: atheromatous and dermoid cysts, periapical and follicular cysts of the jaw, old infarcts, and hematomas (Korthals Altes, 1966). When the granulomas are stained, prominent iron deposits or hemosiderin may be found (Bak-Pederson and Tos, 1972; Nager and Vanderveen, 1976), but not in quantities sufficient to account for the otoscopic appearance of the blue tympanic membrane.

The condition has been reproduced in experimental animals by injecting foreign material into the middle ears of guinea pigs (Friedmann, 1959) and rabbits (Dota et al., 1963), by obstructing the long bones of birds (Ojala, 1957; Beaumont, 1966, 1967), and after chronic obstruction of the eustachian tube in monkeys (Main et al., 1970). The pathogenesis described in the latter experimental model is similar to that known to occur in humans when the eustachian tube was obstructed by a muscle pedicle flap (Linthicum, 1971) or by a tumor (Sheehy et al., 1969). In addition to occurring as an isolated pathologic entity, cholesterol granuloma can be associated with chronic suppurative otitis media with or without cholesteatoma or any inflammation that may obstruct portions of the middle ear or mastoid, or both.

The condition will not respond to medical treatment, middle-ear inflation, or myringotomy with tympanostomy tube insertion. However, when a child is observed to have a tympanic membrane that has a dark-blue appearance and is unresponsive to nonsurgical management, a myringotomy under general anesthesia should be performed, since on occasion, chronic otitis media with effusion may also be associated with a blue tympanic membrane (again, probably as the result of the way light from the otoscope is reflected from the middle-ear effusion). However, if a thick, brown liquid is found during the procedure, successful aspiration of the material will not be possible, and if a tympanostomy tube is inserted, it will become occluded immediately. The treatment of choice for a cholesterol granuloma is middle ear and mastoid surgery. The granuloma in the mastoid can be removed by performing a complete simple mastoidectomy, and the middle-ear portion can be removed by using a tympanomeatal approach. There is no reason to remove the canal wall unless a cholesteatoma is present. A tympanostomy tube should be inserted into the tympanic membrane at the time of the procedure and reinserted as often as needed, that is, until the middle ear remains normally aerated following spontaneous extubation.

It would appear from what is known of the pathogenesis and pathology of cholesterol granuloma that the best management is prevention, which should consist of active treatment and prevention of chronic otitis media with effusion.

INFECTIOUS ECZEMATOID DERMATITIS

Otitis media with perforation (also a patent tympanostomy tube) can be associated with an infection of the external auditory canal (external otitis) secondary to a discharge from the middle ear and mastoid. An infection in the mastoid may also erode the bone of the ear canal or the postauricular area, resulting in a dermatitis (see Fig. 22–1A). The ear canal skin is erythematous, edematous, and filled with purulent drainage, and yellow-crusted plaques may be present. The organisms involved are usually the same as those found in the middle ear–mastoid infection, but the flora of the external canal may contribute to the infectious process. *Pseudomonas* and *Proteus* are frequently present. Fungi may also be present in chronic cases; most commonly, *Aspergillus niger* or *alba* is found. A culture of the external auditory canal should be obtained, and the results should be compared with those of a needle aspiration of the middle ear discharge through the tympanic membrane perforation or the tympanostomy tube, which will aid in determining the offending organisms. Antimicrobial therapy can then be selected by the results of the culture and sensitivity testing. The infection may spread to the auricle, periauricular area, or other parts of the body, possibly as a result of direct implantation of the organisms or possibly as an autosensitivity phenomenon. Coagulase-positive *S. aureus* is the most frequently involved bacterium (Senturia et al., 1980b).

Severe inflammatory stenosis of the external auditory meatus is uncommon and, therefore, can be differentiated from the extreme tenderness and pain that are so commonly present in acute diffuse external otitis. Also included in the differential diagnosis would be impetigo contagiosa and a secondary infection associated with contact, or seborrheic, dermatitis. Management should be directed toward resolving the middle ear–mastoid infection, which may require medical treatment or surgery, or both. If the skin of the ear canal is the only area of involvement, then a combination of an antibiotic with or without hydrocortisone otic drops is usually sufficient to reduce the inflammation (Table 22–2). Polymyxin B, neomycin sulfate with hydrocortisone (Cortisporin Otic Suspension) or colistin sulfate, neomycin sulfate, and thonzonium bromide (Coly-Mycin S Otic) are the most commonly employed drugs; however, the ototopical agents may be ototoxic to the cochlea if they penetrate the middle ear and, therefore, should be used with caution. If a fungal infection is present, M-cresyl acetate eardrops (Cresylate) may need to be prescribed. Irrigation of the ear canal with 2 per cent acetic acid or frequent suctioning of the ear canal may also hasten the resolution of the external canal infection.

If the adjacent skin around the auricle or other parts of the body is involved, the skin should be cleansed with saline solution or aluminum acetate and treated with a local antibiotic-corticosteroid cream. The child should be cautioned about spread of the infection from the ear canal to other parts of the body and should refrain from putting his or her finger in the ear or scratching the infected skin. Cotton in the external ear canal can be helpful if profuse drainage is present but should be changed as frequently as necessary.

SELECTED REFERENCES

McCabe, B. F., Sade, J., and Abramson, M. (eds.) 1977. Cholesteatoma: First International Conference. New York, Aesculapius Pub.

This is the state of knowledge of the epidemiology, pathogenesis, management, and complications of cholesteatoma.

Paparella, M. M., and Meyerhoff, W. L. 1980. Mastoidectomy and tympanoplasty. *In* Paparella, M. M., and Shumrick, D. A. (eds.): Otolaryngology, Vol. 2. Philadelphia, W. B. Saunders Co., pp. 1510–1547.

This chapter has an excellent description of procedures employed for the intratemporal complications and sequelae of otitis media.

Saunders, W. H., Paparella, M. M., and Miglets, A. 1986. Atlas of Ear Surgery, 4th ed. St. Louis, The C. V. Mosby Co.

The current techniques for surgery of the middle ear and mastoid are illustrated and described in detail.

Schuknecht, H. F. 1974. Pathology of the Ear. Cambridge, MA, Harvard University Press, pp. 215–244, 251–254.

This is the best description of the pathology of the intratemporal complications and sequelae of otitis media.

Shambaugh, G. E., and Glasscock, M. E. 1980. Surgery of the Ear, 3rd ed. Philadelphia, W. B. Saunders Co., pp. 251–287, 326–347, 408–453.

The indications for surgery and the techniques for the procedures are described in detail.

REFERENCES

Abramson, M. 1969. Collagenolytic activity in middle ear cholesteatoma. Ann. Otol. Rhinol. Laryngol. 78:112.

Abramson, M. 1985. Open or closed tympanomastoidectomy for cholesteatoma in children. Am. J. Otol. 6:167.

Abramson, M., Lachenbruch, P. A., Press, B. H. J., et al. 1977. Results of conservative surgery for middle ear cholesteatoma. Laryngoscope 87:1281.

Adkins, W. Y., and White, B. 1984. Type I tympanoplasty: Influencing factors. Laryngoscope 94:916.

Allam, A. F., and Schuknecht, H. F. 1968. Pathology of petrositis. Laryngoscope 78:1813.

Andreasson, L., and Harris, S. 1979. Middle ear mechanics and eustachian tube function in tympanoplasty. Acta Otolaryngol. (Suppl.) 360:141.

Armstrong, B. W. 1965. Tympanoplasty in children. Laryngoscope 75:1062.

Austin, D. F. 1976. The retraction pocket in the treatment of cholesteatoma. Arch. Otolaryngol. 102:741.

Avery, A. D., et al. 1976. Quality of Medical Care Assessment Using Outcome Measures: Eight Disease-Specific Applications. Prepared for the Health Resources Administration, Department of Health, Education and Welfare by the Rand Corp., Santa Monica, CA.

Bailey, T. H., Jr. 1976. Absolute and relative contraindications to tympanoplasty. Laryngoscope 86:67.

Bak-Pederson, K., and Tos, M. 1972. The pathogenesis of idiopathic haemotympanum. J. Laryngol. Otol. 86:473.

Baron, S. H. 1969. Management of aural cholesteatoma in children. Otolaryngol. Clin. North Am. 2:71.

Baxter, J. D. 1982. Observations on the evolution of chronic otitis media in the Inuit of the Baffin Zone, N.W.T. J. Otolaryngol. 11:161.

Baxter, J. D., and Ling, D. 1974. Ear disease and hearing loss among the Eskimo population of the Baffin zone. Can. J. Otolaryngol. 3:110.

Beaumont, G. D. 1966. The effects of exclusion of air from pneumatized bones. J. Laryngol. Otol. 80:236.

Beaumont, G. D. 1967. Cholesterol granuloma. J. Laryngol. Soc. Aust. 2:28.

Beery, Q. C., Doyle, W. J., Cantekin, E. I., et al. 1980. Eustachian tube function in an American Indian population. Ann. Otol. Rhinol. Laryngol. 89(68):28.

Bergen, G., Shapira, A., and Marshak, G. 1983. Myringoplasty in children. J. Otolaryngol. 12:228.

Berko-Gleason, J. 1983. Otitis media and language development (workshop on effects of otitis media on the child). Pediatrics 71:639.

Bess, F. H., and Tharpe, A. M. 1984. Unilateral hearing impairment in children. Pediatrics 74:206.

Bezold, F. 1889. Cholesteatom, Perforation der Membrana Flaccida Shrapnelli und Tubenverschluss, eine Atiologische Studie. Ztschrf. Ohrenheilk. 20:5.

Bluestone, C. D. 1971. Eustachian tube obstruction in the infant with cleft palate. Ann. Otol. Rhinol. Laryngol. 80(2):1.

Bluestone, C. D., Beery, Q. C., Cantekin, E. I., et al. 1975. Eustachian tube ventilatory function in relation to cleft palate. Ann. Otol. Rhinol. Laryngol. 84:333.

Bluestone, C. D., Beery, Q. C., and Paradise, J. L. 1973. Audiometry and tympanometry in relation to middle ear effusions in children. Laryngoscope 83:594.

Bluestone, C. D., Cantekin, E. I., Beery, Q. C., et al. 1977. Functional Eustachian tube obstruction in acquired cholesteatoma and related conditions. *In* McCabe, B. F., Sade, J., and Abramson, M. (eds.): Cholesteatoma: First International Conference. New York, Aesculapius Pub., pp. 325–335.

Bluestone, C. D., Cantekin, E. I., Beery, Q. C., et al. 1978. Function of the Eustachian tube related to surgical management of acquired aural cholesteatoma in children. Laryngoscope 88:1155.

Bluestone, C. D., Cantekin, E. I., and Douglas, G. S. 1979. Eustachian tube function related to the results of tympanoplasty in children. Laryngoscope 89:450.

Bluestone, C. D., Casselbrant, M. L., and Cantekin, E. I. 1982. Functional obstruction of the Eustachian tube in the pathogenesis of aural cholesteatoma in children. *In* Sade, J. (ed.): Cholesteatoma and Mastoid Surgery. Proceedings of the Second International Conference on Cholesteatoma and Mastoid Surgery. Amsterdam, Kugler Pub., pp. 211–224.

Bluestone, C. D., Klein, J. O., Paradise, J. L., et al. 1983. Workshop on effects of otitis media on the child. Pediatrics 71:639.

Bluestone, C. D., Wittel, R. A., and Paradise, J. L. 1972. Roentgenographic evaluation of the Eustachian tube function in infants with cleft and normal palates. Cleft Palate J. 9:93.

Brandow, E. C., Jr. 1977. Implant cholesteatoma in the mastoid. In McCabe, B. F., Sade, J., and Abramson, M. (eds.): Cholesteatoma: First International Conference. New York, Aesculapius Pub., pp. 253–256.

Brook, I. 1985. Prevalence of β-lactamase–producing bacteria in chronic suppurative otitis media. Am. J. Dis. Child. 139:280.

Brown, D. T., Marsh, R. R., and Potsic, W. P. 1983. Hearing loss induced by viscous fluids in the middle ear. Int. J. Pediatr. Otorhinolaryngol. 5:39.

Brummet, R. E., Harris, R. F., and Lindgren, J. A. 1976. Detection of ototoxicity from drugs applied topically to the middle ear space. Laryngoscope 86:1177.

Buchwach, K. A., and Birck, H. G. 1980. Serous otitis media and type I tympanoplasties in children. Ann. Otol. Rhinol. Laryngol. 89(68):324.

Buckingham, R. A. 1982. The clinical appearance and natural history of cholesteatoma. In Cholesteatoma and Mastoid Surgery. Amsterdam, Kugler Publications, pp. 13–21.

Buckingham, R. A., and Ferrer, J. L. 1966. Reversibility of chronic adhesive otitis with polyethylene tube. Laryngoscope 76:993.

Cambon, K., Galbreath, J. D., and Kong, G. 1965. Middle ear disease in Indians on the Mount Currie Reservation, British Columia. Can. Med. Assoc. J. 93:1301.

Cantekin, E. I., Saez, C. A., Bluestone, C. D., et al. 1979. Airflow through the Eustachian tube. Ann. Otol. Rhinol. Laryngol. 88:603.

Cawthorne, T., and Griffith, A. 1961. Primary cholesteatoma of the temporal bone. Arch. Otolaryngol. 73:252.

Cody, D. T. 1977. The definition of cholesteatoma. In McCabe, B. F., Sade, J., and Abramson, M. (eds.): Cholesteatoma: First International Conference. New York, Aesculapius Pub., pp. 6–9.

Cohn, A. M., Schwaber, M. K., Anthony, L. S., et al. 1979. Eustachian tube function and tympanoplasty. Ann. Otol. Rhinol. Laryngol. 88:339.

DeBlanc, G. B. 1975. Otologic problems in Navajo Indians of the Southwestern United States. Hear. Instrum. 26:15–16, 40–41.

Derlacki, E. L. 1973. Congenital cholesteatoma of the middle ear and mastoid. A third report. Arch. Otolaryngol. 97:177.

Derlacki, E. L., and Clemis, J. D. 1965. Congenital cholesteatoma of the middle ear and mastoid. Ann. Otol. Rhinol. Laryngol. 74:706.

Diamant, M. 1952. Chronic Otitis. A Critical Analysis. New York, S. Karger.

Dota, T., Nakamura, K., Saheki, M., et al. 1963. Cholesterol granuloma: Experimental observations. Ann. Otol. Rhinol. Laryngol. 72:346.

Downs, M. P. 1975. Hearing loss: Definition, epidemiology and prevention. Pub. Health Rev. 4:255.

Downs, M. P. 1983. Audiologist's overview of sequelae of early otitis media. Pediatrics 71:643.

Doyle, W. J. 1977. A functiono-anatomic description of Eustachian tube vector relations in four ethnic populations: An osteologic study. Microfilm, Ann Arbor, MI, University of Michigan.

Doyle, W. J., Cantekin, E. I., and Bluestone, C. D. 1980. Eustachian tube function in cleft palate children. Ann. Otol. Rhinol. Laryngol. 89(68):34.

Ekvall, L. 1970. Eustachian tube function in tympanoplasty. Acta Otolaryngol. (Stockh.) (Suppl.) 263:33.

Fairbanks, D. N. 1981. Antimicrobial therapy for chronic suppurative otitis media. Ann. Otol. Rhinol. Laryngol. 90(84):58.

Feagans, L. 1986. Otitis media: A model for long-term effects with implications for intervention. In Kavanagh, J. (ed.): Otitis Media and Child Development. Parkton, MD, York Press, pp. 192–208.

Fischler, R. S., Todd, N. W., and Feldman, C. M. 1985. Otitis media and language performance in a cohort of Apache Indian children. Am. J. Dis. Child. 139:355.

Fisher, B. 1966. The social and emotional adjustment of children with impaired hearing attending ordinary classes. Br. J. Educ. Psychol. 36:319.

Fria, T. J., Cantekin, E. I., and Eichler, J. A. 1985. Hearing acuity of children with otitis media with effusion. Arch. Otolaryngol. 111:10.

Friedberg, J., and Gillis, T. 1980. Tympanoplasty in childhood. J. Otolaryngol. 9:165.

Friedmann, I. 1959. Epidermoid cholesteatoma and cholesterol granuloma: Experimental and human. Ann. Otol. Rhinol. Laryngol. 68:57.

Friel-Patti, S., Finitzo-Hieber, T., Conti, G., et al. 1982. Language delay in infants associated with middle-ear disease and mild fluctuating hearing impairment. Pediatr. Infect. Dis. 1:104.

Fry, J., Dillane, J. B., McNab Jones, R. F., et al. 1969. The outcome of acute otitis media. (A report to the Medical Research Council). Br. J. Prev. Soc. Med. 23:205.

Glasscock, M. E. 1969. Middle fossa approach to the temporal bone: An otologic frontier. Arch. Otolaryngol. 90:15.

Glasscock, M. E. 1972. Chronic petrositis: Diagnosis and treatment. Ann. Otol. Rhinol. Laryngol. 81:677.

Glasscock, M. E. 1976. Symposium: Contraindications to tympanoplasty: II. An exercise in clinical judgment. Laryngoscope 86:70.

Glasscock, M. E. 1977. Results in cholesteatoma surgery. In McCabe, B. F., Sade, J., and Abramson, M. (eds.): Cholesteatoma: First International Conference. New York, Aesculapius Pub., pp. 401–403.

Glasscock, M. E., Dickins, J. R. E., and Wiet, R. 1981. Cholesteatoma in children. Laryngoscope 91:1743.

Goetzinger, C. P., Harrison, C., and Baer, C. J. 1964. Small perceptive hearing loss: Its effect in school-age children. Volta Rev. 66:124.

Gonzalez, C., and Bluestone, C. D. 1986. Visualization of a retraction pocket/cholesteatoma: Indications for use of the middle-ear telescope in children. Laryngoscope 96(1):109.

Gonzalez, C., Reilly, J. S., and Bluestone, C. D. 1987. Synchronous airway lesions in infancy. Ann. Otol. Rhinol. Laryngol. 96:77.

Goodey, R. J., and Smyth, G. D. 1972. Combined approach tympanoplasty in children. Laryngoscope 82:166.

Gray, S. W. 1983. Cognitive development in relation to otitis media. Pediatrics 71:645.

Grundfast, K. M., and Bluestone, C. D. 1978. Sudden or fluctuating hearing loss and vertigo in children due to perilymph fistula. Ann. Otol. Rhinol. Laryngol. 87:761.

Habermann, J. 1888. Zur Entstehung des Cholesteatoms des Mittelohrs (Cysten in der Schleimhaut der Paukenhohle, Atrophie der Nerven in der Schnecke). Arch. f. Ohrenh. (Leipz.) 27:42.

Harker, L. A., and Koontz, F. P. 1977. The bacteriology of cholesteatoma. In McCabe, B. F., Sade, J., and Abramson, M. (eds.): Cholesteatoma: First International Conference. New York, Aesculapius Pub., pp. 264–267.

Harker, L. A., and Severeid, L. R. 1982. Cholesteatoma in the cleft palate patient. In Cholesteatoma and Mastoid Surgery. Amsterdam, Kugler Publications, pp. 32–40.

Heermann, J., Jr., Heermann, H., and Kopstein, E. 1970. Fascia and cartilage palisade tympanoplasty. Arch. Otolaryngol. 91:228.

Hellman, K. 1925. Studien uber das Sekundare Cholesteatom des Felsenbeins. Z. Hals. Nas Ohrenheilk. 11:406.

Herzon, F. S. 1980. Tympanostomy tubes: Infectious complications. Arch. Otolaryngol. 106:645.

Hignett, W. 1983. Effect of otitis media on speech, language, and behavior. Ann. Otol. Rhinol. Laryngol. 92:47.

Hildmann, H., Scheerer, W. D., and Meertens, H. J. 1985. Tympanoplasty in children and anatomical variations of the epipharynx. Am. J. Otol. 6:225.

Hinchcliffe, R. 1977. Cholesteatoma: Epidemiological and quantitative aspects. In McCabe, B. F., Sade, J., and Abramson, M. (eds.): Cholesteatoma: First International Conference. New York, Aesculapius Pub., pp. 277–286.

Holm, V. A., and Kunze, L. H. 1969. Effects of chronic otitis media on language and speech development. Pediatrics 43:833.

Holmquist, J. 1968. The role of the Eustachian tube in myringoplasty. Acta Otolaryngol. (Stockh.) 66:289.

Hubbard, T. W., Paradise, J. L., McWilliams, B. J., et al. 1985. Consequences of unremitting middle-ear disease in early life: Otologic, audiologic and developmental findings in children with cleft palate. N. Engl. J. Med. 312:1529.

Igarashi, M., Konishi, S., Alford, B. R., et al. 1970. The pathology of tympanosclerosis. Laryngoscope 80:233.

Ingelstedt, S., Flisberg, K., and Ortegren, U. 1963. On the function of middle ear and Eustachian tube. Acta Otolaryngol. (Stockh.) Suppl. 182.

Jaffe, B. F. 1969. The incidence of ear disease in the Navajo Indians. Laryngoscope 79:2126.

Jansen, C. 1963. Cartilage-tympanoplasty. Laryngoscope 73:1288.

Jeang, M. K., and Fletcher, E. C. 1983. Tuberculous otitis media. J.A.M.A. 249:2231.

Juselius, H., and Kaltiokallio, K. 1972. Complications of acute and chronic otitis media in the antibiotic era. Acta Otolaryngol. (Stockh.) 74:445.

Kaplan, G. J., Fleshman, J. K., Bender, T. R., et al. 1973. Long-term effects of otitis media: A ten-year cohort study of Alaskan Eskimo children. Pediatrics 52:577.

Karma, P., Jokipii, L., Ojala, K., et al. 1978. Bacteriology of the chronically discharging middle ear. Acta Otolaryngol. (Stockh.) 86:110.

Kenna, M., Bluestone, C. D., and Reilly, J. 1986. Medical management of chronic suppurative otitis media without cholesteatoma in children. Laryngoscope 96:146.

Kessner, D., Snow, C. K., and Singer, J. 1974. Assessment of Medical Care for Children. Contrasts in Health Status, Vol. 3. Washington, DC, Institute of Medicine, National Academy of Sciences.

Khanna, S. M., and Tonndorf, J. 1972. Tympanic membrane vibrations in cats studied by time-averaged holography. J. Acoust. Soc. Am. 51:1904.

Kinney, S. E. 1978. Postinflammatory ossicular fixation in tympanoplasty. Laryngoscope 88:821.

Klein, J. O., Chase, C., Teele, D. W., et al. 1988. Otitis media and the development of speech, language, and cognitive abilities at seven years of age. In Lim, D. J., Bluestone, C. D., Klein, J. O., et al. (eds.): Recent Advances in Otitis Media. Toronto, B. C. Decker, pp. 396–397.

Kodman, F. 1963. Educational status of hard of hearing children in the classroom. J. Speech Hear. Disord. 28:297.

Kokko, E. 1974. Chronic secretory otitis media in children. Acta Otolaryngol. (Stockh.) Suppl. 327:7.

Korthals Altes, A. J. 1966. Cholesterol granuloma in the tympanic cavity. J. Laryngol. Otol. 80:691.

Lange, W. 1932. Tief Eingezogene Membrana Flaccida und Cholesteatom. Z. Hals. Nas. Ohrenheilk. 30:575.

Lau, T., and Tos, M. 1986. Tympanoplasty in children: An analysis of late results. Am. J. Otol. 7:55.

Lee, K., and Schuknecht, H. F. 1971. Results of tympanoplasty and mastoidectomy at the Massachusetts Eye and Ear Infirmary. Laryngoscope 81:529.

Levenson, M. J., Parisier, S. C., Chute, P., et al. 1986. A review of twenty congenital cholesteatomas of the middle ear in children. Otolaryngol. Head Neck Surg. 94:560.

Leviton, A., and Bellinger, D. 1985. Consequences of unremitting middle-ear infection in early life. N. Engl. J. Med. 313:1352.

Lewis, N. 1976. Otitis media and linguistic incompetence. Arch. Otolaryngol. 102:387.

Lindeman, P., and Holmquist, J. 1987. Mastoid volume and eustachian tube function in ears with cholesteatoma. Am. J. Otol. 8:5.

Linthicum, F. H., Jr. 1971. Cholesterol granuloma (iatrogenic), further evidence of etiology, a case report. Ann. Otol. Rhinol. Laryngol. 80:207.

Litman, R. S., Parisier, S. C., Hausman, S. A., et al. 1987. Bilateral congenital cholesteatoma: A cause or result of chronic otitis media with effusion? Am. J. Otol. 8:426.

Lous, J., and Fiellau-Nikolajsen, M. 1984. A 5-year prospective case-control study of the influence of early otitis media with effusion on reading achievement. Int. J. Pediatr. Otorhinolaryngol. 8:19.

Lowe, J. F., Bamforth, J. S., and Pracy, R. 1963. Acute otitis media: One year in a general practice. Lancet 2:1129.

Maharaj, D., Jadwat, A., Fernandez, C. M., et al. 1987. Bacteriology in acute mastoiditis. Arch. Otolaryngol. 113:514.

Main, T. S., Shimada, T., and Lim, D. J. 1970. Experimental cholesterol granuloma. Arch. Otolaryngol. 91:356.

Manning, S. C., Cantekin, E. I., Kenna, M. A., et al. 1987. Prognostic value of eustachian tube function in pediatric tympanoplasty. Laryngoscope 97:1012.

Mawson, S. R., and Ludman, H. 1979. Diseases of the Ear: A Textbook of Otology. Chicago, Year Book Medical Pub., pp. 378–380.

Maynard, J. E. 1969. Otitis media in Alaskan Eskimo children: An epidemiological review with observations on control. Alaska Med. 11:93.

McCafferty, G. J., Coman, W. B., Shaw, E., et al. 1977. Cholesteatoma in Australian aboriginal children. In McCabe, B., Sade, J., and Abramson, M. (eds.): Cholesteatoma: First International Conference. New York, Aesculapius Pub., pp. 293–301.

McGuckin, F. 1961. Concerning the pathogenesis of destructive ear disease. J. Laryngol. Otol. 75:949.

McKenzie, D. 1931. The pathogeny of aural cholesteatoma. J. Laryngol. Otol. 46:163.

McLelland, C. A. 1980. Incidence of complications from use of tympanostomy tubes. Arch. Otolaryngol. 106:97.

Menyuk, P. 1977. Effects of hearing loss on language acquisition in the babbling stage. In Jaffee, B. F. (ed.): Hearing Loss in Children. Baltimore, University Park Press, pp. 621–629.

Menyuk, P. 1980. Effect of persistent otitis media on language development. Ann. Otol. Rhinol. Laryngol. 89:257.

Menyuk, P. 1986. Predicting speech and language problems with persistent otitis media. In Kavanaugh, J. (ed.): Otitis Media and Child Development. Parkton, MD, York Press, pp. 83–96.

Meyerhoff, W. L., and Truelson, J. 1986. Cholesteatoma staging. Laryngoscope 96:9.

Meyerhoff, W. L., Morizono, T., Shaddock, L. C., et al. 1983. Tympanostomy tubes and otic drops. Laryngoscope 93:1022.

Miller, G. F., Jr., and Bilodeau, R. 1967. Preoperative evaluation of Eustachian tube function in tympanoplasty. South. Med. J. 60:868.

Morizono, T., Giebink, G. S., Paparella, M. M., et al. 1985. Sensorineural hearing loss in experimental purulent otitis media due to Streptococcus pneumoniae. Arch. Otolaryngol. 111:794.

Muenker, G. 1980. Results after treatment of otitis media with effusion. Ann. Otol. Rhinol. Laryngol. 89:308.

Munzel, M. A. 1978. Tympanoplasty and tuberculosis of the middle ear. Clin. Otolaryngol. 3:311.

Nager, F. 1925. The cholesteatoma of the middle ear. Ann. Otol. Rhinol. Laryngol. 34:1249.

Nager, G. T., and Vanderveen, T. S. 1976. Cholesterol granuloma involving the temporal bone. Ann. Otol. Rhinol. Laryngol. 85:204.

Needleman, H. 1977. Effects of hearing loss from early recurrent otitis media on speech and language development. In Jaffe, B. F. (ed.): Hearing Loss in Children. Baltimore, University Park Press, pp. 640–649.

Neil, J. F., Harrison, S. H., Morbry, R. D., et al. 1966. Deafness in acute otitis media. Br. Med. J. 1:75.

Ojala, L. 1957. Pneumatization of the bone and environmental factors: Experimental studies on chick humerus. Acta Otolaryngol. (Stockh.) Suppl. 133.

Ojala, L., and Saxen, A. 1952. Pathogenesis of middle ear cholesteatoma arising from Shrapnell's membrane (attic cholesteatoma). Acta Otolaryngol. (Stockh.) Suppl. 100:33.

Olmstead, R. W., Alvarez, M. C., Moroney, J. D., et al. 1964. The pattern of hearing following acute otitis media. J. Pediatr. 65:252.

Ophir, D., Porat, M., and Marshak, G. 1987. Myringoplasty in the pediatric population. Arch. Otolaryngol. Head Neck Surg. 113:1288.

Orisek, B. S., and Chole, R. A. 1987. Pressures exerted by experimental cholesteatomas. Arch. Otolaryngol. Head Neck Surg. 113:386.

Palva, A., Karma, P., and Karja, J. 1977. Cholesteatoma in children. Arch. Otolaryngol. 103:74.

Paparella, M. M. 1977. Otologic surgery in children. Otolaryngol. Clin. North Am. 10:145.

Paparella, M. M., and Lim, D. J. 1967. Pathogenesis and pathology of the "idiopathic" blue eardrum. Arch. Otolaryngol. 85:249.

Paparella, M. M., Goycoolea, M. V., and Meyerhoff, W. L. 1980. Inner ear pathology and otitis media: A review. Ann. Otol. Rhinol. Laryngol. 89:249.

Paparella, M. M., Goycoolea, M. V., Meyerhoff, W. L., et al. 1979. Endolymphatic hydrops and otitis media. Laryngoscope 89:43.

Paparella, M. M., Morizono, T., Le, C. T., et al. 1984. Sensorineural hearing loss in otitis media. Ann. Otol. Rhinol. Laryngol. 93:623.

Paparella, M. M., Oda, M., Hiraide, F., et al. 1972. Pathology of sensorineural hearing loss in otitis media. Ann. Otol. Rhinol. Laryngol. 81:632.

Paradise, J. L. 1977. On tympanostomy tubes and rationale, results, reservations, and recommendations. Pediatrics 60:86.

Paradise, J. L. 1983. Long-term effects of short-term hearing loss—menace or myth? Pediatrics 71:647.

Paradise, J. L., Bluestone, C. D., and Felder, H. 1969. The universality of otitis media in fifty infants with cleft palate. Pediatrics 44:35.

Paradise, J. L., and Rogers, K. D. 1986. On otitis media, child development, and tympanostomy tubes; New answers or old questions. Pediatrics 77:88.

Peckham, C. S., Sheridan, M., and Butler, N. R. 1972. School attainment of seven-year-old children with hearing difficulties. Dev. Med. Child. Neurol. 14:592.

Pedersen, C. B., and Zachau-Christiansen, B. 1986. Otitis media in Greenland children: Acute, chronic, and secretory otitis media in three- to eight-year-olds. J. Otolaryngol. 15:332.

Raine, C. H., and Singh, S. D. 1983. Tympanoplasty in children: A review of 114 cases. J. Laryngol. Otol. 97:217.

Ranier, A. 1938. Development and construction of the pyramidal cells. Arch. Ohren.-Nasen-U., Khelkopfh. 145:3.

Rapin, I. 1979. Conductive hearing loss effects on children's language and scholastic skills: A review of the literature. Ann. Otol. Rhinol. Laryngol. 88:3.

Ratnesar, P. 1977. Aeration: A factor in the sequelae of chronic ear disease among the Labrador and Northern Newfoundland coast. In McCabe, B., Sade, J., and Abramson, M. (eds.): Cholesteatoma: First International Conference. New York, Aesculapius Pub., pp. 302–307.

Reed, D., Struve, S., and Maynard, J. E. 1967. Otitis media and hearing deficiency among Eskimo children. A cohort study. Am. J. Public Health 57:1657.

Ritter, F. N. 1977. Complications of cholesteatoma. In McCabe, B. F., Sade, J., and Abramson, M. (eds.): Cholesteatoma: First International Conference. New York, Aesculapius Pub., pp. 430–437.

Roberts, J. E., Sanyal, M. A., Burchinal, M. R., et al. 1986. Otitis media in early childhood and its relationship to later verbal and academic performance. Pediatrics 78:423.

Ruedi, L. 1958. Cholesteatosis of the attic. J. Laryngol. Otol. 72:593.

Sade, J. 1977. Pathogenesis of attic cholesteatoma: The metaplasia theory. In McCabe, B. F., Sade, J., and Abramson, M. (eds.): Cholesteatoma: First International Conference. New York, Aesculapius Pub., pp. 212–232.

Sade, J., Avraham, S., and Brown, M. 1982. Dynamics of atelectasis and retraction pockets. In: Cholesteatoma and Mastoid Surgery. Amsterdam, Kugler Publications, pp. 267–281.

Sade, J., Halevy, A., Klajman, A., et al.: 1980. Cholesterol granuloma. Acta Otolaryngol. (Stockh.) 89:233.

Sak, R. J., and Ruben, R. J. 1982. Recurrent middle-ear effusion in childhood: Implications of temporary auditory deprivation for language and learning. Ann. Otol. Rhinol. Laryngol. 90:546.

Sanna, M., Zini, C., Gamoletti, R., et al. 1987. The surgical management of childhood cholesteatoma. J. Laryngol. Otol. 101:1221.

Saunders, W. H., Paparella, M. M., and Miglets, A. 1986. Atlas of Ear Surgery, 4th ed. St. Louis, The C. V. Mosby Co.

Schiff, M., Poliquin, J. F., Catanzaro, A., et al. 1980. Tympanosclerosis: A theory of pathogenesis. Ann. Otol. Rhinol. Laryngol. 89:1.

Schlieper, A., Kisilevsky, H., Mattingly, H., et al. 1985. Mild conductive hearing loss and language development: A one-year follow-up study. Dev. Behav. Pediatr. 6:65.

Schuknecht, H. F. 1974. Pathology of the Ear. Cambridge, MA, Harvard University Press, pp. 227–233.

Senturia, B. H., Bluestone, C. D., Lim, D. J., et al. 1980a. Recent advances in otitis media with effusion. Ann. Otol. Rhinol. Laryngol. 89, Suppl. 68.

Senturia, B. H., Marcus, M. D., and Lucente, F. E. 1980b. Diseases of the External Ear: An Otologic-Dermatologic Manual, 2nd ed. New York, Grune & Stratton.

Severeid, L. R. 1977. Development of cholesteatoma in children with cleft palate: A longitudinal study. In McCabe, B. F., Sade, J., and Abramson, M. (eds.): Cholesteatoma: First International Conference. New York, Aesculapius Pub., pp. 287–292.

Shambaugh, G. E., and Glasscock, M. E. 1980. Surgery of the Ear, 3rd ed. Philadelphia, W. B. Saunders Co., pp. 432–436.

Sheehy, J. C. 1978. Management of cholesteatoma in children. Adv. Otorhinolaryngol. 23:58.

Sheehy, J. L. 1985. Cholesteatoma surgery in children. Am. J. Otol. 6:170.

Sheehy, J. L., and Anderson, R. G. 1980. Myringoplasty: A review of 472 cases Ann. Otol. Rhinol. Laryngol. 89:331.

Sheehy, J. L., Brachman, D. E., and Graham, M. D. 1977. Complications of cholesteatoma: A report on 1024 cases. In McCabe, B. F., Sade, J., and Abramson, M. (eds.): Cholesteatoma: First International Conference. New York, Aesculapius Pub., pp. 420–429.

Sheehy, J. L., Linthicum, F. H., Jr., and Greenfield, E. C. 1969. Chronic serous mastoiditis, idiopathic hemotympanum and cholesterol granuloma of the mastoid. Laryngoscope 79:1189.

Sheehy, J. L., and Patterson, M. E. 1967. Intact canal wall tympanoplasty with mastoidectomy: A review of 8 years' experience. Laryngoscope 77:1502.

Siedentop, K. H. 1968. Eustachian tube dynamics, size of the mastoid air cell system, and results with tympanoplasty. Otolaryngol. Clin. North Am. 1:33.

Smyth, G. D. 1972. Tympanic reconstruction. Otolaryngol. Clin. North Am. 5:111.

Smyth, G. D. 1977. Postoperative cholesteatoma. In McCabe, B. F., Sade, J., and Abramson, M. (eds.): Cholesteatoma: First International Conference. New York, Aesculapius Pub. pp. 355–362.

Smyth, G. D. L., and Hassard, T. H. 1980. Tympanoplasty in children. Am. J. Otol. 1:119.

Sobol, S. M., Reichert, T. J., Faw, K. D., et al. 1980. Intramembranous and mesotympanic cholesteatomas associated with an intact tympanic membrane in children. Ann. Otol. Rhinol. Laryngol. 89:312.

Solomon, N. E., and Harris, L. J. 1976. Otitis media in children: Assessing the quality of medical care using short-term outcome measures. Quality of medical care assessment using short-term outcome measurement: Eight disease-specific applications. Rand Report R-2021/2-HEW, Rand Corp., Santa Monica, CA, p. 589.

Sorensen, H. 1977. Antibiotics in suppurative otitis media. Otolaryngol. Clin. North Am. 10:45.

Stool, S. E., and Randall, P. 1967. Unexpected ear disease in infants with cleft palate. Cleft Palate J. 4:99.

Storrs, L. A. 1976. Contraindications to tympanoplasty. Laryngoscope 86:79.

Supance, J. S., and Bluestone, C. D. 1983. Perilymph fistulas in infants and children. Otolaryngol. Head Neck Surg. 91:663.

Teed, R. W. 1936. Cholesteatoma verum tympani. Its relationship to first epibranchial placode. Arch. Otolaryngol. 24:455.

Teele, D. W., Klein, J. O., Rosner, B. A., and the Greater Boston Otitis Media Study Group. 1984. Otitis media with effusion during the first three years of life and development of speech and language. Pediatrics 74:282.

Todd, N. W., and Bowman, C. A. 1985. Otitis media at Canyon Day, Arizona: A 16-year follow-up in Apache Indians. Arch. Otolaryngol. 111:606.

Tos, M. 1983. Treatment of cholesteatoma in children. A long-term study of results. Am. J. Otol. 4:189.

Tschopp, C. F. 1977. Chronic otitis media and cholesteatoma in Alaskan native children. In McCabe, B., Sade, J., and Abramson, M. (eds.): Cholesteatoma: First International Conference. New York, Aesculapius Pub., pp. 290–292.

Tumarkin, A. 1938. A contribution to the study of middle ear suppuration with special reference to the pathogeny and treatment of cholesteatoma. J. Laryngol. Otol. 53:685.

Valvassori, G. E., and Buckingham, R. A. 1974. Middle ear masses mimicking glomus tumors: Radiographic and otoscopic recognition. Ann. Otol. Rhinol. Laryngol. 83:606.

Vartiainen, E., and Karjalainen, S. 1987. Factors influencing sensorineural hearing loss in chronic otitis media. Am. J. Otolaryngol. 8:13.

Ventry, I. M. 1983. Research design issues in studies of effects of middle-ear effusion. Pediatrics 71:644.

Virtanen, H., Palva, T., and Jauhiainen, T. 1980. The prognostic value of Eustachian tube function measurements in tympanoplastic surgery. Acta Otolaryngol. (Stockh.) 90:317.

vonTroltsch, A. F. 1869. Handbuch der Ohrenheilkunde. Leipzig, W. Engelmann.

Walby, A. P., Barrera, A., and Schuknecht, H. F. 1983. Cochlear pathology in chronic suppurative otitis media. Ann. Otol. Rhinol. Laryngol. 92 (Suppl. 103).

Watanabe, H., Shin, T., Fukaura, J., et al. 1985. Total actual speaking time in infants and children with otitis media with effusion. Int. J. Pediatr. Otorhinolaryngol. 10:171.

Webster, D. B. 1983. Conductive loss affects auditory neural soma size only during a sensitive postnatal period. In Lim, D. J., Bluestone, C. D., Klein, J. O., et al. (eds.): Recent Advances in Otitis Media with Effusion. Burlington, Ontario, B. C. Decker Inc., pp. 344–346.

Weiderhold, M. L., Zajtchuk, J. T., Vap, J. G., et al. 1980. Hearing loss in relation to physical properties of middle-ear effusions. Ann. Otol. Rhinol. Laryngol. 89:185.

Wendt, H. 1873. Desquamative Entzundung des Mittelohrs (Cholesteatom des Felsenbeins). Arch. Ohren-heilk. (Leipzig) 14:428.

Wiet, R. J. 1979. Patterns of ear disease in the Southwestern American Indian. Arch. Otolaryngol. 105:381.

Wiet, R. J., DeBlanc, G. B., Stewart, J., et al. 1980. Natural history of otitis media in the American native. Ann. Otol. Rhinol. Laryngol. 89(68):14.

Willis, R. 1985. Otitis media and the Australian aboriginal. Am. J. Otol. 6:316.

Wishik, S. M., Kramm, E. R., and Koch, E. M. 1958. Audiometric testing of school children. Public Health Rep. 73:265.

Wittmaack, K. 1933. Wie ensteht ein genuines Cholesteatom? Arch. f. Ohren-Nasen-u. Kehlkopfh. 137:306.

Wolfman, D. E., and Chole, R. A. 1986. Experimental retraction pocket cholesteatoma. Ann. Otol. Rhinol. Laryngol. 95:639.

Young, C., and McConnell, F. 1957. Retardation of vocabulary development in hard of hearing children. Except. Child Ann. 368–370.

Zinkus, P. W., Gottlieb, M. I., and Schapiro, M. 1978. Developmental and psychoeducational sequelae of chronic otitis media. Am. J. Dis. Child. 132:1100.

Zollner, F. 1956. Tympanosclerosis. J. Laryngol. Otol. 70:77.

Zonis, R. D. 1970. Chronic otitis media in the Arizona Indian. Arizona Med. 27:1.

Chapter 23

INTRACRANIAL SUPPURATIVE COMPLICATIONS OF OTITIS MEDIA AND MASTOIDITIS

Charles D. Bluestone, M.D.   Jerome O. Klein, M.D.

There has been an overall decline in the incidence of suppurative intracranial complications of otitis media since the advent of antimicrobial agents. Today, these complications occur more often in association with chronic suppurative otitis media and mastoiditis, with or without cholesteatoma, than in association with acute otitis media (Juselius and Kaltiokallio, 1972).

The middle ear and mastoid air cells are adjacent to important structures, including the dura of the posterior and middle cranial fossa, the sigmoid venous sinus of the brain, and the inner ear. Suppuration in the middle ear or mastoid, or both, may spread to these structures, producing the following suppurative intracranial complications: meningitis, extradural abscess, subdural empyema, focal encephalitis, brain abscess, lateral (sigmoid) sinus thrombosis, and otitic hydrocephalus (Fig. 23–1).

Multiple complications are frequently dependent on the route of infection. Thus, a patient may have meningitis, lateral sinus thrombosis, and a cerebellar abscess or other combinations of suppurative disease involving adjacent areas.

Any child who has acute or chronic otitis media who develops one or more of the following signs or symptoms, especially while receiving medical treatment, should be suspected of having a suppurative intracranial complication: persistent headache, lethargy, malaise, irritability, severe otalgia, onset of fever, nausea, and vomiting. The following would be definitive signs and symptoms demanding an intensive search for an intracranial complication: stiff neck, focal seizures, ataxia, blurred vision, papilledema, diplopia, hemiplegia, aphasia, dysdiadochokinesia, intention tremor, dysmetria, and hemianopsia. Conversely, children

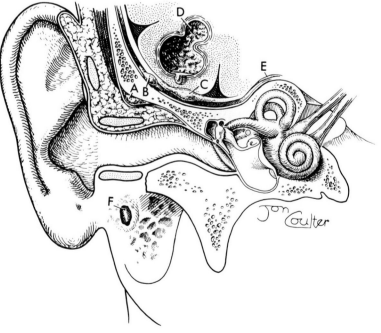

Figure 23–1. Suppurative complications of otitis media and mastoiditis. *A*, Subperiosteal abscess; *B*, extradural abscess; *C*, subdural empyema; *D*, brain abscess; *E*, meningitis; *F*, lateral sinus thrombosis.

with intracranial infection, such as meningitis or a brain abscess, must have middle ear–mastoid disease ruled out as the origin of, or concomitant with, the central nervous system disease.

In children who have acute or chronic suppurative otitis media, the presence of headache, even though a nonspecific symptom, should indicate a potential complication. Irritability, lethargy, or other changes in personality may be secondary to intracranial spread of the infection. Even though fever is common when acute infection of the ear is present, persistent or recurrent fever may be a potentially dangerous sign. Fever is rarely present in children with chronic suppurative otitis media and, when present, may be a hallmark of an impending intracranial complication.

The diagnosis of intracranial complications has been greatly improved since the advent of the widespread availability and use of computed tomography (CT), but when it is not available, arteriography should be used. Magnetic resonance imaging (MRI) is not as widely available as CT but provides excellent resolution of intracranial suppuration and its consequences (edema, thrombosis, hydrocephalus) (Chap. 10).

Intracranial extension of infection may take place because of (1) progressive thrombophlebitis permitting the inflammatory process to spread through the intact bone (osteothrombophlebitis), (2) erosion of the bony walls of the middle ear or mastoid (osteitis), and (3) extension along preformed pathways—the round window, dehiscent sutures, skull fracture, or congenital or surgically acquired bony dehiscences (mastoidectomy with dura exposure).

In this chapter, the incidence, pathogenesis, etiology, diagnosis, management, and outcome for each of these complications as they relate to children will be presented. Following the description of the specific complications, a section on timing and type of otologic surgery appropriate for children is provided, but a detailed description of the operative procedures has not been included, since the latest otologic and neurologic surgical techniques are adequately described and illustrated in currently available texts that are listed at the end of the chapter (see Selected References).

INCIDENCE

Prior to the introduction of antimicrobial agents, 2.3 per cent of all patients with acute and chronic suppurative otitis media developed intracranial complications, and two thirds of the cases were due to chronic disease of the middle ear (Turner and Reynolds, 1931). In the antibiotic era, intracranial complications are uncommon, but approximately two thirds are still caused by chronic ear disease (Jeanes, 1962). However, Dawes (1979) reported that most intracranial complications in children were secondary to acute otitis media. Ritter (1977) reviewed 152 cases of cholesteatoma, about half of which were present in patients younger than 20 years of age. The study, which rep-

resented patients seen between 1965 and 1970, included four cases with suppurative intracranial complications: two patients with sigmoid sinus thrombosis and one patient each with an extradural abscess and a brain abscess. In a review by Sheehy and colleagues (1977), of 1024 operations in 949 patients, 17.7 per cent of whom were 15 years of age or younger, performed during the years 1965 through 1974, only one patient had meningitis, and in only two patients was an extradural abscess present. However, neither of these complications occurred in children. The relative incidence of suppurative intracranial complications of acute and chronic otitis media is indicated in a report of 29 consecutive cases treated at a medical center in Finland during the years 1965 through 1971 (Table 23–1). Meningitis was the most common of these complications even in the antibiotic era (Krajina, 1956; Proctor, 1966). In a more recent report from North Carolina by Gower and associates (1985), 84 infants and children were diagnosed and treated for intracranial complications of ear disease between the years 1963 and 1982. Of the 84 patients, 65 (77 per cent) had otitic meningitis, eight (10 per cent) had either otitic subdural empyema or effusion, four (5 per cent) had brain abscess, four (5 per cent) had otitic hydrocephalus, and three (4 per cent) had lateral sinus thrombosis.

MENINGITIS

Meningitis may be associated with infections of the middle ear in three circumstances: (1) direct invasion, in which a suppurative focus in the middle ear or mastoid spreads through the dura and extends to the pia-arachnoid, causing generalized meningitis; (2) inflammation in an adjacent area, in which the meninges may become inflamed if there is suppuration in an adjacent area such as a subdural abscess, brain abscess, or lateral sinus thrombophlebitis; (3) concurrent infection, in which otitis media arises by contiguous spread from an infectious focus in the upper respiratory tract, and meningitis results from invasion of the blood from the upper respiratory focus. The infections are simul-

TABLE 23–1. Suppurative Intracranial Complications of Acute or Chronic Otitis Media in 29 Children and Adults Treated at the Vasa Center Hospital (Vasa, Finland)

	ACUTE OTITIS MEDIA	CHRONIC OTITIS MEDIA	TOTAL
Meningitis	9	5	14
Extradural or perisinuous abscess	3	5	8
Lateral sinus thrombosis	2	3	5
Temporal lobe abscess	0	2	2
TOTAL	14	15	29

Adapted from Juselius, H., and Kaltiokallio, K. 1972. Complications of acute and chronic otitis media in the antibiotic era. Acta Otolaryngol. (Stockh.) 74:445–450.

taneous, but meningitis does not arise from the middle-ear infection.

The most common route is the third, hematogenous spread. Less common is direct invasion through congenital preformed pathways or by thrombophlebitis, which usually extends to the middle cranial fossa through the petrosquamous suture or to the posterior cranial fossa through the subarcuate fossa, that is, the first route. In the preantibiotic era, Lindsay (1938) examined the histopathology of temporal bones of patients who had acute otitis media and meningitis and found that most of the specimens had evidence of direct spread of the infection through the petrous apex. However, since the advent of the widespread use of antimicrobial agents, extension of the infection has been thought to be along preformed pathways or by direct extension through the dura. Spread of infection from the middle ear and mastoid through the inner ear to the meninges is another pathway but is thought to be rare compared to the other pathogenic mechanisms. More recently, Eavey and coworkers (1985) examined 16 temporal bones from children who had died of meningitis and found otitis media in 14 bones but could not find any evidence that the middle-ear infection had spread to the meninges.

The symptoms of meningitis caused by any of the three mechanisms include fever, headache, neck stiffness, and altered consciousness. A CT scan should be considered prior to lumbar puncture if there are signs of increased intracranial pressure to define the presence of abscess or mass effect. Examination of cerebrospinal fluid reveals pleocytosis and elevation of protein concentration in all routes of infection, but depression of sugar levels is common in only the first and third routes. Polymorphonuclear leukocytes are the predominant cell type in the early phase of meningitis caused by the first and third mechanisms. When infection occurs by the second mechanism, it is likely to be more chronic; therefore, lymphocytes usually predominate. Organisms are usually isolated from the spinal fluid when meningitis is caused by the first and third mechanisms but not by the second one. Thus, meningitis from the second mechanism may be defined as an aseptic meningitis (clinical signs of meningitis associated with cells in the cerebrospinal fluid but without bacteria isolated by usual laboratory techniques). Gower and colleagues (1985) provide information about 65 children and adults with suppurative intracranial complications of acute or chronic otitis media (Table 23–2).

The organisms responsible for meningitis are associated with acute otitis media, and the common agents of meningitis are *Streptococcus pneumoniae* and *Haemophilus influenzae* Type b. About 20 per cent of all cases of acute otitis media are due to *H. influenzae*, but less than 10 per cent of these are Type b (Harding et al., 1973). Feigin (1981) reported that 14 per cent of children with *H. influenzae* Type b otitis media also had meningitis.

Initial management of meningitis involves the

TABLE 23–2. Age of Infants and Children with Meningitic Complication Related to Stage of Ear Disease Treated at the Wake Forest University Medical Center 1963–1982

AGE	ACUTE EAR DISEASE	CHRONIC EAR DISEASE	TOTAL
≤ 12 mo	38	1	39
13–24 mo	15	2	17
2–5 yr	4	0	4
6–10 yr	1	0	1
11–20 yr	0	4	4
TOTAL	58	7	65

Adapted by permission from the Southern Medical Journal (Volume 78, pages 429–434, 1985).

administration of high doses of antimicrobial agents. If the causative agent is unknown, ampicillin and chloramphenicol or a third-generation cephalosporin, ceftriaxone or cefotaxime, are administered (see Chap. 21, Table 21–25). The regimen may be modified after the results of cultures are known. If the cultures are negative and there is concern that a suppurative focus may be producing the aseptic process, diagnostic tests should be performed to identify the focus, to obtain material for culture, and to clear, usually by incision and drainage, the local infection. If acute or chronic otitis media is present, then tympanocentesis, for identification of the causative organism within the middle ear, and myringotomy, for drainage, should be performed immediately. If acute mastoiditis with osteitis is present, a complete simple mastoidectomy is indicated as soon as the child is able to tolerate a general anesthetic. If chronic suppurative otitis media with or without cholesteatoma is present, then a radical mastoidectomy is frequently required and should be performed when the patient's condition is stable. Appropriate management of any of the suppurative intratemporal complications, such as petrositis or labyrinthitis, or intracranial complications, such as an extradural abscess, will also require surgical intervention.

Occasionally, following trauma to the temporal bone, acute otitis media develops that is complicated by meningitis. Tympanocentesis and myringotomy should be performed immediately for culture and drainage or culture of the otorrhea, if present. However, exploration of the middle ear and mastoid may be necessary later to search for and repair possible defects in the dura, especially if cerebrospinal fluid otorrhea is present.

Appropriate management of both the meningitis and the suppurative focus within the temporal bone should result in a favorable outcome, although many studies still report a considerable mortality associated with otitic meningitis. Kessler and coworkers (1970) reported a mortality rate of 33 per cent in their series of 51 cases of otitic meningitis. In the study by Gower and associates (1985), a seven per cent mortality was reported in 58 patients (mostly infants), but a 43 per cent mortality rate was reported in the seven patients who developed meningitis secondary to chronic ear disease. Overall mortality was 10.7 per cent.

EXTRADURAL ABSCESS

Extradural (epidural) abscess usually results from the destruction of bone adjacent to dura by cholesteatoma or infection, or both. This occurs when granulation tissue and purulent material collect between the lateral aspect of the dura and adjacent temporal bone. Dural granulation tissue within a bony defect is much more common than an actual accumulation of pus. When an abscess is present, a dural sinus thrombosis or, less commonly, a subdural or brain abscess may also be present. If extensive bone destruction has occurred when acute mastoid osteitis (acute "coalescent" mastoiditis) is present, an extradural abscess may develop in the area of the sigmoid dural sinus.

Symptoms can include severe earache, low-grade fever, and headache in the temporal region with deep local throbbing pain, but the more common extradural abscess encountered today may produce no signs or symptoms. Frequently, an asymptomatic extradural abscess is found in patients undergoing elective mastoidectomy for cholesteatoma.

When otorrhea accompanies an extradural abscess, it is characteristically profuse, creamy, and pulsatile. Compression of the ipsilateral jugular vein may increase the rate of discharge and the degree of pulsation. Usually there is no accompanying fever, but malaise and anorexia may be observed. Usually, there are no neurologic signs, the intracranial pressure is normal, and it is difficult to detect any displacement of the brain. Cerebrospinal fluid cell count and pressure are normal unless meningitis is also present. Computed tomography may demonstrate a sizable extradural abscess (Fig. 23–2).

Although identification of the infecting organism and appropriate antimicrobial therapy can help prevent the development of an intradural complication from an extradural abscess, the treatment of extradural abscess itself consists of surgical drainage. A mastoidectomy is performed, enough bone is removed so that the dura of the middle and posterior fossae may be inspected directly, the extradural abscess is identified and removed (and in some instances a drain is also inserted), and the otologic procedure that will provide optimal exteriorization of the diseased area is completed by removing all the granulation tissue until normal dura is found.

SUBDURAL EMPYEMA

A subdural empyema is a collection of purulent material within the potential space between the dura externally and arachnoid membrane internally. Since the pus collects in a preformed space, it is correctly termed empyema rather than abscess. Subdural em-

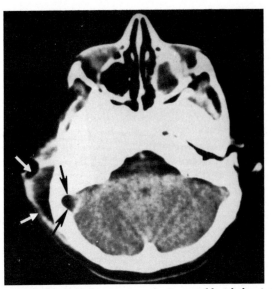

Figure 23–2. Computed tomogram of a 9-year-old girl showing a right perisinuous extradural abscess (black arrows) as a complication of acute mastoiditis with osteitis and a subperiosteal abscess (white arrows). There had been a one-week history of hearing loss, otalgia, and a profuse, foul-smelling otorrhea, and a three-day history of high fever, postauricular swelling, disorientation, and irritability, which persisted in spite of parenterally administered antimicrobial agents. A complete simple mastoidectomy and drainage of the extradural abscess resulted in a favorable outcome.

pyema may develop as a direct extension of infection or, more rarely, by thrombophlebitis through venous channels. It is one of the rarer complications of otitis media and mastoiditis.

Children with subdural empyema are extremely toxic and febrile. There are usually the signs and symptoms of a locally expanding intracranial mass. Severe headache in the temporoparietal area is usually present. Central nervous system findings may include seizures, hemiplegia, dysmetria, belligerent behavior, somnolence, stupor, deviation of the eyes, dysphagia, sensory deficits, stiff neck, and a positive Kernig sign. Hemiplegia and jacksonian epilepsy in a child with suppurative disease of the middle ear and mastoid usually are indicative of a subdural empyema. Computed tomography is often diagnostic of the process. The peripheral white blood cell count is high, and there is a predominance of polymorphonuclear leukocytes. The cerebrospinal fluid glucose concentration is normal, and no microorganisms are seen on smear or culture of the cerebrospinal fluid.

Treatment of subdural empyema includes intensive intravenous antimicrobial therapy, anticonvulsants, and neurosurgical drainage of the empyema through burr holes or craniectomy. Corticosteroids are occasionally needed to diminish severe edema in spite of their effects on the inflammatory response. Mastoid surgery to locate and drain the source of infection is usually delayed until after neurosurgical intervention has yielded some improvement in neurologic status. The condition still has a high mortality rate, and more than half of those children who recover will have some neurologic deficit.

FOCAL OTITIC ENCEPHALITIS

Focal areas of the brain may become edematous and inflamed as a complication of acute or chronic otitis media or of one or more of the suppurative complications of these disorders, such as an extradural abscess or dural sinus thrombophlebitis. This localized inflammation is called focal otitic encephalitis, the signs and symptoms of which may be similar to those that are characteristic of a brain abscess, except that suppuration within the brain is absent. Ataxia, nystagmus, vomiting, and giddiness would indicate a possible focus within the cerebellum, whereas drowsiness, disorientation, restlessness, seizures, and coma may indicate a cerebral focus. In both sites, headache may be present. However, since these signs and symptoms are also commonly associated with a brain abscess or subdural empyema, needle aspiration may be necessary to rule out the presence of an abscess. Computed tomography is helpful in making this distinction. If an abscess is not thought to be present, then the focal encephalitis should be treated by administering therapeutic doses of antimicrobial agents and by an appropriate otologic surgical procedure to remove the infection performed as soon as possible, since failure to control the source of the infection within the temporal bone, as well as the focal encephalitis, may result in the development of a brain abscess. Anticonvulsive medication is given when there is cerebral involvement.

BRAIN ABSCESS

Of all age groups, infants and children have the highest incidence of brain abscess (Brewer et al., 1975). However, the incidence of brain abscess has decreased significantly in the antibiotic era. From 1930 to 1960, there were 89 cases of otogenic brain abscess at the Otolaryngological Hospital of the University of Helsinki, whereas between 1961 and 1969, there were only three cases (Tarkkanen and Kohonen, 1970). Several studies have reported that infection of the middle ear and mastoid was the predominant source of infection when abscess in the brain occurred in children (Beller et al., 1973; Liske and Weikers, 1964; Morgan et al., 1973). However, Jadavji and coworkers (1985) reviewed 74 cases of brain abscess diagnosed at Toronto Hospital for Sick Children between 1960 and 1984 and found cyanotic congenital heart disease (24 per cent) was the most common cause; 10 children (14 per cent) had chronic otitis media with or without mastoiditis. Chronic suppurative otitis media with cholesteatoma is thought to be more commonly the cause when brain abscess is present, but Browning (1984) reviewed 26 consecutive patients with brain abscess and found that 10 of them had chronic ear disease without cholesteatoma.

Otogenic abscess of the brain may follow directly from acute or chronic middle ear and mastoid infection or may follow the development of an adjacent infection, such as lateral sinus thrombophlebitis, petrositis, or meningitis. The dura overlying the infected mastoid is invaded either along vascular pathways or by adherence of the dura to underlying infected bone. Chronic otitis media or mastoiditis with or without cholesteatoma may lead to erosion of the tegmen tympani by pressure necrosis and perforation of the bone with resultant inflammation of the dura and invasion by pathogenic organisms. An extradural abscess occurs with subsequent infiltration of the dura and spreads to the subdural space. A localized subdural abscess or leptomeningitis ensues. Invasion of brain tissue follows, and the various stages of abscess formation take place: inflammatory reaction, suppuration, necrosis and liquefaction, and development of a fibrinous capsule. If delimitation of the abscess does not occur, infection may rarely extend to the meninges or may rupture into the ventricles.

The site of the abscess is the area closest to the primary source of infection. Thus, temporal lobe abscesses occur following invasion through the tegmen tympani or petrous bone. Cerebellar abscesses occur when the infectious focus is the posterior surface of the petrous bone or thrombophlebitis of the lateral sinus. An abscess in the temporal lobe occurs more commonly than does one in the cerebellum, and multiple abscesses are not uncommon.

The natural history of brain abscesses if left untreated includes resorption and healing through gliosis and calcification, spontaneous rupture through a fistulous tract, or spillage into the ventricles or subarachnoid space, producing encephalitis or meningitis.

The bacterial pathogens responsible for brain abscesses include the virulent invasive strains associated with acute disease of the middle ear or the more indolent strains associated with chronic disease (Brewer et al., 1975). These include the following: (1) gram-positive cocci—Group A *Streptococcus*, *S. pneumoniae*, *S. viridans*, and *Staphylococcus aureus*; (2) gram-negative coccobacilli—*H. influenzae* and *H. aphrophilus*; (3) gram-negative enteric bacilli—*Escherichia coli*, *Proteus*, *Enterobacter aerogenes*, *E. cloacae*, and *Pseudomonas aeruginosa*; (4) anaerobic bacteria—*Eubacterium*, *Bacteroides*, *Peptostreptococcus*, and *Propionibacterium acnes* (Heineman and Braude, 1963).

Signs and symptoms of invasion of the central nervous system usually occur about a month after an episode of acute otitis media or an acute exacerbation of chronic otitis media. Most children are febrile, although systemic signs, including fever and chills, are variable and may be absent. Signs of a generalized central nervous system infection include severe headache, vomiting, drowsiness, seizures, irritability, personality changes, altered levels of consciousness, anorexia and weight loss, and meningismus. In addition to these signs of an expanding intracranial lesion, there may be specific signs of involvement of the temporal or cerebellar lobes. Temporal lobe abscesses are associated with seizures in some children and may be associated with visual field deficits (optic radiation involvement) or may be silent. Cerebellar abscesses cause vertigo, nystagmus, ataxia, dysmetria, and symptoms of hydrocephalus. There may be persistent purulent ear drainage, suggesting the primary site of infection. Terminal signs include coma, papilledema, or cardiovascular changes.

Diagnosis is based on development of clinical signs, the results of electroencephalography, and roentgenographic evidence. Computed tomography is an invaluable aid in diagnosis (Fig. 23–3). Radionuclide brain scans can be abnormal when focal encephalitis or a brain abscess is present. Of particular concern is the sudden appearance of signs of acute disease—fever and headache—in a patient with chronic disease of the middle ear.

Lumbar puncture is not recommended owing to the possibility of herniation of the brain and death and should be performed only after a CT scan shows no mass effect or hydrocephalus. However, when it is performed, the cerebrospinal fluid may be normal if the abscess is deep in the tissue and does not produce inflammation of the meninges, or if it does, there may be an increased number of cells, initially a predominance of polymorphonuclear leukocytes, then lymphocytes. The concentration of protein may be high, but the sugar level is not usually reduced unless there is bacterial invasion of the meninges. Cultures of the spinal fluid are usually negative in the absence of suppurative meningitis.

Treatment includes use of antimicrobial agents, drainage or resection of the brain abscess, or both, as well as the surgical débridement of the primary focus, the mastoid, or adjacent infected tissues such as thrombophlebitis of the lateral sinus. The choice of the most appropriate antimicrobial regimen is difficult because

of the varied bacteriology of otogenic brain abscess. Aspiration of the abscess to define the etiology is most helpful (Garfield, 1979). Initial therapy should include administration of a penicillin for gram-positive cocci, an aminoglycoside for gram-negative enteric pathogens, and chloramphenicol to combat gram-negative organisms and, more important, anaerobic bacteria (see Chap. 21, Table 21–25). Even with the administration of antimicrobial agents, the mortality rate of patients with brain abscess has been approximately 30 per cent (McGreal, 1962; Morgan et al., 1973). The best results, a zero mortality rate, were reported in brain abscesses in children treated by catheter drainage (Selker, 1975). More recently, reports have described successful medical treatment of brain abscess without neurosurgical intervention (Berg et al., 1978; Keven and Tyrell, 1984; Rennels et al., 1983).

LATERAL SINUS THROMBOSIS

Lateral and sigmoid sinus thrombosis or thrombophlebitis arises from inflammation in the adjacent mastoid. The superior and petrosal dural sinuses also are intimately associated with the temporal bone, but they are rarely affected. The mastoid infection in contact with the sinus walls produces inflammation of the adventitia, followed by penetration of the venous wall. Formation of a thrombus occurs after the infection has spread to the intima. The mural thrombus may become infected and may propagate, occluding the lumen. Embolization of septic thrombi or extension of infection into the tributary vessels may produce further disease.

This complication is still common in children. Of the 13 patients who had otogenic lateral sinus disease at the Groote Schurr Hospital in South Africa during the period from 1967 to 1970, nine were younger than 20 years of age; six children had chronic ear infections, and three had acute ear infections (Seid and Sellars, 1973). In a more recent report from the same country, Samuel and Fernandes (1987) treated 45 black patients with lateral sinus thrombosis between 1978 and 1984; all but three patients were 20 years of age or younger. Their patients had chronic otorrhea, as did the patients reported by Teichgraeber and associates (1982). However, Gower and McQuirt (1983) reported that 83 per cent of their patients had lateral sinus thrombosis as a complication of acute otitis media. It is apparent that this complication can be caused by both acute and chronic otitis media and mastoiditis.

The clinical signs of lateral sinus thrombosis may be grouped as follows:

1. General—fever, headache, and malaise. With the formation of the infectious mural thrombus, the patient may have spiking fever and chills.

2. Central nervous system—headache, papilledema, signs of increased intracranial pressure, altered states of consciousness, and seizures.

3. Metastatic disease caused by infected thrombi and septic infarcts—pneumonia, septic infarcts, em-

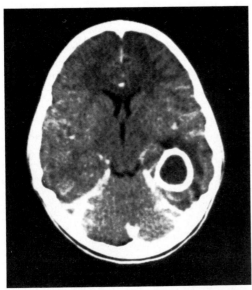

Figure 23–3. Computed tomogram of a 14-year-old boy showing a brain abscess as a complication of chronic suppurative otitis media with an attic cholesteatoma. There had been an eight-week history of persistent aural discharge, lethargy, and progressive hearing loss, and a four-week history of vomiting and headache. Physical examination revealed papilledema and bilateral abducens palsy. Complete recovery followed neurosurgical removal of the abscess and a radical mastoidectomy.

pyema, bone and joint infection, and, less commonly, thyroiditis, endocarditis, ophthalmitis, and abscess of the kidney (Rosenwasser, 1945).

4. Spread to skin and soft tissues—cellulitis or abscess.

5. Signs of intracranial complications, including meningitis, cavernous sinus thrombosis, and brain abscess.

In Rosenwasser's series of 100 patients (1945), the specific years of the cases are not mentioned. However, only 19 patients received sulfonamides, so presumably most were evaluated prior to 1935. Bacteremia was frequent. Eighty to 100 patients had presurgical cultures of the blood that were positive. Eight to 17 patients whose cultures had been negative preoperatively had positive cultures postoperatively. Bacteremia persisted after the operation in 36 patients for a median of 4 to 5 days and a range of 1 to 24 days. The predominant organism was beta-hemolytic streptococci (68 patients), with *Streptococcus pneumoniae* Type 3 (3), *Proteus* species (2), *Staphylococcus aureus* (1), and *P. aeruginosa* (1) also being found.

Computed tomography and, more recently, magnetic resonance imaging are invaluable aids in making the diagnosis and should precede a lumbar puncture (Fig. 23–4). Variations in cerebrospinal fluid pressure occur and can be demonstrated by the Queckenstedt test, which measures changes in cerebrospinal fluid pressure with compression and release of the jugular vein. If the sinus is occluded, there is no rise in pressure when the jugular vein of the affected side is compressed, whereas compression of the contralateral jugular vein results in a brisk rise and fall in pressure. However, if the intracranial pressure is increased, the brain may herniate. In addition to this potential danger, the Queckenstedt test may be negative or inconclusive (Juselius and Kaltiokallio, 1972), and its risks now outweigh its benefits. There are usually no other abnormalities in the cerebrospinal fluid, although in some cases, leakage of red cells and subsequent xanthochromia may occur (Greer and Berk, 1963).

Management includes the use of antimicrobial agents (as described in the section on mastoiditis in Chap. 22) and surgery. The administration of anticoagulant medication has also been advocated. However, some clinicians advise against the use of anticoagulants because of a fear that when a septic thrombophlebitis is present, septic emboli could be released, and the potential complication of uncontrollable hemorrhage in the mastoid (Samuel and Fernandes, 1987). The sinus should be uncovered, and any perisinous abscesses should be drained. The lateral sinus should be opened, and the thrombus removed. If a septic thrombophlebitis is absent, some clinicians believe that the clot should not be evacuated in this, the antibiotic era. On rare occasions, the internal jugular vein may have to be ligated. For a complete description of the surgical technique, see Shambaugh and Glasscock (1980).

The mortality in the Rosenwasser series was 27 per cent, with an increased risk in patients older than 30 years of age. The mortality rate is still high and has been reported in a large series of cases to be between 10 and 40 per cent (Teichgraeber et al., 1982; Samuel and Fernandes, 1987). Not much has changed with regard to mortality resulting from this intracranial complication 40 years after the introduction of antimicrobial agents.

OTITIC HYDROCEPHALUS

The term "otitic hydrocephalus" was introduced by Symonds in 1931 to describe a syndrome of increased intracranial pressure but with no abnormalities of the cerebrospinal fluid complicating acute otitis media. The pathogenesis of the syndrome is unknown, but since the ventricles are not dilated, the term benign intracranial hypertension also seems appropriate. The disease is frequently associated with lateral sinus thrombosis.

Symptoms include a headache that is often intractable, blurring of vision, nausea, vomiting, and diplopia. Signs include a draining ear, abducens paralysis of one or both lateral rectus muscles, and papilledema.

Computed tomography must be performed prior to lumbar puncture to prevent brain herniation. When performed, the cerebrospinal fluid pressure is high, sometimes above 300 mm H_2O, but protein, cells, and sugar concentrations are normal, and the ventricles are of normal or small size. Although thought of as benign, otitic hydrocephalus in some cases has proceeded to loss of vision secondary to optic atrophy.

Treatment includes the use of antimicrobial agents and mastoidectomy, and normalization of intracranial pressure by medications (acetazolamide or furosem-

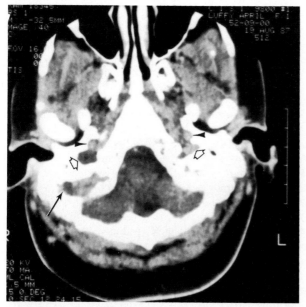

Figure 23–4. Computed tomogram showing a right lateral sinus thrombosis. The bolus intravenous contrast material shows good opacification of the carotid arteries (arrowheads). But the jugulars (open arrows) are asymmetric. The left side enhances normally. The right shows no enhancement, again suggesting thrombosis. The sigmoid sinus (arrow) also shows no opacification.

ide), repeated lumbar punctures, or a lumboperitoneal shunt. An aggressive surgical approach would appear to be warranted because of the possibility of optic atrophy.

TYPE AND TIMING OF OTOLOGIC SURGICAL INTERVENTION

In general, an aggressive approach to surgical management should be taken when a suppurative intracranial complication of otitis media and mastoiditis is present. If an acute or chronic middle-ear effusion is present, an immediate tympanocentesis for culture of the middle-ear effusion and myringotomy for drainage are mandatory. A tympanostomy tube should also be inserted to promote continued drainage of the middle ear and mastoid. The tympanostomy tube can be inserted even though a purulent middle-ear effusion is present. If the tube is subsequently spontaneously extruded owing to profuse otorrhea, it can always be replaced if the perforation closes. However, the insertion of a tympanostomy tube that remains in place will eliminate the need for subsequent myringotomies if the myringotomy incision heals during the course of the illness (when a tube is not inserted). There is no reason to withhold this procedure even in the critically ill child, since a tympanocentesis-myringotomy can be invaluable in the diagnosis and management of the infection. If the child is toxic, the procedure can be performed without general anesthesia. The technique should include a culture of the ear canal followed by sterilization of the external ear canal prior to the tympanocentesis, since an unusual organism may be present (see Chap. 21, section on tympanocentesis and myringotomy).

When more extensive otologic surgery is required to eliminate the infection within the temporal bone, the timing of the surgical intervention will depend on the status of the child. Ideally, the otologic surgery should be performed as soon as the diagnosis of intracranial complication is confirmed. However, this is frequently not possible, since the neurologic status of the patient or the presence of sepsis, or both, may make the child an anesthesia risk. For such patients, otologic surgical intervention may not be possible until the child's condition has stabilized. When neurosurgical intervention is required immediately, as when a brain abscess or subdural empyema is present, the otologic surgery can be performed at the same time if the child's condition is stable at the end of the neurosurgical procedure. However, if the patient's condition does not warrant prolonging the anesthesia, then the otologic surgery should be performed as soon as the child is able to tolerate a second surgical procedure. This usually is within a few days or a week. However, the surgery should not be delayed so long that the primary source of the infection is not controlled, as lack of control of the primary source of infection can interfere with the resolution of the intracranial infec-

tion or can even result in another intracranial complication.

The type of otologic surgical procedure chosen will depend on the type of pathologic process present. If acute mastoid osteitis is present, then a complete simple (cortical) mastoidectomy should be performed and a drain inserted into the mastoid cavity. The middle ear must also be drained, which may be accomplished by inserting a tympanostomy tube if a perforation is not present. If a subperiosteal abscess is present, a drain should also be used. If a child has an ear infection that has resulted in a suppurative intracranial complication, drainage of the mastoid may not be achieved by a myringotomy alone because of an aditus ad antrum obstruction, and, therefore, performance of a mastoidectomy should be considered in order to drain the infection. In these cases, the mastoidectomy is performed as an emergency procedure. Occasionally, when such an obstruction exists between the middle ear and the mastoid air cell system, the middle ear will be found to be free of effusion (as confirmed by a myringotomy), but the mastoid will be infected. In such cases, the mastoid infection must be drained as soon as possible.

When the suppurative intracranial infection is secondary to chronic suppurative otitis media, especially when a cholesteatoma is present, performance of a radical mastoidectomy is invariably indicated. A possible exception to this rule would be the incidental finding of extradural granulation tissue or an abscess during mastoid surgery to remove cholesteatoma. If an intratemporal complication is present, such as petrositis or labyrinthitis, definitive surgery must be performed. A search for a labyrinthine fistula, an extradural abscess, or extension of infection into the sigmoid sinus should always be part of the surgical procedure.

PREVENTION

The life-threatening complications of disease of the middle ear in children are relatively uncommon. Our goal should be to reduce the incidence of these complications still further by effective management of acute and chronic otitis media with effusion and prevention of chronic suppurative otitis media and cholesteatoma. Multiple factors may influence the extension of infection from the middle ear and mastoid to the intracranial cavity, such as the virulence of the bacteria, efficacy of antimicrobial therapy, defects in anatomy, altered host immunity, and surgical drainage. An impending complication may be prevented from developing into a life-threatening condition if tympanocentesis and myringotomy are performed to identify the causative organism and to provide adequate drainage when children with acute otitis media have persistent or recurrent fever, otalgia, or other signs and symptoms of toxicity that are not responding to medical management. In such patients, the results of the culture from the middle-ear effusion should guide the clinician in the selection of the appropriate antimicrobial agent. If persistent or recurrent discharge through a perforation is present, then a culture should be obtained by needle aspiration of the purulent material that is within the middle-ear cavity. The antimicrobial agent chosen should be administered in a dose that is adequate by the route appropriate to prevent a suppurative complication.

In children who have had an episode of meningitis as a complication of acute otitis media, presence of a perilymphatic fistula (cerebrospinal fluid fistula) must be ruled out, especially if more than one episode of meningitis has occurred. The fistula may be in the area of the oval or round window, or both, and may be of congenital origin or may be due to an acquired defect (Grundfast and Bluestone, 1978; Supance and Bluestone, 1983). Suppurative labyrinthitis is usually present, and the fistula must be repaired to prevent recurrence of the intracranial complication. Acute mastoid osteitis and petrositis are other possible intratemporal complications of acute otitis media in which the infection may spread to the intracranial cavity. Early diagnosis and appropriate management of these conditions can prevent intracranial complications.

A suppurative complication should be suspected in children who have the signs and symptoms of acute infection or when preexisting chronic suppurative otitis media is present with or without a cholesteatoma. An acute exacerbation in a chronically infected ear may destroy bone and permit bacteria to enter the intracranial cavity. A persistent aural discharge may indicate the presence of this type of pathologic process.

In children who have chronic suppurative otitis media and in whom the discharge from the ear is persistent in spite of medical treatment, such as ototopical medication and orally administered antimicrobial agents, hospitalization may be required to provide more aggressive therapy. A parenterally administered antimicrobial agent may be necessary, depending on the results of the culture of the discharge, and direct instillation through the tympanic membrane perforation of appropriate ototopical medication after thorough aspiration of the middle ear may be warranted. This procedure is best performed using the otomicroscope. If the suppurative process continues in spite of this type of medical management, then surgical intervention is indicated. Frequently, a cholesteatoma is found in the middle ear and possibly the mastoid, which could not be identified by inspection of the tympanic membrane even when visualized with the aid of the otomicroscope. Even if a cholesteatoma is not present, then middle ear and mastoid surgery is still indicated in such cases in order to drain the ear and decrease the possibility of further complications. Tympanoplasty surgery, which may be performed at the time of the initial procedure or as a second-stage operation, may be required to prevent subsequent episodes of discharge.

When a cholesteatoma is present, the diagnosis should be made as soon as possible, and surgery is indicated, since structural damage to the middle ear and mastoid is usually progressive and suppurative

complications are an ever-present danger. The most important goals of surgery on such ears are complete eradication of the cholesteatoma (or its exteriorization), elimination of the infection, and prevention of potential intratemporal or intracranial complications. If these goals are met, the ear is "safe." Prolonged follow-up of children who have had cholesteatoma is mandatory, since recurrence is common. In patients who have had middle ear and mastoid surgery performed and in whom infection in the middle ear or mastoid cavity, or both, persists in spite of medical management, surgical intervention may again be necessary. In cases in which a radical mastoidectomy has been performed, the middle ear–mastoid discharge may be the result of reflux of nasopharyngeal secretions through a patent eustachian tube into the middle ear. Surgical closure of the middle-ear end of the eustachian tube may be required to eliminate the reflux and chronic infection (see Chap. 22). Likewise, identification of an extradural abscess can prevent spread of the infection further into the intracranial cavity. During surgery, a thorough examination of the tegmen tympani should be performed, since such an abscess may be present as a result of cholesteatoma or infection, or both, being present in the area. If the cholesteatoma is in the area of the lateral semicircular canal, the possibility of a labyrinthine fistula must be ruled out. Juselius and Kaltiokallio (1972) reported that of 42 patients with labyrinthine fistulas, 5 had suppurative labyrinthitis and meningitis.

Antimicrobial agents have greatly reduced the incidence of intracranial complications of infections of the middle ear and mastoid, but the physician must remain alert to the possibility of an unusual event. In less developed areas of the world, where availability of medical facilities is still limited, complications occur with significant morbidity and mortality rates (Raikundalia, 1975).

Acknowledgment: The authors would like to thank Leland Albright, M.D., who provided assistance in the neurological aspects of this chapter.

SELECTED REFERENCES

Alford, B. R., and Cohn, A. M. 1980. Complications of suppurative otitis media and mastoiditis. *In* Paparella, M. M., and Shumrick, D. A. (eds.): Otolaryngology, Vol. 2. Philadelphia, W. B. Saunders Co., pp. 1490–1509.
  The descriptions of the intracranial suppurative complications of otitis media are presented in a clear and concise manner.
Dawes, J. D. K. 1970. Complications of infections of the middle ear. *In* Ballantyne, J., and Groves, J. (eds.): Diseases of the Ear, Nose, and Throat, 4th ed., Vol. 2. London, Butterworth and Co., pp. 305–384.
  This section of an authoritative four-volume otolaryngology text contains a detailed description of the intracranial complications of otitis media by a clinician with extensive experience.
McCabe, B. F., Sade, J., and Abramson, M. (eds.). 1977. Cholesteatoma: First International Conference. New York, Aesculapius Pub., pp. 420–437.
  The papers presented at this meeting on the complications of cholesteatoma represent the current state of our knowledge.

Miglets, A. W., Paparella, M. M., and Saunders, W. H. 1986. Atlas of Ear Surgery, 4th ed. St. Louis, The C. V. Mosby Co., Chap. 3, 6, 9.

This atlas provides clear illustrations of otologic surgical procedures.

Schuknecht, H. F. 1974. Pathology of the Ear. Cambridge, MA, Harvard University Press, pp. 247–251.

This text has the best description of the pathology of intracranial suppurative complications of otitis media written for the otolaryngologist.

Shambaugh, G. E., and Glasscock, M. E. 1980. Surgery of the Ear, 3rd ed. Philadelphia, W. B. Saunders Co., pp. 289–326.

The description in this text of the otologic surgical techniques employed for patients with suppurative disease in the intracranial cavity is excellent.

REFERENCES

Beller, A. J., Sahar, A., and Praiss, I. 1973. Brain abscess: Review of 89 cases over a period of 30 years. J. Neurol. Neurosurg. Psychiatry 36:757.

Berg, B., Franklin, G., Cuneo, R., et al. 1978. Nonsurgical care of brain abscess: Early diagnosis and follow-up with computerized tomography. Ann. Neurol. 3:474.

Brewer, N. S., MacCarty, C. S., and Wellman, W. E. 1975. Brain abscess: A review of recent experience. Ann. Intern. Med. 82:571.

Browning, G. G. 1984. The unsafeness of "safe" ears. J. Laryngol. Otol. 98:23.

Dawes, J. D. K. 1979. Complications of infections of the middle ear. *In* Ballantyne, J., and Groves, J. (eds.): Scott-Brown's Diseases of the Ear, Nose, and Throat, 4th ed., Vol. 2. London, Butterworth and Co., Ltd., pp. 305–384.

du Boulay, G. H. 1979. Current practice in neurosurgical radiology. *In* Symon, L. (ed.): Neurosurgery. *In* Rob, C., and Smith, R. (eds.): Operative Surgery Series, 3rd ed. London, Butterworth and Co., Ltd., pp. 13–45.

Eavey, R. D., Gao, Y. Z., Schuknecht, H. F., et al. 1985. Otologic features of bacterial meningitis of childhood. J. Pediatr. 106:402.

Feigin, R. D. 1981. Bacterial meningitis beyond the neonatal period. *In* Feigin, R. D., and Cherry, J. D. (eds.): Textbook of Infectious Disease, Vol. I. Philadelphia, W. B. Saunders Co., pp. 293–308.

Garfield, J. 1979. Intracranial abscess. *In* Symon, R. (ed.): Neurosurgery. *In* Rob, C., and Smith, R. (eds.): Operative Surgery Series, 3rd ed. London, Butterworth and Co., Ltd., p. 335.

Gower, D., and McQuirt, W. F. 1983. Intracranial complications of acute and chronic infectious ear disease: A problem still with us. Laryngoscope 93:1028.

Gower, D. J., McQuirt, W. F., and Kelly, D. L. 1985. Intracranial complications of ear disease in a pediatric population with special emphasis on subdural effusion and empyema. South. Med. J. 78:429.

Greer, M., and Berk, M. S. 1963. Lateral sinus obstruction and mastoiditis. Pediatrics 31:840.

Grundfast, K. M., and Bluestone, C. D. 1978. Sudden or fluctuating hearing loss and vertigo in children due to perilymph fistula. Ann. Otol. Rhinol. Laryngol. 87:761.

Harding, A. L., Anderson, P., Howie, V. M., et al. 1973. *Haemophilus influenzae* isolated from children with otitis media. *In* Sell, S. H., and Karzon, D. T. (eds.): *Haemophilus influenzae*. Nashville, TN, Vanderbilt University Press, pp. 21–28.

Heineman, H. S., and Braude, A. I. 1963. Anaerobic infection of the brain: Observations on 18 consecutive cases of brain abscess. Am. J. Med. 35:682.

Jadavji, T., Humphreys, R. P., and Prober, C. G. 1985. Brain abscess in infants and children. Pediatr. Infect. Dis. 4:394.

Jeanes, A. 1962. Otogenic intracranial suppuration. J. Laryngol. Otol. 76:388.

Juselius, H., and Kaltiokallio, K. 1972. Complications of acute and chronic otitis media in the antibiotic era. Acta Otolaryngol. (Stockh.) 74:445.

Kessler, L., Dietzmann, K., and Krish, A. 1970. Beitrag zur otogenen meningitis. Z. Laryngol. Rhinol. Otol. 49:93.

Keven, G., and Tyrell, L. J. 1984. Nonsurgical treatment of brain abscess: Report of two cases. Pediatr. Infect. Dis. 3:331.

Krajina, Z. 1956. Observations on endocranial complications of the ear and sinuses in the era of antibiotics. Pract. Otorhinolaryngol. (Basel) 18:1.

Lindsay, J. R. 1938. Suppuration in the petrous pyramid. Ann. Otol. Rhinol. Laryngol. 47:3.

Liske, E., and Weikers, N. J. 1964. Changing aspects of brain abscesses: Review of cases in Wisconsin 1940 through 1962. Neurology 14:294.

McGreal, D. A. 1962. Brain abscess in children. Can. Med. Assoc. J. 86:261.

Morgan, H., Wood, M. W., and Murphey, F. 1973. Experience with 88 consecutive cases of brain abscess. J. Neurosurg. 38:698.

Proctor, C. A. 1966. Intracranial complications of otitic origin. Laryngoscope 76:288.

Raikundalia, K. B. 1975. Analysis of suppurative otitis media in children: Aetiology of non-suppurative otitis media. Med. J. Aust. 1:749.

Rennels, M. B., Woodward, C. L., Robinson, W. L., et al. 1983. Medical cure of apparent brain abcesses. Pediatrics 72:220.

Ritter, F. N. 1977. Complications of cholesteatoma. *In* McCabe, B. F., Sade, J., and Abramson, M. (eds.): Cholesteatoma: First International Conference. New York, Aesculapius Pub., pp. 430–437.

Rosenwasser, H. 1945. Thrombophlebitis of the lateral sinus. Arch. Otolaryngol. 41:117.

Samuel, J., and Fernandes, C. M. C. 1987. Lateral sinus thrombosis: A review of 45 cases. J. Laryngol. Otolaryngol. 101:1227.

Seid, A. B., and Sellars, S. L. 1973. The management of otogenic lateral sinus disease at Groote Schuur Hospital. Laryngoscope 83:397.

Selker, R. G. 1975. Intracranial abscess: Treatment by continuous catheter drainage. Child's Brain 1:368.

Shambaugh, G. E., and Glasscock, M. E. 1980. Surgery of the Ear, 3rd ed. Philadelphia, W. B. Saunders Co., pp. 302–312.

Sheehy, J. L., Brackmann, D. E., and Graham, M. D. 1977. Complications of cholesteatoma: A report on 1024 cases. *In* McCabe, B. F., Sade, J., and Abramson, M. (eds.): Cholesteatoma: First International Conference. New York, Aesculapius Pub., pp. 420–429.

Supance, J. S., and Bluestone, C. D. 1983. Perilymph fistulas in infants and children. Otol. Head Neck Surg. 91:663.

Symonds, C. P. 1931. Otitic hydrocephalus. Brain 54:55.

Tarkkanen, J., and Kohonen, A. 1970. Otogenic brain abscess. Arch. Otolaryngol. 91:91.

Teichgraeber, J. F., Per-Lee, J. H., and Turner, J. S. 1982. Lateral sinus thrombosis: A modern perspective. Laryngoscope 92:744.

Turner, A. L., and Reynolds, E. E. 1931. Intracranial Pyogenic Diseases. Edinburgh, Oliver and Boyd.

Chapter 24

DISEASES OF THE INNER EAR AND SENSORINEURAL DEAFNESS

Robert J. Ruben, M.D.

The diseases of the inner ear can become manifest at any time during childhood. There are no cures for these maladies; the physician can only prevent or care for them. This chapter will discuss the more common and serious of these diseases. The child's physician must know that the condition exists, and the best intervention is dependent on early detection and recognition of a hearing loss. All children affected can be significantly helped by the use of hearing aids and proper education, but unless the hearing loss is recognized, these interventions cannot be instituted. Lack of proper care for these children may condemn them to irreversible loss of language and other cognitive functions.

Congenital sensorineural hearing loss is classified into the types that occur before birth and those that occur after birth. In the area of genetic disease, this is an artificial nosologic distinction because the genetic diseases that phenotypically manifest themselves after birth occur before birth. However, the differentiation between congenital and postnatal disease is important in terms of the management of the child. It is important always to remember that when etiology cannot be established, it also cannot be said that genetic disease has been ruled out. Many of the unknowns will, with further examination or in subsequent children in the same family, prove to be genetic.

Classification of Sensorineural Deafness

I. Congenital
  A. Genetic
  B. Acquired
    1. Infection
    2. Other teratogens
      (e.g., ototoxic drugs)
  C. Unknown
II. Postnatal
  A. Genetic
  B. Acquired
    1. Infection
    2. Trauma
    3. Ototoxic medication
    4. Other
  C. Unknown

CONGENITAL PROBLEMS OF THE INNER EAR

Pathoembryology

Congenital sensorineural deafness can be divided into two histopathologic groups: cases in which the bony labyrinth is normal and the neuroepithelium (organ of Corti) is abnormal (Fig. 24–1) and cases in which the bony labyrinth is abnormal and in which there may or may not be normal neuroepithelium (Fig. 24–2). These two histopathologic types have their origin in the development of the inner ear and also have clinical consequences for the management of the patient.

The types of pathologic change in which there are major malformations of the bony labyrinth are rare and are most probably due to faulty induction of the inner ear. The primary inductor of the bony labyrinth is probably the developing central nervous system, as demonstrated by a number of experimental studies in amblystoma (Yntema, 1950) and mice (Deol, 1964). The surrounding mesenchyme can also contribute to the form of the bony labyrinth (Ruben and Van De Water, 1983). If there is an abnormality in the developing brain stem, it appears that this will result in an abnormal bony labyrinth. The operation of this principle has also been observed in humans (Henke and Lubarsch, 1926). It would appear that human fetuses with anencephaly have abnormal bony labyrinths (Fig. 24–3), a condition that can be detected clinically by the use of various forms of radiographic imaging (Olson et al., 1982). Faulty induction of the bony labyrinth by an abnormally developing central nervous system implies that if a child has an abnormally shaped bony labyrinth, he or she may also have an abnormal central nervous system. This clinical correlation appears to be most constant in children with severe labyrinthine malformations. Radiographic examination of the inner ear of a deaf neonate should lead the physician to suspect a malformation of the central nervous system and to perform appropriate studies. The prognosis for such a neonate may be guarded.

The second general type of histopathologic condition

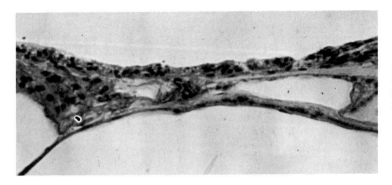

Figure 24–1. Degeneration of the organ of Corti in the temporal bone of a deaf patient. The organ of Corti, tectorial membrane, and nerve fibers are absent. The scala media is collapsed.

of the inner ear is related to the sensory epithelium, most often evidenced by absence of the organ of Corti and pathologic changes in the membranous structures that surround the organ of Corti. The mechanism for this loss of hair cells has been considered to be either lack of development or degeneration. Four separate areas of observation indicate that lack of the organ of Corti is the result of premature cell death:

1. A study of the cell kinetics of the inner ear (Ruben, 1967b) showed that the organ of Corti is composed of end-state cells (i.e., after the cells are formed they are unable to reproduce themselves). Because the cells of the organ of Corti in humans are probably formed during the second month of intra-uterine life, any loss of cells after this time would result in a hearing loss.

2. Malformations of the bony labyrinth still result in labyrinths with sensory epithelia (Fig. 24–2). Thus, even the most severely congenitally malformed ears will have sensory structures.

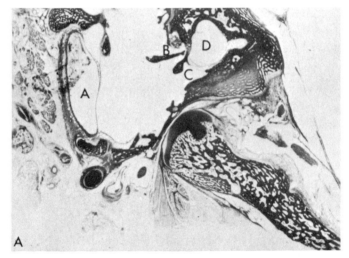

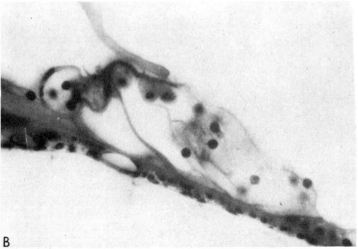

Figure 24–2. A, Cross-section through a malformed human temporal bone. The patient had an associated central nervous system malformation. On the left (A) are the external auditory canal and the tympanic membrane. On the right side of the picture is a large, saclike cochlea (D) in which the round window (C) and the oval window can be seen. There is an abnormal columellalike stapes present (B). B, A higher-power photomicrograph from the same specimen, part A, which shows the organ of Corti in this severely malformed cochlea. Note that three outer hair cells and an inner hair cell can be identified.

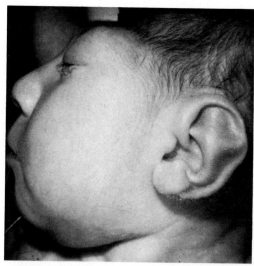

Figure 24–3. Anencephalic child. This patient had a bony labyrinthine abnormality diagnosed by radiography. The patient responded to sound.

3. These data come from observations of the development of genetically determined sensorineural deafness in the cat (Bosher and Hallpike, 1966), mouse (Mikaelian and Ruben, 1965), and dog (Anderson et al., 1968). In all of these instances, hair cells are present during development, and they degenerate either before birth or sometime after birth (Fig. 24–4).

4. Premature cell death as the probable cause of pathologic conditions of the organ of Corti was found in the few studies of human fetuses that had a high probability of being deaf, because they were infected with the rubella virus (Bordley et al., 1968). All of these fetuses were found to have sensory epithelia. The histopathologic characteristics of rubella sensorineural deafness are well known and show, among other findings, a lack of sensory cells (Schuknecht, 1974).

The evidence strongly indicates that an important mechanism for the lack of the organ of Corti in congenital sensorineural hearing loss is premature cell death. This is the most probable explanation of all sensory deafness that occurs after birth, including genetically determined deafness and that which comes about through acquired diseases of the inner ear.

Another aspect of developmental pathologic change of the inner ear with important clinical application is the effect of the loss of the organ of Corti, sound deprivation, or both on the auditory pathways of the central nervous system. One of the earliest studies of this subject showed that when the otocyst was removed from a chick embryo and the embryo was allowed to develop, there was a decrease in the number of the structures composing the auditory pathways (Levi-Montalcini, 1949). These findings were restudied and expanded (Jackson and Rubel, 1976; Parks and Robinson, 1976). It has been shown that there will be structural changes in the central auditory pathways when destruction of the inner ear or sound deprivation

Figure 24–4. A, The organ of Corti of a Dalmatian puppy showing the beginning of the pathologic changes in the organ of Corti (A) and the scala media. The hair cells are present but appear abnormal. The tectorial membrane (B) is adherent to Reissner membrane. B, Organ of Corti from a deaf, mature Dalmatian dog showing the end stage of degeneration of the organ of Corti and a collapsed scala media. The hair cells, nerve fibers, and tectorial membrane are absent.

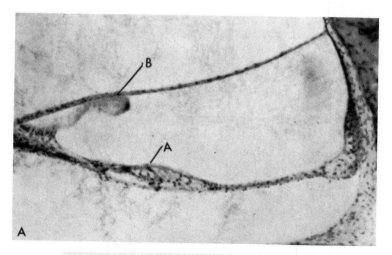

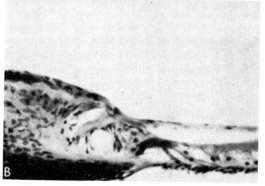

occurs at later stages of development (Webster and Webster, 1977). Behavioral expressions of these probable anatomic changes in the central nervous system as a result of auditory deprivation have also been reported (Gottlieb, 1975; Riesen and Zilbert, 1975).

These observations have two clinical implications. The first is that early loss of the organ of Corti, or of hearing, may induce anatomic changes in the central nervous system in humans. Thus, the normal development of the central nervous system may be impaired. These data have been reviewed (Ruben, 1986; Ruben and Rapin, 1980). Second, some of the central nervous system anatomic changes, with their subsequent behavioral deficits, may be ameliorated by the use of sound stimuli as early as possible. This supposition makes imperative the need for early detection and initiation of hearing aid therapy in deaf infants.

Etiology of Deafness

Determining the etiology of deafness in an individual has particular utility in the management of the patient and his or her family, as will be discussed below. It is thought that, of all congenital deafness, about 50 per cent is due to acquired disease, 15 per cent is due to autosomal dominant inheritance, 34 per cent is due to autosomal recessive inheritance, and 1 per cent is due to X-linked inheritance. When these percentages are based on actual observations of patients, they may include a group of cases, amounting to 40 per cent of the total, in which the etiology is unknown (Ruben and Rozycki, 1971; Parving, 1985). It has been suggested that most of the unknown cases are probably due to autosomal recessive inheritance (Fraser, 1976).

Genetic Deafness

There are more than 70 different genetic syndromes associated with congenital sensorineural deafness. These have been catalogued and described (Fraser, 1976; Konigsmark and Gorlin, 1976; McKusick, 1986), and most of them are rare. The most common or important of the genetically determined sensorineural deafnesses found in humans are Waardenburg syndrome (a dominant gene) and the Jervell and Lange-Nielsen, Pendred, and Usher syndromes (recessive). There are also dominant, recessive, and X-linked genetically transmitted diseases that have no other recognized signs or symptoms than deafness.

Waardenburg syndrome (Fig. 24–5) was first described by Waardenburg (1951). This syndrome is transmitted as an autosomal dominant trait, and it is believed to be responsible for approximately 1 to 2 per cent of all cases of congenital deafness (Fraser, 1976). The description of the syndrome includes six features: (1) lateral development of the internal canthi with dystrophia of the lacrimal punctum and horizontal shortening of the palpebral fissures; (2) a prominent, broad, nasal root; (3) hypertrichosis of the eyebrows;

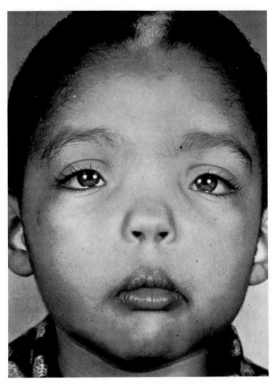

Figure 24–5. This patient is profoundly deaf in both ears, has a white forelock, an increased intercanthal distance, and an antimongoloid slant of both eyes. The patient's family members show other stigmata of the Waardenburg syndrome.

(4) white forelock; (5) heterochromia of the irides; and (6) sensorineural deafness, either total or subtotal. Since the syndrome was identified, several other associated features have been defined, including a cleft lip, cleft palate, or both and high-arched palate (Fisch, 1959); patchy depigmentation of the skin that can best be seen under ultraviolet light; changes in iris pigmentation in one eye during the first year of life (Settlemayer and Hogan, 1961); absent vestibular response (Stoller, 1962); pigmentary heterochromia of the fundus (Goldberg, 1966); and disappearance of the white forelock after the first year of life (Hansen et al., 1965). Occasional patients have been reported to have Hirschsprung disease, which is consistent with the concept that both may be an effect of abnormalities in the organization of the neural tube (Rarey and Davis, 1984; Nutman et al., 1986). Waardenburg syndrome has been found throughout the world and in all races, and the expression of this dominant gene is quite variable. A study of 523 affected individuals in 81 families (Pantke and Cohen, 1971) demonstrated some of the variability of expressivity (Table 24–1). These data were derived from patients who were suspected of having this syndrome and who had profound sensorineural hearing losses. It can be seen that, of the group of families, 44 per cent had profound sensorineural hearing losses and 9 per cent had partial hearing losses. These partial hearing losses included unilateral hearing losses.

The diagnosis of Waardenburg syndrome can be made by observing any of the stigmata of the syndrome

TABLE 24–1. Variability of Expressivity of
Waardenburg Syndrome

FINDING	INCIDENCE
Dystrophic canthus	83
Hypertelorism	17
Laterally displaced lacrimal punctum	59
Dacrocystitis	19
Broad nasal root	68
Hyperplasia of eyebrows	57
Heterochromia of iris	51
White forelock (poliosis)	48
Vitiligo	16
Premature graying of hair	33
Congenital deafness, profound	44
Congenital deafness, partial	9
Cleft lip and palate	10
High-arched palate	27

From Pantke, O. A., and Cohen, M. M., Jr. 1971. The Waardenburg syndrome. *In* Bergsma, D. (ed.): Orofacial Structures, Part XI. Baltimore, Williams & Wilkins for the National Foundation–March of Dimes Birth Defects:OAS 7(7):142–152, with permission.

in the propositi or the family. Dystrophic canthi and an abnormal intercanthal distance are two of the most common expressions of this syndrome. An excellent table of interpupillary distance in various racial groups and at various ages has been compiled by Pryor (1969) and helps determine the normality of this factor. A difference in color of the irides should not be confused with heterochromia, which results from lesions of the cervical sympathetics (Calhoun, 1919).

The degree of penetrance for profound congenital sensorineural deafness in Waardenburg syndrome is about 0.20 and the mutation rate for this syndrome is about 0.5 per 100,000 gametes (Fraser, 1976). There is a possible linkage of the Waardenburg gene to the ABO gene (Simpson et al., 1974).

The histopathologic findings of one case of Waardenburg syndrome has been reported (Fisch, 1959) to show a normal bony labyrinth, lack of the organ of Corti and spiral ganglion cells, and atrophy of the stria vascularis. The vestibular labyrinth was normal.

Usher disease (retinitis pigmentosa) was first described by von Graefe (1858). This disease is transmitted as an autosomal recessive trait and is believed to be responsible for approximately 4 per cent of congenital deafness cases (Fraser, 1976). There is heterogeneity in the syndrome, and it is considered as consisting of three different types (Grondhal and Mjoen, 1986). The syndrome comprises congenital sensorineural deafness, progressive retinitis pigmentosa, night blindness and tunnel vision, cataracts, vestibular impairment, mental retardation, psychosis, spinocerebellar ataxia, and nystagmus (Hallgren, 1959; Nuutila, 1970). Additionally, a decrease in olfaction (Vernon, 1969) and an increased incidence of branchial cleft cysts (Kloepfer et al., 1966) have been noted in these patients. The retinal findings show granular accumulations of pigment that begin at the optic fundus and extend toward the periphery (Fig. 24–6). Although these symptoms are due to an autosomal recessive gene, there is a significant amount of variability in the

expression of the gene (Table 24–2). It appears that most but not all of the individuals homozygotic for Usher disease have a severe to profound sensorineural hearing loss, although some may have only a mild to moderate hearing loss, and there is one report in which the hearing loss was progressive (Sirles and Slasghts, 1943). Almost all these children will not have a vestibular response to caloric test or ice-water irrigation of the external auditory canal. This lack of vestibular response is an important observation in a child who is deaf, without a known etiology. Many of these, in the author's experience, have been children who eventually were diagnosed as having Usher disease. The retinal signs and symptoms are progressive throughout life. Nuutila (1970) showed that night blindness is the first retinal sign in 92 per cent of cases and will be evident before the age of 10 years. At the end of the second decade of life, 2 in 63 people will be blind, 5 in 63 will have tunnel vision, and 34 in 63 will have decreased visual acuity.

The diagnosis of retinitis pigmentosa can be made early in life with an ophthalmoscope or by means of electroretinography (Vernon, 1969). An infant born with sensorineural hearing loss for which there is no definite etiology should be examined with the ophthalmoscope and, if available, by electroretinography. If electroretinography is not available and if there is no history of retinitis pigmentosa, routine fundoscopic examinations should be made throughout the first two decades of life. It is important to determine whether the patient will lose his or her vision, because if the patient is deaf and will then lose his or her vision, special habilitative intervention must be initiated. It is also important for the parents to be aware that they are carrying the gene. The use of electroretinography and audiology has enabled the retrospective identification of some of the heterozygote carriers of the syndrome (Kloepfer et al., 1970). These techniques for identification of heterozygote carriers should be undertaken in all members of the family to determine the carriers of the disease.

The high prevalence of mental retardation and psychosis in this syndrome has, in part, been accounted for by abnormal electroencephalograms and pneumoencephalograms (Nuutila, 1970). Some of the psychoses may be the result of the extreme sensory deprivation occurring with both deafness and blindness.

The histopathologic changes of retinitis pigmentosa were reported by Belal (1975). This report showed that degeneration of the organ of Corti and spiral ganglion cells, mainly in the basal turn, occurs in patients with this disease, although the remainder of the structures of the inner ear were not noticeably diseased. An earlier report described marked degeneration of the organ of Corti and supporting structures, including the stria vascularis in the basal turn, with retinitis pigmentosa (Nager, 1927). The saccular and vestibular apparatuses were abnormal, and atrophy was noted in the primary auditory portion of the central nervous system in the ears studied. These findings

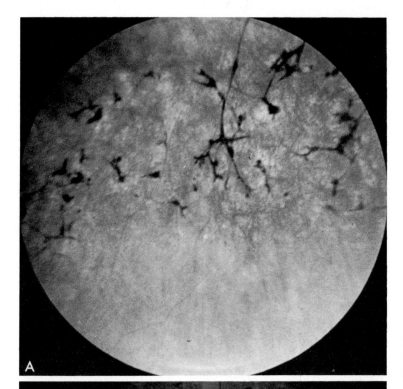

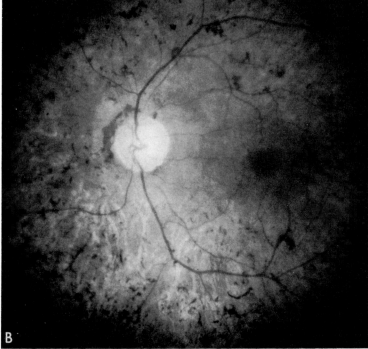

Figure 24–6. *A*, The retina of a patient with Usher disease (retinitis pigmentosa) at the onset of the visual deficits. *B*, The retina of a patient with Usher disease in its late stage. (Courtesy of Dr. Paul Henkind, Professor of Ophthalmology, Albert Einstein College of Medicine and the Montefiore Hospital and Medical Center of New York.)

have been reviewed and an additional case has been assessed with light and electron microscopy (Shinkawa and Nadol, 1986). This case was consistent with other observations in that there was loss of hair cells in the basal turn of the cochlea, a severe loss of spiral ganglion cells, and collections of degenerating supporting cells in the organ of Corti.

The *Jervell and Lange-Nielsen syndrome* involves autosomal recessive sensorineural deafness (Jervell and Lange-Nielsen, 1957). This syndrome consists of hear-

ing impairment associated with syncopal episodes and sudden death. It is one of the genetic syndromes that must be detected early, as there are efficacious interventions to preserve the life of the patient.

The frequency of this disease is variable, perhaps depending on the thoroughness of the diagnostic work-up of the population and the early death of affected individuals. The variability of symptoms and frequency of early death may account for a number of crib deaths in families in which there are other affected members.

TABLE 24–2. Incidence of Defects in 177 Individuals with Retinitis Pigmentosa and 304 Nonaffected Siblings in 102 Families

SIGN OR SYMPTOM	NUMBER	PERCENTAGE
Glaucoma	3/88	3
Nystagmus	11/158	7
Profound to severe deafness	155/177	88
Moderate to severe deafness	22/177	12
Vestibular impairment*	6/7	86
Mental deficiency	41/172	24
Psychosis	26/113	23

*This testing was carried out in children with gait impairment by caloric testing.

With permission from Hallgren, B. 1959. Retinitis pigmentosa combined with congenital deafness; with vestibulo-cerebellar ataxia and mental abnormality in a proportion of cases. Acta Psychiatr. Scand. 34 Suppl. 138. © 1959 Munksgaard International Publishers Ltd., Copenhagen, Denmark.

It is estimated that the frequency may be as high as 1 in 1 million births or 1 per cent of the deaf population (Fraser et al., 1964b). Another survey in Canada showed an incidence of about 1 in 1000 deaf children or 0.1 per cent of severely hearing impaired patients (Fay et al., 1971). The syndrome has been reported to have a wide geographic distribution in North America, Western Europe, and India (Fraser, 1976). It presents as severe congenital sensorineural hearing loss; the average hearing levels for nine cases were 125 Hz, 60 dB; 250 Hz, 65 dB; 500 Hz, 75 dB; 1000 Hz, 85 dB; 2000 Hz, 100 dB; 2000 Hz, no response; 4000 Hz, no response; and 8000 Hz, no response (Fraser et al., 1964a). The electrocardiographic (ECG) anomalies are large T waves, and the QT interval may not be too prolonged (Fraser et al., 1964a). The QT interval has also been found to vary among and within individuals. The most marked feature of the syndrome is the syncopal episodes, which may begin in the second to third year of life or earlier. They may last from five to ten minutes and can vary in frequency from one per day to one per year or less often. Without therapy, approximately half of the patients die before the age of 15 years.

The cardiac abnormalities that appear to result in death can be treated, if diagnosed. There are at least two reports of the effectiveness of propranolol in treating this syndrome. Olley and Fowler (1970) stated that during a syncopal attack, the electrocardiogram shows asystole, followed by ventricular tachycardia, which can lead to ventricular fibrillation. The latter would respond to defibrillation. They recommended that patients with the Jervell and Lange-Nielsen syndrome be given 5 mg of propranolol each day and also discussed the use of phenobarbital in these patients. An implanted cardioverter defibrillator has been successfully used in cases that have been refractory to drug therapy (Platia et al., 1985). It is apparent that all patients with either idiopathic sensorineural hearing loss or autosomal recessive disease in which a specific syndrome has not been identified should have at least one electrocardiogram. One series found that there were 28 abnormal electrocardiograms in a population

of 1126 severely to profoundly deaf children (Fay et al., 1971). The 27 cases included one with the Jervell and Lange-Nielsen syndrome, four with a prolonged QT interval that was not as long as those found in the Jervell and Lange-Nielsen syndrome, five with wandering pacemakers and a predominant sinus rhythm, one with an atrioventricular (A-V) nodal rhythm, two with first-degree heart block, three with an occasional ectopic ventricular premature beat, one with Wolff-Parkinson-White type B pattern, and ten with isolated QRS frontal axis abnormalities.

The possibility of identifying heterozygote carriers by means of a prolonged QT interval has been suggested (Fraser et al., 1964b; Sanchez-Cascos et al., 1969). This technique may have its limitations, and there are some suggestions that the QT interval may normalize in the young adult (James, 1967), but this has not been proved, and the usefulness of identifying heterozygotic carriers is so great that it appears advisable for relatives of known patients with the Jervell and Lange-Nielsen syndrome to have an electrocardiogram.

The histopathologic change in both the inner ear and the heart in this syndrome has been described (Fraser et al., 1964a; Friedmann et al., 1966). The bony labyrinth is normal, the organ of Corti shows degeneration in all turns with a decrease in the number of spiral ganglion cells, and there are large periodic acid–Schiff (PAS) hyaline deposits in a partially atrophic stria vascularis. The macula of the utricle and the three cristae show degeneration and PAS-positive hyaline nodules. The cardiac findings reveal hypertrophy of the tunica intima of the artery of the sinoatrial node, infarction of the sinoatrial node with fibrosis, a marked decrease in the perinuclear clear zone of Purkinje fibers, and abnormalities of the A-V node; the parasympathetic ganglia near the nodes were noted to be hemorrhagic and appeared to be degenerating.

Pendred disease is an autosomal recessive form of sensorineural deafness associated with goiter, first described in 1896 by Pendred. The diagnosis of this disease was further advanced in 1958 by Morgans and Trotter by the use of the perchlorate test, which showed an abnormal organification of nonorganic iodine. The disease is found throughout the world (Fraser, 1976) and may account for deafness in from 1 to 7 per cent of severely to profoundly deaf children (Thould and Scowen, 1964). This author's experience has not confirmed the high frequency, but this may be due to the difference in populations examined.

This disease is clearly inherited in an autosomal recessive manner, with some variability of expressivity of the effect of the gene in the homozygote. The hearing loss is sensorineural and is usually static, but there have been observations of possible progression (Fraser, 1976). The hearing loss is usually severe to profound, mainly affecting the high tones, but there may be some cases of unilateral hearing loss and others in which significant hearing may remain. Thould and Scowen (1964), after reviewing the audiograms of 23 patients with Pendred disease, stated that 1 of 23 had no response; 12 of 23 were very severely deaf; 8 of 23 were less severely deaf; and 2 of 23 had low levels of hearing. Vestibular responses are quite variable in these patients.

The goiters will usually be apparent before the age of 8 years and in some instances may be found at birth (Thould and Scowen, 1964). The patients are usually eurythyroid (Fraser, 1976; Thould and Scowen, 1964). It has been found that the goiter in this syndrome is not associated with cancer and is easily treated with exogenous thyroid hormone. Many patients have undergone multiple and partial thyroidectomies, and the goiter has returned (Smith, 1960). A review of the literature indicates that in almost all cases a total or partial thyroidectomy is contraindicated.

Fraser (1976) believed that the frequency of the allele in this disease is approximately 0.008 and that the mutation rate may be 56 per 1 million loci per gamete (Fraser, 1965a). It has also been noted that heterozygotes may show a decrease in protein-bound iodine (Fraser, 1965a). Statistically this decrease in the protein-bound iodine is significant at the 2 per cent level.

A set of temporal bones from a patient who may have had Pendred disease has been reported (Hvidberg-Hansen and Jorgensen, 1968). The patient had recurrent goiter and an abnormal perchlorate test result. The family history was suggestive of Pendred disease but not pathognomonic, and study of sections of the abnormal thyroids showed findings consistent with but not pathognomonic for Pendred disease. Temporal bone histopathologic studies indicated that the cochlea contained only two turns and that the neuroepithelium of the cochlea and the spiral ganglion cells was absent. The macula was normal, but periotic connective tissue was found with ossification of the endosteum of the labyrinthine wall. Study of an additional six temporal bones from five patients with Pendred disease confirmed the abnormalities in the bony labyrinth (Johnsen et al., 1986).

Pathologic conditions of the thyroid consisted of colloid tissue, and there was fibrous scarring of the nodules in all 14 cases studied; epithelial proliferation was a dominant feature in nine of the cases, while there were focal areas of proliferation in five cases and occasional focal calcifications (Smith, 1960).

There are a number of congenital sensorineural deafness syndromes that are inherited by autosomal recessive, autosomal dominant, or X-linked mechanisms and in which there are no other associated stigmata (Konigsmark and Gorlin, 1976). These cases may account for 16 per cent of the total population of those who have congenital sensorineural deafness. Of this 16 per cent, approximately 66 per cent inherited the disorder by a dominant gene, 33 per cent inherited the gene recessively, and in less than 1 per cent of these cases was the deafness sex linked (Ruben and Rozycki, 1971).

There were two reports of dominantly inherited sensorineural hearing loss without stigmata as early as 1883 and 1898 (Bell, 1969; Fay, 1898). However, even before the acceptance of mendelian genetics, there was an appreciation of the inheritance of deafness that was clinically characterized by consanguinity or familial deafness (Wilde, 1853). The incidence of congenital sensorineural deafness without stigmata has been reported for different populations throughout the world, and there are several aspects of these inherited forms of sensorineural deafness that should be noted. The first is the variability of penetrance in those with a dominant form of transmission; it appears that unilateral sensorineural deafness represents incomplete penetrance of a dominant gene for sensorineural hearing loss (Smith, 1939). Everberg (1960) found that about 25 per cent of unilateral sensorineural deafness was genetic and that the family members of these individuals had varying degrees of sensorineural hearing loss.

X-linked sensorineural hearing loss has frequently been reported (Sataloff et al., 1955). Fraser (1965b) points out that X-linked inheritance with the appearance of the disease in the male may account for the greater percentage of males than females with severe to profound congenital sensorineural hearing loss. It is of interest to note that Wilde (1853) also found a higher percentage of deaf males than females in all of the populations he studied. X-linked inheritance contributes to the difficulty of making a correct genetic diagnosis, because families at the present time are usually small, and many times there may be no further pregnancies after a deaf child is born. In families with only one male child who is deaf, the possibility of X-linked inheritance must be considered when there is no other diagnosis. Fraser (1965b) estimated that this form of inheritance could account for 6.2 per cent of deafness in males and 3.2 per cent of the congenitally sensorineurally deaf population.

The diagnosis of genetically transmitted sensorineural deafness without associated stigmata can be made if there are (1) two or more siblings affected, (2) a consanguineous marriage, (3) a family history of sensorineural deafness, and (4) audiometric indications of sensorineural hearing loss that cannot be attributed to another cause in relatives of the deaf child (Johnsen, 1952a).

The preceding are only some of the most common of the genetic diseases that result in congenital sensorineural hearing loss. Other defined syndromes, when aggregated, account for a larger number of the cases.

Acquired Congenital Diseases

There are two major perinatal types of acquired sensorineural hearing loss. The first is from the ingestion of various ototoxic and teratogenous substances, thalidomides being the best known of the latter group. Maternal ingestion of streptomycin during pregnancy has been found to cause sensorineural hearing loss in the fetus (Robinson and Cambon, 1964); quinine and chloroquine phosphate are also thought to cause congenital sensorineural hearing loss (Fraser, 1976).

The second major cause of acquired congenital sensorineural hearing loss is intrauterine infection. Syphilis, toxoplasmosis, and possibly cytomegalic inclusion disease are relatively infrequent causes of infection, whereas the most common cause of acquired congenital sensorineural hearing loss is maternal infection with rubella. *Congenital rubella infection* as a cause of congenital sensorineural hearing loss was first reported in 1943 (Swan et al.), although perhaps the earliest cases of probable rubella deafness were described by Wardrop in 1813. Fetuses that have been infected with the rubella virus will exhibit a constellation of abnormal findings, and the earlier the infection occurs in intrauterine life, the more severe the effects tend to be. Manifestation of the syndrome varies not only with each child but also in different populations, depending on both the susceptibility of the population and the variability of the virus. Table 24–3 summarizes some of the findings in a group of 41 Australian patients aged 5 to 19 years whose mothers contracted rubella during pregnancy.

Congenital rubella may be diagnosed by means of physical examination and immunologic techniques. The most common and consistent finding is the clumped pigmentary retinitis that may or may not be associated with cataracts (Fig. 24–7). Other abnormal findings are microcephaly, intrauterine growth retardation, jaundice, and lesions of the long bones. Any mother with a history of a rash during pregnancy or who may have been exposed to rubella should be considered as possibly having had a rubella infection. It has been suggested that all pregnant women have rubella titers taken routinely at the beginning of their pregnancies and that follow-up titers be taken as pregnancy progresses (Ruben, 1970). The results of testing an infant for an increase in rubella titers can be misleading, but the presence of rubella-specific IgM antibodies in the cord or the mother's or the infant's serum during the first 6 months of life is diagnostic of congenital rubella (Forrest and Menser, 1975), although the test may not discover all cases of congenital rubella. The diagnosis of congenital rubella in older children may be difficult, as they may have been infected with a wild type of virus or vaccinated.

TABLE 24–3. Frequency of Rubella-Induced Abnormalities in 41 Children

DEFECTS	NUMBER	PERCENTAGE
Ocular defects	37	90
Deafness	31	76
Congenital heart disease	15	37
Central nervous system involvement	13	32
Low birth weight	17	41
Neonatal difficulties	14	34
Skeletal defects	27	66
Small stature	22	54
Dental defects	16	39
Dermatoglyphic changes	18	44

With permission from Forrest, J. M., and Menser, M. A. 1970. Congenital rubella in school children and adolescents. Arch. Dis. Child. 45:66.

If children older than 2 years of age with a low rubella antibody titer do not respond to vaccine, they may have had rubella congenitally (Cooper et al., 1971). A rubella antibody titer should be obtained from all patients and their mothers when etiology for the congenital sensorineural hearing loss cannot be established, unless the child has been immunized with the rubella vaccine.

The hearing loss found in congenital rubella is predominantly sensorineural in nature. Most of the patients will have severe to profound sensorineural hearing losses, although the loss might be different for each ear (Bordley et al., 1968). Other patients will have a lesser loss, and in some cases the hearing loss may be progressive (Alford, 1968; Bordley and Alford, 1970). The hearing loss may also be conductive, owing either to a fixed stapes (Richards, 1964) or to serous otitis media, which is consistent with the frequent finding of a high-arched palate in these patients. The presence of progressive and conductive disease of the middle ear emphasizes the need for constant audiometric and impedance monitoring of all patients with deafness due to congenital rubella.

Another aspect of the rubella syndrome is that a number of patients have been reported to have significant language retardation (Weinberger et al., 1970) without an associated hearing loss. The possibility exists that some cases of language impairment may be attributed to mild or moderate sensorineural hearing loss, a fluctuating conductive hearing loss, or both.

The variability of findings in cases of congenital rubella is thought to have a possible genetic basis. Both Fraser (1976) and Anderson and colleagues (1970) have reported data indicating that there is an increased incidence of sensorineural hearing loss, caused by rubella, in families with a genetic predisposition to sensorineural hearing loss. The hypothesis is that the predisposition to deafness is increased by the presence of both etiologic factors.

Vaccination for rubella is widespread in the United States at present, but the program could be expanded, as it was estimated that in 1975, 19 per cent of children 5 to 9 years of age were not immune to rubella, accounting for not less than 16,000 new cases of rubella in 1975 (Salisbury and Ma, 1976). New cases of congenital sensorineural hearing loss resulting from intrauterine rubella infection may still present to the physician, who must consider this possible etiology in any differential diagnosis of congenital sensorineural hearing loss.

The ears of patients with congenital rubella infection show a normal bony labyrinth, degeneration of the organ of Corti, granulation at the junction of the stria vascularis and Reissner membrane and collapse of the saccule (Bordley and Alford, 1970; Friedmann, 1974; Michaels, 1987). All of these findings are not the same in each case and reflect the clinical variability of the hearing losses found in these patients.

Cytomegalic inclusion disease (CID) is one of the most ubiquitous viral infections of mothers and their offspring. Cytomegalovirus (CMV) can and does infect

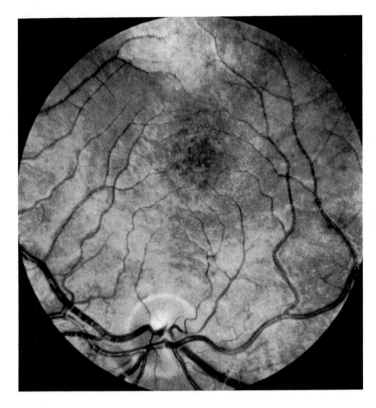

Figure 24–7. The retina of a patient with congenital rubella who has typical "salt and pepper" retinitis. (Courtesy of Dr. Paul Henkind, Professor of Ophthalmology, Albert Einstein College of Medicine and the Montefiore Hospital and Medical Center of New York.)

the neonate when the mother has a primary or subsequent infection. It has been shown that consecutive pregnancies can result in infected children.

The action of CMV as a teratogen for the developing ear is variable and the incidence of detectable pathologic change, considering the virulence of rubella, is low. The neonate who is infected during the mother's primary infection appears to have a more severe morbidity and to be more likely to be infected than those who are affected in later pregnancies (Stagno et al., 1982).

Numerous authors have studied the association of CMV infection with sensorineural hearing loss and evaluated its pathologic consequences in the inner ear (Strauss, 1982). The hearing losses are variable in their severity and can be progressive. The possibility that a progressive sensorineural hearing loss in a child may be due to a CMV perinatal infection must be considered when attempting to establish its etiology.

Because of the high prevalence of CMV infection, a large portion of the population has positive CMV titers. Between 55 and 72 per cent of pregnant women, depending on their social class, will have positive CMV titers, and approximately 10 per cent of their offspring will have CMV infection, most probably acquired *in utero*. It is estimated that there may be as many as 2000 infants born each year with hearing loss caused by CMV.

Diagnosis of hearing loss as a result of CMV infection relies on the demonstration of positive titers in both mother and child. Maternal infection and positive CMV titers before the pregnancy that resulted in the birth of the hearing-impaired child does not preclude, as in the case of congenital rubella, the possibility that

the child's hearing loss results from CMV. The demonstration of positive CMV titers in the mother and the child are not, by themselves, enough to make a secure diagnosis of CMV-caused hearing loss. Some of the children with proven CMV infections and hearing losses are severely stigmatized, with other signs of congenital CMV infection (e.g., microcephaly, hydrocephaly, mental retardation, palatal abnormalities, and intracerebral calcifications). Others who have little or no other signs of infection besides their hearing loss have positive CMV cultures from the urine or, in the absence of a urine culture, a Reye CMV titer. The diagnosis in a nonstigmatized child is somewhat more secure if a positive urine culture for CMV was obtained, especially if it was obtained in early infancy.

Genetic Counseling

Auditory habilitation must be instituted as soon as possible for each patient with congenital sensorineural hearing loss. The physician must also be able to offer the family guidance concerning the risks of having other deaf children. The previous paragraphs have stressed the need for exact delineation of the etiology of the hearing loss, although when this is done in a clinical setting about 40 per cent of the cases will not be found to have a known cause. In all of these "idiopathic" cases, the relatives should be further examined; a review of the family history should be made; and a search for consanguinity, physical examination of the family members for the stigmata of known genetic syndromes, and audiometric examination of the family members should be performed. The audiometric examination appears to be the best, albeit a far from satisfactory, way to detect heterozygotes in recessive disease and partial penetrance in dominant disease (Deraemaeker, 1960; Anderson and Wedenberg, 1968). The age of the parents must also be taken into account, as children born to older parents may be affected through new, dominant mutations (Fraser, 1976).

The risk in proved cases of autosomal dominant deafness of having other children with the same problem is 50 per cent; for having other children with autosomal recessive deafness, the risk is 25 per cent. Those cases of deafness for which there is no known etiology must be presumed to be genetic (dominant, recessive, or X-linked). The possibility of having another affected child in such a family is greater than 1 in 1000 and less than 1 in 2 or 1 in 4, depending on the mode of transmission of the deafness (Fraser, 1976). Some probable recurrence rates, based on a number of different factors, have been calculated by Fraser (1976), who states that the overall risk of deafness for another child is approximately 10 per cent, a figure that varies according to the birth order. For the first child born after an affected sibling, the risk of recurrence is 12.5 per cent; the recurrence risk for the second child is 10 per cent; for the third child it is 7.5 per cent; and for the fourth child it is 5 per cent. These figures, although they are only estimations, are useful in informing parents of the risks of having other affected children.

POSTNATAL DEAFNESS

There are no adequate data on the frequency of postnatal sensorineural hearing loss in children, although it is a common clinical finding. Many of the children have a moderate to severe hearing loss, not severe to profound. Thus, the diagnosis may be delayed, and the presenting problems, especially in a younger child, may not be recognized. The importance of early diagnosis of postnatal sensorineural hearing loss is twofold. First, a habilitation program should be instituted so that the child's auditory ability will be improved. This is even more important in the progressive types of sensorineural hearing loss. If the deficit is recognized early, habilitation may be instituted before the sensorineural hearing loss becomes profound, and the child will have the advantage of a period of auditory learning while there is still useful hearing. The second major reason why early diagnosis is important is that a number of sensorineural hearing losses are associated with life-threatening diseases for which effective medical and surgical interventions are available. The hearing loss may be the first clinical symptom of these disease states.

Genetic Causes of Deafness

There are over 30 different genetically determined syndromes in which sensorineural hearing loss is in-

volved, either wholly or in part, most of which are characterized by progressive sensorineural hearing loss.

Alport disease, probably the most common of these, is an inherited condition that consists of progressive sensorineural hearing loss and progressive nephritis. It was first described in 1927 by Alport and is one of a series of genetically transmitted renal diseases associated with sensorineural hearing loss. The disease has been found throughout the world and in many different racial groups.

Some of the other syndromes in which genetic sensorineural hearing losses are associated with renal disease are hypertension, renal failure, abnormal steroidogenesis, hypogenitalism, and sensorineural deafness; Charcot-Marie-Tooth syndrome with nephritis and sensorineural deafness; macrothrombocytopathia, nephritis, and sensorineural deafness; infantile renal tubular acidosis and congenital sensorineural deafness; adolescent or young adult renal tubular acidosis and slowly progressive sensorineural deafness; renal disease, hyperprolinuria, ichthyosis, and sensorineural deafness; and nephritis, urticaria, amyloidosis, and sensorineural deafness.

Alport disease is more severe in males than in females, although the symptoms are variable in a given patient. Conditions characteristic of Alport disease include hematuria, pyuria, uremia, sensorineural hearing loss, and ocular pathologic changes (consisting of myopia, cataracts, lenticonus, and spherophakia). The age of onset of sensorineural hearing loss is usually after the first decade of life, although the renal symptoms have been found, retrospectively, in infants and have been characterized by the appearance of a "red diaper" as a consequence of the hematuria. If the disease is untreated, affected males usually die by the third decade of life. Females usually have a longer or normal life span but will have toxemia during pregnancy. The advanced renal lesions can be noted by an intravenous pyelogram that shows atrophy, a lobulated kidney, or both. Occasionally there may be ureteral abnormalities.

The possibility of Alport disease should be considered in any child with a sensorineural hearing loss of recent onset, regardless of sex. Urinalysis and either a serum creatinine or blood urea nitrogen level should be obtained. More than three red blood cells or five white blood cells per high-power field, or protein in the urine, is considered abnormal.

The hearing loss characteristic of Alport disease progresses with age, as demonstrated by the data of Cassidy and associates (1965) (Table 24–4). The sensorineural hearing loss is predominant in the higher frequencies, showing characteristics of a cochlear lesion (positive short increment sensitivity index [SISI], recruitment, and a lack of tone decay). There appears to be some direct correlation between the severity of the hearing loss and the severity of the renal disease. Patients seldom have more than a severe hearing loss and can usually be helped significantly with a hearing aid. There are two reports that have shown an improve-

TABLE 24–4. Frequency of Sensorineural Hearing Loss in Alport Disease

	PERCENTAGE WITH SIGNIFICANT HEARING LOSS	
AGE (YEARS)	Male	Female
0–19	25	10
20–39	74	33
40–59	64	55
>60	86	83

From Cassidy, G., Brown, K., Cohen, M., and DeMaria, W. 1965. Reproduced by permission of Pediatrics Vol. 35 page 967 copyright 1965.

ment in the hearing levels of patients with Alport disease after renal dialysis or renal transplantation (Johnsen et al., 1976; Mitschke et al., 1975).

The ocular abnormalities occurring in Alport disease are important in that, as in Usher disease and congenital rubella, there is a possibility that the patient may have impairment of two sensory modalities, hearing and vision. Ocular defects, as reported by Faggioni and associates (1972), can occur in 23 per cent of the cases and are four times more frequent in males than in females. They involve the lens in 14 per cent of patients, and lenticonus is a feature in 6 per cent, cataracts in 7 per cent, and spherophakia in 1 per cent of patients.

The classic forms of mendelian inheritance do not explain the inheritance of Alport disease: There is a propensity for sons of affected mothers to be more affected than sons of affected fathers (Preus and Fraser, 1971). A hypothesis at this time to explain the transmission of Alport disease is that it is an autosomal dominant with decreased penetrance in sons of affected fathers. Another hypothesis is that there is genetic heterogeneity of different modes of inheritance, which include autosomal dominant, autosomal recessive, and an X-linked dominant form (Feingold et al., 1985). Table 24–5 presents the risks of renal failure developing in the offspring of affected parents: Renal failure will develop in about 50 per cent of sons and daughters of affected females, in about 50 per cent of daughters of affected males, and in 13 per cent of sons of affected males.

The disease can also be transmitted by an apparently asymptomatic parent, although it is probable that with a more precise definition of the phenotype the asymptomatic parents can be shown to be affected. Inheri-

TABLE 24–5. Risks of Development of Microscopic Signs of Kidney Disease for Offspring of Parents with Symptoms of Alport Disease

AFFECTED PARENT	SONS	DAUGHTERS
Mother	42	45
Father	13	53

With permission from Preus, M., and Fraser, F. G. 1971. Genetics of hereditary nephropathy with deafness (Alport's disease). Clin. Genet. 2:331. © 1971 Munksgaard International Publishers Ltd., Copenhagen, Denmark.

tance of Alport disease by the offspring of asymptomatic parents follows the same pattern as inheritance from symptomatic parents.

The histopathologic condition of the ears and kidneys in Alport disease has often been reported; there was no consistent temporal bone pathologic change, although in all cases the middle ears and bony labyrinths were normal. The pathologic findings in four pairs of temporal bones ranged from minor changes in the macula (Fujita and Hayden, 1969) to degeneration of the organ of Corti, atrophy of the spiral ligament, and foam cells in the endolymphatic sac (Crawfurd and Toghill, 1968). Fujita and Hayden (1969) reported on a number of patients who had severe sensorineural hearing loss as evidenced on audiograms; even though in another instance the patient had had good cochlear microphonics and acoustic nerve action potentials, as recorded from the round window, he had a significant high-frequency hearing loss with a speech reception threshold of 40 dB (Ruben, 1967a).

The renal lesions occurring in Alport disease have been examined by light and electron microscopy (Kaufman et al., 1970; Spear and Gussen, 1972) and show thickening of the basement membrane of the glomerulus, flocculent precipitates in the basilar membrane, extrinsic thickening of the lamina densa, focal sclerosis, interstitial fibrosis (which was progressive in serially studied cases), interstitial infiltration, centrolobular proliferation, epithelial proliferation, glomerular hyalinization, tubular atrophy, and a variable appearance of foam cells, both within and between patients. There also appears to be a decrease in the dense deposits in the glomeruli that is correlated with a decrease in immunoglobulins.

Hicks disease is one of more than 15 different genetic diseases that have central and peripheral nervous system degeneration associated with progressive sensorineural hearing loss (Konigsmark and Gorlin, 1976). Hicks disease—sensory radicular neuropathy and sensorineural deafness—has been reported to be associated with sensorineural hearing loss developing in the second decade (Fitzpatrick et al., 1976) and must be considered to be one of the progressive sensorineural disease syndromes of childhood.

Refsum disease, consisting of retinitis pigmentosa, hypertrophic peripheral neuropathy, motor and sensory deficits, ataxia, ichthyosis, and sensorineural hearing loss, is the only sensorineural hearing disease in which the biochemical abnormality is known. It was first described by Refsum in 1946. The disease is transmitted as an autosomal recessive trait and is rare; approximately 50 cases have been reported in the world literature from Western Europe and North America.

The disease usually manifests itself during the first decade of life or at the beginning of the second decade. The patient will usually have night blindness that is progressive and results in severe visual difficulties due to decreased visual fields and posterior cataracts (Richterich et al., 1965). The patients develop weakness, especially in the limbs, and moderate to marked muscle wasting. There will be associated cerebral ataxia, and in about 80 per cent of the patients electrocardiographic changes are found, including an increased PQ interval and nodal and auricular extrasystoles. Clinically these changes are evidenced by tachycardia, gallop rhythm, and cardiac insufficiency. In many patients there are bony changes, including spondylitis, kyphoscoliosis, hammer toes, and pes cavus. These bony changes are probably caused by the peripheral neuropathy that is similar to that seen in Hicks disease. More than half of these patients will have mild ichthyosis.

The hearing loss accompanying Refsum disease usually begins in the second decade. Bergsmark and Djupesland (1968) noted a clinical hearing loss in 34 of their 44 patients with this disease. Audiometric data were obtained in 34 of the patients with a hearing loss, and, of these, 22 had a sensorineural hearing loss as shown by the presence of recruitment, a decreased middle ear reflex threshold, and a lack of tone decay. Vestibular testing, consisting of cold water caloric testing, was performed in only a few patients, and the results were normal.

The biochemical basis of Refsum disease was reported in 1963 (Klenk and Kahlke) to be an accumulation of phytic acid. Patients were placed on diets free of phytic acid, phytol, and phytanic acid (eliminating all chlorophyll, butterfat, and so forth), and the phytic acid levels fell, in seven to eight months, to within 25 or 30 per cent of the prediet levels (Eldjarn et al., 1966). None of the patients' conditions worsened, and the peripheral nerve conduction time of one patient improved. Another report on two patients showed a considerable improvement in ulnar nerve conduction time, increased strength of muscle groups, return of reflexes, lessened pain, and improvement in light touch, position sense, and coordination. There was no improvement in vision or hearing (Steinberg et al., 1970).

Hernoon and Steinberg (1969) defined the enzymatic defect in cultured fibroblasts of patients with Refsum disease: deficiency in the enzyme involved in the alpha hydroxylation of phytanate. The enzymes for subsequent steps in the degradation of phytic acid appear to be normal or near normal.

Temporal bone pathologic change has been reported in two cases of Refsum disease (Friedmann, 1974; Hallpike, 1967). Both reports describe a normal middle ear and bony labyrinth but note degeneration of the organ of Corti and of the saccule. In one case there was a marked decrease in spiral ganglion cells, and in the other they were normal. The cristae and maculae were normal in both specimens, but in one (Hallpike, 1967) the disease was associated with a sudden hearing loss.

The neuropathologic findings in Refsum disease (Refsum, 1952) include fibrous thickening of the leptomeninges and infiltration by lipid macrophages, moderate degeneration of the peripheral nerve, axonal changes in the anterior horn cells of the spinal cord, degeneration of the fiber tracts from the pontobulbar region to the cerebellar white matter, and Sudan-positive fat in moderate amounts in the nerve cells and ependyma. Electron microscopic studies of the nerves (Fardeau and Engel, 1969) showed frequent nonspecific lipid deposits in Schwann cell cytoplasm.

Sensorineural hearing loss without other stigmata, which is genetically transmitted, occurs in a large group of patients. This group includes patients with bilateral acoustic neuromas that are inherited as an autosomal dominant trait. Such cases have been described by Feiling and Ward (1920) and by Gardner and Frazier (1930). This disease entity may be different from von Recklinghausen neurofibromatosis in that it is less frequently associated with pigmentary changes and cutaneous neurofibromatosis (Alliez et al., 1975). This form of acoustic neuroma may account for 1 to 4 per cent of all patients with acoustic neuromas and has been found in Western Europe and North America.

Young and coworkers (1971) studied the relatives of the patients studied by Gardner and Frazier (1930) and obtained information on 1500 family members, of which 648 were alive at the time of the study. The onset of the symptoms of hearing loss or unsteadiness can be as early as 2 years of age, with a mean age of 21 years. The initial symptoms were decreased hearing in 11 of 21 patients, tinnitus in 6 of 21, unsteadiness in 3 of 21, and facial weakness in 1 of 21 patients. Café au lait spots were usually small and solitary. Autopsy findings in 4 of 14 cases showed that there were other asymptomatic central nervous system tumors. Those individuals who were not operated on lived an average of 18.5 years, and those who were operated on lived for an average of 9.2 years after the operation.

The hearing loss associated with congenital acoustic neuromas can initially be unilateral and progress to a bilateral loss. There is some variability in the nature of the loss, and the audiometric characteristics appear to be similar to those of other cerebropontine angle tumors. Most tumors, when of sufficient size, will lead to tone decay, a high-frequency hearing loss, difficulty in speech discrimination, and absent middle ear reflexes.

Individuals with acoustic neuromas have abnormal or absent vestibular responses. It has been noted that the numbers of drownings and near drownings in the children of these patients were remarkably high (Young et al., 1971); three individuals nearly drowned as a result of losing their sense of direction while under water, and three teenagers did drown. They were all children of affected parents. It seems reasonable to assume that the pathologic change of congenital acoustic neuroma is similar to that of other acoustic neuromas and that growth of the tumor begins on the superior vestibular nerve. Thus, one might also assume that the patients who drowned had vestibular deficits. Because the author's clinical experience has shown that children with vestibular impairment have a greater propensity for drowning than others, tests of vestibular function should be performed on all children with sensorineural hearing loss. If an impairment of the vestibular system is found, the parent and the child should be warned about the risk of swimming, especially underwater, and precautions, such as close supervision, use of life jackets, and avoidance of underwater swimming, should be instituted.

The diagnosis of acoustic neuroma in a child should be made by means of audiometric, vestibular, electrophysiologic and radiographic examinations. The tumors can be detailed with imaging techniques.

The histopathologic condition in acoustic neuromas is similar to that in other neuromas (Nager, 1964), with bundles of elongated cells forming palisades. Acoustic neuromas invade the internal auditory meatus, infiltrate the modiolus and scala tympani of the basal turn, and leave proteinaceous precipitate in the scalae tympani and vestibuli. A typical case of bilateral acoustic neuroma is illustrated in Figure 24–8. The patient first had symptoms at 10 years of age and died at age 15.

There are numerous other genetically transmitted sensorineural hearing losses that have their onset after birth with no associated stigmata (Konigsmark and Gorlin, 1976). Most of these are progressive and seldom result in profound deafness. They are inherited as autosomal dominant, autosomal recessive, or X-linked characteristics. Children with progressive sensorineural hearing loss can present a diagnostic problem in that they may not have symptoms directly referable to their hearing. This is especially true of younger children, who may exhibit social and psychologic changes. Another indication of possible sensorineural hearing loss may be marked changes in school achievement. Many of these children are hard of hearing. Most will have significant language retardation (Ruben et al., 1982). The histopathologic findings and expressivity of the gene for such sensorineural loss are variable (Rapoport and Ruben, 1974).

Acquired Sensorineural Hearing Loss

Acquired sensorineural hearing losses in children occur mainly during the perinatal period, the most common cause being prematurity. Prematurity is defined in many ways and is really nothing more than a statement about the gestational age of an infant. A number of different factors associated with prematurity could result in sensorineural hearing loss: anoxia; kernicterus, which probably acts through anoxia; ototoxic medication; labyrinthitis; meningitis; and temporal bone fractures. The last four will be discussed under separate headings because they contribute in large part to postnatal acquired sensorineural hearing loss in children.

The incidence of prematurity as a factor in sensorineural hearing loss has been reported in a clinical outpatient population to be approximately 10 per cent (Ruben and Rozycki, 1970) and as high as 23 per cent in a total population of deaf children (Johnsen, 1952b). It has been established that about 2 per cent of children with birth weights under 1.36 kg (3 lb) may have significant sensorineural hearing loss (Fraser, 1976). The chance of a premature infant's being deaf is 20 times greater than that of the child with a normal birth weight.

Premature sensorineural hearing-impaired children will usually have a severe sensorineural hearing loss, a high-frequency hearing loss, or both. These children have been found to have a high percentage of multiple handicaps: Vernon (1967) found in a deaf school population that 33 per cent of premature children had one other handicap, 27 per cent had two other handicaps, and 8 per cent had three other handicaps. Thus, 68 per cent of the children had multiple handicaps, which included aphasia, mental retardation, visual pathologic changes, emotional disturbance, and orthopedic abnormalities. Table 24–6 presents comparable data concerning multiple handicaps compared with other etiologic factors. It may be noted from Table 24–6 that those children who were premature had the highest percentage of single handicaps in three of the six categories and were the only group that had the highest percentage in more than one category. These data indicate that a premature child who has sensorineural deafness may be expected to have other difficulties, and this information must be considered in planning any habilitative program for the child. This also means that, in general, the prognosis for normal development

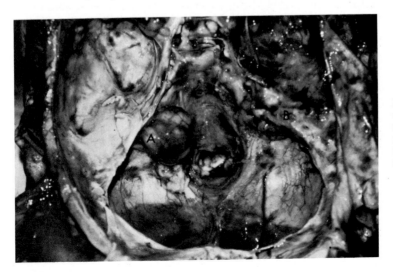

Figure 24–8. The base of the cranium of a 14-year-old child who died of multiple brain tumors. A large acoustic neuroma can be seen on the left (A). On the right in the region of the temporal bone there is a surgical deficit (B) where another acoustic neuroma was successfully removed three years before death.

TABLE 24–6. Prevalence of Other Abnormalities with Sensorineural Deafness Due to Five Causes

ETIOLOGY	CEREBRAL PALSY OR HEMIPLEGIA (%)	MENTAL RETARDATION (IQ BELOW 70) (%)	APHASIC DISORDERS (%)	VISUAL DEFECTS (%)	ORTHOPEDIC— EXCLUDING CEREBRAL PALSY (%)	SEIZURE (%)
Prematurity	18	17	36	28	9	2
Heredity	0	0	2	21	2	0
Meningitis	10	14	16	6	5	3
Rubella	4	8	22	30	5	0
Rh incompatibility	51	5	23	24	2	7

From Prematurity and deafness: The magnitude and nature of the problem among deaf children, by M. Vernon, Except. Child., volume 33, 1967, pages 289–298. Copyright 1967 by The Council for Exceptional Children. Reprinted with permission.

of a premature sensorineural hearing-impaired child must be more guarded than that for other children.

There are a number of factors that may bring about sensorineural hearing loss in the premature infant, of which anoxia is probably the most important. Hall (1964) examined the inner ears and cochlear nuclei of 39 children who had undergone prolonged periods of neonatal anoxia; 32 could be considered premature. The findings revealed that the inner ears were either normal or showed changes compatible with histologic or postmortem artifacts. The changes found in the inner ears were not similar to those found in experimental anoxia. The cochlear nuclei showed a decrease in cell number and a decrease in volume proportional to the length of time of the anoxia. The cochlear nuclei, both dorsal and ventral, showed a decrease in cell population of 20 per cent after 10 hours of anoxia, 40 per cent after 24 hours of anoxia, and 45 per cent after 2 days of anoxia. These findings agree with the histopathologic observations of kernicterus; in prematurity associated with anoxia, they suggest that the pathologic lesion resulting in sensorineural hearing loss may not lie in the cochlea but in the cochlear nucleus complex and perhaps in other portions of the central nervous system. This information also agrees with the observation that premature infants with respiratory distress syndrome develop more neurologic anomalies than weight-controlled premature infants who do not have the respiratory distress syndrome (Fisch et al., 1968). The hypothesis that a central nervous system pathologic condition is the underlying mechanism for sensorineural hearing loss in the premature infant is also congruent with the high rate of multiple central nervous system handicaps found in these children (Vernon, 1967).

The problems encountered with kernicterus are similar to those seen with prematurity, and many children with kernicterus are also premature. The frequency of a history of kernicterus in a population of sensorineurally deaf children today is about 0.5 to 1.5 per cent (Ruben and Rozycki, 1970; Vernon, 1967). Owing to improved perinatal care, fewer cases of Rh incompatibility are seen, but ABO and other blood group incompatibilities are found to be associated with kernicterus and sensorineural hearing loss. The hearing loss in these cases is usually a high-frequency loss with little loss of speech discrimination. The acoustic

characteristics are those of a cochlear loss (Matkin and Carhart, 1966), but in one study a number of the subjects heard the signals in the binaural median plane localization tests as separate signals and not as a fused signal. This was thought to be a possible indication of central auditory pathologic changes (Matkin and Carhart, 1966).

A long-term follow-up study of children with kernicterus (Walker et al., 1974) found that 22 per cent of the children had severe sensorineural hearing loss consistent with the severity of the hemolytic disease. This report noted that children with the greatest sensorineural hearing losses had multiple handicaps as well.

Histopathologic examination of the ears and brains of patients with kernicterus shows the middle and inner ears to be normal, with the abnormalities occurring in the central nervous system (Dublin, 1976). Changes are noted throughout the central nervous system, and, whereas the auditory system shows the greatest amount of nerve cell injury in the ventrocochlear nucleus, there appears to be a sparing of the dorsal cochlear nucleus. The dorsal olivary complex, inferior colliculus, medial geniculate body, and auditory cortex show variable degrees of pathologic findings.

Meningitis is one of the common causes of postnatal sensorineural hearing loss and may account for 4 to 7 per cent of the cases seen in a clinical setting (Barr and Wedenberg, 1965; Ruben and Rozycki, 1970). Meningitis may also play a role in the sensorineural hearing loss associated with prematurity in infancy, as the incidence of meningitis appears to be higher in the premature than in the full-term infant. A serial autopsy study of 101 infants showed that of five infants with meningitis who died, three had bacterial labyrinthitis that probably would have resulted in a severe to profound sensorineural hearing loss (Johnson, 1961). Only one of the three patients had pathologic evidence of otitis media, although otitis media was found in 55 per cent of the total population studied. Meningitis occurs throughout the pediatric age range, and the incidence of bilateral sensorineural hearing loss may be as high as 3 per cent of cases (Dahnsjo et al., 1976). Unilateral sensorineural hearing loss may also result from meningitis, and, in the report mentioned, this was found in 8 per cent of the patients. The hearing loss following meningitis can either remain static or be

TABLE 24–7. Mean Pure Tone Loss, From 512 to 2048 Hz, ASA, in Deafness Due to Five Causes, 1951

ETIOLOGY	MEAN HEARING LOSS (dB)
Kernicterus	76
Rubella	82
Prematurity	83
Genetic	88
Meningitis	93

From Prematurity and deafness. The magnitude and nature of the problem among deaf children, by M. Vernon, Except. Child., volume 33, 1967, pages 289–298. Copyright 1967 by The Council for Exceptional Children. Reprinted with permission.

progressive. The author has observed that the onset of severe to profound sensorineural hearing loss has also been noted to be delayed several weeks or months after the meningitis has resolved. Improvement in hearing has been reported after meningococcal meningitis (Liebman and Ronis, 1963) and *Haemophilus influenzae* meningitis (Roeser et al., 1975).

Children with deafness resulting from meningitis show symptoms similar to those with deafness due to prematurity. Vernon (1967) states that 28 per cent of such children will have one other significant handicap, 4 per cent will have two handicaps, 4.3 per cent will have three handicaps, and 1 per cent will have four handicaps. Overall, 38 per cent of the group will have one or more additional handicaps, including cerebral palsy, aphasia, mental retardation, visual pathologic abnormalities, emotional disturbance, and orthopedic pathologic conditions. The severity of the deafness is, on the average, greater in these children than in those who are deaf from other causes (Table 24–7). Patients with meningitic sensorineural hearing loss almost invariably have an absence of vestibular function. Thus, the same precautions apply concerning swimming that were cited for patients with acoustic neuromas.

The histopathologic characteristics of hearing loss following meningitis have been well described (Friedmann, 1974; Schuknecht, 1974). This results in a labyrinthitis that destroys the neuroepithelium. The inner ear is then replaced by granulation tissue, fibrous

scars, and new bone (Fig. 24–9). Occasionally the diagnosis of postmeningitis deafness can be made radiographically, because part of the membranous labyrinth will be replaced by bone; this abnormal bone can be detected by suitable radiographic techniques.

Labyrinthitis without meningitis may be of viral origin and is only infrequently due to bacterial or fungal infection. The incidence of labyrinthitis without meningitis, in a clinical population of patients with deafness, has been reported as about 2 per cent (Ruben and Rozycki, 1970). Various viruses, including mumps (Vuori et al., 1962), herpes zoster (Blackley et al., 1967), perhaps the coxsackievirus, and others have been implicated in sensorineural hearing loss (Rowson et al., 1975). The incidence of significant hearing loss attributable to viral labyrinthitis in the childhood population is probably less than 1 per cent. The hearing losses are usually unilateral, but, as previously mentioned (Everberg, 1960), many unilateral hearing losses are genetic in origin. A study of an epidemic of mumps in 298 Finnish servicemen revealed that 13 men, or 4 per cent, developed sensorineural hearing loss (Vuori et al., 1962). The hearing returned to normal or near normal in 13 of the 14 affected patients, and only one, or less than 1 per cent of the total population, had a persistent, unilateral, significant sensorineural hearing loss.

The histopathologic characteristics of viral infection have been reported. One of the more accurately documented cases is that reported by Blackley and colleagues (1967) in which the patient had a history of herpes zoster infection associated with the Ramsay Hunt syndrome (facial paralysis, herpetic eruption on the face, and sensorineural hearing loss). The histopathologic examination in this case showed perivascular, perineural, and intraneural round cell aggregations in the facial nerve, cochlea, and mastoid process. The organ of Corti was absent, and the scala media was collapsed.

Patients with sickle cell anemia have been found to have sensorineural hearing loss (Todd et al., 1973; Urban, 1973). Todd and associates (1973) showed that 15 per cent of patients with this disorder between the

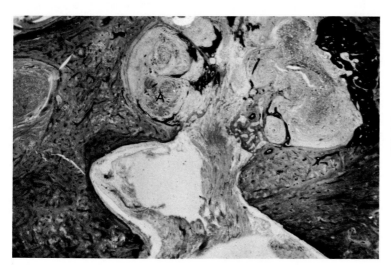

Figure 24–9. A cross-section through the temporal bone demonstrating the end stage of labyrinthitis. The entire cochlea has been replaced by granulation tissue and new bone formation (A).

ages of 10 and 19 years had sensorineural hearing losses of more than 25 dB at one or more frequencies from 500 to 8000 Hz International Standards Organization (ISO). However, some of these hearing losses may be spontaneously reversible (Urban, 1973). The ears of one 10-year-old boy with sickle cell disease and sensorineural hearing loss, with a pure tone audiogram of 35 dB and a positive SISI at 1000 and 4000 Hz, showed degenerative changes in the organ of Corti and stria vascularis but normal spiral ganglion cells (Morgenstein and Manace, 1969). The changes were thought to be due to repeated hypoxic episodes during sickle cell crises.

There are numerous other causes of sensorineural hearing loss in children, perhaps the most prevalent of which are head trauma, ototoxic drugs, and noise trauma. Patients with head injury may have fractures of the temporal bone, which may result in conductive, mixed, or sensorineural hearing loss with or without associated facial paralysis. If the fracture goes through the bony labyrinth, there will usually be a profound sensorineural hearing loss. Fractures of the bony labyrinth heal by a nonbony fibrous union. If the fracture extends into the middle ear, for the rest of their lives these patients will be at risk for developing meningitis from otitis media, as the infection can spread from the middle ear cleft via the fibrous fracture line to the meninges. It has been suggested that some of the sensorineural hearing loss following head trauma may be the result of hemorrhage into the statoacoustic nerve (Makishima and Snow, 1975). These cases would not show radiographic signs of temporal bone fracture, and they may have no otologic signs of fracture, such as hemotympanum or ruptured tympanic membrane.

Sound trauma is another cause of sensorineural hearing loss and is usually associated with workers exposed to sudden, loud noises, such as explosions. Occasionally a child will be seen who has had a firecracker explode next to his or her ear. Such a child may have a tympanic membrane perforation and may also exhibit a temporary threshold shift. Another possible cause of sound trauma is the high sound levels in incubators (American Academy of Pediatrics, 1974). These sound levels have not been proved to be harmful but may be a contributing factor to deafness in a premature infant who is also receiving ototoxic medication. It has been noted that young guinea pigs are more susceptible to noise trauma than are adult guinea pigs (Douek et al., 1976).

Another cause of sensorineural hearing loss is ototoxic medications, the most common of which are the aminoglycosides, including neomycin, kanamycin, streptomycin, dihydrostreptomycin, vancomycin, and gentamicin, and ethacrynic acid and furosemide (Worthington, 1973). Most of these drugs are excreted by the kidneys, to which they may also be toxic. A patient who is administered any of these drugs must have his or her renal function carefully monitored. The most common situations in which sensorineural deafness is observed with the use of these drugs are when an overdose is inadvertently given, when there is unrec-

ognized renal impairment, and when the drug is used to preserve life, even with the knowledge of the possibility of sensorineural hearing loss. If possible, all patients taking these medications should have serial audiometric and vestibular studies performed. If these patients have symptoms of auditory or vestibular impairment or if the objective testing shows a deficit in either the auditory or vestibular system, then the treatment plan should be reconsidered. Some of the medications (e.g., neomycin) will continue to cause irreversible hearing loss after the first signs of deficiency are noted and the drug is discontinued. Others, such as ethacrynic acid, will usually cause a hearing loss that is resolved when the medication is stopped. Experimental evidence shows a synergistic effect with ethacrynic acid and some of the aminoglycosides.

Perilymphatic fistulas occur in children with static or progressive hearing losses. These occur in three different ways. The first is a sudden hearing loss, with or without vertigo, which is associated in time with trauma or exertion such as lifting weights. These cases were similar to those first described by Goodhill and colleagues (1973). The second group of patients, with or without hearing losses, have vertigo associated with middle ear effusion. The vertigo and autonomic symptoms can be so severe as to result in dehydration, which requires hospitalization for fluid replacement. These children may have a severe head tilt, usually toward the affected side. Other than the head tilt, there are few localizing signs to indicate the affected side. Evoked potential testing and imaging have not been definitive in disclosing the affected ear. Electronystagmographic analysis of vestibular function, when combined with the fistula test, has in some instances indicated which ear has the fistula. However, there are cases in which the fistula test result with electronystagmographic analysis of vestibular function has been normal. Such cases may require exploration of the middle ear to determine if there is a fistula. These fistulas are usually found in the oval window; their closure usually results in a cessation of symptoms. The fistula may recur in the repaired ear. Hearing in children whose hearing was normal remains normal; hearing may have been stabilized in those with a progressive loss. The third group of children with perilymphatic fistulas comprises those with sensorineural hearing losses who have sudden additional loss or marked threshold fluctuation, with or without vertigo. These children are similar to those described by Healy and coworkers (1978) and Supance and Bluestone (1983). Such children may have a malformation of the bony labyrinth, ossicular chain, or both. They may or may not have vestibular signs; electronystagmographic analysis is helpful only if the fistula test result is abnormal. Normal vestibular responses have been found in patients with fistulas. Not all hearing-impaired children with sudden loss or fluctuation should be explored for a fistula, as there are other causes for this type of change in hearing. Children with labyrinthitis resulting from bacterial meningitis or congenital infections may have progressive losses.

These children should have other evidence of a fistula before exploration is undertaken. Other vestibular signs such as nystagmus, feeling of dizziness or vertigo, head tilt, clumsiness, or radiologic findings of abnormalities of the middle or inner ear may be present. Closure of the fistula may stabilize hearing; in an occasional case there is a significant recovery of hearing function.

There are numerous causes of sensorineural hearing loss in children, each of which accounts for only a small portion of the total number of those affected with this condition. The physician must be able to establish the cause of the sensorineural hearing loss, because a knowledge of the cause will, in many instances, mandate a specific form of intervention. Whether the intervention is genetic counseling, renal dialysis, or intensive aural habilitation is dependent on knowledge of the etiology of deafness or impairment.

DIAGNOSIS AND MANAGEMENT OF SENSORINEURAL DEAFNESS

Diagnosis

The prompt diagnosis of sensorineural deafness in the infant or child is one of the most important interventions a physician can make. If the diagnosis is delayed, the result may be irreversible abnormal patterns of speech, language cognition, and socialization. Figures 24–10 and 24–11 give some strategies for diagnosis and management of sensorineural deafness in children.

There are three ways in which a child can be identified as being at risk for sensorineural hearing loss: by referral from an infant or school screening program, by identification of the child through a high-risk registry, or, perhaps the most common, by parental identification of a possible hearing problem. All too often this last method of possible identification is ignored by the physician (Ruben, 1978); the physician should assume in all cases that the parent is probably correct and should investigate the child thoroughly for a sensorineural hearing loss.

It is possible, through the use of electrocochleography, brain stem evoked potentials, cortex evoked potentials, acoustic reflexes, and various behavioral techniques, to make a diagnosis of significant hearing loss in any child at any age. The differential diagnosis of sensorineural hearing loss in an infant or child who does not respond to sound or in one with delayed or abnormal language development must include peripheral hearing loss, central auditory processing abnormality, mental retardation, and, in some instances, maturational delay in responsiveness to sound. In many cases, the final diagnosis may include both peripheral hearing loss and mental retardation. After a diagnosis of the site of the deficit is made, the etiology of the hearing loss should be determined, and the child should be further evaluated to determine what other organ systems may be affected. It is im-

portant to establish the etiology of the deafness for genetic counseling of the parents and the child, to assess other organ systems that may be involved, to determine the possible medical treatment, and to provide for optimal habilitation of the patient.

The etiologic diagnosis of a sensorineural hearing loss in infants and children begins with the medical history. This must include a family history, and special inquiries should be made to elicit the possibility of consanguinity, even if it is not readily apparent. This will, in the usual American family, involve tracing the origins of both sides of the family for three or four generations. Careful attention should be given to any history of hearing impairment in other family members and to evidence of any other stigmata of genetic disease. If the family history is normal and no acquired etiology is evident, then audiometric assessment of the parents, siblings, and grandparents should be undertaken to determine if there are any carriers of a deafness gene that may lead to a diagnosis of genetic hearing loss.

The prenatal history is examined to determine whether there is any history of possible infection (viral or bacterial), administration of ototoxic medication, or attempted abortion. The perinatal history is obtained to determine if the child was premature or had kernicterus or if there was significant birth trauma or anoxia. The past history of the child is obtained to determine whether the child had meningitis, ototoxic medication, labyrinthitis, or head trauma.

In about half of the cases, a probable cause may be established from the history and physical examination; in the remainder the cause will remain unknown. Almost all infants with a diagnosis of sensorineural hearing loss will undergo further laboratory investigation to determine the etiology and to ascertain the integrity of other organ systems. Each patient should have mastoid computed tomography (CT) scanning to determine if the bony labyrinth is normal. If it is abnormal, other neurologic deficits may be expected. Vestibular testing is performed in all cases to assess the integrity of the vestibular system. As previously mentioned, an absent vestibular response can be dangerous if the child goes swimming and it may be an indication that the child has Usher disease. Also of importance is the observation that patients with decreased vestibular responses will have delayed motor development, which can be confused with early signs of developmental delay (Rapin, 1974).

The high incidence of neurologic, ophthalmologic, cardiac, and renal diseases in children with sensorineural deafness makes it imperative that each patient also undergo appropriate evaluation of these other organ systems.

All patients should undergo a pediatric neurologic, developmental, and ophthalmologic examination. Additionally, all those with hearing loss other than mild conductive losses should have imaging of the temporal bone, vestibular assessment, evaluation of brain stem responses, and speech and language evaluation. Other studies will be requested on an individual basis and

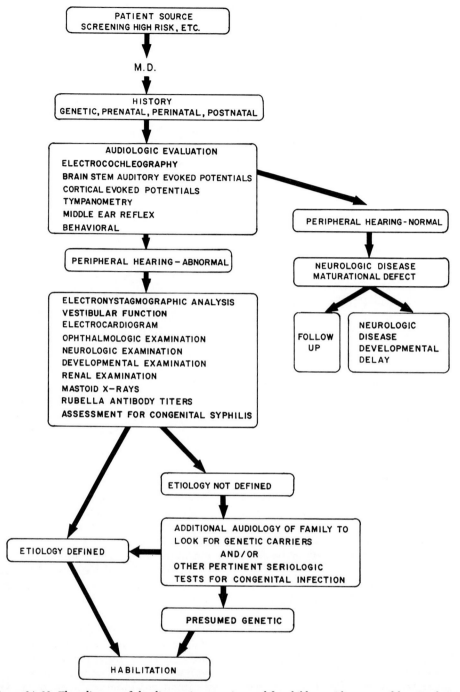

Figure 24–10. Flow diagram of the diagnostic strategies used for children with suspected hearing losses.

may include urinalysis, culture of the urine for CMV, electrocardiogram, TORCH titers, testing of the parents' and siblings' hearing to look for other affected individuals or gene carriers, and other tests as appropriate. These examinations have been useful in making a diagnosis and in defining other systemic abnormalities.

Congenital infection by rubella is still a primary cause of sensorineural deafness, even though many times the infection in the mother may be subclinical. Because of the importance of being able to diagnose the cause of deafness, all mothers and children should

have rubella antibody titers obtained if there is no history of previous immunization. Other intrauterine infections, such as toxoplasmosis and cytomegalic inclusion disease, are assessed by serum studies and physical examination if the history indicates that this may be a cause. Congenital syphilis resulting in sensorineural hearing loss in infants has been, in the author's experience, an uncommon occurrence. However, owing to the increase in the incidence of venereal disease in the general population, this source of congenital deafness should not be disregarded. Most often, syphilis can be ruled out by examining the obstetric

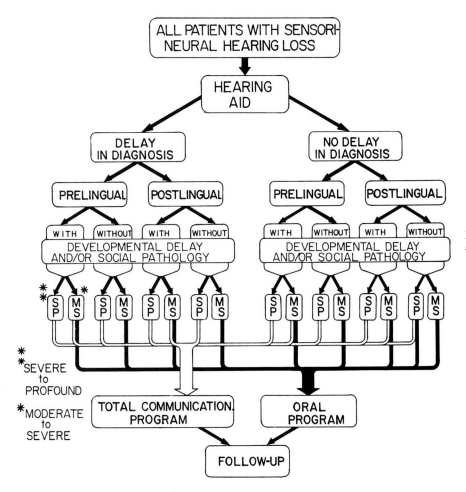

Figure 24–11. Flow diagram for the management of children with hearing loss.

and birth records, in which there is usually a report of at least one test for syphilis performed on the mother, the umbilical cord blood, or both. The infant with congenital syphilis will usually, but not invariably, be stigmatized, and the diagnosis can then be confirmed.

The older child is investigated in a similar manner, but more emphasis should be placed on the renal, ophthalmologic, and neurologic examinations.

Intervention and Health Maintenance

After the diagnosis of a sensorineural hearing loss has been made, the otorhinolaryngologist has only begun his or her task of caring for the patient. The diagnosis of the degree and type of hearing loss must be considered in its relationship to the patient's general health and psychologic and social status. Those patients who are diagnosed prelingually as having severe to profound hearing loss need at least three interventions. The first is proper amplification, usually a binaural hearing aid, at the earliest possible time. The second necessary intervention is an infant auditory training program. There is wide debate concerning two types of auditory habilitation. There are those who believe that habilitation should be based solely on oral training, perhaps reinforced with speech reading (lipreading).

The other group advises a total communication program that includes both sign language and oral training with the aid of speech reading. Based on experiences gathered over a number of years, in most instances, total communication habilitative therapy is recommended if it is available (Dee et al., 1982). This advice is given to the parent, for it is strongly believed that it is most important for the infant to learn language. Experience with infant auditory programs, both oral training and total communication, has shown that those infants with total communication develop better language skills as they mature. There is a second and perhaps equally compelling reason for recommending the total communication program: The child's social relations appear to be better when she or he is involved in this program. It becomes easier for the parents and child to communicate, and they can more clearly demonstrate their love and affection for each other.

The recommendation for a total communication program is made even more strongly when the patient has or is suspected of having a developmental delay. It is thought that these patients need all the communicative input available to learn the maximum amount of language. Additionally, those children from families in which there is significant social stress will also need the additional help in the development of language and socialization that a total communication program can afford.

A total communication program is also advocated for all patients for whom there has been a significant delay in diagnosis. Many times the diagnosis may not be made until the patient is 2 to 5 years of age, and these children have lost what may be the most critical and important years for language formation and will have great difficulty in acquiring language. Every means should be employed to optimize their acquisition of language.

The recommendation for an oral program is usually reserved only for those children with moderate to severe hearing losses who have no developmental delays and no significant social problems. The oral program is also recommended for children who are postlingually deaf and who have no developmental delay or significant social function deficits.

There are many communities in which there is no choice between a total communication program and an oral program. In these communities, attempts should be made to provide a comprehensive program for infant auditory training that allows all patients to be exposed to an optimal educational program.

The third intervention is to inform the parents about the child's disability (i.e., why the child has the problem and how the child is to be cared for). This is usually done in an informing interview. The parents, with or without the child, depending on the child's age, meet with the professionals who have performed the diagnostic assessment of the child. This group should, before the meeting with the parents, review the material and decide among themselves the best plan for the child. One to two hours should be allowed for the interview, for the professionals must explain to the parents in understandable terms what has been ascertained and the rationale for habilitation of the child. One member of this group should then become the responsible professional for the continued long-term care of the child. The parents will contact this person to ask questions and seek advice concerning the development of the child for many years after the diagnosis and plan for management have been made. This person should also reassess the child continually as he or she develops. This is done by means of a hearing test, given at least once a year, and by reassessment of cognitive, language, and social development (Ruben et al., 1984). The long-term care of the child must also include a careful assessment for serous otitis media; if this develops in addition to the sensorineural hearing loss, there will be even greater impairment (Ruben and Math, 1978). The patient must also be followed for possible progression of the sensorineural hearing loss. All patients wearing hearing aids need to have their aids checked frequently, and molds for the hearing aids will need to be remade often for infants, as the size and shape of the external auditory canal will change rapidly. Occasionally an external otitis will occur, which must be treated properly so the child can wear the aid and not be deprived of hearing (Ruben and Fishman, 1980).

There is one special category of patients, those in whom no etiologic diagnosis is made and in whom the possible cause may be a recessive genetic gene. Some of these patients will have Usher disease (retinitis pigmentosa), and the possibility of this diagnosis must always be considered so that a proper habilitative program can be instituted for a child who is deaf and will become blind. The development of blindness in a child who has been taught to depend on visual cues will cause the child to lose much of what he or she has learned. All children with deafness of unknown etiology should be routinely examined ophthalmologically to detect impending blindness as soon as possible.

Periodic assessment of the child should be undertaken, for there is always a possibility that the original diagnosis was incorrect. One can be sure of the diagnosis if, over time, the clinical and laboratory findings are consistent. Although there have been substantive advances in the diagnosis of communication disorders in infants and young children, there is still the possibility of error. If an error has been made, the habilitative therapy should be corrected as soon as possible.

SELECTED REFERENCES

Fraser, G. R. 1976. The Causes of Profound Deafness in Childhood. Baltimore, Johns Hopkins University Press.

This is an excellent book that reviews the genetic components of deafness and evaluates them in terms of the other causes of this impairment. This is probably the best book in the field of deafness etiology.

Konigsmark, B. W., and Gorlin, R. J. 1976. Genetic and Metabolic Deafness. Philadelphia, W. B. Saunders Co.

This book is a catalog of different types of genetic deafness. It contains many illustrations that will help to identify various syndromes.

McKusick, V. A. 1986. Mendelian Inheritance in Man, 7th ed. Baltimore, Johns Hopkins University Press.

This is an up-to-date cataloging of known genetic syndromes, which include those of deafness. It is essential for the care of patients with congenital genetically based hearing loss.

Michaels, L. 1987. Ear Nose and Throat Histopathology. London, Springer-Verlag.

This is an excellent book on pathologic conditions of the ear containing many valuable references and an excellent systematization of the pathologic entities.

Ruben, R. J., and Rapin, I. 1988. Management of hearing impaired deaf infant and child. *In* Alberti, P., and Ruben, R. J. (eds.): Otological Medicine and Surgery. New York, Churchill Livingstone.

This is a detailed presentation of additional aspects of diagnosis, evaluation, and forms of intervention.

Schuknecht, H. 1974. Pathology of the Ear. Boston, Harvard University Press.

This is an excellent text of pathology of the ear that lists many of the types of congenital hearing losses. There is also an excellent treatment of the pathophysiology underlying the various sensorineural hearing losses. The illustrations in this work are of the highest caliber.

REFERENCES

Alford, B. R. 1968. La bête noire de la medecine. Laryngoscope 78:1623.

Alliez, J., Masse, J. L., and Alliez, B. 1975. Tumeurs bilaterales de l'acoustique et maladie de Recklinghausen observées dans plusieurs generations. Rev. Neurol. (Paris) 131:545.

Alport, A. C. 1927. Hereditary familial, congenital, hemorrhagic nephritis. Br. J. Med. 1:504.

American Academy of Pediatrics Committee on Environmental Hazards. 1974. Noise pollution: Neonatal aspects. Pediatrics 54:476.

Anderson, H., and Wedenberg, E. 1968. Audiometric identification of normal hearing carriers of genes for deafness. Acta Otolaryngol. 65:535.

Anderson, H., Barr, B., and Wedenberg, E. 1970. Genetic disposition as a prerequisite for maternal rubella deafness. Arch. Otolaryngol. 91:141.

Anderson, H., Henricson, B., Lundquist, P. G., et al. 1968. Genetic hearing impairment in the Dalmatian dog. Acta Otolaryngol. Suppl. 232.

Barr, B., and Wedenberg, E. 1965. Prognosis of perceptive hearing loss in children with respect to genesis and use of hearing aid. Acta Otolaryngol. 59:462.

Belal, A. 1975. Usher's syndrome (retinitis pigmentosa and deafness). J. Laryngol. Otol. 89:175.

Bell, A. G. 1969. Memoirs upon the Formation of a Deaf Variety of the Human Race. Report to the National Academy of Science, 1883. Washington, DC, A. G. Bell Association for the Deaf.

Bergsmark, J., and Djupesland, G. 1968. Heredopathia atactica polyneuritiformis (Refsum's disease). Eur. Neurol. 1:122.

Blackley, B., Friedmann, I., and Wright, I. 1967. Herpes zoster auris associated with facial nerve palsy and auditory nerve symptoms. Acta Otolaryngol. 63:531.

Bordley, J. E., and Alford, B. R. 1970. The pathology of rubella deafness. Int. Audiol. 9:58.

Bordley, J. E., Brookhouser, P. E., Hardy, J., et al. 1968. Prenatal rubella. Acta Otolaryngol. 66:1.

Bosher, S. K., and Hallpike, C. S. 1966. Observations of the histogenesis of the inner ear degeneration of the deaf white cat and its possible relationship to the aetiology of certain unexplained varieties of human congenital deafness. J. Laryngol. Otol. 80:222.

Calhoun, F. P. 1919. Causes of heterochromic irides with special reference to paralysis of the cervical sympathetics. Am. J. Ophthalmol. 2:255.

Cassidy, G., Brown, K., Cohen, M., et al. 1965. Hereditary renal dysfunction and deafness. Pediatrics 35:967.

Cooper, L. Z., Florman, A. L., Ziring, P. R., et al. 1971. Loss of rubella hemagglutination inhibition antibody in congenital rubella. Am. J. Dis. Child. 122:397.

Crawfurd, M. D., and Toghill, P. J. 1968. Alport's syndrome of hereditary nephritis and deafness. Q. J. Med. 37:563.

Dahnsjo, H., Andersson, H., Hallander, H. O., and Rudberg, R. D. 1976. Tone audiometry control of children treated for meningitis with large intravenous doses of ampicillin. Acta Paediatr. Scand. 65:733.

Dee, A., Rapin, I., and Ruben, R. J. 1982. Speech and language development in a parent-infant communication program. Ann. Otol. Rhinol. Laryngol. 9:62.

Deol, M. S. 1964. Abnormalities of inner ear in Kreisler mice. J. Embryol. Exp. Morphol. 12:475.

Deraemaeker, R. 1960. Recessive congenital deafness in a North Belgian province. Acta Genet. (Basel) 10:295.

Douek, E., Bannister, L. H., Dodson, H. C., et al. 1976. Effects of incubator noise on the cochlea of the newborn. Lancet 2:1110.

Dublin, W. B. 1976. Fundamentals of Sensorineural Auditory Pathology. Springfield, IL, Charles C Thomas.

Eldjarn, L., Try, K., Stokke, O., et al. 1966. Dietary effects on serum–phytanic acid levels and on clinical manifestations in heredopathia atactica polyneuritformis. Lancet 1:691.

Everberg, A. 1960. Unilateral anacusis: Clinical, radiological and genetic investigations. Acta Otolaryngol. Suppl. 158:366.

Faggioni, R., Scouras, J., and Streiff, E. B. 1972. Alport's syndrome: Clinicopathological considerations. Ophthalmologica (Basel) 165:1.

Fardeau, M., and Engel, W. K. 1969. Ultrastructural study of a peripheral nerve biopsy in Refsum's disease. J. Neuropathol. Exp. Neurol. 28:278.

Fay, E. A. 1898. Marriages of the Deaf in America. Washington, DC, Volta Bureau.

Fay, J. E., Olley, P. M., Partington, M. W., et al. 1971. Surdo-cardiac syndrome: Incidence among children in schools for the deaf. Can. Med. Assoc. J. 105:718.

Feiling, A., and Ward, E. A. 1920. A familial form of acoustic tumor. Br. Med. J. 1:496.

Feingold, J., Bois, E., Chompert, A., et al. 1985. Genetic heterogeneity of Alport syndrome. Kidney Int. 27:672.

Fisch, L. 1959. Deafness as part of an hereditary syndrome. J. Laryngol. Otol. 73:355.

Fisch, R. O., Gravem, H. J., and Engel, R. R. 1968. Neurological status of survivors of neonatal respiratory distress syndrome. J. Pediatr. 73:395.

Fitzpatrick, D. B., Hooper, R. E., and Seife, B. 1976. Hereditary deafness and sensory radicular neuropathy. Arch. Otolaryngol. 102:552.

Forrest, J. M., and Menser, M. A. 1970. Congenital rubella in school children and adolescents. Arch. Dis. Child. 45:66.

Fraser, G. R. 1965a. Association of congenital deafness with goitre (syndrome of Pendred)—study of 207 families. Ann. Hum. Genet. 28:201.

Fraser, G. R. 1965b. Sex-linked recessive congenital deafness and the excess of males in profound childhood deafness. Ann. Hum. Genet. 29:171.

Fraser, G. R. 1976. The Causes of Profound Deafness in Childhood. Baltimore, Johns Hopkins University Press.

Fraser, G. R., Froggatt, P., and James, T. N. 1964a. Congenital deafness associated with electrocardiographic abnormalities, fainting attacks and sudden death—a recessive syndrome. Q. J. Med. 33:361.

Fraser, G. R., Froggatt, P., and Murphy, T. 1964b. Genetic aspects of the cardioauditory syndrome of Jervell and Lange-Nielsen. Ann. Hum. Genet. 28:133.

Forrest, J. M., and Menser, M. A. 1975. Recent implications of intrauterine and postnatal rubella. Aust. Paediatr. J. 11:65.

Friedmann, I. 1974. Pathology of the Ear. London, Blackwell Scientific Publications.

Friedmann, I., Fraser, G. R., and Froggatt, P. 1966. Pathology of the ear in the cardio-auditory syndrome of Jervell and Lange-Nielsen (recessive deafness with electrocardiographic abnormalities). J. Laryngol. 80:451.

Fujita, S., and Hayden, R. C. 1969. Alport's syndrome. Arch. Otolaryngol. 90:453.

Gardner, W. J., and Frazier, C. H. 1930. Bilateral acoustic neurofibromas: A clinical study and field survey of a family of five generations with bilateral deafness in 38 members. Arch. Neurol. Psychiatr. 23:266.

Goldberg, M. F. 1966. Waardenburg's syndrome with fundus and other anomalies. Arch. Ophthalmol. 76:797.

Goodhill, V., Harris, I., and Brockman, S. J., 1973. Sudden deafness in labyrinthine window ruptures. Ann. Otol. Rhinol. Laryngol. 73:2.

Gottlieb, G. 1975. Development of species identification in ducklings. (1) Nature of perceptual deficit caused by embryonic auditory deprivation. J. Comp. Physiol. Psychol. 89:387.

Grondahl, J., and Mjoen, S. 1986. Usher's syndrome in four Norwegian counties. Clin. Genet. 30:14.

Hall, J. G. 1964. The cochlea and the cochlear nuclei in neonatal asphyxia. Acta Otolaryngol. Suppl. 194.

Hallgren, B. 1959. Retinitis pigmentosa combined with congenital deafness; with vestibulo-cerebellar ataxia and mental abnormality in a proportion of cases. Acta Psychiatr. Scand. 34, Suppl. 138.

Hallpike, C. S. 1967. Observations on the structural basis of two rare varieties of hereditary deafness. In de Reuck, A. V., and Knight, J. (eds.): Myotatic, Kinesthetic and Vestibular Mechanisms. Ciba Foundation Symposium. Boston, Little, Brown and Co.

Hansen, A. C., Ackouy, G., and Crump, E. P. 1965. Waardenburg's syndrome: Report of a pedigree. J. Natl. Med. Assoc. 57:8.

Healy, G., Friedman, J. M., and Toria, A., 1978. Ataxia and hearing loss secondary to perilymph fistula. Pediatrics 61:238.

Henke, F., and Lubarsch, O., 1926. Handbuch der Speziellen Pathologischen Anatomie und Histologie. Berlin, Springer-Verlag.

Hernoon, J. H., and Steinberg, D. 1969. Refsum disease—characterization of enzyme defect in cell culture. J. Clin. Immunol. 58:1017.

Hvidberg-Hansen, J., and Jorgensen, M. B. 1968. The inner ear in Pendred's syndrome. Acta Otolaryngol. 66:129.

Jackson, J. R., and Rubel, E. W. 1976. Rapid transneuronal degeneration following cochlear removal in the chick. Anat. Rec. 184:434.

James, T. N. 1967. Congenital deafness and cardiac arrhythmias. Am. J. Cardiol. 19:627.

Jervell, A., and Lange-Nielsen, F. 1957. Congenital deaf-mutism, functional heart disease with prolongation of Q-T interval and sudden death. Am. Heart J. 54:59.

Johnsen, S. 1952a. Natal causes of perceptive deafness. Acta Oto-laryngol. 42:51.

Johnsen, S. 1952b. The heredity of perceptive deafness. Acta Otolaryngol. 42:439.

Johnsen, T., Jorgensen, M. B., Jonsen, S. 1986. Mondini cochlea in Pendred's syndrome. A histological study. Acta Otolaryngol. (Stock.) 102:239.

Johnson, D. W., Wathen, R. L., and Mathog, R. H. 1976. Effects of hemodialysis on hearing threshold. ORL 38:129.

Johnson, W. W. 1961. A survey of middle ears: 101 autopsies of infants. Ann. Otol. Rhinol. Laryngol. 70:377.

Kaufman, D. B., McIntosh, R. M., and Smith, F. G. 1970. Diffuse familial nephropathy: A clinical pathological study. J. Pediatr. 97:37.

Klenk, E., and Kahlke, W. 1963. Uber das Vorkommen der 3, 7, 11, 15-Tetramethylhexadecansaure in den Cholesterinestern und anderen Lipoidfraktionen der Organe bei einem Krankheitsfall unbekannter Genese. Hoppe-Seyler's Z. Phys. Chem. 333:133.

Kloepfer, H. W., Hallpike, C. S., De Hass, E. B., et al. 1970. Usher's syndrome with special reference to heterozygote manifestations. Docum. Ophthalmol. 28:166.

Kloepfer, H. W., Laguaite, J. K., and McLaurin, J. W. 1966. The hereditary syndrome of deafness in retinitis pigmentosa. Laryngoscope 76:850.

Konigsmark, B. W., and Gorlin, R. J. 1976. Genetic and Metabolic Deafness. Philadelphia, W. B. Saunders Co.

Levi-Montalcini, R. 1949. Development of the acousticovestibular centers in chick embryo in the absence of the afferent root fibers and descending fiber tracts. J. Comp. Neurol. 91:209.

Liebman, E., and Ronis, M. L. 1963. Hearing improvement following meningitis deafness. Arch. Otolaryngol. 90:470.

Makishima, K., and Snow, J. B. 1975. Pathogenesis of hearing loss in head injury. Arch. Otolaryngol. 102:426.

Matkin, N. D., and Carhart, R. 1966. Auditory profiles associated with Rh incompatibility. Arch. Otolaryngol. 84:502.

McKusick, V. A. 1986. Mendelian Inheritance in Man (Catalogs of Autosomal Dominant, Autosomal Recessive and X-linked Phenotypes). Baltimore, Johns Hopkins University Press.

Mikaelian, D., and Ruben, R. J. 1965. Development of hearing in the normal CBA-J mouse. Acta Otolaryngol. 59:451.

Mitschke, H., Schmidt, P., Kopsa, H., and Zazgornik, J. 1975. Reversible uremic deafness after successful renal transplantation. N. Engl. J. Med. 292:1062.

Morgans, M. E., and Trotter, W. R. 1958. Association of congenital deafness with goitre. Lancet 1:607.

Morgenstein, K. M., and Manace, E. D. 1969. Temporal bone histopathology in sickle cell disease. Laryngoscope 79:2172.

Nager, F. R. 1927. Zur Histologie der Taubstummheit bei Retinitis pigmentosa. Beitr. Path. Anat. 77:288.

Nager, G. T. 1964. Association of bilateral VIIIth nerve tumors with meningiomas in von Recklinghausen's disease. Laryngoscope 74:1220.

Nutman, J., Steinherc, R., Sivan, Y., and Goodman, R. M., 1986. Possible Waardenburg syndrome with gastrointestinal anomalies. J. Med. Genet. 23:175.

Nuutila, A. 1970. Dystrophia retinae pigmentosa-dysacusis syndrome (DRD). A study of the Usher or Hallgren syndrome. J. Genet. Hum. 18:57.

Olley, P. M., and Fowler, R. S. 1970. The surdo-cardiac syndrome and therapeutic observations. Br. Heart J. 32:467.

Olson, J. E., Dowrat, R. H., and Brant, W. E. 1982. Use of high resolution thin section CT scanning of the petrous bone in temporal bone anomalies. Laryngoscope 92:1274.

Pantke, O. A., and Cohen, M. M. J. 1971. The Waardenburg syndrome. Birth Defects 7:147.

Parks, T. N., and Robinson, J. 1976. The effects of otocyst removal on the development of chick brain stem auditory nuclei. Anat. Rec. 184:497.

Parving, A. 1985. Hearing disorders in children: Some procedures for detection, identification and diagnostic evaluation. Int. J. Pediatr. Otorhinolaryngol. 9:31.

Pendred, V. 1896. Deaf mutism and goitre. Lancet 2:532.

Platia, E. V., Griffith, L., Watkins, L., et al. 1985. Management of the prolonged QT syndrome and recurrent ventricular fibrillation with an implantable automatic cardioverter-defibrillator. Clin. Cardiol. 8:490.

Preus, M., and Fraser, F. G. 1971. Genetics of hereditary nephropathy with deafness (Alport's disease). Clin. Genet. 2:331.

Pryor, H. B. 1969. Objective measurement of interpupillary distance. Pediatrics 44:973.

Rapin, I. 1974. Hypoactive labyrinth and motor development. Clin. Pediatr. 13:922.

Rapoport, Y., and Ruben, R. J. 1974. Dominant neurosensory hearing loss: Genetic, audiologic and histopathologic correlates. Trans. Am. Acad. Ophthalmol. Otol. 78:423.

Rarey, K. E., and Davis, L. E. 1984. Inner ear anomalies in Waardenburg's syndrome associated with Hirschsprung's disease. Int. J. Pediatr. Otorhinolaryngol. 8:181.

Refsum, S. 1946. Heredopathia atactica polyneuritiformis. Acta Psychiatr. Neurol. Scand. Suppl. 38.

Refsum, S. 1952. Heredopathia atactica polyneuritiformis. J. Nerv. Mental Dis. 116:1046.

Richards, C. S. 1964. Middle ear changes in rubella deafness. Arch. Otolaryngol. 80:48.

Richterich, R., Moser, H., and Rossi, E. 1965. Refsum's disease (heredopathia atactica polyneuritiformis). Humangenetik 1:322.

Riesen, A. H., and Zilbert, D. E. 1975. Developmental Neuropsychology of Sensory Deprivation. New York, Academic Press.

Robinson, G. C., and Cambon, K. G. 1964. Hearing loss in infants of tuberculous mothers treated with streptomycin during pregnancy. N. Engl. J. Med. 271:949.

Roeser, R. J., Campbell, J. D., and Daly, D. D. 1975. Recovery of auditory function following meningitic deafness. J. Speech Hear. Disord. 40:405.

Rowson, K. E. K., Hinchcliffe, R., and Gamble, D. R. 1975. A virological and epidemiological study of patients with acute hearing loss. Lancet 1:471.

Ruben, R. J. 1967a. Cochlear potentials as a diagnostic test in deafness. Symposium on Sensory Neural Hearing Processes and Disorder. Boston, Little, Brown and Co., pp. 313–338.

Ruben, R. J. 1967b. Development of the inner ear of the mouse: A radioautographic study of terminal mitosis. Acta Otolaryngol. Suppl. 220.

Ruben, R. J. 1970. Screening for rubella during pregnancy. N. Engl. J. Med. 283:1292.

Ruben, R. J. 1978. Delay in diagnosis (editorial). Volta Review #4, 80:201.

Ruben, R. J. 1984. An inquiry into the minimal amount of auditory deprivation which results in a cognitive effect in man. Presented in Umea, Sweden, 1983. Acta Otolaryngol. (Stockh.) 414:157.

Ruben, R. J. 1986. Unsolved problems around critical periods with emphasis on clinical applications. Acta Otolaryngol. (Stockh.) 429:61.

Ruben, R. J. and Fishman, G. 1980. Otological care of the hearing impaired child. In Proceedings of the Third Elk's International Conference: Early Management of Hearing Loss. New York, Grune & Stratton, pp. 106–119.

Ruben, R. J., and Math, S, 1978. Serous otitis media associated with sensorineural hearing loss in children. Laryngoscope 7:1139.

Ruben, R. J., and Rapin, I. 1980. Plasticity of the developing auditory system. Ann. Otol. Rhinol. Laryngol. 89:303.

Ruben, R. J., and Rozycki, D. 1970. Diagnostic screening for the deaf child. Arch. Otolaryngol. 91:429.

Ruben, R. J., and Rozycki, D. 1971. Clinical aspects of genetic deafness. Ann. Otol. Rhinol. Laryngol. 80:255.

Ruben, R. J., and Van De Water, T. R. 1983. Recent advances in the developmental biology of the ear. In Gerber, S. C., and Menchner, G. T. (eds.): Development of Auditory Behavior. New York, Grune & Stratton, pp. 3–35.

Ruben, R. J., Levine, R., Fishman, G., et al. 1982. The moderate to severe sensorineural hearing impaired child: An analysis of etiology, intervention and outcome. Laryngoscope 92:38.

Ruben, R. J., Silver, M., and Umano, H. 1984. Assessment of

efficacy of intervention in hearing impaired children with speech and language deficits. Laryngoscope 94:10.

Salisbury, A. J., and Ma, P. 1976. Reported rubella in the United States, 1975. National Foundation—March of Dimes.

Sanchez-Cascos, A., Sanchez-Harguindey, L., and de Rabago, P. 1969. Cardio-auditory syndromes. Br. Heart J. 31:26.

Sataloff, J., Pastore, P. N., and Bloom, E. 1955. Sex-linked hereditary deafness. Am. J. Hum. Genet. 7:201.

Schuknecht, H. 1974. Pathology of the Ear. Boston, Harvard University Press.

Settlemayer, J. R., and Hogan, M. 1961. Waardenburg syndrome—Report of a case in a non-Dutch family. N. Engl. J. Med. 261:500.

Shinkawa, H., and Nadol, J. B., Jr. 1986. Histopathology of the inner ear and Usher's syndrome as observed by light and electromicroscopy. Ann. Otol. Rhinol. Laryngol. 95:313.

Simpson, J. L., Falk, C. T., Morillo-Cucci, et al. 1974. Analysis for possible linkage between loci for the Waardenburg syndrome and various blood groups and serological traits. Am. J. Hum. Genet. 13:45.

Sirles, W. A., and Slasghts, H. 1943. Pigmentary deafness of retina and neural type deafness. Am. J. Ophthalmol. 26:961.

Smith, A. B. 1939. Unilateral hereditary deafness. Lancet 2:1172.

Smith, J. F. 1960. The pathology of the thyroid in the syndrome of sporadic goitre and congenital deafness. Quart. J. Med. 29:297.

Spear, G. S., and Gussen, R. 1972. Alport's syndrome, emphasizing electron microscopic studies of the glomeruli. Am. J. Pathol. 69:213.

Stagno, S., Pass, R. F., Dworsky, M. E., et al. 1982. Congenital cytomegalovirus infection: The relative importance of primary and recurrent maternal infection. N. Engl. J. Med. 306:945.

Steinberg, D., Mize, C. E., Hernoon, J. H., et al. 1970. Phytic acid in patients with Refsum's syndrome and response to dietary treatment. Arch. Intern. Med. 125:75.

Stoller, F. M. 1962. A deaf mute with two congenital syndromes. Arch. Otolaryngol. 76:42.

Strauss, M. 1982. A clinical and pathological study of hearing loss in the congenital cytomegalic virus infection. Laryngoscope 95:951.

Supance, J. S., and Bluestone, C. D. 1983. Perilymph fistuli in Infants and Children. Otolaryngol. Head Neck Surg. 91:663.

Swan, C., Tostevin, A. L., Moore, B., et al. 1943. Congenital defects in infants following infectious diseases during pregnancy. With special reference to the relationship between German measles and cataract, deaf-mutism, heart disease and microcephaly, and to the period of pregnancy in which the occurrence of rubella is followed by congenital abnormalities. Med. J. Aust. 2:201.

Thould, A. K., and Scowen, E. F. 1964. The syndrome of congenital deafness and simple goiter. J. Endocrinol. 30:69.

Todd, G. B., Serjeant, F. R., and Larson, M. R. 1973. Sensorineural hearing loss in Jamaicans with sickle cell disease. Acta Otolaryngol. 76:268.

Urban, G. E. 1973. Reversible sensorineural hearing loss associated with sickle cell crisis. Laryngoscope 83:633.

Vernon, M. 1967. Prematurity and deafness: The magnitude and nature of the problem among deaf children. Except. Child. 33:289.

Vernon, M. 1969. Usher's syndrome—deafness and progressive blindness. Clinical cases, prevention, theory and literature survey. J. Chronic Dis. 22:133.

von Graefe, A. 1858. Vereinzelte Beobachtungen und Bemerkungen. Exceptionelles Verhalten des Gesichtsfeldes bei Pigmentenartung der Netzhaut. Albrecht von Graefe's Arch. Klin. Ophthalmol. 4:250.

Vuori, M., Lahikainen, E. A., and Peltonen, T. 1962. Perceptive deafness in connection with mumps. Acta Otolaryngol. 55:232.

Waardenburg, P. J. 1951. A new syndrome combining developmental anomalies of the eyelids, eyebrows and nose root with pigmentary defects of the iris and head hair and with congenital deafness. Am. J. Hum. Genet. 3:195.

Walker, W., Ellis, M. I., Ellis, E., et al. 1974. A follow-up study of survivors of Rh hemolytic disease. Dev. Med. Child Neurol. 16:592.

Wardrop, J. 1813. History of James Mitchell, a Boy Born Blind and Deaf with an Account of the Operation Performed for Recovery of His Sight. London, Murray.

Webster, D. G., and Webster, M. 1977. Neonatal sound deprivation affects brain stem auditory nuclei. Arch. Otolaryngol. 103:392.

Weinberger, M. M., Masland, M. W., Asbed, R. A., et al. 1970. Congenital rubella presenting as retarded language development. Am. J. Dis. Child. 120:125.

Wilde, W. R. 1853. Practical Observations on Aural Surgery and the Nature and Diagnosis of Diseases of the Ear. Philadelphia, Blanchard and Lea.

Worthington, E. L. 1973. Index-Handbook of Ototoxic Agents, 1966–1971. Baltimore, Johns Hopkins University Press.

Yntema, C. L. 1950. Analysis of induction of the ear from foreign ectoderm in the salamander embryo. J. Exp. Zool. 113:211.

Young, D. F., Eldridge, R., Nager, G. T., et al. 1971. Hereditary bilateral acoustic neuroma—central neurofibromatosis. Birth Defects 7:73.

Chapter 25

DISEASES OF THE LABYRINTHINE CAPSULE

LaVonne Bergstrom, M.D.

The labyrinthine or otic capsule consists of persistent or primary bone overlaid both internally and externally with perichondrial or lamellar bone. The ossicles, although of branchial origin, have a similar composition. Most diseases of the otic capsule also affect the skeleton generally; only one, otosclerosis, seems to occur only in the otic capsule. Many of these disorders are seen in the preadult years; some are present at birth. When they occur in the temporal bone they may be silent or latent, but when symptomatic they profoundly affect a child's school and social life.

OSTOSCLEROSIS (OTOSPONGIOSIS)

Clinical otosclerosis is rare under the age of 5 years and is extremely rare in people of Asian or African heritage (McKenzie, 1948; Larsson, 1960; Friedmann, 1974; Schuknecht, 1974). Symptoms begin between the ages of 11 and 30 years in 70 per cent of individuals but in only 2 to 3 per cent prior to age 15 years. The youngest recorded patient was 1 year of age (Nager, 1969). Otosclerosis is genetic, probably of autosomal dominant inheritance with reduced penetrance, although this may be more apparent than real, as histologic otosclerosis may occur in "silent" areas of the labyrinthine capsule. Polygenic inheritance, possibly involving genes affecting collagen, calcium, parathormone, and bony structure, has also been postulated (Mendlowitz and Hirschhorn, 1976). Low fluoride content in drinking water has been hypothesized to contribute to the development of otosclerosis (Daniel, 1969), but its relationship to genetic factors has yet to be clarified. Otosclerotic foci occurred in only 0.6 per cent of temporal bones in patients under age 5 years and 4 per cent over age 5 years, rising to an incidence of 10 per cent in males and 18 per cent in females between the ages of 30 and 50 years. However, stapes ankylosis occurred in only 15 per cent of bones with histologic findings of otosclerosis (Guild, 1944). Clinically, the otosclerosis patient experiences insidious, usually bilaterally symmetric, progressive hearing loss. Tinnitus and vertigo are unusual in young individuals. On examination, the tympanic membranes of these patients are intact and mobile, and the results of nose and throat examination are normal. The patient's articulation and voice quality are good unless the hearing loss occurred early and was rapidly progressive. Bone conduction may be louder than air conduction as measured by tuning fork tests, but in early cases only audiometry may demonstrate an air-bone gap. The acoustic impedance instrument will show normal middle-ear pressure, but the acoustic reflex will either show a peculiar on-off negative deflection in early cases or will be absent, and impedance may be high (Terkildsen et al., 1973; Van Wagoner and Campbell, 1976). Concurrent sensorineural hearing loss may also occur. The accelerating effects of pregnancy and possibly of birth control pills on the symptomatic onset of otosclerosis in about 25 per cent of cases must be noted, as more teen-age girls are using contraceptives or becoming pregnant.

Otosclerosis often begins in the endochondral bone anterior to the oval window. An active or immature focus, often thought to represent an earlier phase in the evolution of the lesion (Nager, 1969), is sometimes visible through an intact tympanic membrane as an area of reddish glow on the promontory, referred to as Schwartze sign. When examined during surgery such a focus is soft and bleeds readily; histologically it stains blue with hematoxylin and eosin and is quite vascular and spongiotic. Nager reported an extensive, active lesion in the temporal bone of an 8½-year-old girl with normal hearing (Nager, 1969). In young patients with otosclerosis, otologic surgeons may encounter active vascular lesions that tend to refix the stapes after mobilization or to obliterate the oval window. Mature, inactive, or "healed" foci are grossly white and avascular, stain red or pink with hematoxylin and eosin, and more closely resemble normal compact bone than otosclerotic bone. Active and inactive foci may be seen at different locations in the same individual. Circumferential confluent or multiple lesions have been described in these types of bones (Black et al., 1969).

Ankylosis of the stapes may involve only the fibrous annulus; if the ankylosis is bony, it may involve only the anterior footplate, or if it is obliterative it may bury the crura and footplate in a mound of otosclerosis. An otosclerotic focus may invade labyrinthine spaces and may be associated with spiral ligament and strial atrophy, organ of Corti hair cell loss, neural atrophy, and vestibular pathologic changes (Sando et al., 1968, 1974). Rüedi and Spoendlin believe that blood shunts from the middle-ear circulation to the spiral ligament, causing congestion of its vessels and resultant cochlear neuroepithelial damage (Rüedi and Spoendlin, 1966). Other theories are that an otosclerotic focus releases toxic substances into the inner ear or that its effect is purely mechanical, distorting basilar membrane movement or propagation of the traveling wave (Altmann et al., 1966; Sando et al., 1968).

The differential diagnosis of otosclerosis is congenital ossicular fixation, which may present identical clinical findings and a positive family history. Petrous pyramid polytomography may demonstrate gross congenital ossicular lesions or large, active otosclerotic lesions. Ossicular discontinuity, which may be congenital or postinflammatory, may cause increased compliance on the tympanogram and may be demonstrable by tomography. Most sequelae of otitis media are evident on otologic examination, and other disorders of the otic capsule have systemic or regional manifestations.

The treatment of significant hearing loss due to otosclerosis in early life deserves special consideration, although little authoritative information on this subject is available. Some clinicians believe that surgery should be postponed until active foci become inactive to decrease the risk of inner ear damage or recurrent stapes fixation. Amplification of hearing could tide over the individual until the disease stabilizes and surgery is indicated. Some espouse treatment with fluoride, calcium, and vitamin D for adults who develop progressive sensorineural hearing loss and who show roentgenographic evidence of labyrinthine invasion by otosclerosis (Shambaugh and Causse, 1974; Parkins, 1974). Such a regimen should probably be undertaken only after consultation with an endocrinologist because no longitudinal data on children or adolescents treated in this manner are available. Stapes surgery may give good long-term results in those patients whose otosclerosis seems mature and inactive, but long-term hearing improvement is maintained at a 10-dB or smaller air-bone gap in less than 70 per cent of patients of all ages (Schuknecht, 1974). It would seem wise to avoid operating on the only ear through which the patient can hear or on unilaterally involved ears and to reserve operating on the second ear until adult life, because operative techniques may improve. A child or teen-ager who may not be capable of fully informed consent deserves consultation with the most experienced and skillful otologic surgeon available before a decision for or against surgery is made. Complications of stapes surgery include sensorineural hearing loss, oval window fistula (Hemenway et al., 1968), granuloma (Gacek, 1970), and suppurative labyrinthitis (Schuknecht, 1974). The child operated on for otosclerosis might be particularly at risk for this last complication, because the incidence of upper respiratory tract infections and otitis media is highest in the early school years.

OSTEOGENESIS IMPERFECTA

Osteogenesis imperfecta occurs in two forms. The more severe congenital type is distinguished by craniotabes, multiple wormian bones of the skull, and congenital and many postnatal fractures that cause stunting and deformities of the torso and limbs (Fig. 25–1). Affected neonates may not survive. In the less severe form, osteogenesis imperfecta tarda, congenital fractures may occur, but deformity is less pronounced. Hearing loss, which may be sensorineural, conductive, or mixed, typically begins in the second or third decade of life. Three types of pathologic findings in the middle ear have been described. The ossicles, especially the stapes, are fragile, with such thinning of the structures that ossicular discontinuity or fracture occurs. A second finding has been that of a bulky, soft, crumbly stapes footplate that may be lightly ankylosed. Occasionally, thin crura and a bulky footplate occur together. Because there is abundant histologic, biochemical, and other evidence to show that osteogenesis imperfecta and otosclerosis are distinct dysplasias of the temporal bone, it is of considerable interest that they may occur together. Lesions compatible with congenital conductive hearing loss have been reported. Lopping, outward slanting, posterior rotation, or notching of the posterosuperior helical margin of the pinnae and salmon-pink flush of the promontory are other otologic features of interest. Other head and neck findings may include blue sclerae, dentinogenesis imperfecta, and epistaxis. These children, who may undergo many surgical procedures, are at risk for hemorrhage, malignant hyperthermia, hypertrophic scar formation, incompetent or floppy heart valves, and cor pulmonale (Bergstrom, 1977).

Older children and teen-agers may develop enough hearing loss to require treatment. Measures such as preferential seating in school and speech reading training may suffice, but amplification or middle-ear surgery might be desirable.

When examined histologically, osteogenesis imperfecta bone appears to be porous and has poor matrix surrounding a few cancellous trabeculae containing numerous osteocytes. There is an increased amount of osteoid and woven bone; microfractures may be seen, and the collagen of this type of bone is defective in some way. In the temporal bone there is widespread deficiency of ossification of the ossicles and the area around membranous labyrinthine end organs and nerves. As a result of deficient laying down of bone the internal auditory canal may appear to be widened and the mastoid air cells to be unusually well pneumatized. Fractures may occur. Inner ear pathologic changes includes calcific deposits in, and acute degeneration of, the cochlear vascular stria; swelling and distortion of the tectorial membrane; and degeneration of the organ of Corti and vestibular neuroepithelium. Petrous pyramid polytomography duplicates some of the above findings. In addition, a widened cochlea or "cochlea within a cochlea" may be seen (Bergstrom, 1977) (Fig. 25–2).

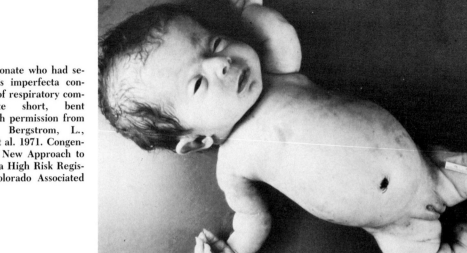

Figure 25–1. Neonate who had severe osteogenesis imperfecta congenita and died of respiratory complications. Note short, bent extremities. (With permission from Black, F. O., Bergstrom, L., Downs, M. P., et al. 1971. Congenital Deafness: A New Approach to Diagnosis Using a High Risk Register. Boulder, Colorado Associated Univ. Press.)

There appear to be fewer fractures of facial bones than of the skeleton generally, but there is some evidence to suggest that facial fractures may occur more frequently in osteogenesis imperfecta than had heretofore been suspected (Bergstrom, 1977).

The inheritance of osteogenesis imperfecta tarda may be dominant or recessive. Subclinically affected parents may have affected children. Osteogenesis imperfecta congenita offspring have been born to normal parents, to carriers of the trait, and to those affected by the tarda form.

OSTEOPETROSIS (ALBERS–SCHÖNBERG DISEASE)

Osteopetrosis, also called marble bone or chalk bone disease, is a sporadic or recessively inherited general

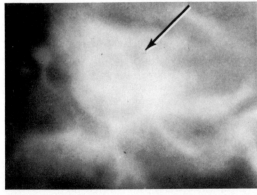

Figure 25–2. Petrous polytomogram of patient who has van der Hoeve syndrome of osteogenesis imperfecta tarda and hearing loss. Note widened appearance of the cochlea owing to deficient laying down of bone, giving a "cochlea within a cochlea" appearance (arrow). (Used by permission of W. Hanafee, M.D.)

bone dyscrasia characterized by hard, brittle bones. There is no race, sex, or geographic predisposition to the disease, and two clinical forms exist. The malignant form is characterized by progressive cranial compression, causing blindness, deafness, facial palsy, anosmia, mental retardation, and medullary compression (Fig. 25–3). These and severe anemia, hepatosplenomegaly, long-bone fractures, and hypocalcemic tetany cause death in the early months or years of life. The benign variant of this disease is compatible with a normal life span and normal intelligence but is expressed clinically in excessive height, a leonine appearance, conductive or mixed hearing loss, and facial palsy that may begin in the teen-age years (Fig. 25–4). Headaches, optic atrophy, clubbing of long bones, genu valgum, coxa vara, proptosis, and osteomyelitis may become manifest later in life (Klintworth, 1963; Hamersma, 1970, 1973).

The pathophysiologic characteristics of this disease are based on the observation that primitive fetal bone does not resorb, and the resulting increase in bone density that characterizes osteopetrosis may be seen on late prenatal roentgenograms. Calcium salts are deposited in the bone in large quantities, but the resultant hard bone lacks the adult structure designed to withstand stress and hence breaks readily at right angles to the long axis (Myers and Stool, 1969). The bone has small haversian canals and a relatively poor blood supply; hematopoietic marrow encroachment, neutropenia, and poor vascular supply predispose to osteomyelitis (Sofferman et al., 1971). Cranial foramina, including the foramen magnum, fail to enlarge during growth.

Roentgenograms are essential to the diagnosis of osteopetrosis. They show homogeneous bone density, loss of the diploë, and thickening of the base and dome of the skull. Mastoid and petrous pyramid films show

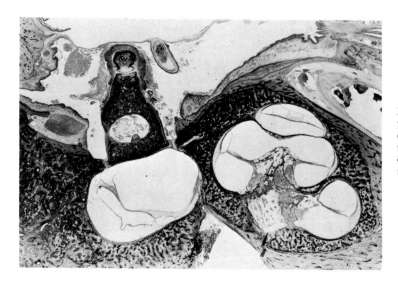

Figure 25–3. Horizontal temporal bone section from a young child who, prior to death, had been blind and deaf owing to the malignant form of osteopetrosis. Note the stapes, the bulk of which is due to lack of resorption of cartilage, thus preventing remodeling into the adult form. (× 12) (Courtesy of S. E. Stool, M.D.)

obliteration of the air cell system and may show narrowed external and internal auditory canals, oval and round windows, middle-ear space, and dense bone engulfing the malleus and incus in the epitympanum. Cholesteatoma may form behind bony external auditory canal masses.

Examination of postmortem temporal bone specimens of patients with osteopetrosis has shown shallow middle-ear spaces, dehiscent fallopian canals, a bulky

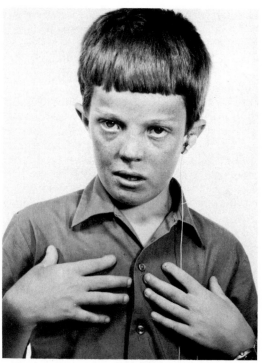

Figure 25–4. Twelve-year-old boy with the benign form of osteopetrosis. He had several episodes of facial palsy with nerve degeneration prior to undergoing facial nerve decompression at age 6 years. Note his relatively expressionless, somewhat asymmetric face. He also underwent surgical widening of narrowed external auditory canals and exploratory tympanotomy for fixation of malleus and incus in the epitympanum. Subsequently the stapes has fixed. He also has syndactyly, absent fingernails, and an enlarging skull. (Courtesy of H. Hamersma, M.D.)

stapes of fetal form, and cochlear and saccular endolymphatic hydrops (Myers and Stool, 1969). Other postmortem temporal bone findings include exostoses of the middle-ear cavity and downgrowth of a greatly thickened epitympanic plate, narrowed internal autitory canal, and incomplete temporal bone fractures (Hamersma, 1970, 1973; Suga and Lindsay, 1976).

CRANIOMETAPHYSEAL DYSPLASIA (PYLE DISEASE)

This autosomal, dominantly inherited disorder affects the temporal bone in childhood. Its overall features include widening of the metaphyseal part of the long bones and overgrowth of the craniofacial bones (leontiasis ossea) (Fig. 25–5). Progressive conductive and/or sensorineural hearing loss, eustachian tube obstruction, nasal deformity, obliteration of nasal passages and paranasal sinuses, nasolacrimal duct obstruction, mandibular overgrowth, defective dentition and occlusion, hypertelorism, facial paralysis, other cranial nerve palsies, cerebellar tonsil compression with resultant nystagmus, and brain stem compression due to narrowing of the foramen magnum complete the clinical picture. Physical findings include narrow external auditory canals and hypoactive vestibular responses. Roentgenograms may show narrowing of the middle ear, internal carotid canal, jugular foramen, and internal auditory canal; encroachment on the cochlea and oval and round windows; fusion of ossicles; and obliteration of mastoid air cells. These more detailed findings are best delineated by petrous pyramid polytomography (Kietzer and Paparella, 1969; Kim, 1974).

Microscopically, these temporal bones show increased amounts of subperiosteal and subendosteal bone that produce a compact laminar bone, the dilated haversian canals that contain osteoblasts and osteocytes but no osteoclasts. There is an increased amount of intercellular ground substance in these bones (Kietzer and Paparella, 1969).

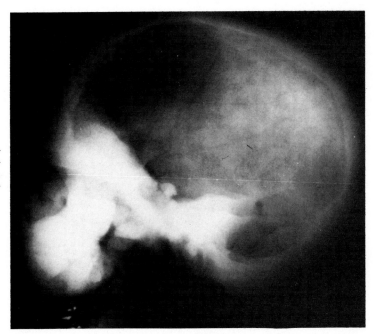

Figure 25–5. Skull film of patient with far-advanced craniometaphyseal dysplasia. The overgrowth of facial and cranial bones, especially around the cranial base, is extreme. Note obliteration of labyrinthine spaces. (Used by permission of Dr. Lorraine Smith.)

FRONTOMETAPHYSEAL DYSPLASIA (GORLIN–HOLT SYNDROME)

This entity is thought to be due to failure to absorb secondary spongy bone, and a number of features distinguish it from craniometaphyseal dysplasia. Cases may be sporadic or may result from a rare autosomal recessive gene. Patients with this dysplasia exhibit severe overgrowth of the supraorbital ridges, especially laterally, agenesis of the frontal sinuses, hypodevelopment of the mandible, defective dentition, a high-arched palate, decreased vision, and a conductive or mixed hearing loss. Also seen are hirsutism, winged scapulae, flaring of the iliac bones, a limited range of motion of the joints (especially in elbow extension), and poorly developed muscles. However, these individuals seem to be of normal intellect (Gorlin et al., 1976).

Roentgenograms show metaphyseal splaying of tubular bone, internal hyperostosis, perisutural sclerosis, thoracic scoliosis, irregular rib and vertebral contours, disproportionately long limbs and digits, and absence or atrophy of temporal muscles. Frequently in these patients the frontal ridge is hyperostotic, the frontal sinuses are absent, the foramen magnum is enlarged, and the cervical vertebrae may be abnormal (Arenberg et al., 1974; Gorlin et al., 1976). Petrous pyramid polytomography may show fused and/or fixed malleus and incus, a malformed stapes, and irregular thickness of the cochlear capsule (Arenberg et al., 1974). No temporal bone histopathologic condition has been reported in these cases.

FIBROUS DYSPLASIA (OSSIFYING FIBROMA)

Fibrous dysplasia occurs in three forms, any one of which may involve the temporal bone: (1) monostotic, in which, as the name implies, bony involvement is confined to one bone, usually in the craniofacial region; (2) polyostotic, in which multiple bones are involved; however, the disorder is nonsyndromal and affects only bony tissue; and (3) polyostotic, or the McCune-Albright syndrome (Talbot et al., 1974; Rimoin and Hollister, 1973). Common associated abnormalities include precocious sexual development and café au lait spots. The proportion of females with this disease exceeds that of males for all forms of the disease.

The clinical symptoms of temporal bone involvement are external hard swelling in the temporal and periauricular area, sometimes with associated pain and fever; external auditory stenosis; hearing loss that is usually conductive, although total sensorineural hearing loss has been reported; and facial nerve paresis or paralysis. Characteristically, bone swelling begins in childhood or adolescence, may progress to grotesque proportions, and tends to become quiescent after general skeletal growth stops, although it does not regress spontaneously. Cases of adult onset have been reported. Hearing loss may be present for some time before bone swelling, and it is not clear from published reports whether in all such instances the hearing loss was due to fibrous dysplasia or an unrelated cause. Otorrhea may occur and may herald the development of cholesteatoma behind an occluding mass of fibrous dysplastic bone in the external auditory canal, the middle ear, or the mastoid. Postauricular fistula has been reported, and, although vestibular symptoms have not been emphasized in published reports, in one patient the lateral semicircular canal was eroded (Cohen and Rosenwasser, 1969; Sharp, 1970; Tembe, 1970; Chatterji, 1974).

General roentgenographic findings in these cases may be categorized as follows: (1) cystic changes (21 per cent); if teeth are involved the lamina dura may be absent and tooth roots separated; (2) sclerotic (23 per cent); and (3) pagetoid (56 per cent), characterized by a cotton-wool appearance. This last symptom tends to be found in older patients. The mastoid air cell system, middle-ear space, and internal auditory canal may be obliterated (Talbot et al., 1974) (Fig. 25–6).

When these patients are examined during surgery, dense sclerotic bone or gritty vascular tissue is found to be eroding the otic capsule or invading and filling available spaces, including the external ear canal, the mastoid, and the labyrinthine cavities (Cohen and Rosenwasser, 1969). Cholesteatoma may be found in nearly 50 per cent of cases (Sharp, 1970).

The pathologic picture of this disease varies. In its active form, cellular connective tissue composed of stellate or fusiform cells and numerous mitoses is seen. The margin between the connective tissue matrix and the bony islands is marked by a scroll edge to the bone, and the bone has been likened to the pieces of a jigsaw puzzle. The quiescent stage shows more mature fibrous tissue with few mitoses and more bone, but osteoblasts, osteoclasts, and osteoid are not present. The inactive stage shows degeneration of the connective tissue matrix and no bone islands (Batsakis, 1974). The underlying etiology of these histologic changes is unknown.

OTHER DYSPLASIAS

Hearing loss of varying degrees and types has been reported in other disorders, including craniofacial dysostosis (Crouzon) (Baldwin, 1968), diastrophic dwarfism (Bergstrom, 1971), and an unclassified bone dysplasia associated with retinal detachment and deafness (Roaf et al., 1967).

NEOPLASMS

Primary and metastatic tumors are rare in children but may infrequently invade the otic capsule and the labyrinth. Osteogenic sarcoma may invade by direct extension or metastasize from a distant site (Schuknecht, 1974).

Histiocytosis X usually appears in the mastoid and middle ear and can simulate otitis media. This disorder usually affects children under the age of 2 years. Temporal bone involvement may be found in approximately 60 per cent of patients. It has been reported in adults and may involve the otic capsule and labyrinth (McCullough, 1980; Cohn et al., 1970).

EVALUATION AND THERAPY

Many of the dysplasias can be differentiated by characteristic radiographic findings. The extent and type of involvement of the middle ear, mastoid, fallopian canal, or labyrinthine capsule can be demonstrated best by computed tomography, using horizontal cuts, and with bone reconstruction techniques (Lambert and Brackmann, 1984). Occasionally, as in fibrous dysplasia, biopsy of the affected bone may be necessary for confirmation of the diagnosis. Functional disturbances can be detected and quantified by the use of tuning forks, audiometry, tympanometry, vestibular testing, and facial nerve conduction studies. Occasionally, retrocochlear testing may be indicated.

Conductive hearing loss in these cases may be caused by surgically correctable external ear canal or middle ear lesions. If cholesteatoma is known or suspected, surgery to exteriorize or remove it along with obstructing bony masses is essential, regardless of the

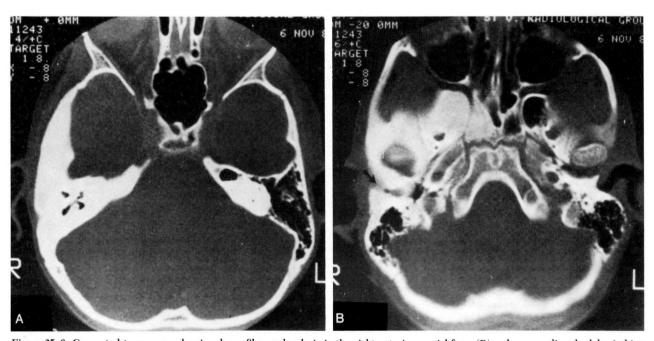

Figure 25–6. Computed tomograms showing dense fibrous dysplasia in the right anterior cranial fossa (B) and surrounding the labyrinthine structures (A). (Used by permission of W. Hanafee, M.D.)

state of the hearing. If bony compression of the fallopian or internal auditory canal exists and has caused facial weakness or seems likely to be a cause of sensorineural hearing loss, surgical decompression may be feasible but should be preceded by thorough neurosurgical and roentgenographic evaluation.

When surgery is not possible or has been unsuccessful, hearing amplification and other measures to improve communication should be instituted. In young children in whom surgery can be deferred, amplification should be used if hearing loss interfering with normal language development exists. Hearing conservation measures should be urged for sensorineural losses, and genetic counseling should be offered to individuals and families affected by inherited bony disorders. Every attempt to detect hearing loss early should be made in those children at risk for the disorder or already known to have it.

There is no acceptable chemotherapy for any of the known bony dysplasias affecting the labyrinthine capsule in childhood or adolescence.

SELECTED REFERENCES

Gorlin, R. J., Pindborg, J. J., and Cohen, M. M. 1976. Syndromes of the Head and Neck. New York, McGraw-Hill Book Co.
This edition of a by now classic reference work is notable for its systematic presentation of syndromes, a few of which are included in this chapter. The illustrations of pertinent craniofacial features are excellent.
Schuknecht, H. F. 1974. Pathology of the Ear. Cambridge, MA, Harvard University Press, pp. 351–364, 378–383.
A large format, superb illustrations from the author's large collection of temporal bone specimens, and a writing style that clearly communicates years of careful study and observation of an extensive otologic patient population make this reference unique and indispensable for an understanding of the pathology of some of the entities described in this chapter.

REFERENCES

Altmann, F., Kornfeld, M., and Shea, J. 1966. Inner ear changes in otosclerosis. Ann. Otol. Rhinol. Laryngol. 75:5.
Arenberg, I. K., Shambaugh, G. E., Jr., and Valvassori, G. E. 1974. Otolaryngologic manifestations of frontometaphyseal dysplasia. The Gorlin-Holt syndrome. Arch. Otolaryngol. 99:52.
Baldwin, J. L. 1968. Dysostosis craniofacialis of Crouzon. Laryngoscope 78:1660–1676.
Batsakis, J. G. 1974. Tumors of the Head and Neck. Baltimore, Williams & Wilkins Co., pp. 306–308.
Bergstrom, L. 1971. A high risk register to find congenital deafness. Otolaryngol. Clin. North Am. 4:369.
Bergstrom, L. 1977. Osteogenesis imperfecta: Otologic and maxillofacial aspects. Laryngoscope 87 Suppl. 6.
Black, F. O., Sando, I., Hildyard, V. H. et al. 1969. Bilateral multiple otosclerotic foci and endolymphatic hydrops. Ann. Otol. Rhinol. Laryngol. 78:1062.
Chatterji, P. 1974. Massive fibrous dysplasia of the temporal bone. J. Laryngol. Otol. 88:179.
Cohen, A., and Rosenwasser, H. 1969. Fibrous dysplasia of the temporal bone. Arch. Otolaryngol. 89:447.
Cohn, A. M., Sataloff, J., and Lindsay, J. R. 1970. Histiocytosis X (Letterer-Siwe disease) with involvement of the inner ear. Arch. Otolaryngol. 91:24.
Daniel, H. J., III. 1969. Stapedial otosclerosis and fluorine in drinking water. Arch. Otolaryngol. 90:585.

Friedmann, I. 1974. Pathology of the Ear. London, Blackwell Scientific Publications, pp. 245–278.
Gacek, R. R. 1970. The diagnosis and treatment of poststapedectomy granuloma. Ann. Otol. Rhinol. Laryngol. 79:970.
Gorlin, R. J., Pindborg, J. J., and Cohen, M. M. 1976. Syndromes of the Head and Neck. New York, McGraw-Hill Book Co., pp. 315–318.
Guild, S. R. 1944. Histologic otosclerosis. Ann. Otol. Rhinol. Laryngol. 53:246.
Hamersma, H. 1970. Osteopetrosis (marble bone disease) of the temporal bone. Laryngoscope 80:1518.
Hamersma, H. 1973. Total decompression of the facial nerve in osteopetrosis. ORL 36:21.
Hemenway, W. G., Hildyard, V. H., and Black, F. O. 1968. Poststapedectomy perilymph fistulas in the Rocky Mountain area. Laryngoscope 78:1687.
Kietzer, G., and Paparella, M. M. 1969. Otolaryngological disorders in craniometaphyseal dysplasia. Laryngoscope 79:921.
Kim, B. H. 1974. Roentgenography of the ear and eye in Pyle disease. Arch. Otolaryngol. 99:458.
Klintworth, G. K. 1963. The neurologic manifestations of osteopetrosis (Albers-Schönberg's disease). Neurology 13:512.
Lambert, P. R., and Brackmann, D. E. 1984. Fibrous dysplasia of the temporal bone: The use of computerized tomography. Otolaryngol. Head Neck Surg. 92:461.
Larsson, A. 1960. Otosclerosis, a genetic and clinical study. Acta Otolaryngol. Suppl. 154.
McCullough, C. J. 1980. Eosinophilic granuloma of bone. Acta Orthop. Scand. 51:389.
McKenzie, W. 1948. Otosclerosis in childhood. J. Laryngol. Otol. 62:661.
Mendlowitz, J. C., and Hirschhorn, K. 1976. Polygenic inheritance of otosclerosis. Ann. Otol. Rhinol. Laryngol. 85:281.
Myers, E. N., and Stool, S. E. 1969. The temporal bone in osteopetrosis. Arch. Otolaryngol. 89:460.
Nager, G. T. 1969. Histopathology of otosclerosis. Arch. Otolaryngol. 89:341.
Parkins, F. M. 1974. Fluoride therapy for osteoporotic lesions. Ann. Otol. Rhinol. Laryngol. 83:626.
Rimoin, D. L., and Hollister, D. W. 1973. Polyostotic fibrous dysplasia. In Birth Defects. Atlas and Compendium. Baltimore, Williams & Wilkins Co., pp. 739–740.
Roaf, R., Longmore, J. B., and Forrester, R. M. 1967. A childhood syndrome of bone dysplasia, retinal detachment and deafness. Dev. Med. Child. Neurol. 9:464.
Rüedi, L., and Spoendlin, H. 1966. Pathogenesis of sensorineural deafness in otosclerosis. Ann. Otol. Rhinol. Laryngol. 75:525.
Sando, I., Hemenway, W. G., Hildyard, V. H., et al. 1968. Cochlear otosclerosis: A human temporal bone report. Ann. Otol. Rhinol. Laryngol. 77:23.
Sando, I., Hemenway, W. G., Miller, D. R., et al. 1974. Vestibular pathology in otosclerosis, temporal bone histopathological report. Laryngoscope 84:593.
Schuknecht, H. F. 1974. Pathology of the Ear. Cambridge, MA, Harvard University Press, pp. 351–364, 421.
Shambaugh, G. E., and Causse, J. 1974. Ten years' experience with fluoride in otosclerotic (otospongiotic) patients. Ann. Otol. Rhinol. Laryngol. 83:635.
Sharp, M. 1970. Monostotic fibrous dysplasia of the temporal bone. J. Laryngol. Otol. 84:697.
Sofferman, R. A., Smith, R. O., and English, G. M. 1971. Albers-Schönberg's disease (osteopetrosis), a case with osteomyelitis of the maxilla. Laryngoscope 81:36.
Suga, F., and Lindsay, J. R. 1976. Temporal bone histopathology of osteopetrosis. Ann. Otol. Rhinol. Laryngol. 85:15.
Talbot, I. C., Keith, D. A., and Lord, I. J. 1974. Fibrous dysplasia of the craniofacial bones. J. Laryngol. Otol. 88:429.
Tembe, D. 1970. Fibro-osseous dysplasia of temporal bone. J. Laryngol. Otol. 84:107.
Terkildsen, K., Osterhammel, P., and Bretlau, P. 1973. Acoustic middle ear muscle reflexes in patients with otosclerosis. Arch. Otolaryngol. 98:152.
Van Wagoner, R. S., and Campbell, J. D. 1976. The use of electroacoustic impedance measurements in detecting early clinical otosclerosis. J. Otolaryngol. 5:33.

Chapter 26

INJURIES OF THE EAR AND TEMPORAL BONE

Simon C. Parisier, M.D.

Accidental injuries have become a major problem in modern mechanized society. Vehicular or pedestrian accidents account for more than 50 per cent of the deaths of persons in the first two decades of life (Vital Statistics, 1974). Falls continue to be a leading cause of injuries to children under 5 years of age (Hendrick et al., 1965). Moreover, the head injuries that commonly occur in such accidents are often accompanied by damage to the ear (Podoshin and Fradis, 1975; Hough and Stuart, 1968). The popularity of scuba diving, water skiing, and other sports has exposed an additional number of young people to possible ear injuries. When the above hazards are added to such existing problems as the fetish of cleaning wax from the ear canals of infants, or the apparent sensual satisfaction which young children experience when playing with their ears, the extent of the problem becomes apparent. This chapter reviews the variety of injuries that involve the ear and temporal bone. Trauma to the auricle is covered in Chapter 20.

THE PHYSICIAN AND THE INJURED CHILD

Traumatic injuries to the ear and temporal bone occur more commonly to children and adolescents than to adults (Hough and Stuart, 1968; Tos, 1973). In dealing with children, the physician must establish himself or herself as a gentle, concerned person. Any examination, no matter how routine, should be explained or demonstrated beforehand so that it can be understood, thus eliminating fear of the unknown. For example, the otoscope or ear speculum can be introduced to the child by examining the child's hand with it before placing it in his or her ear. The patient can be familiarized with the wax curette by first tickling his or her hand with it, then touching the auditory meatus, before using the metal instrument to clean the canal. The child can be prepared for the loud noise of the suction aspirator by a demonstration of its function with a cup of water. When a procedure is expected to be painful, a general anesthetic is recommended, even in small infants who can be restrained

effectively. The child who is confident that the physician will not cause unnecessary pain is usually a cooperative patient.

Trauma to the ear, even a minor scratch that causes bleeding from the external canal, will generally seem catastrophic to the injured patient and the parents. The physician treating the child must enroll the family's full cooperation by explaining the problem in terms the family understands. It must be remembered that the attitude of the parent toward the physician is transmitted to the injured child.

INJURIES AND FOREIGN BODIES OF THE EXTERNAL AUDITORY CANAL

The cleaning of wax from the ears seems to be a cultural phenomenon. To gain access to the ear canal, a variety of objects, ranging from bobby pins to match sticks, are used. It is not uncommon for a new mother in this country to be given free samples of products for her newborn. Included in the gift package may be cotton-tipped applicators, which are often used to clean the baby's ear canals. Thus, from infancy, the individual is taught that the ever-present cerumen is a form of dirt and must be removed regularly.

During the ear-cleansing ritual, the mother's manipulations may be painful, causing the child to jerk his head, and the ear may be injured. Ordinarily, only a minor laceration of the ear canal will result. Although the bleeding may be profuse at the onset, it usually stops spontaneously, forming a clot that may obstruct the external canal. To determine if the tympanic membrane has been damaged, the debris should be removed gently. It may not be possible to clean the canal if a child is unable to cooperate adequately or if the blood has formed a tenacious crust that is firmly attached to the skin of the canal wall or to the drum. In such instances, rather than risk inflicting further damage by traumatic manipulations, the physician should observe the child's progress. To prevent infection, the ear must be kept dry. When bathing the child, the parents are instructed to prevent water from getting into the auditory canal by occluding the meatus with a nonabsorbent cotton (lamb's wool) impregnated with petroleum jelly.

During play, young children between 1 and 3 years of age will frequently place small beads, paper, peanuts, or other foreign bodies into their external ear canals. Even an older child may innocently stick something into a friend's ear canal. If the child does not complain, the presence of a foreign body may be detected only later, during a routine examination or because the ear has become secondarily infected.

Removal of these foreign bodies can be both technically difficult for the physician and painful to the child, especially when the foreign body is wedged in the ear canal. The problem may be compounded if an unskilled person has unsuccessfully attempted to remove the material, thereby producing local trauma and swelling within the ear canal. Should a secondary infection be present, the problem would be complicated by inflammatory changes characterized by swelling of the canal wall skin, otorrhea, and, if the inflammation is severe, granulation tissue. These findings, which can mimic a chronic mastoid infection, generally will not respond to local or systemic antibiotics and will completely resolve only after the offending object is removed.

As a rule, the removal of a foreign body requires that the patient be extremely cooperative, as an inappropriate movement can result in further injury with damage to the eardrum and the ossicular chain. Therefore, the use of a general anesthetic for removal of the foreign body should be considered if the physician anticipates that the process may be technically difficult and painful, or if the child is not able to hold still without being restrained.

TRAUMATIC MIDDLE-EAR INJURIES

Trauma to the delicate tympanic membrane resulting in a tympanic membrane perforation occurs quite often and may be caused by a variety of injuries (Silverstein et al., 1973; Wright et al., 1969). An explosive blast, such as a firecracker going off near an ear, will produce a violent shock wave capable of rupturing the drum (Sudderth, 1974; Singh and Ahluwalia, 1968). A damaging shock wave can be produced if a child is slapped with an open hand across the ear (e.g., by an angry parent or when fighting with another child). If the blow occludes the external auditory meatus, the resulting inward displacement of the air column contained in the external canal will cause a rupture of the membrane. A similar type of injury occurs during dives or falls into swimming pools, during water skiing, while surfboarding, or while tumbling in a rough surf. A perforation may occur if the ear hits the water in such a way that the column of air contained within the external canal is forcibly displaced, or if the water strikes the ear with considerable impact.

Tympanic membrane lacerations frequently occur when a cotton-tipped applicator or other object being used to relieve an itch or clean out wax is accidentally pushed through the drum. Iatrogenic tears of the drum have occurred in the process of removing foreign bodies from the ear of a struggling child. Additionally, the tympanic membrane can be perforated during ear syringing to remove wax. Occasionally, the pressure of the water being instilled into the external canal is enough to drive a hard waxy pellet through the drum.

Following an uncomplicated tympanic membrane perforation, a mild conductive hearing loss will be observed on audiometric testing (10 to 35 dB). Although small children rarely complain of loss of acuity, occasionally a tympanic membrane laceration will occur in a child who has an unrecognized preexisting hearing loss in the opposite ear, thus causing a bilateral loss. In such cases, behavioral changes may reveal the change in hearing.

When a traumatic tympanic membrane perforation occurs, there is generally considerable pain, accompanied by bleeding from the ear that stops spontaneously. If water gets into the ear, a secondary infection may occur that should be treated with systemic antibiotics (e.g., ampicillin) and local nonirritating acidified eardrops.

Injuries severe enough to rupture the tympanic membrane may also damage the ossicular chain (Silverstein et al., 1973; Wright et al., 1969). A dislocation of the incus is the most commonly observed injury. Usually, the incudostapedial joint will be separated, the stapes arch is fractured (Sadé, 1964), or both occur. This trauma may cause a transient subluxation of the stapes into the inner ear vestibule, resulting in a tear of the annular ligament and a perilymphatic fluid leak into the middle ear space (Silverstein et al., 1973; Fee, 1968). Generally, this fluid leak produces a significant sensory hearing loss, severe vertigo, or both (Fig. 26–1).

Traumatic perilymph fistulas can also occur without ossicular involvement. The force of an injury sufficient to cause a tympanic membrane perforation may result in an accompanying rupture of the round window membrane. Such a defect will allow the leakage of perilymph into the middle ear, producing the characteristic symptoms of sensory hearing loss and vertigo (Fig. 26–2).

Ear injuries that result in the production of excessive stapedial vibrations can also produce intracochlear damage (Igarashi et al., 1964). Such trauma may be caused by a sudden explosive noise, an excessive excursion of the intact tympanic membrane, or a direct force applied to the stapes. These injuries cause a damaging pistonlike movement of the stapes that produces a forceful perilymphatic fluid wave. This movement results in traumatic excursions of the basilar membrane that can lead to a loss of hair cells and even avulsion of the organ of Corti (Fig. 26–3).

Treatment of Middle-Ear Injuries

Most traumatic tympanic membrane perforations will heal spontaneously. Small perforations may repair

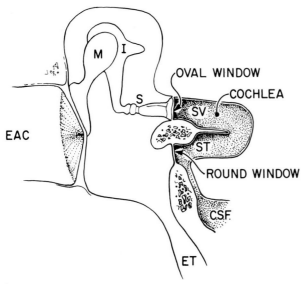

Figure 26–1. Diagrammatic representation of the ear. Movement of the stapes (S) in the oval window produces a perilymphatic fluid wave that travels from the scala vestibuli (SV) through the scala tympani (ST) and causes a displacement of the round window membrane. The perilymph communicates with the cerebrospinal fluid (CSF) through the cochlear aqueduct. EAC, external auditory canal; M, malleus; I, incus; ET, eustachian tube.

themselves within a few weeks. Occasionally, however, a large perforation will persist. In such cases, the lacerated epithelial margins of the defect do not grow across the drum defect to bridge the existing gap. Instead, the edges curl under the remaining drum remnant, forming a healed epithelial rim; thus, the perforation becomes a permanent one.

If the child is seen shortly after suffering a tympanic membrane perforation, an attempt can be made to realign the torn edges. The procedure can be performed either using general anesthesia or, in a coop-

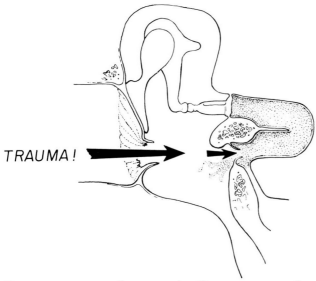

Figure 26–2. Trauma (large arrow) sufficient to rupture the tympanic membrane may also cause a round window membrane rupture (small arrow) with a resulting leak of perilymph (stippling) into the middle ear.

erative child, under local anesthesia. The edges of the perforation, which frequently become inverted below the residual drum remnant, should be approximated and the fragments supported by absorbable gelatin sponge (Gelfoam) placed in the middle ear.

A persistent tympanic membrane perforation can often be encouraged to heal. The epithelialized edge of the drum remnant can be debrided chemically by cauterization, using minute quantities of 50 per cent trichloroacetic acid. A mildly irritating topical medication is prescribed to stimulate spontaneous reparative processes (Juers, 1963; Derlacki, 1973). Generally, the treatment has to be repeated several times; it is somewhat painful and therefore may not be well tolerated by young children.

Although most traumatic tympanic membrane perforations will heal spontaneously, in certain specific instances immediate surgery is necessary (Silverstein et al., 1973). If, following a middle ear injury, the patient suffers a sensorineural hearing loss and vertigo, the middle ear should be explored for a possible perilymphatic leak (Fig. 26–4). If a stapedial subluxation is present, it should be corrected by returning the stapes to its original position. Additionally, the oval window area should be sealed with a tissue graft. The possibility of round window membrane rupture should be explored; the presence of this condition is confirmed by the observation of clear fluid welling up from the round window niche or by the visualization of an actual tear in the round window membrane. In such cases, the area should be packed with a tissue graft. Another indication for immediate surgery would be a complete facial paralysis, the onset of which was noted immediately following the middle ear trauma. This problem is discussed in the section on temporal bone fractures in this chapter.

Should ossicular chain involvement be suspected following injury to the middle ear, elective surgery to correct the hearing mechanism may be advantageous (Armstrong, 1970). Generally, patients who have a tympanic membrane perforation will have a 30- to 40-dB conductive hearing loss. In these situations, a patch test may be useful in determining whether the hearing loss is due to the existing tympanic membrane perforation. This test is performed by first documenting the existing hearing loss with a preliminary audiogram. Next, a patch made of cigarette paper is placed over the entire drum defect. If the perforation is large, it may not be possible to cover it entirely; moreover, in some cases, the anterior edge of the defect may be obscured by a prominent overhang of the canal wall. After the patch is applied, a repeat audiogram is obtained. A significant improvement in hearing indicates that the ossicular chain is intact and that the hearing loss is due to the perforation. However, when the hearing acuity is unchanged or is worse, the presence of a coexisting ossicular discontinuity should be suspected.

The radiologic examination of the ossicular chain using computed tomography (CT) has superseded polytomography in evaluating patients with trauma to the

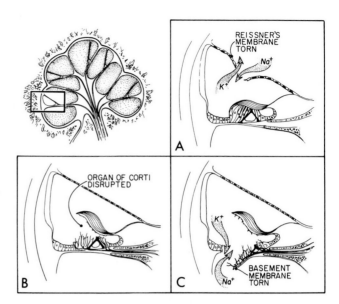

Figure 26–3. Excessive vibrations of the stapes can produce a forceful perilymphatic fluid wave that may result in intracochlear damage. *A,* Reissner membrane, which normally separates the endolymph (high potassium–low sodium) from the perilymph (low potassium–high sodium), may be torn. The resulting changes in the K^+–Na^+ concentration damage the affected hair cells, producing a sensory hearing loss. *B,* Excessive vibrations of the basilar membrane may produce a disruption of the organ of Corti. *C,* Tears of the basilar membrane will be associated with severe injuries to the organ of Corti and a profound hearing loss.

middle ear (Chakeres and Weider, 1985; Wright et al., 1969). This technique will reveal a dislocated incus or malleus 90 per cent of the time. However, it should be noted that the delicately structured stapes cannot be adequately visualized (Fig. 26–5).

When the ossicular chain is disrupted, elective surgical correction may be considered. The immediate repair of traumatic injuries to the ossicular chain allows the surgeon to reduce an existing dislocation and to restore an essentially normal condition before fibrotic adhesions form. Additionally, at the time of the ossicular repair, the tympanic membrane perforation may be grafted to restore hearing to a normal level.

Prior to undertaking elective repair of a traumatic middle ear defect, one must carefully evaluate the child's ability to cooperate with the surgeon who will care for the ear postoperatively. In younger children particularly, the past medical background must be

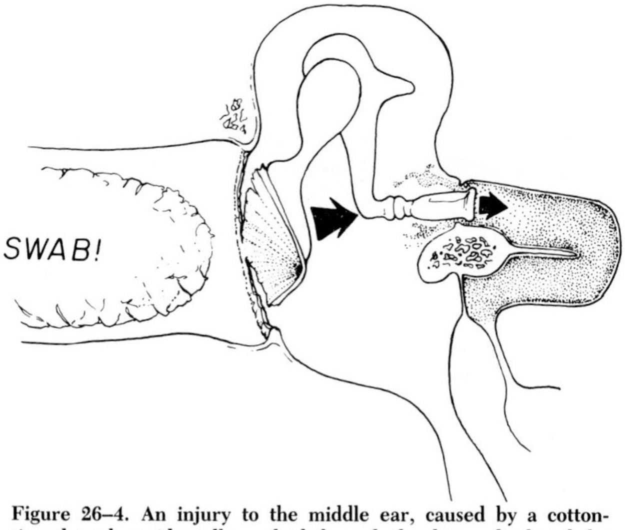

Figure 26–4. An injury to the middle ear, caused by a cotton-tipped swab accidentally pushed through the drum, displaced the stapes (larger arrow) into the vestibule and produced an oval window perilymphatic leak (stippled area, smaller arrow).

reviewed for problems suggestive of an underlying eustachian tube dysfunction that would jeopardize the chances for successful otologic surgery. A history of recurrent serous or purulent otitis media, an allergic background, symptoms suggestive of chronic nasal congestion, and a history of frequent upper respiratory tract infections with otalgia would indicate that the child is not a suitable candidate for elective middle ear reconstructive surgery (Chap. 22). In such children, especially if they are very young, the most suitable therapeutic alternative may be to temporize and accept the presence of a chronic tympanic membrane perforation. One must not overlook the clinical reality that the treatment for many children with eustachian tube dysfunction and serous otitis media is a myringotomy (i.e., creation of a perforation that is kept open by insertion of a middle ear ventilating tube).

When a child has a tympanic membrane perforation, it is essential that water be prevented from entering the ear. Water irritates the exposed middle ear mucosa, producing a profuse seromucinous otorrhea. When infection supervenes, an acute bacterial otitis media will occur. Fungi, whose growth is stimulated by the moist environment of these draining ears, are a common cause of superficial infections. These problems can be avoided by occluding the external ear canal with either lamb's wool and petroleum jelly or waxlike commercially available plugs when there is any chance that water may get into the ear. When swimming, the child should wear a bathing cap to assure that the plug sealing the ear canal is not displaced. Definitive surgery to close the tympanic membrane perforation may be performed when the child has "outgrown" the frequent ear problems associated with respiratory tract infections.

Surgical Repair of Middle-Ear Injuries

Fracture of the ossicles can be corrected by tympanoplastic surgery in which the conductive mechanism

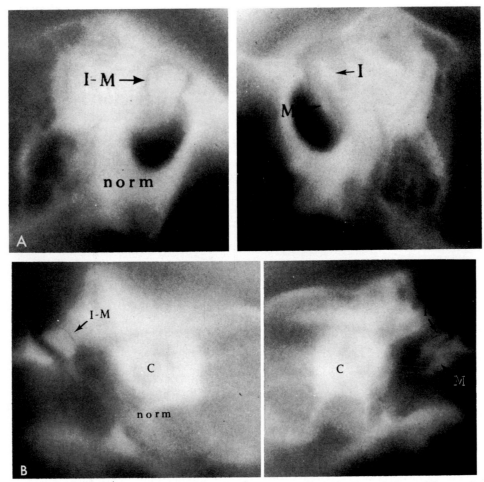

Figure 26–5. Ossicular dislocation demonstrated using polytomography, A, Lateral section through the middle ear. On the normal side (norm), the incus-malleus complex (I-M) has a molar tooth appearance. A dislocation of the ossicles produces a separation of the incus (I) from the malleus (M). B, Frontal section. On the normal side (norm), the incus and malleus produce a single density (I-M). On the opposite side a traumatic ossicular discontinuity is present. The malleus (M) and incus (I) are seen as individual structures. The malleus is rotated laterally, with its head in the external canal and its long process pointing to the promontory. C, Cochlea.

is reconstructed, often dramatically improving the hearing level. Thus, when the long process of the incus has been fractured, the continuity of the ossicular chain can be restored by appropriately reshaping the incus and interposing it between the malleus handle and the stapes capitulum (Pennington, 1973). An alternative technique would be to use a stainless steel wire to connect these two structures (Bellucci, 1966). When both the stapes superstructure and the long process of the incus are fractured, the body of the incus can be sculpted so as to extend from the malleus handle to the stapes footplate. Malleolar fractures are usually associated with fracture or dislocation of the incus. In such cases, the sound-conducting mechanism can be reconstituted by placing a strut of cartilage onto the stapes capitulum or the footplate, thereby enabling it to make contact with the tympanic membrane.

In comminuted temporal bone fractures, the patient's incus may have been shattered and therefore may not be available for ossicular reconstruction. In such cases, homograft incudi (Wehrs, 1974) and conchal cartilage have been utilized. In children the use of cortical bone for ossicular replacement is discour-

aged because there is a tendency for a bony ankylosis to form, with fixation to adjacent bony structures that results in recurrence of the conductive hearing loss.

Tympanic membrane defects can be repaired by grafting. The most common type of tissue used is the fascia that covers the temporalis muscle. The perichondrium obtained from the tragal cartilage is also a useful material for closing small defects or for reconstructing the ossicular mechanism when cartilage is required.

OTITIC BAROTRAUMA

As has been previously noted, snorkeling and scuba diving have become popular, with many adolescents participating in underwater diving as a recreational activity. Even more common is travel by plane. These activities, however, require that the individual be able to adapt to rapid changes in pressures (Graves and Edwards 1944; Elner et al., 1971).

During ascent in an airplane, the pressure in the middle ear increases until it reaches a point at which the eustachian tube is forced open. On descent, as the plane prepares to land, a negative middle-ear pressure builds. Because the eustachian tube is normally closed while at rest, this pressure difference will persist until the person swallows. With the muscular activity of swallowing, the tensor veli palatini muscle contracts, the tubal lumen is opened, and the tympanic pressure is equalized. When diving underwater, the reverse sequence occurs: positive pressure is experienced on descent and negative pressure occurs on ascent.

If the eustachian tube fails to open, the resulting negative middle-ear pressure causes a retraction of the tympanic membrane. To equilibrate the induced negative pressure, a transudation of serous fluid from the mucosal surface fills the middle ear (Flisberg et al., 1963). If the pressure changes are sudden, bleeding into the middle-ear space may result or the tympanic membrane may rupture (Schuknecht, 1974). In adults, these pressure changes have been known to produce traumatic perilymphatic leaks due to round or oval window ruptures or both (Pullen, 1972; Goodhill et al., 1973) (Fig. 26–6).

Eustachian tube function is generally compromised when a person has an upper respiratory tract disorder. Thus, diving or flying—both of which require good eustachian tube function to equilibrate the middle-ear pressure—may cause certain individuals to experience the difficulties described in the preceding paragraph. Many young children have borderline eustachian tube function and should not fly when they have a cold. Even on commercial airlines, as descent takes place, a negative middle-ear pressure will result that may produce severe pain and a hearing loss. These problems can be minimized by using both oral and topical nasal decongestants to shrink the nasal and the eusta-

chian tube mucosal linings before the plane begins to descend. Encouraging the child to swallow repeatedly or giving him chewing gum or giving an infant a bottle will keep the normal forces that are necessary to open the eustachian tube operating. Additionally, the child should be kept in an erect position with his or her head elevated to decrease the passive venous mucosal congestion that tends to further compromise eustachian tube patency (Rundcrantz, 1970).

TEMPORAL BONE FRACTURES

Care of the Accident Victim

Head trauma is frequently associated with a simultaneous injury to the ear. In a motor vehicle or pedestrian accident, the victim may suffer multiple injuries that are life threatening and may require urgent medical attention. When treating these patients, primary consideration must be given to assuring an adequate airway, preventing shock due to blood loss, controlling bleeding, and maintaining a stable neurologic state.

In treating the unconscious patient, the first priority must be to establish an unobstructed airway. Oral and tracheal secretions must be cleared; tracheal toilet must be carried out if there is a suggestion of aspiration. Assisted ventilation must be provided when respirations are inadequate. If there is evidence of a chest injury, such as a pneumothorax, a flail chest, or a cardiac tamponade, the condition must be immediately corrected.

After adequate ventilation is assured, the patient should be evaluated for bleeding. It must be empha-

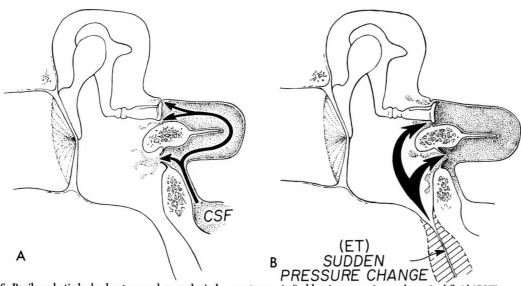

Figure 26–6. Perilymphatic leaks due to round or oval window ruptures. *A,* Sudden increases in cerebrospinal fluid (CSF) pressures (arrows) occur during vigorous physical activity, sneezing, and so on. The cerebrospinal and perilymph fluid spaces communicate through the cochlear aqueduct. Abrupt increases in cerebrospinal fluid pressure may be transmitted to the labyrinth, producing ruptures and leakage of perilymph into the middle ear (Explosive Route; Goodhill, 1971). *B,* Sudden air pressure changes transmitted through the eustachian tube (ET) (arrows) into the middle ear space can produce ruptures of the round window membrane or of the annular ligament in the oval window and leakage of perilymph into the middle ear (Implosive Route; Goodhill, 1971).

sized that hypotensive shock is rarely caused by a head injury alone. The common signs and symptoms of acute blood loss are a rising pulse rate and falling blood pressure. Generally, the opposite findings are seen with increased intracranial pressure—the pulse rate slows and the blood pressure rises. The treatment for hypovolemic shock is immediate replacement of the intravascular volume. Initially, an appropriate intravenous solution should be given until compatible whole-blood transfusions are obtained. The source of bleeding, whether it is a ruptured spleen or kidney, a lacerated liver, or a pelvic fracture, must be identified and the hemorrhage controlled.

After stabilizing the patient's respiratory and circulatory systems, the neurologic status should be evaluated. It is important that the patient's level of consciousness be explicitly documented. The fundi should be evaluated for papilledema as an indication of increased intracranial pressure. Pupil size, equality, and reactivity and corneal reflexes should be recorded. Spontaneous or induced extraocular movements and the presence of nystagmus should be noted. Facial movements, either spontaneous or provoked by painful stimuli, should be documented. Moreover, symmetry of limb movements, muscle tone, and reflexes must be evaluated. Additionally, the possibility of a vertebral fracture should be considered, and, if it is suspected, special care must be taken to prevent possible spinal cord injury.

The initial neurologic evaluation establishes a baseline. The patient's clinical status will be determined by any changes in these primary observations. Thus, an improving level of consciousness and the absence of asymmetric lateralizing findings are hopeful signs. Increasing coma, dilatation of a pupil, and hemiparesis suggest a deteriorating condition that may be caused by cerebral edema or an expanding intracranial hematoma that may require neurosurgical intervention.

The care of accident victims suffering from head and other bodily injuries requires the specialized attention of physicians from various disciplines who must work as a team in a cooperative endeavor. Generally, the otolaryngologist has the dual responsibilities of establishing and maintaining proper ventilation, as well as evaluating the otoneurologic status.

The radiologic examination of a patient with head injury should be performed only after the patient's acute problems have been stabilized. The computed tomographic study of the head is useful for demonstrating the presence of intracranial damage, such as an intracerebral or subdural hematoma and pneumocephalus (Fig. 26–7). Additionally, it may clearly demonstrate a fracture of the skull, temporal bone, or both (Fig. 26–8). Skull radiographs should be obtained to observe for sutural splitting, a linear or depressed skull fracture, and the existence of pneumocephalus.

Classification of Temporal Bone Fractures

Temporal bone fractures were thoroughly studied and categorized during the end of the 19th and begin-

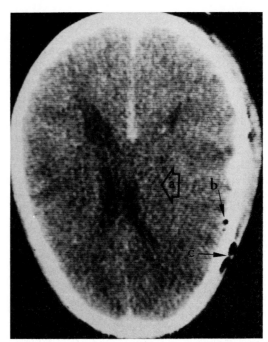

Figure 26–7. Computed tomography performed because of a head injury. Intracerebral edema with compression of the lateral ventricle (a), pneumocephalus (b), subcutaneous emphysema (arrowhead) (c).

ning of the 20th centuries (Grove, 1928). The fractures, which occasionally may be bilateral, are classified according to their course relative to the axis of the temporal bone (Grove, 1939; Proctor et al., 1956; Hardwood-Nash, 1970; Ward, 1969). The longitudinal fracture that follows a course parallel to the long axis of the petrous apex is the most common; it accounts for 80 per cent of the temporal bone fractures seen (Fig. 26–9). Clinically, this type of fracture occurs following a circumscribed blow delivered to the tem-

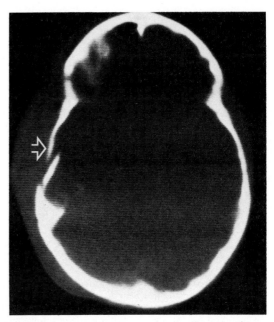

Figure 26–8. Computed tomogram showing fracture of temporal squama (arrow).

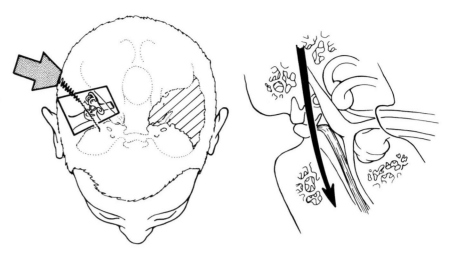

Figure 26–9. Longitudinal fractures of the temporal bone usually occur as a result of a circumscribed blow delivered to the temporoparietal area (shaded arrow). The fracture line follows a course parallel to the long axis of the petrous apex (solid arrow).

poroparietal region. The individual may not be knocked unconscious. However, the injury causes a bending inward of the skull and results in a fracture that follows a characteristic pathway. The separation extends from the squama to involve the posterior superior bony canal wall, lacerating the attached skin and causing bleeding from the ear. Evidence of the defect can sometimes be seen otoscopically, appearing as a steplike deformity with notching of the tympanic ring. The fracture continues anteriorly through the area of the tegmen. The bony rent that involves the roof of the middle ear causes mucosal bleeding that produces a hemotympanum. When the force of the impact is sufficient to cause a separation of the bony segments, significant middle ear injuries can result. In such a case, the tympanic membrane may be torn and the ossicles may be dislocated, fractured, or both. The facial nerve is involved in 25 to 30 per cent of patients with longitudinal temporal bone fractures. Injury to the facial nerve generally occurs in its horizontal portion between the geniculate ganglion and the second genu (McHugh, 1963). The fracture line continues anteriorly and parallel to the eustachian tube toward the foramen lacerum.

Transverse fractures, which run perpendicular to the long axis of the temporal bone, are much less common (Fig. 26–10). They occur as a result of forceful blows that usually produce serious head injury and loss of consciousness. Such blows may be fatal. Generally, the impact is exerted over the occipital or frontal area, which causes a compression of the calvarium in an anteroposterior direction. This results in a fracture where the skull is structurally weakest (i.e., in the area of the foramen magnum and at the base of the petrous bone, where it is perforated by many canals and foramina). The resulting bony rent characteristically crosses the pyramid at a right angle, extending into the area of the internal auditory canal, the cochlea, and the vestibule. This injury to the auditory and vestibular system immediately produces profound sensorineural hearing loss and vertigo. In 50 per cent of these cases, a severe facial nerve injury occurs that results in an immediate facial paralysis.

The fracture may or may not extend into the middle ear. If the promontory surface is involved, rupture of the round and oval windows may occur, accompanied by dislodgement of the stapes.

Because the tympanic membrane generally remains intact, a hemotympanum may also be observed. Moreover, the fracture can extend to involve the jugular bulb area and other structures of the base of the skull.

The classification of temporal bone fractures into longitudinal and transverse is useful in that it emphasizes the various important anatomic structures likely to be injured (Table 26–1). However, radiographically the fracture may not fall into either classification (Yamaki et al., 1986). The small child's skull is elastic, and, following significant head trauma, inward compression of the convex surface can result in extensive lines of fracture. This may produce a comminuted type of fracture having both a longitudinal temporoparietal component and a transverse base-of-skull component (Hardwood-Nash, 1970; Potter, 1971) (Fig. 26–11). Additionally, in spite of the presence of cerebrospinal otorrhea, a temporal bone fracture may not be seen radiographically (Hardwood-Nash, 1970; Potter, 1972). Occasionally, even with CT scans or polytomography, when the fragments are not greatly displaced or separated, it may not be possible to demonstrate a fracture (Mitchell and Stone, 1973). Therefore, it should be emphasized that serious damage can occur to the tympanic membrane, ossicular chain, and cochleovestibular systems without radiographic evidence of either a skull or a temporal bone fracture. Furthermore, it may be difficult to keep a small child properly positioned for the length of time necessary for adequate radiographic examination of the temporal bone without using sedation or a general anesthetic (see Chapter 10 for a complete discussion of temporal bone radiography). In spite of these inherent difficulties, radiographs of the temporal bones will be useful to the clinician because they may show an ossicular dislocation. Furthermore, in the presence of a facial paralysis, visualization of the responsible fracture may help determine the operative approach and also may indicate the complexity of the existing problem. Thus, if a trans-

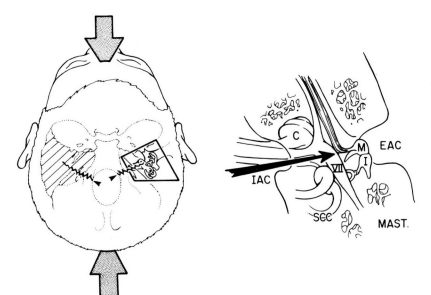

Figure 26–10. Transverse fractures of the temporal bone usually occur as a result of a forceful blow, the impact of which is exerted over the frontal or occipital area (shaded arrows). This causes a compression of the calvarium in an anteroposterior direction with a fracture where the skull is weakest, i.e., the foramen magnum and the foramen within the petrous bone. The fracture line crosses the long axis (zigzag line and arrowheads) of the petrous apex at right angles and may be bilateral (solid arrow). C, Cochlea; M, malleus; I, incus; IAC, internal auditory canal; EAC, external auditory canal; MAST, mastoid; SCC, superior semicircular canal.

verse fracture is observed, the surgeon will be alerted preoperatively that the facial nerve may have been torn and will be prepared for the possibility of nerve grafting. Nevertheless, it must be stressed that, although the radiographic studies can be useful, the demonstration of a temporal fracture in itself does not mean treatment is required.

Treatment of Temporal Bone Fractures

The comprehensive care of the accident victim has been discussed. However, depending on the severity of any coexisting trauma, it may be necessary to postpone such diagnostic procedures as audiometric evaluation, caloric tests, radiography, and facial nerve testing. Even minor operative procedures may have to be deferred until the patient's condition is stable, especially with small children who require general anesthesia. Occasionally, when a serious concomitant condition requires operative intervention with general anesthesia, it may be possible to evaluate and treat existing otologic problems at the same time. For example, while the child is under general anesthesia, the external ear canal can be cleaned of blood clots and ceruminous debris and the tympanic membrane can be examined. If there has been a perforation, the edges can be reapproximated and the drum defect repaired. At the same time, minor ossicular defects can be corrected.

Evaluation and Management of Signs and Symptoms Associated with Temporal Bone Injuries

When considering the management of temporal bone fractures, the saying "It's what's inside that counts" is appropriate. Therapy is aimed at restoring the function of the injured structures. Therefore, treatment must be guided by the individual victim's signs and symptoms.

TABLE 26–1. Classification of Temporal Bone Fractures

	LONGITUDINAL FRACTURES	TRANSVERSE FRACTURES
Percentage of temporal bone fractures	80%	20%
Point of impact	Temporoparietal area	Frontal or occipital area
Force of impact	Moderate to severe	Severe
Loss of consciousness	Not always present	Present
Associated Otologic Findings		
Ear canal bleeding	Frequent	Infrequent
Tympanic membrane perforation	Frequent	Infrequent
Hemotympanum	Common	Less common
Hearing loss	Variable: conductive, mixed, and sensorineural	Profound sensorineural loss
Vertigo	Variable frequency and severity	Frequent; severe
Facial nerve:		
Injury	Variable severity	Severe
Incidence	25%	50%
Paralysis	May be incomplete; onset may be delayed	Immediate onset; complete paralysis

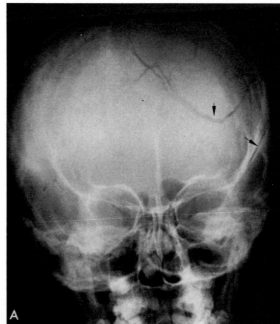

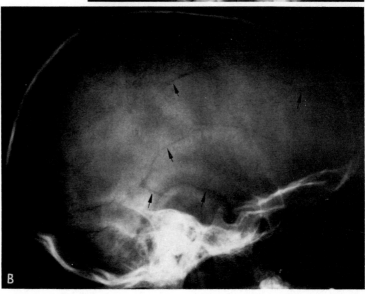

Figure 26–11. Frontal (A) and lateral (B) views of 9-year-old boy involved in a bicycle-automobile accident; he suffered a head injury with a period of unconsciousness. An extensive comminuted skull fracture that involves the temporal bone is present (arrows).

Bleeding

Bleeding from the ear commonly occurs following acute trauma to the temporal area (Grove, 1939; Proctor et al., 1956; Mitchell and Stone, 1973; Røhrt, 1973). To determine its significance, the exact source of the hemorrhage must be identified. Glancing blows that displace the pinna from its soft tissue attachments to the scalp can produce a shearing effect that may lacerate the skin of the bony external canal and produce bleeding even with an intact tympanic membrane. Injuries of sufficient violence to produce a temporal bone fracture will frequently be associated with a tear of the external canal that extends to and perforates the adjacent drum. Finally, severe trauma to the chin can cause the mandibular condyle to fracture through the anterior wall of the external auditory canal, causing

bleeding from the ear and severe otalgia when the mouth is opened. Generally, the bleeding noted is self-limiting and requires no active therapy. Instilling a few drops of a sterile vasoconstrictor (1:100,000 adrenaline, 1 per cent phenylephrine [Neo-Synephrine]) can usually control the bleeding. Only rarely will significant hemorrhaging result, with bleeding coming from the ear as well as going through the eustachian tube into the nose and pharynx. In such cases, packing for hemostasis is required.

Following an ear injury, the external ear canal should be cleansed of ceruminous debris and blood clots. As soon as the more pressing injuries have been treated and the child is stable, the extent of injury to the ossicles and drum should be assessed. Admittedly, this task may be extremely difficult when dealing with a frightened child who is unable to cooperate. As discussed above, if an associated injury has required general anesthesia, the ear can be evaluated and treated efficiently while the child is asleep.

It is not unusual for an ecchymotic area to appear in the area of the mastoid process (Battle sign) 4 or 5 days after a base-of-skull fracture. This is caused by the extravasation of blood pigments into the area and is evidence of an existing fracture but, in itself, is not an indication for any therapy.

Cerebrospinal Fluid Otorrhea

A cerebrospinal fluid (CSF) otorrhea noted after head trauma is a definite sign that the skull has been fractured and a meningeal tear has occurred. This traumatic communication can be the pathway for bacterial contamination and the cause of meningitis. Cerebrospinal fluid otorrhea has been reported as occurring much more frequently in children than in adults following a temporal bone fracture (Hardwood-Nash, 1970; Mitchell and Stone, 1973). The higher incidence of this clinical sign in youngsters is probably related to the elastic properties of the child's skull. Following significant trauma, the displacement of the highly malleable bony structures results in a stretching, with tearing of the underlying attached meningeal structures.

A cerebrospinal fluid leak may be obscured by active bleeding coming from the injured ear. When a cerebrospinal fluid leak is suspected, the bloody material from the ear should be collected and a sample placed on a filter paper. If cerebrospinal fluid is present, it will separate from the blood, forming a clear ring around the central hemorrhagic spot. As the coexisting bleeding ceases, the character of the otorrhea changes. Moreover, as the fluid becomes more watery and clearer, the presence of a cerebrospinal fluid leak becomes more obvious. In cases in which the tympanic membrane has remained intact, the presence of cerebrospinal fluid behind the drum will mimic the otoscopic findings observed in serous otitis media (i.e., a dull, immobile drum). In such cases, if the patient is instructed to bend over or is held upside down, clear fluid may pass down the eustachian tube and drip out the nose. An alternative way of obtaining a sample of the fluid is to perform a myringotomy and to collect the fluid directly from the middle ear. The material obtained should be analyzed for glucose. A glucose concentration of greater than 40 gm/100 ml, or two thirds of the simultaneously determined blood glucose value, suggests that the material is cerebrospinal fluid.

In most cases, traumatic cerebrospinal fluid otorrhea will stop spontaneously within 2 weeks and rarely requires surgical intervention. The use of prophylactic antibiotics to prevent meningitis is controversial (Mac Gee et al., 1970; Klastersky et al., 1976). Bed rest, avoidance of activity, and elevation of the head to decrease the intracranial cerebrospinal fluid pressure are recommended.

A persistent or recurrent cerebrospinal fluid leak is a common cause for recurrent meningitis. When this possibility is suspected, the presence of the leak should be documented and its exact location identified. The area from which the contrast material extravasates into the temporal bone may be pinpointed by performing a posterior fossa contrast study (Schultz and Stool, 1970; Kaufman et al., 1969). The presence of a cerebrospinal fluid leak may also be detected by using radioisotopes (Parisier and Birken, 1976). Indium diethylenetriamine pentaacetic acid (^{111}In DTPA) is injected into the cerebrospinal fluid spaces, and if a tympanic membrane perforation is present, a cottonball is placed adjacent to the drum opening. Additional cottonballs are inserted intranasally to absorb any cerebrospinal fluid leaking down the eustachian tube. Serial scans of the patient's head area are performed to observe suspected extravasation into the temporal bone. If the cerebrospinal fluid leak persists for more than 4 weeks, or, if it recurs, surgery should be considered. Using an appropriate temporal bone operative technique, the area from which the cerebrospinal fluid is leaking must be identified and securely packed off using temporalis fascia and a free muscle plug. Occasionally, in refractory cases, a neurosurgical approach to seal the leak from within the cranial cavity may be required.

Hearing Loss

Following a significant head injury, the focus of medical attention is directed toward controlling life-threatening problems and closely monitoring the patient's neurologic status. When there is no bleeding from the ear and the tympanic membrane is intact, it may be erroneously concluded that no significant ear damage has occurred. Indeed, infants and young children generally will not complain of a hearing loss. As a result, traumatic hearing losses may not be detected at the time of the injury, especially when they are unilateral and the child suffers no functional impairment. Thus, it is common for the effect of the trauma not to be recognized until much later. For example, it may first be detected when the child's hearing acuity is screened in school, or even later during a military preinduction or a preemployment physical examination when the individual is noted to have an unusual hearing loss of undetermined origin. Therefore, following significant head injury, an attempt should be made to establish accurate auditory thresholds. In infants, this may require repeated evaluations performed over many months, until reliable thresholds can be obtained (see the discussion of audiologic assessment in Chapter 9).

The hearing losses that occur as a result of head trauma vary considerably (Table 26–2). The most common type of hearing impairment following head and temporal bone trauma is a sensorineural hearing loss (Table 26–3), which has been reported in from 13 to 83 per cent of patients with these injuries (Podoshin and Fradis, 1975; Hough and Stuart, 1968; Tos, 1973; Grove, 1947; Mitchell and Stone, 1973; Røhrt, 1973; Barber, 1969). Audiometric analysis of the hearing loss

TABLE 26–2. Incidence of Traumatic Conductive Hearing Loss Due to Ossicular Disruption

REFERENCE	FRACTURE OF TEMPORAL BONE (%)	HEAD INJURY (%)
Podoshin and Fradis, 1975		1.4
Cremin, 1969		1
Røhrt, 1973	1	
Mitchell and Stone, 1973*	6	
Proctor et al., 1956	32	
Hough and Stuart, 1968	37	

*Pediatric series.

by complete site-of-lesion tests has demonstrated that some patients develop a cochlear loss, whereas others exhibit a retrocochlear loss. Additionally, even when a conductive hearing disorder is present, a coexisting sensorineural type of loss will frequently be observed.

PATHOGENESIS OF COCHLEAR HEARING LOSS. When significant trauma occurs to the head, with or without fracture, the force of the impact will momentarily compress the child's relatively elastic skull, which rapidly regains its original configuration. The pressure wave involves the encased cochlear structures and is thought to cause an excessive displacement of the basilar membrane (Igarashi et al., 1964; Schuknecht, 1969; 1950). This displacement produces a hearing loss similar to that caused by intense acoustic stimulation (i.e., a discrete drop in acuity in the 4000- to 8000-Hz range). Generally, the discrimination scores will be good, recruitment may be present, and there will not be any abnormal tone decay. Similar hearing losses were produced experimentally in animals (Schuknecht et al., 1951). A powerful blow to a cat's head held in a fixed position, produced a loss of acuity confined to the 3000- to 8000-Hz range. The pathologic findings observed in these temporal bones resembled those of patients with a history of head trauma. Histologically, there were varying degrees of damage to the organ of Corti. This damage was most marked in the midbasal cochlear turn.

A traumatic cochlear-type hearing loss may occur as a result of leakage of perilymph from the inner ear vestibule (Fee, 1968) (Fig. 26–12). A blow to the skull may produce a shock wave that will distort the area of the round window niche and disrupt the attachment

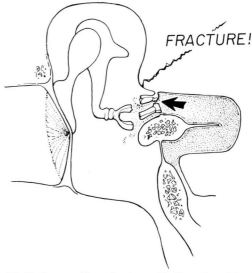

Figure 26–12. Temporal bone fracture with disruption of the stapes and a perilymph leak (arrow) producing a sensory hearing loss.

of the round window membrane, thereby causing it to tear. Following a significant head injury, the stapes, which is suspended within the air-containing middle ear cleft, will be exposed to a different compressional force than will the surrounding temporal bone. Moreover, the trauma may stimulate the simultaneous contraction of the stapedius muscle, which acts to rotate the stapes posteriorly and laterally out of the oval window. As a result of these forces, a subluxation of the stapes occurs that produces a tear of the annular ligament. Following either of these injuries involving the round or oval window, there is a resulting perilymphatic fluid leak that is associated with a hearing loss of varying severity. Furthermore, the traumatic distortion of the cochlear configuration following a blow to the head can produce a rupture of the relatively delicate basilar or Reissner membrane. This results in a disruption of the partition between the cochlear duct and the scala tympani or vestibuli. As a consequence, the potassium-rich endolymph mixes with the sodium-rich perilymph, producing biochemical changes that cause a significant labyrinthine disorder (see Fig. 26–3).

Symptomatically, vertigo usually occurs following cochlear membrane tears, perilymphatic leaks, or both. The spinning and accompanying nausea with vomiting may be so unpleasant that the patient will not immediately be aware of the associated hearing loss. The treatment of traumatic perilymphatic leaks was discussed in the consideration of treatment of middle ear injuries.

PATHOGENESIS OF A TRAUMATIC RETROCOCHLEAR HEARING LOSS. Following a head injury, the patient may have a hearing loss characterized audiometrically by a discrimination score that is surprisingly low and the presence of pathologic tone decay. These findings indicate the existence of a retrocochlear process. Animal experiments have demonstrated that, following trauma to the freely mobile head, a retrocochlear or

TABLE 26–3. Incidence of Traumatic Neurosensory Hearing Loss

REFERENCE	FRACTURE OF TEMPORAL BONE (%)	HEAD INJURY (%)
Hough and Stuart, 1968	62	
Barber, 1969	63	46
Proctor et al., 1956	56	83
Tos, 1973	27	
Røhrt, 1973	14	
Mitchell and Stone, 1973*	13	
Grove, 1939	63	24 to 45
Podoshin and Fradis, 1975		19

*Pediatric series.

central auditory hearing loss occurs (Makishima and Snow, 1975a; 1975b; 1976). At the moment of impact, the brain, which is suspended in cerebrospinal fluid, moves independently within the rigid skull, causing a substantial amount of swirling. This rotational displacement of the brain around the brain stem frequently results in a contrecoup cerebral injury. Moreover, this movement can severely stretch the cranial nerves where they leave the brain to enter their respective foramina (Strich, 1961). The abducens and the auditory-vestibular nerves seem to be particularly susceptible to this type of shearing force. As a result of this type of injury, multiple unilateral or bilateral cranial nerve deficits may occur even without skull fractures.

Pathologic examination of temporal bones obtained from persons who died as a result of head trauma have shown hemorrhages of the eighth cranial nerve at the fundi of the internal auditory canal (Grove, 1928; Makishima and Snow, 1975a). Animal experiments were performed that were designed to simulate the kind of injury that occurs to human (Makishima and Snow, 1975a; 1976): Guinea pigs with freely mobile heads were shaken within a padded cell. None of the experimental animals suffered a skull fracture. Nevertheless, the experiments did produce retrocochlear, central, or both types of hearing losses. The pathologic findings were similar to those observed in human temporal bones. Areas of hemorrhage were present in the cerebrum, cerebellum, brain stem, eighth nerve, and seventh nerve.

The extent of the sensorineural hearing loss that occurs following head trauma is not always consistent with the severity of the blow or with the extent of the resulting neurologic trauma. Occasionally, a patient who has had a mild head injury will have a surprisingly severe sensorineural hearing loss, whereas the victim with a serious concussion may not experience a significant loss of acuity. In addition, the sensorineural hearing loss observed following trauma is not always permanent. Frequently, there is some return of hearing acuity. Low-frequency losses, for instance, have a greater tendency to resolve than do higher-frequency losses. Indeed, depending on the mechanism of the injury, spontaneous improvement of hearing may occur. The hemorrhage and edema within a nerve that is caused by stretching may also resolve, leaving little permanent damage. Finally, the healing of intracochlear membrane tears and the sealing off of traumatic oval or round window leaks may be accompanied by the recovery of hearing.

CONDUCTIVE HEARING LOSS. A longitudinal fracture of the temporal bone is often associated with middle ear injuries because bleeding into the middle ear space frequently occurs as a result of the trauma. When the drum remains intact, a hemotympanum results (Podoshin and Fradis, 1975; Hendrick et al., 1965). This has been estimated to occur in 3 to 5 per cent of patients with skull fractures and in 20 per cent of patients with temporal bone fractures (Mitchell and Stone, 1973). The condition is usually temporary, improving spontaneously when the blood is either resorbed from the tympanic cavity or evacuated from the area through the eustachian tube into the nasopharynx. Occasionally, the fluid collection persists for many weeks. In these cases, when a myringotomy is performed, the fluid aspirated will resemble serum. In such cases, a tube should be inserted to ventilate the middle ear cleft.

When the force of an injury fractures the temporal bone, a gap results between the fragments as they momentarily separate. Characteristically this rent will extend through the posterior superior canal wall and will produce a rupture of the tympanic membrane, with bleeding from the ear canal. Tympanic membrane perforations occur in about 50 per cent of patients with temporal bone fractures (Grove, 1939; Mitchell and Stone, 1973). Often, the traumatic drum defect will heal spontaneously. In some cases, the traumatic fragmentation of the temporal bone can damage the contained ossicles (Hough, 1959; Hough and Stuart, 1968; Wright et al., 1969; Spector et al., 1973; Elbrond and Aastrup, 1973; Cremin, 1969) (Fig. 26–13). Usually, this type of injury occurs with head trauma of sufficient intensity to cause unconsciousness (see Table 26–3). The most common type of ossicular injury associated with temporal bone fractures is a separation of the incudostapedial joint (Fig. 26–14). Dislocation of the incus occurs almost as often. In fact, it is not unusual for these two types of injuries to occur simultaneously. Stapedial crural fractures are less common (Fig. 26–15), with the malleus being the ossicle least likely to be injured (Fig. 26–16).

There are several anatomic reasons that may explain these observations (Hough, 1959; Hough and Stuart, 1968). The malleus and stapes have firmer points of attachment than the incus. Moreover, the malleolar handle is supported by the tympanic membrane and has attachments to the anterior malleolar ligament and to the tensor tympani muscle, which give this ossicle ample support. The stapes is also anchored in the oval

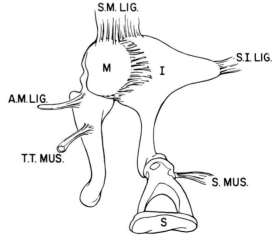

Figure 26–13. Ossicular chain—malleus (M), incus (I), stapes (S). Middle ear muscles—tensor tympani muscle (T.T. MUS.), stapedius muscle (S. MUS.). Ossicular ligaments—anterior malleolar ligament (A.M. LIG.), superior malleolar ligament (S.M. LIG.), short incudal ligament (S.I. LIG.).

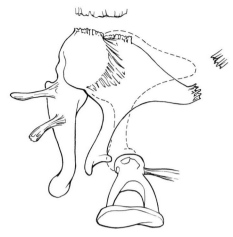

Figure 26–14. Dislocation of the incus with a separation of the incudostapedial joint is the most common type of ossicular injury.

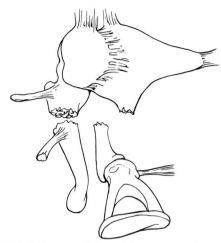

Figure 26–16. A fracture of the malleus is generally accompanied by other ossicular injuries.

window niche by the annular ligament, and it gains further support from the attachment of the stapes muscle. Therefore, of the three ossicles, the incus is the most vulnerable to traumatic injuries because it is suspended between the malleus and stapes with only one firm point of attachment—the posterior incudal ligament.

The vulnerability of the incus is compounded by the contraction of the middle ear muscles. A traumatic blow causes an abrupt reflex muscular contraction. The stapedius muscle rotates the stapes posteriorly and laterally out of the oval window. The tensor tympani muscle contraction simultaneously pulls the malleus handle and the attached incus medially toward the promontory. Following a severe blow to the head, the uncontrolled reflex muscular contraction may produce an unstable ossicular situation, making the incudostapedial joint the most vulnerable link in the ossicular chain (Fig. 26–17).

In many case reports describing the surgical correction of traumatic ossicular disruptions in adults, the damage actually occurred in childhood (Hough, 1959; Hough and Stuart, 1968; Spector et al., 1973; Wright et al., 1969). Such an ear injury may not be detected,

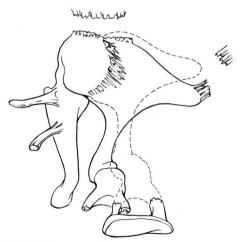

Figure 26–15. Dislocation of the incus; fracture of the stapes crura.

as most small children will not complain of the resulting loss of hearing. Therefore, following any otologic trauma, an audiometric evaluation should be obtained routinely.

Vertigo

The trauma that produces a sensorineural hearing loss may simultaneously cause vertigo (Podoshin and Fradis, 1975; Silverstein et al., 1973; Grove, 1939; Proctor et al., 1956; Barber, 1969; Schuknecht, 1969). The pathogenesis of traumatic vestibular and auditory injuries involves common sensory organ and neural innervation. Thus, for example, when the eighth nerve is damaged by a shearing force or when a perilymph leak occurs, vestibular symptoms as well as hearing loss may occur.

A labyrinthine concussion may result from a head injury, especially when the otic capsule is fractured. The victim, if conscious, will immediately experience a violent spinning sensation, which will be accompanied by a sensorineural hearing loss, nausea, and vomiting. Characteristically, following a peripheral labyrinthine injury, the patient will be more comfortable when positioned with the head turned so that the injured ear is up. The rapid phase of nystagmus will beat toward the uninvolved ear. However, in many instances, in spite of the patient's subjective complaint of vertigo, the observer will fail to see the expected nystagmus. In such cases, the absence of nystagmus is due to its suppression by visual fixation: when the patient is examined with eyes open, nystagmus due to a peripheral labyrinthine disorder may be markedly suppressed or abolished by visual fixation. This effect of the visual system may be abolished by examining the patient with eyes closed using electronystagmography (Chap. 15). Another way of overcoming visual fixation is by using Frenzel glasses, which contain +20 diopter lenses embedded in a gogglelike frame (Cohen, 1966). Within the frame are small light bulbs. The purpose of these glasses is to blur the vision and effectively prevent visual fixation. Additionally, they

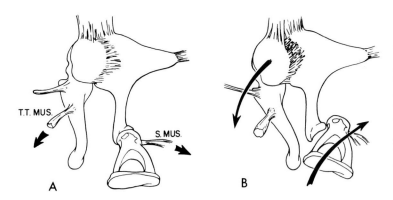

Figure 26–17. A traumatic blow to the head causes an abrupt contraction of the middle-ear muscles. *A*, The stapedius rotates the stapes laterally and posteriorly out of the oval window (S. MUS arrow). The tensor tympani pulls the malleus handle medially toward the promontory (T.T. MUS arrow). T.T., tensor tympani muscle; S. MUS., stapedius muscle. *B*, The simultaneous reflex contraction of these two muscles creates a tension that pulls the malleus in an opposite direction from the stapes (arrows) and that may be a factor in producing a dislocation of the incus.

magnify and illuminate the patient's eyes, making it easier for the examiner to detect even a fine nystagmus. The Frenzel glasses can easily be carried in a medical bag, and are extremely useful when the physician is required to perform a bedside evaluation of the vertiginous patient who either cannot be transported to a vestibular laboratory for electronystagmography because of associated injuries or who is unwilling to move because the slightest change in position produces violent spinning and vomiting.

Following a traumatic labyrinthine injury, the patient generally will be unwilling to move. The central nervous system gradually compensates for the injury and a characteristic recovery phase occurs. For the first 2 to 4 days, the vertigo will be constantly present. After a few days the patient will be dizzy with any movement. Slowly, the vertigo diminishes so that it only occurs transiently during head movement. After a few weeks, it will be present only when the head is turned so that the affected ear is facing downward. In children, complete symptomatic recovery usually occurs within 3 to 6 weeks.

An otoneurologic evaluation should be performed routinely to differentiate between imbalance and vertigo caused by injury to the brain stem or cerebellum, and that due to damage of the peripheral end organ (Chap. 11). Following an ear injury, when vestibular damage is suspected, the caloric test is useful in evaluating the functional status of a traumatized labyrinth. Caloric testing should not be performed when a perilymphatic or a cerebrospinal fluid leak is suspected. When a tympanic membrane perforation is present, unless air is used for the caloric test, special precautions must be taken before water is instilled into the ear. In cooperative children and adolescents with external canals of adequate size, finger cots are inserted into both the ear canals. This will prevent water from getting into the middle-ear space through a drum defect. An equal volume of ice water is instilled into each finger cot; the nystagmus produced by the caloric stimulation can then be evaluated. Sterile saline can be used to perform a caloric examination in smaller children with a perforated eardrum in whom a finger cot cannot be inserted. A 30-cc sterile saline vial is chilled in a beaker of iced water, the ear canal is carefully cleaned of any wax or debris, and then the minimum amount of iced sterile saline that will pro-

duce a definite nystagmus is instilled into the normal ear (0.2 to 0.6 cc). The volume of the same solution necessary to induce nystagmus in the affected ear is determined for comparison. The functional status of both labyrinths is qualitatively evaluated by comparing the volume of iced saline required in each ear to produce nystagmus.

Posttraumatic positional vertigo has been reported to occur in children (Eviatar and Eviatar, 1974). In this condition, the vertigo is induced when the head is placed in a supine or hyperextended position. When the patient is placed in this position, the nystagmus appears after a latency period of a few seconds, builds to a crescendo, and then disappears. Clinically, the Frenzel glasses are extremely helpful in observing these characteristic eye movements. If the patient's head is moved and then returned to the original position, the nystagmus will not occur because it is fatigable. In adults, this condition is common. It has been attributed to the jarring loose of the utricular otoliths, which gravitate to the most dependent portion of the vestibular system and come to rest on the ampullated end of the posterior semicircular canal (Schuknecht, 1969). Clinically, however, this condition seldom seems to occur in children.

Facial Paralysis

Overall, a facial paralysis occurs in 21 to 33 per cent of children with temporal bone fractures (Hardwood-Nash, 1970; Mitchell and Stone, 1973; Alberti and Biagioni, 1972). A facial paralysis occurs in half of the patients who have a transverse type of fracture (Grove, 1939; Proctor et al., 1956). However, because 75 to 80 per cent of temporal bone fractures are of the longitudinal type, the majority of facial nerve injuries occur as a result of this latter injury. Anatomically, the facial nerve is most commonly injured where it is most vulnerable (McHugh, 1963). Regardless of the type of temporal bone fracture, damage to the facial nerve usually occurs in its horizontal portion between the geniculate ganglion and the second genu, where it turns to assume a vertical course. In this area, the thin, relatively fragile bone that covers the facial nerve affords little protection. In longitudinal fractures, the damage to the facial nerve is frequently mild, and most patients recover spontaneously. The more serious transverse fractures of the temporal bone that are caused by violent head trauma occur infrequently; 50 per cent of persons with these fractures sustain a severely traumatized or torn facial nerve.

When examining a patient following significant head trauma, the physician must evaluate facial movement. Specific detailed observations describing the movements of the upper and lower face, including eye closure, should be recorded when the patient is initially seen. Admittedly, this may be extremely difficult when severe facial lacerations, ecchymotic changes, and swelling are present. If the patient is unconscious, an attempt to produce facial grimacing should be made by using a painful stimulus. The symmetry of facial muscle tone should be assessed. When a facial paralysis is present, it must be determined whether the paralysis is complete or partial. Even in the unconscious patient, an assessment of tear production should be attempted by performing the Schirmer test. When the patient is conscious, complete topographic testing should be performed to try, anatomically, to localize the site of injury to the facial nerve (Chap. 17). Thus, when a patient with a facial paralysis does not tear on the affected side, this indicates that the facial nerve has been injured at, or proximal to, the geniculate ganglion.

The facial paralysis following severe head injury may be caused by an injury to the central nervous system rather than to the peripheral nerve. In one study of 115 cases of traumatic facial paralysis occurring in children, 55 per cent were attributable to upper motor neuron injury (Hendrick et al., 1965). Frequently, but not invariably, the central type of facial paralysis will be more marked in the lower two thirds of the face. Additionally, in spite of the paralysis, movement on the affected side may occur in association with involuntary emotional expressions.

If a patient is noted to have a complete facial paralysis immediately following a temporal bone injury, it is necessary to perform only topographic testing to determine the site of injury. Additionally, a complete CT examination may help to pinpoint the site and extent of involvement. In these patients, electric testing is unnecessary, as the results observed will be misleading for at least 48 to 72 hours after the acute injury. As soon as the patient is able to tolerate surgery, the facial nerve should be explored to determine the cause of injury. Bony fragments impinging on the nerve should be removed. Because damage to the nerve is frequently caused by edema, the neurolemmal sheath should be incised. If the nerve is lacerated, immediate nerve grafting should be performed. When topographic tests demonstrate that tearing is absent on the affected side, a complete exploration with decompression of the facial nerve into the internal auditory canal is indicated.

When the facial paralysis is of delayed onset or is incomplete, the prognosis for spontaneous recovery is better. The status of the facial nerve should be monitored carefully using the tests of facial function described in Chapter 17. If, on serial testing, nerve degeneration is observed, exploration of the facial nerve with decompression should be performed.

FACIAL PARALYSIS IN NEONATES

Infrequently, a newborn infant is noted to have a peripheral facial paralysis, which may be due to several causes (Alberti and Biagioni, 1972; Miehlke, 1973; Hepner, 1951; Kornblut, 1974). During the last months of pregnancy, the increased intrauterine pressure may continuously press the side of the embryo's face against its own shoulder, resulting in a facial paralysis. During delivery, damage to the facial nerve can occur either when the neonate's head is squeezed against the mother's sacral prominence or when obstetric forceps are applied traumatically. In such cases, the nerve may be injured by direct pressure either in the facial-parotid area or within the temporal bone. In the latter instance, the trauma may occur as a result of either a forceful indentation of the elastic skull or an actual fracture. Frequently, the intrapartum traumatic facial paralysis will improve spontaneously (Alberti and Biagioni, 1972). However, facial nerve decompression has been required in selected cases (McHugh, 1963; Kornblut, 1977). Facial paralysis is discussed in Chapter 17.

ACOUSTIC TRAUMA

One of the most common causes of loss of hearing is acoustic trauma. An explosive blast near a child's ear, such as the detonation of a firecracker, cap gun, or weapon, can produce an immediate loss of hearing that occasionally is severe. Repeated, frequent exposure to the loud noises produced by snowmobiles, motorcycle engines, power tools, or model gasoline engines can also damage the inner ear. The popularity of loudly amplified music has made headphone amplifiers and loud electronic rock music a part of youth culture. However, it has been suggested that this fad can damage hearing.

A loud, explosive blast produces a sound wave causing a large excursion of the tympanic membrane, which is translated through the ossicular chain into a forceful inner ear perilymphatic traveling fluid wave. As a result, an excessive displacement of the basilar membrane occurs that causes a shearing force that damages the hair cells.

Prolonged exposure to loud noises produces enzymatic and biochemical activity within the organ of Corti. Moderate auditory stimuli produce increased metabolism of the hair cells, which after a period of time leads to exhaustion of energy sources and results in a loss of auditory acuity. Although these changes are initially reversible, a permanent hearing loss will occur when a person is repeatedly exposed to loud noises (Schuknecht, 1974).

The severity of the hearing loss following chronic noise exposure is related to the intensity of the sound and daily duration of exposure; for example, exposure to a constant noise of 100 dB for 2 hours is equivalent to exposure to a noise of 115 dB for 15 minutes. Thus, it has been estimated that 41.5 per cent of individuals 50 years of age who have been habitually exposed to a 100-dB noise will suffer a noise-induced hearing handicap (Guide for Conservation of Hearing in Noise, 1969).

Noise-induced hearing losses can be prevented by use of ear protectors that reduce the exposure of the inner ear to traumatic acoustic stimuli. Earplugs designed to occlude the ear canal are an inexpensive way of obtaining personal protection. Contrary to popular opinion, filling the ear canal with dry cotton is not effective, as it does little to attenuate sound levels. Another approach is to control noise exposure environmentally—preventing children from playing with cap guns or exploding firecrackers and controlling the intensity of amplified music.

SELECTED REFERENCES

Hardwood-Nash, D. C. 1970. Fractures of the petrous and tympanic parts of the temporal bone in children: A tomographic study of 35 cases. Am. J. Roentgenol. Radium Ther. Nucl. Med. 110:598.

Hough, J. V. D., and Stuart, W. D. 1968. Middle ear injuries in skull trauma. Laryngoscope 78:899.

A comprehensive, well-organized clinical review that describes the authors' experiences with 31 cases of temporal bone fractures with accompanying middle ear damage.

Mitchell, D. P., and Stone, P. 1973. Temporal bone fractures in children. Can. J. Otolaryngol. 2:156.

Hardwood-Nash's and Mitchell's articles review the clinical experience with temporal bone fractures at the Hospital for Sick Children, Toronto, Canada. Unlike most reports, which are based on patients of all ages, these authors' observations are derived exclusively from a pediatric population.

REFERENCES

Alberti, P. W., and Biagioni, E. 1972. Facial paralysis in children. A review of 150 cases. Laryngoscope 82:1013.

Armstrong, B. W. 1970. Traumatic perforations of the tympanic membrane: Observe or repair? Laryngoscope 82:1822.

Barber, H. O. 1969. Head injury. Audiological and vestibular findings. Ann. Otol. Rhinol. Laryngol. 78:239.

Bellucci, R. J. 1966. Tympanoplasty, the malleus stapes wire and total defect skin graft. Laryngoscope 76:1439.

Chakeres, D. W., and Weider, D. J. 1985. Computed tomography of the ossicles. Neuroradiology 27:99.

Cohen, B. C. 1966. The examination of vestibulooculomotor function. Mt. Sinai J. Med. N.Y. 33:243.

Cremin, M. D. 1969. Injuries of the ossicular chain. J. Laryngol. Otol. 83:845.

Derlacki, E. L. 1973. Office closure of central tympanic membrane perforations: A quarter century of experience. Trans. Am. Acad. Ophthalmol. Otolaryngol. ORL 77:53.

Elbrond, E., and Aastrup, J. E. 1973. Isolated fractures of the stapedial arch. Acta Otolaryngol. 75:357.

Elner, A., Ingelstedt, S., and Ivarsson, A. 1971. Normal function of the eustachian tube. Acta Otolaryngol. 72:320.

Eviatar, L., and Eviatar, A. 1974. Vertigo in childhood. Clin. Pediatr. 13:940.

Fee, G. A. 1968. Traumatic perilymphatic fistulas. Arch. Otolaryngol. 88:477.

Flisberg, K., Ingelstedt, S., and Ortegren, V. 1963. On middle ear pressure. Acta Otolaryngol. (Suppl.) 182:43.

Goodhill, V., Harris, I., Brockman, S. J., and Hantz, O. 1973. Sudden deafness and labyrinthine window ruptures. Ann. Otol. Rhinol. Laryngol. 82:2.

Goodhill, V. 1974. Sudden deafness and round window rupture. Laryngoscope 81:1462.

Graves, G. O., and Edwards, E. F. 1944. The eustachian tube. Arch. Otolaryngol. 39:359.

Grove, W. E. 1928. Otological observations in trauma of the head. A clinical study based on 42 cases. Arch. Otolaryngol. 8:249.

Grove, W. E. 1939. Skull fractures involving the ear. A clinical study of 211 cases. Laryngoscope 49:678, 833.

Grove, W. E. 1947. Hearing impairment due to craniocerebral trauma. Ann. Otol. Rhinol. Laryngol. 56:264.

Guide for Conservation of Hearing in Noise. 1969. Rochester, MN, American Academy of Ophthalmology and Otolaryngology.

Hardwood-Nash, D. C., 1970. Fractures of the petrous and tympanic parts of the temporal bone in children: A tomographic study of 35 cases. Am. J. Roentgenol. Radium Ther. Nucl. Med. 110:598.

Hendrick, E. B., Hardwood-Nash, D. C., and Hudson, A. R. 1965. Head injuries in children: Survey of 4,465 consecutive cases at Hospital for Sick Children, Toronto, Canada. Clin. Neurosurg. 11:46.

Hepner, W. R., Jr. 1951. Some observations of facial paresis in the newborn infant: Etiology and incidence. Pediatrics 8:494.

Hough, J. V. D. 1959. Incudostapedial joint separation: Etiology, treatment and significance. Laryngoscope 69:644.

Hough, J. V. D., and Stuart, W. D. 1968. Middle ear injuries in skull trauma. Laryngoscope 78:899.

Igarashi, M., Schuknecht, H., and Myers, E. 1964. Cochlear pathology in humans with stimulation deafness. J. Laryngol. 78:115.

Juers, A. L. 1963. Perforation closure by marginal eversion. Arch. Otolaryngol. 77:76.

Kaufman, B., Jordan, V. M., and Pratt, L. L. 1969. Positive contrast demonstration of a cerebrospinal fluid fistula through the fundus on the internal auditory meatus. Acta Radiol. 9:83.

Klastersky, J., Sadeghi, M., and Brihaye, J. 1976. Antimicrobial prophylaxis in patients with rhinorrhea or otorrhea: A double blind study. Surg. Neurol. 6:111.

Kornblut, A. D. 1974. Facial nerve injuries in children. J. Laryngol. Otol. 88:717.

Kornblut, A. D. 1977. Facial nerve injuries in children. Ear Nose Throat J. 56:369.

Mac Gee, E. E., Cauthen, J. C., and Brackett, C. E. 1970. Meningitis following acute traumatic cerebrospinal fluid fistula. J. Neurosurg. 33:312.

Makishima, K., and Snow, J. B., Jr. 1975a. Pathogenesis of hearing loss in head injury. Arch. Otolaryngol. 101:426.

Makishima, K., and Snow, J. B., Jr. 1975b. Electrophysiological responses from the cochlea and inferior colliculus in guinea pigs after head injury. Laryngoscope 85:1947.

Makishima, K., and Snow, J. B., Jr. 1976. Effect of head blow on the development of hearing loss. Laryngoscope 86:971.

McHugh, H. F. 1963. Facial paralysis in birth injury and skull fractures. Arch. Otolaryngol. 78:443.

Miehlke, A. 1973. Surgery of the Facial Nerve, 2nd ed. Philadelphia, W. B. Saunders Co., pp. 86–87.

Mitchell, D. P., and Stone, P. 1973. Temporal bone fractures in children. Can. J. Otolaryngol. 2:156.

Parisier, S. C., and Birken, E. A. 1976. Recurrent meningitis secondary to idiopathic oval window CSF leak. Laryngoscope 86:1503.

Pennington, C. L. 1973. Incus interposition techniques. Ann. Otol. Rhinol. Laryngol. 82:518.

Podoshin, L., and Fradis, M. 1975. Hearing loss after head injury. Arch. Otolaryngol. 101:15.

Potter, G. D. 1971. Fractures of the temporal bone. In Jensen, J., and Roysing, H.: Fundamentals of Ear Tomography. Springfield, IL, Charles C Thomas, pp. 106–118.

Potter, G. D. 1972. Temporal bone fractures. Problems in radiologic diagnosis. Laryngoscope 82:408.

Proctor, B., Gurdjian, E. S., and Webster J. E. 1956. The ear in head trauma. Laryngoscope 66:16.

Pullen, F. W., II. 1972. Round window membrane rupture: A cause of sudden deafness. Trans. Am. Acad. Ophthalmol. Otolaryngol. 76:1444.

Røhrt, T. 1973. Fracture of temporal bone, early or retrospective diagnosis and surgical hearing reconstruction. Acta Otolaryngol. 75:355.

Rundcrantz, H. 1970. The effects of position change on eustachian tube function. Otolaryngol. Clin. North Am. 3:103.

Sadé, J. 1964. Traumatic fractures of the stapes. Arch. Otolaryngol. 80:258.

Schuknecht, H. F. 1950. A clinical study of auditory damage following blows to the head. Ann. Otol. Rhinol. Laryngol. 59:330.

Schuknecht, H. F. 1969. Mechanism of inner ear injury from blows to the head. Ann. Otol. Rhinol. Laryngol. 78:253.

Schuknecht, H. F. 1974. Pathology of the Ear. Cambridge, MA, Harvard University Press, pp. 309–310.

Schuknecht, H. F., Neff, W. D., and Perlman, H. B. 1951. An experimental study of auditory damage following blows to the head. Ann. Otol. Rhinol. Laryngol. 60:275.

Schultz, P., and Stool, S. E. 1970. Recurrent meningitis due to a congenital fistula through the stapes footplate. Am. J. Dis. Child. 120:553.

Silverstein, H., Fabian, R. L., Stool, S. E., and Hong, S. W. 1973. Penetrating wounds of the tympanic membrane and ossicular chain. Trans. Am. Acad. Ophthalmol. Otolaryngol. ORL 77:125.

Singh, D., and Ahluwalia, K. S. 1968. Blast injuries of the ear. J. Laryngol. Otol. 82:1017.

Spector, G. J., Pratt, L. L., and Randall, G. 1973. A clinical study of delayed reconstruction in ossicular fractures. Laryngoscope 83:837.

Strich, S. J. 1961. Shearing of nerve fibers as a cause of brain damage due to head injury. A pathological study of 20 cases. Lancet 2:442.

Sudderth, M. F. 1974. Tympanoplasty in blast induced perforation. Arch. Otolaryngol. 99:157.

Tos, M. 1974. Course of sequelae of 248 petrosal fractures. Acta Otolaryngol. 75:353.

Vital Statistics of the United States 1974, Vol. II, Mortality Part B. Rockville, MD, 1976. National Center for Health Statistics.

Ward, P. H. 1969. Histopathology of auditory and vestibular disorders in head trauma. Ann. Otol. Rhinol. Laryngol. 78:227.

Wehrs, R. E. 1974. The homograft notched incus in tympanoplasty. Arch. Otolaryngol. 100:251.

Wright, J. W., Jr., Taylor, C. E., and Bizal, J. A. 1969. Tomography of the vulnerable incus. Ann. Otol. Rhinol. Laryngol. 78:263.

Yamaki, T., Yoshino, E., Higuchi, T., et al. 1986. Value of high-resolution computed tomography in diagnosis of petrous bone fracture. Surg. Neurol. 26:551.

Chapter 27

TUMORS OF THE EAR AND TEMPORAL BONE

John R. Stram, M.D.

Tumors of the external ear and temporal bone constitute a relatively small percentage of tumors of the head and neck seen in the pediatric patient. Of 25,000 cases of pediatric neoplasms on file at the Armed Forces Institute of Pathology (AFIP), there are approximately 100 examples of primary involvement of the temporal bone. Textbooks of pediatric otolaryngology by Ferguson and Kendig (1972) and by Jaffe (1977) have only briefly discussed the more common neoplasms that occur in this region, apparently because there was insufficient material available from which to develop a more extensive presentation. In a review of 54 neoplasms of the temporal bone and middle ear, Bradley and Maxwell (1954) identified only four tumor examples in pediatric patients. Of the 38 cases of malignant tumors of the middle ear and mastoid process reported by Figi and Hempstead (1943), only one tumor in the temporal bone occurred in a child.

It is unfortunate that temporal bone neoplasms in children are often diagnosed late in the course of disease and usually only after treatment for another suspected illness has failed. Early, accurate diagnosis, confirmed by histologic evaluation of a biopsy specimen, is essential to the planning of effective treatment for such tumors. Once the correct diagnosis has been made, improved surgical and anesthesia techniques, radiotherapy control, and an expanding inventory of chemotherapeutic agents make control of these neoplasms possible.

As Chapter 6 of this text indicates, the temporal bone contains structures that are fully developed at birth, whereas other parts are vestigial at birth and assume their adult configurations through later growth and development. Tremble's observations (1977) suggest that little growth occurs in the membranous labyrinth following birth. In his publications on meningioma and temporal bone epidermoids, Nager (1964, 1975) demonstrated that neither the tympanic membrane nor the fibrous annulus undergoes significant postnatal growth. Therefore, it is not surprising that mesenchymal tumors of these structures are not reported. Nager has demonstrated that the centers of most active growth in the temporal bone include the suture lines of the temporal bone, the tympanic bone, and the tympanic annulus, as well as the soft parts of the auricle, the ear canal, and the vascular and nerve supplies to these areas. Most tumors in pediatric patients develop in these anatomic areas of greatest growth activity. Rhabdomyosarcoma, plexiform neurofibroma, mesenchymoma, osteosarcoma, chondrosarcoma, and fibrosarcoma are tumor types commonly associated with growing tissue and are also the types of tumors most frequently reported to occur in the temporal bones of children (Bradley and Maxwell, 1954; Figi and Hempstead, 1943).

The temporal bone develops as an enlarging tissue mass that either invests or displaces adjacent organs and tissues. This mode of development helps explain the occurrence of choristomas and meningiomas in the temporal bone. A popular theory of tumor development is that tissue anlagen of organs adjacent to the temporal bone become separated from their normal tissue masses and are included in the developing temporal bone. With growth, this tissue becomes a recognizable tumor mass of histologically normal tissue in an alien location. Frequent literature reports of the presence of arachnoid villi, central nervous system tissue, primitive neurectoderm, and salivary gland tissue in the temporal bone support this theory of temporal bone tumor formation (Guzowski and Paparella, 1976; Nager, 1964). This heterotopic tissue is benign, and its anatomic location in the temporal bone, as well as the size of the mass, will govern the presenting signs and symptoms and dictate the therapeutic approach. Occasionally, heterotopic arachnoid tissue may give rise to primary meningiomas of the temporal bone as described by Nager (1964) and Guzowski and Paparella (1976). In discussing the pathophysiology of a yolk sac tumor in the temporal bone, Stanley has also postulated a mechanism whereby ectopic germinal cells from the primitive streak and remnants of the midline germinal ridge can migrate laterally as far as the temporal bone (Wick and Siegal, 1980; Teilum, 1978).

An understanding of the embryology of tissues contained within the temporal bone is essential to an understanding of the histologic variations possible in a biopsy specimen of a tumor of this region. The accurate diagnosis of neoplasms of the temporal bone requires that histologic material be examined by experienced pathologists who are familiar with the histology of developing tissues of this region. Frequently, sophisticated diagnostic techniques, such as electron microscopy, and tissue culture techniques, such as those described by Wigger and Mitsudo in their 1976 report of a congenital malignant fibrous histiocytoma, may be necessary to arrive at an accurate diagnosis.

EXOSTOSES

Benign bony occlusion of the external auditory canal (exostosis) has been associated by Van Gilse (1938) and by Fowler and Osmun (1942) with cold water entering the external auditory canal. Exostoses are hard, bony masses that have either a sessile or pedunculated configuration and that commonly occur in the suture lines of the external auditory canal. They are seldom seen before the age of 10 years. According to Mawson (1963), they are often bilateral and are three times more common in males than in females. They are probably the most common bony proliferation found in the external ear canal. Ash (1960) distinguishes between this lesion and a true osteoma, the latter being considered rare, usually presenting in the inferior aspect of the ear canal at the junction of bone and cartilage of the external auditory canal. There are reports in the literature of giant cell tumors occurring in the temporal bones of newborn infants (Japanese) and of chondrosarcomas occurring in the first decade of life (Leedham, 1972), but these represent single case reports and are quite uncommon.

FIBROUS DYSPLASIA

In a 1970 review of monostotic fibrous dysplasia, Sharp states that this entity has been known to occur in the temporal bones of pediatric patients since 1946. Five of the 11 cases reviewed and reported in the world literature occurred in children, in whom the tumor developed at the beginning of the second decade of life. Histologically, the tumor tissue was sclerotic, with expansion in size of the involved bone in all cases reported. Occlusion of the external auditory meatus was a common finding, and in half the cases in which the dysplastic bone occluded the external auditory canal, cholesteatomas were also present. The differential diagnosis of this entity includes osteoblastoma, osteoma, osteomyelitis, and local reaction to a meningioma. Conservative local therapy provided control in the cases reported. In only one of these 11 cases of monostotic fibrous dysplasia was trauma associated with the recognition of this tumor. A hearing loss was a common primary complaint in these cases. Confusion exists in the literature as to whether or not valid clinical and histologic distinctions can be made between monostotic fibrous dysplasia and a benign fibroosseous lesion, ossifying fibroma (juvenile ossifying fibroma), which can involve the temporal bones in children. Respected authorities feel that there are grounds for separation of the two entities, particularly on clinical, radiologic, therapeutic, and prognostic grounds (Hyams, 1976; Lichtenstein and Jaffe, 1942; Lichtenstein, 1972).

TUMORS OF BONE AND CARTILAGE

There are no pediatric case reports of cartilaginous neoplasms of the external ear or external auditory canal; there is but one reference, by Piepgras (1972), to a chondroblastoma occurring in the temporal bone of a patient who was close to the second decade of life. Coltrera and colleagues (1986) have included a chondrosarcoma of the temporal bone in a 19-year-old female in their series of 13 cases. In 1974, Ronis reported on the incidence of osteoblastoma of the temporal bone in the pediatric age group. This histologically bizarre but benign osteoid-producing tumor, although rare, has been reported specifically in the temporal bone by Lichtenstein and Sawyer (1964), Dahlin and Johnson (1954), and Byers (1968). Although they occur more commonly in the vertebrae and the long bones, 15 to 20 per cent of these lesions involve the calvarium. Two thirds of the cases reported by Lichtenstein and Sawyer (1964) were in children between 6 and 12 years of age, and there were no racial or sexual predilections. Osteoblastomas presented clinically as radiologically osteolytic lesions associated with primary complaints of vascular tinnitus or a conductive hearing loss. Surgical removal of the tumor provided relief of these symptoms in the cases reported.

Ewing sarcoma, the second most common primary bone malignancy in children and the most common bone tumor in the first decade of life, has been described in the temporal bone by Carroll and Miketic (1987). This tumor, which has an incidence of skull involvement in less than 4 per cent (Falk and Alpert, 1965; Ewing, 1921), has now been described in the temporal bone and computed tomography (CT) findings are those of a bone-replacing and bone-deforming bony neoplasm.

METASTATIC TUMORS

Metastatic tumors and secondary malignant tumors of the temporal bone were reported by Schuknecht and colleagues in 1968, but none of the tumors reported occurred in children. However, these tumors may occur in the pediatric age group. The primary tumors include renal cell carcinomas; adenoid cystic carcinomas of the parotid; carcinomas of the larynx, thyroid, and nasopharynx; meningeal sarcomas; gliomas of the pons; lymphosarcomas; and melanosarcomas. The metastatic forms of these tumors in the temporal bone were characterized by bone destruction and scattered involvement throughout the temporal bone.

SOFT TISSUE TUMORS

Rhabdomyosarcomas

By far the most common tumor of mesenchymal origin in the temporal bone is rhabdomyosarcoma. A review of the world literature prior to 1973 by Deutsch and Felder (1974) revealed 73 cases that presented in the ear or mastoid region. In 1958, in what is essentially a histologic classification, Horn and Enterline divided rhabdomyosarcomas of the head and neck, including the temporal bone, into embryonal rhabdomyosarcoma, alveolar rhabdomyosarcoma, and sarcoma botryoides. In a 1976 review of AFIP otolaryngologic pathology material, Hyams reported that the majority of cases with involvement of the temporal bone by rhabdomyosarcoma occurred in the pediatric age group. From a review of a published series of case reports, there appears to be no difference in the clinical presentations of the different histologic types of this entity. The mean age for establishment of the diagnosis is 6.1 years; the age range is 16 months to 16 years. Approximately half the individuals reported in the literature sought medical care and examination after sustaining trauma to the region of the ear and mastoid. The average interval between initial symptoms and establishment of the diagnosis and institution of therapy was 3.5 months. The most common presenting sign was a tumor or swelling; the most common presenting symptom was pain. Physical findings usually revealed the tumors to be in the ear canal or postauricular region. On gross examination there was a characteristic, superficial blood vessel dilatation over the tumor mass. It is unfortunate that these entities have frequently been initially diagnosed as hematomas, otitis media, or aural polyps. Subsequently, at the time of definitive diagnosis, the tumor had already spread to the nasopharynx, pharynx, cranial cavity, dura, cervical lymph nodes and orbit, thus lessening the chances of cure. The majority of the patients reported in the literature and in the AFIP otolaryngologic pathology registry died as a result of uncontrolled primary tumor. A 1973 report by Jaffe and coworkers and a 1976 report by Liebner support the effectiveness of the current philosophy of treating the primary tumor and its most common sites of spread initially with intensive radiotherapy or combining radiotherapy with surgical debulking and chemotherapy.

TUMORS OF HEMATOPOIETIC ORIGIN

Histiocytosis

Histiocytosis X is the term used to identify a composite common to eosinophilic granuloma, Hand-Schüller-Christian disease, and Letterer-Siwe disease. The common single or multiple bone lesions appear to be lytic on radiography and are histologically benign, with a proliferation of lipid-laden histiocytes, giant cells, and eosinophils. Eosinophilic granuloma is the most probable of these entities to present as a solitary lesion and is, therefore, reported as a tumor that occurs in the temporal bone. In a review of 16 cases of eosinophilic granuloma of the temporal bone by Toohill in 1973, 14 occurred in the pediatric age group. The age range was 1 to 12 years, with a male predominance. In four cases, the temporal bone lesions were bilateral. The most common presenting symptoms were otorrhea, pain, and postauricular swelling; one patient presented with facial paralysis. The most common physical findings were granulation tissue polyps of the external ear canal with evidence of bone erosion primarily involving the posterosuperior external canal wall. The majority of patients responded to either surgical or radiation therapy. A review of the AFIP Temporal Bone Inventory by Hyams in 1976 identified ten cases of histiocytosis X in children aged 1 to 10 years, with an equal distribution in males and females.

The etiology of histiocytosis is unknown. Clinicians can draw few clues to aid in management of the disease from the philosophic arguments for differentiation of acute disseminated and localized multifocal histiocytosis or from the arguments that morphologically the acute and chronic forms are the same. However, clinicians should be encouraged that this condition responds well to supportive treatment, whether it be radiation therapy or surgical extirpation.

LYMPHORETICULAR NEOPLASMS (LYMPHOMA AND LEUKEMIA)

Lymphomatous involvement of the temporal bone has been comprehensively reported on by Shambron and Finch (1958), Zechner and Altman (1969), and Paparella (1973). These authors suggest that the incidence of temporal bone involvement by this malignant neoplastic entity ranges from 16 to 35 per cent. Histologically, acute leukemic infiltration of the temporal bone is manifested as perivascular infiltration of the submucosal stroma of the mucous membrane of the middle ear and of the pneumatized cells of the mastoid. Temporal bone studies have demonstrated similar infiltration of the external auditory canal, the tympanic membrane, the mucosa of the middle ear, the facial nerve, the eustachian tube, and the mastoid air cell system. Occasionally, the membranous labyrinth may be involved by the leukemic infiltrate or at least by hemorrhage precipitated by the disease. Paparella (1973) points out that approximately 28 per cent of the clinical problems in leukemic patients were directly attributable to leukemic infiltrates of the ear and temporal bone. It is interesting to note that 48 per cent of the leukemic patients studied had otologic signs and symptoms in the course of their disease that were not directly attributable to postmortem temporal bone involvement by the leukemic process. Paparella (1973) recommends routine otologic, audiologic, and vestibular evaluation of all patients with leukemia. The common presenting signs and symptoms of leukemic involvement of the temporal bone include ulceration and hemorrhage of the ear canal and the middle ear, thickened mucosa of the tympanic membrane and middle ear, and lesions of the major nerve trunks in the temporal bone, producing hearing loss, facial paralysis, and vertigo. Acute lymphocytic leukemia, acute myelogenous leukemia, and erythroleukemia are the diagnoses associated with temporal bone involvement.

Although no clinical reports of a lymphoma involving the temporal bone of a child by metastatic spread or by contiguous spread could be found in the literature, it should be understood that lymphosarcoma and Hodgkin disease are forms of lymphoma commonly found in children. These entities rarely occur primarily in the temporal bone but may encroach on the temporal bone from without, particularly from the region of the parotid gland and parotid lymph nodes.

TUMORS OF NERVE TISSUE ORIGIN

Tumors of nerve tissue origin are rare in the pediatric age group, although peripheral nerve schwannomas (neurilemomas) and neurofibromas (plexiform neuromas) have been recognized in the external ear canal and the middle ear. Tumors of the eighth nerve, either in association with neurofibromatosis (von Recklinghausen disease) or as primary neurilemomas of the eighth nerve, are rare in children but must be considered in the differential diagnosis of retrocochlear hearing loss. Previous mention has been made of the presence of heterotopic brain tissue in the middle ear, the so-called glioma. Extensive reviews by Nager (1964), Guzowski and Paparella (1976), and Buehrle (1972) have identified arachnoid tissue in the petrous apex, along the course of the greater superficial petrosal nerve, in the semicanal of the tensor tympani muscle, in the anterior middle ear, in the genu of the facial nerve, in the internal auditory meatus, and in the jugular foramen. The potential for aberrant meningeal tissue in these locations to develop into meningiomas is supported in the extensive review of this tumor by Nager (1964). Histologically, this tumor can be mistaken for a glomus jugulare tumor (jugulotemporal extraadrenal paraganglioma), but the problem of differential diagnosis has not presented itself in the pediatric age group because glomus jugulare tumors rarely occur before the end of the second decade of life.

TUMORS OF THE SKIN AND SKIN APPENDAGES

The tissue components of the external ear and the temporal bone are those of the body in general. Squamous cell carcinomas, squamous papillomas, sweat gland tumors, melanomas, basal cell carcinomas, sebaceous gland tumors, and hair follicle tumors all have been reported to occur in the skin of the external ear and the ear canal by Ash and Raum (1956) and Batsakis (1974), but essentially only single case reports occur in the pediatric population. In general, the observations of Bradley and Maxwell (1954) are supported: Tumors of the temporal bone in children are more often sarcomas. However, a 1976 report by Conley and Schuller indicates that 6.5 per cent of all ear canal malignancies occur in children under the age of 20 years; cerumen gland adenocarcinomas predominate in this series. MacComb and Fletcher (1968) reported that melanomas rarely occur before the age of 16 years but that 20 to 30 per cent of pediatric melanomas involve the head and neck. Xeroderma pigmentosa most often involves the skin of the head and neck in the pediatric patient and is a precursor of squamous cell and basal cell carcinoma. This entity tends to be more common in blacks.

EPIDERMOID TUMORS (CONGENITAL CHOLESTEATOMA)

Congenital cholesteatomas or epidermoids of the temporal bone are considered aberrant epithelial tissue or teratomatous malformations found in the temporal bone from birth to the eighth decade (Nager, 1975). The peak age for symptom development is 15 years. These lesions are pearly or shiny epithelial masses, usually developing behind an intact tympanic membrane in the petrotympanic suture line. They tend to expand with general body growth toward the cerebellopontine angle. There is a characteristic absence of a history of chronic disease of the middle ear in these patients. The recommended management is surgery, with protracted follow-up care.

MISCELLANEOUS ENTITIES

Tumors of blood vessels and superficial lymphatics have not been reported as temporal bone entities. The observed regression of these entities with total body growth should govern the decision for timing of surgical therapy, if any is performed.

Toward the end of the second decade of life, adenocarcinoma (Goebel et al., 1987) and carcinoid tumor (Stanley et al., 1987a, 1987b) have been described. These entities present as a middle ear mass clinically confused with chronic inflammation and present with external ear discharge, pain, hearing loss, and, on occasion, facial nerve paralysis. A low index of suspicion and less than optimum biopsy techniques delay the accurate diagnoses of these rare neoplasms of the middle ear.

Nodular fasciitis and fibromatosis are histologic entities that present as postauricular swellings and are difficult to classify accurately. When found in a neonate or a very young child, they may have benign courses, but fibromatosis may be persistently aggressive and destructive despite its benign histology. Electron microscopy and tissue culture techniques, as well as careful histologic study, may be necessary to establish the cell or origin of this entity. A review of the subject by Vogel and Karmody (1979) emphasizes the difficulty in predicting the clinical course and response to therapy of this lesion.

Table 27–1 is a compilation of the neoplasms seen in the temporal bone area in the pediatric age group in the AFIP material from 1955 to 1975 (Hyams, 1976). Because of the relatively small number of cases in the entire study, statistical analysis by sex or age is not possible.

CLINICAL CORRELATIONS

A review of the literature shows that temporal bone neoplasms have been recorded as presenting with the following signs and symptoms: (1) external auditory canal obstruction, (2) discharge, (3) recognizable tumor in the ear canal, (4) ulceration, (5) a fixed mass over the mastoid process or canal wall, (6) facial paralysis, (7) mastoid tenderness, and (8) chronic and unremitting pain.

With the exception of facial paralysis, any clinician recognizes these as the primary complaints of a multiplicity of inflammatory disorders involving the ear and the mastoid. Even the most sophisticated outpatient department would soon tire of comprehensively evaluating each case with this symptom complex to detect possible temporal bone neoplasms at the initial clinical evaluation. Table 27–2 attempts to identify the tumor types found in the temporal bone by signs and

symptoms associated with neoplasms in this anatomic region. It is hoped that this presentation will help the clinician identify these tumors by their clinical presentations.

BIOPSY DIAGNOSIS

The 1962 study by Dito and Batsakis, as well as a more recent work by Liebner (1976), suggests that an inverse relationship exists between duration of symptoms and survival after therapy. There is a lack of reassurance in their observation that the initial tissue biopsy report was possibly neither accurate nor tumor specific in a large number of the cases that presented as ear canal masses and later were proved to be primary neoplasms of the temporal bone. The cases reported in the literature are also characterized by a significant delay in obtaining surgical biopsy specimens. A thorough knowledge of the expected courses of inflammatory disease and familiarity with the expected responses to therapy of each of these inflammatory entities will serve to alert the clinician to a disease process that is quite different from an inflammatory disease. The fact that these tumors were not identified in the initial specimens may be explained by inaccuracies or deficiencies in the biopsy procedure or by artifacts in the specimen submitted to the pathologist for sectioning; inflammation and granulation tissue play a role in the pathologic appearance of any tumor that presents to an external surface with ulceration or superficial necrosis. Biopsy specimens that are too small or that fail to sample tissue deep to the surface

TABLE 27–1. Neoplasms of the Temporal Bone Area in the Pediatric Age Group (AFIP 1955–1975)

NEOPLASMS	EXTERNAL EAR	MIDDLE EAR	TEMPORAL BONE
Squamous papilloma	1 (10 yr) M*	—	—
Squamous cell carcinoma	1 (6 yr) M	1 (10 yr) F	—
Pilomatrixoma	4 (4–14 yr) 2F, 2M	—	—
Basal cell carcinoma	1 (12 yr) M	—	—
Ceruminoma	—	1 (10 yr) M	—
Juvenile xanthogranuloma	3 (1–6 yr) 1F, 2M	—	—
Nodular fasciitis	2 (4, 5 yr) 2M	—	—
Dermatofibroma	2 (8, 10 yr) 1F, 1M	—	—
Fibromatosis	2 (6, 8 yr) 2M	—	—
Fibromyxoma (sarcoma)	—	—	1 (? yr) M
Lymphangioma	1 (6 yr) M	—	—
Embryonal rhabdomyosarcoma	10 (2–11 yr) 3F, 7M	6 (2–11 yr) 3F, 3M	10 (2–12 yr) 5F, 5M
Lymphoma	—	1 (8 yr) F	—
Neurilemoma	—	1 (13 yr) M	—
Neurofibroma	2 (1, 7 yr) 2M	—	—
Glioma	—	1 (11 yr) M	—
Meningioma	—	1 (8 yr) M	—
Giant cell tumor	—	—	1 (4 yr) M
Histiocytosis X	—	—	10 (1–10 yr) 5F, 5M
Ossifying fibroma	—	—	8 (5–12 yr) 3F, 5M
Chondrosarcoma	—	—	1 (4 yr) M
Hamartoma	—	1 (11 yr) F	—

*The first number is the number of cases reported, the age in parentheses is the age or ages of the patients reported, and M and F denote the sex of the patients.

Data from Hyams, V. J. 1976. AFIP symposium: Pediatric neoplasms of the temporal bone in the pediatric age group. Otolaryngologic Pathology, December 6–8.

TABLE 27–2. Symptoms of Various Tumors of the Temporal Bone

	CHRONIC, UNREMITTING PAIN	MASTOID TENDERNESS	FACIAL PARALYSIS	MASTOID OR CANAL SWELLING	ULCERATION	EAR CANAL TUMOR	EAR DISCHARGE	EAR CANAL OBSTRUCTION	HEARING LOSS	TINNITUS	VERTIGO	POSTAURICULAR DEFORMITY
Tumors of bone and cartilage	X		X	X	X	X	X	X	X	X		X
Tumors of blood and lymph vessels				X	X			X				
Tumors of nerve tissue			X	X					X	X	X	X
Tumors of skin and appendages	X	X		X	X	X	X					
Leukemia and lymphoma	X	X	X	X	X		X	X	X	X	X	
Tumors of mesenchymal tissue	X	X	X	X	X	X	X	X	X	X		X
Metastatic tumors	X	X	X	X					X	X	X	

ulceration and inflammation may not include tissue characteristic of these tumor types. The use of cupbiting forceps or mechanical compression of a biopsy fragment after it is obtained may introduce crushing artifacts that mask the true morphology of the tissue. The last, and perhaps most common, artifact in small tissue biopsies is dessication artifacts produced by drying of very small tissue specimens between the time they are obtained and the time they are placed in formalin. Three guidelines for maximizing the amount of information that can be obtained from specimens follow.

1. Obtain a biopsy specimen from deep enough in the tumor that it is representative of the tumor.

2. Avoid crushing the biopsy specimen in cupbiting forceps or compressing it mechanically.

3. Avoid dessicating the specimen. Place the biopsy specimen in tissue cassettes or on filter paper and then into formalin as rapidly as possible after the biopsy specimen is obtained.

Pathologists should be alerted to the clinical differential diagnosis of the tissue mass biopsied. Special histologic stains and additional pathology consultations should be obtained for any case in which the morphology of the lesion is less than characteristic of an entity that explains the patient's clinical course. With the advent of polytomography, computed tomography, and magnetic resonance imaging radiographic evaluation of the temporal bone can be carried out with great precision. Mastoid survey radiographs are indicated in every patient with facial paralysis and in patients presenting with periauricular tumor masses. Complete audiometric studies with tympanometry will alert the clinician to the presence of middle-ear tissue masses associated with a conductive hearing loss. The recognition of a middle-ear mass should be followed by a comprehensive radiologic evaluation of the temporal bone in order to plan definitive surgical biopsy procedures.

MANAGEMENT

The treatment modalities available to the clinician treating neoplasms of the temporal bone are surgery, radiation therapy, and chemotherapy. Solitary lesions that lend themselves to surgical extirpation include monostotic fibrous dysplasias, eosinophilic granulomas, epidermoids, meningiomas, choristomas, neurilemomas, and gliomas. Radiation therapy alone, or combined radiation therapy and surgical debulking procedures, are the recommended approaches to rhabdomyosarcoma, cerumen gland carcinoma, and extensive eosinophilic granuloma. It should be emphasized that in treating sarcomatous lesions, radiation therapy should include the sites to which the tumors commonly spread as part of the initial therapy. The addition to the treatment possibilities of acute and chronic chemotherapy with an ever-expanding inventory of drugs has led to a major increase in the survival of these tumor patients. Drug regimens change too rapidly to be included in a textbook, but their significance in treating tumors of the temporal bone cannot be overlooked. Thus, the management of a child with a malignancy or mass should always be handled by a team that includes a chemotherapist.

Tumors of the temporal bone in children are rare. They are seen more commonly in the muscle, blood vessels, and growing bone than in the skin and nerve tissue of the temporal bone. These entities should be suspected whenever more common disease entities fail to respond to conventional therapy.

Accurate, early diagnosis is facilitated by anatomically appropriate biopsy material properly fixed and processed by a pathologist alerted to the clinical suspicion of these entities.

SELECTED REFERENCES

Batsakis, J. G. 1979. Tumors of the Head and Neck. Baltimore, Williams and Wilkins Co. 2nd ed.
This anatomically specific work provides concise, current information as well as a comprehensive bibliography for further reading.
Nager, G. T. 1975. Epidermoids of the temporal bone. Laryngoscope 85, Suppl. 2.
This is an excellent source of information on temporal bone development and growth as well as an excellent reference source on this subject.
Sharp, M. 1970. Monostotic fibrous dysplasia of the temporal bone. J. Laryngol. Otol. 84:697.
This is a comprehensive clinical review of this subject.
Kinney, S. E., and Wood, B. G. 1987. Malignancies of the external ear canal and temporal bone: Surgical techniques and results. Laryngoscope 97:158.
For the surgeon and nonsurgeon, this is a good technical review and introduction to combined therapy of this region.

REFERENCES

Ash, J. E. 1960. Pathology of the ear. *In* Schenk, H. P. (ed.): Otolaryngology, Vol. I. Hagerstown, MD, Harper & Row, Chap. 4.
Ash, J. E. and Raum, M. 1956. An Atlas of Otolaryngologic Pathology. Washington, DC, American Registry of Pathology.
Batsakis, J. G. 1974. Tumors of the Head and Neck. Baltimore, Williams & Wilkins Co.
Bradley, W., and Maxwell, N. J. 1954. Neoplasms of the middle ear and mastoid. Laryngoscope 64:533.
Buehrle, R. 1972. Meningioma in the temporal bone. Can. J. Otol. 1:16.
Byers, P. D. 1968. Benign osteoblastic lesions of bone. Cancer 22:43.
Carroll, R., and Miketic L. M. 1987. Ewing sarcoma of the temporal bone: CT appearance. J. Comput. Assist. Tomogr. 11:362.
Coltrera, M. D., Googe, P. B., Harrist, T. J., et al. 1986. Chondrosarcoma of the temporal bone: Diagnosis and treatment of 13 cases and review of the literature. Cancer 58:2689.
Conley, J., and Schuller, D. 1976. Malignancies of the ear. Laryngoscope 86:1147.
Dahlin, D. C., and Johnson, E. W., Jr. 1954. Giant osteoid osteoma. J. Bone Joint Surg. 36A:559.
Deutsch, M., and Felder, H. 1974. Rhabdomyosarcoma of the ear and mastoid. Laryngoscope 84:586.
Dito, W. R., and Batsakis, J. G. 1962. Rhabdomyosarcoma of the head and neck: An appraisal of the biologic behavior in 170 cases. Arch. Surg. 84:582.
Ewing, J. 1921. Diffuse endothelioma of bone. Proc. NY Pathol. Soc. 21:17.
Falk, S., and Alpert M.: 1965. The clinical and roentgen aspects of Ewing's sarcoma. Am. J. Med. Sci. 250:492.
Ferguson, C. F., and Kendig, E. L. 1972. Pediatric Otolaryngology. Philadelphia, W. B. Saunders Co.
Figi, F. A., and Hempstead, B. E. 1943. Malignant tumors of middle ear and mastoid. Arch. Otolaryngol. 37:149.
Fowler, E. P., Jr., and Osmun, P. M. 1942. New bone growth due to cold water in ears. Arch. Otolaryngol. 36:455.

Goebel, J. A., Smith, P. G., Kemink, J. L., et al. 1987. Primary adenocarcinoma of the temporal bone mimicking paragangliomas: Radiographic and clinical recognition. Otolaryngol. Head Neck Surg. 96:231.
Guzowski, J., and Paparella, M. M. 1976. Meningiomas of the temporal bone. Laryngoscope 86:1141.
Horn, R. C., Jr., and Enterline, H. T. 1958. Rhabdomyosarcoma, a clinical pathological study and classification of 39 cases. Cancer 11:181.
Hyams, V. J. 1976. AFIP symposium: Pediatric neoplasms of the temporal bone in the pediatric age group. Otolaryngologic Pathology, December 6–8.
Jaffe, B. F. 1977. Hearing Loss in Children. Baltimore, University Park Press.
Jaffe, N., Filler, R. M., Farber, S., et al. 1973. Rhabdomyosarcoma in children: Improved outlook with a multidisciplinary approach. Am. J. Surg. 125:482.
Leedham, P. W. 1972. Chondrosarcoma with subarachnoid dissemination. J. Pathol. 107:59.
Lichtenstein, L. 1972. Bone Tumors, 4th ed. St. Louis, C. V. Mosby Co.
Lichtenstein, L., and Jaffe, H. L. 1942. Fibrous dysplasia of bone. Arch. Pathol. 33:777.
Lichtenstein, L., and Sawyer, W. R. 1964. Benign osteoblastoma, further observations and report of 20 additional cases. J. Bone Joint Surg. 46A:755.
Liebner, E. J. 1976. Embryonal rhabdomyosarcoma of head and neck in children: Correlation of stage, radiation dose, local control and survival. Cancer 37:2777.
MacComb, W. S., and Fletcher, G. H. 1968. Cancer of the Head and Neck. Baltimore, Williams & Wilkins Co.
Mawson, S. R. 1963. Diseases of the Ear. Baltimore, Williams & Wilkins Co.
Nager, G. T. 1964. Meningiomas involving the temporal bone. Springfield, IL, Charles C Thomas.
Nager, G. T. 1975. Epidermoids of the temporal bone. Laryngoscope 85, Suppl. 2.
Paparella, M. M. 1973. Otologic manifestations of leukemia. Laryngoscope 83:1510.
Piepgras, U. 1972. Chondroblastoma of the temporal bone, an unusual cause of increasing intracranial pressure. Neuroradiology 4:25.
Ronis, M. L. 1974. Benign osteoblastoma of the temporal bone. Laryngoscope 84:857.
Schuknecht, H. F., Allam, A. F., and Murakami, Y. 1968. Pathology of secondary malignant tumors of the temporal bone. Ann. Otol. Rhinol. Laryngol. 77:5.
Shambron, E., and Finch, S. C. 1958. The auditory manifestations of leukemia. Yale J. Biol. Med. 31:144.
Sharp, M. 1970. Monostotic fibrous dysplasia of the temporal bone. J. Laryngol. Otol. 84:697.
Stanley, M. W., Horwitz, C. A., Levinson, R. M., et al. 1987a. Carcinoid tumors of the middle ear. Am. J. Clin. Pathol. 5:592.
Stanley, R. J., Scheithauer, B. W., Thompson, E. I., et al. 1987b. Endodermal sinus tumor (yolk sac tumor) of the ear. Arch. Otolaryngol. Head Neck Surg. 113:200.
Teilum, G., cited by Kempson, R. L., and Hendrickson, J. R. 1978. The female reproductive system. *In* Coulson, W. F. (ed.): Surgical Pathology. Philadelphia, J. B. Lippincott, p. 718.
Toohill, R. 1973. Eosinophilic granuloma of the temporal bone. Laryngoscope 83:877.
Tremble, G. E. 1977. Observations made in the labyrinths of adults. J. Otolaryngol. 6:327.
Van Gilse, P. H. G. 1938. Des observations ultereures sur la genese des exostoses du conduit externe par l'irritation d'eau froide. Acta Otolaryngol. 26:343.
Vogel, D. H., and Karmody, C. S. 1979. Congenital fibrous lesion of the temporal bone. Arch. Otolaryngol. 105:215.
Wick, M. R., and Siegal, G. P. 1980. Primary mediastinal embryonal carcinoma. Minn. Med. 63:723.
Wigger, H. J., and Mitsudo, S. M. 1976. Fibrous histiocytoma simulating congenital fibromatosis. Virchows Arch. (Pathol. Anat.) 370:255.
Zechner, G., and Altman, F. 1969. Histological studies of the temporal bone in leukemia. Ann. Otol. Rhinol. Laryngol. 78:375.

Section III

THE NOSE, PARANASAL SINUSES, FACE, AND ORBIT

Chapter 28

EMBRYOLOGY AND ANATOMY

David N. F. Fairbanks, M.D.

CHRONOLOGY

The period of development of the nose and paranasal sinuses is a continuum spanning from the third week of gestation, when the primordia of these structures first appear, through early adulthood, when sinus pneumatization and nasal bony growth cease. The events and the timing of development of these structures may be outlined in the following manner.

Fetus at three weeks:	Olfactory placodes appear in frontonasal process.
Fetus at four weeks:	Olfactory placodes become nasal pits.
	Maxillary processes appear.
Fetus at five weeks:	Nasal pits deepen into clefts separated by primitive septum (frontonasal process). Vomeronasal organ appears.
Fetus at six weeks:	Oronasal membranes rupture, forming primitive choanae.
	Primitive palate forms by fusion of maxillary process with medial and lateral nasal processes.
	Upper lip forms by fusion of medial nasal and lateral nasal maxillary processes.
	Nasooptic furrow (to become lacrimal apparatus) disappears.
	Maxillary and ethmoidal folds appear (to become turbinates).
Fetus at seven weeks:	Definitive septum begins growth.
	Second ethmoidal fold appears.
Fetus at eight weeks:	Olfactory nerve bundles appear.
	Palatine processes fuse in midline anteriorly.
	Uncinate process and ethmoidal infundibulum appear.
Fetus at three months:	Palate fusion completed.
	Maxillary sinus outpouching appears.
	Cartilaginous nasal capsule forms from mesenchymal condensation.
	Nasal glands appear.
Fetus at four months:	Ethmoidal sinus outpouching appears.
	Sphenoidal sinus outpouching appears.
	Bulla ethmoidalis becomes well defined.
Fetus at five months:	Vomeronasal organ begins degeneration.
Fetus at six months:	Cartilaginous nasal capsule divides into alar, lateral, and septal cartilages.
	Maxillary ossification begins.
Fetus at seven months:	Maximal development of ethmoidal turbinates (up to five) occurs; turbinates begin coalescence.
BIRTH:	Frontal sinus furrows appear.
	Only two to three ethmoidal turbinates remain.
	Craniofacial ratio is 8:1.
six months:	Nares double their birth dimensions.
one year:	Maxillary sinus reaches infraorbital nerve.
two years:	Frontal sinuses reach frontal bone.
	Ethmoidal sinuses approximate each other and lamina papyracea.
three years:	Nasal growth spurt occurs.
	Ossified union occurs between perpendicular plate of ethmoid, lamina papyracea, cribriform plate, and vomer.
four years:	Sphenoidal sinus begins invasion of sphenoid bone.
five years:	Craniofacial ratio is 4:1.
six years:	Frontal sinuses are visible on radiographs in frontal bone.
	Sphenoidal sinus is pneumatized to vidian canal.
	Nasal growth spurt occurs.
seven years:	Nose doubles its birth length.
	Maxillary sinus begins inferiorly directed growth.
	Ethmoidal sinuses extend beyond boundaries of ethmoids.
eight years:	Maxillary sinus approximates inferior nasal meatus.

nine years: Frontal sinus reaches level of orbital roof in 50 per cent of children.

nine years: Maxillary sinus pneumatizes zygomatic process.

12 years: Floor of maxillary sinus is level with floor of nose.

Puberty: Accelerated nasal and maxillary growth occurs.

  Nose triples its birth length.

End of puberty: Sphenoidal sinus growth ceases.

  Frontal sinus growth ceases.

  Ethmoidal sinus growth ceases.

  Maxillary sinus growth ceases except at area of third molar, which will become pneumatized when the molar erupts.

Adulthood: Closure of sphenooccipital synchondrosis occurs.

  Craniofacial ratio is 2:1.

50 years: Fusion of perpendicular plate of ethmoid with vomer is completed.

THE NOSE AND FACE

Early Development

The nose originates in the cranial ectoderm near the embryonic anterior neuropore. The cellular thickening of sensory epithelium that becomes the paired olfactory placodes is recognizable as early as the third fetal week. As the surrounding mesoderm increases in thickness, the nasal placodes become passively depressed, forming the nasal pits in a broad mass of tissue, the frontonasal process (Fig. 28–1).

Further deepening of the pits separates the frontonasal process into paired medial and lateral boundaries of the nasal walls. The medial processes fuse in the formation of the central portion of the upper lip, the premaxillary process, and the primitive nasal septum. By the fifth week, the nasal pits are cleftlike, blindly ending epithelial pouches with smooth lateral nasal walls and a thick "septum" of frontonasal process showing the early vomeronasal organ of Jacobson.

The inferior boundary of the nasal cavity is deficient until the paired maxillary processes of the first (mandibular) arches grow anteriorly and medially to abut against, and later fuse with, the medial nasal processes. Fusion also takes place laterally between the maxillary and lateral nasal processes to obliterate the nasooptic furrow.

Posterior extension of the nasal cavities thins out the membrane separating them from the oral cavity. By the 38th day this bucconasal membrane is so thin that it has only two layers, the nasal and oral epithelia. It becomes so attenuated that rupture ensues, forming the choanae. Failure of rupture results in choanal atresia. These early choanae do not correspond in position to the definitive choanae, which will ulti-

mately be more posterior and are not established until the third month, when the definitive palate is completed. This accounts for the observation that the anterior extent of choanal atresia is unexpectedly far anterior in the nasal cavity.

Between the 40th and 60th fetal days, the nares are temporarily obstructed by proliferating epithelial cells. These cells must later degenerate and shed, and if they fail to do so, atresia of the nares with bony and membranous closure occurs.

Details of the formation of the lips and palate are covered in Section I in this text. It is sufficient to say that the primitive choanae become elongated by posterior extension and then by progressive posteriorly directed fusion of the palatal processes. In formation of the definitive palate, the final position of the choanae is established. During this process, a portion of the buccal cavity becomes incorporated into the nose on the nasal side of the hard palate and in the inferior nasal meatus. The palatal processes fuse not only with each other but also with the definitive nasal septum, which is concurrently growing posteriorly from the primitive septum toward the buccal pituitary outpouching.

During the third fetal month, condensation of mesenchyme results in formation of the primitive nasal capsule (Fig. 28–2), a cartilaginous structure from which, or on which, will develop all the bony and cartilaginous nasal and paranasal structures. Just as Meckel's cartilage is the primary skeleton of the lower face, so is the nasal capsule the primary skeleton of the upper face. Its continuity is short-lived. In the sixth fetal month, ingrowth of connective tissue divides it into individual alar (lower lateral) cartilages, septal, and (upper) lateral cartilages. The greater part of the posterior capsule becomes ossified as the ethmoid bone, encompassing the ethmoidal turbinates, sinus walls, and perpendicular plate. Portions of the sphenoid bone ossify from this capsule. Upon its lateral surfaces form the nasal bones and maxillae. Ossification and absorption of this capsule is a process that begins early in fetal life, progresses well into adulthood, and is never completed (inasmuch as the cartilage of the anterior nose and septum persists as remnants of the capsule).

The Internal Nose, Lateral Wall

Simultaneous with palatal formation, the nasal walls begin to develop the complex configuration that ultimately characterizes them. There is an inherent tendency for the nasal cavity to increase its surface area. The 40-day-old embryo shows shallow grooves, which will become inferior and middle meatuses. The intervening tissue proliferates, bulges into the nasal cavity, and becomes the inferior or maxillary turbinate. The ethmoidal turbinates (e.g., middle, superior, and supreme) initially arise on the nasal septum, but the direction of growth in the nasal cavity shifts them to the lateral wall. Initially, there is a single ethmoidal

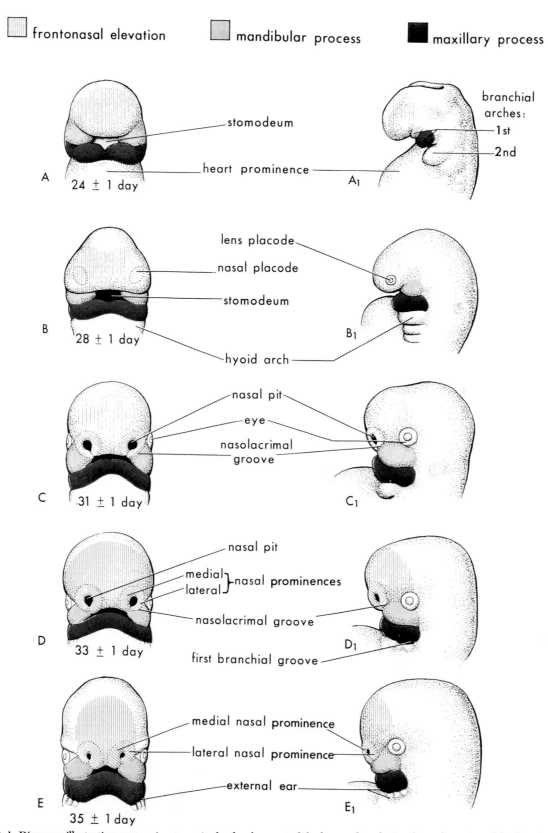

frontonasal elevation   mandibular process   maxillary process

Figure 28–1. Diagrams illustrating progressive stages in the development of the human face during the embryonic and fetal periods. (From Moore, K. L. 1988. The Developing Human, 4th ed. Philadelphia, W. B. Saunders Co.)

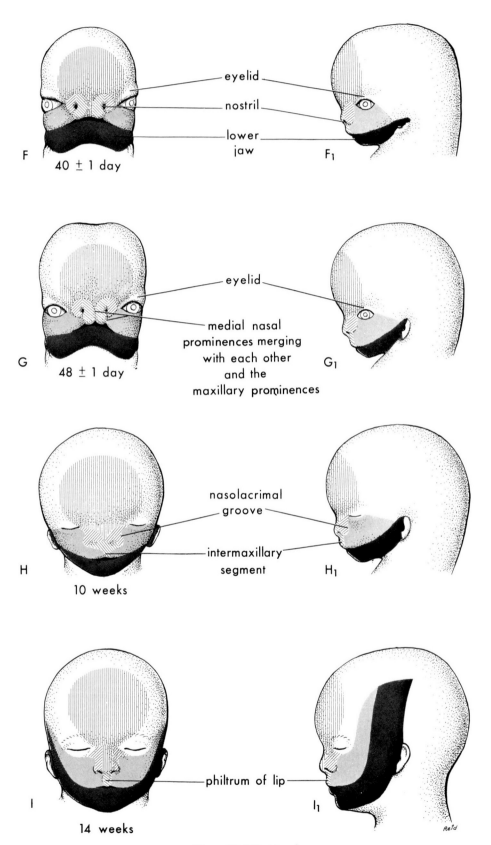

eyelid

nostril

lower jaw

F   40 ± 1 day   F₁

eyelid

medial nasal prominences merging with each other and the maxillary prominences

G   48 ± 1 day   G₁

nasolacrimal groove

intermaxillary segment

H   10 weeks   H₁

philtrum of lip

I   14 weeks   I₁

Figure 28–1 *Continued*

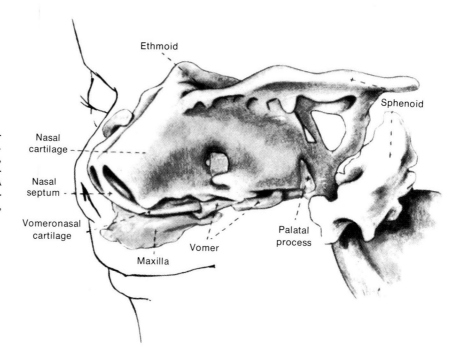

Figure 28–2. The cartilaginous nasal capsule from a human fetus aged 4 months. (From Schaeffer, J. P. 1920. The Nose, Paranasal Sinuses, Nasolacrimal Passageways, and Olfactory Organ in Man. A Genetic, Developmental and Anatomico-Physiological Consideration. Philadelphia, Blakiston Co.)

fold in each nasal cavity. By 48 days, there is a second; by 100 days, a third. By the seventh to ninth fetal months, there may be as many as five ethmoidal turbinates with intervening meatuses, but after birth the uppermost and less developed ones coalesce and disappear (Schaeffer, 1920).

The typical number of ethmoidal turbinates is three: middle, superior, and supreme. The supreme turbinate has been identified in 88 per cent of fetuses, 73 per cent of 9-year-old children, and 26 per cent of adults (Zimmerman, 1938). Rarely, an even higher turbinate persists.

Posterior and superior to the highest ethmoidal turbinate lies the sphenoethmoidal recess, which is limited by the angle formed by the cribriform plate superiorly and the anterior surface of the sphenoid posteriorly. In the recess is found the ostium of the sphenoid sinus.

The agger nasi is a slight elevation above the inferior turbinate and anterior to the middle turbinate that develops more or less parallel to the bridge of the nose. The olfactory sulcus is a channellike space anterior and superior to the agger nasi, limited by the arched confluences of the medial and lateral nasal walls. It leads from the nasal vestibule to the olfactory area in the roof of the nose and then posteriorly into the sphenoethmoidal recess.

Under cover of the middle turbinate, the middle meatus of the nose begins its complex development. As early as the 60th day of fetal life, a crescent-shaped fold (the uncinate process) appears with a furrow (the ethmoid infundibulum) immediately above it. Shortly thereafter, another bulge (the ethmoid bulla) arises above the furrow. Above the bulla appears the suprabullar furrow, from which anterior ethmoid air cells will develop. In ensuing weeks, a variety of folds and furrows develop as if the nose would develop into a complex turbinate–meatus system as in other mammals, but by birth or shortly thereafter, most of them have coalesced and disappeared. However, the uncinate process, ethmoid bulla, and ethmoid infundibulum remain constant and prominent (Fig. 28–3).

From the infundibulum the maxillary sinus will develop, as will some ethmoid air cells, including those that pneumatize the ethmoid bulla. The frontal sinus forms from the superior extent of the infundibulum or, more commonly, from separate furrows superior to the infundibulum.

Continued development of the ethmoid bulla and the uncinate process so narrows the communication of the infundibulum with the nose that it becomes a slitlike opening, the hiatus semilunaris.

The superior nasal meatus contains ostia of the posterior ethmoid cells and is much less complicated than the middle meatus. Occasionally, however, various recesses and folds are present. When a supreme meatus is found, it usually contains an ostium of a posterior ethmoid air cell.

The Nasal Septum

The nasal septum is first apparent as the thick, fused, medial processes of the frontonasal process between the nasal pits. By the third month of fetal life, mesenchymal condensation occurs, and cartilage grows in from the body of the sphenoid to form two adjacent plates. These plates subsequently fuse with one another (except in the case of the bifid nose) and fuse ventrally with the lateral nasal walls to complete the primitive nasal capsule.

The cartilaginous septum is formed by the septal (quadrilateral) cartilage, the vomeronasal cartilages, and the medial crura of the alar (lower lateral) cartilages

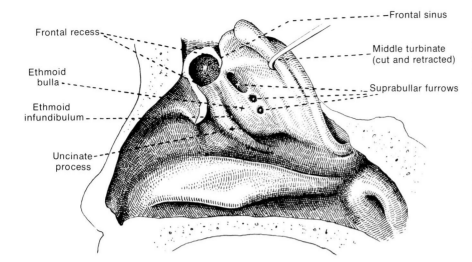

Figure 28–3. The lateral wall of a 14-month-old child with the middle turbinate turned aside. The whole frontal recess is expanding toward the frontal region in the establishment of the frontal sinus. The infundibulum and the frontal recess are discontinuous. The suprabullar furrow is represented by a series of depressions, rudimentary ethmoidal cells. (From Schaeffer, J. P. 1920. The Nose, Paranasal Sinuses, Nasolacrimal Passageways, and Olfactory Organ in Man. A Genetic, Developmental and Anatomico-Physiological Consideration. Philadelphia, Blakiston Co.)

(Fig. 28–4). The septal cartilage is roughly quadrangular with a taillike posterior extension, the sphenoidal process. In infancy, the sphenoidal process is in continuity with the sphenoid bone, completely separating the vomer and perpendicular plate of the ethmoid (Fig. 28–5). Fusion between the latter two bones begins posteriorly and extends forward by progressive absorption of the sphenoidal process or sometimes by displacement of it to one side.

Superiorly, the septal cartilage is continuous with the (upper) lateral cartilages, which extend like wings from it. As it projects anteriorly, it separates from them and extends between the alar cartilages to within 1 cm of the tip of the nose.

The vomeronasal cartilages are two narrow, longitudinal strips, 7 to 15 mm long, lying along the inferior margin of the septal cartilage, attached to the vomer posteriorly and to the maxillary crest anteriorly. They

are not always differentiated from the septal cartilage and may appear only as lateral processes or spurs from its inferior border.

The membranous septum (mobile septum) is the portion anterior to the end of the septal cartilage. It is formed by skin and subcutaneous tissue of the nasal columella.

The bony septum is composed of two major elements: the vomer and the perpendicular plate of the ethmoid, and their articulating points with the nasal spine of the frontal bone, the rostrum of the sphenoid, and the crests of the nasal, maxillary, and palate bones, as shown in Figure 28–4.

The perpendicular plate of the ethmoid (mesoethmoid) is the ossified upper to midline portion of the primitive nasal capsule. Ossification begins in the fifth fetal month and is not completed until the 17th year. Ossification means replacement of thick, infantile car-

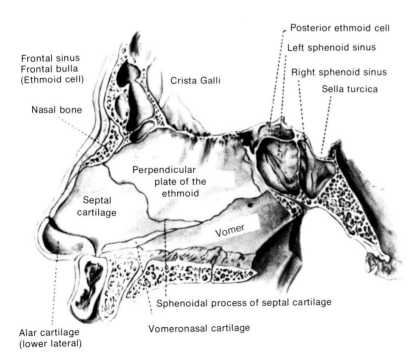

Figure 28–4. The osseous and cartilaginous septum of the nose. (From Schaeffer, J. P. 1920. The Nose, Paranasal Sinuses, Nasolacrimal Passageways, and Olfactory Organ in Man. A Genetic, Developmental and Anatomico-Physiological Consideration. Philadelphia, Blakiston Co.)

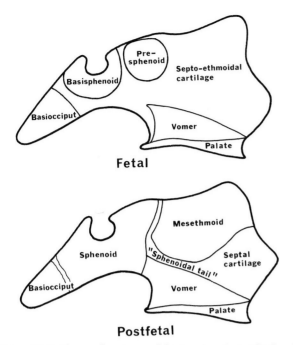

Figure 28–5. The nasal septum and basicranium during fetal and early postnatal life. Not to scale. (From Moore, W. J., and Lavelle, C. L. 1974. Growth of the Facial Skeleton in the Hominoidea. London, Academic Press, Inc.)

tilaginous septum with thin bone. The perpendicular plate is thin except at points of articulation with adjacent bone and septal cartilage, where it remains thick and may even contain marrow spaces.

At the nasal roof it articulates with the cribriform plate and even extends above it into the cranial cavity as the crista galli (Fig. 28–4). The cribriform plate is a fibrous structure until it becomes ossified in the third year, providing a firm union between the lateral and medial ethmoidal elements. The anterior extent of ossification of the perpendicular plate is quite variable. It may extend no further forward than the anterior extent of the nasal spine of the frontal bone, or as far forward as the distal border of the nasal bones, or any distance in between. Obviously, its size is reciprocally related to the size of the septal cartilage.

The vomer, by contrast, develops not by ossification of cartilage but rather from connective tissue membrane on each side of the septal cartilage. For the opposing lamellae of the vomer to fuse, the intervening cartilage must be absorbed, a process that begins about the third fetal month and may not be completed until midadulthood. The lamellae grow upward toward the perpendicular plate of the ethmoid, imprisoning the sphenoid process (tail) of the septal cartilage. Ideally, absorption and fusion proceed in an orderly fashion, and the remaining cartilage lies in a V-shaped groove on top of the two plates of the vomer. However, any inequality of growth between the plates will allow the cartilage to escape its imprisoned position and to buckle laterally, creating the posterior septal spur, a common irregularity of the septal surface.

Even on the normal, fully matured septum, elevations and ridgelike protuberances interrupt the smooth surface. The most constant is the tuberculum septi, an area of thickened mucosa appearing opposite the anterior end of the middle nasal turbinate. Occasionally, oblique mucosal ridges are notable on the posteroinferior septum. These are septal plicae, remnants of mucosal folds prominent up to eight months of fetal age, which generally regress and disappear in infancy. They may persist and may even hypertrophy into tumorlike obstructing masses.

Anomalies and Variations, The Internal Nose

Asymmetry of the Nasal Septum

Approximately 80 per cent of humans have some deformity of the nasal septum. The asymmetry may affect any or all parts of the septum except for the posterior free border at the choanae, where it is always midline. A common area of deflection is along the articulation between the vomer and the perpendicular plate of the ethmoid, especially when these two bones are separated for a considerable distance by the sphenoidal process of the septal cartilage. Ridgelike deflections and spurs may occur there, even if the rest of the septum is straight. Sometimes the septum bows entirely into one nasal cavity; at other times, a double buckling occurs with an S-shaped deformity affecting both cavities. The septal cartilage is often dislocated out of the midline groove of the maxillary crest (Fig. 28–6).

No one hypothesis is adequate to explain all cases of septal deformity. Twin studies do not suggest that septal deformity is genetically determined. However, it is a trait that is characteristic of the family of humans and some other primates, species that exhibit a prominent forward extension of the cranial cavity above the face. Even prehistoric *Australopithecus boiseii*, who lived 1,750,000 years ago, appears to have had the deformity. Gray (1978) studied more than 3000 skulls of various mammals and found only one case (in a Pekingese dog) of septal deformity in 642 nonprimates. He found septal deformities in 7 per cent of lower apes (baboons and mandrills), 37 per cent of higher apes (chimpanzees and gorillas), and 73 to 87 per cent of humans of various races. Two theories are postulated to explain these observations:

1. The erect posture of the gravid female results in a lengthy period during which the fetus' head is engaged in the pelvis, which creates external pressures against the nose and face.

2. Vertical growth of the septum is impeded by its fixed position between an unyielding hard palate below and an overhanging cranial cavity above, which causes the growing septum to buckle.

Even passage of the head through the birth canal causes significant nasal injury. Gray (1978) found nasal and septal deformities in 4 per cent of infants born of normal vaginal deliveries and in 13 per cent of difficult

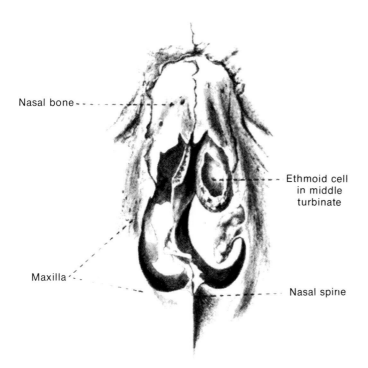

Figure 28–6. Septal deformity with compensatory turbinate hypertrophy. Note the ethmoid air cell in the middle turbinate. (From Schaeffer, J. P. 1920. The Nose, Paranasal Sinuses, Nasolacrimal Passageways, and Olfactory Organ in Man. A Genetic, Developmental and Anatomico-Physiological Consideration. Philadelphia, Blakiston Co.)

deliveries (e.g., occipitoposterior presentations), but only rarely in infants delivered by cesarean section. Although most newborn nasal deformities can be corrected easily by gentle, close reduction, occasionally the deformed pyramid is immobile and resistant to corrective manipulations. Kirchner (1955) and Cottle (1951) observed that such solid deformities are self-correcting and that the nose will return to the midline position within the first year, sometimes even within the first few months. This solid deformity is probably due to a long-standing intrauterine position where some unusual pressure is placed against one side of the face (such as an arm or a shoulder) during development. Gray regards this type of pressure against the maxilla as responsible not only for nasal and septal deformities but also for deformities of the palate and teeth. He notes that when the deformity of the septum results in shortening of its height, the palate will fail to grow downward, and a high-arched palate with abnormalities in dental occlusion will occur.

Nasal injury accounts for most cases of nasal and septal deformity, but the injury may be remote in time and often not remembered. Indeed, the prominent, unprotected position of the nose on the face makes injury almost impossible to avoid throughout life. Frequently, a deformity resulting from a childhood injury may appear to be insignificant, but it becomes prominent during adolescence when asymmetries become exaggerated under the pressure of accelerated septal growth.

Turbinate Deformity

Extra space available in one nasal cavity, due to long-standing displacement of the septum into the other, is likely to become occupied by overdeveloped inferior or middle turbinates (Fig. 28–6). Both bone and mucosal elements participate in this compensatory hypertrophy. Additionally, an ethmoid air cell may invade the middle turbinate, giving it a rounded, bullous look, often creating airway obstruction. Whether the turbinate enlargement forces the septum to become deformed or the turbinate simply enlarges to fill the space created by the septal deformity is a developmental puzzle. Although such turbinate invasion by ethmoid air cells is common in adults (12 per cent or more), it is only occasionally seen in children (see the section on ethmoid sinuses).

The Vomeronasal Organ

The vomeronasal organ (organ of Jacobson) is an accessory olfactory organ in some mammalian species, but it is rudimentary in man. It reaches its maximal development in the 20th fetal week and usually degenerates in late fetal life. It is sometimes detectable even in adulthood as a blind mucosal pocket 2 to 6 mm deep on each side of the septum just above the orifice of the nasopalatine canal.

Other anomalies of the internal nose, such as nasopalatine cysts and choanal atresia, are described in other chapters of this text. The nasal encephalocele is described in the section on surgical hazards.

The External Nose

Nasal landmarks are illustrated in Figure 28–7. It should be noted that the superoanterior surface of the nose is termed the nasal dorsum even though it

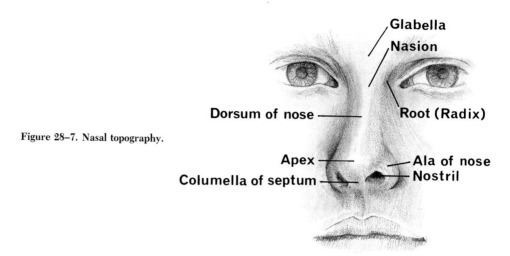

Figure 28–7. Nasal topography.

occupies a ventral position with respect to the rest of the body. The glabella is the point between the eyebrows, or more specifically, the smooth body triangular portion of frontal bone between the supraorbital ridges. The nasion is the point where the internasal suture meets the frontal bone.

Three paired bones form the external nasal skeleton: the nasal bones, the frontal processes of the maxillae, and the nasal portions of the frontal bones (Fig. 28–8). The last named articulate with and project beneath the nasal bones (Fig. 28–4) and frontal processes of the maxilla so that both frontal and maxillary bones lend support to the nasal bridge. The point of articulation is named the nasal root, or radix. When the nasal bones grow unequally or are absent, the frontal processes of the maxillae grow anteriorly to fill in the defect. The nasal bones are paired, arched structures that articulate with each other at their apex, where they also articulate with the frontal spine of the frontal bone and the perpendicular plate of the ethmoid. They are thickest at this point and are narrowed laterally where they articulate with the frontal processes of the maxillae. Their free anterior margins articulate with and overlie the fused (upper) lateral and septal cartilages. That they must overlie the lateral cartilages is a developmental imperative. They develop in membrane on the surface of the cartilaginous nasal capsule. The

cartilage of the capsule can be demonstrated as late as the first postfetal month before it is absorbed. The lacrimal bone forms in a similar manner.

Maxillary ossification begins at about the sixth fetal week from a center above the canine tooth germ and spreads in all directions. At about the fourth fetal month, the maxilla invades the cartilaginous nasal capsule and participates in formation of the lateral nasal wall and ethmoidal boundaries. The cartilaginous capsule is absorbed beneath the maxilla so that the latter receives the evaginating maxillary sinus pouch. Cartilaginous masses that are occasionally seen in the alveolar processes of the developing maxilla may represent cartilaginous capsule remnants.

Four major cartilages and a variable number of minor or accessory cartilages participate in the formation of the external nose (Fig. 28–8). The septum also participates, as described in previous paragraphs. The lateral nasal cartilage (also termed upper lateral, or triangular, cartilage) is a flattened triangular plate in the middle of the nose. It is fused in the midline with the septum and with its fellow of the opposite side. The paired alar cartilages (also termed greater alar, lobular, or lower lateral cartilages) partially encircle the nares and assist in keeping them open and in giving shape to the base of the nose. Each consists of two crura, which are continuous at the apex, giving

Figure 28–8. Cartilaginous and bony nasal skeleton.

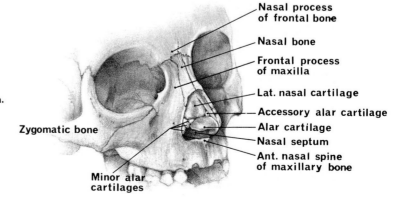

the nasal tip an arched contour. The medial crura approximate each other, bounding a deep median groove, extend posteroinferiorly in the nasal columella, and end in a free out-turned border.

Each lateral crus extends posterolaterally in the ala toward the maxilla but does not reach it, the interval being filled with a strong sheet of fibrous tissue in which are embedded the minor nasal cartilages. In some cases, the lateral crus is so prolonged that it replaces the minor (lesser, accessory) cartilages.

The lateral crura are bound by fibrous tissue to the septum anteriorly and to the lateral cartilages superiorly. At the connection between lateral and alar cartilages, the latter overlies the former in most instances (77 per cent), and they are often interlocked by their scroll-like curling margins. Occasionally (in 17 per cent of cases), they do not overlap at all, or the lateral may overlie the alar cartilage at the articulation (11 per cent) (Dion et al., 1978).

Postnatal Growth and Development

At birth, the face is small relative to the cranium, as illustrated in Figure 28–9. The craniofacial ratio is 8:1 compared to 4:1 at 5 years and 2:1 in adulthood. At birth, the nasal fossae are as wide as they are high, and their lower border is just below the plane of the orbit. The ethmoidal part of the nasal fossa is twice as high as the maxillary portion, but since the latter grows faster after birth, the two portions are equal by the time dentition is completed in the late teens.

The nares are small at birth, measuring 5 to 7 mm vertically and 7 to 8 mm horizontally. By 6 months of age, they have doubled their dimensions, but they retain their roughly circular shape until puberty when the vertical diameter becomes greater and the nares become oval or oblong in shape (Fig. 28–10). The nose

grows in several spurts, with maxima at ages 3, 6, and 7 years, and then from puberty to age 20 (Reichert, 1963). The nose reaches twice its birth length by 7 years, and at 14 years it is triple its birth length.

The maxilla grows forward and downward at a rate of 1 mm per year in childhood, slowing to 0.25 mm in the 11th year, then accelerating to 1.5 mm per year in adolescence, eventually ceasing at about age 17. Its direction of growth is 51 degrees forward and downward from an imaginary line between the nasion and the sella (Moore and Lavelle, 1974).

As early as 1857, it was recognized that a major force in the projection and growth of the upper face is the thrust of the growing nasal septum (Scott, 1953). Facial growth occurs as a complex interaction of four processes: (1) cartilaginous expansion, specifically the septal cartilage, which grows as a sheet, creates forward projection of the nose, and forces the maxilla and palate forward and downward (Fig. 28–11); (2) conversion of cartilage into bone at bony–cartilaginous junctions, a process most active in the fetal period and first three years; (3) intersutural periosteal bone deposition, which is stimulated by external forces (e.g., the force of the expanding septum) that create intersutural separation; (4) surface periosteal bone deposition, which is a constant remodeling process in which, for the most part, internal surfaces are resorbed and new bone is deposited on outer surfaces. The outer deposition accounts for facial growth and the internal resorption allows the sinuses to invade the facial bones (Enlow, 1978).

Anomalies and Variations, The External Nose

The external nose characteristically exhibits individual, familial, and racial variability. These differences are not pronounced in the early childhood years. Even

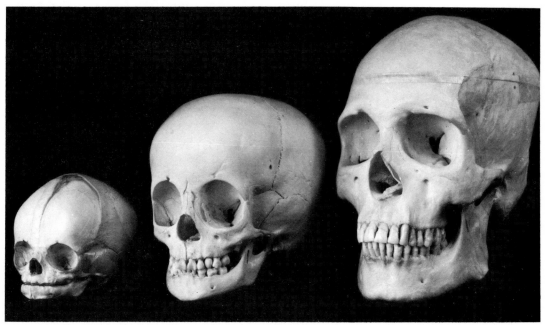

Figure 28–9. Skulls of newborn, 5-year-old child, and adult demonstrate decreasing craniofacial ratios.

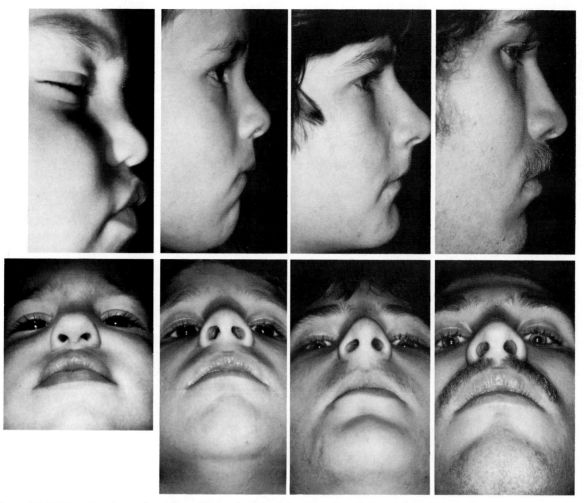

Figure 28–10. Changing shape of nose from infancy through adolescence. From left to right: Infant, 7 years, 13 years, 17 years.

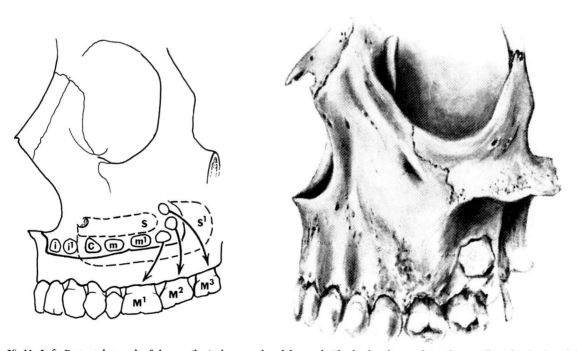

Figure 28–11. *Left*, Postnatal growth of the maxilla is downward and forward. The broken line outlines the maxilla at birth; the adult bone is shown in solid lines. c, Deciduous canine; i and i_1, deciduous incisors; m and m_1, deciduous molars; M_1, M_2, and M_3, permanent molars; s, maxillary sinus at birth; s_1, maxillary sinus at maturity. *Right*, Arrested development in rotation may result in an impacted third molar, high and posterior in the maxilla. (From Schaeffer, J. P. 1920. The Nose, Paranasal Sinuses, Nasolacrimal Passageways, and Olfactory Organ in Man. A Genetic, Developmental and Anatomico-Physiological Consideration. Philadelphia, Blakiston Co.)

in persons destined to have prominent noses with "hump" deformities, the dorsum is usually straight or concave during childhood. Not until the period of rapid nasal (especially septal) growth in puberty does the nose assume its individual characteristics, which are the result of a combination of genetic and traumatic influences.

A common developmental defect is the nasal dermoid cyst, a hair-bearing epidermal inclusion cyst appearing in the midline over the nasal dorsum (Pratt, 1965). Its surface opening is usually a pinpoint depression, but it may be deep and long, even as a midline cleft or fissure. It represents a failure of fusion of the medial processes. Other manifestations of that failure include the bifid nasal tip and the median nasal cleft.

Developmental failures can lead to unilateral or bilateral nasal absences, deficient cartilage and bone formation, and other abnormalities. Nasal deformity always accompanies a cleft lip, since development of the upper lip and nares is a process of fusion of portions of the frontonasal process with the maxillary process, all occurring simultaneously.

These and other deformities are detailed in other chapters of this volume.

Surgical Hazards

The primary hazard of nasal surgery in children is interruption of nasal growth. In early puberty nasal growth outdistances that of the face and produces exaggerated nasal features that tempt both patient and surgeon to correct them. Since the final result of growth is difficult to predict, premature surgery may produce a nose disproportionately small with respect to the fully grown face.

Bony growth occurs on subperiosteal surfaces as well as at all points of union between the various osseous and cartilaginous elements of the nose. Disruption of these suture lines and periosteal coverings can hardly be avoided during rhinoplastic procedures. For the same reason, nasal fractures in children should be reduced by the closed method.

Cartilaginous growth occurs throughout the entire plate of the quadrilateral cartilage. Therefore, removal of any portion of that plate reduces the total growth capacity of the septum, which is the determining factor for projection not only of the nasal profile but also of the facial profile. Gilbert and Segal (1958) suggest that the degree of saddle formation is proportional to the amount of resected cartilage and that when surgery is required for nasal obstruction in a child, only small buttons of cartilage should be removed, only at the point of maximal obstruction. Furthermore, the mucoperichondrial incision and elevation should be made close to the resection site so that there is minimal interference with the blood supply that the mucoperichondrium provides to surrounding cartilage. They also warn against disrupting the attachments of the upper and lower lateral cartilages to the septum or maxillae.

Elective surgery on the external nose is generally avoided until full facial growth is achieved, usually by age 16 for females and 18 for males. Certain exceptions to this rule are notable. Severe congenital deformities, such as those associated with cleft lip, should be corrected early, lest growth exaggerate the deformity (Farrior and Connolly, 1970). The same applies to severe traumatic deformities.

Intracranial complications are also a hazard in nasal surgery. The perpendicular plate of the ethmoid at the nasal roof articulates with the cribriform plate, then extends into the floor of the cranial cavity to form the crista galli (Fig. 28–4). This structure should not be subjected to vigorous manipulations such as twisting and pulling during a septal resection for fear that hazardous communications into the intracranial cavity will be opened. Another potential pathway to the intracranial space is presented by the nasal encephalocele, a rare congenital intranasal mass that masquerades as a polyp. True nasal polyps occur rarely in children (except in those with cystic fibrosis), so a single unilateral polyplike structure in a child should be considered to be an encephalocele until proven otherwise.

Septal perforations usually occur in the cartilaginous septum. The cartilage is entirely dependent on overlying mucosa for its blood supply, and it will disintegrate if mucosa is damaged on both sides of the septum in corresponding areas. Simultaneous bilateral nasal cautery for epistaxis is inadvisable for this reason. Septal surgery is the most common cause of perforations (Fairbanks and Chen, 1970).

THE MAXILLARY SINUSES

Growth and Development

The maxillary sinus is first evident about the 70th fetal day as an evagination in the lateral wall of the ethmoidal infundibulum. Although usually a single pouch, it may be two pouches that develop into two sinus cavities that later fuse but leave two ostia.

The fetal maxillary sinus is a slitlike space in the middle meatus between the lateral wall of the nose and the inferior turbinate. Even before birth, enough resorption of the cartilaginous capsule takes place so that the sinus comes into contact with the maxilla and pneumatization commences. At birth, the sinus is 7 to 8 mm deep (anterior to posterior), half as wide, and slightly more than half that dimension in height. It is a tubular sac, the lower margin of which lies slightly below the level of the upper border of the interior meatus. Anteriorly, it extends to the lacrimal duct. It is not always demonstrable on radiographs, although it is of considerable size. Facial growth and maxillary sinus growth proceed together.

Not until the end of the first year has the sinus extended laterally below the orbit to the position of the infraorbital nerve. Growth in width lags behind growth in other dimensions, for until the teeth erupt there is little room in the maxilla into which the sinus can grow (Fig. 28–12). During the third and fourth years, conspicuous growth in width occurs. At 5 years, the sinus reaches considerably beyond the infraorbital canal, and by 9 years it has pneumatized the zygomatic process of the maxilla (Figs. 28–13 through 28–16).

Inferiorly directed expansion accelerates between the seventh and ninth years with the eruption of the permanent teeth, particularly the canines and the molars, which leaves vacant spaces that the sinus pneumatizes. This growth brings the sinus in proximity to the inferior nasal meatus by age 8 years. It reaches the level of the nasal floor variably between ages 8 and 12 years.

By the 15th year, the sinus reaches its adult size except for some expansion that will occur in height. The lowest extension of the cavity occurs when the third molar erupts and the space is pneumatized by the sinus.

As the sinus expands posteriorly, the posterior part of the maxilla, which contains the rudiments of the permanent molar teeth, undergoes a rotation inferiorly, as illustrated in Figure 28–11. What was located posteriorly ultimately comes to occupy a position on the alveolar border of the maxilla. An impacted third molar, placed high posteriorly on the posterior maxilla, is due to arrested development in rotation.

Anomalies and Variations

The walls of the maxillary sinus are often smooth and even. Yet almost 50 per cent of adult maxillary sinuses have ridges, crescentic projections, and septa incompletely dividing the cavity into various-sized compartments. They are probably due to uneven bone resorption during pneumatization or possibly may have been duplicated cavities that failed to fuse completely.

True duplication of the maxillary sinus (with two separate ostia, both of which enter the nasal infundibulum) is developmentally explainable, as mentioned in previous paragraphs. However, more often, the ostium of the superior or posterior compartment enters the superior meatus, and the cell is actually a posterior ethmoid sinus that invaded the maxilla. Considering true duplications and maxillary ethmoid cells together, Schaeffer (1920) described the incidence of this phenomenon as 2.5 per cent of specimens.

The clinical significance of these separated compartments is that during irrigations and surgical explorations, the surgeon may enter one cavity and neglect disease in an adjacent one.

The maxillary sinus ostium lies in the ethmoid infundibulum, which is reached by traversing the hiatus semilunaris deep in the middle meatus of the

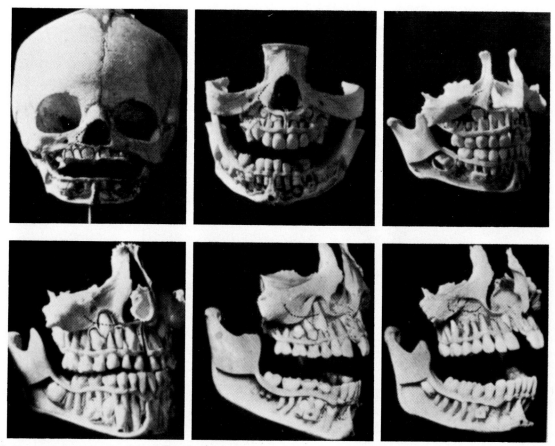

Figure 28–12. Dissections showing the relationship of the teeth to the developing maxillary sinus, indicated by a dotted line. (From Schaeffer, J. P. 1920. The Nose, Paranasal Sinuses, Nasolacrimal Passageways, and Olfactory Organ in Man. A Genetic, Developmental and Anatomico-Physiological Consideration. Philadelphia, Blakiston Co.)

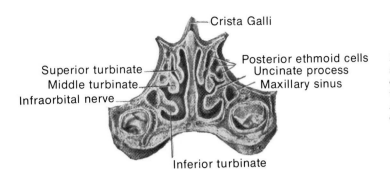

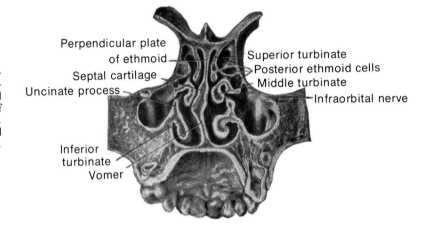

Figure 28–13. Coronal section from a 38-day-old child showing extent of superoinferior and lateral development of the maxillary sinus and proximity of the developing teeth to the orbital floor. (From Davis, W. B. 1918. Anatomy of the nasal accessory sinuses in infancy and childhood. Ann. Otol. Rhinol. Laryngol. 27:940–967.)

Figure 28–14. Coronal section from a 3½-year-old child showing the extent of lateral and superoinferior development of the maxillary sinus and the posterior ethmoid cells. Note the deflection of the septum and its influence on the turbinates. (From Davis, W. B. 1918. Anatomy of the nasal accessory sinuses in infancy and childhood. Ann. Otol. Rhinol. Laryngol. 27:940–967.)

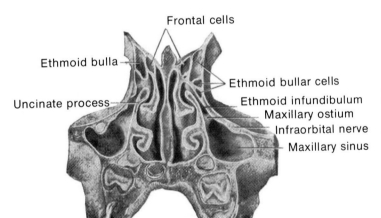

Figure 28–15. Coronal section from a 4½-year-old child showing the extent of lateral and superoinferior development of the maxillary sinus and its relation to developing teeth. Note the ridge beneath the left infraorbital nerve. (From Davis, W. B. 1918. Anatomy of the nasal accessory sinuses in infancy and childhood. Ann. Otol. Rhinol. Laryngol. 27:940–967.)

Figure 28–16. Coronal section from a 10-year-old child showing the size and relations of the maxillary sinus, the maxillary ostium, and its relationship with the ethmoid infundibulum, the bulla, the uncinate process, and the anterior ethmoid cells. (From Davis, W. B. 1918. Anatomy of the nasal accessory sinuses in infancy and childhood. Ann. Otol. Rhinol. Laryngol. 27:940–967.)

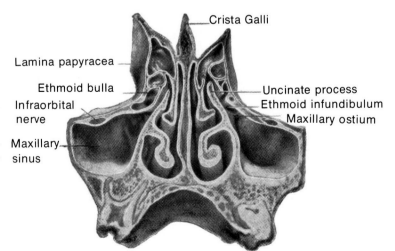

nose (Figs. 28–14 through 28–16). Bounding the hiatus is the ethmoid bulla above and the uncinate process below. These structures are often pneumatized by ethmoid air cells. When enlarged, they narrow the hiatus to slitlike dimensions and not only impede maxillary sinus drainage but also direct frontal and anterior ethmoid sinus drainage into the maxillary sinus ostium.

When the uncinate ridge is high (25 per cent of cases), or the ethmoid bulla is low and overhanging (11 per cent), or the middle turbinate is low and bulky (17 per cent), cannulation of the natural ostium is difficult or impossible (Van Alyea, 1951). Indeed, Schaeffer (1920) concluded, after dissecting a large number of specimens, that cannulation of the natural ostium in the live patient would have been anatomically impossible in the vast majority of cases. But Van Alyea (1951) claimed that the ostium was easily accessible in 40 per cent of cases, and both authors conceded that the cannula may succeed in entering the sinus, not through the natural ostium but rather by penetrating the lateral nasal wall posterior to the hiatus in an area of thin or absent bone termed the "undefended area."

This area is in the medial wall of the maxillary sinus where the perpendicular plate of the palate bone, the uncinate process of the ethmoid bone, the maxillary process of the inferior turbinate, and a portion of the lacrimal bone are all loosely and incompletely articulated. There are numerous dehiscences and defects there; the area is held intact only by membrane on the sinus and nasal side. In dried skulls, the area is usually found devoid of bone, as a large dehiscence.

The accessory maxillary ostium (or ostia) that is so common in adults occurs in this "undefended area." It drains directly into the middle meatus of the nose and not into the ethmoid infundibulum, which distinguishes it from the natural or the duplicated maxillary sinus ostium. It develops by the gradual thinning of bone in the advanced stages of maxillary sinus pneumatization until the bone is finally absorbed and the

thinned membranes rupture spontaneously (a situation analogous to the rupture of the bucconasal membrane in the formation of the choana). This accounts for the frequency of accessory ostia in adulthood (variously reported at 25 to 50 per cent) and the rarity before the age of 15 years (15 per cent in children) (Van Alyea, 1951) (Fig. 28–17).

The size of the maxillary sinus varies considerably among patients of the same age and even from side to side in the same patient. Small sinuses occur when there is deficient absorption of cancellous bone in the sinus floor, a deep canine fossa with encroachment of the anterior sinus wall, excessive bulging of the nasal wall, or imperfect dentition. Minor differences in size and shape between the right and left maxillary sinuses are commonplace. Dixon (1959) claims that true absence of the sinus never occurs, but in his series of 200 dissections he found one sinus with a capacity of only 1 cc, and Maresh (1940) reports the incidence of hypoplasia to be 6.3 per cent.

Sinuses can be unusually large when pneumatization extends into the alveolar, frontal, or zygomatic processes of the maxilla, the orbital process of the palatine bone, or underneath the nasal floor into the palatal recess.

Thickness of sinus walls varies from 5 to 8 mm down to a papery thin delicacy or absence, especially on the nasal wall and in the canine fossa. There are many exceptions to the idea that large sinuses have the thinnest walls and vice versa.

Ectopic teeth in the maxillary sinuses are regularly reported, especially in the dental literature. Developmental errors may be causative but so also could injuries to the maxilla, such as facial trauma or difficult dental manipulations. Any absent tooth in the maxilla with unusually long delayed eruption should suggest eruption into the nose or sinus. Ectopic incisors and canines may appear in the nasal floor. Ectopic molars are found in the floor of the maxillary sinus; the third molar is most frequently involved, as explained in a previous paragraph.

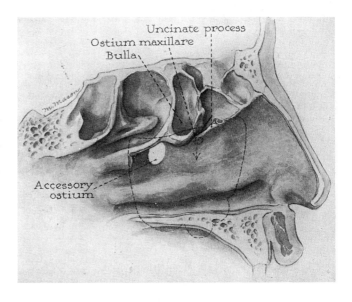

Figure 28–17. Low overhanging ethmoid bulla makes the maxillary ostium inaccessible. However, a large accessory ostium is available for cannulation. (From Van Alyea, O. E. 1951. Maxillary sinus. *In* Nasal Sinuses, An Anatomic and Clinical Consideration, 2nd ed. Copyright 1951, The Williams & Wilkins Company. Reproduced by permission.)

Anatomic Relationships and Surgical Hazards

The floor of the maxillary sinus is the alveolar process of the maxilla. Spongy bone separates the sinus cavity from the roots of the teeth and their sockets. Even though this is the thickest of the sinus walls, it is frequently thin enough to show irregular elevations in the sinus floor overlying the tooth roots. Thinning to the point of direct communication of tooth roots with the maxillary sinus sometimes occurs in young adulthood, but usually not until advanced age.

Dr. Nathaniel Highmore, after whom this antrum has been called, gave a detailed description of the cavity as early as 1651. He had a patient whose abscess in the sinus was drained by extraction of the canine tooth. That particular sinus must have been exceptionally large because the canine tooth does not usually come into close relationship with the sinus; neither do the incisors. Even the first and second premolars are often not in close proximity to the floor of the cavity. The three molar teeth are most constantly and intimately related to the sinus, but in small sinuses even the first molar may be omitted.

In children, surgical procedures through the canine fossa should be done with great consideration for developing teeth. Injury to them leads to either death of the teeth or ultimate eruption of deformed teeth. Radiographs should locate their position, and the approach should be high and lateral enough to avoid them. Endonasal approaches to the sinus in children are best carried out through the middle meatus, since the floor of the sinus may not reach the level of the nasal floor until the 12th year. Furthermore, the inferior meatus is exceedingly narrow because of the relatively large inferior turbinate and its heavy mucosa.

The anterior wall of the sinus contains the infraorbital foramen at the upper aspect of the canine fossa. It is approximately the same distance from the midline as the palpable supraorbital notch, and it is 0.5 cm or less below the infraorbital rim. The nerve and vessel that exit through this foramen should be protected during periosteal elevation in the Caldwell-Luc approach. Damage to the nerve results in sensory loss to the cheek and upper lip and occasionally neuroma formation that can be painful.

The roof of the maxillary sinus is the thin plate of bone forming the orbital floor. Not infrequently it is modeled into a ridge by the infraorbital canal (Fig. 28–15). In some instances, the ridge is replaced by a groove covered only by thin membrane.

The infraorbital nerve and artery are in jeopardy when curettage is performed on the roof of the sinus cavity. The orbital periosteum is a sufficiently thick and recognizable barrier between the orbital contents and the sinus. However, in orbital floor fractures, the periosteum is often lacerated and orbital fat protrudes into the roof of the sinus, mimicking a mucosal polyp. It should not be removed lest enophthalmus be exaggerated by a further loss of orbital contents.

Innervation of the maxillary teeth may also be jeopardized by sinus surgery. The posterosuperior dental nerves, branches of the maxillary nerve, enter the maxilla posteriorly through tiny foramina and run through spongy bone covering the tooth roots of the molars and premolars. They may be immediately submucosal; thus, curettage of the sinus floor leaves the teeth numb.

Canine and incisor teeth are innervated by the anterosuperior dental nerve, which branches off the infraorbital nerve midway in its canal. In some instances, it runs obliquely (anteromedially) across the roof of the maxillary sinus in a raised, thin bony canal, but often it is covered only by mucous membrane. Otherwise, it remains in the infraorbital canal until it reaches the anterior sinus wall, where it turns medially. In the medial wall of the sinus, at the level of the anterior end of the inferior turbinate, the nerve turns downward toward the nasal spine and gives off its branches to the teeth. When surgery requires removal of the anterior wall of the sinus high and medially or removal of the antral roof, injury to this nerve may occur.

The posterior boundary of the sinus is the anterior wall of the pterygopalatine fossa, which contains the ramifying maxillary nerve and artery. One branch of that artery, the greater palatine, courses toward the palate through a canal in the posteroinferior medial wall of the maxillary sinus. It may be encountered by the surgeon as he or she takes down the posteroinferior bony ridge during nasoantral fenestration. Bleeding can be troublesome.

Sometimes the posterior or superior wall is divided into two plates separated by an invading ethmoid air cell. Indeed, the ethmoid sinus field is the most medial superior boundary of the maxillary sinus cavity. It requires only gentle pressure to crack through the thin, shell-like bone to perform the transantral ethmoidectomy, an operation that affords good, safe visualization of the posterior ethmoid complex.

THE SPHENOID SINUSES

Growth and Development

The sphenoid sinus arises in the posterior cupola, or dome, of the cartilaginous nasal capsule; its origin is suggested as early as the fourth fetal month. It develops as a constricted portion of the nasal fossa, its ostium always to remain cephalic to the highest nasal concha.

Although this sinus remains in its nasal position until the fourth postnatal year, it may be large enough to retain infectious material in its cavity. During the fourth year, the nasal capsule resorbs and the sinus comes in contact with the sphenoid bone, allowing ingrowth and sphenoid pneumatization. Its early growth is posterolateral rather than ventral, leading to early thinning of the lateral walls and an early intimate relationship with the ophthalmic and maxillary nerves. By the age of 6 or 7 years, it establishes a close relationship with the pterygoid (vidian) canal and its

Figure 28–18. Sagittal section from an 8-day-old child shows the left lateral nasal wall and the extent of development of the sphenoid sinus. Note the anteroinferior wall of the sphenoid sinus, termed the sphenoid concha or ossiculum Bertini. (From Davis, W. B. 1918. Anatomy of the nasal accessory sinuses in infancy and childhood. Ann. Otol. Rhinol. Laryngol. 27:940–967.)

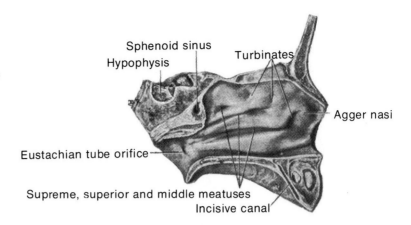

vessels and nerve. The growth rate averages 0.25 mm per year in the posterior direction, but it progresses in irregular spurts (Hinck and Hopkins, 1965).

Sphenoid sinuses have been classified into three categories that reflect the degree of pneumatization into the sphenoid bone.

1. *Conchal type.* Pneumatization does not extend into the body of the sphenoid bone but is arrested in its infantile position (Figs. 28–18 and 28–19). The small right and left sinuses are widely separated by a thick bony septum. Persistence of this type of sinus into late childhood is rare and is observed in only 2.5 per cent of adults (Hammer and Radberg, 1961).

2. *Presellar type.* Pneumatization extends only as far posteriorly as the sella turcica, or more specifically not beyond the vertical plane of the tuberculum sella (Fig. 28–20). This is the usual condition of childhood (Table 28–1). However, pneumatization proceeds with age, and by adulthood the frequency of this type drops below 10 per cent.

3. *Sellar type.* Pneumatization advances beyond the tuberculum sella in 90 per cent of cases by the end of adolescence, underneath the sella in over 20 per cent of cases (Fig. 28–21), and even posterior to the sella in up to 10 per cent of cases (Fig. 28–22).

The sphenoid is the first of all the paranasal sinuses to achieve full development. Growth ceases in early adulthood; 50 per cent are mature at age 15 years.

Anomalies and Variations

The sinus cavity is generally limited to the anterosuperior part of the sphenoid bone, although extensive sinuses have been described with pneumatization of the entire sphenoid bone, lesser and greater wings, basilar process of the occipital bone, supermedial aspect of the orbit, and orbital process of the palatal bone, and otherwise crowding spaces ordinarily occupied by posterior ethmoid cells.

In a small sinus, the interior walls are usually even and regular. However, of all the paranasal sinuses, the sphenoid is most likely to have the most irregular internal topography. Partial septa and recesses vary from slight elevations to bridgelike osseous barriers incompletely dividing the sinus into subcompartments. Diverticula may extend into outlying portions of the sphenoid, even into the epidural spaces of the hypophysis, cavernous sinus, and optic nerves. Mounds and raised areas give evidence and warning of externally bordering neural and vascular structures (Fig. 28–22).

The intersinus septum is variable in both thickness and location. It is midline only at its anterior origin, where it is in line with the nasal septum. Elsewhere, it deviates to one side or the other or may even be situated in an oblique semihorizontal plane, so that the sinus of one side may seem to rest on top of the

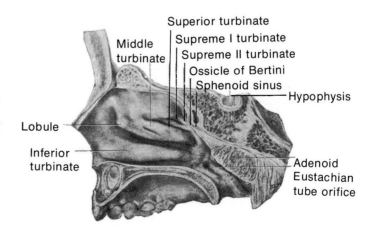

Figure 28–19. Sagittal section from a child nearly 2 years old. The sphenoid sinus appears small, but in a more lateral plane it was developed more extensively in the posterolateral direction, its inferolateral wall being only 1 mm from the pterygopalatine fossa. (From Davis, W. B. 1918. Anatomy of the nasal accessory sinuses in infancy and childhood. Ann. Otol. Rhinol. Laryngol. 27:940–967.)

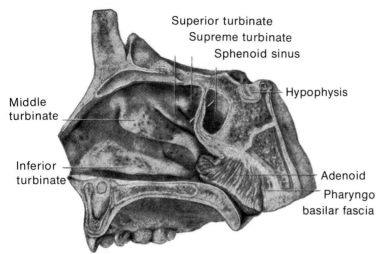

Figure 28–20. Sagittal section from a 6-year-old child showing presellar sphenoidal pneumatization. (From Davis, W. B. 1918. Anatomy of the nasal accessory sinuses in infancy and childhood. Ann. Otol. Rhinol. Laryngol. 27:940–967.)

other. The sphenoid sinuses do not communicate with each other. If there appears to be no septum at all, it is probably due to agenesis of one sinus with compensatory pneumatization of the other with only one ostium.

The size and the location of the sphenoid ostia are quite variable, even from one side to the other in the same specimen. However, they are always located in the sphenoethmoidal recess, cephalic to the uppermost turbinate that is present. Usually, they are slightly superior to the midplane of the anterior sinus wall and 35 to 40 mm above the floor of the nasal cavity at maturity. The usual ostium is 2 by 3 mm in diameter, is placed 2 mm lateral to the nasal septum, and is hidden from anterior view by the superior turbinate. Large ostia, up to 6 mm in diameter, are occasionally seen opening immediately lateral to the septum. The ostium may be as far as 7 mm distant from the septum and may be as small as 1 by 1.5 mm in diameter (Fig. 28–23).

Anatomic Relationships and Surgical Hazards

The paired sphenoid sinuses are located in what has been termed the danger position in the skull, owing to their proximity to important vascular and neurologic structures, as listed in Table 28–2 (Fig. 28–22).

Van Alyea's studies (1941, 1951) were from obser-

vations on mature sinuses, which exhibit more advanced pneumatization than do those of children. The interior of the sinus lumen often exhibited elevated ridges or mounds, which indicated important underlying neurovascular structures, separated from the sinus by as little as 0.2 mm of bone. Occasionally, bone was even dehiscent (absent) in the adult specimens. More often in children, however, the bone is thicker, and there may be no landmarks on the interior sinus walls to suggest the position of such structures.

THE ETHMOID SINUSES

Growth and Development

The ethmoid air cells are evaginations of nasal mucosa from the middle, superior, and first supreme nasal meatuses. As dimplelike depressions, they are in evidence as early as the fourth fetal month. By the seventh fetal month, they are hollowed-out blind sacs with ostia into their respective meatuses.

Ethmoid cells grow relatively rapidly in the early years. At birth, they all are present as widely separated, rounded epithelial recesses. During the second year, they approach each other and alter their shape by mutual compression and become flattened laterally by the lamina papyracea. Growth is then directed upward toward the cribriform plate. There is little uniformity of development in what has been termed a "struggle for space." Even though one cell may have its origin inferior to another, it may outgrow its neighbor and force it to progress in a direction other than that in which it was primarily growing. But each cell will always communicate with the meatus from which it originated; cells from unlike meatuses never communicate with each other.

By the seventh year, the enlarged ethmoid cells begin to pneumatize all available space, extending into the turbinates and the frontal and sphenoid bones. Between the 12th and 14th years, they attain their final forms.

TABLE 28–1. The Occurrence of Different Types of Sphenoid Sinuses among Various Age Groups

TYPE OF SINUS	0–3 YR (%)	4–12 YR (%)	13–20 YR (%)	21–30 YR (%)
Presellar	100	57	13	6
Sellar	0	43	65	72
Sellar–extensive	0	0	22	22

Modified from B. Vidic, 1968. The postnatal development of the sphenoidal sinus and its spread into the dorsum sellae and posterior clinoid processes. Am. J. Roentgenol 104:177–183, 1968, © by American Roentgen Ray Society.

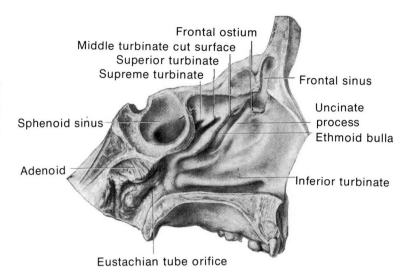

Figure 28–21. Sagittal section from a 10-year-old child showing sellar-type pneumatization, which has extended beneath the anterior portion of the sella turcica. The anterior portion of the middle turbinate and a portion of the medial wall of the frontal sinus have been removed to demonstrate continuity from the sinus into the ethmoid infundibulum. (From Davis, W. B. 1918. Anatomy of the nasal accessory sinuses in infancy and childhood. Ann. Otol. Rhinol. Laryngol. 27:940–967.)

There is an early division of the ethmoid labyrinth into anterior and posterior groups. Anterior cells arise inferior to the attachment of the middle turbinate, and posterior cells arise superior to it. The anterior ethmoid cells develop from three areas in the middle meatus (Fig. 28–3).

1. *Frontal recess.* The most ventral and cephalic of the anterior group develop from furrows on the lateral wall of the frontal recess. They vary in number; one or more may become frontal cells, or the group may be absent altogether. The agger nasi is commonly pneumatized by the most ventral of these cells.

2. *Infundibulum.* From the ventral end of the ethmoid infundibulum grow the infundibular cells, which may number as many as seven but usually are not more than three. They variably pneumatize the agger nasi and the uncinate process and may grow sufficiently into the frontal bone to become frontal sinuses or frontal bullae. It should be recalled that the maxillary sinus ostium also drains into the infundibulum. This explains why suppurative disease may coexist in the frontal, maxillary, and infundibular ethmoid sinuses yet not involve the bullar and posterior ethmoid cells, which have separate ostia.

3. *Bullar furrows.* The ethmoid bulla, also termed the accessory concha, is hollowed out by cells originating in the furrows above and below it. Such bullar cells frequently also pneumatize the supraorbital plate of the frontal bone and the infraorbital plate of the maxilla. Their size greatly influences the width of the hiatus semilunaris and, therefore, the natural drainage channel of the maxillary sinus.

The posterior ethmoid cells gradually pneumatize and make the superior and supreme turbinates appear as shell-like structures. They may extend into the supraorbital plate of the frontal bone, the infraorbital plate of the maxilla, the middle nasal turbinate, and the orbital process of the palate.

Figure 28–22. Irregularities of the sphenoid walls. Prominences are caused by underlying neural and vascular structures. Note recesses caused by pneumatization of the lesser wing (superior lateral recess) and the pterygoid process and greater wing (pterygoid recess) of the sphenoid. (From Van Alyea, O. E. 1951. Sphenoid sinus. *In* Nasal Sinuses, An Anatomic and Clinical Consideration, 2nd ed. Copyright 1951, The Williams & Wilkins Company. Reproduced by permission.)

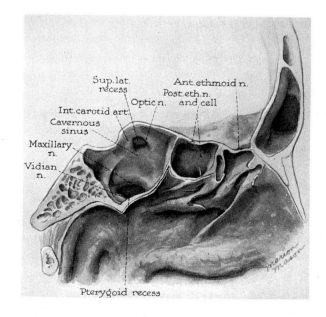

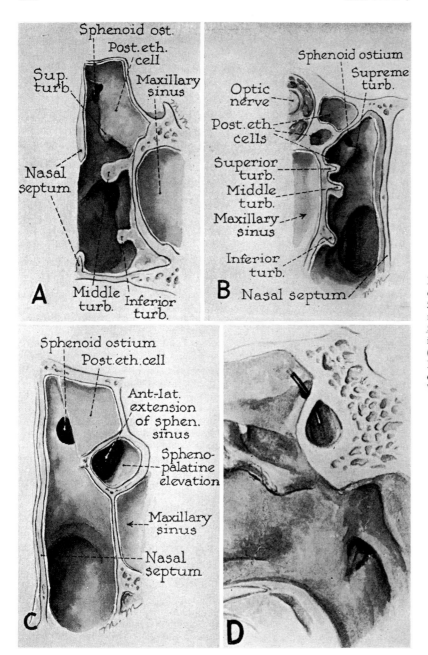

Figure 28–23. Types of sphenoid ostium. *A,* Average type. The orifice shown measures 3.5 by 2.5 mm. It is located in a shallow sphenoethmoid recess less than 2 mm from the nasal septum. *B,* Small ostium deep in the recess. *C,* Large opening in typical location. *D,* Ostium in roof of sinus. (From Van Alyea, O. E. 1951. Sphenoid sinus. *In* Nasal Sinuses, An Anatomic and Clinical Consideration, 2nd ed. Copyright 1951, The Williams & Wilkins Company. Reproduced by permission.)

TABLE 28–2. Elevations in the Sphenoid Sinus Wall

STRUCTURE	INCIDENCE (%)	ANATOMIC POSITION
Hypophysis	87	Midline, posterior (presellar sinus) Midline, superior (sellar sinus)
Internal carotid artery*	53	Lateral wall, as a raised serpentine mound
Optic nerve and artery	40	Superolateral (chiasm is anterior to hypophysis in roof)
Maxillary nerve*	40	Lateral wall
Vidian nerve and artery	36	Floor
Nerves of superior orbital fissure	35	Lateral wall
Sphenopalatine artery and ganglion	30	Anterior floor
Mandibular nerve*	4	Lateral wall

*Several of the above structures actually course through or lateral to the cavernous sinus, which lies between them and the sinus lumen on the lateral wall of the sphenoid sinus.

Modified from Van Alyea, O. E. 1941. Sphenoid sinus, anatomic study, with consideration of the clinical significance of the structural characteristics of sphenoid sinus. Arch. Otolaryngol. 34:225–253, and Van Alyea, O. E. 1951. Nasal Sinuses, An Anatomic and Clinical Consideration, 2nd ed. Baltimore, Williams & Wilkins Co.

Pneumatization of the ethmoid bulla is the most constant feature of ethmoid sinus development; it can be demonstrated in all anatomic dissections. Posterior ethmoid cells were found in 96 per cent of Van Alyea's (1951) specimens and pneumatization of the agger nasi in 89 per cent (Figs. 28–24 and 28–25).

Anomalies and Variations

By adulthood the ethmoid labyrinth is seldom entirely confined within the ethmoid bone. Even before puberty, significant encroachments into neighboring areas can be demonstrated. Particularly common are supraorbital extensions into the frontal bone (15 per cent of cases studied) and infraorbital extensions into the maxilla (11 per cent). An extension into the maxilla could be termed a supernumerary maxillary sinus, but, in fact, it is a posterior ethmoid cell with its natural ostium draining into the superior meatus.

Posterior ethmoid cells may encroach on the sphenoid sinus lumen (9 per cent) and may erode into the palate bone (the inappropriately named palatal sinus).

Anterior cells may crowd the lacrimal bone, encroach on the frontal sinus lumen as frontal bullae (see section on frontal sinuses), and invade the middle turbinate (concha), hollowing it out and making it shell-like (Fig. 28–6). These conchal cells develop from either anterior or posterior ethmoid cells. They are quite common in adults (12 per cent of skulls dissected by Schaeffer, 1920). Although such extensions have been demonstrated in fetal and childhood specimens, their development is not pronounced until puberty or

later. Other than their location, they do not differ from other ethmoid cells. However, their dependent position with respect to their ostia makes them disadvantageously placed for natural drainage; hence, they are frequently involved in suppurative disease. Their ostia may be located in either the superior or middle meatus (in approximately equal proportions) according to their origins.

Dehiscences (deficient osseous boundaries) occur frequently, particularly in the lamina papyracea (orbital plate) and occasionally in the floor of the anterior cranial fossa. Thus, ethmoid membrane may be contiguous with periorbitum and dura mater, respectively. Likewise, ethmoid membranes may be in actual contact with the lacrimal sac.

Anatomic Relationships and Surgical Hazards

The anatomic position of the ethmoidal field accounts for not only surgical hazards but also the hazard of extension of uncontrolled infection. The ethmoid sinus complex is a roughly pyramid-shaped mass, wide posteriorly, narrowed anteriorly, inconstantly contained within the following boundaries.

Superiorly: The fovea ethmoidalis is a plate of bone separating the floor of the anterior cranial fossa from the ethmoid complex. This plate descends in a posterior to inferior direction at an angle of 15 degrees from horizontal. Therefore, anterior ethmoid cells extend higher than posterior cells even when they do not encroach upon the frontal sinuses. The superior boundary of the most anterior cells is the floor of the frontal sinus.

Anteriorly: The lacrimal bone houses the lacrimal sac on its anterolateral surface and the agger nasi medially.

Inferiorly: The most medial aspect of the roof of the maxillary sinus is adjacent to the ethmoid sinus complex. The relationship is narrow anteriorly, but it widens posteriorly.

Laterally: The lamina papyracea (orbital plate, or *os planum*) separates the orbit from the ethmoid complex. It articulates with the lacrimal bone anteriorly, the maxilla inferiorly, the frontal bone superiorly, and the lesser wing of the sphenoid posteriorly.

Medially: The nasal turbinates and meatuses form the lateral wall of the nose and medial boundaries of the sinuses.

Posteriorly: The posterior ethmoid cells share a common wall with the sphenoid sinuses anterolaterally.

It is common for ethmoid cells in their pneumatization to push their boundaries beyond the usual anatomic positions.

Separating the ethmoid field from the orbit is the lamina papyracea, which is, as its name implies, of paper-thin delicacy and which may even be dehiscent in places. The optic nerve at the optic foramen is separated from the most posterior and superior eth-

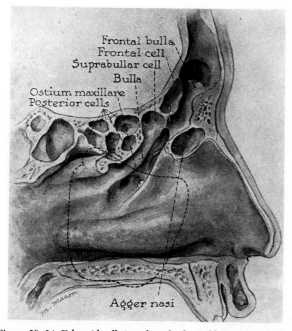

Figure 28–24. Ethmoid cells invading the frontal bone, encroaching upon the frontal sinus (frontal bulla). Note also the large cell in the agger nasi. (From Van Alyea, O. E. 1951. Ethmoid sinus. *In* Nasal Sinuses, An Anatomic and Clinical Consideration, 2nd ed. Copyright 1951, The Williams & Wilkins Company. Reproduced by permission.)

Frontal bulla
Frontal cell
Suprabullar cell
Bulla
Ostium maxillare
Posterior cells

Agger nasi

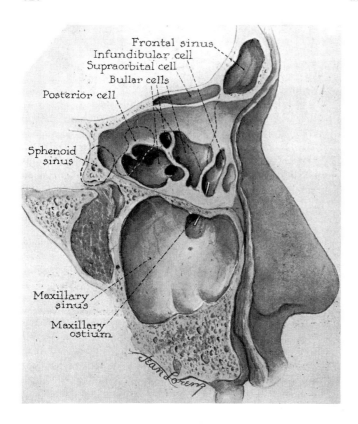

Figure 28–25. Large bullar cells crowd other ethmoid cells. Note also the supraorbital ethmoid cell. (From Van Alyea, O. E. 1951. Ethmoid sinus. *In* Nasal Sinuses, An Anatomic and Clinical Consideration, 2nd ed. Copyright 1951, The Williams & Wilkins Company. Reproduced by permission.)

moid cells by bone of only 2 to 5 mm thickness, and it may be seen prominently in 4 per cent of specimens (Dixon, 1959) (Fig. 28–26). Sometimes, aggressive posterior ethmoid cells pneumatize the body and lesser wing of the sphenoid bone at the expense of the sphenoid sinus (ethmosphenoidal cell). Then, the proximity of these cells to the optic nerve exists for much of its distance from the orbital foramen to the optic chiasm. The intervening bone may be of tissue-paper thickness, or it may be absent.

Such an ethmosphenoidal cell will replace the sphenoid as the superior and posterior boundary of the pterygomaxillary fossa with its neurovascular contents. A "supernumerary maxillary sinus," which is, in fact, an extended posterior ethmoid sinus, will replace the maxillary sinus as the anterior boundary of the same fossa.

Two small neurovascular bundles penetrate the lamina papyracea to supply the ethmoid complex: the anterior and posterior ethmoidal arteries and branches

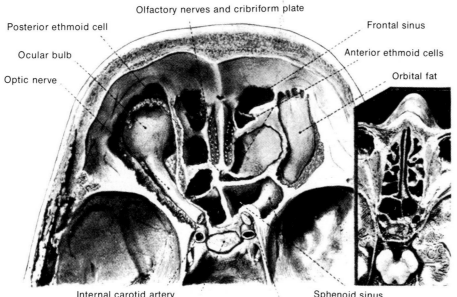

Figure 28–26. Exposure of the ethmoid and sphenoid sinuses, optic nerves, and eyeballs by removal of the floor of the anterior cranial fossa. Note the right optic nerve in the sphenoid sinus, which extends above and below it. The left optic nerve bears a more common relationship to the posterior ethmoid and sphenoid sinuses. The insert is a transection of the ethmoid and sphenoid sinuses showing a larger number of ethmoid cells and the relationship of the optic nerve to the posterior ethmoid cells and sphenoid sinuses. (From Schaeffer, J. P. 1920. The Nose, Paranasal Sinuses, Nasolacrimal Passageways, and Olfactory Organ in Man. A Genetic, Developmental and Anatomico-Physiological Consideration. Philadelphia, Blakiston Co.)

of the trigeminal nerve (Fig. 28–27). They will be encountered during an external surgical approach to the ethmoid. The anterior is the larger of the two arteries and may require ligation or application of a surgical clip to achieve hemostasis. The ligature should be placed on the orbital side of any anticipated division since arterial flow is from lateral to medial. The posterior branch should be the posterior limit of dissection, for it lies only a few millimeters in front of the optic nerve (3 to 8 mm in an adult). A line connecting these two foramina is on a parallel with and is just inferior to the floor of the anterior cranial fossa and the cribriform plate. The anterior and posterior ethmoidal arteries arise from the ophthalmic artery as it courses along the medial wall of the orbit. Although the posterior branch passes directly into the ethmoid sinuses and nasal fossa, the anterior branch takes a more circuitous route. It courses through its foramen to enter the anterior cranial fossa. It then passes forward on top of the cribriform plate to a slitlike foramen at the side of the crista galli, where it enters the nasal fossa. It descends on the interior lateral nasal wall and finally exits between the nasal bone and the lateral cartilage to reach the tip of the nose. Coursing with the arteries are corresponding ethmoidal veins that communicate freely with the dural veins, including the superior sagittal sinus, as well as the ophthalmic vein, which empties into the cavernous sinus. These pathways afford easy extension of nasal and sinus infection into periorbital and intracranial areas (Fairbanks et al., 1975).

During ethmoid surgery, the cribriform plate is at a risk. Damage to it not only jeopardizes the olfactory sense but also can cause cerebrospinal fluid leakage and intracranial spread of infection. The cribriform plate actually lies lower than the roof of the ethmoid labyrinth. In fact, in 70 per cent of specimens, it lies 4 to 7 mm below the level of the orbital roof.

To avoid injury to the cribriform plate, surgeons are usually admonished to dissect no further medially than the origin of the middle turbinate, which is the safe surgical landmark. Actually, the posterior ethmoid cells arise medial to the middle turbinate, but they are lateral to the origin of the superior turbinate,

which becomes the landmark in the deeper recesses of the nasal cavity.

The external ethmoidectomy carries an added risk of disrupting the attachment of the medial canthal ligament of the orbit, which leads to unilateral widening of the intercanthal distance. However, since surgical exposure is limited in children and since the surgical hazard to the optic nerve is so great with poor exposure, the external approach is most widely recommended in children. Furthermore, the usual indication for ethmoidectomy in children is orbital cellulitis or abscess, which requires an external approach in any instance.

THE FRONTAL SINUSES

Growth and Development

The frontal sinuses originate as outgrowths of the ventral cephalic ends of the middle meatuses in an area termed the frontal recess. This area, operculated by the middle turbinate, is identifiable in the late third to early fourth fetal month. Both the frontal sinuses and the anterior ethmoid cells develop in this area.

By the time of birth, the area has developed only to the stage of pits or furrows in that recess (Fig. 28–28). It is from one or more of these furrows that the sinuses will develop. They develop variously:

1. By direct extension of the whole frontal recess (Fig. 28–3).

2. From one or more of the anterior ethmoid cells, which originate in the frontal furrows (Fig. 28–29).

3. Occasionally, from the ventral end of the ethmoid infundibulum.

In the first instance there will be no true nasal duct but instead a wide communication with the nose anterior and superior to the hiatus semilunaris. This is the most common finding. In the latter two instances, a frontal duct will develop, the tortuosity of which will depend on the cell from which the sinus originated and the degree of development and disposition of neighboring ethmoid cells. Furthermore, the relation-

Figure 28–27. Medial view of the orbit demonstrates foramina of the anterior and posterior ethmoid neurovascular bundles, which serve as surgical landmarks, indicating the proximity of the optic nerve and cribriform plate.

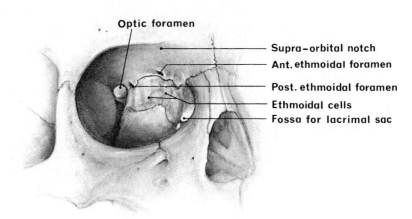

Optic foramen

Supra-orbital notch
Ant. ethmoidal foramen
Post. ethmoidal foramen
Ethmoidal cells
Fossa for lacrimal sac

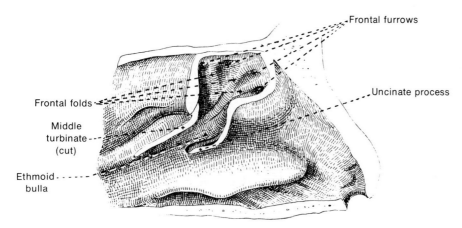

Figure 28–28. Lateral nasal wall of a full-term fetus. The middle turbinate has been removed, which exposes the accessory folds and furrows of the frontal recess. (From Schaeffer, J. P. 1920. The Nose, Paranasal Sinuses, Nasolacrimal Passageways, and Olfactory Organ in Man. A Genetic, Developmental and Anatomico-Physiological Consideration. Philadelphia, Blakiston Co.)

ship of that duct to the ethmoid infundibulum may be so intimate that drainage from the duct could find its way into the infundibulum and from there through the maxillary ostium into the maxillary sinus (Fig. 28–24). This may explain the old clinical dictum that the maxillary sinus is a cesspool for frontal sinus drainage. Anatomically, however, that should be the case in less than 50 per cent of cases.

At birth, the frontal sinuses still may not be demonstrable. Although the rudiments are advanced, they are not topically frontal. The appearance of the frontal sinus is not certain until the sixth to 12th postfetal month. By the 20th month, the frontal sinus has eroded into and begun to ascend the vertical portion of the frontal bone. By the middle of the third year, the cupola of the sinus is visible above the level of the nasion, and by the eighth year, at least one frontal sinus reaches the level of the orbital roof in 50 per cent of subjects (Maresh, 1940). The sinus grows vertically at an average rate of 1.5 mm per year (Davis, 1918), more slowly in early years and more rapidly after the seventh or eighth year (Fig. 28–30). It reaches its mature size during puberty and thereafter grows a small amount into old age.

Anatomists agree that there is no constant or so-called "normal" type anatomy of the sinuses. According to Schaeffer (1920), "adherence to a single fixed and arbitrary normal is fraught with danger since with variations come altered size, altered shape, altered

anatomic relations." Maresh's longitudinal radiographic study of 100 children demonstrates this variability in Figures 28–31 and 28–32; he noted that growth proceeds at an irregular pace. In many instances, a cell would begin to bud upward and after reaching a point above the nasion would fail to increase for several years. Later, it would increase in size again very rapidly and either equal the size of the other frontal sinus or even become larger in a comparatively short time.

Early vertical invasion is nearer the inner plate of the frontal bone than the outer. This leads to a thin inner plate of almost entirely compact bone as opposed to the thick outer (anterior) wall of both compact and cancellous bone. Invasion is, from the outset, variable and asymmetric. The intersinus septum is midline only at its base. Although it becomes paper-thin, it is not normally perforated.

Anomalies and Variations

In many instances, the frontal sinus never invades far into the vertical portion but grows extensively into the horizontal portion of the frontal bone, forming large air spaces over the orbits. This leads to the erroneous belief that there is frequently an agenesis of the frontal sinus. True bilateral agenesis occurs in no more than 4 per cent of skulls, but unilateral absence

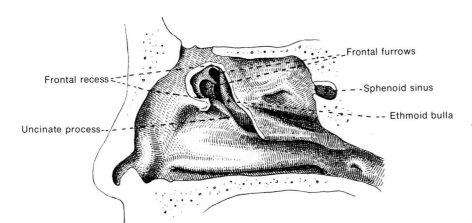

Figure 28–29. The frontal recess of a 5-month-old child. Note the pouching of the frontal furrows and the frontal recess in the formation of the anterior ethmoidal cells and the frontal sinus. The sphenoid sinus is also well established. (From Schaeffer, J. P. 1920. The Nose, Paranasal Sinuses, Nasolacrimal Passageways, and Olfactory Organ in Man. A Genetic, Developmental and Anatomico-Physiological Consideration. Philadelphia, Blakiston Co.)

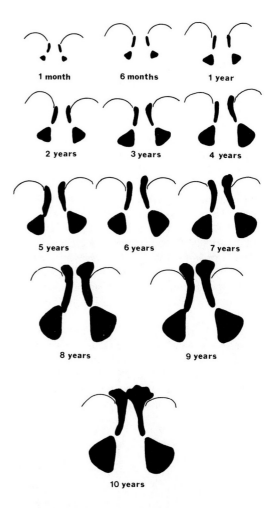

Figure 28–30. The development of the sinuses in a series of radiographs of one child over a 10-year period. (From Maresh, M. M. 1940. Paranasal sinuses from birth to late adolescence. Am. J. Dis. Child. 60:58–75. Copyright 1940, American Medical Association.)

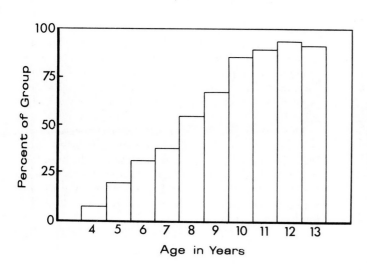

Figure 28–31. Percentage of children who had one or both frontal sinuses at the level of or above the orbital roof in the radiographs made at the indicated ages. (From Maresh, M. M. 1940. Paranasal sinuses from birth to late adolescence. Am. J. Dis. Child. 60:58–75. Copyright 1940, American Medical Association.)

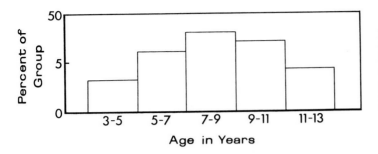

Figure 28–32. Time of appearance of frontal sinuses above the orbital roofs as shown by radiographs taken at the age intervals indicated, when one or both frontal sinuses first reached the level of the orbital roof. (From Maresh, M. M. 1940. Paranasal sinuses from birth to late adolescence. Am. J. Dis. Child. 60:58–75. Copyright 1940, American Medical Association.)

is seen in 11 per cent (Dixon, 1959). In as many as 30 per cent of skulls, the frontal sinuses are considered to be underdeveloped or hypoplastic (Maresh, 1940).

Supernumerary frontal sinuses are common in both the horizontal and the vertical portions of the frontal bone. They can be placed side by side or one posterior to the other, a confusing situation for the surgeon. Schaeffer (1920) has described as many as six frontal sinuses in one skull, two on one side and four on the other. Each sinus is normally independent of another (developed from a different furrow) and has its own ostium of communication with the anterior middle meatus.

Not infrequently, an anterior ethmoid cell encroaches upon the frontal sinus floor, pushing it upward, balloonlike, into the sinus lumen. This is called a frontal bulla (Figs. 28–24 and 28–33). At times, several such cells will arrange themselves, tierlike, in the floor of the frontal sinus. Bullae may be so prominent and so located that the usual trephine operation could enter a bulla instead of the frontal sinus.

Asymmetry between right and left frontal sinuses is the rule rather than the exception, and asymmetry of the intersinus septum may be so exaggerated that one frontal sinus overlies the other, the latter appearing as a bulla. Extensive pneumatization of the sinus is described as far laterally as the temporal bones and into the nasal bones, but this condition occurs in adulthood.

Anatomic Relationships and Surgical Hazards

Only the thin layer of compact bone of the inner (posterior) table of the frontal sinus separates it from the dura mater and frontal lobe of the brain. The floor of the sinus overlies the orbit and some of the anterior ethmoid cells (Fig. 28–33). If the horizontal portion of the frontal bone has been extensively pneumatized, the sinus can overlie posterior ethmoid cells as well. Posteromedially, a mound may be seen that overlies the olfactory area. Infection spreads readily from the frontal sinuses to the orbit and intracranial space, either by osteitis of their common walls or through the thrombophlebitic intercommunications. The proximity of these structures to the frontal sinus should be considered during surgery to avoid entering and spreading disease into uninvolved areas.

In the diseased state, especially when a mucocele is present, any of the bony walls may be eroded (Fairbanks et al., 1975). However, dura and periorbita are usually recognizable if the surgical exposure is wide enough. When the sinuses are extremely small, finding the lumen may represent the greatest challenge of the surgical procedure. Preoperative tomography is helpful.

The supraorbital and supratrochlear nerves and vessels, branches of the ophthalmic nerve and artery, exit the orbit superficial to the periosteum of the supraorbital ridge. If a brow incision requires penetration of the periosteum and is carried as far laterally as the supraorbital notch, numbness and paresthesia of the forehead will result.

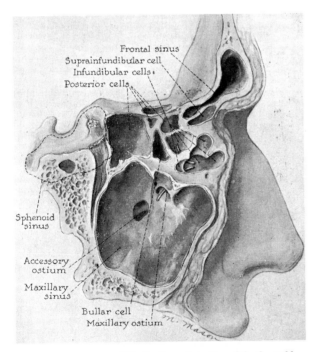

Figure 28–33. Invasion of the horizontal portion of the frontal bone by both frontal and ethmoid air cells. Note supraorbital extension of frontal sinus and bulge in its floor by ethmoid cell. (From Van Alyea, O. E. 1951. Ethmoid sinus. In Nasal Sinuses, An Anatomic and Clinical Consideration, 2nd ed. Copyright 1951, The Williams & Wilkins Company. Reproduced by permission.)

REFERENCES

Cottle, M. H. 1951. Nasal surgery in children. E.E.N.T. Monthly 30:32.

Davis, W. B. 1918. Anatomy of the nasal accessory sinuses in infancy and childhood. Ann. Otol. Rhinol. Laryngol. 27:940.

Dion, M. C., Jafek, B. W., and Tobin, C. E. 1978. The anatomy of the nose, external support. Arch. Otolaryngol. 104:145.

Dixon, F. W. 1959. Clinical significance of anatomical arrangement of paranasal sinuses. Ann. Otol. Rhinol. Laryngol. 67:736.

Enlow, D. H. 1978. Handbook of Facial Growth. Philadelphia, W. B. Saunders Co.

Fairbanks, D. N. F., and Chen, S. C. A. 1970. Closure of large nasal septum perforations. Arch. Otolaryngol. 91:403.

Fairbanks, D. N. F., Vanderveen, T. S., and Bordley, J. E. 1975. Intracranial complications of sinusitis. In Maloney, W. H. (ed.): Otolaryngology, Vol. III. Hagerstown, Md., Harper & Row, Chap. 19.

Farrior, R. T., and Connolly, M. E. 1970. Septorhinoplasty in Children. Otolaryngol. Clin. North Am. 3:345.

Gilbert, J. G., and Segal, S. 1958. Growth of the nose and the septorhinoplastic problems in youth. Arch. Otolaryngol. 68:673.

Gray, L. P. 1978. Deviated nasal septum, incidence and etiology. Ann. Otol. Rhinol. Laryngol. 87, Suppl. 50.

Hammer, G., and Radberg, C. 1961. Sphenoidal sinus: Anatomical and roentgenologic study with reference to transsphenoid hypophysectomy. Acta Radiol. 56:401.

Hinck, V. C., and Hopkins, C. E. 1965. Concerning growth of the sphenoid sinus. Arch. Otolaryngol. 82:62.

Kirchner, J. A. 1955. Traumatic nasal deformity in the newborn. Arch. Otolaryngol. 62:139.

Maresh, M. M. 1940. Paranasal sinuses from birth to late adolescence. Am. J. Dis. Child. 60:58.

Moore, K. L. 1973. The Developing Human. Philadelphia, W. B. Saunders Co., pp. 150–151.

Moore, W. J., and Lavelle, C. L. 1974. Growth of the Facial Skeleton in the Hominoidea. London, Academic Press, Inc.

Pratt, L. W. 1965. Midline cysts of the nasal dorsum: Embryologic origin and treatment. Laryngoscope 75:968.

Reichert, H. 1963. Plastic Surgery of the nose in children. Plast. Reconstr. Surg. 31:51.

Ritter, F. N. 1973. The Paranasal Sinuses: Anatomy and Surgical Technique. St. Louis, The C. V. Mosby Co.

Schaeffer, J. P. 1920. The Nose, Paranasal Sinuses, Nasolacrimal Passageways, and Olfactory Organ in Man. A Genetic, Developmental and Anatomico-Physiological Consideration. Philadelphia, Blakiston Co.

Scott, J. H. 1953. The cartilage of the nasal septum. Br. Dent. J. 95:37.

Van Alyea, O. E. 1941. Sphenoid sinus, anatomic study, with consideration of the clinical significance of the structural characteristics of sphenoid sinus. Arch. Otolaryngol. 34:225.

Van Alyea, O. E. 1951. Nasal Sinuses, An Anatomic and Clinical Consideration, 2nd ed. Baltimore, Williams & Wilkins Co.

Vidic, B. 1968. The postnatal development of the sphenoidal sinus and its spread into the dorsum sellae and posterior clinoid processes. Am. J. Roentgenol. 104:177.

Zimmerman, A. A. 1938. Development of the paranasal sinuses. Arch. Otolaryngol. 27:793.

Chapter 29

NASAL PHYSIOLOGY

Timothy P. McBride, M.D.

From birth onward, the nose is uniquely positioned to perform certain physiologic functions that enhance the airway and buttress the body's defense against infectious and environmental intrusion. Not only is the nose the primary airway of infancy, but deformation of this air conduit may cause enough symptomatic obstruction that surgical intervention, in the form of a tracheotomy or nasal surgery, is needed to sustain life. The nose humidifies the air and adjusts the temperature closer to that of the internal milieu. Its cycle resistance patterns are integrated via a neural network into the overall pulmonary system and provide a needed control area to optimize lung function.

The nasal hairs and the rich mucous blanket provide a highly efficient filter mechanism that removes inspired particulate matter. A mucociliary clearance action continually sweeps the accumulated debris into the gullet and removes any of the sinus discharge that drips from the various sinus ostia located in the midnose. Immunoglobulins can be secreted in the nose and begin an early neutralization of infectious particles prior to their widespread seeding of the pulmonary tract. The nose also contains specialized nerve cell endings that provide the sense of smell.

PHYSIOLOGIC ANATOMY

Spatial Relationships

It is simplest to think of the nose as a protruding midface structure that is centered above the oropharynx. This location allows the back-up oral airway to be economically used when there is primary nasal obstruction. Additionally, the nasal airway intake port is always under the watch of the eyes during periods of environmental danger. Anatomically, it is composed of three parts: the bony pyramid, the upper lateral cartilages, and the septum.

The nasal valve is the area of greatest airway resistance throughout the entire pulmonary tract; thus, the valve may be considered a choke point for control purposes. It lies between the upper and the lower lateral cartilages. The stiffness of the nasal cartilages is of absolute importance in preventing inspiratory collapse of the nasal soft tissues and resultant obstruction.

The septum, which divides the nose into right and left compartments, is made up of the quadrangular cartilage and the vomer. The columella is the portion of the quadrangular cartilage that extends the nose out from above the upper lip and provides the medial boundary of the right and left nostrils.

The internal structure of the nose is complex and consistent with the varied functions the nose is required to perform. The walls and floor of the nose are rigid. The roof arches upward from the nasal tip to the cribriform plate. The floor is level, or slightly downsloping, as it comes to the superior surface of the soft palate. The interior nose opens posteriorly into the nasopharynx through the two choanae. The shape of the internal structures serves to modify and direct the nasal airflow.

The septum, in its posterior portion, becomes bony as it joins with the rigid skeletal frame of the nasopharynx. The posterior septum is composed of the perpendicular plate of the ethmoid superiorly, the vomer and the rostrum of the sphenoid bone posteriorly, and the crests of the maxillary and palatine bones inferiorly. Congenital septal deformities are common, particularly along the maxillary crest, and if they are severe enough, they may cause symptomatic nasal obstruction. It is important to note that the vast majority of nontraumatic deformities are minor and do not cause nasal obstruction. The presence of an abnormality itself is not sufficient reason to perform surgery, unless there is symptomatic obstruction and the subject is of an appropriate age with regard to the cartilage growth centers.

There are three turbinates attached to each lateral wall. The inferior turbinate is the most prominent and contains its own skeletal bone, the concha. The middle and the superior turbinates are extensions of the ethmoid bone. The turbinates enlarge in diameter as they extend in a posterior direction, and they also cover the entire lateral nasal wall from the anterior nares to the choanae.

The paranasal sinuses are hollow, air-filled structures that lie immediately adjacent to the nose and are connected to the nose via small ostia that are located on the lateral nasal wall. It is important to realize that all of the paranasal sinus secretions must drain into the nose, for there is no other outlet for these anatomic cul-de-sacs except these ostia. Various degrees of nasal inflammation may narrow the ostia and predispose a patient to infection. The ostia are grouped into three meati: the superior, the middle, and the inferior. The middle meatus, which lies between the middle and the inferior turbinates, is the most important. The middle meatus ostia from anterior to posterior drain sequentially the frontal sinus, the maxillary sinus, and the anterior ethmoid cells. The superior meatus, under the superior turbinate, drains the posterior ethmoid cells. The inferior meatus, which lies under the inferior portion of the inferior turbinate, does not drain a sinus but rather is the orifice for the nasolacrimal duct. This is essential for draining the large volume of normal tears from the eyes.

The anatomic development of the nose reviewed in the previous chapter notes that the nasal airway undergoes significant change in shape during early infancy, but at the end of the first year of life, the shape and the function are similar to those of an adult nose (Negus, 1958). The nose continues to enlarge in size until puberty, and similarly its total resistance will decrease as its size increases. However, because of autoregulation of the mucosal surface thickness and neural arc influences on the same tissue, the skeletal diameters do not form a one-to-one correlation with the total resistance patterns and age. It is important to understand that in spite of the higher nasal resistance of the infant, the infant is reluctant to use the oropharyngeal airway until the seventh to ninth month (Cole, 1982). This observation is not well understood.

The Mucous Membranes

The bones and the cartilage that form the framework of the nose are covered by periosteum or perichondrium. Overlying this on the inside of the nose is a highly specialized thick, rich vascular mucous membrane. This membrane is similar to the respiratory epithelium that lines the paranasal sinuses, the eustachian tube, and the tracheobronchial tree. However, the nasal membrane differs in that there is a greater density of ciliated cells and mucous glands.

The respiratory epithelium is composed of pseudostratified columnar cells with cilia. The actual shape of the ciliated cell varies with the cell's position in the nasal cavity. Along the surface of the turbinates and septum, one finds short irregular surface cilia, while near the ostia of the sinuses, one finds short columnar cells with long cilia. The cells of the membrane on the anterior portion of the turbinate and the nasal vestibule resemble squamous cells rather than columnar cells and do not contain cilia. The sinuses, by contrast, are lined by cuboidal cells and scanty cilia.

The dense vascularity and many glands in the submucosa of the nose warm and humidify the inspired air. The glands are racemose in that they contain both serum-producing and mucus-producing cell types. Additionally, there are varying numbers of goblet cells interspersed among the surface columnar cells that contribute to the total nasal secretion. The number and the density of the goblet cells are not constant and may vary with conditions that alter airflow patterns, such as septal deflections and chronic inflammation.

The ciliated cells that are concentrated in the nose blend into the upper nasopharynx. There is no district border where the ciliated cells change over to stratified squamous epithelium of the oropharynx, but autopsy studies show that the change occurs in the area where the soft palate touches the lateral and posterior wall of the pharynx during the act of swallowing. It is important to note that the ciliated cells extend through the nasal opening of the eustachian tube and line the tubal surface into the cavity of the middle ear, where the concentration of ciliated cells begins to thin out.

Surface Histology and Microanatomy

The types of epithelial cells that have been identified in the nose are basal cells, goblet cells, and columnar cells (both ciliated and nonciliated). The typical microscopic section shows pseudostratified columnar cells in contact with the basement membrane, but not all the cells reach out to the surface. A thin basement membrane lies under the epithelial cells, and below this is a connective tissue layer of collagen fibrils that averages 8 microns in depth. The basement membrane layer together with the connective tissue separates the epithelium from the submucosal structures (Fig. 29–1).

Basal cells lie on the basement membrane. These cells are short, flat cells that have electron-dense cytoplasm and are thought of as replacement cells for

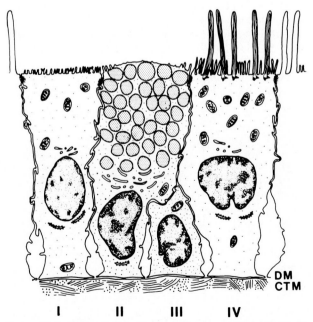

Figure 29–1. Transmission electron microscope diagram of cell types in the pseudostratified ciliated columnar epithelium. I, Nonciliated columnar cell with microvilli. II, Goblet cell with mucous granules. III, Basal cell. IV, Ciliated columnar cell. DM, Basement membrane; CTM, connective tissue membrane. (With permission from Mygind, N. 1979. Nasal Allergy. Oxford, Blackwell Scientific Publications.)

the respiratory epithelium. Mitosis has been observed in these stem cells, and it is thought that they can differentiate into either ciliated or goblet cells after they pass through an intermediate cell phase. The turnover rate for the basal cells is not known.

The goblet cells together with the nasal glands in the submucosa produce the mucous secretions of the nose. The goblet cells are arranged perpendicular to the epithelial surface and in direct contact with the basement membrane. Autoradiographic studies have shown that the synthesis and release of mucus takes place continuously. The secretion of mucus occurs when the internal mucin droplet membrane fuses with the stomal membrane.

Unlike the goblet cells of the intestinal tract, which have a lifetime of about three days, the nasal goblet cells last beyond 14 days. Studies of the fetal distribution of the goblet cells first note their presence in the anterior nares at the 13th week. There is a progressive posterior migration of the cells along the floor of the nose, and they are found in the nasopharynx by the 17th week. After that, a gradual migration superiorly over the septum and the turbinates will cover the entire nasal surface by the 30th week.

The goblet cell distribution measured by density measurement is not entirely uniform. Areas of greater airflow show a fewer number of cells, whereas areas of airflow obstruction show a greater number of cells. Infection increases the number of goblet cells associated with an increased number of basal cells. The interplay of these factors is poorly understood at this time (Tos and Poulsen, 1975).

The columnar ciliated cells are positioned on the basement membrane and are joined together by tight cell junctions. The lumenal surface of these cells is covered by 50 to 100 cilia and 300 to 400 microvilli that are unrelated to the cilia. Their function is reviewed below with the mucous blanket physiology. In contrast with the goblet cells, to our knowledge there are no studies of the density patterns of fetal nasal cilia.

Nasal Glands

The nasal glands produce the greatest proportion of the nasal secretions. They are located in the submucosal stroma below the basement membrane. There are three major types of nasal glands: (1) anterior serous glands, (2) seromucous glands, and (3) Bowman glands. There are many glands distributed throughout each nasal cavity, particularly of the seromucous type, whereas there are only a scattered few found in the paranasal sinuses.

The anterior serous glands are located near the nasal vestibule. Each of these glands has ducts 2 to 20 mm in length that empty into small crypts. It is thought that their strategic placement in the vestibule plays an important part in keeping the nasal mucosa moist. The forces of nasal breathing spread the serous secretions backward like a nasal spray. Their total contribution to nasal secretion, however, is thought to be minimal.

There is only a small number of these gland types, and the serous secretions that drip from the nose from colds or allergies do not originate from these glands.

The smaller seromucous glands are distributed throughout the entire nose and are present in large numbers. These glands are the primary secretory glands of the nose. The glands have a short duct and contain both serum-secreting and mucin-secreting cells. They are similar to the glands found in the trachea and secrete a varying seromucous mixture. Their control mechanism is not understood, but there appear to be both neural and mediator components of secretion control. These glands lie in the immediate submucosal area and are found in fetal nasal preparations by the 11th week. The glands migrate posteriorly and superiorly to all areas of the nose by the 18th week. The distribution density is greatest in the anterior third of the nose.

Bowman glands are very small, serous glands found in the olfactory region. They have short tubules and are lined with cubical serous cells. First noted in the 15th week, the density of the glands is three times greater than the density of the seromucous respiratory glands. Their function is not understood, but the assumption is that they play a role in the sense of smell (Tos and Poulsen, 1975).

In contrast to the nose, the paranasal sinuses have far fewer glands. Except for the 30-mm² area around the sinus ostia, there is no glandular layer in the sinus mucosa. A few isolated glands are found widely scattered in the mucosa, but there are large areas without glands. Because of this, the mucus-producing capacity of the sinuses is small compared with that of the nose. It is thought that, because there is no airflow, the mucosa needs little protection from drying. In addition, the small amount of evaporation that takes place from the mucosa is easily compensated for by the goblet cells.

Cilia

Cilia are phylogenetically old structures that are found in many unicellular organisms and in some cells of almost all multicellular animals. They are structures that project from the cell surface and exhibit an intrinsic rhythmic movement that propels the cell, or the fluid lying over the cell if the cell is fixed in place. All motile cilia have the same basic structure, but the motion may be modified to fit the needs of the particular organ or organism.

Cilia in the human nose are thought to have a beat frequency of 1000 beats per minute and a velocity of 0.8 cm per minute. They have the characteristic "biphasic motion" that all cilia possess, consisting of a rapid "effective stroke" and a slow "recovery stroke." The whiplike recoil of the "recovery stroke" occurs in the periciliary layer below the layer of the mucous blanket. When the cilium has returned to its starting position, the fully extended cilium's tip reaches up into the mucous layer; thus, when the "effective stroke" begins, the calcium propels the mucous layer in the direction of the stroke.

The cilium is made up of an external shaft and an intracellular basal body. The shaft has the standard 9 + 2 pattern: 9 peripheral microtubule doublets and 2 central single microtubules. The outer doublets are connected to each other by nexin links, while the A microtubule of each doublet contains 2 dynein arms. The basal body, to which the shaft is rooted, is just under the cell surface. It is thought that the basal body is identical to the mitotic centriole of the cell nucleus. It has a small projection known as the basal foot. This structure points in the direction of the shaft's "effective stroke."

There is an amazing degree of coordination between the cilia. When the surface of a nasal membrane is observed under a microscope, wavelike motions are observed. It stands to reason that if the mucous blanket is to be moved in one direction, then synchrony must be present. It is not known how this synchrony is achieved, but mechanical impulses transferred from one cell to the next provide both the stimulus and the coordination. Neural control has not been observed, and hormonal control is thought to be limited to parasympathetic alteration of the viscosity of the mucus or the total amount of mucous production (Sleigh, 1977).

The Mucociliary Clearance System

The mucociliary clearance system provides a basic function for the nasal airway. Through the actions of the ciliary transport system, the interior nasal surface is kept clean, moist, and fresh. The clearance system is made up of the mucous blanket, the periciliary fluid layers, and the ciliated cells. It is important to understand that all three components of the transport system are needed for the mucociliary clearance system to function.

The Mucous Blanket

The mucous blanket is a thin, sticky, continuous, highly viscid secretion that covers all the surfaces of the nose, ear, sinuses, and tracheobronchial tree. It is propelled continuously, along with any particles trapped in it, by the ciliated cells. The mucous blanket in the nose moves posteriorly through the nasal choanae into the pharynx, where it is swallowed.

The mucous layer is commonly referred to as a carpet or blanket. It is made up of secretions from the goblet cells and the material secreted from the nasal glands. The blanket is found superficial to the periciliary layer, which is the watery fluid bath surrounding the beating cilia. The depth of the mucous blanket is approximately 20 microns, but it is not always uniform and, in some areas, may be temporarily absent (Adler et al., 1973). The mucous blanket is secreted through the periciliary layer and then, through its viscoelastic properties, forms into partial islands and incomplete sheets.

The sticky, slimy characteristics of mucus have been studied for many years. Glycoproteins contribute 70 to 80 per cent of the dry weight of mucus; the remaining portions are made up from immunoglobulins and albumin. Ninety-seven per cent of its biological weight is due to water, but variations in the water content change in response to the control mechanisms, the state of hydration, and the presence of nasal pathology. Mucus is a nonnewtonian viscoelastic substance; therefore, its flow properties are time dependent rather than linear. Depending on the rate of ciliary beat, the elasticity of the mucus may affect the rate of transit time to a greater extent than the viscosity does.

The Periciliary Fluid

Although the mucus layer has long been recognized, histologic sections have consistently shown that the mucous blanket lies above the cilia and is not interspersed among them. The fluid that surrounds the beating cilia has a different ionic and viscous consistency. It is called the periciliary fluid layer. Little is known about its origins and what is known is derived from studies on the trachea rather than the nasal mucosa.

The periciliary layer is thought to be created through the actions of a chloride pump located on the cellular surface. The fluid has a higher chloride and sodium concentration than does plasma and also has a greater osmolality. Although the depth control of the periciliary fluid is important for effective transport, it is unknown how the depth is regulated.

The ciliary motion creates currents in the superficial layer of the periciliary fluid. In certain situations, particles and solubilized dyes in the periciliary fluid stream are transported entirely through the stream independent of the mucous blanket, and at a different rate of speed than that of the surface mucous blanket (Fig. 29–2).

Measures of Clearance Times

Although a number of different methods have been developed to measure mucociliary clearance times, these are mostly of a basic research nature and have found little clinical application (Lippman, 1970). The earliest methods used colored or highly visible materials. Small disks, dyes, iron filings, radioisotope-labeled resin particles, and saccharin all have been tested and found to have some validity. It has been observed that the size, density, and consistency of the particle have little effect on the actual transport time of the marker.

One criticism of these methods, however, is that they do not differentiate between surface clearance and periciliary clearance. It has proved difficult to separate these two phases of transport. While the determination of a normal clearance range has been

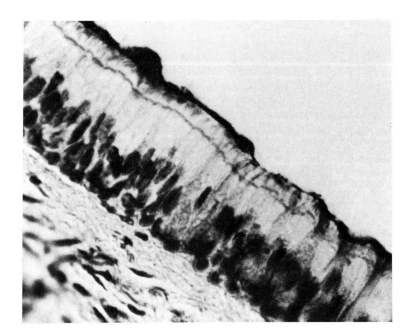

Figure 29–2. Frozen section of mucosa. Mucus is seen overlying the clear periciliary fluid layer above the pseudostratified respiratory epithelium. (With permission from Proctor, D. F., and Anderson, I. B. [eds.]. 1982. The Nose: Upper Airway Physiology and the Atmospheric Environment. Amsterdam, Elsevier Science Publishers.)

accomplished, 20 per cent of otherwise normal subjects lie outside of the range. This makes it difficult to apply the physiologic measures to disease states of individual patients who are seen after symptoms are developed.

The average rate of transit is 8 mm per minute. Slow clearance (less than 1 mm per minute) is not understood, but it is thought to be due to variations in secretions rather than differences in frequencies of ciliary beats. During the nasal transit period, some subject, for unknown reasons, will have episodic stasis during which particle movement is halted, but most subjects will show a constant steady particle passage. There is good agreement regarding rate of transit within the passage time in each individual when the tests are done sequentially or when the right passage is compared with the left passage. Some investigators have found a modest increase in the transit time during exercise. To some extent, the transit system is under the influence of the autonomic system via the secretion control system. Pharmacologic agents (e.g., beta-adrenergic agonists, which enhance the clearance time) may affect the total transit time (Camner et al, 1976). Epinephrine hydrochloride, when applied to ciliated cells, causes 20 minutes of reversible inhibition. Alterations in the pH, temperature, and ambient humidity have been shown to affect the transit time.

In some persons with known structural ciliary defects, such as patients with Kartagener syndrome, in whom there is a known absence of the dynein arms, there is a total lack of nasal mucociliary transport. The influenza virus that destroys the ciliated cells is known to disrupt ciliary transport for up to six weeks after infection. Rhinovirus infections, which cause 40 per cent of common colds, do not destroy the ciliated cells but nonetheless prolong transit time for three weeks after infection. The site of the lesion is not known for the common cold, but there is the possibility that the depth of the periciliary fluid is altered, leading to a decoupling of the mucous blanket from the cilia. It is not known how allergies affect nasal transit times.

We depend on the clearance system to remove and filter particulate matter in the nose. The efficiency of this system is optimized through the coordination of the beating cilia and the correct depth and consistency of the fluids lining the nasal surface.

Nasal Blood Supply and Lymphatic Drainage

The first well-done studies of the nasal vasculature were done in the 1850's. The subepithelial capillary network and the cavernous plexus in the turbinates were identified (Kolliker, 1852). The nasal glands were noted, and erectile tissue was demonstrated through air injection into the cavernous plexi of the turbinates (Kohlrausch, 1853).

The nasal surface receives its blood supply from the maxillary, ophthalmic, and facial arteries. The sphenopalatine branch of the internal maxillary artery supplies the turbinates, meatus, and septum. The anterior and the posterior ethmoid branches of the ophthalmic artery supply the ethmoid and the frontal sinuses and the roof of the nose. A branch of the superior labial artery supplies the nasal vestibule, anterior septum, and parts of the maxillary sinus. One septal branch, the nasopalatine artery, extends to the vermonasal organ and the incisive canal through which it anastomoses with the greater palatine artery. The septal branches of the sphenopalatine artery form multiple anastomoses with terminal branches of the anterior ethmoidal and facial arteries in the Kiesselbach triangle.

The arterioles of the nasal respiratory mucosa are distinctive because they lack an internal elastic layer, and the vascular endothelial basement membrane is continuous with smooth muscle cells in the walls of the arterioles. Because of this, it is thought that the subendothelial musculature of these vessels is more readily influenced than other vessels by agents such as histamine and pharmacologic vasoconstrictors.

Veins accompanying the branches of the sphenopalatine artery drain into the pterygoid plexus. The ethmoidal veins join with the ophthalmic plexus in the orbit. From there, the venous blood proceeds to the cavernous sinus. There are also many anastomoses with the veins of the face, pharynx, palate, and the superficial cerebral veins that drain through the cribriform plate.

There are multiple venous plexi and venous lakes underneath the mucous membrane. The plexi receive their blood from the capillaries and through arteriovenous anastomosis. The plexi are particularly well developed over the middle and the inferior turbinates (Fig. 29–3). The venous system of the nose, sinuses, and orbit communicates freely through valveless veins. Venous stasis related to nasal congestion is thought to be responsible for dark circles under the eyes, otherwise known as allergic shiners.

Small regular capillaries are found in the submucosa, but in the next layer down the capillaries are larger and have many fenestrations. These larger capillaries are very porous and allow for rapid passage of fluid through the vascular walls. It is interesting to note that the fenestrations of the deep capillary layer are always oriented to the nasal lumenal surface. It had been thought that the source of humidification for the nasal airflow came from the nasal glands, but since higher secretory production of these glands does not increase the degree of humidification some observers think that the fenestrations are the source of the humidification fluid (Cauna et al., 1972).

The lymphatic drainage of the nose is divided into an anterior and a posterior network. The anterior network drains along the facial vessels to the nodes of the submaxillary glands. Most of the anterior nose, the vestibule, and the preturbinal area is drained in this way. The posterior network drains the major portion of the nose, and it forms three channels. The superior group, from the middle and the superior turbinates, and adjacent septum, forms channels passing above the eustachian tube to drain into the retropharyngeal nodes. The middle group, passing below the eustachian tube, serves the inferior turbinate, the inferior meatus, and a portion of the floor, and drains into the external jugular system of nodes. The inferior group, from the septum and a part of the floor, drains through lymph nodes along the internal jugular vein.

Innervation of the Nose

The innervation of the nose consists of the olfactory nerve (the first cranial nerve), branches of the trigeminal nerve (the fifth cranial nerve), and autonomic nerves. The nerves enter the nose by three tracts and foramen: the cribriform plate, the sphenopalatine foramen, and the ethmoidal foramen.

Sensory innervation is provided by the olfactory and the trigeminal nerves. The paired olfactory nerves enter through the cribriform plate located in the superior nasal vault. This nerve is mainly concerned with the sense of smell, described later. The remaining nerves that supply sensation to the nasal mucosa are derived from the upper two divisions of the trigeminal nerve: the ophthalmic and the maxillary nerves. These two branches enter through the ethmoidal and sphenopalatine foramina, respectively. The sphenopalatine ganglion is found near the sphenopalatine foramen. There the postganglionic parasympathetic fibers from the ganglion and the postganglionic sympathetic fibers

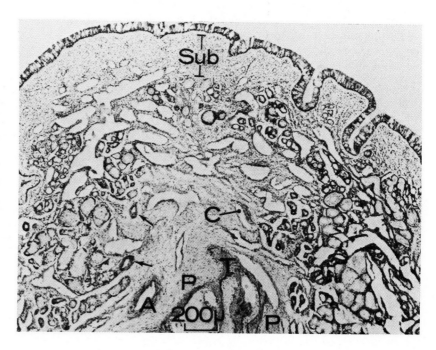

Figure 29–3. Respiratory mucosa from the lower border of the inferior turbinate. The subepithelial zone (Sub) is well developed. The glandular zone is overlapped by the cavernous plexus (C), and both extend down to the periosteum (P), which covers the turbinate (T). A stem artery (A) is seen near the periosteum. (With permission from Proctor, D. F., and Anderson, I. B. [eds.]. 1982. The Nose: Upper Airway Physiology and the Atmospheric Environment. Amsterdam, Elsevier Science Publishers.)

from the cervical sympathetic ganglia join with the posterior (maxillary) nasal sensory nerve to enter the nose.

A major function of the parasympathetic fibers is to control glandular nasal secretions. As early as 1898, it was shown that stimulation of the dog's sphenopalatine ganglia causes profuse watery nasal discharge (Prevost, 1898). Sympathetic nerves are not thought to influence nasal secretions except through indirect actions on the nasal vasculature (Anggard and Densert, 1974).

UPPER RESPIRATORY AIRFLOW

Although the vast body of pulmonary literature has focused on the lower airway, clinical observation has repeatedly noted that an obstruction in any of the flow segments of the airway can cause significant debility. An increase in pulmonary resistance, together with changes in blood gas measures and decreased lung compliance, has been reported in subjects with artificial nasal obstruction (Wyllie et al., 1976). Distant reflexes that cause decreased pulmonary resistance have been elicited when vasoconstrictors were applied to the nasal mucosa. It is clear that the nose is an integral part of the airway and cannot be divorced from the dynamics of the whole airway, but the examination of nasal function does require special attention, in order to understand the pulmonary inputs of this uniquely designed organ.

Infants are obligatory nasal breathers, and nasal obstruction in the infant is a life-threatening condition. Bilateral choanal atresia requires immediate surgical intervention, and partial nasal obstruction is a matter of great concern. Nasal resistance is greater in infants than adults, but the ratio of nasal resistance to total airway resistance is less. Additionally, the location of the larynx in the infant is higher in the neck, with the soft palate in close proximity with the epiglottis, and a velopharyngeal sphincter has been described. These observations in themselves do not explain the infant's dependence on the nasal airway, but it is clear that the nasal airway is critical for the first six months of life (Purcell, 1976).

The Nasal Valve and Mucosa

Air enters the nose through the nasal valve, which is an inverted trumpet-shaped orifice. Each passage narrows from a 90-mm^2 area to a 30-mm^2 triangular slit called the nasal valve. The nasal valve has the smallest cross-sectional diameter and greatest resistance of the airway that is proximal to the alveoli. The shape and the size of the nasal valve is modified through the actions of small alar muscles and by the airflow pressures generated by airflow rates. The muscle activity prevents alar collapse during inspiration. Electromyographic studies show muscle dilator activity occurring with inspiration (Mann et al., 1977). This activity is important, because even at rest, there is a

differential pressure of at least 2 cm H$_2$O. Alar dilator activity is synchronous with that of the pharyngeal and laryngeal dilators and precedes diaphragmatic activity.

Air, after passing through the valve, is streamlined into a column 1 to 3 mm thick and flows along the floor between the turbinates and the septum. The nasal mucosa is approximately 160 cm^2 and the volume is about 20 ml. The cross-sectional area of the main nasal cavity is 130 mm^2. The transit time of a portion of air, while in a basal resting state, is less than one twentieth of a second. Resistance in this segment is created by the turbinate size, which is altered by the vascular tone and blood volume of the nasal sinusoids. Changes in the nasal resistance are noted in the nasal cycle shifts, which is described later, and are induced by exercise, posture changes, and hyperventilation. Chemical irritants, medications, pain, and emotion are also thought to influence nasal resistance. Changes in mucosal volume occur rapidly and can fluctuate synchronously with inspiration and expiration.

Airflow

On inspiration, air passes vertically upward in the nose at a velocity of 2 to 3 meters per second. At the nasal valve, the airflow becomes horizontal and laminar. Airspeeds at the nasal valve reach 12 to 18 meters per second, which is equivalent to gale force winds. Hurricane airspeeds are attained during sniffs and snorts. When the airstream enters the nasal cavity proper, where the cross-sectional area is greater, the resulting decrease in velocity and altered direction cause disruption of the laminar flow. The disruption allows for humidification and warming of the inspired air. Most of the air continues horizontally parallel to the middle turbinate for 8 cm to where it joins the air from the other nostril in the nasopharynx (Swift and Proctor, 1977).

In addition to the rates of airflow, the volume flow measures are of interest. Pressure recordings are characteristic for the section of the airway from which they were obtained. Resistance is a pressure-flow ratio that can be obtained by using an X-Y plot of the flow and pressure (Fig. 29–4). Individual breaths across the nasal cavity produce a sigmoid tracing, the points of which represent the instantaneous nasal resistance, that is used to assess the degree of nasal patency. Through the use of microprocessors, bounded derivatives such as work and power can be obtained and studied (Cole et al., 1980).

Rhinomanometry is the measurement of the nasal respiratory function. Nasal pressures and flow studies have been performed for many years. Both mechanical and hydrostatic methods were used almost a century ago. There are four methods: anterior active, anterior passive, posterior active, and posterior passive. In each of these methods, an X-Y pressure-versus-flow graph is generated, and the nasal resistance is derived. There are many ways to describe obstruction in mathematical

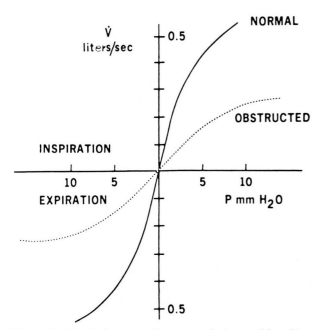

Figure 29–4. Typical pressure-flow curves during nasal breathing at rest. (With permission from Proctor, D. F., and Anderson, I. B. [eds.]. 1982. The Nose: Upper Airway Physiology and the Atmospheric Environment. Amsterdam, Elsevier Science Publishers.)

terms, but their variety has made it difficult to compare them.

These attempts to standardize nasal air flow measures were spurred by the need for a valid clinical tool to take the place of simple nasal inspection. Structural abnormalities are present in approximately 75 per cent of noses, and the dynamic irregularities, such as alar collapse, are difficult to document. Measurements show that only a small number of the structurally abnormal noses have abnormal nasal resistances. Conversely, the patients with symptomatic obstruction frequently show obstruction on rhinomanometry.

In the last decade, the use of microcomputers has led to more practical methods of measures. The research that has been done in the pediatric age group has focused on the normal child. It has been possible to document the presence of an altered nasal cycle and the inherently higher nasal resistance in the child using computer-assisted techniques.

The Nasal Cycle

The term nasal cycle refers to the alternating changes in patency of the right and the left nasal cavities (Fig. 29–5). The nose is divided into two nasal passages by the septum, and the nasal mucosa of each side has a separate autonomic innervation. Congestion and decongestion of the erectile tissues of the nasal mucosa of the lateral nasal wall and septum occur in rhythmic sequence in about 80 per cent of normal individuals. As one nasal chamber opens and the mucosal glands secrete, the erectile tissues of the opposite chamber fill with blood. The presence of this

periodic congestion-decongestion was first described by Kayser in 1895 and labeled the "nasal cycle."

The average person is completely unaware of the alternation of nasal airflow because the total resistance to the nasal airflow remains constant. The cycle is controlled through the autonomic adrenergic centers, and investigators have postulated a hypothalamic control center. If the cervical ganglion is sectioned, there is abolition of the nasal cycle on the side on which the sympathetic ganglion was cut. The cycle oscillates every three to four hours and is exaggerated during periods of inflammation. Head position and body posture, through their effects on hydrostatic pressure, can influence the intensity and duration of the cycle. Vasoconstrictive medications can temporarily interrupt the cycle.

Children do not have a fully functioning nasal cycle, but rather a cycle in which both nares are simultaneously obstructed. This "solid" cycle was observed in children 3 to 6 years of age and lasted one hour instead of three hours. This may be due to an incompletely developed adrenergic system and offers an explanation

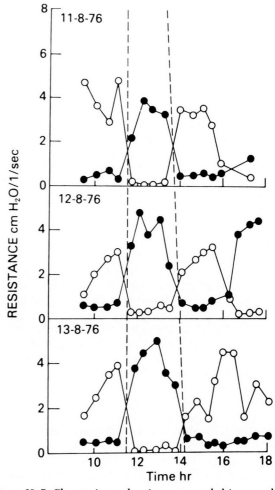

Figure 29–5. Changes in nasal resistance recorded in one subject on three consecutive days. The clear circles indicate the left nasal passage, and the black circles indicate the right nasal passage. (With permission from Eccles, R. The domestic pig as an experimental animal for studies on the nasal cycle. Acta Otolaryngol. [Stockh.] 85[5–6]:431–436, May–June.)

for the child who mouth breathes in the absence of adenoidal hypertrophy or allergies (Van Cauwenberge and Deleye, 1984).

It is unfortunate that there are no satisfactory explanations for the existence of the nasal cycle. It has been observed in other animals such as the rabbit and the pig. Some guesses include that of a nasal lymphatic pump, humidification control, air-conditioning maintenance down time, and a distant reflection of the periodicity inherent in the adrenergic control system.

Nasal Pharmacology

The nasal vasculature is extremely sensitive to pharmacologic intervention. Antihistamines and sympathomimetics are the most commonly used drugs in the treatment of nasal congestion, and occasionally anticholinergics are used for this condition.

Epinephrine and pseudoephedrine administered into the circulation or applied topically to the nasal mucosa result in pronounced vasoconstriction of the erectile tissue. Rebound vasodilation occurs with cessation of these drugs and is thought to be due to the prolonged tissue hypoxia incurred by the decreased blood flow through the turbinate sinusoids. Alpha-antagonists, when used as antihypertensive medications, block the effect of endogenous sympathomimetics and may cause annoying nasal congestion (Malm, 1974).

Parasympathetics cause a watery nasal secretion and some tissue congestion. Atropine can reduce nasal discharge when administered in small doses. There are conditions under which atropine has no effect on the amount of nasal discharge. It is postulated that these conditions occur when the inflammation is due to particular mediators such as vasoactive peptides and prostaglandins.

Histamine causes vasodilatation when it comes into contact with the nasal mucosa and stimulates sneezing. Histamine also activates a reflex arc that causes stimulation of the parasympathetic nerves and results in a watery discharge. It is thought that in nasal allergies histamine is released from mast cells near or in the nasal mucosa. Antihistamines are widely used in the treatment of nasal allergies, but their efficacy has been disputed. Their actions are poorly understood, and some investigators doubt that they affect the surface release of histamine in the nose.

Corticosteroids have shown some effect in the treatment of nasal allergies through their local application to the nasal mucosa. They seem to dampen the nasal inflammatory response through the suppression of inflammatory mediator release, but, in truth, their complex effects are poorly understood (Mygind, 1979).

Hormonal influences appear to affect the nose as nasal obstruction is often observed with puberty, pregnancy, hypothyroidism, and menstruation (Sorri et al., 1980). High levels of circulating estrogen are associated with a hypertrophic rhinitis, and experimentally used estrogens cause nasal edema and congestion in guinea pigs. This "nasogenital" relationship seems to be mediated through the sphenopalatine ganglion in that it is abolished when the ganglion is removed. The nasal symptoms seen with hypothyroidism resemble that of vasomotor rhinitis. In this condition, the nasal tissues accumulate acid mucopolysaccharides, which leads to tissue congestion.

OLFACTION

Even though much is unknown about the sense of smell, the ability of the nose to discriminate between odorous compounds is quite remarkable. The smell sense organ can analyze a wide variety of compounds and frequently can detect odor substances that are measured in the parts-per-billion range. Although the sense of smell is of less importance in humans than in other species, odors still play a part in everyday life. They are important in food choices and in social interaction; they can be a warning sign for toxic gases and spoiled foods.

To smell a substance, the molecules of that substance must somehow reach the olfactory mucosa located in the roof of the nose (Fig. 29–6). The odor sensation is then determined by the number of odorant particles that reach the olfactory receptor at a given time. The odor-producing substance must have a vapor pressure and must be relatively water- and lipid-soluble in order to be sensed. The final perception is the result of processing mechanisms of the central nervous system that have eluded our understanding.

The olfactory mucosa is approximately 200 to 400 mm^2. In the rabbit, there are 50,000 receptor cells per square millimeter, each of which is a specialized neural cell with dendrites that project into the nasal mucus. The odorous compound is thought to combine with the dendritic membrane, causing a temporary change in the membrane structure. This alteration generates a potential that is sent through unmyelinated nerve fibers to the olfactory bulb located on the cortical side of the cribriform plate.

In the olfactory bulb, fibers are bunched topographically and are wrapped in myelin sheets. Once the fibers are parceled into the myelin bundles, they are routed to one of the "glomeruli" found in the bulb. In the rabbit, there are about 2000 glomeruli, and each of these glomeruli receives 25,000 fibers. Signals from the bulb are sent to the cortex for further processing. The mechanism of odor recognition and identification is not known (Berglund and Lindvall, 1982).

It is thought that odor sensation is never immediate, but requires a build-up phase for the odor to reach its full intensity. This process of temporal integration is not found in the senses of vision or hearing. The sense of smell is easily fatigued with prolonged exposure to a substance, but rapid recovery of recognition is the rule after the termination of the exposure. It is not known whether recovery is a central or a peripheral phenomenon. The detection of an odor has been measured using threshold techniques. It is known that

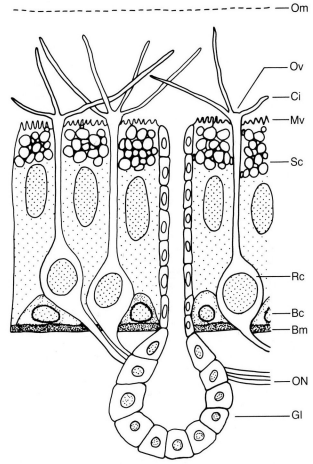

Figure 29–6. A schematic diagram of olfactory epithelium. Om, Surface of the olfactory mucus; Ov, olfactory vesicle; Ci, olfactory cilia; Mv, microvilli; Sc, supporting cell; Rc, olfactory receptor cell; Bc, basal cell; Bm, basement membrane; ON, olfactory nerve; Gl, olfactory gland. (With permission from Takagi, S. F. 1978. Biophysics of smell. *In* Carterette, E. C., and Friedman, M. P. [eds.]: Handbook of Perception. Vol. VI A: Tasting and Smelling. New York, Academic Press.)

there is a wide variability in interindividual and intraindividual sensitivity of smell detection for each particular substance (Engen, 1971). Of note, the threshold level of detection for hydrogen sulfide is 1 ppb. Although there are many variables to consider, the strongest correlation with loss of smell is an individual's increasing age. Temperature and humidity may alter the individual's smell detection, but there is only contradictory evidence for claims of sexual and hormonal differences (Lindvall, 1970).

Anosmia, or the lack of smell, is found in conditions of nasal obstruction and nasal infection. It seems obvious that the receptor molecule cannot reach the olfactory mucosa to stimulate a response. Nasal polyposis and nasal deformities are reversible conditions in adults. Infections and allergies cause temporary interruption of smell, and olfactory capability returns when the conditions resolve. Some investigators have reported that smell can trigger an asthmatic attack and can worsen emphysema. Others have thought that this phenomenon is a trigeminal reflex, which is induced by a chemical irritant stimulating the nasal mucosa,

and leads to reflex bronchial constriction (Alarie, 1973). As with much of what is known about the olfactory sense, it is at best poorly understood and remains mostly a mystery.

IMMUNOLOGY

The nose, because of its unique position at the portal of the airway, assumes an immunologic interest. Not only is it particularly exposed to infectious particles, but it can be viewed by the body's immunologic defenses as the first zone of engagement. It is not surprising that the body uses both local and systemic mechanisms to combat infectious and allergic invasion.

Secretory immunoglobulin A (IgA) is the major immunoglobulin found in nasal secretions and accounts for 10 to 50 per cent of the total protein content of nasal secretions (Bellanti et al., 1965). This dimeric version of the plasma IgA is produced locally in the nose by the plasma cells found in the submucosa near the seromucous glands. The secretory component is produced by the nasal glands and allows the IgA to be actively extruded onto the nasal surface. The concentration of IgG (3 per cent) and IgM (1 per cent) increases during actual infections, but this may be due to transudation of plasma resulting from mucosal injury. It has also been noticed that chronic nasal infections lead to a higher concentration of IgG-producing plasma cells in the submucosa.

Virus-neutralizing activity is greatest with the IgA fraction of nasal secretions, and the secretory type of IgA is thought to have a greater neutralizing effect than that of serum IgA. Levels of virus-specific IgA begin to rise in the nasal secretions two weeks after the initial infection in nonimmune persons. These levels peak three to four weeks after the initial infection. In persons who have circulating antibody present, the IgA level begins to rise at the end of the first week. Because the actual symptomatic infection may resolve at the end of five to seven days, the secretory antibody is not able to modify the infection in the nonimmune person (Butler et al., 1970).

In bacterial infections, the IgA coats the bacterial surface and prevents adherence to the nasal mucosa. This may explain the lack of colonization by certain types of bacteria. It has been shown in animal models that intraimmunization can prevent invasive infection in spite of the lack of serum immunity.

Immunoglobulin E is also produced in the nasal mucosa near the seromucous glands. IgE binds to tissue mast cells in the mucosa and submucosa. Its role in defense is poorly understood, but in allergic subjects, antigen degranulates the IgE–mast cell complex and causes the release of inflammatory mediators. These include histamine, prostaglandins, bradykinin, and leukotrienes. This release initiates the allergy cascade and can lead to the development of symptoms in varying degrees of severity (Riott, 1980).

Interferons are also found in the nasal secretions and are thought to derive from sensitized T-lymphocytes. They exhibit an antiviral activity that is indirect and seem to inhibit translation of viral RNA. Interferon is found one to two days after viral shedding occurs, and the level continues to rise throughout an infection (Jao et al., 1970). Interferon is not found in all infections, and exogenously applied interferon only sporadically reduces the severity of symptoms and the occurrence of infection.

SELECTED REFERENCES

Proctor, D. F., and Anderson, I. B. 1982. The Nose—Upper Airway Physiology and the Atmospheric environment. Amsterdam, Elsevier Biomedical Press.
This book is a wonderful textbook and sourcebook of nasal physiology and is highly recommended for students who wish more detail.
Sleigh, M. A. 1977. The nature and action of respiratory tract cilia. *In* Brain, J. D., Proctor, D. F., and Reid, L. M. (eds.): Respiratory Defense Mechanisms. New York, Marcel Dekker.
A comprehensive review of ciliary anatomy and physiology.
Swift, D. L., and Proctor, D. F. 1977. Access of air to the respiratory tract. *In* Brain, J. D., Proctor, D. F., and Reid, L. M. (eds.): Respiratory Defense Mechanisms. New York, Marcel Dekker.
A fine treatment of the study of nasal airflow with many interesting insights.

REFERENCES

Adler, K. B., Wooten, O., and Dulfano, M. J. 1973. Mammalian respiratory mucociliary clearance. Arch. Environ. Health 27:364.
Alarie, Y. 1973. Sensory irritation by airborne chemicals. CRC Crit. Rev. Toxicol. 2:299.
Anggard, A., and Densert, O. 1974. Adrenergic innervation of the nasal mucosa in the cat. Acta Otolaryngol. (Stockh.) 78:323.
Bellanti, J. A., Artenstein, M. S., and Beuscher, E. L. 1965. Characterization of virus-neutralizing antibodies in human serum and nasal secretions. J. Immunol. 94:344.
Berglund, B., and Lindvall, T. 1982. Olfaction. *In* Proctor, D. F., and Anderson I. B. (eds.): The Nose. Amsterdam, Elsevier Biomedical Press, pp. 279–305.
Butler, W. T., Waldmann, T. A., and Rossen, R. D. 1970. Changes in IgA and IgG concentrations in nasal secretions prior to the appearance of antibody during viral respiratory infection in man. J. Immunol. 105:584.
Camner, P., Strandberg, K., and Philipson, K. 1976. Increased mucociliary transport by adrenergic stimulation. Arch. Environ. Health 31:79.
Cauna, N., Cauna, D., and Hinderer, K. H. 1972. Innervation of the human nasal glands. J. Neurocytol. 1:49.

Cole, P. 1982. Upper respiratory airflow. *In* Proctor, D. F., and Anderson, I. B. (eds.): The Nose. New York, Elsevier Science Publishing Co., Inc., pp. 163–214.
Cole, P., Fastag, O., and Niiminaa, V. 1980. Computer-aided rhinometry. Acta Otolaryngol. 90:139.
Engen, T. 1971. Psychophysics 1. Discrimination and detection. *In* Kling, J. W., and Riggs, L. A. (eds.): Woodworth and Schlosberg's Experimental Psychology. New York, Holt, Rinehart & Winston, pp 11–46.
Jao, R. L., Wheelock, F., and Jackson, G. G. 1970. Production of interferon in volunteers infected with Asian influenza. J. Infect. Dis. 121:419.
Kayser, R. 1895. Die exacte messung der luftdurchgangikeit der nase. Arch. Laryngol. 3:101.
Kohlrausch, O. 1853. Ueber das Schwellgewebe an den Muscheln der Nasenschleimhout. Arch. Anat. Physiol., pp. 149–150.
Kolliker, A. 1852. Handbuch der Gewebelehre des Menchen. Liepzig, Wilhelm Engelman.
Lindvall, T. 1970. On sensory evaluation of odorous air pollutant intensities. Nord. Hyg. Tidskr. (Suppl.) 2:1.
Lippman, A. M. 1970. Deposition and clearance of inhaled particles in the human nose. Ann. Otol. Rhinol. Laryngol. 79:518.
Malm, L. 1974. Respones of resistance and capacitance vessels in the feline nasal mucosa to vasoactive agents. Acta Otolaryngol. (Stockh.) 78:90.
Mann, D. G., Sasaki, C. T., and Suzuki, M. 1977. Dilator nares muscle. Ann. Otol. Rhinol. Laryngol. 86:362.
Mygind, N. 1979. Nasal Allergy. Oxford, Blackwell Scientific Publications.
Negus, V. E. 1958. The Comparative Anatomy and Physiology of the Nose and Paranasal Sinuses. Edinburgh, E. & S. Livingstone, Ltd.
Prevost, J. L. 1898. Recherches anatomiques et physiologiques ser le ganglion spheno-palatin. II. Physiologie du ganglion spheno-palatin. Arch. Physiol. Norm. Path. Par. 1:207.
Purcell, M. 1976. Response in the newborn to raised upper airway resistance. Arch. Dis. Child. 51:602.
Riott, I. 1980. Essential Immunology. Oxford, Blackwell Scientific Publications.
Sleigh, M. A. 1977. The nature and action of respiratory tract cilia. *In* Brain, J. D., Proctor, D. F., and Reid, L. M. (eds.): Respiratory Defense Mechanisms. New York, Marcel Dekker, Inc., Part 1, pp. 247–288.
Sorri, M., Sorri, A., and Karja, J. 1980. Rhinitis during pregnancy. Rhinology 18:83.
Swift, D. L., and Proctor, D. F. 1977. Access of air to the respiratory tract. *In* Brain, J. D., Proctor, D. F., and Reid, L. M. (eds.): Respiratory Defense Mechanisms. New York, Marcel Dekker, Inc.
Tos, M., and Poulsen, J. 1975. Mucous glands in the developing human nose. Arch. Otolaryngol. 101:367.
Van Cauwenberge, P. B., and Deleye, L. 1984. Nasal cycle in children. Arch. Otolaryngol. 110:108.
Wyllie, J. W., Kern, E. B., O'Brien, P. C., et al. 1976. Alteration of pulmonary function associated with artificial nasal obstruction. Surg. Forum Mayo Clin. (Rochester) 27:535.

Chapter 30

METHODS OF EXAMINATION

Gerald B. Healy, M.D.

Examination of the pediatric patient requires a careful, gentle approach. One must remember that the child is usually apprehensive and afraid when approaching any physician. This is probably due to strange surroundings filled with multiple gadgets. This fear can frequently be alleviated by placing familiar objects, such as puppets, toys, and cartoon characters, in the examining area.

One of the essential parts of the examination is the time spent talking to the patient. Obviously, with the infant, this may not be rewarding, but with the older child it will help alleviate some of his or her fears. Time should be taken to show the patient the various objects to be used in the examination, such as the head mirror or nasal speculum. In fact, it is wise to allow the child to handle the instruments and perhaps even to let him or her examine a toy animal. If a head mirror will be used, the child should be allowed to see his or her reflection in the mirror to alleviate the fear of this large, awesome object sitting on the physician's head. It is a matter of tell, show, and do!

It is essential that the physician be truthful with the patient regarding what is going to be done. If the examination will be uncomfortable, the physician should tell the patient. The child should never be confronted by sudden, unexpected maneuvers. Each part of the examination should be explained to the child. This will play a large role in gaining the patient's trust.

Parental participation is most important. The physician must take time to obtain a good history and display genuine concern and interest when speaking with the parents. A complete history, including questions about other organ systems, as well as a family history, is frequently invaluable in arriving at a precise diagnosis.

General anesthesia may be required to do an adequate examination of the nose and paranasal sinus region. This often occurs in cases in which foreign bodies are present or with uncontrollable epistaxis, when absolute cooperation is required. The physician should not hesitate to use this mode of examination if the individual problem warrants it.

Palpation plays a very important role in examining the nose, sinuses, and face, and at times the examination can be done without the use of any instruments whatsoever.

EQUIPMENT

A head light, the hand-held otoscope, and the hands of the examiner are the primary pieces of examining equipment. Other sources of illumination, such as the electric head lamp or flashlight, may be used when circumstances warrant it. A nasal speculum may occasionally be required in the examination. The nasopharyngeal mirror and tongue depressor are also essential.

Topical vasoconstrictors with various means of application, including aerosol delivery systems, cotton-tipped applicators, and cotton pledgets, should be available.

Sinus transillumination is of limited value in the pediatric patient, but the completely equipped examining area should have this means of evaluation available.

The operating microscope may be required for more precise examination, and, when it is available, it is helpful. An ordinary ear speculum used with the microscope may well allow examination of the entire length of the nasal passage, especially in the very small child.

Positioning of the patient is most important. The patient must feel as comfortable and secure as possible. Often, this requires the parent to hold the child in his or her lap and provide reassurance frequently during the examination (Fig. 30–1). It is usually not advisable to hold the child down on the table and restrain him or her, as most children can be examined in the upright position. However, infants may need to be placed in the supine position for evaluation. It is advisable that the infant be adequately restrained, so that there will be no unexpected movement.

CLINICAL EXAMINATION

The Face

Examination of the face must be preceded by an adequate history. Mass lesions in the region of the face and orbit should prompt questions regarding their duration, changes in size, the presence or absence of pain, or any evidence of infection. A history of trauma is most important in the evaluation of facial swelling. History of exposure to infectious disease, such as

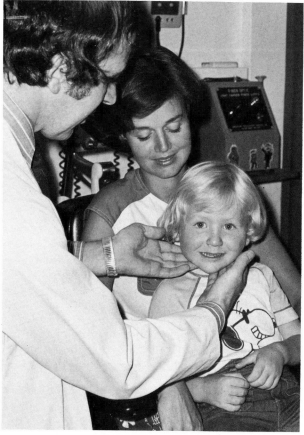

Figure 30–1. Positioning of child in mother's lap is most appropriate for examining pediatric patients.

tuberculosis, is quite important. When the orbital region is involved, questions regarding vision must be asked, and the presence or absence of diplopia must be ascertained, especially in cases related to trauma.

Facial asymmetry should lead to questions regarding facial function or evidence of muscular weakness. Asymmetry of the face secondary to seventh cranial nerve dysfunction should obviously prompt a search into the patient's neurologic and otologic history. Any swelling of the parotid or submaxillary regions requires questioning regarding a possible relationship of eating to fluctuation in size of the swelling. The dental history must also be considered when determining the cause of swellings around the face and upper neck.

Clinical examination of this region begins by careful observation. Any asymmetry or masses should be noted. Attention should be given to the location of the masses, which frequently will be helpful in the differential diagnosis. The examiner should also be aware of any draining sinuses, as this can be indicative of congenital defects. Such a sinus, occurring on the dorsum of the nose, may be indicative of a dermoid cyst.

Sinuses occurring on the lateral portion of the face or neck may indicate first or second branchial groove anomalies. These anomalies in the neck may also lead to cystic defects of the branchial cleft system.

The punctum of the lacrimal sac should be inspected to rule out the presence or absence of debris or purulence in this region.

Any patient with periorbital swelling or pain should have a complete ophthalmologic examination, as well as radiographic evaluation of the sinuses.

Examination of the face should also include the region of the salivary glands. This requires gentle palpation to determine the relationship of the gland in question to underlying structures. A finger cot is placed over the index finger, and then the finger is placed into the oral cavity over the gland in question. The first and second fingers of the opposite hand are placed on the outside, and bimanual palpation is undertaken. This allows for estimation of the presence or absence of a mass, as well as tenderness and mobility. External massage of the glands should always be undertaken to determine flow from the salivary ducts. The appearance and consistency of the secretions should be noted carefully (Chap. 57).

Evaluation of facial swelling should include examination of the teeth, oral cavity, pharynx, and nasopharynx. Note should be made of any distortion of the parapharyngeal structures, as this may indicate extension of disease from the deep facial structures. The examiner must inspect the tonsils and observe for any medial displacement secondary to such underlying pathologic conditions. The presence or absence of trismus should be noted, as this may indicate pathologic conditions involving the pterygoid muscles.

The presence of facial masses often requires a search for systemic disease. Any nodular mass, especially if associated with drainage, should prompt a suspicion of tuberculosis or atypical microbacteria. No biopsy specimen should be obtained from a mass until a thorough search for systemic disease has been carried out. Skin testing, as well as hematologic evaluation, may be necessary. Rapidly changing masses deserve immediate attention because of the ever-present possibility of neoplasm.

Trauma can present a puzzling and challenging problem to the examiner. Distortion and asymmetry due to swelling can confuse the issue and prevent absolute definition of underlying pathologic states. Observation, palpation, and the help of roentgenograms may be necessary to delineate completely the extent of the problem.

Bimanual palpation of the bony structures of the face should be undertaken in an attempt to ascertain defects. This should be done simultaneously on both sides of the face. Trauma to the maxillary or mandibular region should prompt an evaluation of occlusion. Any question of maxillary fracture requires digital palpation of the palate to assess the presence or absence of mobility (Fig. 30–2). A finger cot is placed on the examiner's index finger and thumb, and the upper alveolus is firmly grasped and rocked with a to-and-fro motion to establish the presence or absence of freely floating components.

Injuries to the cervical spine often accompany severe facial trauma. The patient should not be manipulated needlessly until this possibility has been ruled out.

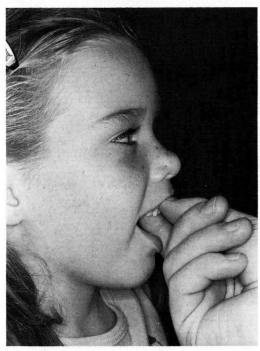

Figure 30–2. Digital palpation of the maxilla to establish the presence of fracture.

The Nose

Evaluation of the nose must be done in a systematic and organized fashion. One method of examination should be adopted, and a mental checklist should be employed so that no area is left out.

History should be sought from the parents, and, if the age of the child warrants, it is frequently possible to get useful information by merely asking the patient. Questions related to trauma, prior nasal disease, pain, nasal obstruction, nasal discharge, allergy, and distortion of olfaction should be asked. It is most important to ascertain sleeping habits and breathing patterns during sleep. Snoring and mouth breathing may signal nasal obstruction. This may warrant further examination of the nasopharynx.

Syndromes related to the cardiovascular system have had their origins traced directly to nasal obstruction. Therefore, the patient with a history suggesting severe obstruction may require more investigation, including cardiopulmonary evaluation, in addition to examination of the nasopharynx.

EXTERNAL EXAMINATION. Inspection plays an important role in examining the external nose. This will give an indication of the relative size and contour of the nose, which may be important in assessing breathing capabilities. Visible deformities, such as skin lesions, fistulae, swellings, and deviations, should be noted. The presence or absence of a supratip crease should be noted. This may indicate the "nasal salute" of allergy (Chap. 42).

The bony and cartilaginous framework must be carefully examined not only for their relationships to each other but also for their relationships to the rest of the face. Such observations may explain the cause of nasal obstruction. The nasal bones should be palpated carefully, and the junction of the nasal bones with the upper lateral cartilages, as well as the junction of the cartilages with each other, should be noted.

The vestibular region should be inspected for gross lesions and for patency of the air passage. This is particularly important in the newborn infant, in whom evaluation of airflow is very critical inasmuch as these children are obligate nose breathers. A small wisp of cotton may be placed under the naris on each side to test for airflow. It is also possible to place a small nasopharyngeal mirror under each naris to watch for "fogging," which will indicate the presence or absence of airflow.

INTERNAL EXAMINATION. The internal examination of the nose begins with careful inspection of the vestibular region. This is frequently overlooked by the passage of a nasal speculum, which obscures the first 1.0 to 1.5 cm of the nose.

Examination of the internal nose may be accomplished in a number of ways. Gentle upward rotation of the tip of the nose by the thumb of the examiner gives access to the vestibular region as well as to the anterior portion of the septum and the anterior segment of the inferior turbinates (Fig. 30–3). Illumination must be adequate and can be provided by a head mirror, head light, an otoscope with a nasal speculum attached, or even a flashlight.

Location of the septum is a critical element in evaluating the nose for nasal obstruction. The caudal septum must be evaluated carefully for discoloration,

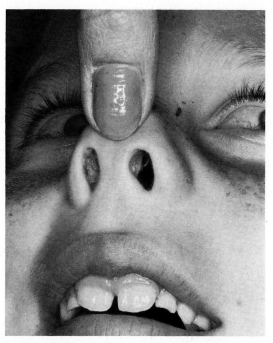

Figure 30–3. Elevation of the nasal tip by the examiner for inspection of the vestibule and septum. This maneuver avoids the need for nasal speculum.

as it may play a major role in impeding free breathing. This portion is frequently bypassed by the insertion of a nasal speculum or the nasal head of the otoscope.

Inspection of the distal portion of the septum is important in evaluating the patient with epistaxis. The anterior portion has a rich vascular supply and is frequently the site of bleeding. This is also the site of septal perforation, which occasionally can be hidden by small crusts. If crusts are present in this area, they must be removed gently with a bayonet forceps or similar instrument to gain complete visualization of the internal nose.

Palpation of the septum is often necessary, especially after trauma. A small cotton swab may be used to compress the mucosa delicately in order to decide whether or not hematoma or abscess is present. These usually present as soft, doughy swellings either with or without tenderness.

Adequate examination of the nasal passage must be undertaken in any neonate with respiratory distress. These children are obligate nose breathers, and conditions such as choanal atresia or subluxation of the septum must be ruled out (Chap. 36).

This examination begins by an estimation of the amount of airflow through the nasal passage. A small, no. 8 catheter is gently passed along the floor of the nose into the pharynx. Frequently, it is necessary to apply a vasoconstrictor to the nasal mucous membrane in the form of 0.125 per cent phenylephrine hydrochloride solution. This is especially true in the newborn, in whom mucous membrane swelling is quite common. After appropriate shrinkage, it is possible to examine the internal nose by the use of an appropriately small ear speculum on the head of the hand-held otoscope.

Neonatal evaluation requires adequate illumination so that the entire internal framework of the nose can be inspected. An adequate evaluation of the septum must be undertaken to determine the presence or absence of dislocation.

Evaluation of the mucous membrane is an important part of the internal examination. Healthy mucosa is usually pink and moist, while pale, cyanotic, excessively moist mucosa may signal allergy or some other pathologic condition. Usually, the neonate has slightly more edematous and moist mucosa than the older child.

In the presence of severely swollen mucosa, an adequate assessment of the internal nose cannot be undertaken without the use of vasoconstrictors. The use of a rapid aerosol spray is probably the most advisable way of obtaining vasoconstriction. A 0.125 or 0.25 per cent solution of phenylephrine hydrochloride is usually adequate to obtain this. Occasionally, 1 or 2 per cent cocaine can be used when topical anesthesia is required. It is not advisable to pack the nose of a very young child with cotton pledgets, as this may frighten and alienate the patient.

Full lateral examination of the internal nose is frequently overlooked. This involves a visualization of the turbinates, noting their size, color, and shape. Often, patients with a severe nasal septal deviation will present with compensatory hypertrophy of the turbinate facing the concavity of the deviation.

The middle turbinate region should be observed for the presence of a discharge and, if one is present, its appearance and location should be recorded. The anterior nasal sinuses (maxillary and anterior ethmoid) open into the middle meatus, and discharges from infections in these regions will present themselves in this area (Fig. 30–4). Posterior sinuses (the sphenoid and posterior ethmoid) drain into the superior meatus. The swollen, edematous mucosa associated with sinusitis must be shrunken in order to get an adequate

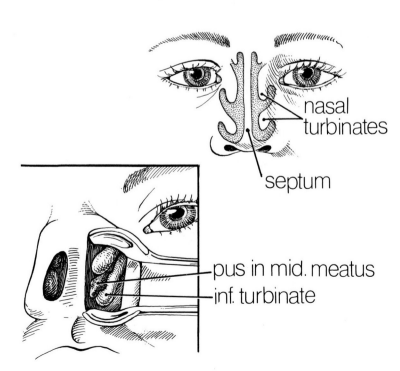

Figure 30–4. Internal nasal anatomy showing location of discharge in infections of the anterior sinuses (middle meatus).

estimation of the type and location of discharge. This material should be cultured, although the value of these cultures is somewhat controversial.

Clear, watery discharge may signify a vasomotor condition, or, on occasion, can represent cerebrospinal fluid. This is especially true after trauma or in patients with recurrent meningitis. If one suspects the presence of cerebrospinal fluid, analysis of the fluid is necessary. Radioisotope studies can be helpful in ruling out the presence or absence of a cerebrospinal fluid leak in the region of the cribriform plate. A computed tomography (CT) scan may also be employed to identify defects in the sinus region.

Mucosa should be observed for other changes. A polypoid appearance or frank polyps may signal an allergic condition. Cystic fibrosis often presents with nasal polyps or polypoid changes in the nose, and thus, any child presenting with nasal polyps should have a sweat test to rule out the possibility of this disease (Chap. 41).

Mass lesions, such as gliomas and encephaloceles, can be mistaken for nasal polyps in the young child, and their presence must be considered in any patient with a nasal mass. A biopsy specimen of mass lesions in the nose should not be taken without consideration of this diagnosis. If one entertains the diagnosis, radiographic (including CT scan) and radioisotopic studies should be undertaken to confirm its presence or absence.

Unilateral nasal discharge may signal the presence of a foreign body or unilateral choanal atresia. If one suspects a foreign body, it may be unwise to attempt its removal without the use of general anesthesia. In this instance especially, this adjunct to examination becomes important and should not be overlooked.

If possible, an estimation of the adequacy of olfactory function should be made. An easy and accurate method has yet to be developed, but gross testing should be attempted whenever possible. Any condition causing mucosal changes in the nose may well distort the sense of smell.

If precise examination of the nose is required, the surgical microscope and an ear speculum may be used (Fig. 30–5). This will give an excellent view after appropriate vasoconstriction and is especially useful in the cooperative patient.

The Sinuses

The development of the sinuses is variable in the pediatric patient. The ethmoids represent the most often clinically involved sinus in the patient younger than 10 years of age. The ethmoids and extremely small maxillary sinuses are present at birth. The frontal sinus does not begin to develop until approximately the age of 8 years. It never develops in approximately 5 per cent of the population and has only unilateral development in about 15 per cent. The sphenoid sinus begins to pneumatize at approximately 3 years of age, but full pneumatization is not complete until adolescence.

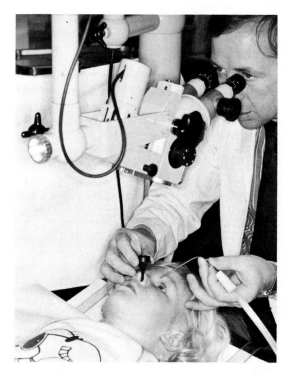

Figure 30–5. Use of the surgical microscope for detailed examination of the nose.

History of disease of the paranasal sinuses should be taken in conjunction with the history of the nasal status. Prior history of allergy is not uncommon. Perhaps the most common symptoms of acute sinus pathology are pain and nasal obstruction. The patient may often complain of nasal discharge as well. Occasionally, the only presenting manifestation of the disease in children will be a history of progressive swelling in the periorbital region; this can occur early with ethmoid sinusitis, especially in the young patient.

EXAMINATION. Palpation plays a large role in examination of the sinuses of any young child. The supraorbital region must be palpated carefully, and gentle tapping with the index finger should be undertaken to determine the presence or absence of tenderness. The ascending process of the maxilla and the canine fossa must be inspected. After gloving, the index finger is placed in the gingivobuccal sulcus, and gentle pressure is applied over the anterior and lateral walls of the maxillary sinus. However, these maneuvers may be unrewarding in the very young infant, and reliance on other clinical signs may be necessary.

Transillumination of the sinuses plays no significant role in examination of the pediatric patient, although it may be helpful in the adolescent.

Diagnostic surgical procedures involving the sinuses may occasionally be indicated in the pediatric patient. This may include sinoscopy, as well as irrigation and biopsy. Cytologic specimens may be obtained as well. Radiographic studies of the maxillary sinuses to ascertain their size and relationship to erupted and unerupted teeth are necessary as a first step. Sinoscopy may be undertaken either transnasally, to examine the ethmoid sinuses, or transfacially, to examine the maxillary sinus, provided it has developed adequately.

The Hopkins rod lens system may be utilized for this purpose. In most patients, examination using this system should be performed with the patient under general anesthesia. After topical vasoconstriction, the ethmoids may be examined via the transnasal route. The maxillary sinus is best evaluated by passing the trocar and lens system through the anterior wall of the maxilla. This is done via the gingivobuccal sulcus (Fig. 30–6).

Antral puncture always requires general anesthesia in children. An appropriate vasoconstrictor is applied, and the sinus is entered with a trocar and cannula. Puncture is made through the inferior meatus, approximately 1.5 cm posterior to the anterior tip of the inferior turbinate (Fig. 30–7). The needle is gently advanced until the posterior wall is reached, then gently withdrawn approximately 0.5 cm. A syringe is attached and saline solution is gently instilled into the sinus. Fluid should be observed entering the nasal cavity through the natural ostium of the sinus. If this is not observed, the procedure should be immediately stopped, as the needle may not be in the proper position. In the young child with unerupted teeth, entrance may need to be made through the middle meatus rather than through the inferior meatus.

Other methods of sinus irrigation have been advocated in the past. The technique described by Proetz

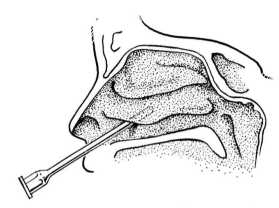

Figure 30–7. Position of trocar in inferior meatus for antral puncture.

(1939) uses the principle of displacement, whereby air is drawn from the sinuses by suction and the fluid to be introduced into the sinus lies over the ostium when pressure is returned to normal. This will allow the fluid to flow into the sinus from which the air has been withdrawn. This technique is rarely used now because of the fear that infection may be transferred to previously healthy sinuses. It should be used only after cultures of the sinus have been obtained and appropriate antimicrobial therapy has been instituted. On occasion, it can be of great value in treating subacute or chronic ethmoiditis.

The Proetz method requires vasoconstriction. The patient's head is held back so that the chin and the external auditory canal are in the same vertical plane. The nose is then filled with a solution of ephedrine and saline. Negative pressure is applied to one nostril while the other is closed by a finger, and the patient is asked to occlude his pharynx by repeating the letter "k-k-k-k-k" or "kitty-kitty-kitty."

Exploratory sinus surgery may on rare occasion be required, especially if the presence of a neoplasm is suspected. Any bony destruction noted on roentgenograms of the sinuses requires further investigation in the form of surgical exploration. This may well represent either chronic infection or the presence of malignancy.

Nasopharynx

Roentgenography and rhinoscopy are the two primary means of evaluating the nasopharynx (see section on diagnostic procedures). Digital examination is not advocated because bleeding may be precipitated, which can be frightening to the patient and difficult to control. However, palpation of the soft palate is advised to ascertain the presence or absence of a submucous cleft. The presence of such a defect would obviously alert the physician against removing any of the lymphoid tissue in the nasopharynx.

The nasopharynx should be observed for the presence or absence of any mass lesion, which in children commonly represents adenoid tissue. The possible

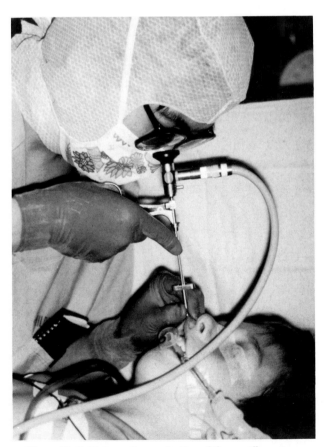

Figure 30–6. Endoscopic examination of the maxillary sinus.

presence of lesions such as angiofibromas and neoplasms of other types must be kept in mind during the examination. The size, configuration, and surface appearance of all masses must be noted. Posterior rhinoscopy by the direct or indirect method should be attempted on all patients in whom a lesion might be present. If the patient is unable to tolerate this procedure, then direct examination under general anesthesia is required. This is accomplished by placing small catheters through the nose into the pharynx. The palate is then gently retracted laterally, and a large mirror is used to give a full panoramic view of the nasopharyngeal vault and the eustachian tube orifices.

Radiographic evaluation may also determine the presence or absence of a mass lesion when posterior rhinoscopy is not possible.

DIAGNOSTIC PROCEDURES

POSTERIOR RHINOSCOPY. Posterior rhinoscopy is often overlooked in young children because many believe it cannot be accomplished. Contrary to this opinion, young children will frequently cooperate for this examination if they are reassured and if time is spent to gain their confidence. The use of a 00 or 000 mirror with gentle tongue depression will accomplish this. The child may be distracted by asking him or her to "breathe like a doggy" while the physician proceeds with the examination (Fig. 30–8).

Fiberoptic flexible or rigid endoscopic equipment may be used but frequently requires the use of topical or general anesthesia. Obtaining the cooperation of the child may be difficult, especially if he or she is very young. The advent of the small, flexible rhinolaryngoscope is making this evaluation somewhat more feasible. This instrument is gently passed over the floor of the nose while the examiner carefully observes the nasopharynx (Fig. 30–9).

ROENTGENOGRAPHY. A radiographic evaluation is part of any comprehensive examination of the sinuses. Radiographic evaluation of the nose is somewhat less informative, except in cases in which the presence of a foreign body is suspected. All children with periorbital cellulitis or swelling, nasal discharge, or edema of the nasal mucosa who do not respond to conventional therapy should have radiographic evaluation of their sinuses.

A dental view of the nasal bones may be helpful in estimating the degree of trauma to the nasal framework. The gross appearance of the external nose, as well as estimation of the internal framework, is far more valuable than questionable roentgenograms of the nasal bones.

Roentgenographic evaluation of the paranasal sinuses is somewhat more valuable, however. The four traditional views—Caldwell, Waters, lateral, and submentovertical—are the most helpful in the estimation of diseases of the sinuses and facial bones.

The Caldwell, or occipitofrontal, view best delineates the ethmoid and frontal sinuses. The temporal bones and base of the skull are projected onto the maxillary antrum, thereby concealing it and making this an undesirable view for evaluating the maxillary sinuses (Fig. 30–10).

The Waters, or occipitomental, view best delineates the maxillary sinus and the orbital floor. It is an important view in the estimation of facial trauma, as it gives a fairly panoramic view of the facial bones (Fig. 30–11).

The lateral view gives good visualization of the anterior and posterior ethmoid cells, as well as of the frontal and sphenoid sinuses. It also shows the thickness of the antral walls and the relationship of the antral floor to the teeth (Fig. 30–12). This is especially

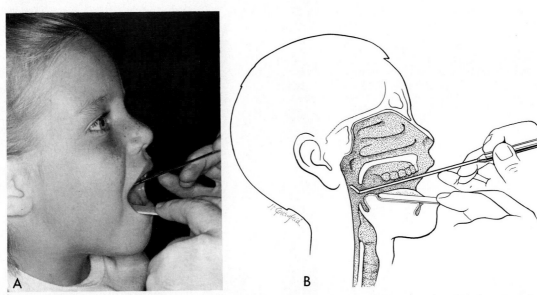

A   B

Figure 30–8. A, Posterior indirect rhinoscopy in the young child. B, Schematic drawing of the proper location of a mirror for view of the nasopharyngeal vault.

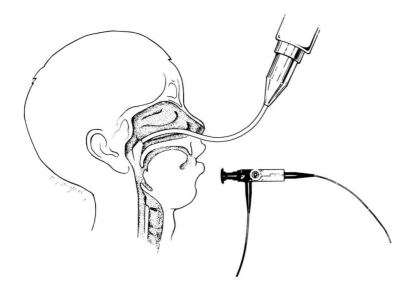

Figure 30–9. Location of the flexible fiberoptic na-sopharyngoscope along the floor of the nose for view of the nasopharynx and pharynx. (A full view of the instrument is also shown.)

Figure 30–10. A, Photograph of the dried skull in the Caldwell projection. B, Caldwell view: A, frontal sinus; B, crista galli; C, superior orbital margin; D, optic foramen; E, ethmoid sinus; F, foramen rotundum; G, maxillary sinus; H, pyriform aperture; I, nasal cavity; J, nasal septum; K, floor of the nose; L, lesser wing of the sphenoid bone; M, greater wing of the sphenoid bone; N, zygomatic-frontal suture; O, temporal line; P, zygo-matic bone; Q, petrous ridge of temporal bone; R, infraorbital foramen; S, lateral wall of maxillary sinus; T, floor of posterior cranial fossa. (From Yanagisawa, E., and Smith, H. M. 1968. Radiographic anatomy of the paranasal sinuses. IV. Caldwell view. Arch. Otolar-yngol. 87:311–322. Copyright 1968, American Medical Association.)

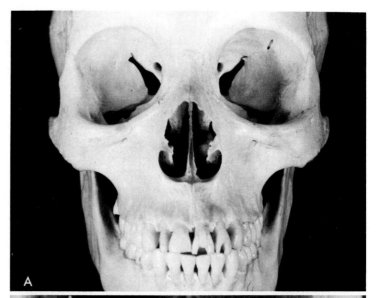

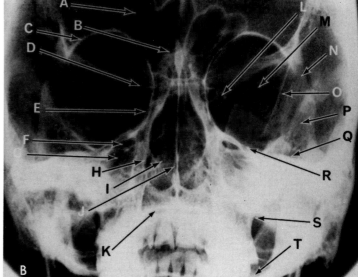

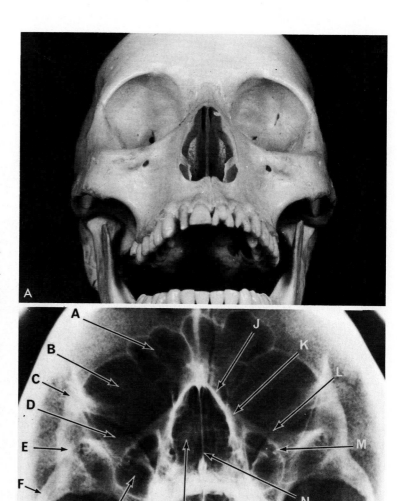

Figure 30–11. *A*, Dried skull in Water projection. *B*, Waters view: A, frontal sinus; B, orbit; C, zygomatic-frontal suture; D, inferior orbital rim; E, zygoma; F, zygomatic arch; G, infratemporal fossa; H, maxillary sinus; I, nasal cavity; J, nasal bone; K, frontal process of maxilla; L, superior orbital fissure; M, infraorbital foramen; N, nasal septum; O, petrous ridge of temporal bone; P, sphenoid sinus. (From Merrell, R. A., Jr., and Yanagisawa, E. 1968. Radiographic anatomy of the paranasal sinuses. II. Lateral view. Arch. Otolaryngol. 87:184–195. Copyright 1968, American Medical Association.)

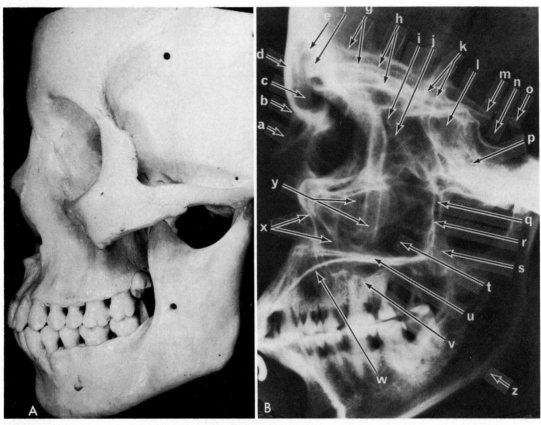

Figure 30–12. *A,* Dried skull on lateral projection. *B,* Lateral view showing: a, nasal bone; b, nasofrontal suture; c, frontal sinus; d, anterior wall of frontal sinus; e, posterior wall of frontal sinus; f, supraorbital margin; g, cerebral surface orbital plate; h, orbital surface of orbital plate; i, cribriform plate; j, anterior ethmoid air cells; k, anterior wall of middle cranial fossa (greater wing of sphenoid bone); l, posterior ethmoid cells; m, anterior clinoid process; n, sella turcica; o, posterior clinoid process; p, sphenoid sinus; q, turgomaxillary fissure; r, posterior wall of maxillary sinus; s, pterygoid plates; t, maxillary sinus; u, floor of the nose; v, floor of the maxillary sinus; w, roof of the mouth; x, anterior wall of the maxillary sinus; y, zygomatic process of the maxilla; z, mandible. (From Yanagisawa, E., Smith, H. W., and Thaler, S. 1968. Radiographic anatomy of the paranasal sinuses. II. Lateral view. Arch. Otolaryngol. 87:196–209. Copyright 1968, American Medical Association.)

important in the young patient. This view can be used conveniently to estimate the presence or absence of a nasopharyngeal mass lesion.

A submentovertical view estimates the extent of the posterior ethmoid and sphenoid sinuses and gives an excellent panoramic view of the base of the skull (Fig. 30–13).

POLYTOMOGRAPHY. Polytomography of the paranasal sinus region can, on occasion, give useful information, especially if there is a possibility of fracture or bony destruction (Fig. 30–14). Defects in the region of the cribriform plate can occasionally be demonstrated with this technique as well.

RADIOPAQUE MEDIA. Special studies with radiopaque materials are rarely, if ever, used in the nose any more. This technique was once used to diagnose such lesions as choanal atresia. Today, however, CT scans have replaced this method in the diagnosis of such lesions.

SIALOGRAPHY. Sialography may be used to study both the parotid and the submaxillary glands. With this technique, radiopaque material is gently injected into the duct of the salivary gland to be studied, and films are taken of the gland in question (Fig. 30–15). Occasionally, the use of fluoroscopy is helpful as an adjunct to this study. Preliminary films include stereoposteroanterior and lateral films of the mandibular region. After these are reviewed and the contrast material is injected, the same views are repeated.

The analysis of the sialogram includes a detailed examination of the main secretory ducts (Wharton or Stensen), the smaller ducts branching within the gland, and the parenchyma of the gland itself. Deep sedation or even general anesthesia may be required in the very young child in order to undertake this study (Gates, 1977).

RADIOISOTOPIC EXAMINATION. The use of radioisotopic evaluation in the region of the face has its greatest

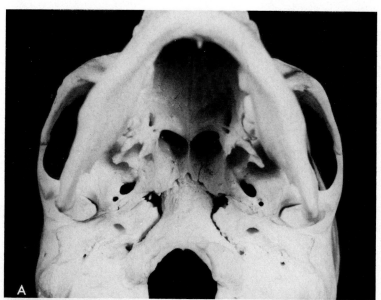

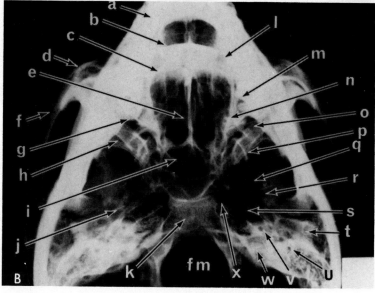

Figure 30–13. *A,* Dried skull in submentovertical projection. *B,* Submentovertical view: a, mandible; b, anterior wall of frontal bone; c, posterior wall of frontal bone; d, zygoma; e, nasal septum; f, zygomatic arch; g, lateral wall of antrum; h, lateral wall of orbit; i, sphenoid sinus; j, eustachian tube; k, clivus; l, lacrimal canal; m, maxillary sinus; n, greater palatine foramen; o, inferior orbital fissure; p, pterygoid plates; q, foramen ovale; r, foramen spinosum; s, carotid canal; t, external auditory canal; u, stylomastoid foramen; v, cochlea; w, internal auditory canal; x, foramen lacerum; fm, foramen magnum. (From Yanagisawa, E., Smith, H. W., and Merrell, R. A., Jr. 1968. Radiographic anatomy of the paranasal sinuses. II. Submentovertebral view. Arch. Otolaryngol. 87:299–310. Copyright 1968, American Medical Association.)

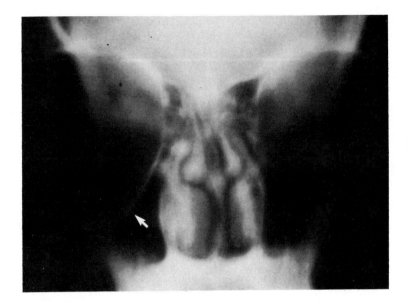

Figure 30–14. Polytomograph of maxillary sinuses showing orbital floor fracture (*arrow*).

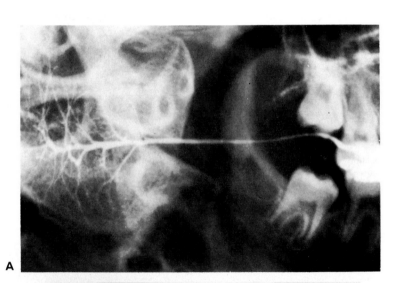

A

Figure 30–15. *A*, Normal parotid sialogram (lateral view); *B*, Normal parotid sialogram (AP view).

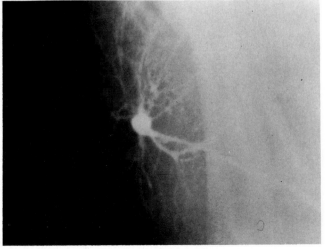

B

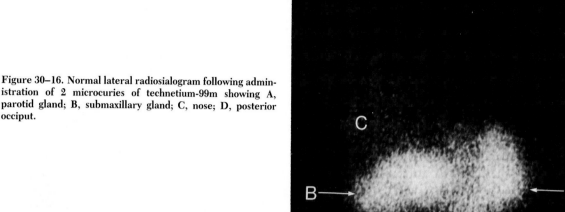

Figure 30–16. Normal lateral radiosialogram following administration of 2 microcuries of technetium-99m showing A, parotid gland; B, submaxillary gland; C, nose; D, posterior occiput.

application in examination of the salivary glands. The ductal cells of these structures have the ability to extract iodide from the peritubular capillaries and to secrete it into the ductal lumen. Iodine-125 or technetium-99m can be recorded from salivary gland tissue, thus providing the basis for salivary gland scanning (Gates, 1977).

The material is injected intravenously, and then the structures to be examined are scanned at varying intervals thereafter. Normal outlines of the glandular structures can be seen easily and the presence of mass lesions can be detected (Figs. 30–16 and 30–17).

COMPUTED TOMOGRAPHY. Computed tomography (CT) was introduced in 1972. This method of evaluation makes it possible to identify different soft tissue structures that vary by 1 to 2 per cent in their absorption of x-rays. This equipment is much more sensitive than radiographic film in the differentiation of various anatomic structures. The images are made in a transverse plane rather than in the traditional coronal or sagittal planes.

The computed tomographic scanner is a roentgenographic machine capable of producing a cross-sectional image on a television monitor. Mathematical formulas are used to calculate very slight differences in absorption coefficients of different tissue to an x-ray beam that passes through the body from a number of directions around a parallel to the transverse axis. The computer is then utilized to sort out the large number of equations presented by this technique (Carter et al., 1977).

The use of CT in examination of the region of the nose and paranasal sinuses is widely employed. Various anatomic structures can be delineated in the nose and paranasal sinus region by this computer examination technique (Figs. 30–18 and 30–19).

Contrast material (enhancement technique) has been used frequently in conjunction with CT scans of the head. Its major value is in delineating lesions of the brain, and it has limited usefulness in the discovery of pathologic conditions of the nose and paranasal sinuses, unless they are vascular in nature.

ULTRASONOGRAPHY. Ultrasonography is a technique for examining the acoustic properties of tissues. Sound waves are generated by a piezoelectric crystal placed in close contact with the skin, and a short pulse of ultrasound (usually 1 to 5 MHz) is transmitted. A

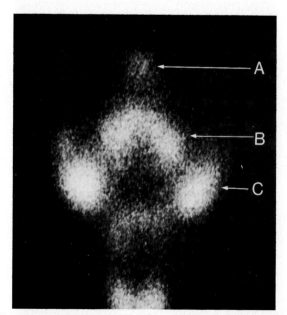

Figure 30–17. Normal AP radiosialogram following administration of 2 microcuries of technetium-99m, showing: A, nose; B, submaxillary gland; C, parotid gland.

returning echo is then received by the crystal. Inasmuch as the velocity of sound through most tissues is fairly uniform (1500 m per sec), it is possible to compute the distance of the echo from the transducer. This is done by means of a cathode ray tube, which displays both the starting point of the signal and the location of the echo on an oscilloscope screen.

A linear recording showing the amplitude and time relationship of the echo to the original pulse is called an *A Scan*. If the echo is stored, it can be assimilated to produce a composite picture called a *B Scan* (Noyek et al., 1977).

This technique has been shown to be quite useful in delineating orbital lesions (Chap. 34). Its usefulness in the remainder of the face and sinus region is somewhat limited, although it has been used to differentiate solid from cystic lesions in the parotid gland and thyroid.

MISCELLANEOUS PROCEDURES. Other helpful diagnostic procedures in the region of the nose and paranasal sinuses may occasionally be required. The use of nasal smears for cytologic evaluation is often helpful in ascertaining the presence or absence of an allergic state. A specimen of nasal mucus is obtained by swabbing with a cotton-tipped applicator just below the inferior turbinate and along the floor of the nose. The material is then gently rolled onto a glass slide and immediately sprayed with fixative solution. Wright stain is then applied for approximately 15 seconds, followed by a buffered solution for 15 seconds. The slide is then rinsed with distilled water and allowed to dry. It is then ready for examination under the oil immersion microscope. The relative numbers and types of cells seen on the slide are tabulated in a *cytogram* (Bryan and Bryan, 1974).

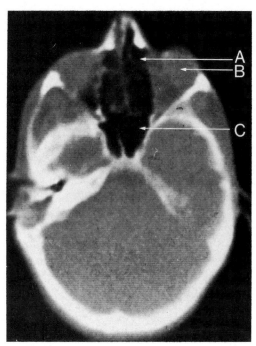

Figure 30–19. Normal transverse computed tomograph showing: A, ethmoid sinuses; B, orbit; C, sphenoid sinus. (Courtesy of Barbara Carter, M.D.)

Large numbers of eosinophils may be indicative of an allergic state. However, patients with vasomotor rhinitis may occasionally have eosinophilia as well. Eosinophilia is also seen on the nasal smears of infants younger than 3 months of age.

A negative cytogram does not necessarily rule out allergy. Serial cytograms may be necessary. This test is just one in the armamentarium of the examiner, and it should be coupled with the assessment of the history and appearance of the nose and sinuses before an allergy is diagnosed or ruled out.

Cultures of the nasopharynx can occasionally be helpful in treating patients with persistent rhinitis or chronic sinusitis. These may be obtained by gently passing a small wire nasopharyngeal swab along the floor of the nose into the nasopharynx after the mucous membrane has been treated with appropriate vasoconstrictors.

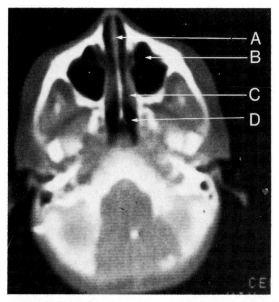

Figure 30–18. Normal transverse computed tomograph showing: A, nasal septum; B, maxillary sinus; C, turbinates; D, nasopharynx. (Courtesy of Barbara Carter, M.D.)

REFERENCES

Bryan, M. P., and Bryan, W. T. K. 1974. Cytologic diagnosis in allergic disorders. Otolaryngol. Clin. North Am. 7(3):637.

Carter, G., et al. 1977. Cross-Sectional Anatomy—Computed Tomography and Ultrasound Correlation. New York, Appleton-Century-Crofts.

Gates, G. A. 1977. Sialography and scanning of salivary glands. Otolaryngol. Clin. North Am. 10(2):379.

Noyek, A. M., Holgate, R. C., Wortzman, G., et al. 1977. Sophisticated radiology in otolaryngology. J. Otolaryngol. (Supp. 3) 6:95.

Proetz, A. W. 1939. The Displacement Method. St. Louis, Annals Pub. Co.

Chapter 31

NASAL OBSTRUCTION AND RHINORRHEA

Walter M. Belenky, M.D.

INTRODUCTION

The importance of nasal obstruction and rhinorrhea in nasal function and disease was well known by, and the concern of, many physicians in ancient times. Among the earliest writing on this subject, the Hindu Arthava-Veda Sanhita (1500–800 B.C.) (Wise, 1898) listed causes of nasal discharge. Although Hippocrates described nasal discharge in his humoral theory in 415 B.C., and this problem was again mentioned by Celsus (c. 30 A.D.), Galen was the first to postulate on the etiology of rhinorrhea around 160 A.D.. He suggested that nasal discharge contained waste products from the brain that had been filtered by the pituitary and entered the nose by the cribriform and ethmoid plates. This theory was accepted for 1500 years until Schneider in 1600 A.D. pronounced that nasal discharge is a product of the membrane lining of the nose (cited by Schaeffer in 1932).

This concern of the ancient physicians with nasal discharge was well taken, as the obstructed or draining nose is the most common complaint the otolaryngologist faces in evaluating nasal problems in all patients, including the pediatric patient. The nose acts as the "guardian of the lower respiratory tract" and the "initiator of the immune response to inhaled antigens and pathogens" (Taylor, 1979). Nasal obstruction and rhinorrhea may appear as both symptoms and signs, reflecting the anatomic and physiologic importance of the nose in both health and disease. Frequently occurring together, they may vary sufficiently in their characteristics to aid the observant clinician in his or her diagnosis. The presence of one without the other may be equally significant.

Nasal obstruction and rhinorrhea present in a variety of ways. The onset of symptoms may be acute, as in the common cold, or chronic, as in the older child's suffering from the stuffy, runny nose of perennial allergic rhinitis. These complaints may be the symptoms of a life-threatening disease, such as bilateral choanal atresia, or they may be due simply to the bothersome but normal physiologic changes that occur in the nose during puberty. The symptoms of nasal obstruction and rhinorrhea that may prompt parents to bring a child to the physician for treatment are often accompanied by the nonnasal symptoms of a dry, coated tongue, bad breath, snoring, mouth-breathing, and postnasal drip.

The clinician must recognize the symptoms of nasal obstruction and rhinorrhea and, through the taking of a thorough history and the performance of a complete physical examination, must assess the entire patient, particularly the internal and external nose and related structures, in order to determine whether the condition is of local or systemic origin, pathologic or physiologic. In evaluating nasal obstruction, the clinician must first determine whether it is unilateral or bilateral, complete or partial, intermittent or constant, congenital or acquired, acute or chronic, and of sudden or gradual onset. Examination of the nose may determine the anatomic site of obstruction. Cottle (1968) described five areas of the nose where abnormalities may occur: (1) the vestibular area; (2) the "liminal valve" area, or the relationship of the caudal end of the upper lateral cartilage to the nasal septum, the os internum, the narrowest portion of the nasal passage; (3) the attic, or area of the septum under the bony vault; (4) the anterior turbinates; and (5) the posterior turbinates and posterior choanae. For completeness, a sixth area, the nasopharynx, might be added (Chap. 30).

Physiologically, certain areas appear to be more important during nasal inspiration and have been described by Bridger (1970) and others (Bridger and Proctor, 1970) as nasal valves. These include the "liminal valve," considered by many to be the most important part during inspiration in the nose of the white patient (Bridger, 1970; von Dishoeck, 1942, 1965); the erectile tissue of the nasal turbinates (turbinate valve); and the nasal septum (septal valve). Fanous (1986) states, "The nasal valve consists of a circular obstruction formed inferiorly by the pyriform crest, superiorly by the limen nasi and medially by the corresponding strip of nasal septum." Internal displacement of any of these components will affect the nasal airway. Structures immediately anterior (alar cartilage) or posterior (anterior tip of the inferior turbinate) can influence this area and nasal resistance. Haight and Cole (1983) concluded that "the main air flow resistance of the whole respiratory tract is confined to a short nasal segment of a few millimeters which is situated in close proximity with the junction of the compliant cartilaginous vestibule with the rigid bony cavity of the nose." In their studies of the "flow limiting segment," the greater portion of the resistance was situated at the level of the anterior end of the inferior turbinate, and resistance could vary as much as fourfold by the adjusted state of this structure.

To aid the clinician and the researcher in measuring the degree of obstruction objectively and in quantifying nasal functions, rhinomanometry procedures have been developed to measure the air pressure gradient and the rate of airflow through the nasal channel during respiration. These procedures have been helpful in substantiating clinical findings of nasal obstruction; for example, significant airway obstruction may occur with minimal anatomic abnormality in areas 1 and 2, while larger deformities in areas 3, 4, and 5 may cause minimal obstructive symptoms (Bridger, 1970; Bridger and Proctor, 1970). Further, such data have highlighted the importance of the streamlined airflow in the nose with reduction of eddy currents and resistance. Anterior active and passive rhinomanometry (van Cauwenberge and Deleye, 1984) and posterior rhinomanometry (Timms, 1986; Cole et al., 1983), along with "head out" body plethysmography (Niinimaa et al., 1979), have been utilized to more completely understand and measure nasal resistance. However, because of difficulties in performing the various procedures, especially in young children, variability in the nasal airway, such as the congestion of erectile tissue, and disturbance of the nasal airway from the instrumentation, the research and clinical value of such studies, though improved, must still be critically interpreted as to its importance in pediatric otolaryngology (Chap. 29).

However, some conclusions with regard to the pediatric nasal airway, especially in comparison with the adult nasal airway, are self-evident or have been determined. The nasal airway is obviously smaller in the newborn than in the adult. The resistance to airflow is approximately four times that in the adult, and the variability in resistance is much greater (Lacourt and Polgar, 1971).

In the past, the clinical impression of nasal obstruction could be confirmed by lateral radiographs of the nose and the nasopharynx. Such radiographs, if taken with the mouth closed, were especially useful in showing the obstruction of the airway by hypertrophic adenoids. Contrast-enhanced nasograms were also helpful in demonstrating choanal atresia.

In the last decade, computed tomography (CT) scanning became the first objective method of obtaining true cross-sectional imaging of the nose, nasopharynx, and allied structures. It is still the best mechanism for visualization of the bony dimensions and abnormalities of the area. Slovis and colleagues (1985) were the first to show its value in the diagnosis and classification of choanal atresia. Recently, magnetic resonance imaging (MRI), which is noninvasive and uses no ionizing radiation, has been a further advancement in this area and is especially useful in soft tissue lesions producing obstruction (Lusk and Lee, 1986). Axial, coronal, sagittal, and even three-dimensional imaging can now be obtained for further evaluation of the nose, nasopharynx, and surrounding structures.

Furthermore, more direct evaluation of nasal and nasopharyngeal anatomy and etiologies of obstruction has been enhanced by the development of both rigid and fiberoptic nasoscope and nasopharyngoscopes. The simplicity of utilizing these instruments even in children, along with the ability to evaluate both static and dynamic states of the areas, is a significant advancement and has become a basic part of the nasal and nasopharyngeal examination of children.

Endoscopy of the area progressed with the development of sinus endoscopy equipment and techniques (Kennedy et al., 1985). Stammberger (1986) and Kennedy and associates (1985), with sinus endoscopy evaluations, showed the rhinogenic origin of many sinus infections and the importance of the lateral wall and especially the anterior ethmoid region in the pathogenesis of sinusitis.

As with nasal obstruction, rhinorrhea must first be evaluated by the clinician as to extent, frequency, duration, time and nature of onset, and quantity. By classic definition, rhinorrhea is the "free discharge of a thin nasal mucus" (Dorland, 1988). The vasomotor reaction is the primary response of the nasal mucosa to a variety of stimuli and is an etiologic factor in many cases of nasal obstruction and rhinorrhea. The ratio of acetylcholine production to acetylcholine enzymatic destruction is important in determining the intensity and the duration of the vasomotor reaction. Numerous factors influence this ratio, but primary control is exerted by the hypothalamus by direct stimulation via the autonomic system to release acetylcholine, and indirect control is established via the hypothalamic pituitary axis and estrogen release, which inhibits acetylcholinesterase function. As is well documented (Stoksted, 1952; Chladek et al., 1972; Taylor, 1961b, 1973, 1979), the control of nasal respiration regulates the oxygen intake of the lungs and thus influences cellular respiration throughout the body. This control is neuroendocrine in nature, originating in the hypothalamus in response to afferent stimuli from body receptors monitoring the internal and external environments of the body. Control is effected via chemical mediators working directly at cell surface nerve endings or indirectly via hormonal activity.

The primary target site effecting control of nasal respiration is the nasal mucosa, which is in a dynamic state, changing constantly under normal and abnormal conditions in response to internal and external stimuli. This complex, integrated neuroendocrine pathway utilizes the autonomic nervous system efferent nerves and hormonal mediators of the pituitary axis to effect a primary functional response of the nasal mucosa, known as the vasomotor reaction.

The vasomotor reaction is the end result of these multiple interactions and is characterized by increased nasal mucosal surface area, increased nasal obstruction, and increased nasal secretions (Taylor, 1973, 1979). The vasomotor reaction is chemically initiated at the end organ by vasodilating agents; the most important and powerful dilating agent in normal and disease states is acetylcholine, which is produced at parasympathetic nerve endings. Its action, in turn, is regulated by acetylcholinesterase activity at the nerve endings.

Nasal obstruction is produced by vasomotor reaction and, in many diseases, is controlled by the autonomic nervous system, which acts on the erectile tissue of the nasal lining.

The increased nasal secretions of the vasomotor reaction are largely composed of mucus from the nasal mucosa. Nasal mucus is the basic ingredient of nasal discharge and consists of 2.3 to 3 per cent nonsulfated and sulfated mucoproteins and mucopolysaccharides, 1 to 2 per cent inorganic salts, and 96 per cent water (Taylor, 1979). It is produced by nasal mucosa, from goblet cells, stromal mucosa, serous glands, and duct cells. Transudation can quickly occur via the semipermeable basement membrane and from the capillary loops that pierce the membrane, thus bringing fluid and debris directly onto the surface epithelium and contributing to mucus formation (Taylor, 1974). This fluid may be seen as the sudden, diffuse, watery discharge occurring in several diseases.

Excessive mucus formation or increased viscosity in response to internal and external stimuli may lead to stasis and poor drainage from the nose. Such stasis frequently leads to secondary infections, chronic changes in the nasal mucosa, or both. The normal nasal secretion rate is 0.1 to 0.3 ml per kg per day.

The significance of the mucus and increased nasal secretions that are a part of the vasomotor reaction and that accompany nasal disease lies in the relationship of the specific physiochemical qualities of mucus to nasal function. Along with the erectile nature of the nasal mucosa, nasal mucus provides temperature regulation of the internal environment and inspired air, humidification of inspired air, and vasorespiration control. The peculiar adhesiveness and surface electric activity of nasal mucosa, the result of sulfated mucins, combines with the vibrissae to keep particulate matter from the lower airway. Mucus acts as a primary defense mechanism in inflammatory disease by retaining immunoglobulins and bacteriolytic enzymes (lysozymes) as well as agents or allergens to which this response is directed. Taylor (1973, 1974, 1979) has written excellent reviews of nasal physiology, for the reader who wishes to obtain further information on the subject.

NORMAL PHYSIOLOGIC STATE

The clinician is at times confronted with infants and children who complain of nasal obstruction and rhinorrhea but who exhibit no signs of local or systemic disease. In these cases, obstruction and rhinorrhea may represent a normal physiologic nasal function or may be symptoms of a pathologic condition. The frequency of such complaints increases as the child approaches adolescence, and this fact must be taken into consideration when making a differential diagno-

sis. Table 31–1 lists a number of normal physiologic states in which increased rhinorrhea and nasal obstruction may occur.

The Nasal Cycle

The nasal cycle is a rhythmic, alternating side-to-side congestion and decongestion of the cavernous tissue of the nasal turbinates. Although it occurs in 80 per cent of the population, it is usually unnoticed because the total nasal resistance remains constant. Occasionally, the cycle will increase in intensity and produce signs of obstruction without any significant increase in nasal secretions (Taylor, 1979).

As mentioned, there is a greater variability in nasal air resistance exhibited by young children (Lacourt and Polgar, 1971). This variability suggests an immaturity of the vasomotor reaction in the nasal mucosa of children. This is further exhibited by the apparent lack of an established nasal cycle in children (Van Cauwenberge and Deleye, 1984). In young children, instead of the usual alternation of nasal air resistance from side to side as seen in the adult, the total nasal airway resistance does vary, with changes occurring simultaneously in both sides of the nose.

Paradoxic Nasal Obstruction

The older child and the adolescent with long-standing, severe unilateral obstruction (such as that due to a septal deformity) will often complain of intermittent obstruction of the patent nasal airway. The patent side has functioned as the entire nasal airway, and complaints are elicited only when factors such as the nasal cycle intermittently obstruct the patent side (Arbour and Kern, 1975).

The Nasopulmonary Reflex

Often, older children with a common cold will complain of breathlessness out of proportion to the degree of nasal obstruction observed by the examiner. This is probably the result of reduced vital capacity secondary to stimulation of a nasopulmonary reflex by increased nasal obstruction (Taylor, 1973). Similarly, hypothalamus-mediated nasopulmonary reflexes account for a common complaint of dependent nasal

TABLE 31–1. Normal Physiologic Causes of Increased Nasal Obstruction and Rhinorrhea

Nasal cycle
Paradoxic nasal obstruction
Nasopulmonary reflex
Puberty
Menses
Psychosomatic factors
External environmental stimuli

obstruction in the recumbent position; compression of the dependent lung elicits an ipsilateral nasal obstruction (Sercer, 1930). Ogura and others have studied the nasopulmonary reflexes and have documented a relationship between nasal resistance and pulmonary resistance. They found that increased nasal resistance produces increased pulmonary resistance and decreased pulmonary compliance with probable decreased alveolar ventilation (Ogura et al., 1964, 1966, 1968, 1973); Ogura and Nelson, 1968; Ogura and Harvey, 1971). This may result in aberration of blood gases, in acid-base imbalance, and in tissue hypoxemia, which may account for the generalized symptoms of fatigue, restlessness, and irritability seen in children with severe upper airway obstruction (Ohnishi and Ogura, 1969; Ohnishi et al., 1972).

In contrast, in newborns, Lacourt and Polgar (1971) found that there are reciprocal changes in nasal and pulmonary resistance. "Changes observed in nasal resistance were in opposite direction to pulmonary resistance changes resulting in stabilization of total air resistance."

Puberty and Menses

Adolescent females, and even males, will occasionally complain of intermittent nasal obstruction and rhinorrhea during the pubescent period, resulting from increases in the level of estrogen and, in part, testosterone, which increase the normal vasomotor reaction by decreasing the activity of acetylcholinesterase. Similarly, periodic complaints will occur in the postpubescent female, regarding menstruation (Taylor, 1973, 1979; Mortimer et al., 1936; Parkes and Zuckerman, 1931).

Psychosomatic Factors

Teenagers especially may present with symptoms of intense vasomotor reactions related to emotional states such as anxiety, stress, fatigue, and anger. These are mediated through reflexes centered in the hypothalamus. These symptoms may be accompanied by unilateral migraine headaches, which are mediated by similar reflexes (Taylor, 1973, 1979; Holmes et al., 1950).

External Environmental Stimuli

Numerous complaints of obstruction and rhinorrhea are nothing more than an expression of the nasal vasomotor reaction to external stimuli and reflect the nasal mucosa's normal function as an interface between the body's internal and external environments. Thus, such symptoms may be dependent on the composition of gases and particulate matter (e.g., dust, fur, and smog) or on the temperature and water content of the inspired air. The watery discharge one experiences on

going outside during the winter is a good example of this type of vasomotor reaction (Taylor, 1973).

NASAL OBSTRUCTION AND RHINORRHEA IN DISEASE

The significance of nasal obstruction and rhinorrhea in nasal disease that may occur in the pediatric patient cannot be stressed too greatly. As discussed, both may be manifestations of the basic vasomotor reaction to abnormal internal or external stimuli. However, obstruction may occur with little contribution from the vasomotor reaction but from a single mass blockage of the nasal airway as seen in choanal atresia. Similarly, rhinorrhea may lack the usual mucous component and instead may be distinctly pathologic in nature, as when it is composed of cerebrospinal fluid.

Nasal obstruction and rhinorrhea vary in nature according to their etiology. Table 31–2 classifies these according to their pathogenesis.

Unique to the newborn and the infant airways is the impact of nasal obstruction on the physiologic status of the child. It has been well established that most newborns and infants up to many months of age are obligatory nasal breathers and depend almost entirely on this mode of respiration. Bilateral complete obstruction usually produces a significant respiratory distress state with intermittent cyanosis, apnea, failure to thrive, and, in some cases, life-threatening situations. Even unilateral obstruction may produce some respiratory distress or at least a significant feeding problem (Masing and Horbasch, 1969). The reason for such obligation has been postulated on a number of factors, including (1) "a high cephalic position of cervical viscera with close opposition of the soft palate to the tongue and epiglottis" (Taylor, 1979; Swift and Emery, 1973); (2) the safety provided by the rigid nasal airway in one who spends most of the time recumbent and sleeping; (3) an aid to suckling; and (4) nature's way of ensuring maximum exposure of nasal and nasopharyngeal lymphoid tissue to inspired pathogens and allergens, thus promoting the early development of the immune response (Taylor, 1979; McCaffrey, 1986).

The degree and the duration of obligatory nasal breathing is quite variable. Indeed, some newborns, although distressed by bilateral nasal obstruction, quickly adapt to oral respiration, while others become oral breathers only after a number of months.

In general, as mentioned, nasal resistance is higher in children than in adults, and pediatric nasal resistance is much more variable (Lacourt and Polgar, 1971). The sleeping child will show patterns of rapid eye movement (REM) sleep with increased episodes of periodic breathing with decreased amplitude, accompanied by apnea (Taylor, 1979). Unilateral nasal obstruction in a sleeping child will also reflect sleep-produced periodic major body movements, seemingly attempting to decrease the airway obstruction (Masing and Horbasch, 1969). Nasal obstruction in obligatory nasal breathers, such as infants, along with delays in

TABLE 31–2. Nasal Obstruction and Rhinorrhea in Disease

CONGENITAL
Total nasal agenesis
Proboscis lateralis
Congenital occlusion of anterior nares
Posterior choanal atresia
Choanal stenosis
Mandibulofacial dysostoses
  Treacher Collins syndrome
  Crouzon disease
Coronal craniosynostosis
Cleft palate
Congenital cysts of nasal cavity
  Dermoid
  Nasoalveolar
  Dentigerous
  Mucous cysts of floor of nose
  Jacobson organ cysts
Meningoencephalocele
Encephalocele
Pharyngeal bursa (Tornwaldt)
Hamartomas
Craniopharyngiomas
Chordomas
Teratoid tumors
Epignathus
  Possible third branchial cleft cyst (Frazer, 1940)
    (presenting in Rosenmüller fossa)
Congenital squamous cell carcinoma of nasopharynx

INFLAMMATORY
Infectious
Bacterial
  Secondary invaders
    Haemophilus influenzae
    Streptococcus pneumoniae
    Other streptococci
    Staphylococcus
    Branhamella catarrhalis
  Primary agent
    Diphtheria
    Pertussis
    Tuberculosis
    Rhinoscleroma
    Leprosy
    Chlamydia
Viral
  Primary agent
    Acute viral rhinonasopharyngitis
    Rhinovirus
    Adenovirus
    Coxsackieviruses A and B
    Myxoviruses
      Influenza
      Parainfluenza
      Respiratory syncytial virus
  Prodromal stage of virus disease
    Mumps
    Poliomyelitis
    Measles (rubella, rubeola)
    Roseola infantum
    Erythema infectiosus
    Infectious mononucleosis
    Hepatitis
AIDS
Spirochetal
  Congenital "snuffles"
  Acquired snuffles

Protozoan
  Leishmaniasis
Fungal
  Moniliasis
  Mucormycosis (immunocompromised children)
  Aspergillosis (immunocompromised children)
Parasitic
Allergic
Acute—Type I (anaphylactic, reagin-dependent)
Chronic—Nasal polyposis
Toxic
External stimuli
  Inhalants (e.g., urban pollutants)
  Ingested (hormones, iodides, bromides, aspirin)
  Topically applied (nose drops, cocaine) (rhinitis
    medicamentosa)
Nasopharyngeal
Adenoid hyperplasia
Nasopharyngeal and/or gastroesophageal reflux

TRAUMATIC
External deformity
In utero
Neonatal
Acquired in childhood
Internal deformity
Neonatal
Septal hematoma acquired in childhood
Septal abscess acquired in childhood
Foreign bodies
Rhinolith
Cerebrospinal fluid rhinorrhea
Traumatic
Spontaneous

NEOPLASTIC
Ectodermal origin
Mesodermal origin
Neurogenic origin
  Olfactory neuroblastoma
Odontogenic origin
Idiopathic origin
  Juvenile angiofibroma
  Nasopharyngeal carcinoma

METABOLIC
Cystic fibrosis
Calcium abnormalities
Thyroid disease
  Hypothyroidism
  Hyperthyroidism
Diabetes mellitus
Immunodeficiency disease

IDIOPATHIC
Ciliary dyskinesia (Kartagener syndrome, congenital and
  acquired immotile cilia syndrome)
Atrophic rhinitis
Chronic catarrhal rhinitis
Granulomatosis and vasculitis diseases
  Lupus erythematosus
  Rheumatoid arthritis
  Psoriatic arthritis
  Scleroderma
  Sarcoidosis
  Wegener granulomatosis
  Midline lethal granuloma
  Churg-Strauss syndrome
  Pemphigoid—cicatricial or benign mucoid pemphigoid

body movement may lead to sufficient hypoxia to produce apnea during REM sleep (Taylor, 1979).

Significant nasal obstruction, especially of some chronicity in older developing children, may lead to chronic mouth breathing, abnormal tongue posturing, and resultant dental arch changes with concomitant craniofacial changes (McCaffrey, 1986). The resultant long-face syndrome (adenoid facies) presents with vertical excess in the lower third of the facial height, lip incompetence, narrow maxillary arch with high palate, and steep mandibular plane angle (Klein, 1986). Many feel that there is no conclusive evidence that nasal obstruction alters facial growth and development (Klein, 1986; Gwynn-Evans and Ballard, 1959; Martin et al., 1981). Others (Linder-Aronson, 1975; Solow and Greve, 1979; Principato et al., 1986; Richter, 1987) in their studies and writings report at least a closer correlation, if not a direct cause-and-effect relation, albeit acknowledging that other factors may be present.

Concurrently, the effect of nasal or nasopharyngeal obstruction on obstructed and sleep apnea syndrome in children is being studied extensively (Lavie et al., 1983; Heimer et al., 1983). It has been well accepted that both nasal and oropharyngeal obstruction together may lead, via hypoxia, alveolar hypoventilation, and pulmonary hypertension, to cor pulmonale (Levy et al., 1967). However, this syndrome may occur with nasal obstruction, nasopharyngeal obstruction, or both (McCaffrey, 1986). Either or both nasal and nasopharyngeal obstruction can cause a significant increase in the number of apneic episodes during sleep (Lavie et al., 1983). The whole spectrum of obstructive sleep apnea syndrome, with snoring, enuresis, hypersomnia, decreased mental and physical performance, and daytime hypersomnolence, can occur with nasal or nasopharyngeal obstruction (Laurikainen et al., 1987). It is interesting to note that it is difficult, however, to obtain a correlation between sleep apnea and measured parameters of nasopharyngeal shape or volume of adenoids and dimensions of the nasopharynx (Laurikainen et al., 1987).

Congenital

In view of the varied and complicated plications and involutions that tissues involved in the formation of the face and nose undergo, it is remarkable how infrequently congenital abnormalities of the nose occur. Such abnormalities are most probably due to a combination of exogenous teratogenic factors and inherited gene patterns. In some cases in which nasal development is limited, the cause of the symptoms of obstruction is obvious. Total nose agenesis, although rare, has been reported (Wilson, 1962). Proboscis lateralis similarly is an extreme congenital anomaly (Wilson, 1962; Biber, 1949). Congenital occlusion of the anterior nares seldom occurs. However, when it does, it may be unilateral or bilateral and complete or partial, and nasal obstruction may vary accordingly (Wilson, 1962). Rhinorrhea plays a limited role in the

complaints that result from these rare anomalies (Chap. 36).

The almost total dependency of neonates and infants on nasal respiration is highlighted by the acuteness and severity of the symptoms of nasal obstruction in these children with congenital nasal anomalies, especially as seen in choanal atresia, the most common congenital nasal anomaly. The incidence of congenital choanal atresia ranges from 1 in 5000 births to 1 in 8000 births (Theogaraj et al., 1983). It may be unilateral or bilateral, complete or incomplete, and bony or membranous. Unilateral presentation is more common, 2:1, and is often diagnosed later in life. Bony atresia appears more commonly than membranous (Skolnik et al., 1973). The high incidence of associated anomalies, up to 50 per cent in some series, has been characterized by the acronym, CHARGE, derived from the first letters of the six major categories of associated anomalies occurring in patients with coloboma or choanal atresia (Pagon et al., 1982). The term, CHARGE, is utilized when malformations are present in at least four of the six categories (Dobrowski et al., 1985). The six categories are coloboma, heart disease, atresia choanae, retarded development of central nervous system, genital hypoplasia, and ear anomalies or deafness.

Newborns with bilateral, complete choanal atresia present in acute respiratory distress, as might be expected with complete nasal obstruction in an obligatory nasal breather. The severity and the duration of the unattended distress may vary according to the adaptability of the neonate in acquiring oral respiration. The nasal mucosa of such children may secrete glary mucus. Unilateral atresia, although producing a persistent unilateral discharge, may remain asymptomatic from an obstructive standpoint until later in life, although occlusion of the normal side by acquired disease may produce marked symptoms, especially in infancy.

The diagnosis is confirmed and evaluation of atresia best completed by utilization of horizontal computed tomography in a plane paralleling the posterior hard palate (Slovis et al., 1985). This advancement has led to documentation of the importance of the vomer bone width, degree of medial pterygoid bowing, and the resultant lateral wall of the nasal cavity to vomer (LWNC-V) dimension. Also documented is the presence of nasal obstruction due to posterior choanal stenosis in some neonates.

More recently (Usowicz et al., 1986), neonates with fetal alcohol syndrome have been shown to present with nasal obstruction and rhinorrhea secondary to upper airway anomalies. The latter include nasal hypoplasia, choanal stenosis, and contracted nasopharyngeal vault. Midfacial growth deficiencies have been shown in the past to be a common feature of fetal alcohol syndrome, with maxillary hypoplasia occurring in 64 per cent of infants in a series by Jones and Smith (1975).

Congenital nasal deformity and obstruction may occur as part of the various mandibulofacial dysostoses (e.g., Treacher Collins syndrome and Crouzon disease) secondary to intrauterine disturbance in the development of the first and second branchial arch. There may be associated hypoplasia of the external nose or nasal obstruction secondary to malar, maxillary, and palatal hypoplasia. Coronal craniosynostosis, accompanied by a brachycephalic skull with shortened anterior-posterior dimensions, may result in midface contracture and subsequent nasal and nasopharyngeal airway obstruction. Cleft palate deformities also alter the structure of the nasal cavity, as they are accompanied by nasoseptal deformities (Longacre, 1968) (Chap. 4).

Congenital cysts may occur in the nasal cavity and, depending on their size and location, may present with degrees of nasal obstruction. Such cysts may be dermoid, nasoalveolar (incisive canal cysts), or dentigerous and mucous cysts of the floor of the nose and Jacobson organ. Nasal discharge may be present from a draining sinus tract and may consist of epithelial debris and ectodermal gland secretions (Furstenberg, 1936; Proctor and Proctor, 1979). Nasal obstruction in the neonatal period may occur secondary to congenital cerebral herniation into the nose in the form of a meningocele (meninges alone), meningoencephalocele (meninges and a portion of the brain), or encephalocele (glial tissue with no persistent brain connection). Rhinorrhea may be present as a vasomotor response to altered airflow with a purulent component from secondary bacterial infection; however, in herniations with central connections, clear, watery cerebrospinal fluid rhinorrhea may occur spontaneously (Furstenberg, 1936; Proctor and Proctor, 1979).

Nasopharyngeal lesions may present at birth with obstruction, minimal rhinorrhea, mucopurulent crusting, and postnasal discharge secondary to mucostasis. The pharyngeal bursa (Tornwaldt bursa) in the midline of the nasopharynx may be patulous at birth, although this is rarely noted, but later may become cystic, inflamed, and symptomatic (Proctor and Proctor, 1979; Dorrance, 1931). Other uncommon lesions of the nasopharynx include hamartomas, craniopharyngiomas, chordomas, congenital squamous cell carcinomas (Chang et al., 1983), and teratoid tumors (embryomas and epignathus). Frazer and others have even postulated that a third branchial cleft cyst could present in the fossa of Rosenmüller (Dorrance, 1931).

Inflammatory Nasal Disease

By far, the most common nasal disease in children is that due to inflammatory responses of the nasal mucosa to infectious, allergic, or toxic agents. Obstruction and rhinorrhea occur in response to the nasal vasomotor reaction, which is initiated as a specific defense mechanism to dilute the offending agents and to bring specific antibodies into action. Since the majority of offending agents are airborne, the nasal vasomotor reaction is the first line of body defense. Typically, the reaction works to increase the nasal surface area and increase nasal secretions, which results in increased obstruction; the total effect represents the prodromal symptoms of many common illnesses in children (Chaps. 37 and 42).

The obstruction produced enhances the retention of the offending agents in the nose and allows for appropriate sensitization and antibody response from cells in the nasal mucosa.

In acute inflammation, vascular dilatation, along with arteriolar constriction, occurs, accompanied by exudation of protein-rich fluid and the emigration of polymorphonuclear leukocytes and monocytes into the inflamed tissues (Taylor, 1979). Immunoglobulin A (IgA), the major immunoglobulin in nasal secretions, is synthesized by plasma cells in the mucosa and nasal lymphoid tissues (Ogra and Karzon, 1970). It is produced locally to a variety of bacterial antigens. It is virus-neutralizing and may be active in promoting phagocytosis and intracellular destruction of organisms by macrophages.

Following acute inflammation, one may find a variable onset of mucosal damage to the epithelial and basal membranes and underlying structures that may be quite extensive, especially in those with recurrent infection. Mucosal appearance on examination is variable and noncharacteristic, being pale and swollen or red and swollen. With recurrent episodes of nasal infection, along with abnormal mucociliary transport due to decreased ciliated cells or ultrastructural deficiencies, one may see increased goblet cell or submucosal glands, altered periciliary fluid due to increased tissue fluid leak, and increased purulent secretions due to microabscesses (Petruson and Hansson, 1987). These changes may take up to three to four weeks to heal after resolution of the inflammatory process. Chronic inflammation may occur with prolongation of the symptoms of rhinorrhea and infection.

Bacterial infection in the nose is most commonly a secondary infection, often a result of the prolongation of the vasomotor reaction with obstruction and mucostasis. With the continuity of nasal and sinus mucosa, acute and chronic sinusitis may subsequently develop for similar reasons. Rhinorrhea becomes more purulent, reflecting the increased inflammatory exudate. Obstruction persists from the swollen turbines and mucosa. Offending organisms include *Haemophilus influenzae*, *Streptococcus pneumoniae*, other streptococcal species, *Staphylococcus*, and frequently *Branhamella catarrhalis* (Taylor, 1979; Wilson, 1962; Rachelefsky et al., 1984; Friedman et al., 1984; Lew et al., 1983). With continued sinus orifice obstruction and reduced sinus cavity oxygen saturation, anaerobic organisms proliferate and become a feature of both acute and chronic sinusitis. Often rhinorrhea and obstruction may be the only symptoms and signs of acute, and especially chronic, sinusitis. Careful nasal examination for evidence of purulent exudate in middle and supreme meati along with sinus radiographs is needed to confirm the diagnosis. Sphenoid sinusitis may present with such subtle signs (Lew et al., 1983). Bacterial culture of nasal, nasopharyngeal, and pharyngeal secretions may not be indicative of the true sinus pathogen (Rachelefsky et al., 1984; Friedman et al., 1984).

Recurrent active airway disease (asthma) unresponsive to control and treatment may be aggravated by recurrent acute or chronic sinusitis in children (Friedman et al., 1984). In the last few years, the otolaryngologist has had to be alert to the fact that chronic sinusitis or recurrent otitis media often precedes development of opportunistic processes in children affected with acquired immunodeficiency syndrome (AIDS) (Church, 1987).

Special mention must be made of diphtheritic rhinitis. Although uncommon today, it is a grave disease that, if untreated, may be fatal. Caused by *Corynebacterium diphtheriae*, acute nasal diphtheria may present with a foul, possibly bilateral nasal discharge that often excoriates the upper lip and nostrils. Chronic nasal diphtheria also occurs and is often called membranous rhinitis. A thin, glary discharge is frequently seen. Nasal obstruction is found in both diseases. The classic pale-yellow or whitish membranous exudate of diphtheria may be seen covering the mucous membranes of the nose, and the nasal discharge may contain shreds of membranes along with blood (Wilson, 1962).

Other specific bacterial infections producing nasal symptoms in children include pertussis, tuberculosis, rhinoscleroma, and leprosy. The first stage of pertussis is called the catarrhal phase, with symptoms similar to those of the common cold (Wilson, 1962; Lederer, 1952).

In tuberculosis of the skin (lupus vulgaris), involvement of the nasal vestibule and subcutaneous structures of the nose, including cartilage, may be present. This is usually endogenic, with bacilli of *Mycobacterium tuberculosis* produced via the blood, although the organisms may be introduced externally. Obstruction and mucopurulent secretions may characterize the presence of the disease in the nose (Lederer, 1952).

Primary tuberculosis of the nose is rare, but it may occur as a result of direct contamination by bacilli in the air or from fingers and instruments or via blood and lymphatic routes. The primary granulomas formed by reaction to the bacilli may ulcerate and obstruct the nose. The symptoms of primary tuberculosis of the nose are related to the degree of nasal ulceration present. When ulceration occurs, the resultant rhinorrhea is usually mucopurulent and blood-tinged (Lederer, 1952).

Other causes of chronic granulomatous disease of the nose include rhinoscleroma and leprosy. However, the obstruction that occurs as a result of these illnesses is usually the first sign of the disease, with mucopurulent and semisanguineous discharge developing later secondary to tissue necrosis (Lederer, 1952).

Chlamydia infection in newborns and infants may be acquired during passage through the birth canal of infected mothers, with a transmission rate of 50 per cent. *Chlamydia trachomatis* is best classified as a bacteria, although it is an obligate intracellular parasite, with approximately one fifth of contaminated infants developing nasopharyngeal involvement. The latter is usually asymptomatic. Conjunctivitis and pneumonia are common manifestations of the disease process. However, some infected newborns present with obstructions, rhinorrhea, and a fiery red nasal mucosa with positive cell culture for *Chlamydia trachomatis* (Hammerschlag, 1985).

Viruses may be present but remain inactive in the nasal cavities of children. Under the proper circumstances, such as cooling of the limbs, a decrease in nasal temperature may occur, which may activate the virus and produce symptoms of infection. Viruses present extracellularly, stimulating a vasomotor reaction, and may take part in antigen-antibody reactions (Taylor, 1979).

Acute viral rhinitis or rhinonasal pharyngitis, the "common cold," is the most frequently seen cause of nasal obstruction and rhinorrhea in children. This self-limiting disease is caused by a number of different viruses, including rhinovirus (the most common), adenovirus, coxsackie A, and coxsackie B (Nelson, 1975). The myxoviruses, including influenza, parainfluenza, and respiratory syncytial virus (RSV), may also cause colds. Respiratory syncytial virus has been recognized as the most important cause of severe respiratory tract disease in infants and preschool children (Hoekstra, 1970). It is especially prevalent in infants younger than 2 months of age, although newborns may have a high concentration of antibodies to RSV from their mother (Taylor, 1979; Kim et al., 1969). The nasal obstruction resulting from infection by RSV may cause problems in these obligatory nasal breathers, but such infection may help them develop early active immunity to the virus.

Nasal obstruction and rhinorrhea may appear in the prodromal periods of a variety of other childhood viral illnesses, including mumps, poliomyelitis, measles (both rubella and rubeola), roseola infantum, erythema infectiosum, infectious mononucleosis, and hepatitis (Nelson, 1975).

Spirochetal disease, although rare nowadays, may also occur in the nasal cavity of children with treponemal diseases, particularly *Treponema pallidum*, which causes syphilis, the most common. Syphilis may be congenital or acquired. The nasal symptoms of congenital syphilis may appear in two stages. Symptoms of the early stage develop between the second week to third month of life and resemble those of acute viral rhinitis. There is a thin, watery discharge that becomes mucopurulent. Marked nasal obstruction develops, with characteristic noisy breathing, termed "snuffles." The later stage of congenital syphilis occurs in children aged 3 years or older and is marked by gummatous involvement of the nose, with persistent obstruction and purulent, sanguineous discharge. In acquired syphilis, the primary stage seldom involves the nose. The secondary stage presents with acute rhinitis, while tertiary stage symptoms are secondary to tissue destruction and may include nasoseptal perforations, cartilage collapse, and subsequent saddle nose deformity resulting from gummatous involvement (Wilson, 1962; Lederer, 1952; Martinez and Mouney,

1982). Other treponemes causing bejel, yaws, and pinta are nonvenereal in nature and may but rarely involve the nasal cavities.

In tropical environments, leishmaniasis from the protozoa *Leishmania tropica* may produce symptoms similar to those of syphilis (Lederer, 1952).

Although fungal infection of the nose and the paranasal sinuses was considered to be rare in children and to usually occur secondary to injury of the nasal mucosa (Lederer, 1952), more recently, the presence of fungal infection must be suspected in the debilitated, immunodeficient, or immunosuppressed child presenting even with the most subtle symptoms of nasal obstruction and rhinorrhea (Landoy et al., 1985). Mucormycosis (Abedi et al., 1984) and aspergillosis (Landoy et al., 1985) are the two most common infections, and diagnosis must be established by biopsy, culture, or both. Early diagnosis and treatment are essential to offset this often fatal complication in the immunocompromised patient.

In children, parasitic diseases cause nasal reactions similar to those seen when an organic foreign body is present in the nose. Parasites that may infect the nose include leeches and maggots.

Allergic rhinitis is another common cause of obstruction and rhinorrhea in the pediatric patient. Although there are four basic types of allergic rhinitis, Type I (anaphylactic-reagin–dependent) hypersensitivity is predominant in most inhalant allergies and allergic rhinitis (Gell and Coombs, 1968). A vasomotor reaction occurs in response to an antigen (allergen)-antibody (IgE) reaction in the nasal mucosa. In genetically predisposed individuals, continuous exposure to an inhalant allergen results in the production of antibodies of the reagin type (IgE) from plasma cells in the nasal tissue. Immunoglobulin E becomes attached to mast cells. When additional antigen is inhaled, it is trapped by the nasal mucosa and is passed to the tissue level, where the reaction occurs. Subsequently, there is a release of chemical mediators (called vasoactive amines) from the mast cells. These mediators include histamine, serotonin, slow-reacting substances of anaphylaxis (SRS-A), and eosinophilic chemostatic factor (ECF-A). These, in turn, produce vasodilatation, increased capillary permeability, and an intense vasomotor reaction (Taylor, 1979; Stahl, 1974).

Clinically, the result of such an intensive vasomotor response is nasal obstruction and a profuse watery rhinorrhea, often associated with sneezing and nasal pruritus. Mucostasis can occur, with resultant secondary bacterial infection. The symptoms usually occur chronically with a specific periodicity.

With chronic inflammation of the mucous membrane of the nose and paranasal sinuses, manifested by hypersecretion and hyperplasia, nasal and sinus polyps can form. They represent a focal exaggeration of hyperplastic rhinosinusitis in which stromal binding of the intracellular fluid results in the formation of tissue polyps. The obstruction increases, and both water and mucoid secretions are more abundant (Stahl, 1974). Nasal polyps not only can occur with allergy, especially in aspirin-intolerant and intrinsic-asthma patients, but also can occur in Young syndrome, cystic fibrosis, and Kartagener and ciliary motility dyskinesis syndrome, along with those conditions secondary to chronic infection and mucostasis (Settipane, 1987). Their underlying etiology can, in part, be differentiated histologically. Chemical mediators that can be found in nasal polyps include histamine, serotonin, leukotriene, ECF-A, norepinephrine, kinen, esterase, and possibly prostaglandin D_2 (Settipane, 1987).

Nasopharyngeal adenoid hyperplasia is another common cause of nasal obstruction in the pediatric patient. As part of Waldeyer ring, the adenoids occupy a key position in the development of the immune process. Adenoids are minimal in size at birth and increase in size, usually from 1 to 2 years of age, after immunity has been established. They may recede at puberty (Taylor, 1979; Hollender, 1959), although some evidence suggests a more frequent persistence of size into adulthood than was previously thought. In the nasopharynx, they are in constant contact with inspired air and are continually bathed by nasal mucus cleared from the posterior choanae by the nasal ciliary mechanism. Thus, they are continually exposed to antigens (bacterial, viral, or allergens) inhaled by the individual. They react by forming their own complement of antibodies to these antigens, and it has been postulated that "they modify the microorganisms encountered and release them or their toxins into the reticuloendothelial system of the body as an antigen stimulus for exciting active immunization" (Taylor, 1979). This activity may account for the increase in size of adenoidal tissue with increasing antigen stimulation, often seen in the allergic patient, and may explain the occurrence of adenoid hypertrophy. Nasal obstruction and chronic purulent rhinorrhea may result from such hypertrophy.

The severest form of nasal obstruction may occur in the presence of marked hypertrophy of adenoid tissue with or without tonsil enlargement. As mentioned previously, increased nasal airway resistance may lead to increased pulmonary resistance and alveolar hypoventilation, which is mediated by nasopulmonary reflexes. The result may be hypoxia, causing secondary pulmonary vasoconstriction with increased pulmonary vascular resistance. Eventually, prolongation of these symptoms may lead to cor pulmonale (Levy et al., 1967; Luke et al., 1966).

In newborns and young infants, especially those with central nervous system immaturity, nasal obstruction and rhinorrhea along with recurrent respiratory disorders, oropharyngeal dysphagia, chronic regurgitation, and hematemesis may be secondary to the irritative and inflammatory response of the nasal and nasopharyngeal mucosa and an indicator of either or both nasopharyngeal and gastroesophageal reflux. Formula or gastric contents in the nasopharynx produces a vasomotor reaction to these chronic irritative stimuli. This is enhanced by the infant receiving a bottle in the crib or being placed in the supine position immediately after feeding (Hellemans et al., 1981).

A similar pathogenesis of rhinorrhea and obstruction may be seen in children with oropharyngeal dysphagia, with resultant nasal regurgitation secondary to cerebral disease, peripheral neuropathies, inherited or degenerative muscular disorders, cricopharyngeal dysfunctions and local factors such as tumors of the oropharynx or hypopharynx. Nasopharyngeal reflux due to delayed opening of the cricopharyngeal sphincter in children with familial dysautonomia is a typical example.

A toxic nasal inflammatory response may occur in children in response to stimulation by a variety of external substances, both inhaled and ingested. Inhaled substances may act as chemical irritants and react with the nasal mucosa to cause defensive vasomotor responses. Such responses may be difficult to distinguish from those occurring as part of Type I–mediated allergic reactions (Taylor, 1979).

Children may inhale from 10,000 to 15,000 liters of air per day, much of this polluted, in our present environment. The urban pollutants may include oxides of nitrogen, carbon monoxide, ozone, aldehydes, ketones, chlorine, sulfur dioxide, ammonia, and hydrocarbons. These plus cigarette smoke may lead to increased nasal discharge as a result of the vasomotor reaction (Taylor, 1973, 1979).

Locally applied prescribed and over-the-counter preparations including sympathomimetic agents may produce a quick nasal toxic reaction owing to the rebound phenomenon of rhinitis medicamentosa. Although such a phenomenon is less commonly seen in children than in adults, it may account for the persistent obstruction and rhinorrhea following a cold. Currently, adolescents are being seen with nasal problems resulting from cocaine and other illicit drug usage. The local vasoconstriction with subsequent reactive hyperemia that occurs when cocaine is snuffed may produce mucoid rhinorrhea. Prolonged use of the drug results in tissue necrosis, and the mucoid drainage may become purulent (Blue, 1969; May and West, 1973).

Ingested substances that may produce rhinorrhea and symptoms of nasal obstruction include hormones, iodides, and bromides. Aspirin sensitivity may be the cause of intermittent, profuse watery rhinorrhea and nasal obstruction in adolescents, especially those with polyp formation. Such sensitivity may be the result of the inability of some individuals to counteract the effects of prostaglandin release or inhibition (Stahl, 1974).

Traumatic Disease

The necessity to diagnose traumatic nasal disease in children early has been emphasized in recent years owing to the recognition of the importance of nasal respiration and the nasopulmonary reflex on lung physiology and the realization of the influence of abnormal nasal functions on subsequent facial, dental arch, and palatal growth, as previously mentioned. Conservative management of abnormal nasal function or deformities

of the nose is still advocated, but treatment should not be delayed if "marked disturbance in function or distortion exists that also interferes with growth and facial development" (Farrior and Connolly, 1970).

Nasal obstruction is the primary symptom of external and internal nasal trauma. The severity of the effects of such obstruction is dependent on the extent and the location of the injury and the age of the child. Obstruction may be evident and total or more subtle and intermittent, depending on such factors as "paradoxical nasal obstruction" and the nasal cycle (Chap. 40).

Alteration of the normal "streamlined" flow of air through the nose may lead to turbulence and eddies in airflow and a resultant vasomotor reaction. Mucosal injury and mucostasis may lead to bacterial invasion, which could result in mucopurulent nasal discharge. This may be further aggravated by mucociliary damage. Atrophic mucosa may be the end result, with further accentuation of rhinorrhea and obstructive symptoms.

With increased turbulence and stasis of air in the nose, particulate matter and allergens accumulate in the mucosa, causing more intense vasomotor, allergic, and inflammatory reactions.

This pathogenesis has led to the treatment maxim of restoring the normal streamlining of nasal respirations in order to improve alveolar ventilation and to avoid interference with nasal mucosal function, especially in children.

Nasal obstruction from traumatic deformities may occur at any age but may not be symptomatic in the young infant or the neonate unless it is severe enough to cause respiratory distress in the obligatory nasal breather. Such obstruction may be obvious in cases of severe external trauma but more occult in the younger patient with only septal trauma. Nasal trauma can be classified as to its time of origin. The recent advent of frequent ultrasonic examinations in the prenatal and perinatal periods has shown that nasal abnormalities may occur *in utero* owing to fetal head presentation. Nasal trauma may also occur at birth during vaginal deliveries, with or without forceps. Some septal deformities may be evident on careful examination in as many as 70 per cent of newborns, secondary to intrauterine or birth trauma (Kirchner, 1955; Hinderer, 1976). Additional nasal trauma may occur at any time from birth onward in childhood but often will be subtle. Such subtle injuries may affect the main "growth center" of the nose, the septovomerine angle, and may be asymptomatic until adolescence, when the deformity is accentuated by nasal growth. The symptoms at that time will depend on the age of the child and the degree and location of the deformity.

In the acute traumatic period, intermittent bleeding and the development of nasal obstruction suggest development of a septal hematoma. This occurs more commonly in children than in adults because of a thicker and more elastic mucoperichondrium in children (Pirsig, 1984). Trauma disrupts septal vessels, but not the mucoperichondrium, with the subsequent development of a septal hematoma. Subsequent throbbing pain and elevated temperature may indicate the presence of a septal abscess. Untreated, this abscess may lead to septal perforation with resultant airway turbulence and subsequent increased obstruction and rhinorrhea.

Internal trauma may be the result of the introduction of foreign materials into the nasal cavity, which would cause an intensive vasomotor reaction, rhinorrhea, and obstruction. Such trauma characteristically is seen in children 3 years of age or younger, who frequently stuff foreign objects into their nostrils. Less frequently, foreign material enters the nose through the posterior choanae secondary to regurgitation (Lederer, 1952) (Chap. 39).

The symptoms of a foreign body in the nose are dependent on the nature of the foreign material, its size, the number of objects, and the location of the foreign body. However, unilateral purulent, fetid nasal drainage in a child is highly suggestive of a foreign body. Symptoms of a foreign body reaction may be delayed but are earlier in onset when the foreign body is organic. Long-standing symptoms of obstruction may indicate that calcareous deposits have formed about the foreign body and a rhinolith has developed (Lederer, 1952) (Chap. 39).

In traumatic nasal disease, special attention must be paid to determining the presence or absence of rhinorrhea or cerebrospinal fluid. Cerebrospinal fluid rhinorrhea is most commonly seen after skull trauma, although it may occur spontaneously either with or without increased intracranial pressure. It may also be a manifestation of cerebrospinal fluid otorrhea presenting in the nasal cavity via the eustachian tube. Spontaneous cerebrospinal fluid rhinorrhea has been seen with a variety of intracranial lesions, especially intrasellar tumors, but it may also be present in young infants, secondary to congenital bone dehiscences (Montgomery, 1973; Briant and Snell, 1967; Kaufman, 1909; Duckert and Mathog, 1977).

The presence of cerebrospinal fluid rhinorrhea is first suggested by history and the gross nature of the nasal discharge. A clear, salty, often unilateral drainage from the nose, especially after a head injury, is highly suggestive of cerebrospinal fluid rhinorrhea. When such fluid flows profusely from the nose and when the discharge increases in quantity with changes in position of the head, during a Valsalva maneuver, and with jugular compression, the possibility that the rhinorrhea is cerebrospinal fluid is significant. A rapid method of analyzing such nasal drainage is to test it with glucose oxidase–impregnated test sticks. However, since these sticks react to as little as 10 mg per 100 ml of glucose, they may give a false-positive reaction because of the presence of lacrimal secretions or the products of an allergic reaction or infectious rhinosinusitis in the nasal secretions. A negative test result is highly significant in ruling out the presence of cerebrospinal fluid rhinorrhea, while a strongly positive reaction to nasal secretions shows the presence of 50 mg per 100 ml or more of glucose, indicating that the presence of cerebrospinal fluid in the nasal discharge is quite probable (Kaufman, 1909). If sufficient fluid can be collected, biochemical analysis for the presence of protein, glucose, and electrolytes will confirm the diagnosis of cerebrospinal fluid rhinorrhea. Demonstration of the area of the fistula is best achieved by evaluating the results of radiography, enhanced computed tomography, placement of an intrathecal tracer with intranasal pledgets, and cisternography (Duckert and Mathog, 1977).

Neoplastic Disease

Primary neoplasms of the nasal cavity are rare; they account for as few as 0.3 per cent of tumors of the body (Axtell et al., 1972). When they do occur, they may be of ectodermal, mesodermal, neurogenic, or odontogenic origin (Bortnick, 1973). Any tumor that occurs in adults may also occur in children, but a few are more commonly seen in and, indeed, tend to be specific to the pediatric patient (Chap. 41).

Nasal obstruction and rhinorrhea are the two most common symptoms of nasal tumors. These symptoms are related to the increasing size of the neoplastic mass and the effect of the tumor on the nasal mucosa. In neoplasms primary to the nasal cavity, symptoms arise early but are delayed in tumors of the nasopharynx and sinuses until nasal cavity invasion occurs (Bortnick, 1973).

Rhinorrhea may occur as a typical vasomotor reaction to nasal airway invasion. Such nasal discharge may become purulent with stasis and secondary infection or sanguineous with tissue necrosis and eventually may contain cerebrospinal fluid as a result of extension of the pathologic lesion into the cranial cavity. The triad of symptoms, including nasal obstruction, rhinorrhea, and epistaxis, is common in neoplasms. Nasal polyposis may also arise as a secondary sign of nasal neoplasm.

Juvenile nasopharyngeal angiofibromas are specific to the adolescent male, with symptoms usually arising between 7 and 17 years of age, at an average age of 14. The symptoms are progressive, partial unilateral obstruction followed by progressive obstruction of the involved side and then partial obstruction on the opposite side. Epistaxis attacks occur with increasing frequency along with pathologic symptoms in adjacent structures (Patterson, 1965, 1973).

The nose may be the first site of symptoms of nasopharyngeal carcinoma. Twenty-one per cent of patients with nasopharyngeal carcinoma present with symptoms of rhinorrhea, obstruction, or loss of smell. Epstein-Barr virus (EBV) serologic testing may be helpful in the diagnosis and prognosis with certain types of nasopharyngeal carcinomas.

Olfactory neuroblastoma is another uncommon neoplasm, but one that may present in the pediatric patient. Originating primarily in the area of the olfactory mucosa, it may not produce signs of obstruction until it has grown to considerable size. Epistaxis due to tissue destruction is the usual presenting sign (Cantrell et al., 1977; Schenck and Ogura, 1972; Ogura and Schenck, 1973). In children, neoplasms of the hematopoietic system rarely present in the nasal cavity, but when they do, they are usually secondary to metastatic invasion from leukemic disease (Sanford and Becker, 1967).

Metabolic Disease in the Nasal Cavity

Nasal symptoms of obstruction and rhinorrhea may be important in the early diagnosis of cystic fibrosis or mucoviscidosis. In mucoviscidosis, an inherited systemic disease in which the alimentary and respiratory tracts are involved, abnormally viscid mucus is produced. Histologically, the nasal submucosal glands are hypoplastic and appear to be dilated with eosinophilic staining material. Nasal mucous secretions exhibit marked adhesiveness and a changed water-binding capacity and permeability related to an increased calcium concentration (Gharib et al., 1964). The viscid, tenacious mucus and nasal obstruction characteristic of mucoviscidosis lead to stasis and secondary infection by *Staphylococcus aureus, Pseudomonas, Streptococcus viridans, Haemophilus influenzae,* or *Branhamella catarrhalis.* Nasal polyps frequently occur in association with mucoviscidosis and secondary infections (Baker and Smith, 1970).

The nasal obstruction of mucoviscidosis is produced by (1) the thick, tenacious mucus; (2) the chronic, thickened nasal mucosa; and (3) nasal polyps. Chronic sinusitis may aggravate the situation: as many as 90 per cent of children with cystic fibrosis have evidence of severe opacification of the sinuses on radiographic examination (Baker and Smith, 1970; Gharib et al., 1964). The result is that a child presenting with thick, foul-smelling, purulent, bilateral nasal secretions, chronic nasal obstruction, nasal polyps, and a broad nasal bridge must be considered to have mucoviscidosis until it is proved otherwise.

In other metabolic diseases, obstruction and rhinorrhea are produced as a result of modification of the normal vasomotor reaction. The effects of endogenous hormones on nasal mucosa have been discussed earlier. Exogenous hormones may have a similar effect on the vasomotor reaction (Schreiber, 1973).

Calcium and magnesium potentiate the action of acetylcholinesterase in nasal mucosa, and the former modifies the permeability of the basement membrane. Deficiencies of these elements may intensify the vasomotor reaction, while exogenous calcium has been used to alleviate symptoms of vasomotor rhinitis (Taylor, 1973, 1979).

In hypothyroid states, low levels of ionic calcium will be seen and can modify the vasomotor reaction. In hyperthyroidism, thyroxine, through its influence on lung dynamics, may hypothalamically influence the nasal mucosa and produce symptoms of vasomotor rhinitis (Taylor, 1979; May and West, 1973).

Disorders of carbohydrate metabolism often lead to chronic nasal infection in children. This may be the result of impairment of the system by which carbohydrate metabolism releases antibodies from cells in the nasal mucosa (Taylor, 1979; May and West, 1973).

In immunodeficiency diseases, there is a general increased incidence of infections. However, with isolated IgA deficiency, these infections are confined mostly to the upper respiratory tract. In response to pathogens, a more intensive and prolonged vasomotor reaction will be seen, as the lack of IgA allows the invasion of the nasal mucosa by the pathogens (Taylor, 1979).

Idiopathic Nasal Disease

There are a number of idiopathic systemic diseases that, although uncommon in childhood, may present with nasal symptoms and signs. Mucopurulent or serosanguineous rhinorrhea, obstruction, crusting, and epistaxis, are characteristic nasal signs of a number of granulomatosis and vasculitis entities. Nasal septal perforation has been a well-known diagnostic criterion of systemic lupus erythematosus (Reiter and Myers, 1980). Similar lesions have been described in patients with rheumatoid arthritis, psoriatic arthritis, and scleroderma. Sarcoid noncaseating granulomas may present as tiny, 1-mm, yellow nodules on the nasal mucosa surrounded by hyperemic boggy mucosa. Although these lesions are often self-limiting, they may lead to fibrosis, synechiae, and atrophic rhinitis (Gordon et al., 1976).

More destructive granulomatosis and vasculitis type lesions of the nasal cavity and sinuses can be found with Wegener granulomatosis, midline lethal granuloma, and Churg-Strauss syndrome. Their clinical and morphologic appearances are similar to each other and to certain fungal diseases such as *Sporothrix schenckii* and *Coccidioides* and highlight the importance of biopsy, culture, special staining, and overall organ system evaluation to differentiate the diseases that these entities involve (McDonald and DeRemee, 1983; Fauci et al., 1983).

Cicatricial pemphigoid or benign mucous pemphigoid, a chronic blistering disease of mucosal epithelium, may present with nasal lesions (Person and Rogers, 1977).

Among primary nasal diseases of unknown etiology, there are several that may present in the pediatric patient with characteristic symptoms of obstruction and rhinorrhea. The first is a rapidly evolving syndrome of mucociliary dysfunction or ciliary immotility syndrome. Although much of this syndrome is known to occur on an inherited or on an acquired basis, the rapid assimilation of new knowledge and new case reports prevent the proper classification of this entity. In 1933, Kartagener reported a triad of sinusitis, situs inversus, and bronchiectasis. In 1976, Afzelius identified the cause of the defect as of genetic origin, producing immotile cilia and spermatozoa. Acquired defects of ciliary motility were also discovered, and now these lesions can be properly classified as ciliary dyskinesias. Ciliary dyskinesia is now divided into primary and secondary ciliary dyskinesia. Primary ciliary dyskinesia is an inherited disorder such as Kartagener syndrome with axonemal defects including defective dynein arms, absence of radial spokes, microtubular transposition, and disorientation of the central pair of microtubules. Some of these anomalies may occur in other disorders of the respiratory epithelium, indeed even in normal, healthy subjects.

In secondary ciliary dyskinesia, the noninherited type, these ultrastructural abnormalities are variable and even less specific (Burgersdijk et al., 1986). Studies utilized to determine the nature of the ciliary motility must include biopsy with transmission electronmicroscopy, phase contrast microscopy, and technetium-99m mucociliary clearance testing. When children present with chronic rhinorrhea and obstruction accompanied by chronic bronchitis, sinusitis, otitis media, and nasal polyposis, thought must be given to possible ciliary dyskinesia (immotile cilia syndrome) and Kartagener syndrome if the patient also has situs inversus.

Atrophic rhinitis (ozena, rhinitis fetida, rhinitis crustosa) is a chronic nasal disease with onset in childhood that features progressive atrophy in nasal mucosa and underlying bone. The presenting symptoms are obstruction of the nasal airway due to enlargement of the nasal cavity and disturbance of normal streamlined airflow. Characteristically, the nasal mucosa is foulsmelling, green, and crusted, although there is minimal purulent discharge. The secretions are characteristically composed of exfoliated nasal mucosal cells. Vitamin, iron, endocrine, and nutritional deficiencies have been implicated. The principal organisms that are responsible for the purulence of the secretions are *Klebsiella ozaenae*, a form of *Corynebacterium diphtheriae*, and the *Perez-Hofer bacillus* (Wilson, 1962; Goodman and DeSouza, 1973). The isolation of *Klebsiella ozaenae* from the nasal cavity is considered a *sine qua non* for diagnosis of allergic rhinitis (Dudley, 1987).

Chronic catarrhal rhinitis is a chronic nasal disease of children, occurring most commonly in the lower socioeconomic groups. This disease is characterized by chronic mucopurulent discharge. It tends to resolve spontaneously at puberty and has been thought to be a basement membrane disease, metabolic in origin, with an endocrine defect as its underlying etiology (Taylor, 1961a, 1979; Wilson, 1962).

REFERENCES

Abedi, S., Sismanis, A., Choi, K., et al. 1984. Twenty-five years experience in treating cerebro-rhino-orbital mucormycosis. Laryngoscope 94:1060.

Afzelius, B. A. 1976. A human syndrome caused by immotile cilia. Science 193:317.

Arbour, P. L., and Kern, E. B. 1975. Paradoxical nasal obstruction. Can. J. Otolaryngol. 4:333.

Axtell, L. M., Cutter, S. J., and Meyers, M. H. 1972. End results in cancer. Report no. 4. Washington, D.C., U.S. Dept. of Health, Education, and Welfare, Public Health Service, N.I.H., 85–88.

Baker, D. C., and Smith, J. T. 1970. Nasal symptoms of mucoviscidosis. Otolaryngol. Clin. North Am. 3:257.

Biber, J. J. 1949. Proboscis lateralis: Rare malformation of nose; its genesis and treatment. J. Laryngol. Otol. 63:734.

Bickmore, J. T., and Marshall, M. L. 1976. Cytology in nasal secretions: Further diagnostic help. Laryngoscope 86:516.

Blue, J. A. 1969. Over-medication of nasal mucosa. Mod. Med. 37:90.

Bortnick, E. 1973. Neoplasms of the nasal cavity. Otolaryngol. Clin. North Am. 6:801.

Briant, T. D. R., and Snell, D. 1967. Diagnosis of cerebrospinal fluid rhinorrhea and the rhinology approach to its repair. Laryngoscope 7:1390.

Bridger, G. P. 1970. Physiology of the nasal valve. Arch. Otolaryngol. 92:543.

Bridger, G. P., and Proctor, D. F. 1970. Maximum nasal inspiratory flow and nasal resistance. Ann. Otol. Rhinol. Laryngol. 79:481.

Bryan, M. P., and Bryan, W. T. K. 1969. Cytologic and cytochemical aspects of ciliated epithelium in differentiation of nasal inflammatory diseases. Acta Cytol. 13:515.

Bryan, W. T. K., and Bryan, M. P. 1959. Cytologic diagnosis in otolaryngology. Trans. Am. Acad. Ophthalmol. Otolaryngol. 63:597.

Burgersdijk, F. J., DeGroot, J. C., Graamans, K., et al. 1986. Testing ciliary activity in patients with chronic and recurrent infections of the upper airways: Experiences in 68 cases. Laryngoscope 96:1029.

Cantrell, R. W., Ghorayeb, B. Y., and Fitz-Hugh, G. S. 1977. Esthesioneuroblastoma: Diagnosis and treatment. Ann. Otol. Rhinol. Otolaryngol. 86:760.

Celsus, A. C. *De Medicina*, trans. Spencer, W. G.

Chang, C., Berrios, J. A., Strong, D. D., et al. 1983. Squamous cell proliferative lesions of the nasopharynx: A distinct clinicopathologic entity. Pediatr. Pathol. 1:362.

Chladek, V., Pihrt, J., and Engler, V. 1972. Vasomotor reactions in nasal mucosa in adolescents. Cesk. Hyg. 17:241.

Church, J. A. 1987. Human immunodeficiency virus (HIV) infections at Children's Hospital of Los Angeles: Recurrent otitis media or chronic sinusitis as the presenting process in pediatric AIDS. Immunol. Allergy Pract. IX:25.

Cole, P., Forsythe, R., and Haight, J. S. J. 1983. Effects of cold air and exercise on nasal patency. Ann. Otol. Rhinol. Laryngol. 92:196.

Cottle, M. H. 1968. Rhino-manometry: An aid in physical diagnosis. Int. Rhinol. 6:7.

De Catarrhis Libri, Vol. I (cited by Schaeffer, 1932).

Dobrowski, J. M., Grundfast, K. M., Rosenbaum, K. N., et al. 1985. Otorhinolaryngic manifestations of CHARGE association. Otolaryngol. Head Neck Surg. 93:798.

Dorland's Illustrated Medical Dictionary, 27th ed. 1988. Philadelphia, W. B. Saunders Co.

Dorrance, G. M. 1931. The so-called bursa pharyngea in man. Arch. Otolaryngol. 13:187.

Duckert, L. G., and Mathog, R. H. 1977. Diagnosis in persistent cerebrospinal fluid fistulas. Laryngoscope 87:18.

Dudley, J. P. 1987. Atrophic rhinitis: Antibiotic treatment. Am. J. Otolaryngol. 8:387.

Fanous, N. 1986. Anterior turbinectomy. Arch. Otolaryngol. Head Neck Surg. 112:850.

Farrior, R. T., and Connolly, M. E. 1970. Septorhinoplasty in children. Otolaryngol. Clin. North Am. 3:545.

Fauci, A. S., Haynes, B. F., Katz, P., et al. 1983. Wegener's granulomatosis: Prospective clinical and therapeutic experience with 85 patients in 21 years. Ann. Intern. Med. 98:76.

Frazer, J. E. 1940. A Manual of Embryology, 2nd ed. London, Bailliere, Tindall and Cox.

Friedman, R., Ackerman, M., Wald, E., et al. 1984. Asthma and bacterial sinusitis in children. J. Allergy Clin. Immunol. 74:185.

Furstenberg, A. C. 1936. A Clinical and Pathological Study of Tumors and Cysts of the Nose, Pharynx, Mouth and Neck of Teratological Origin. Ann Arbor, Edward Brothers.

Galen, C. 1916. On the Natural Faculties, trans. Brock, A. J. London, W. Heinemann Ltd.

Gell, P. G. H., and Coombs, R. R. A. 1968. Clinical Aspects of Immunology, 2nd ed. Philadelphia, F. A. Davis Co.

Gharib, R., Allen, R. P., Joos, H. A., et al. 1964. Paranasal sinuses in cystic fibrosis. Am. J. Dis. Child. 108:499.

Goodman, W. S., and DeSouza, F. M. 1973. Atrophic rhinitis. Otolaryngol. Clin. North Am. 6:773.

Gordon, W. W., Cohn, A. M., Greenberg, S. D., et al. 1976. Nasal sarcoidosis. Arch. Otolaryngol. 102:11.

Gwynn-Evans, E., and Ballard, C. F. 1959. Discussion on the mouth-breather. Proc. R. Soc. Med. 51:279.

Haight, J. S. J., and Cole, P. 1983. The site and function of the nasal valve. Laryngoscope 93:49.

Hammerschlag, M. R. 1985. *Chlamydia trachomatis.* Birth Defects: Original Article Series. 21:93.

Heimer, D., Scharf, S. M., Lieberman, A., et al. 1983. Sleep apnea syndrome treated by repair of deviated nasal septum. Chest 84:184.

Hellemans, J., Pelemans, W., and Vantrappen, G. 1981. Pharyngoesophageal swelling disorders and the pharyngoesophageal sphincter. Med. Clin. North Am. 65:1149.

Hinderer, K. H. 1976. Nasal problems in children. Pediatr. Ann. 52:499.

Hippocrates. The Aphorisms, trans. Jones, W. H. S., and Withington, E. T. 1922. London, W. Heinemann Ltd.

Hoekstra, R. E., Herrman, E. C., Jr., and O'Connell, E. J. 1970. Virus infections in children. Am. J. Dis. Child. 12:14.

Hollender, A. R. 1959. The lymphoid tissue of the nasopharynx. Laryngoscope 69:529.

Holmes, T. H., Goodell, H., Wolf, S., et al. 1950. The Nose: An experimental study of the reactions within the nose in human subjects during varying life experiences. Springfield, IL, Charles C Thomas.

Jones, K. L., and Smith, D. W. 1975. The fetal alcohol syndrome. Teratology 12:1.

Kartagener, M. 1933. Zur Pathogenese die Bronchiecktarien bei situs viscerum inversus. Bietr. Klin. Tuherk. 83:489.

Kaufman, H. H. 1909. Non-traumatic cerebrospinal fluid rhinorrhea. Arch. Neurol. 21:59.

Kennedy, D. W., Zinreich, S. J., Rosenbaum, A. E., et al. 1985. Functional endoscopic sinus surgery. Arch. Otolaryngol. 111:576.

Kern, E. B. 1973. Rhinomanometry. Otolaryngol. Clin. North Am. 6:863.

Kim, H. W., Bellanti, J. A., Arrobio, J. O., et al. 1969. Respiratory syncytial virus neutralizing activity in nasal secretions following natural infection. Proc. Soc. Exp. Biol. Med. 131:658.

Kirchner, J. A. 1955. Traumatic nasal deformity in the newborn. Arch. Otolaryngol. 62:139.

Klein, J. C. 1986. Nasal respiratory functional and craniofacial growth. Arch. Otolaryngol. Head Neck Surg. 112:843.

Lacourt, G., and Polgar, G. 1971. Interaction between nasal and pulmonary resistance in newborn infants. J. Appl. Physiol. 30:870.

Landoy, Z., Rotstein, C., and Shedd, D. 1985. Aspergillosis of the nose and paranasal sinuses in neutropenic patients at an oncology center. Head Neck Surg. 8:83.

Laurikainen, E., Erkinjuntii, M., Alihanka, J., et al. 1987. Radiological parameters of the bony nasopharynx and the adenotonsillar size compared with sleep apnea episodes in children. J. Pediatr. Otolaryngol. 12:303.

Lavie, P., Fischel, N., Zomer, J., et al. 1983. The effects of partial and complete mechanical occlusion of the nasal passages on sleep structure and breathing in sleep. Acta Otolaryngol. 95:161.

Lederer, F. L. 1952. Diseases of the Ear, Nose and Throat, 6th ed. Philadelphia, F. A. Davis Co.

Levy, A. M., Tabakin, B. S., and Hanson, J. S. 1967. Hypertrophied adenoids causing pulmonary hypertension and severe congestive heart failure. N. Engl. J. Med. 277:506.

Lew, D., Southwick, F. S., Montgomery, W. W., et al. 1983. Sphenoid sinusitis. A review of 30 cases. N. Engl. J. Med. 309:1149.

Linder-Aronson, S. 1975. Effects of adenoidectomy on the dentition and facial skeleton over a period of 5 years. *In* Cook, J. T. (ed.): Transactions of the Third International Orthodontic Congress. St. Louis, C. V. Mosby Co. pp. 85–100.

Longacre, J. J. 1968. Craniofacial Anomalies: Pathogenesis and Repair. Philadelphia, J. B. Lippincott Co.

Lorin, M. I., Pureza, F. G., Irwin, D. M., et al. 1976. Composition of nasal secretions with cystic fibrosis. J. Lab. Clin. Med. 88:114.

Luke, M. J., Mehrizi, A., Folger, G. M., Jr., et al. 1966. Chronic nasal obstruction as a cause of cardiomegaly, cor pulmonale and pulmonary edema. Pediatrics 37:762.

Lusk, R. P., and Lee, P. C. 1986. Magnetic resonance imaging of congenital midline nasal masses. Otolaryngol. Head Neck Surg. 95:303.

Martin, R., Vig, P. S., Warren, D. W. 1981. Nasal resistance and vertical dentofacial features. Int. Am. Dent. Res. Abstract.

Martinez, S. A., and Mouney, D. F. 1982. Treponemal infections of the head and neck. Otolaryngol. Clin. North Am. 15:613.

Masing, H., and Horbasch, G. 1969. The influence of the nose on the sleeping habits of infants. Int. Rhinol. 7:41.

May, M., and West, J. W. 1973. The stuffy nose. Otolaryngol. Clin. North Am. 6:655.

McCaffrey, R. V. 1986. Nasal physiology in children. Rhinology 24:7.

McDonald, T. J., and DeRemee, R. A. 1983. Wegener's granulomatosis. Laryngoscope 93:220.

Montgomery, W. W. 1973. Cerebrospinal fluid rhinorrhea. Otolaryngol. Clin. North Am. 6:757.

Mortimer, H., Wright, R. P., Bachman, C., et al. 1936. Effect of estrogenic hormones on nasal mucosa of monkeys. Proc. Soc. Exp. Biol. Med. 34:535.

Nelson, W. E. 1975. Textbook of Pediatrics, 10th ed. Philadelphia, W. B. Saunders Co.

Niinimaa, V., Cole, P., Mintz, S., et al. 1979. A head-out body plethysmograph. J. Appl. Physiol. 47:1336.

Ogra, P. L., and Karzon, D. T. 1970. The role of immunoglobulins in the mechanism of mucosal immunity to virus infection. Pediatr. Clin. North Am. 17:385.

Ogura, J. H., and Harvey, J. E. 1971. Nasopulmonary mechanics—experimental evidence of the influence of the upper airway upon the lower. Acta Otolaryngol. 71:123.

Ogura, J. H., and Nelson, J. R. 1968. Nasal surgery: Physiologic considerations of nasal obstruction. Arch. Otolaryngol. 88:288.

Ogura, J. H., and Schenck, N. L. 1973. Unusual nasal tumors. Otolaryngol. Clin. North Am. 6:813.

Ogura, J. H., Dammkuehler, R., and Nelson, J. R. 1966. Nasal obstruction and the mechanics of breathing. Arch. Otolaryngol. 83:135.

Ogura, J. H., Nelson, J. R., Dammkuehler, R., et al. 1964. Experimental observations on the relationships between upper airway obstruction and pulmonary function. Ann. Otol. Rhinol. Laryngol. 73:381.

Ogura, J. H., Nelson, J. R., Suemitsu, M., et al. 1973. Relationship between pulmonary resistance and changes in arterial blood gas tensions in dogs with nasal obstruction and partial laryngeal obstruction. Ann. Otol. Rhinol. Laryngol. 82:668.

Ogura, J. H., Unno, T., and Nelson, J. R. 1968. Baseline values in pulmonary mechanics for physiologic surgery of the nose: Preliminary report. Ann. Otol. Rhinol. Laryngol. 77:367.

Ohnishi, T., and Ogura, J. H. 1969. Partitioning of pulmonary resistance in the dog. Laryngoscope 79:1847.

Ohnishi, T., Ogura, J. H., and Nelson, J. R. 1972. Effects of nasal obstruction upon the mechanics of the lung in the dog. Laryngoscope 82:712.

Pagon, R. A., Graham, J. M., Zonana, J., et al. 1981. Coloboma, congenital heart disease and choanal atresia with multiple anomalies: CHARGE association. J. Pediatr. 99:223.

Parkes, A. S., and Zuckerman, S. 1931. Menstrual cycle of primates: II. Some effects of oestin on baboons and macaques. J. Anthropol. 65:272.

Patterson, C. N. 1965. Juvenile nasopharyngeal angiofibroma. Arch. Otolaryngol. 81:270.

Patterson, C. N. 1973. Juvenile nasopharyngeal angiofibroma. Otolaryngol. Clin. North Am. 6:839.

Person, J. R., and Rogers, R. S., III. 1977. Bullous and cicatricial pemphigoid. Clinical, histopathologic, and immunopathologic correlations. Mayo Clin. Proc. 52:54.

Petruson, B., and Hansson, H. 1987. Nasal mucosal changes in children with frequent infections. Arch. Otolaryngol. Head Neck Surg. 113:1294.

Pirsig, W. 1984. Historical notes and actual observations on the nasal septal abscess especially in children. Int. J. Pediatr. Otorhinolaryngol. 8:43.

Principato, J. J., Kerrigan, J. P., Wolf, P. 1986. Pediatric nasal resistance and lower anterior vertical face height. Otolaryngol. Head Neck Surg. 95:226.

Proctor, B., and Proctor, C. 1979. Congenital lesions of the head and neck. Otolaryngol. Clin. North Am. 3:221.

Rachelefsky, G. S., Katz, R. M., and Sheldon, S. C. 1984. Chronic sinus disease with associated reactive airway disease in children. Pediatrics 73:526.

Reiter, D., and Myers, A. R. 1980. Asymptomatic nasal septal perforations in systemic lupus erythematosus. Ann. Otol. Rhinol. Laryngol. 89:78.

Richter, H. J. 1987. Obstruction of the Pediatric Upper Airway. Ear Nose Throat J. 66:40.

Sanford, D. M., and Becker, G. D. 1967. Acute leukemia presenting as nasal obstruction. Arch. Otolaryngol. 85:102.

Schenck, N. L., and Ogura, J. H. 1972. Esthesioneuroblastoma: An enigma in diagnosis, a dilemma in treatment. Arch. Otolaryngol. 96:322.

Schreiber, U. 1973. Vasomotor rhinitis with hormonal contraception. H.N.O. 21:180.

Sercer, A. 1930. Researches on the reflex influence of each lung from its corresponding nasal cavity. Acta Otolaryngol. 14:99.

Settipane, G. A. 1987. Nasal Polyps: Epidemiology, pathology, immunology and treatment. Am. J. Rhinol. 1:119.

Skolnik, E. M., Kotler, R., and Hanna, W. A. 1973. Choanal atresia. Otolaryngol. Clin. North Am. 6:83.

Slovis, T. L., Renfro, B., Watts, F. B., et al. 1985. Choanal atresia: Precise CT evaluation. Radiology 155:345.

Solow, B., and Greve, E. 1979. Craniocervical angulation and nasal respiratory resistance. In McNamara, J. A., Jr. (ed.): Nasal Respiratory Function and Craniofacial Growth Symposium, monograph 9, Craniofacial Growth Series. Ann Arbor, University of Michigan, Center for Human Growth and Development, pp. 87–119.

Stahl, R. H. 1974. Allergic disorders of the nose and paranasal sinuses. Otolaryngol. Clin. North Am. 7:703.

Stammberger, H. 1986. Endoscopic endonasal surgery—concepts in treatment of recurring rhinosinusitis. Part I. Anatomic and pathophysiologic considerations. Otolaryngol. Head Neck Surg. 94:143.

Stoksted, P. 1952. The physiologic cycle of the nose under normal and pathologic conditions. Acta Otolaryngol. 42:175.

Swift, P. G., and Emery, J. L. 1973. Clinical observations on response to nasal occlusion in infancy. Arch. Dis. Child 48:947.

Taylor, M. 1961a. Catarrhal rhinitis in children. Proc. R. Soc. Med. 54:1961.

Taylor, M. 1961b. An experimental study of the influence of the endocrine system on nasal respiratory mucosa. J. Laryngol. Otol. 75:972.

Taylor, M. 1973. The nasal vasomotor reaction. Otolaryngol. Clin. North Am. 6:645.

Taylor, M. 1974. The origin and function of nasal mucus. Laryngoscope 84:612.

Taylor, M. 1979. Physiology of the nose, paranasal sinuses and nasopharynx. In English, G. M. (ed.): Otolaryngology, Vol. 2. Hagerstown, MD, Harper & Row.

Theogaraj, S. D., Hoehn, J. G., and Hagan, K. F. 1983. Practical management of congenital choanal atresia. Plast. Reconstr. Surg. 72:634.

Timms, D. J. 1986. The effect of rapid maxillary expansion on nasal airway resistance. Br. J. Orthodon. 13:221.

Usowicz, A. G., Golabi, M., and Curry, C. 1986. Upper airway obstruction with fetal alcohol syndrome. Am. J. Dis. Child. 140:1039.

Van Cauwenberge, P. B., and Deleye, L. 1984. Nasal cycle in children. Arch. Otolaryngol. 110:108.

von Dishoeck, H. A. E. 1942. Inspiratory nasal resistance. Arch. Otolaryngol. 30:31.

von Dishoeck, H. A. E. 1965. The part of the valve and the turbinate in total nasal resistance. Int. Rhinol. 3:19.

Wilson, T. G. 1962. Diseases of the Ear, Nose and Throat in Children, 2nd ed., Ch. 10. London, W. Heinemann Ltd.

Wise, T. A. 1898. Arthava Veda Sanhita. In Commentary on the Hindu System of Medicine. Calcutta.

Chapter 32

EPISTAXIS

M. C. Culbertson, Jr., M.D.   **Scott C. Manning, M.D.**

The respiratory system is widely discussed in the writings of ancient philosophers and medical practitioners; only the poorly understood vascular system receives more attention from these early writers. Pre-Hippocrates references to rhinologic subjects include such topics as removal of foreign bodies from the respiratory passages, pain of inflammatory diseases, and the inconvenience of catarrhs. The "Corpus Hippocraticum" frequently mentions epistaxis specifically.

Although epistaxis may occur at any age, at any time, and in any season, nosebleed is a common complaint in the pediatric population and occurs more frequently in the winter months. In a major study of 1734 patients, 175 cases of epistaxis were recorded in the worst winter month and 110 cases occurred in July (Juselius, 1974). A nosebleed may result from nasal trauma at birth or in infancy, but children aged 2 to 10 years are more commonly affected than are infants.

Epistaxis in children often produces parental concern out of proportion to the actual danger to the child, although the bleeding may herald a serious illness, such as a nasopharyngeal angiofibroma or leukemia. Usually epistaxis is associated with no more than a mild irritation or excoriation of the mucosa. The alert physician, when procuring a history and conducting an examination of the nose while firmly quieting the patient and relatives, can assess the seriousness of the episode of bleeding.

ANATOMY

In children the bleeding site is almost always the anterior portion of the nose, usually on the septum in the area of Little or adjacent to this site. The nose receives terminal branches from both the internal and external carotid artery systems (Figs. 32–1 and 32–2). The internal carotid artery supplies blood to the nose through the anterior and posterior ethmoid arteries, which arise in the posterior orbit from the ophthalmic artery. The anterior ethmoid artery, the larger of the two, supplies the lateral wall of the nose, the nasal septum, and the nasal tip; and the posterior ethmoid artery supplies the posterior lateral wall of the nose, including the superior turbinate and the superior portion of the septum. The sphenopalatine artery, which

is a branch of the internal maxillary artery, is the major terminal artery of the external carotid artery system supplying the nose. The major branch enters the nose through the sphenopalatine foramen, and another exits the greater palatine foramen to the palate and into the nose through the incisive canal. The sphenopalatine artery supplies the posterior septum and the inferior and middle turbinate area of the lateral nasal wall. The anterior portion of the upper lip is supplied by a branch of the labial artery. These all coalesce in an area of the septum known as Kiesselbach plexus. The nasal epithelium, especially that of the cartilaginous septum, has little cushioning submucosal tissue so that vessels are offered little protection, and contraction of an injured vessel to close its lumen may be quite limited owing to the lack of an elastic submucosal layer.

Protruding as it does, the nose is a common target for traumatic injury, and by its very function the nasal mucosa is traumatized. In a distance of about 7 cm the nose conditions inspired air. The air entering the nose may be $-20°C$ with a relative humidity of 20 per cent, and when the air reaches the posterior pharynx it is almost free of particulate matter, its temperature is about 37°C, and its relative humidity is approximately 100 per cent (Chaps. 28 and 29).

ETIOLOGY

Inflammation

As noted in Table 32–1, inflammation or infection of the upper respiratory tract is probably the most common cause of epistaxis. Increased vascularity of the nasal mucosa and crusting in the anterior nares occur during an upper respiratory tract infection, so it is not surprising that childhood exanthems are associated with epistaxis. In fact, epistaxis is a common accompaniment to rubella and varicella (Chap. 37).

Children with nasal allergies experience nasal congestion, discharge, and at times superimposed infections of the nose. In addition, occasionally epistaxis will accompany allergic rhinitis (Chap. 42).

672

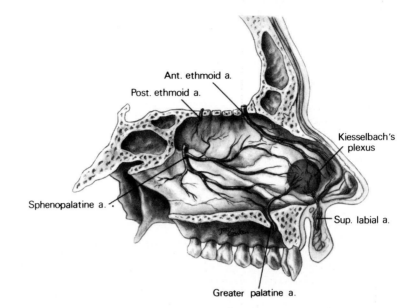

Figure 32–1. Arteries supplying the nasal septum.

Trauma

Trauma to the nose is a principal cause of epistaxis in children and adults. Dry air, as well as physical injury, are sources of nasal trauma. In fact, forced-air central heating systems reduce the humidity in homes to levels below those of the driest deserts, and excessive cooling of air can produce the same lowering of relative humidity. Modern lifestyle could be more a source of nasal trauma than actual physical injury.

Foreign bodies in the nose are discussed fully in Chapter 39. Epistaxis is a common presenting symptom in cases of foreign body obstruction of the nose, and attempts to remove the foreign body without proper patient preparation and restraint, illumination, and adequate instrumentation can result in more severe nasal bleeding (Chap. 40).

Although nasal surgery in children is not common, bleeding can occur after surgery. Surgical procedures in contiguous areas, including adenoidectomy and dacryocystorhinostomy, can result in epistaxis postoperatively (Brenner, 1974).

Trauma to the face and nose with or without nasal bone fracture is a common cause of epistaxis. However, it is important to beware of repeated epistaxis following head trauma without visual evidence of damage to the nose or an obvious bleeding site (Pathak, 1972), as this may indicate more extensive damage of nonnasal structures, requiring more aggressive management.

Barotrauma of the paranasal sinuses, septal perforations, and exposure of the nose to chemicals and caustics, although uncommon, can all cause nasal bleeding. Parasites of the nasal cavity are rarely seen in the United States, but in Southeast Asia their

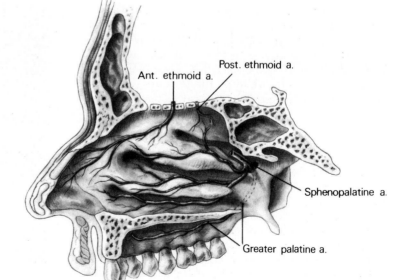

Figure 32–2. Arterial supply of the lateral wall of the nasal cavity.

TABLE 32–1. Etiology of Epistaxis in Children

I. Common causes
  A. Inflammation
    1. Upper respiratory tract infections
      a. Viral
      b. Bacterial
    2. Childhood exanthems
    3. Rheumatic fever
  B. Trauma
    1. Dry air
    2. Injury, external, with or without fracture
    3. Patient induced (nose picking)
    4. Foreign body
  C. Allergic rhinitis with or without accompanying inflammation
II. Uncommon causes
  A. Alterations of intravascular factors of hemostasis
    1. Platelet abnormalities
      a. Idiopathic thrombocytopenic purpura (quantitative change in platelets)
      b. Thrombocytopathic purpuras (qualitative change in the platelets, such as occurs with von Willebrand disease or Glanzmann thrombasthenia)
    2. Coagulation defects
      a. Hemophilia A and B (Christmas disease)
      b. Bleeding caused by anticoagulant drugs such as coumadin
  B. Hypertension (not in the author's experience)
  C. Idiopathic
    1. Polymorphic reticulosis
    2. Pyogenic granuloma
  D. Neoplasms
    1. Benign
      a. Juvenile nasopharyngeal angiofibroma
      b. Polyps
      c. Meningocele and meningomyelocele
    2. Malignant leukemias
  E. Parasite in nasal or nasopharyngeal space
  F. Structural
    1. Deviation of the septum
    2. Adhesions between septum and lateral nasal wall
  G. Trauma
    1. Postsurgical bleeding
    2. Chemical and caustic agents

presence in the nose is a common cause of epistaxis. Granulomas of the nose are seldom encountered in pediatric patients (Roback et al., 1969), but when they occur the presenting symptom is usually epistaxis. Rare inflammatory conditions that cause nosebleeds are leprosy, atrophic rhinitis, tuberculosis, glanders, and certain fungus infections such as rhinosporidiosis.

Other (Rare) Causes

Changes in the blood vessels that occur with hereditary hemorrhagic telangiectasia result in epistaxis. In a series of 80 patients studied from 1962 through 1976, the median age of onset of this familial disease was 17 years, and the earliest incidence of associated epistaxis occurred at 2 years of age (Letson and Birck, 1973).

Tumors can rarely cause epistaxis in children. In newborns and infants, meningoceles and encephaloceles may present initially as nasal bleeding. Likewise,

papillomas, polyps, and malignant tumors may be the cause of recurrent nosebleeds. Epistaxis is the most frequent presenting symptom in patients with juvenile angiofibroma (Chap. 31).

Hypertension is a possible cause of epistaxis, and in older adult patients the severity of the epistaxis may be related to the degree of hypertension.

Epistaxis may be a manifestation of a bleeding disorder. However, one author concluded that, "If on careful history and physical examination and family history, epistaxis proves to be the only manifestation of bleeding, it is most likely that the child does not have an underlying hemorrhagic disorder" (Schulman, 1959).

One must remember to include the ingestion of drugs, especially aspirin, as a possible cause of epistaxis.

Other rare causes of epistaxis in childhood include spontaneous intracavernous (infraclinoid) aneurysm of the internal carotid artery, aneurysm of the vein of Galen communicating with dilated arterioles derived from the posterior cerebral arteries, and primary idiopathic thrombocytopenic purpura. Aplastic anemia associated with drugs and other toxic agents and leukemias are other rare causes of epistaxis.

MANAGEMENT

Proper management of the child with nosebleed begins with the attitude toward the child and her or his relatives. A quick assessment of the patient's general condition (the degree of blood loss) and history

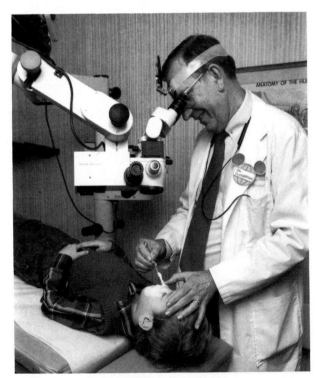

Figure 32–3. Use of the otomicroscope for illumination and magnification of the bleeding site.

from the parents or the child (the circumstances surrounding the onset, cause, past history of epistaxis, and family history) will help to reassure all parties (Stool and Kemper, 1969).

At the time of the initial visit and treatment of the epistaxis or later during follow-up treatment, hematologic evaluation should be considered. This may involve simple laboratory procedures such as complete blood count (CBC), prothrombin time, and partial thromboplastin time. Consultation with the child's primary physician or referral to a pediatric hematologist for further studies is possible. These further steps depend on the cause and the course of the nosebleed in the past and as the child is treated.

Many times the bleeding has stopped by the time the physician sees the child, but these patients should still be examined carefully. If the area from which the bleeding occurred is obvious and it appears that active bleeding could recur, cauterization and packing might be indicated.

Active bleeding from the anterior nose can often be stopped by the application of pressure of the thumb and index finger over the soft parts of the nose for about 5 minutes. If bleeding persists, the nose should carefully be cleaned of blood clots, using suction with adequate illumination (the magnification of the otologic operating microscope is often helpful) (Fig. 32–3), and irrigated with a weak vasoconstrictor such as 0.125 per cent phenylephrine (Neo-Synephrine) isotonic. After such cleansing, examination usually reveals bleeding in or around Kiesselbach plexus area on one side. A cotton pledget dampened with 4 per cent lidocaine (Xylocaine), with or without a vasoconstrictor such as epinephrine 1:10,000, may be placed against the bleeding point and left in place with pressure applied for 5 minutes. Immobilization of the patient and good illumination of the bleeding area during these procedures are essential.

If it appears that the bleeding will recur after these measures have been taken, the offending vessel may be cauterized. In children electrocautery is usually not recommended. A silver nitrate stick may be used, but for very small nares a small-diameter metal applicator sparingly tipped with cotton dipped in trichloroacetic acid is usually safer. Care must be used to place the damp cotton wisp only on the specific area. Petrolatum can be used to cover adjacent mucosa and skin to localize the cauterized area. Repeated cauterizations may be complicated by septal perforations.

In some patients, the bleeding point cannot be found, and simple pressure or cauterization will not control the bleeding. In these children, packing of one or both sides of the nose should be the next step.

For most children, sedation or, on occasion, general anesthesia is necessary for complete examination, reduction of a fracture, or for packing procedures. Chloral hydrate (Noctec) has been found to be superior to barbiturates, tranquilizers, or narcotics, used singly or in combination, for this purpose. The initial oral dose given is 40 mg/kg of body weight, and 15 to 20 mg/kg may be added in 30 to 40 minutes if the child is not tranquil.

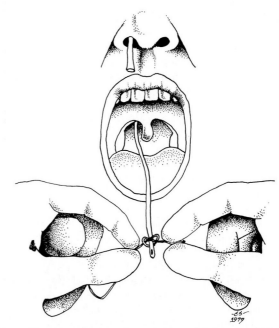

Figure 32–4. Insertion into the nasopharynx of the adenoid hemostatic sponge. A rubber catheter is threaded through the nasal cavity into the pharynx and out of the mouth. The double string on the sponge is tied to the catheter and drawn retrograde through the nose and tied securely but with little pressure over a flexible tube.

The rare cases in which nasal packing is necessary to control epistaxis occur as the result of trauma, with or without a fracture, or in children with blood dyscrasias. When nasal packing must be done, long-fiber or rayon cotton soaked in a mild vasoconstrictor can be fashioned into any length or width pack and placed in the nasal cavity. If the cotton is to be left for any period of time, it should be impregnated with an

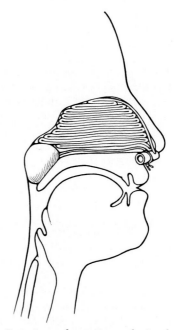

Figure 32–5. Posterior and anterior packs in place. The string holding the posterior pack is illustrated.

antibiotic ointment. Gauze can be placed more tightly in the nasal space than can cotton, as it is packed in layers from the anterior opening of the nose posteriorly to the posterior border of the middle turbinate, and from the floor of the nose to the superior extent of the nasal vault. Oxidized regenerated cellulose gauze or cotton (Oxycel) microfibrillar collagen preparations may be put in the area of active bleeding and then supported. If this absorbable material is used alone it need not be removed later. Packing of other material is usually removed within 3 days, and, even when the nose has not been infected, the patient is given an antibiotic prophylactically.

If packing of both anterior nasal chambers does not suffice to stop the bleeding, then a posterior pack may be used. This may consist of a carefully inflated Foley catheter, which should be inflated with a measured amount of liquid outside the nose to judge its size before insertion. Alternatively, one of the specially prepared postnasal balloons (such as the Gottschalk Nasostat) may be used for the posterior portion of the combined anterior and posterior packing. These newly designed, prefabricated, latex rubber balloons may be obtained in small sizes. The use of a tonsil-adenoid hemostatic sponge passed through the mouth to the nasopharynx with ties through one nostril to the anterior nares is illustrated in Figure 32–4. The posterior pack provides a stable mass against which the carefully placed anterior packing may provide pressure to stop the bleeding (Fig. 32–5). The nasal packing should be impregnated with an antibiotic ointment (without steroid), and antibiotics should be administered parenterally or orally while the packs are in place and for a few days after removal of the packs.

Careful examination of the nasal cavity under general anesthesia using the otomicroscope (lowest power) and suction can help to isolate a bleeding point otherwise inaccessible to view (see Fig. 32–3). Bleeding from an ostium of the maxillary antrum, a vessel hidden by the inferior turbinate, or one high in the vault can better be identified and treated in this manner. Nasal bleeding that persists despite the treatment described may come from a sinus cavity. In these cases further studies to exclude the possibility of bleeding from the sinuses must include radiographic evaluation.

Special care must be undertaken by the clinician in the approach to children with epistaxis in the intensive care unit setting. These patients often have anemia and quantitative or qualitative platelet abnormalities, and they frequently have diffuse mucosal oozing. In addition, they are subject to repeated nasal trauma by the placement of nasogastric and nasotracheal tubes. The approach to these patients should begin with removal (if possible) of any indwelling nasal tubes followed by careful inspection and suctioning of the nasal cavity utilizing a portable light source, a nasal speculum, and a soft suction catheter. Vasoconstriction and local anesthesia can be obtained by placing cotton pledgets soaked in 0.025 per cent oxymetazoline and 4 per cent lidocaine solutions into the nasal cavities for a few minutes. This measure, along with head of

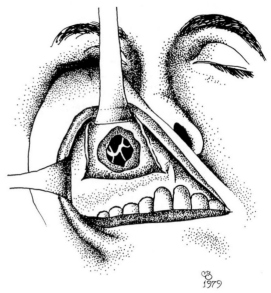

Figure 32–6. View of the internal carotid artery through a fenestra of the posterior wall of the antrum via a Caldwell-Luc approach.

bed elevation and 5 minutes of pressure applied by squeezing the anterior nose, will control a large percentage of nosebleeds. When anterior packs are required, oxidized cellulose or microfibrillar collagen preparations are preferable to gauze, as they promote coagulation and do not further irritate already traumatized mucosal surfaces.

The clinician should keep in mind that nasal packs can themselves result in severe morbidity and should be avoided when possible, especially in very ill patients. In nonintubated patients, bilateral nasal packs can cause an iatrogenic sleep apnea syndrome, which can lead to hypoxia and possibly death. Immunocompromised patients are especially at risk for infectious complications of nasal packing, including sinusitis due to blocked sinus ostia, bacteremia and sepsis, and even toxic shock syndrome (Hull et al., 1983). Mechanical complications of nasal packs include injury to the columella or septum from ischemic necrosis and asphyxiation from aspiration of a loose pack (Fairbanks, 1986).

The measures just discussed will almost always be adequate to control bleeding in the majority of children with epistaxis. Bleeding from extensive fractures, tumors, telangiectasia, surgical procedures, and bleeding disorders can be exceptions.

Nasal septal surgery may be necessary to stop bleeding in rare instances. Septoplasty with replacement of cartilage is an acceptable procedure even in preadolescent patients. Repair of a septum that blocks the airway and also is the cause of recurrent nasal bleeding is an effective and reasonable treatment.

Arterial ligation for epistaxis in children is rarely indicated (Chandler and Serrins, 1965). For anterior and superior bleeding, occlusion of the anterior and posterior ethmoid arteries is employed. For bleeding arising from the posterior portion of the nose, occlusion

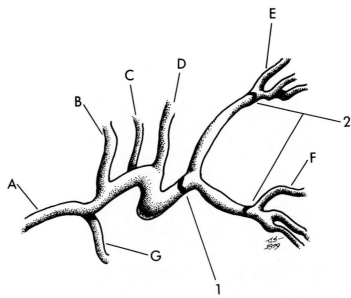

Figure 32–7. Diagram of the third part of the course of the left internal maxillary artery (pterygopalatine portion). A, Internal maxillary artery. B, Artery of the pterygoid canal (vidian). C, Infraorbital artery. D, Pharyngeal artery. E, Sphenopalatine artery. F, Descending palatine artery. G, Dental artery. The areas labeled 1 and 2 are locations of clip application.

of the appropriate branches of the internal maxillary artery is the preferred procedure (Figs. 32–6 and 32–7).

Arterial ligation is carried out if other measures discussed previously have not proved successful in stopping the epistaxis. Septal dermoplasty (Sanders, 1970) is a surgical procedure that may be indicated in children with recurrent epistaxis in hereditary telangiectasia and von Willebrand disease (Letson and Birck, 1973). Likewise, the carbon dioxide laser has been used by some authors to control septal bleeding in these patients. Cryosurgery has been used to treat epistaxis on occasion (Bluestone and Smith, 1967).

Arterial embolization has been reported by some authors as treatment for severe epistaxis refractory to other therapeutic measures (Merland et al., 1980). Potential indications might rarely include Rendu-Osler-Weber disease, uncontrolled coagulopathies, and diffuse angiomas. Advantages to the technique include the ability to visualize the exact site of bleeding on arteriogram and to control it nonsurgically. Disadvantages include the inability to embolize the ethmoid arteries from the internal carotid system and the potential for complications such as trismus and facial paralysis.

PREVENTION

The treatment of a bleeding episode should be extended to measures designed to prevent recurrence of the bleeding. These measures consist of educational and common-sense advice given to the patient and his or her family by the treating physician.

One of the simplest and most effective of these measures is humidification of the child's home environment. In homes in past years, humidity levels were controlled by evaporation of water from vessels placed on radiators and space heaters. In addition, house-plants played a real part in providing humidity in living quarters (Fig. 32–8).

Year-round control of temperature in large numbers of homes began in the warmer climates in the 1950's. Changes in methods of home temperature conditioning, particularly heating, have led to the need for humidity control also. In dwellings with forced-air central heat furnaces, the relative humidity level in

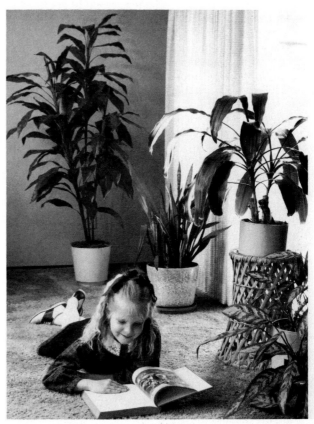

Figure 32–8. Houseplants—humidification by natural means.

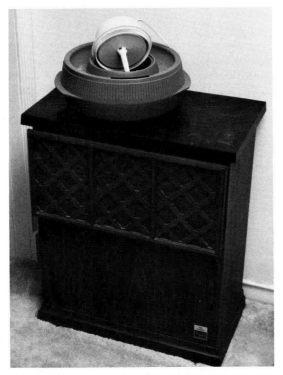

Figure 32–9. Two types of portable humidifiers—"cool mist" and forced air evaporative.

dry cold weather can drop to 5 per cent; the relative humidity level in the heating season *should* be between 40 and 50 per cent. In the heating season, proper insulation and mechanical humidifiers are important to maintain a proper humidity level (Fig. 32–9).

Humidifiers come in a variety of types, but almost all central heating units can be provided with one of two basic types of humidifiers: the most efficient and trouble free are evaporative humidifiers; the spray type is less desirable for homes. These humidifiers are usually controlled by a humidistat. Portable humidifiers, which are filled with water automatically or manually, vary in capacity from many liters to as little as 2 liters. Because humidified air travels about a space rapidly without air circulation, one or several of these portable units can serve a home quite well.

Some humidifiers operate by air forced through water-soaked material, supplying the humidity. Another type produces cool mist by breaking the water into small particles. Portable boiling water humidifiers (steam) are not recommended because of the danger of injury from the hot water and their greater use of fuel. Too great a difference between inside and outside temperatures in summer cooling can drop the humidity below the healthful level. A temperature spread of no more than 12°C is probably optimal.

When dry crusts occlude the nasal airway, petroleum jelly or a similar substance may be put in the anterior nares at bedtime. If an infection is present, an antibiotic or antibiotic-steroid ophthalmic ointment (not water miscible) may be used. Steroid-containing ointments should be used no longer than 2 weeks without follow-up care by the physician.

Prevention of epistaxis also includes the control of nasal and paranasal sinus infections, treatment of allergies affecting the nose, and prevention of nose picking. All of these measures require the cooperation of parents and patients but are worthwhile to prevent an annoying and sometimes frightening episode of bleeding from the nose.

SELECTED REFERENCES

Hansen, J. 1974. Disorders of nasal septum and related structures. *In* Otolaryngology, Vol. 3, Chap. 9. New York, Harper & Row.
    Hansen gives a good review of coagulation and platelet disorders, as well as an extensive table listing causes of epistaxis.
Stool, S. E., and Kemper, B. 1969. Nose and paranasal sinuses. *In* Brenneman's Practice of Pediatrics, Vol. 4, Chap. 54. New York, Harper & Row.
    This chapter is written for the pediatrician and gives an overview of epistaxis in children.
    For further information on this subject, see the following references.

REFERENCES

Adams, D. M. 1973. Transantral internal maxillary artery ligation in prolonged or severe posterior epistaxis. J. La. State Med. Soc. 125:389.
Alavi, K. 1969. Epistaxis and hemoptysis due to Hirudo medicinalis (medical leech). Arch. Otolaryngol. 90:178.
Bell, M., Hawke, M., and Jahn, A. 1974. New device for the management of postnasal epistaxis. Balloon tamponade. Arch. Otolaryngol. 99:373.
Bluestone, C. D., and Smith, H. C. 1967. Intranasal freezing for severe epistaxis. Arch. Otolaryngol. 85:445.
Blumfeld, R., and Skolnik, E. M. 1965. Intranasal encephaloceles. Arch. Otolaryngol. 82:527.
Brenner, R. L. 1974. Dacryocystorhinostomy in children. Tex. Med. 70:71.
Briant, T. D. R., Fitzpatrick, P. J., and Book, H. 1970. The radiological treatment of juvenile nasopharyngeal angiofibromas. Ann. Otol. Rhinol. Laryngol. 79:1108.
Chandler, J. R., and Serrins, A. 1965. Transantral ligation of the internal maxillary artery for epistaxis. Laryngoscope 75:1151.
Coleman, C. C., Jr. 1973. Diagnosis and treatment of congenital arteriovenous fistulas of the head and neck. Am. J. Surg. 126:557.
El bitar, H. 1971. The etiology and management of epistaxis. A review of 300 cases. Practitioner 207:800.
English, G. M., Hemenway, W. G., and Cundy, R. L. 1972. Surgical treatment of invasive angiofibroma. Arch. Otolaryngol. 96:312.
Fairbanks, D. F. 1986. Complications of nasal packing. Otolaryngol. Head Neck Surg. 94:412.
Falter, M. S., and Kaufman, M. F. 1971. Congenital factor VII deficiency. J. Pediatr. 79:298.
Goldstein, A. 1970. Postvaricella bleeding presenting as epistaxis. Arch. Otolaryngol. 92:173.
Goode, R. L., and Spooner, T. R. 1972. Management of nasal fractures in children. A review of current practices. Clin. Pediatr. 119:526.
Hansen, J. 1974. Disorders of nasal septum and related structures. *In* Otolaryngology, Vol. 3, Chap. 9. New York, Harper & Row.
Huggins, S. 1969. Control of hemorrhage in otorhinolaryngologic surgery with oxidized regenerated cellulose. EENT Mo. 48:420.
Hull, H. F., Mann, J. M., Sands, C. J., et al. 1983. Toxic shock syndrome related to nasal packing. Arch. Otolaryngol. 109:627.
Iwamura, S., Sugiura, S., and Nomura, Y. 1972. Schwannoma of the nasal cavity. Arch. Otolaryngol. 96:176.
Jafek, B. 1978. Personal communication.

Jafek, B., Nahum, A., Butler, R., et al. 1973. Surgical treatment of juvenile nasopharyngeal angiofibroma. Laryngoscope 83:707.

Juselius, H. 1974. Epistaxis. A clinical study of 1,734 patients. J. Laryngol. Otol. 88:317.

Kadish, S. P. 1971. Epistaxis in a teen-age boy. J.A.M.A. 216:508.

Kahn, A. A., Khaleque, K. A., and Huda, M. N. 1969. Rhinosporidiosis of the nose. J. Laryngol. Otol. 83:461.

Koltai, P. J. 1984. Nose bleeds in the hematologically and immunologically compromised child. Laryngoscope 94:1114.

Leslie, J., and Ingram, G. I. 1971. The diagnosis of long-standing bleeding disorders. Semin. Hematol. 8:140.

Letson, J. A., Jr., and Birck, H. G. 1973. Septal dermoplasty for von Willebrand's disease in children. Laryngoscope 83:1078.

Malcomson, K. G. 1963. The surgical management of massive epistaxis. J. Laryngol. Otol. 77:299.

Merland, J. J., Melki, J. P., Chiras, J., et al. 1980. Place of embolization in the treatment of severe epistaxis. Laryngoscope 90:1694.

Mettler, C. C. 1947. History of Medicine. Philadelphia, Blakiston Co.

Montgomery, W. W., Lofgren, R. H., and Chasin, W. D. 1970. Analysis of pterygopalatine space surgery. Laryngoscope 80:1179.

Pathak, P. N. 1972. Epistaxis—due to ruptured aneurysm of the internal carotid artery. J. Laryngol. Otol. 86:395.

Pearson, B. W., MacKenzie, R. G., and Goodman, W. S. 1969. The anatomical basis of transantral ligation of the maxillary artery in severe epistaxis. Laryngoscope 79:969.

Pinsker, O. T., and Holdcraft, J. 1971. Surgical management of anterior epistaxis. Trans. Am. Acad. Ophthalmol. Otol. 75:492.

Quick, A. J. 1967. Telangiectasia: Its relationship to the Minot-von Willebrand syndrome. Am. J. Med. Sci. 254:585.

Roback, S. A., Herdman, R. C., Hoyer, J., et al. 1969. Wegner's treatment. Am. J. Dis. Child. 118:608.

Rowe, N. L. 1968. Fractures of the facial skeleton in children. J. Oral Surg. 26:505.

Sanders, W. H. 1970. Septal dermoplasty—its several uses. Laryngoscope 80:1342.

Schulman, I. 1959. The significance of epistaxis in children. Pediatrics 24:489.

Stool, S. E., and Kemper, B. 1969. Nose and paranasal sinuses. In Brenneman's Practice of Pediatrics, Vol. 4, Chap. 54. New York, Harper & Row.

Chapter 33

FACIAL PAIN AND HEADACHE

Frank E. Lucente, M.D.   **Robert L. Pincus, M.D.**

Headache is common in children and adolescents. It is often an incidental finding with systemic illness or fever but can be an important symptom of grave central nervous system disease. By age 7 years, 40 per cent of children will have had one or more headaches. By age 15 years, 75 per cent will have had at least one headache. Twenty per cent of 15-year-old adolescents have frequent headaches, one fourth of these are migrainous (Bille, 1962).

Complaints of facial pain and headache in the child are often difficult to assess if one cannot obtain an accurate history or establish the precise location of the pain. Many of these complaints will disappear quickly and do not require evaluation by a physician. However, patients with persistent or recurrent symptoms should have complete head and neck examinations. Such evaluation may require a multidisciplinary approach by the otolaryngologist, pediatrician, neurologist, ophthalmologist, dentist, psychiatrist, and social worker. It is the responsibility of the otolaryngologist to explore the potential etiologic role of otolaryngologic structures in facial pain and headache.

Pain in the head may result from stimulation, traction, or pressure on any of the pain-sensitive structures of the head, which include the trigeminal, glossopharyngeal, vagal, and upper cervical nerves; the large arteries at the base of the brain and their major branches; the dura mater at the base of the skull; the cranial sinuses and afferent veins; the arteries of the dura mater; and some extracranial structures such as the scalp, arteries, and muscles (Diamond and Dalessio, 1982).

Headache may be a recognizable symptom in children 3 years of age and older. The infant or younger child may have irritability or unusual behavior rather than complaints of headache when experiencing the pathologic processes described below.

Although most pains in the head and neck region result from a pathologic process at or close to the area indicated by the patient, the physician might consider the phenomenon of referred pain when no abnormalities are found in this area. A common example of referred pain is the otalgia produced by inflammatory, infectious, and neoplastic lesions of the pharynx. The external ear and middle ear receive sensory innervation from the fifth, seventh, ninth, and tenth cranial nerves and from the second and third cervical nerves. An irritative process anywhere along the distribution of any of these nerves can cause a referred otalgia.

A thorough history will often provide the diagnosis for the pain. It should include questions about severity, duration, location, character, circumstances of onset, exacerbating or remitting factors, repetition, frequency, and associated symptoms in the head and neck region and elsewhere (Table 33–1). In taking the history the physician should also attempt to become more familiar with the child as a social being by inquiring about his or her family, social, and educational settings. It is often helpful to talk with the child in the absence of the parents, particularly when psychologic factors appear to cause, exacerbate, or modify the headache symptoms. The patient should have a complete head and neck examination, including skull, facial bones, eyes, ears, temporomandibular joint, nose, nasopharynx, oral cavity, teeth, oropharynx, larynx, cervical muscles, and associated soft tissues. In palpating the head and neck region, one should begin in asymptomatic areas and move slowly toward symptomatic or tender areas to avoid frightening or hurting the child any more than necessary. Percussion of the teeth, sinuses, and mastoids should also be included. Cervical muscles should be palpated for spasm. One should listen for bruits over the temples and orbits. A thorough neurologic examination should also be performed with particular attention to the cranial nerves.

The performance of ancillary laboratory tests and radiography is guided by the clinical impression obtained from the history and physical examination. There are few, if any, mandatory screening tests, and indiscriminate ordering of tests should be avoided.

This chapter presents a differential diagnosis for headache and facial pain (Tables 33–2 through 33–4) and considers a few of the more common causes or conditions associated with these complaints. (More extensive discussion is found in related chapters.)

The authors gratefully acknowledge the assistance in critically reviewing the text of Kevin C. Greenidge, M.D. (Department of Ophthalmology, New York Eye and Ear Infirmary) and Jonathan Z. Charney, M.D. (Department of Neurology, Mount Sinai School of Medicine).

680

TABLE 33–1. Sample Questions in the Headache Interview

Age of onset?	Triggering events?
Events surrounding onset?	stress
Duration of significant	school
headaches?	family
Prodrome?	illness
general malaise	exertion
visual aura	fatigue
other	food intake
Characteristics of attack?	medications
frequency	Behavior between attacks?
localization	normal?
duration	irritable?
type of pain	clumsy?
time of day	personality change?
Severity of attacks?	Recent changes in patient
Does it require interruption	weight loss?
of normal activity?	disturbed sleep pattern?
Associated autonomic	school performance?
symptoms?	appetite?
pallor	Family history?
nausea and vomiting	migraine
abdominal pain	tension headache
Associated neurologic deficits?	epilepsy
type	psychiatric disorders
temporal relation to	neurologic disease
headache	Medications?
duration	analgesics
does localization of	birth control pills
neurological deficit	other
correspond to that of	Motion sickness?
headache?	
Postictal state?	
What makes it better?	
What makes it worse?	

Modified with permission from Shinnar, S., and D'Souza, B. J. 1981. The diagnosis and management of headaches in childhood. Pediatr. Clin. North Am. 29:79.

MUSCULAR CONTRACTION HEADACHE (TENSION HEADACHE)

This is probably the most common headache in childhood. It is usually bilateral, steady, nonpulsatile, and less intense than a migraine. The pain tends to present in the occipital region or as a band around the head. Because it probably results from prolonged contraction of muscles of the head and neck, it generally occurs later in the day and after periods of physical or emotional stress or intense intellectual activity. Although less common in children than in adults, it is sometimes seen in hard-working students. The failure of the pain to be intensified by coughing, straining at stool, or placing the head in a dependent position distinguishes this type of headache from those due to intracranial causes. It must also be differentiated from depression, school phobia syndrome, and a conversion syndrome (Gascon, 1984).

On examination, one may find restriction and pain with movement of the neck and tenderness over the occipital nerves. Tenderness in the upper border of the trapezius and intrinsic cervical muscles is also found.

Management varies with the underlying cause. Oral analgesics and local treatment with heat may help, but elimination of the underlying physical or psychologic strain is most important. As with other headaches in children, complete and repeated explanation and reassurance are most important.

MIGRAINE HEADACHE

Migraine headaches commonly begin during adolescence, but this syndrome may occasionally be seen in younger children. Although uncommon before the age of 4 years, migraine has been reported in infants under 1 year of age (Woody and Blaw, 1986).

Although the adolescent may experience classic migraine headaches similar to those found in adults—with prodromal anorexia and scotomas, severe unilateral pulsatile headache lasting 4 to 8 hours and followed by diffuse head pain, photophobia, abdominal discomfort, nausea, vomiting, and postical lethargy—younger children more frequently have common (atypical) migraines, which lack the prodromal signs and which may last from hours to days. For this reason, the diagnosis may be elusive until symptoms have been present for several months. A family history of mi-

TABLE 33–2. Etiologic Classification of Headache

Environmental	**Toxic-Metabolic**
Heat	"Pseudotumor"
Humidity	Steroids
Noxious fumes	Tetracycline
Noise	Vitamin A
Infectious	Other drugs
Extracranial	Sulfa
Teeth	Indomethacin
Sinus	Heavy metals
Pharynx	Lead
Ear	Arsenic
Septicemia	Mercury
Viral exanthems	Hypoglycemia
Musculoskeletal	Hyperammonemia
Intracranial	Metabolic acidosis
Meningitis	Hypoxia
Encephalitis	Anemia
Brain abscess	CO poisoning
Vascular	Hypercarbia
Migraine	Porphyria
Hypertension	**Congenital**
Aneurysm	Arnold-Chiari syndrome
Vascular malformation	**Cervical**
Horton syndrome (histamine	**Neuralgic**
cephalgia)	Herpetic
Traumatic	Postherpetic
Neoplastic	Idiopathic
Extracranial	**Psychologic**
Intracranial	Depression
Epileptic	School phobia syndrome
Psychomotor	Conversion symptom
Postical	Prolonged postconcussive
Ocular	syndrome
Allergic	

Modified with permission from Meloff, K. L. 1973. Headache in pediatric practice. Headache 13:125.

TABLE 33–3. Anatomic-Etiologic Classification of Facial Pain

Forehead	Midfacial (cheek)
Frontal sinus	Maxillary sinus
Ocular	Maxillary teeth
	Periodontal structures
Periorbital	Intranasal
Ocular	Parotid gland
Ethmoid sinus	
	Nasal
Preauricular	Nasal bones
Temporomandibular joint	Ethmoid sinus
External ear canal	Intranasal
Parotid gland	
	Jaw
Periauricular	Mandibular teeth
Middle ear	Periodontal structures
External ear (auricle)	Submandibular gland

graine or convulsive disorders is obtained in 70 to 80 per cent of cases (Prensky and Sommer, 1979).

Occasionally the child will present only with paroxysmal vomiting, hemiparesis, diplopia, or ataxia. Headache may appear later in the clinical course. The attacks usually last 2 to 3 hours but may last up to 48 hours. They are often followed by a period of sleep and tend to recur at irregular intervals.

There is an equal sex incidence in young children, but in adolescents and adults migraine occurs more frequently in females. The patients are often compulsive, intense, hard-working perfectionists. Although

emotional stress may precipitate a migraine episode, it should not be considered a psychiatric disorder. There can be significant vestibulocochlear derangements in children with migraine. Forty-five per cent have a history of motion sickness, seven times the incidence of other groups (Barabas et al., 1983). Vestibular symptoms and phonophobia are major symptoms during the majority of migraine attacks (Kayan and Hood, 1984). The pathogenesis of migraine is thought to involve initial cerebral vasoconstriction followed by rapid vasodilatation.

Mild attacks may be relieved with salicylates or codeine taken at the onset. Ergot preparations used in treating adult migraines may produce more intense and prolonged effects, possibly resulting in cerebral ischemia. Minor tranquilizers may interrupt the headache if given over a period of several months. The child should also be reassured that there is no neoplastic or psychologic cause for the headaches. When frequent attacks are present prophylaxis with agents that inhibit vasoactive substances such as antihistamines, nonsteroidal anti-inflammatory drugs, and beta-adrenergic blockers is indicated (Dehkharghani and Condrey, 1984).

Ophthalmoplegic migraine is a rare variant of this clinical picture, in which partial or complete third-nerve palsy appears 6 to 24 hours after the onset of the headache. Although the ophthalmoplegia generally subsides within a few days, repeated episodes may leave the patient with some residual paralysis.

TABLE 33–4. Clinical Summary of Facial Pain and Headache

DISEASE OR DISORDER	LOCATION	CHARACTER	USUAL FREQUENCY	ACCOMPANYING SYMPTOMS	USUAL TIME OF DAY	GENERAL THERAPY	DURATION
Sinusitis	Frontal Midfacial Periorbital	Dull	Inconsistent	Nasal congestion Nasal drainage	Morning Evening	Decongestant Antibiotic	More than 1 day
Migraine Classic Common	Unilateral Frontotemporal Periorbital	Severe Throbbing	Weekly or monthly	Nausea Vomiting Scotomas	Any time	Ergotamine Tranquilizer Anticonvulsant	Classic: Less than 8 hours Common: Hours to days
Psychogenic (tension)	Frontal Occipital Bandlike	Inconsistent	Daily	Nervousness Anxiety Withdrawn behavior	During or after stress	Analgesic Tranquilizer	Variable
Brain tumor	Frontal Parietal Occipital	Dull	Daily	Ataxia Behavior change Visual disturbance	Morning Evening	Relief of intracranial pressure	More than 1 day
Ocular disorders	Ocular Frontal	Dull	Daily	Squint Refractive errors	Afternoon Evening	Visual correction	Several hours
Convulsive equivalent	Frontal Temporal	Dull	Daily or weekly	Vomiting Staring episodes Hyperactivity	Any time	Anticonvulsant	Minutes to hours
Meningitis Encephalitis	Frontal Occipital	Dull	Constant	Fever Nuchal rigidity Convulsions	Any time	Antibiotics	Constant

Modified and reprinted by permission of Elsevier Science Publishing Co., Inc. from Pediatric Neurology Handbook, by Jabbour, J. T., et al. Copyright 1976 by Medical Examination Publishing Company, Inc.

CONVULSIVE EQUIVALENT

Headaches may be associated with a paroxysmal cerebral dysrhythmia or psychomotor seizure. They usually have an acute onset during the day or night and last several minutes to several hours. They are characteristically dull and are located in the frontotemporal region. Pallor, abdominal discomfort, nausea, and vomiting follow onset of the headache. The pain may disappear after a brief period of sleep, and the child then usually feels quite well. Anticonvulsant medications, such as diphenylhydantoin (Dilantin) or barbiturates, usually produce a dramatic response.

TRACTION HEADACHE (BRAIN MASS HEADACHE)

Traction on intracranial pain-sensitive structures caused by brain tumor, hematoma, aneurysm, or abscess will result in a traction headache. Brain tumors usually produce a steady, aching headache that may be more severe in the early morning. It rarely has the pulsatile pattern of the vascular headache. Brain tumor headache tends to be more severe when the child is lying down and may awaken the child from sleep.

VASCULAR MALFORMATION HEADACHE

Vascular malformation is an uncommon cause of a headache, which usually lasts several days and which may be accompanied by seizures or periods of decreased levels of consciousness. Scotomas may also be present, but they are concomitant rather than antecedent as with migraine. The headache reaches its maximum intensity more quickly than the migraine headache, usually within seconds. In determining the etiology of the headache, it is important to look for coincident neurologic abnormalities that may persist long after the headache has disappeared. This type of headache is also associated with seizures and with cerebral hemorrhage.

HYPERTENSION HEADACHE

Hypertension is rarely seen in childhood and is consequently a rare cause of headaches among children. The headaches tend to resemble the hypertension headaches experienced by adults and the brain mass headache. They occur more commonly in the morning and fluctuate rapidly in intensity during the day, sometimes in relationship to the amount or intensity of physical activity. Among the disorders that may be associated with hypertensive headaches are acute and chronic renal disease, neuroblastoma, pheochromocytoma, and adrenal adenomas. Diagnosis is usually simple if the blood pressure is monitored. Therapy involves analgesics and correction of the hypertension.

NEURALGIAS

The severe pain of trigeminal or glossopharyngeal neuralgia that is seen in adults is extremely rare in children.

NASAL AND PARANASAL SINUS DISEASE

The common viral upper respiratory tract infection is a frequent cause of headache, which may be diffuse or limited to the midfacial region. The pain is usually a dull ache that is exacerbated by placing the head in a dependent position. Associated symptoms and signs, including sneezing, nasal congestion, serous drainage, sore throat, malaise, cough, mild fever, and boggy nasal mucous membranes, will usually confirm the diagnosis. Recovery is usually spontaneous within 4 to 5 days if there are no bacterial complications (Chap. 37).

If the nasal drainage becomes cloudy and the nasal mucous membranes become markedly inflamed, purulent rhinitis should be suspected. It is usually caused by hemolytic *Staphylococcus aureus, Haemophilus influenzae,* or *Diplococcus pneumoniae.* When nasal drainage is persistently unilateral, the presence of a foreign body must be excluded (Chap. 39).

Inflammation, infection, or tumors in the paranasal sinuses produce localized or diffuse facial pain more commonly than headache. Pain from the maxillary sinus is experienced in the midface, cheek, or maxillary teeth. Ethmoid pain is felt between the eyes, and frontal pain is felt in the supraorbital region. Pain from the sphenoid sinus is poorly localized, occasionally being described as coming from deep within the head or at the cranial vertex. The frontal and sphenoid sinuses develop slowly and are usually not of clinical significance until adolescence (Strome, 1976).

Inflammation of the paranasal sinus probably causes far fewer headaches and facial pains than is commonly thought by patients. The sinus ostia, turbinates, and septum are more pain sensitive than the sinus mucosa itself, and, before ascribing midfacial pain to the sinuses, the physician should find corroborative clinical evidence, such as purulent or watery nasal drainage, marked erythema of the nasal mucosa, or tenderness to percussion over the sinuses. Imaging of the sinuses will be helpful in evaluating puzzling patients or in determining therapy. Some think that septal deformation may cause referred pain and chronic headache by exerting pressure on the lateral nasal wall (Schønsted-Madsen et al., 1986).

Sinus disease in the child can be considerably more serious than in the adult owing to the incomplete development in children of the bony walls of the sinuses. The thinness of the lamina papyracea allows rapid extension of ethmoid infection into the orbit with production of orbital cellulitis or orbital abscess. Localized osteomyelitis may appear with spread of infection from any sinus into contiguous bone. Extension of infection through the posterior wall of the frontal sinus, roof of the ethmoid sinus, or any wall of the sphenoid sinus may lead to intracranial complications, such as extradural abscess, meningitis, or brain abscess. Persistent or severe headache in the child with clinical evidence of sinusitis mandates a thorough examination of areas adjacent to the sinuses.

OCULAR HEADACHE

When examining the patient complaining of headache or facial pain, it is important to consider ocular causes, to examine the eyes, and to obtain an ophthalmologic consultation when indicated. Extensive discussion of ocular causes of pain in this region will not be given here. However, several important disorders should be mentioned.

Refractive errors and eye imbalance only rarely cause headache. They usually cause a dull periorbital or frontal pain and can be clearly related to prolonged eye strain.

Acute glaucoma, which is rare in children, is characterized by sudden, severe pain in the eye and the supraorbital region. The pain is accompanied by blurring of vision, increased intraocular pressure, dilated pupil, and a cloudy cornea. The glaucoma occurring in infancy has an insidious onset and may be associated with tearing, photophobia, blurred vision, and less severe pain. Glaucoma occurring in childhood is usually asymptomatic. If symptoms are present, they consist of dull periorbital pain, which may only be noticed at night.

Acute iritis (anterior uveitis) is usually associated with photophobia, blurring, and extreme pain radiating from the eye to the forehead and temporal region. The eye is red (circumcorneal flush) and the pupil is small. Iritis in the child with juvenile rheumatoid arthritis may have an insidious onset and is essentially painless (Chap. 34).

Acute retrobulbar neuritis may be associated with unilateral pain deep in the orbit. The pain occurs before blurring and is increased by rapid eye movement. The patient may complain of sudden loss of central vision. This disorder may be seen in teen-agers but is uncommon in the young child.

Another rare childhood disorder is herpes zoster ophthalmicus, which begins with severe pain in the region of distribution of the ophthalmic division of the trigeminal nerve. Several days later vesicles appear on the forehead and eyelids. Pain may persist after the acute infectious stage has passed.

Among the other ocular disorders to be considered with pain around the eyes are foreign bodies and inflammation of the lid or cornea (chronic blepharitis, conjunctivitis, or allergic reactions).

OTOLOGIC PAIN

Inflammatory, infectious, and neoplastic diseases in the external, middle, and inner ears may produce pain

that the child may interpret or describe as headache or, rarely, facial pain. The numerous otologic causes for headache and facial pain are considered in Chapters 12, 20 through 23, 26, and 27. However, it is appropriate to reemphasize the need for complete otologic and audiometric evaluation of any child with headache, even without associated otologic symptoms (Chap. 12).

DERMATOLOGIC INFECTIONS

Infections of the skin of the head and neck may produce pain. The areas involved can be overlooked in a cursory examination because they are often hidden. Among the bacterial infections that occur in children are facial cellulitis, nasal vestibulitis, and furunculosis of the external ear canal.

DENTAL DISEASE

Inflammation or infection of the teeth or their supporting structures may cause the child to complain of localized, diffuse pain. Inspection, palpation, and percussion of the teeth should be performed carefully and supplemented with radiographic examination when indicated. The condition of the gingivae should also be noted. Among the dental diseases that may present with headache or facial pain are caries, periapical abscess, periodontal disease, eruption of deciduous or permanent teeth, loss of deciduous teeth, dental impaction, infected dental cyst, and aphthous or herpetic stomatitis.

TEMPOROMANDIBULAR JOINT DISEASE

Pain from masticatory dysfunctions involving the temporomandibular joint is usually a dull ache experienced in the preauricular region. It is sometimes more diffuse and may be described by the patient as an earache. The pain is usually steady and is exacerbated by chewing or vigorous jaw motion. It may be seen in conjunction with any generalized or localized disease of synovial joints, such as rheumatoid arthritis.

HEAD TRAUMA

The elicitation of a history of cranial or maxillofacial trauma from the child or parent may be difficult. However, the presence of contusions, ecchymoses, abrasions, or bony tenderness may support the clinical suspicions. Thorough head and neck examination may disclose signs of trauma in regions less visible than the face and the skull. Inconsistencies between the histories given by the child and parents may be noted. Radiographic evaluation should be performed if any trauma is suspected.

SYSTEMIC DISEASES

Headaches occur in association with fever, hypoxemia, hypercapnia, poisoning, systemic viral or bacterial infections, and postictal states. Distention of cerebral and pial vessels is the postulated mechanism for the pain. Headaches associated with systemic infections are often accompanied by fever, nausea, and vomiting.

PSYCHOGENIC HEADACHES

It is impossible to detail the psychologic significance with which the head, face, and neck are invested. However, the role of psychologic factors in the production, modification, and communication of painful sensations in this region cannot be overemphasized. Children learn early that "headache" is a common somatic complaint used by adults to describe a discomfort that may have no relation to physical problems in or around the head. They may use the same phrases, "I have a headache," or "My head hurts," to describe their own experience of that same discomfort experienced by adults or to provide an excuse for their unwillingness to perform a certain act (for instance, going to school, visiting a neighbor, and doing household chores).

They may seek the secondary gain of increased attention that is usually given the sick child, or they may use this somatic complaint as a tool to manipulate parents, teachers, or other associates. It is hoped that careful questioning about both the circumstances of the pain and coincident factors will help to identify those patients in whom psychologic factors must be explored.

When the history is obtained from a parent, the physician should also be aware of the possibility that the parent is projecting his or her own concerns onto the patient, misstating the history or interpreting it prematurely, or seeking attention for his or her own problems. Inconsistencies in the history or the failure to find physical evidence for an abnormality (evidence of a physical abnormality) may suggest this situation.

However, just as one should not make psychogenic headache a diagnosis by exclusion, so also should one be careful not to eliminate physical causes before a thorough evaluation has been made. In ascribing pain in the head or face to a psychologic cause, one should be certain of both the absence of demonstrable organic disease and the presence of detectable emotional disturbance.

SELECTED REFERENCES

Alling, C. C., and Mahan, P. E. (eds.) 1977. Facial Pain. Philadelphia, Lea & Febiger.
   This excellent text discusses the etiology and management of many types of facial pain. Among the subjects covered are functional anatomy, pharmacodynamics, vascular pain, paranasal sinuses, masticatory pain, occlusal disorders, psychosomatics, pain syndromes, and general patient examination.
Dalessio, D. J., and Wolff, H. G. (eds.) 1980. Headache and Other Head Pain. New York, N.Y.U. Press.
   This classic text provides a tremendous amount of clinical and experimental material relevant to the many causes of headache. Although headaches in infants and children are not discussed apart from adult disorders, the coverage of each condition includes pertinent aspects of the pediatric problems.

REFERENCES

Alling, C. C., and Mahan, P. E. (eds.) 1977. Facial Pain. Philadelphia, Lea & Febiger.
Barabas, G., Matthews, W. S., and Ferrari, M. 1983. Childhood migraine and motion sickness. Pediatrics 72:188.
Bille, B. 1962. Migraine in school children. Acta Paediatr. Scand. 51(Suppl. 136):1.
Dalessio, D. J., and Wolff, H. G. (eds.) 1980. Headache and Other Head Pain. New York, N.Y.U. Press.
Dehkharghani, F., and Condrey, Y. A., 1984. Headache: An approach to the pediatric patient. J. Ark. Med. Soc. 86:252.
Diamond, S., and Dalessio, D. J. 1982. The Practicing Physician's Approach to Headache. Baltimore, Williams & Wilkins Co.
Dyken, P. R. 1975. Headaches in children. Arch. Fam. Pract. 11:106.
Gascon, G. C. 1984. Chronic and recurrent headaches in children and adolescents. Pediatr. Clin. North Am. 31:1027.
Jabbour, J. T., Duenas, D. A., Gilmartin, R. C., Jr., et al. 1976. Pediatric Neurology Handbook. Flushing, NY, Medical Examination Publishing Co.
Kayan, A., and Hood, J. D. 1984. Neuro-otologic manifestations of migraine. Brain 107:1123.
Lagos, J. C. 1971. Differential Diagnosis in Pediatric Neurology. Boston, Little, Brown and Co.
Meloff, K. L. 1973. Headache in pediatric practice. Headache 13:125.
Prensky, A. L., and Sommer, D. 1979. Prognosis and treatment of migraine in children. Neurology 29:506.
Schønsted-Madsen, U., Stoksted, P., Christensen, P. H., and Koch-Henrichsen, N. 1986. Chronic headache related to nasal obstruction. J. Laryngol. Otol. 100:165.
Shinnar, S., and D'Souza, B. J. 1981. The diagnosis and management of headaches in childhood. Pediatr. Clin. North Am. 29:79.
Strome, M. 1976. Rhino-sinusitis and midfacial pain in adolescents. Practitioner 217:914.
Woody, R. C., and Blaw, M. E. 1986. Ophthalmoplegic migraine in infancy. Clin. Pediatr. 25:82.

Chapter 34

ORBITAL SWELLINGS

Thomas C. Calcaterra, M.D.

The child with an orbital swelling often represents a diagnostic challenge that may require the expertise of several medical specialists. The otolaryngologist is frequently consulted because many cases of orbital swelling are caused by extracranial disease processes occurring adjacent to the orbit. It is important for the otolaryngologist to be familiar with the spectrum of diseases that may cause orbital swelling, the basic methods of orbital examination, and diagnostic studies applicable to the orbit.

The orbit is a pyramid-shaped space, open anteriorly, but otherwise surrounded by thin bone. Any expansive disease, either within the orbit or from an adjacent site, may cause protrusion of the globe, a condition termed exophthalmos or proptosis. Accordingly, diseases that can cause exophthalmos may be classified into two major groups: intraorbital, lesions arising within the orbital space; and extraorbital, lesions involving the orbit by direct extension from adjacent structures or by metastasis from distant sites. The latter group can be subdivided into categories of intracranial and extracranial lesions. This latter group of extraorbital lesions, the extracranial lesions, are of major interest to the otolaryngologist because they frequently arise within the nose, paranasal sinuses, nasopharynx, or temporal fossa (see Table 34–1).

HISTORY

A comprehensive history is important to an evaluation of unilateral exophthalmos. The mode of onset and progression of the exophthalmos, the status of vision, and the presence of pain should be established. The patient should be questioned about previous sinus infections, allergies, nasal discharge, and facial numbness. Slow progression of proptosis suggests a benign tumor or cyst, whereas rapidly developing proptosis implies the presence of a primary or metastatic malignant tumor. Early loss of vision points to a lesion within the muscle cone involving the optic nerve, such as a glioma. Severe pain is generally symptomatic of an acute infection or hemorrhage.

PHYSICAL EXAMINATION

Direction of Displacement

The direction of displacement often indicates the site of the lesion (Fig. 34–1). Tumors within the muscle cone, such as an optic nerve glioma, may cause pure axial displacement. Acute inflammation or chronic mucopyocele arising from the frontal or ethmoid sinuses displaces the eye downward, laterally, or in both directions (Fig. 34–2). Displacement of the eye in a medial direction often denotes tumors of the lacrimal gland or the temporal fossa. Lesions arising in the maxillary sinus may push the globe upward.

Vertical displacement can be assessed by holding a ruler across both lateral canthi and determining the relationship of the pupils to this straight line. Horizontal displacement is determined by comparing the dis-

TABLE 34–1. Diseases Causing Orbital Swellings: Anatomic Classification

Intraorbital Lesions
Hyperthyroidism
Histiocytosis
Dermoid and teratoma
Optic nerve glioma
Rhabdomyosarcoma
Melanoma
Retinoblastoma
Lacrimal gland tumors
Hemangioma
Metastatic tumors
Extraorbital—Extracranial Lesions
Acute inflammation of any paranasal sinus
Mucocele of any paranasal sinus
Fibrous dysplasia
Osteoma
Angiofibroma of nasopharynx
Nasopharyngeal cancer
Extraorbital—Intracranial Lesions
Meningocele and encephalocele
Cavernous sinus thrombosis
Cavernous sinus fistula
Anterior cranial fossa tumors
Middle cranial fossa tumors

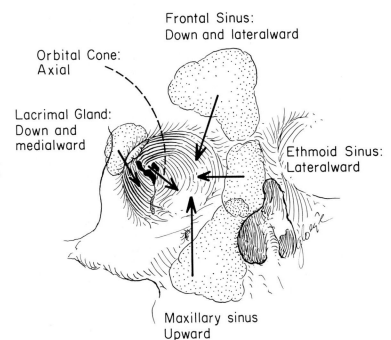

Figure 34–1. The arrows depict the direction of displacement typically encountered by a disease process within each paranasal sinus.

tance from a mark on the center of the bridge of the nose to each limbus (Ophthalmologic Staff, 1967).

External Examination

Examination of the anterior aspect of the globe and eyelids should be performed. While the child is quiet and the radial or carotid pulse is being monitored, any synchronous pulsation of the globe indicates loss of the bony partition between the frontal or temporal lobe and the orbital contents, allowing intracranial pulsations to be transmitted to the eye. Synchronous pulsations may also be observed with a carotid–cavernous sinus fistula. Auscultation over the closed eyelid or

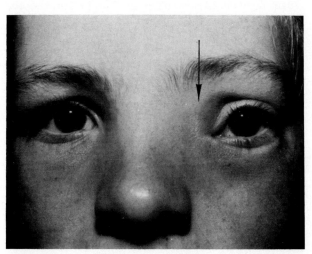

Figure 34–2. The arrow indicates fullness in the canthal region caused by an ethmoid mucocele, which displaces the left eye in a lateral direction.

temporal region may reveal a bruit suggestive of an arteriovenous vascular malformation. Increased proptosis that becomes apparent while the child is crying suggests an orbital varix, particularly if there is concomitant dilatation of the conjunctival veins. A palpable impulse that occurs when the child coughs suggests an encephalocele.

Chemosis, cellulitis, and fluctuation of the eyelids are signals of an inflammatory process, usually transmitted from the paranasal sinuses. Transillumination of the eyelid may disclose an underlying cyst. Although not as common in children as in adults, lid retraction, lid lag on upward gaze, lid restriction on elevation of the globe, and injection of the blood vessels over the lateral rectus muscle all imply the presence of endocrine exophthalmos.

Severe proptosis may prevent the lids from closing and thereby allow the cornea to dry (Calcaterra et al., 1974). The earliest sign of corneal exposure is the loss of normal corneal brightness. Moreover, persistent exposure can lead to ulceration, infection, and permanent scarring.

Palpation

Palpation of the orbital contents may yield important information, particularly regarding anteriorly located lesions such as mucoceles and lacrimal gland tumors. Ballottement of each globe should be performed to compare orbital resilience in each eye. Inflammatory lesions and tumors tend to feel resistant, whereas less resistance is noted with hemangiomas and endocrine exophthalmos (Fig. 34–3). Fullness in the infratemporal fossa suggests lateral extension of the disease process and irregularities of the orbital rim may represent bony destruction.

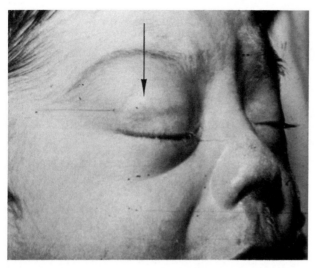

Figure 34–3. Infant with orbital and upper lid hemangioma. On palpation the hemangioma produced minimal resistance.

Ophthalmologic Examination

A complete ophthalmologic evaluation is mandatory. Decreased visual acuity is not characteristic of most intraorbital expansive processes unless the degree of proptosis is great or there is direct pressure on the optic nerve. A tumor directly behind the globe may indent the posterior wall of the retina in such a way as to induce a refractive error. A visual field defect suggests involvement of the optic chiasm. Fundoscopic examination may show the presence of retinal stria or scleral flattening, which usually indicates a discrete intraorbital tumor. Papilledema and optic atrophy generally imply direct involvement of the optic nerve by tumor pressure or infiltration (Kroll and Casten, 1966).

Limitation of ocular movement may reflect either direct mechanical infringement of the muscles or globe or involvement of the third, fourth, or sixth cranial nerves as they pass through the cavernous sinus or superior orbital fissure. The nature of this limitation of motion may be resolved by the forced duction test: after topical or general anesthesia, the limbus is grasped with conjunctival forceps. If the eye can be moved fully in the direction of limited motion, paralysis is the likeliest cause of the abnormal ocular movement, whereas if movement is restricted, mechanical infringement by tumor or inflammation probably is present.

Exophthalmometry

Exophthalmos may be established either by an absolute measurement that relates the distance of the corneal apex to a reference point on the skull, or by a relative measurement that compares the position of one cornea with the other (Calcaterra et al., 1974). Proptosis can be discerned easily by visualizing the eyes from above, over the forehead, or from below,

over the malar eminences. Absolute measurements can be obtained with various instruments, the most common of which is the Hertle exophthalmometer, which uses the lateral orbital rim as a bony reference and projects a lateral view of the cornea on a millimeter scale. Testing variability may range between 1 and 2 mm, depending on the consistent location of the instrument on the edge of the orbital rim, facial asymmetry, and thickness of the subcutaneous tissue over the bone. This instrument is especially useful in detecting smaller degrees of proptosis and for making objective measurements in serial examinations.

Proptosis is considered to be present when one globe is displaced 2 mm farther forward than the other. This difference is usually accompanied by a widened palpebral fissure. However, a misleading appearance of proptosis may be present in patients with unilateral enophthalmos, lid retraction, or unilateral myopia.

Otolaryngologic Examination

Specific attention must be directed toward the nose, paranasal sinuses, nasopharynx, and neck. Inflammatory mucosal changes, purulent exudate, and polyps in the nose or nasopharynx all indicate possible sinusitis and a mucopyocele. Palpation and pressure over the sinuses may indicate inflammation or an underlying neoplasm.

The ears should be checked for a serous effusion inasmuch as it is well known that neoplasia and inflammation of the ethmoid sinuses and nasopharynx can impair function of the eustachian tube. The neck should be palpated carefully for the presence of enlarged lymph nodes that may harbor metastatic cells from a primary tumor in the region of the eye. An enlarged thyroid gland suggests hyperthyroidism and thus an endocrine basis for the exophthalmos.

An evaluation of cranial nerve function should be completed, particularly of the first and fifth cranial nerves. Lesions near the cribriform plate or sphenoid ridge may compromise olfaction. The first and second divisions of the fifth cranial nerve course behind, above, and below the orbital cavity, and adjacent lesions may cause deficient sensation over the forehead, cornea, or cheek.

DIAGNOSTIC STUDIES

Basic laboratory studies should include a complete blood count to ascertain possible evidence of inflammation or blood dyscrasia, as well as a chest radiograph to rule out granulomatous or metastatic disease. Other studies may include thyroid hormone assays to determine thyroid function, serum alkaline phosphatase level to determine possible bone disease, and bone marrow aspiration if blood dyscrasia seems to be a possibility.

Radiologic Plain Films and Tomography

To provide a preliminary survey of more specific radiologic studies, routine films of the orbits and paranasal sinuses consisting of posteroanterior, Waters, lateral, basal, and optic foramina views should be taken. Occasionally such films can be diagnostic.

Tomography enables a three-dimensional perspective of the orbits to be studied, and it gives more precise information regarding their size, extent, and relationship to adjoining structures (Potter, 1972). Anteroposterior tomographic examination usually sections the orbital area every 5 mm, but narrower sections of 1 to 2 mm may be made if necessary. Basal-view tomography is particularly useful in evaluating the lateral walls of the orbit and optic canal.

Increased vertical distances greater than 2 mm between the infraorbital and supraorbital rims signify a space-occupying lesion. This concentric enlargement without bone erosion is typical of benign tumors (e.g., hemangiomas). Likewise, localized bone displacement without destruction of bone margin suggests a slow-growing benign tumor. Widening of the superior orbital fissure is mainly seen with tumors of neural origin (e.g., neurofibroma or glioma). Increased density of bone, particularly along the sphenoid wing, strongly suggests meningioma, whereas diffuse osteolysis or bone destruction is seen when there are malignant tumors such as metastatic lesions or primary orbital malignancies. Calcifications within the orbit are frequently encountered with retinoblastomas but are uncommon with hemangiomas or other venous malformations.

Tomography is especially helpful in precise delineation of osseous anatomy, whereas the computed tomography (CT) scan provides more information regarding soft tissue disease. Osseous structures, which can usually be seen well, include foramen rotundum, pterygopalatine fossa, inferior and superior orbital fissures, and lacrimal fossa.

Computed Tomography

The advent of computed tomography has considerably improved the diagnosis of orbital lesions and is now the most important diagnostic radiologic test employed. In this procedure, the attainment of orbital detail is aided by the relatively large value differences in the absorption rates of fat, bone, and orbital soft tissue structures. When undergoing computed tomography, children usually require general anesthesia (Bozzao et al., 1982).

The chief value of this type of scan is its reliability in localizing intraorbital lesions (Fig. 34–4). Both the optic nerves and extraocular muscles can be visualized readily, and any associated lesions can be outlined. Another advantage is the concomitant assessment of other anatomic sites, such as the ethmoid and sphenoid sinuses, nasopharynx, cranial cavity, and skull walls, thereby providing information about the origin and extent of the disease (Forbes et al., 1982).

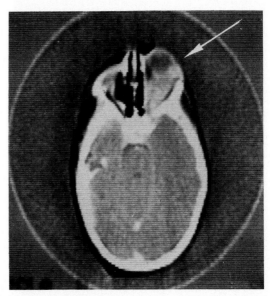

Figure 34–4. A computed tomogram showing an intraorbital neurofibroma in a 1-year-old infant. The arrow indicates proptosis and soft tissue density behind the globe.

Arteriography and Venography

The study of the arterial blood supply can be advantageous in evaluating certain orbital lesions (Vignaud et al., 1972). Selective contrast injection of the internal carotid artery delineates the ophthalmic arterial complex, and visualization is further enhanced by the subtraction technique, which eliminates surrounding osseous shadows (Fig. 34–5). Helpful information is also supplied by the capillary or late arterial phase of the arteriogram, which may outline pathologic vascularity of the lesion itself. Malignant lesions often demonstrate vascular lakes, tangles of tiny vessels, and arteriovenous shunts. However, hemangiomas and venous malformation are typically not visualized (Vignaud et al., 1972).

Venography is particularly valuable in cases of venous malformations and cavernous sinus inflammation or thrombosis (Hanafee, 1972) (Fig. 34–6). Access to the orbital venous system is usually gained via one of

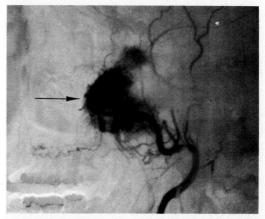

Figure 34–5. An arteriogram in a male adolescent with a nasopharyngeal angiofibroma extending to the orbit. The arrow points to the typical tangle of vessels feeding the tumor.

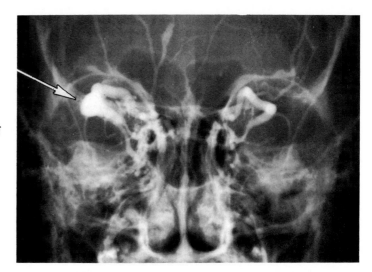

Figure 34–6. An orbital venogram demonstrating a varix of the superior ophthalmic vein as indicated by the arrow.

the forehead veins, although catheterization of the internal jugular vein and retrograde injection into the inferior petrosal sinus may be used. The lesion-localizing capability of this study is predicated on the relatively constant anatomy of the superior ophthalmic vein as it passes near the trochlea, under the medial rectus, and above the optic nerve to enter the cavernous sinus through the superior orbital fissure.

Ultrasonography

The orbital contents may also be scanned by the reflection of ultrasonic echoes (Motolese et al., 1982). These tracings can be recorded on an oscilloscope as a linear display recording the amplitude and time relationship of the echo to the original pulse (A scan) or the storage of the echo pattern to produce a composite picture (B scan) (Fig. 34–7). The latter method pro-

vides two-dimensional acoustic sections of the orbit, which may be photographed. Information is obtained regarding the location, size, and margins of the lesion. Infiltrative lesions can often be distinguished from well-circumscribed lesions by this technique.

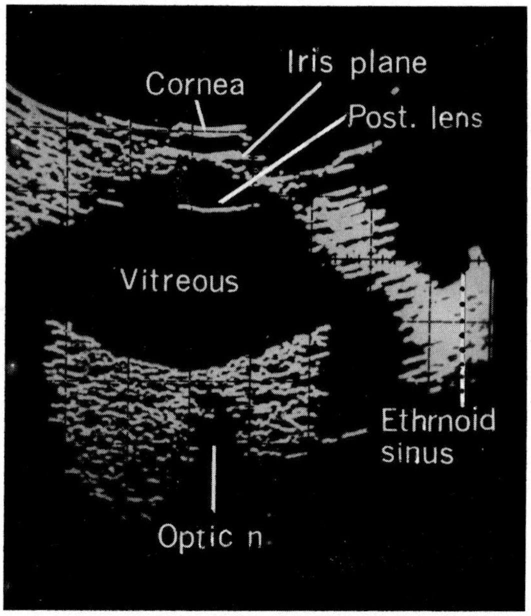

CLINICAL FEATURES OF ORBITAL SWELLINGS

Arbitrarily the origin of proptosis in children can be categorized as being developmental, inflammatory, vascular, neoplastic, or metabolic. It is not the intent of this chapter to give details about each disease but rather to provide an overview of the types of diseases that may affect the orbit in the pediatric patient. Many of these diseases will be covered in the other chapters inasmuch as the orbit can be involved with disease in contiguous structures.

Developmental Anomalies

Various developmental anomalies of the bony orbit produce proptosis simply by insufficient volume of the orbit, which causes the soft tissue of the eye to protrude. These include several types of craniostenosis (oxycephaly, turricephaly) owing to premature closure of one or more cranial sutures. Hereditary craniofacial dysostosis (Crouzon syndrome) also may produce proptosis due to foreshortening of the orbital floors and hypoplasia of the maxillae (Fig. 34–8).

Developmental defects in the orbital roof may allow a herniation of intracranial contents into the orbit. These are termed a meningocele, encephalocele, or hydroencephalocele, depending on what tissues are encompassed in the herniated sac (Kroll and Casten, 1966).

Dermoid cysts and teratomas may occur in the orbit. Dermoids consist entirely of ectodermal tissue and generally appear in the upper half of the orbit. On the other hand, teratomas, consisting of all three germ layers, are quite rare, although they may be large and are occasionally subject to malignant changes.

Figure 34–7. B scan obtained through the midportion of the orbit. The most echo-dense anatomy appears opaque.

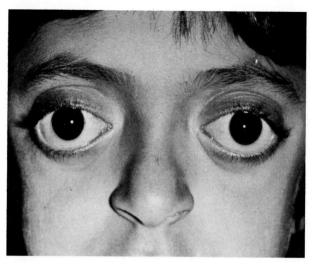

Figure 34–8. A child with Crouzon syndrome exhibiting bilateral proptosis resulting from hypoplasia of the maxillae.

Inflammatory Disease

Acute inflammatory disease of the orbit in children is likely to result from infection in the paranasal sinuses. In children under the age of 10 years, the most common source is acute ethmoiditis (Fig. 34–9). In adolescents the frontal sinus may be the original site of the infection because at that stage it has reached nearly full development. Maxillary sinusitis less commonly produces orbital cellulitis. A more insidious inflammatory swelling may develop with mucocele erosion from any of the adjacent sinuses (Chap. 37).

On occasion, orbital inflammation arises from infections of the face or nose that extend to the orbit by retrograde thrombophlebitis. The dreaded complication in these instances is cavernous sinus thrombosis, which produces severe orbital pain, proptosis, and ophthalmoplegia.

Lacrimal sac infections can occur in children if the nasolacrimal duct is obstructed, causing an inflammatory swelling in the medial quadrant of the orbit. The lacrimal gland involvement may accompany mumps in children, and the inflammatory swelling is usually confined to the upper temporal portion of the orbit.

Several specific organisms may be responsible for chronic infection of the orbit. For example, tuberculosis may involve the orbital bone in the form of periostitis; mycotic infection such as mucormycosis and aspergillosis may affect the orbit in the juvenile diabetic patient as well as in those undergoing intensive chemotherapy for blood dyscrasias.

Vascular Abnormalities

Cavernous hemangioma is the most commonly seen vascular lesion of the orbit (Savoiardo et al., 1983) (Fig. 34–10). Although frequently congenital, this tumor may not grow noticeably until well after birth. Associated hemangiomas of the face, neck, and larynx may occur. Other related disorders are the lymphangiomas that are also seen in infancy and the orbital varices observed more frequently in older children. However, aneurysms of the ophthalmic artery and carotid cavernous sinus fistulas that produce pulsatile proptosis are rare in children.

Neoplasms

Orbital neoplasms may be primary within the orbit, caused by direct extension from neighboring structures, or metastatic from a distant primary malignancy (Augsburger, 1983). The most common primary orbital neoplasms in children are optic nerve glioma and rhabdomyosarcoma. A large proportion of children with glioma will prove to have von Recklinghausen disease, which is characterized by slow growth and early loss of vision (Fig. 34–11). Rhabdomyosarcoma usually grows quite rapidly and appears during the first decade of life (Fig. 34–12). Other primary tumors

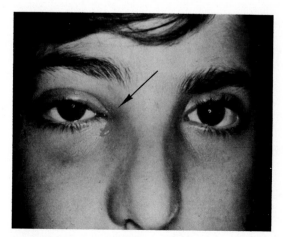

Figure 34–9. The arrow points to orbital cellulitis and proptosis caused by acute ethmoiditis.

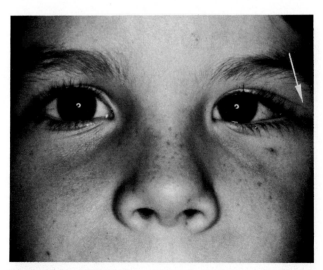

Figure 34–10. A child with a cavernous hemangioma occupying the lateral aspect of the left orbit.

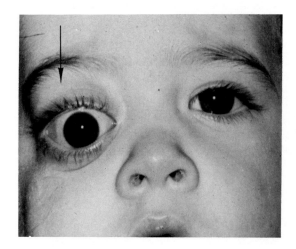

Figure 34–11. An infant with a large neurofibroma of the right posterior-superior aspect of the orbit with obvious proptosis and downward displacement of the eye.

are melanoma, retinoblastoma, and lacrimal gland tumors.

Secondary invasion of tumors from the paranasal sinuses and nasopharynx is much less frequent in children than in adults. Extension of nasopharyngeal angiofibroma to the orbit is well known in male children. Sarcomas of the sinuses and adjacent structures involving the orbit are more common than squamous cell carcinomas in the pediatric age group. Fibrous dysplasia may involve the orbital bone and may decrease orbital volume, thus producing proptosis (Chap. 41) (Moore et al., 1985).

The most common metastatic tumor found in the eye is a neuroblastoma from the adrenal gland, which usually occurs in children under 5 years of age (Kroll and Casten, 1966). Hematopoietic malignancies that may involve the orbit are lymphoma, Hodgkin disease, and chloroma (solid infiltration of cells in leukemia).

Surgical exploration of the orbit is usually required to provide precise histologic identification of a neoplasm. The surgical approach is mainly related to the location of the tumor (Migliavacca et al., 1982).

Metabolic Disease

Hyperthyroidism occurs much more commonly in adults, although several pediatric patients with Graves disease have been reported. The orbital involvement is usually bilateral and is characterized by early lid retraction and eye fullness; eventually chemosis and diplopia may develop.

Other histiocytic diseases that may involve the orbit include eosinophilic granuloma, Hand-Schüller-Christian disease, and Letterer-Siwe disease.

SELECTED REFERENCES

Calcaterra, T. C., Hepler, R. S., and Hanafee, W. N. 1974. The diagnostic evaluation of unilateral exophthalmos. Laryngoscope 84:231.

This article emphasizes those diseases that are otolaryngologic in origin but may present initially as unilateral exophthalmos. The steps in the diagnostic workup are summarized.

Ophthalmologic Staff of the Hospital for Sick Children. 1967.

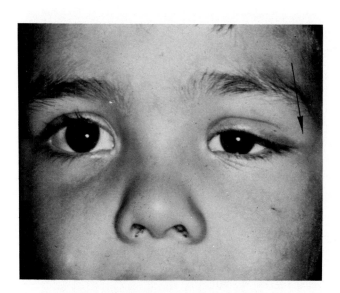

Figure 34–12. A child with a rhabdomyosarcoma involving the left lateral orbital space and temporal fossa.

Diseases of the orbit, Chap. 15. *In* The Eye in Childhood. Chicago, Year Book Medical Publishers.

This chapter provides a comprehensive review of diseases that may cause proptosis in children. The hospital's experiences with 257 cases serve as the source for the review.

Kroll, A. J., and Casten, V. G. 1966. Diseases of the orbit. *In* Liebman, G., and Gillis, P. (eds.): The Pediatrician's Ophthalmology. St. Louis, C. V. Mosby Co.

This chapter discusses orbital disease in children from the standpoint of general disease categories (i.e., developmental, trauma, inflammation, and neoplasm). There is an excellent discussion of differential diagnosis.

REFERENCES

Augsburger, J. J. 1983. Ocular tumors in children. Pediatr. Clin. North Am. 30:1071.

Bozzao, L., Fantossi, L. M., and Rosa, M. 1982. Childhood orbital pathology: Investigation by computed tomography. J. Neurosurg. Sci. 26:25.

Calcaterra, T. C., Hepler, R. S., and Hanafee, W. N. 1974. The diagnostic evaluation of unilateral exophthalmos. Laryngoscope 84:231.

Forbes, G. S., Earnest, F., and Waller, R. R. 1982. Computer tomography of orbital tumors, including late generation scanning techniques. Radiology 142:387.

Hanafee, W. N. 1972. Orbital venography. Radiol. Clin. North Am. 10:63.

Kroll, A. J., and Casten, V. G. 1966. Diseases of the orbit. *In* Liebman, G., and Gillis, P. (eds.): The Pediatrician's Ophthalmology. St. Louis, C. V. Mosby Co.

Migliavacca, F., Furnari, M., Moise, A., and Della Grottague, B. 1982. The surgical approach to intraorbital tumors in children. J. Neurosurg. Sci. 26:29.

Moore, A. T., Bunck, J. R., and Munro, I. R. 1985. Fibrous dysplasia of the orbit in childhood. Clinical features and management. Ophthalmology 92:12.

Motolese, E., Esposti, P., Bardelli, A. M., and Frezzotti, R. 1982. Echographic study of exophthalmos and neoformative endocular pathology in childhood, V. Neurosurg. Sci. 26:17.

Ophthalmologic Staff of the Hospital for Sick Children. 1967. Diseases of the orbit, Chap. 15. *In* The Eye in Childhood. Chicago, Year Book Medical Publishers.

Potter, G. D. 1972. Tomography of the orbit. Radiol. Clin. North Am. 10:21.

Savoiardo, M., Strada, L., and Passerini, A. 1983. Cavernous hemangiomas of the orbit: Value of CT, angiography, and phlebography. Am. J. Neuroradiol. 4:741.

Vignaud, J., Clay, C., and Aubin, M. D. 1972. Orbital arteriography. Radiol. Clin. North Am. 10:39.

Wright, J. E., Lloyd, G. A., and Ambrose, J. 1975. Computerized axial tomography in the detection of orbital space-occupying lesions. Am. J. Ophthalmol. 80:78.

Chapter 35

PEDIATRIC PLASTIC AND RECONSTRUCTIVE SURGERY OF THE HEAD AND NECK

Janusz Bardach, M.D.

Pediatric plastic and reconstructive surgery of the head and neck encompasses a variety of procedures performed by different specialists. Repair of cleft lip and palate and other craniofacial deformities typically has been in the domain of plastic surgeons. Management of facial trauma and subsequent defects has been shared by head and neck surgeons, plastic surgeons, and oral surgeons. Treatment of tumors of the head and neck usually has been dominated by head and neck surgeons. Acute burns and resultant head and neck deformities have been treated by general surgeons, plastic surgeons, and head and neck surgeons. Multiple reconstructive procedures and various facets of aesthetic surgery have been performed by both plastic surgeons and head and neck surgeons.

Currently, it is difficult to define specific areas of competence for plastic surgeons, head and neck surgeons, and oral surgeons because of the vast developments within each specialty during the past decades. New surgical techniques (e.g., microvascular surgery, free and myocutaneous flaps, and craniofacial surgery) have been readily adopted by plastic surgeons, head and neck surgeons, and oral surgeons. Improved training programs and postresidency fellowships have provided better education in specialized areas. Therefore, facility in specific areas cannot be limited to one specialty, as different specialists, plastic surgeons, head and neck surgeons, and oral surgeons are competent in the treatment of various head and neck problems.

Plastic surgery, as well as head and neck surgery, departments have training programs for residents and fellows that focus on various aspects of head and neck treatment. Close cooperation among different specialists is indicated in many cases, contributing to the better care of patients. Craniofacial deformities, head and neck oncology, and maxillofacial trauma are areas in which a team approach and cooperation among specialists is especially advantageous for patient care and research.

Based on this philosophy, knowledge of pediatric plastic and reconstructive surgery by pediatric specialists will enhance communication and cooperation among specialists and will promote a better under-standing of the challenges that both pediatric plastic surgeons and pediatric otolaryngologists may face in their practices. A great variety of problems are encountered in pediatric plastic and reconstructive surgery. Obviously, only a few of these can be addressed in this chapter. The selection of topics was based on the relative magnitude of the problem and on the experience of the author.

CLEFT LIP AND PALATE

Incidence of Clefts

Of the craniofacial deformities of the head and neck, cleft lip and palate is the most common. The incidence of clefting varies among races and nations. According to the statistics based on birth records, the highest incidence was recorded in North American Indians and in the Japanese population (1 in 300 to 400). The lowest occurrence (1 in 1300 to 1800) was noted in the black race. There is a relatively high incidence of clefting in Scandinavia and the middle European countries. For example, in Denmark and Finland, the rate is 1 in 550; in Poland, the incidence was found to be 1 in 575; and in Czechoslovakia, 1 in 665. In Iowa, the incidence of clefts is approximately 1 in 700 (Van-Demark, 1987). Only a few countries have a reliable registry of birth defects. Therefore, these statistics should be discussed with caution.

According to many studies, males are more often affected than are females. The many types of clefts vary in incidence. Oldfield and Tate (1964) reported the following rates of occurrence for the different cleft types: cleft lip only, 22.9 per cent; cleft palate only, 34.6 per cent; and cleft lip, alveolus, and palate, 42.5 per cent. Bardach (1967) reported slightly different rates: cleft lip only, 19.8 per cent; cleft palate only, 30.6 per cent; and cleft lip, alveolus, and palate, 49.5 per cent. In Bardach's study, it was also found that most unilateral clefts occur on the left side (1:2.3). Furthermore, there are more unilateral clefts than bilateral clefts (1:2.9).

Types of Clefts

There are a great variety of cleft forms and associated maxillofacial and nasal deformities (Fig. 35–1A through D). Many systems have been introduced to categorize the various cleft types. Some classifications are based on embryologic development, whereas others focus on morphologic changes. A classification system like that developed by the American Cleft Palate Association includes so many details that it is useful for research but is too cumbersome for clinical use. Many cleft palate centers have developed their own classification methods, which makes comparative studies difficult. The classification system used at The University of Iowa Cleft Palate Center is simple, yet clinically useful because it is based on morphologic characteristics. This system is listed below.

I. CLEFT LIP ONLY
A. Unilateral
B. Bilateral
II. CLEFT LIP AND ALVEOLUS (PARTIAL OR INCOMPLETE)
A. Unilateral
B. Bilateral
III. CLEFT PALATE ONLY
A. Submucous
B. Partial
C. Complete
IV. CLEFT LIP, ALVEOLUS, AND PALATE
A. Unilateral
B. Bilateral
V. ATYPICAL CLEFTS. A combination of clefts listed in the above four groups (e.g., partial bilateral cleft lip and partial cleft palate; complete cleft lip and palate on the left side and cleft lip only on the right side).

In planning surgical treatment, the severity of the cleft must be considered with regard to cleft width, positioning and development of the lip elements and maxillary segment, and the nasal deformity (Bardach and Salyer, 1987). Each cleft must be analyzed because the degree of deformity and congenital hypoplasia may vary considerably in a given cleft form. The most severe deformities are found in complete unilateral or bilateral clefts. These cleft types disrupt the skeletal and soft tissue continuity in the midfacial region.

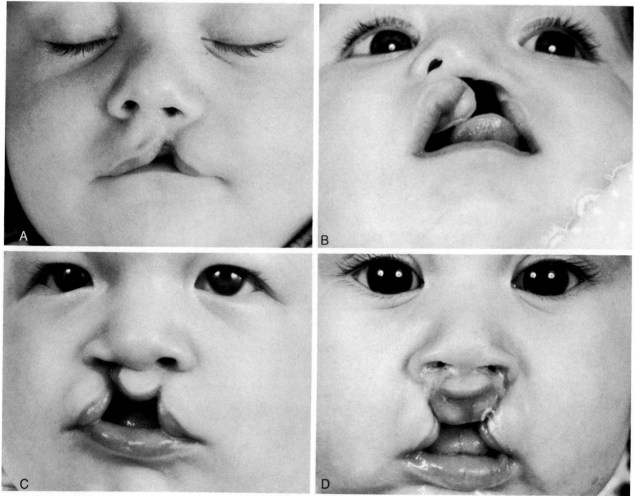

Figure 35–1. *A,* Unilateral incomplete cleft. *B,* Unilateral complete cleft lip, alveolus, and palate. Note severe nasal deformity. *C,* Bilateral cleft of the lip, alveolus, and palate. Complete on the right side and incomplete on the left side. *D,* Bilateral cleft lip, alveolus, and palate with protruding premaxilla.

Congenital dysmorphogenesis and hypoplasia of the soft tissue and bony structures create a functional imbalance, which adversely affects facial growth. The complete cleft also severely affects dentition, occlusion, speech production, and eustachian tube function. The wide communication between the oral and the nasal cavities also may contribute to upper respiratory tract infections. The incomplete bilateral cleft with a protruding premaxilla and small prolabium presents the most difficult treatment problem because of the severity of the initial deformity and the resulting morphologic and functional changes.

Multidisciplinary Management

More than one treatment specialist is needed for successful management of cleft lip and palate because it is a multifaceted problem. The basic goals of multidisciplinary management for cleft lip and palate are to assure a good aesthetic result, satisfactory facial growth, and normal speech production before the child reaches school age. Orthodontic treatment and the correction of secondary nasal deformities, including septoplasty, may continue throughout the school years.

Team Approach

Treatment of cleft lip and palate requires a multidisciplinary approach owing to the variety of impairments caused by this craniofacial deformity. The exclusive use of surgical treatment has often failed and has resulted in severe secondary maxillofacial deformities caused primarily by midfacial growth inhibition. Dental and speech problems are often not corrected. For these reasons, the team approach has become essential in coordinating effective multidisciplinary treatment.

The cornerstones of the multidisciplinary team are the surgeon, the speech pathologist, and the orthodontist. The pediatric otolaryngologist should participate in the treatment of any ear and nasal airway problems associated with the cleft deformity. Cooperation of this team of specialists serves the basic needs of the patient in any multidisciplinary treatment. At some cleft palate centers, the team may also include pediatricians, geneticists, pedodontists, prosthodontists, psychologists, psychiatrists, social workers, audiologists, and nurse specialists. This type of team offers greater expertise, as well as a broad base for clinical research.

The team of specialists is most effective when all members are within one institution and can communicate on a daily basis. Weekly sessions with all members provide the diagnosis, planning of treatment, evaluation of each stage of treatment, and indications for the actual needs of the patients. These meetings also provide a forum for exchange of ideas in regard to a particular patient and for the discussion of various viewpoints and experiences. Close contact among team members, especially between the plastic surgeon and orthodontist, and/or between plastic surgeon and speech pathologist, has been effective in achieving

highly satisfactory results in all phases of treatment. Close cooperation among specialists is also necessary for critically evaluating short- and long-term results and for determining directions for improved treatment strategies. The team approach not only is important in the development of treatment strategies, but also is invaluable in conducting comprehensive clinical research on the various treatment techniques.

Obviously, not all cleft palate centers have teams of the same human resources or competence. Groups of specialists with adequate training who intend to participate in cleft treatment should organize a cleft palate team consisting of the four basic specialists to provide adequate care for the cleft patient. Treatment of cleft patients without an established and functioning cleft palate team is inefficient and often results in secondary maxillofacial deformities, dental problems, and speech problems that are difficult to correct.

Cleft Palate Team

The cleft palate team makes possible a diagnosis derived from broader and more accurate sources of information, and it allows for representative judgments and decisions. The treatment resulting from a group plan is more likely to assume a proper sequence and balance, with techniques approved by most specialists. The team also facilitates proper ordering, sequencing, and timing of each specialist's effort in the process of multidisciplinary treatment.

The type of specialists ordinarily involved in the management program for patients with cleft lip and palate deformities varies according to different situations. The *minimum* cleft palate team consists of the following:

1. Surgeon.
2. Speech pathologist.
3. Orthodontist.

The *ideal* team of cleft palate specialists includes the following:

1. Team coordinator.
2. Surgeon.
3. Speech pathologist.
4. Dental specialists—orthodontist, prosthodontist, pedodontist, general dentist.
5. Otolaryngologist.
6. Pediatrician.
7. Audiologist.
8. Psychologist.
9. Psychiatrist.
10. Social worker.
11. Physical anthropologist.
12. Radiologist.
13. Geneticist.
14. Statistician.
15. Nursing specialists.
16. Anesthesiologist.

Treatment Procedures

There may be differences in the philosophy of cleft management and in the timing of particular treatment procedures. To exemplify this, a summary of treatment procedures and their timing, as used at The University of Iowa Cleft Palate Center, is presented (Table 35–1).

EVALUATION. Most cleft palate centers use different evaluation forms to monitor and document changes following the various treatment procedures. It would be highly beneficial if a standard method of evaluation could be adopted to facilitate comparative studies of management techniques and results.

The University of Iowa Cleft Palate Center and the Dallas Center for Craniofacial Deformities carried out comparative studies that used the same evaluation forms and procedures. The results of these studies indicated a need for further comparative clinical research to critically evaluate current treatment techniques and to explore ways of improving management for cleft patients. More well-designed investigations and statistical data are needed to justify or negate various treatment techniques. Currently, many clinical methods are based on personal experience, with no scientific justification. Cleft lip and palate is a multifaceted problem and must be approached from the viewpoints of many specialists. Because prevention of clefts does not appear possible in the near future, perfection of current treatment techniques remains a primary goal of cleft palate teams.

PLANNING. There is a great variety of cleft forms. Therefore, planning of specific treatment procedures depends on an analysis of the initial deformity. In cleft lip only, the extent of the cleft and degree of the associated nasal deformity are determining factors for the choice of surgical procedure. For cleft lip and alveolus with an intact palate, there may be a severe nasal deformity and displacement of the maxillary segments. Cases of wide clefts with severe nasal and alveolar displacement require more than just surgical treatment. Surgery must be accompanied by orthodontic treatment, sometimes even at the presurgical stage if protrusion of the premaxilla is extremely severe. In the complete cleft lip, alveolus, and palate, the width of the cleft, position of the maxillary segments, degree of soft tissue and bony hypoplasia, distance between the alveolar segments, and width of the palatal cleft must be considered in the choice of timing and the type of surgical procedure used.

It is difficult to anticipate final results in a particular patient because this birth defect must be evaluated in light of the dynamics of the growth and development of the maxillofacial structures. A general management strategy (as presented in Table 35–1) should be adopted. However, evaluation subsequent to each treatment phase is needed before the next treatment steps are undertaken. Various surgical techniques may be used successfully for treatment of similar cleft deformities. The contributions of the speech pathologist, orthodontist, pediatric otolaryngologist, and the other specialists during the various phases of treatment are most successful when they are well coordinated and when results are monitored by all team members.

Psychosocial Aspects of Cleft Lip and Palate

The birth of an infant with a cleft is always shocking and depressing, especially for the mother. The reaction of the father and immediate family may vary from disappointment, resentment, rejection, and high anxiety to immediate acceptance and continuous support. Experience with thousands of families treated and observed by the author indicates that disintegration of the family as a result of the birth of a cleft baby seldom occurs. More typically, first the mother and then the father and immediate family adopt positive and protective attitudes toward the newborn. It is extremely helpful when, during the first 24 hours after the birth of a cleft baby, the mother and immediate family are informed of the highly effective treatment techniques for clefts of the lip and palate.

When the first contact is made by a professional from a cleft palate team, the goal is to leave the mother and family assured that the baby will develop and grow normally with the continued treatment indicated during his or her school years. Booklets, schematic drawings, and photographs of similar deformities before and after treatment have a tremendous impact on family and friends because they demonstrate how successful treatment can be.

The stigma of a cleft is much less pronounced in today's society than in the past. People born with a cleft deformity are not discriminated against in their social and professional environments. An important condition for normal emotional development and growth is the absence of differential treatment for the cleft child. It has been observed that cleft children treated in the same manner as their normal siblings and peers usually develop healthy attitudes and a positive self-image.

EAR DEFORMITIES

Congenital Ear Deformities

Congenital ear deformities in children may cause psychologic problems, no matter how inconspicuous the deformity of the ear may be. Even a slight deformity of the ear is apparent, especially in boys. The child may be teased and ridiculed by his or her peers. Parents usually are sensitive to this and are eager for the defect to be corrected as soon as possible. Some deformities may be corrected successfully before the child goes to school; others may require multistage reconstructive procedures.

The psychologic impact of an existing deformity cannot be underestimated because behavioral problems, which may need to be treated by a pediatric psychologist, could develop. This point must be emphasized because currently treatment of some ear deformities (e.g., prominent ear and cup ear) is considered by insurers to be cosmetic surgery. In the author's opinion, the decision of whether or not a deformity is cosmetic should be made on an individual

TABLE 35–1. Summary of Treatment Procedures*

	TIMING	TECHNIQUE
Surgical Procedures		
Unilateral cleft lip repair	3 months of age	Modification of triangular flap technique
Bilateral cleft lip repair	Two stage: first at 3 months; second at 4.5 months of age	Modification of triangular flap technique or straight-line closure
Palate repair	12–18 months of age	Two-flap palatoplasty
Primary correction for nasal deformity	3 months (at the time of primary lip repair)	Construction of floor of the nose; repositioning of alar base (limited correction)
Correction for secondary nasal deformity	8–12 years of age	Bardach technique, external approach
Septoplasty	14 years and older	
Correction for secondary lip deformity	Before 5 years of age	Various techniques
Pharyngeal flap	4–6 years of age	Superiorly based pharyngeal flap technique (Hogan modification)
Alveolar bone grafting	4–6 years of age	
Premaxillary recession	4–6 years of age	Bilateral alveolar bone grafting with closure of oronasal and nasolabial fistulas
Orthognathic surgery	14 years and older	Mandibular or maxillary osteotomy
Speech Pathology Procedures		
Initial parent counseling about expected speech/language development, and about relationship among cleft palate, surgery, and speech production and importance of verbal stimulation	2–3 months of age	
Follow-up examination and parent counseling	6-month intervals until normal speech/language is developed	
Velopharyngeal function evaluation during speech	Beginning at age 3 years; then at 6-month intervals until adequate velopharyngeal function is established, with examination in later years if indications of developing velopharyngeal disorder	
Language therapy, if needed	Preschool years, if available	
Speech therapy, if needed; continued language therapy, if indicated	Early primary school years	
Definitive diagnosis of velopharyngeal function during speech; referral for secondary surgery if needed	4–7 years of age	
Determine whether audiologic evaluation is needed and make appropriate referrals	Birth to 6 years of age	
During follow-up evaluation, determine extent to which dental-occlusal status influences speech production	Beginning at age 3 years, and at yearly intervals until dental occlusal status is not influencing speech production	
Orthodontic Procedures		
Presurgical orthopaedic treatment	Not performed	
Maxillary expansion	At 3–5 years of age	
Mixed dentition treatment	At 6–9 years of age	Correction of molar relationships; alignment of maxillary teeth; serial extraction when indicated
Final orthodontic correction	At 10 years of age and older	Possible appliances or combination of orthodontic treatment and surgery
Otolaryngologic Procedures		
Myringotomy and ventilating tubes	When indicated	
Adenoidectomy prior to pharyngeal flap surgery	When there is significant adenoid hypertrophy	
Modification of the lateral port size after pharyngeal flap surgery		1. Enlargement of ports using lasers 2. Teflon injection to narrow port size 3. Disconnection of pharyngeal flap from posterior pharyngeal wall
Nasal-septal reconstruction	When there is nasal airway obstruction; performed between 14 and 16 years of age	
Inferior turbinate surgery	1. Partial turbinectomy in severe cases at 7–8 years of age 2. Submucous resection in severe cases at 7–8 years of age	
Cryotherapy for the nasal mucosa	For mucosal disease; performed at 14–16 years of age	
Cleft septorhinoplasty	For airway obstruction; performed at 14–16 years of age	

*Procedures used at The University of Iowa Cleft Palate Center for management of cleft patients. The approach, used at The Hospital for Sick Children, Toronto, is found in Chapter 4.

basis, depending on the ear deformity, the psychologic impact of the existing deformity, and how it influences the child's emotional stability.

Prominent Ear

Normal protrusion of the ear measured by the distance between the rim of the helix and mastoid plane ranges from 15 to 20 mm. Prominence of the ear may also be measured by the angle between the dorsal surface of the upper helical rim and the mastoid plane. An angle of 20 to 30 degrees is considered to be within normal limits. When the angle is greater than 40 degrees or the distance between the helical rim and mastoid plane is greater than 20 mm, the ear is classified as prominent (Farkas, 1974). The degree of prominence varies. The most severe prominent ear appears to be perpendicular to the mastoid plane with an angle of up to 90 degrees.

The prominent ear deformity results from a failure of the anthelix to fold, or from an enlarged and malpositioned concha. When an infant is born with protruding ears, it may seem that by applying pressure, this deformity could be reversed. However, only slight improvement or none at all is typically achieved. In many cases, the deformity remains and requires surgical intervention.

Prominent ears, depending on the severity of the deformity, may cause a serious psychologic problem. Even in mild deformities, particularly in boys, the ears are easily visible and may evoke ridicule and teasing from the child's friends. Surgical correction of protruding ears does not inhibit normal growth. Therefore, it is strongly recommended that surgical correction be performed before the child reaches school age.

Several factors should be considered in planning surgical treatment. It is necessary to determine if the size of the ears is equal and within normal limits and to establish if the prominence is of the same degree bilaterally. In many cases, one ear may be more prominent than the other and the ears may also vary in size. There is an additional need to choose the surgical technique that is best suited to the particular deformity.

When the cause of the prominence is an unfolded anthelix and the concha is normal, weakening of the cartilage, combined with skin reduction on the dorsal side, may suffice. Weakening of the cartilage, using diamond burrs, works best because it facilitates the creation of the anthelical fold without leaving sharp contours that usually occur after incisions through the cartilage.

The suture technique, used frequently in the past, is not recommended because of failures and associated complications. Over time, some sutures cut through the cartilage, becoming prominent and apparent through the skin. Usually, some degree of protrusion recurs. These complications can be avoided if the suture technique is not used.

Protrusion, when caused by a large concha, may require reduction of conchal cartilage with skin reduc-tion on the dorsal surface of the ear. It is necessary to emphasize that after skin reduction, both edges of the skin should be sutured to the periosteum with vertical mattress sutures in the postauricular crease—they should not be sutured to each other. Suturing the skin edge to edge creates a tent effect that may result in hematoma. By suturing each edge to the periosteum, leaving approximately 1 to 2 mm between the skin edges, dead space is avoided. In addition, this facilitates scar formation between the skin edges, which helps to stabilize the ear in the desired position. Reduction of the conchal cartilage, in contrast to through-and-through incisions in the cartilage in the anthelical area, does not leave sharp edges when well approximated and sutured.

Surgeons performing otoplasty should be aware that repositioning of the concha may cause some occlusion of the cartilaginous portion of the ear canal. This must be avoided, especially when using the suture technique. The appearance of a child who had otoplasty before (Fig. 35–2A) and 1 year postoperatively (Fig. 35–2B) is illustrated.

Cup Ear Deformity

There is a great variety of cup ear deformities. These differ in severity. These deformities may occur in combination with severe protrusion of the entire ear or a portion of it. In most cases, the cup ear deformity affects the upper and middle portion of the auricle, while the lobule is usually positioned normally. Bending the upper and middle portions of the auricle downward and forward may reveal that there is a skin deficiency in the anteroposterior dimension. The cartilage may also be deficient, especially in the upper portion.

The size of the cup ear varies. It is usually smaller than normal rather than larger. Hooding of the upper portion of the auricle may be so severe that it covers the entire concha and external auditory meatus. The concha is abnormally large and is usually positioned at an angle of 90 degrees relative to the mastoid plane. This position creates an exaggerated prominence of the concha, which, combined with constriction of the upper portion of the auricle, forms the characteristic cup ear deformity.

During examination, the surgeon must realize that correction of the cup ear deformity is extremely difficult because various forms of cup ear require different approaches to achieve successful results. It helps to analyze each portion of the deformed auricle to define the existing deficiencies of tissue (skin and cartilage) and the degree of malpositioning of the deformed parts. In some cases, more than one operation may be indicated by the severity of the deformity or the deficiency of tissue. It is also helpful to use a template from the normal ear for reconstruction of the affected ear so that it is the same size and in the same position as the normal ear. In some cases, the degree of skin and cartilage deficiency can be estimated accurately only in the operating room, following the release of

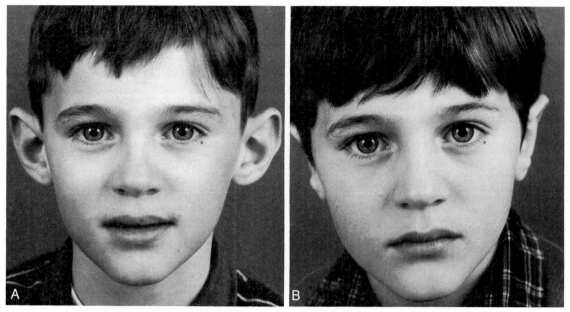

Figure 35–2. *A*, Bilateral severely protruding ears before otoplasty. *B*, One year after otoplasty.

the constricted portion of the auricle (Fig. 35–3*A* and *B*).

Among the various techniques described for correction of the cup ear deformity, the one used most successfully starts with release of the constricted upper auricle. This is followed by transposition of the skin in Z plasty fashion. Reduction or weakening of the conchal cartilage or both and simultaneous reduction of the skin on the dorsal surface of the ear is then

performed. Depending on the severity of the cup ear deformity, one or two operative stages may be needed.

Cryptotia

The main characteristic of this congenital deformity is that the upper portion of the cartilaginous framework adheres to the mastoid bone and is covered with skin, hence the name pocket ear. This abnormality may also

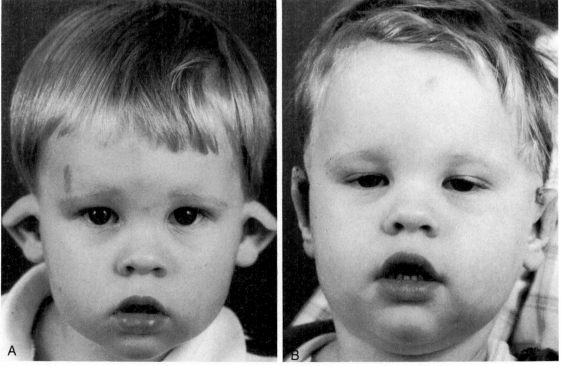

Figure 35–3. *A*, Bilateral severe cup ear deformity before surgical correction. *B*, After surgical correction before the sutures were removed.

involve the size and shape of the upper portion of the cartilaginous framework or the entire ear.

On examination, it may seem that simple elevation of the buried portion of the auricle beneath the skin would correct the problem. This is unfortunately rarely the case. This approach will fail if there is insufficient skin to cover the posterior surface of the upper portion of the elevated auricle and to create a postauricular crease of adequate depth. Usually, local transposition flaps suffice for this purpose. However, when the hairline is near, a free skin graft may be needed to accomplish successful reconstruction. In cases in which the cryptotic ear is smaller than the normal ear, augmentation with a cartilage implant may be performed during the same stage.

Microtia

Reconstruction of the microtic auricle continues to be a most difficult problem. The intricate shape, location, protrusion, and inclination of the auricle necessitates complex procedures. There are various degrees of hypoplasia of the external ear associated with the absence of the external meatus and auditory canal. Typically, the rudimentary auricle forms a longitudinal skin fold that includes misshapen remnants of cartilage. The skin fold is positioned vertically; the lobule is usually preserved, although it is displaced. The rudimentary microtic ear may contain sinus tracts that must be removed completely during surgery. In some rare cases, the entire auricle is absent and there is no tissue available for lobule reconstruction.

Microtia may occur as an ear deformity accompanied by normal growth and development of the craniofacial complex, or it may be a component of hemifacial or bilateral microsomia. In cases of microsomia, changes in the auricle are accompanied by hypoplasia of the mandible, maxilla, malar and temporal bones, soft tissue, and the muscles of mastication. Treatment of microsomia combined with microtia includes extensive bone grafting to create facial symmetry with subsequent ear reconstruction. Partial facial nerve paralysis is not uncommon in children with unilateral microsomia. In cases of unilateral microsomia, reconstruction of the auricle becomes a part of the total facial reconstruction and is far more successful when performed subsequent to the reconstructive procedure on the facial skeleton and soft tissue of the affected side.

Microtia, when not associated with microsomia, can be treated successfully before the child starts school. However, it is usually delayed until the normal ear is almost fully developed. Farkas (1974) indicated that after 7 to 9 years of age, no substantial growth of the auricle occurs. By age 6 to 7 years, the auricle is seven eighths of its mature size. The only treatment stage performed early in microtia is the reconstruction of the lobule when the child is 3 to 4 years of age.

In unilateral microtia, canalplasty to correct hearing loss in the affected ear is not recommended if there is normal hearing acuity in the opposite ear. The author's long-term experience indicates that patients with normal hearing in one ear and bone conduction in the affected ear do well in all aspects of daily life. Experienced otologists (McCabe, Gantz) believe that unilateral microtia does not cause a hearing impairment severe enough to justify canalplasty at an early age because this operation is not always successful.

In planning reconstruction, the surgeon should analyze the existing remnants of the auricle and decide which parts can be used for reconstruction (Bardach, 1974). Precise evaluation of the size and location of the ear to be reconstructed is necessary because, in some cases, the hairline may be close, resulting in an insufficient amount of hairless skin for reconstruction. If the hairline is too close and there is not enough hairless skin to cover the implant, the area may be augmented by rolling up the hair-bearing skin and closing the defect with a full-thickness free skin graft.

The choice of material for the implant, and the decision of how to cover the posterior surface of the ear to be reconstructed to create protrusion, must be made during the planning stage. Autogenous rib cartilage currently is considered to be the most reliable implant material. Silastic implants are an alternative material used by many surgeons. When the child is aged 7 to 8 years, an implant that matches the size of the fully developed normal ear is used. Homogenous, preserved rib cartilage has shown a high resorption rate and is therefore used only as a temporary implant for skin expansion.

After insertion of an implant, the next stage—the elevation of the auricle to create protrusion—is the most difficult step. This may require a full-thickness free skin graft in the area of hair-bearing skin behind the implant to provide enough skin for lining the posterior surface of the elevated auricle and for creating the postauricular crease (Fig. 35–4A through D).

Some refinements may follow basic reconstruction to simulate the external auditory meatus, define the concha (and other auricular contours), and increase protrusion. The author tries to limit reconstructive surgery to two stages: creation of a lobule in the first stage, and use of an implant in the second stage, designed to create a postauricular crease and protrusion without additional operations. Results in this difficult reconstructive surgery obtained by Tanzer (1971), Brent (1971), and others are encouraging.

Posttraumatic Ear Deformities

Trauma to the auricle may result in hematoma, disfigurement, or loss of tissue. In partial auricular defects, local flaps and cartilage implants may be used for reconstruction (Converse and Brent, 1977). When dealing with an acute loss of tissue, the recommended procedure is to suture the edge of the auricular defect to the postauricular skin. This not only enhances healing, but also allows use of postauricular skin for reconstruction of the missing part of the ear. When planning the reconstruction of various parts of the ear, postauricular skin or skin flaps from the nearest area

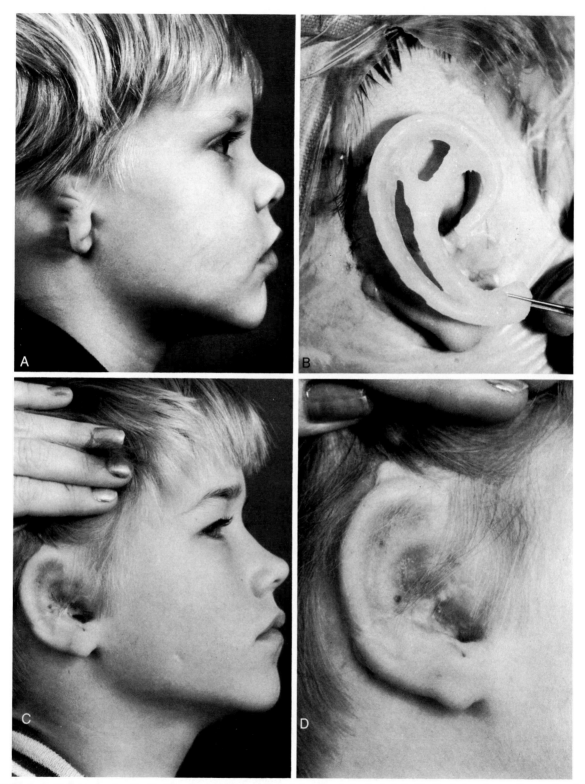

Figure 35–4. *A*, Unilateral microtia. *B*, After transposition of the lobule. Silastic implant, individually designed according to the shape of the opposite normal ear. *C* and *D*, Two years after total ear reconstruction.

are the best materials for repair. Typically, for enlarged defects, additional implant material is needed to achieve the proper shape and size of the ear.

When the entire auricle is lost as a result of trauma or surgery, reconstruction is much more complex and may require a regional or distant tube pedicle flap. This may be supplemented by a cartilage or Silastic implant.

Subsequent to trauma, partial or total avulsion of the auricle may occur. If the avulsed portion of the ear is available, if it has not been mutilated, and if less than 6 hours have elapsed since the time of trauma, reattachment is definitely indicated. The completely detached auricle may be reattached by the method described by Clemons and Connelly (1973).

FACIAL BURN INJURIES

Thermal injuries in the head and neck area are relatively common and may cause various facial deformities. The severity of burns is determined by the size of the exposed area and depth of injury. The size of the burn depends on how much body surface is exposed to the source of heat. The depth depends on the intensity and duration of exposure to the heat source.

In first-degree burns, only the epidermis is involved and healing is usually completed without superficial scar formation. Secondary burns are more severe because the heat penetrates into the dermis, but does not damage it. Erythema, blisters, and swelling may occur. Secondary burns are also painful because the nerve endings are exposed. In third-degree burns, the injury penetrates the dermis down to the soft tissue and bone (scalp), resulting in a charred appearance. The wound usually is dry, and the patient does not experience pain because the nerve endings are damaged.

Healing of second- and third-degree burns, which in recent nomenclature are referred to as partial- and full-thickness burns (based on the degree of skin damage), results in scarring, which may be hypertrophic or contracted and could even lead to formation of keloids. Free skin grafting in the initial stage enhances healing and minimizes subsequent scar contracture and further facial deformities. Secondary deformities may involve disfigurement due to hypertrophic scars, keloids, and scar contracture, causing possible ectropion of the eyelids, impairment of mouth opening, and eversion of the lower lip, as well as defects that usually include the ears and nose (Fig. 35–5A and B). Burns on the scalp leave hairless scars, which may involve a large area.

Timing of Reconstructive Procedures

Subsequent to primary treatment in the burn unit, reconstructive procedures usually are not indicated immediately. Conservative treatment measures are initially tried to improve the appearance of the scars, decrease the deformity, and facilitate further reconstructive surgery. Pressure masks are an effective way of minimizing development of hypertrophic scars and keloids. In cases in which these already exist, the mask helps to flatten and soften the scars. Exercises may help when dealing with scar contracture of the neck that restricts head movements or with scars around the mouth that limit its opening. Hypertrophic scars, keloids, or both in a small area may be treated successfully with steroid injections or massage with vita-

min E cream or a combination of these two. These treatment techniques must always be used when planning reconstructive procedures.

There is another reason to delay surgical management in children. When operating on young patients, it is usually expected that further surgical corrections will be indicated. Therefore, when the deformity is not severe and does not cause psychologic problems or functional impairments, the number of surgical procedures may be reduced by waiting for the patient to grow more. Parents may be eager to begin reconstructive procedures immediately, anticipating that "plastic surgery" will produce miraculous results (i.e., that the child will look the same as before the burn injury). The surgeon, while being supportive, must also be open in discussing realistic expectations, which may not always be optimistic.

The surgeon must be frank in presenting the possibilities and limitations for surgical reconstruction for each patient. Treatment of young patients after burns in the head and neck area is difficult. Reconstruction may continue for a long time, may require multiple surgical procedures, and may result in an appearance that is not totally satisfactory. Understanding the emotional stress on the child and parents is essential for providing the needed support and encouragement. Sometimes, this may require the assistance of a pediatric psychologist.

Reconstructive Techniques

Each patient with burns and their resultant variety of scars and deformities must be treated according to his or her specific condition. Usually, no reconstruction is started in the first year following the injury. During this time, use of the previously described procedures is recommended. However, in some cases, the length of the interim period may vary. If reconstruction is started less than 1 year after the injury, it is for functional reasons (e.g., prevention of exposure of the cornea due to severe ectropion; severe perioral scar contracture restricting food intake; eversion of the lower lip causing drooling; or adduction on the chin due to severe neck scarring). In all these cases, surgery is recommended to improve the functional capabilities and comfort of the patient.

If there is functional impairment and reconstructive surgery is indicated soon after a burn injury, a lower rate of success can be expected than if the same procedure were performed after the scars have matured and a longer period of time has elapsed. In evaluating the damage after a burn in the head and neck area, each region must be examined carefully to assess the existing deformities and plan the timing and sequence of surgical procedures and other treatment techniques.

Reconstructive procedures may seem to be highly successful after they have been completed in the operating room. However, severe scar contracture may recur, destroying the reconstructive effort. This may also happen when free skin grafts or skin flaps are

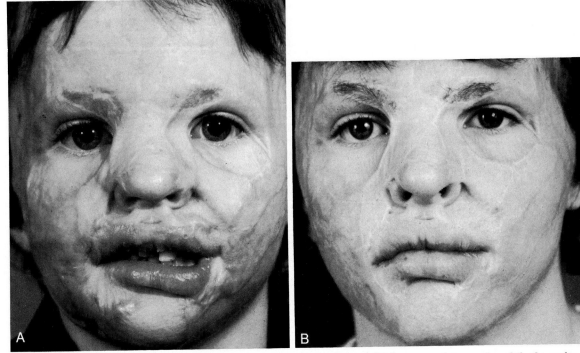

Figure 35–5. *A*, Extensive burn to the entire face. Note severe scarring in periorbital area causing eversion of the lower lip. Multiple hypertrophic scars over the entire face. *B*, Nine years later, after several operations using local transposition flaps and free skin grafting.

used to close a defect. Secondary scar contracture and hypertrophic scarring are especially common in burn patients who display abnormal wound healing.

Measures taken to prevent these complications are not always successful. It is still not known how to prevent the formation of hypertrophic scars or keloids. The surgeon tries to minimize these secondary complications after reconstructive surgery by using pressure dressings, pressure masks, exercises, massage, and steroid injections. At various stages of healing, one technique may work better than another for a given patient. It is important to understand that excision of hypertrophic scars or keloids may be unsuccessful if not accompanied by other treatment techniques. The recurrence rate for hypertrophic scars and keloids is high, especially in young burned patients. Simple excision may seem easiest; however, this is not always the best procedure.

Deformities subsequent to burn injuries in the various regions of the head and neck must be analyzed to determine the need for reconstruction, feasibility of procedures, timing, and choice of surgical technique. In some cases, there may be a large scarred area and the experienced surgeon may decide that reconstructive surgery would not improve the patient's appearance. In other cases, delay may be indicated to allow the scars and grafts to mature or to allow the child to grow and become more cooperative.

The deformities that occur after burns require different treatment techniques depending on the location of the injury. The following deformities are difficult to treat:

1. Hypertrophic scars and keloids.
2. Contracted scars that cause functional impairment.
3. Large scars that preclude use of local flaps.
4. Large scars in the scalp that cause baldness.

When dealing with hypertrophic scars, early excision is not recommended, owing to the high incidence of recurrence in burned patients. Prior to excision of hypertrophic scars, all conservative treatment techniques (pressure masks, steroid injections, massage, and so on) must be tried to reduce the probability of recurrence. If a hypertrophic scar is excised in an area surrounded by scar tissue, it is best to close the defect with a free skin graft. Local flaps that contain scar tissue may result in wound tension and contribute to further development of hypertrophic scars. The optimal depth of excision for hypertrophic scars has not yet been determined. In the author's opinion, the entire scar should be removed, up to the point of normal tissue. This type of excision, combined with wound closure using no tension, usually prevents the recurrence of hypertrophic scars (Fig. 35–6A and B).

Excision of keloids in the head and neck area is performed in one of two ways, depending on the size and location of the keloid. For example, a keloid covering the entire upper or lower lip should be removed completely and the defect should be covered with a full-thickness free skin graft. A keloid on the ear lobe also is totally excised; however, the epidermal layer attached by a pedicle to the normal skin is saved and used for closure of the defect. Use of the epidermis, which is easily dissected from the keloid mass, is

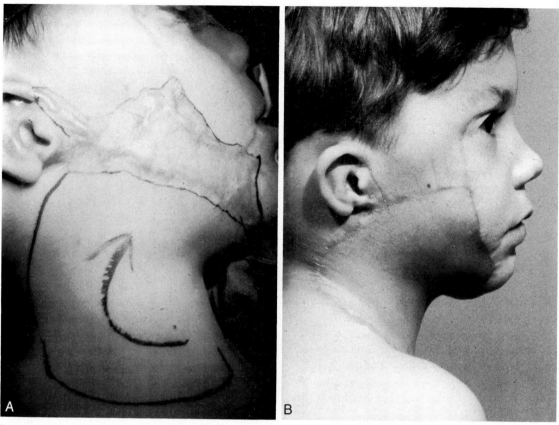

Figure 35–6. *A*, Large contracted scar on the cheek following burn. Design of rotation-advancement flap to close the defect following total excision of the existing scar. *B*, Several months later.

not indicated for defects of the lips because it is not thick enough to close the wound and it tends to contract when applied to a large area.

When there is a severe, large deformity on the forehead, cheeks, or nose with hypertrophic scars or keloids, it is important to keep in mind the aesthetics of the face when planning reconstruction. In the author's experience, full- or split-thickness free skin grafts covering an entire particular facial unit result in much better aesthetic and functional results than more than one skin graft. Excision of scars in an entire aesthetic region and resurfacing the defect with a free skin graft produce good results. Soft, flat atrophic scars present over a large area of the face may not require excision or replacement with a free skin graft, as improvement of the patient's appearance cannot always be achieved. In such cases, the light use of cosmetics is recommended to hide any scars.

Special attention should be given to the eyelids, lips, nose, and neck because deformities in these areas also cause functional impairment. A combination of scar excision, free skin grafting, and local flaps may be used to correct the existing deformity and achieve better functional and aesthetic results. The treatment choice depends on the existing deformity in the specific area of the head and neck. In some cases, use of local flaps or free skin grafts may suffice. For some patients, a combination of all the treatment techniques discussed above may be indicated.

Ectropion of the eyelids may be treated successfully with full- and split-thickness free skin grafts. Eversion of the lip may require total scar excision with free skin grafting. Rarely is the upper or lower lip alone everted owing to scar contracture. In most cases, the surrounding skin is also scarred. If normal, unaffected skin is available in the perioral region, transposition flaps may be used for closure of the defect after scar excision and lip reconstruction.

Large, contracted scars of the neck present difficult treatment problems because only complete excision with total resurfacing of the raw area is effective in releasing the scar contracture. Usually after wide excision of the contracted scars, a large defect remains and closure with local flaps may not be feasible. Free skin grafts, distant flaps, or free flaps with microvascular anastomosis are used for closure of the wound. If free skin grafts or free flaps are used, extension of the patient's neck must be maintained. This is done with individually prepared collars and special exercises. If these measures are not taken, secondary contracture may occur, requiring another surgical procedure.

Scar bands may cause some restriction of movement in various areas of the head and neck. Tension along the line of the scar band can be released by using single or multiple Z plasties. This technique has been successful, especially in the perioral and neck areas.

Scalp defects may present difficult problems when

a large area of hair-bearing skin is damaged. When 10 to 15 per cent of hair-bearing skin is replaced with scars, successful reconstruction is usually achieved in one surgical procedure using a single rotation-advancement flap. Success depends on the location of the defect. When the defect is surrounded by hair-bearing skin, reconstruction is accomplished in one operation. If the defect is not adjacent to hair-bearing skin, more than one reconstructive procedure may be required. For defects that include 15 to 25 per cent of the hair-bearing skin, multiple surgeries may be indicated.

When scar tissue covers 25 to 50 per cent of the scalp, more than one surgery and multiple flaps typically are needed to transpose hair-bearing skin to the frontal area, leaving some hairless areas in the occipital region. Use of single or multiple rotation-advancement flaps in the scalp area requires precise planning because of the poor elastic properties of the scalp and the difficulty of closure of the secondary defects. One technique that is useful is leaving the excised scar on a pedicle, removing it only after the rotation-advancement flap has been raised and the surgeon knows how much of the defect can be covered. The flap is used to cover the area of the excised scar, and the saved scar is used as a free skin graft to cover the secondary defect.

Use of distant skin flaps is indicated when burn defects cause not only scarring, but also loss of tissue that cannot be reconstructed with local flaps because of the damage to and scarring of the surrounding skin. Major tissue loss in the area of the nose, ears, and lips may necessitate use of distant skin flaps depending on the extent of the defect, existing deformity, and scarring in the surrounding tissue. If scars preclude the use of local flaps or if the extent of the defect requires more tissue than local flaps can provide, distant flaps may be necessary. Deltopectoral, pectoralis major, or tube pedicle flaps may be used for nasal reconstruction. Supraclavicular or infraclavicular tube flaps are frequently used for ear reconstruction.

Electric Burns

Electric burns in infants and young children usually occur because the child put an electric plug or cord in his or her mouth. Electric burns of the lips, commissures, and tongue may be quite severe, depending on the area of contact with the electric source and the duration of contact. Immediately after an accident, the area of necrosis from the burn is usually not apparent. Until the demarcation is obvious, surgical débridement or reconstructive procedures are contraindicated.

Special acrylic or Silastic appliances placed in the commissures after a burn to prevent adhesion of the upper and lower lips are not recommended. Proper management in the postinjury stage is limited to the prevention of infection by using antibiotic ointments. Healing may result in deformities owing to tissue loss and contracted scarring. At this stage, massage with vitamin E cream is recommended for at least 6 months.

Usually, reconstructive surgery is not performed until at least 1 year after the burn injury occurred. By then the scar has matured and softened. Reconstruction of the upper or lower lip and especially of the commissure is difficult, requiring the skills of an experienced surgeon (Fig. 35–7A through D). In all cases of electric burns in the oral and perioral areas, successful reconstructive results are achieved by using local mucosal skin flaps or both. In the majority of cases, a combination of both types of flaps may be needed.

HYPERTROPHIC SCARS AND KELOIDS

Excessive scarring subsequent to surgery or injury presents major complications for the healing process. This occurs more frequently in children and adolescents than in adults. In adults, hypertrophic scars and keloids are not as common and rarely do these occur in people older than age 55 to 60 years. Hypertrophic scars and keloids occur more frequently in black and yellow-skinned races than in the white race. Southern Europeans have a greater tendency to develop hypertrophic scars and keloids than people in the Northern European countries.

Hypertrophic scars and keloids result from an imbalance between collagen synthesis and deposition and from collagenolysis (Peacock, 1984, 1981a, 1981b). When excess synthesis and deposition of collagen prevail in a scar, hypertrophic scars and keloids form. In contrast, when collagenolysis occurs, atrophic scars form. Equilibrium between accelerated collagen deposition and its lysis results in stable scars. It seems that hypertrophic scars and keloids reflect a process in which collagen synthesis and deposition prevail.

Hypertrophic scars and keloids are thought to represent different stages of the same abnormality with distinct clinical characteristics. Hypertrophic scars may be considered the initial stage of the existing imbalance, whereas keloids are an advanced and mature stage of impaired wound healing. It is not currently known how to prevent hypertrophic scars and keloids and how to cure them effectively because control of collagen metabolism is not understood.

Hypertrophic scars typically appear soon after surgery or injury and retain the shape of the original scar or defect. The scar is usually red, is elevated, and may be sensitive. Hypertrophic scars may continue to grow and retain their red color for a long period of time.

Keloids may have various shapes and sizes bearing no resemblance to the primary wounds from which they were derived. They may develop after surgery, after injury, or even following a mild injury such as ear piercing, vaccination, or injection. The wound size seems to have no correlation to the size, shape, or growth potential of the keloid. There is also no time frame that is considered typical for the development of keloids. Keloids may follow the development and growth of hypertrophic scars; however, keloids have also been observed to develop several years after an

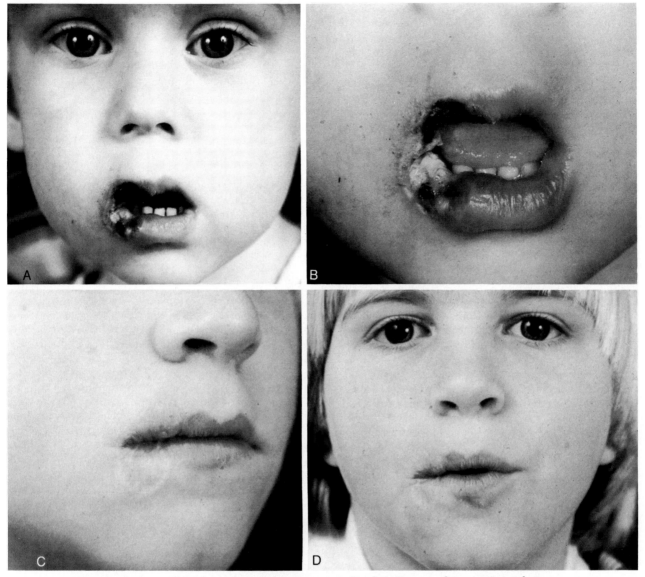

Figure 35–7. *A* and *B*, Electric burn of the commissure. *C* and *D*, Six years after commissuroplasty.

injury. This phenomenon can be attributed to stress (e.g., pregnancy, disease, and surgery) that triggers an abnormal collagen metabolism and starts excessive scar formation in an old scar. Keloids may cause itching, tenderness, and pain.

Clinically, keloids vary in size, shape, surface texture, and attachment to the skin. The base of the keloid may be broad, or it may be attached by a pedicle. It may have a smooth surface covered with a thin, epithelial layer that can be peeled off, thus exposing its mass. This epithelium, left partially attached to the skin, may be used for closure of the defect created by total excision of the keloid. In some cases, the keloid may develop a botryoid surface with deep fissures and fingerlike extensions far beyond the initial wound size and shape. The botryoid keloid is usually attached by a broad base and its excision may create a large defect. The epithelial layer may be so

difficult to peel away that it cannot be used for closure of the defect after excision of the keloid.

Scar Revision

The question of when scar revision is appropriate must be considered in terms of the following:
1. Appearance of the scar.
2. Type of scar.
3. Time elapsed since the injury.
4. Location of the scar.
5. Functional impairment caused by the scar.

A great variety of scars can result from injuries or surgeries. Scars in the facial area are especially apparent, and consequently there is a great demand for scar revision to improve the appearance and minimize the deformity.

In planning reconstructive procedures, even in the

simplest scar revision and especially in young patients, it is necessary to consider the possibility for postoperative complications, in this case, hypertrophic scarring or keloid development. When parents are eager for scar revision to decrease the visibility of a child's scar, it must be emphasized that any scar revision may result in impaired healing with excessive scarring, which may be red, elevated, and worse in appearance than the original scar. It is important not to treat scar revision lightly. Parents should always be advised of the possibility of abnormal collagen metabolism that could lead to postoperative complications.

Delaying scar revision until the child is older is always better if the parents are willing to wait. If parents are eager to achieve the best results as early as possible, they may pressure the surgeon to operate too soon. A surgeon must be able to withstand this pressure because early and frequent scar revisions may be counterproductive in the long run if there is any postoperative development of hypertrophic scars and keloids.

In children, scar revision in the facial region should be delayed for at least 1 year after the injury so that the scar may mature (Peacock [1984] recommends at least 18 months). No surgery should be performed while a scar is changing in growth or color. When hypertrophic scars or keloids persist for a long time, surgery combined with irradiation (900 to 1200 rad, postoperatively) may prevent a recurrence. In the author's experience with this combined approach, keloids have been treated successfully in 50 to 60 per cent of cases (Figs. 35–8A and B and 35–9A and B).

Various surgical techniques are available for scar revision. Release of contracted scars may be achieved using Z plasty or multiple W plasties. Simple excision with perfect approximation of the edges may suffice when neither change in the direction of the scar nor creation of a broken scar line is planned. Breaking the line of a scar is beneficial because a zigzag line is less obvious than a straight line, especially if the scar runs across lines of minimal tension on the face.

VASCULAR LESIONS IN THE HEAD AND NECK

Vascular lesions in the head and neck area vary in origin, clinical symptoms, and course of development. The multiplicity of forms of vascular tumors is reflected by their many classifications. They are somewhat confusing because different characteristics are used to group and define particular lesions.

Batsakis (1979) classifies hemangiomas as (1) capillary, (2) cavernous, (3) mixed, and (4) proliferative ("juvenile"). Mulliken (1984) uses a cell-based classification system that divides vascular lesions into two major categories: hemangiomas and vascular malformations. Hemangiomas are described as vascular tumors with increased endothelial turnover during the proliferative phase. Mast cell production increases in the proliferative phase, but then the number of cells returns to normal levels as involution of the tumor progresses. Vascular malformations are considered to be vascular anomalies with normal endothelial cell cycles. In vascular malformations, the number of mast cells is not elevated as it is in hemangiomas.

Hemangiomas are the most common single vascular tumor in the head and neck area in children. They

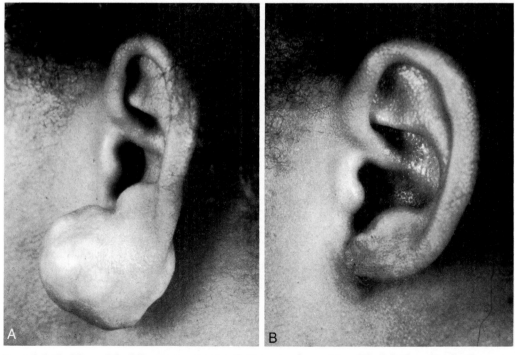

Figure 35–8. Large keloid of the earlobe following ear piercing. *B,* One year after excision of the keloid combined with pre- and postsurgical irradiation.

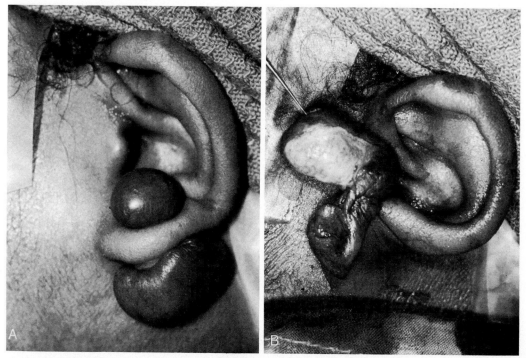

Figure 35–9. *A*, Large keloid on the anterior and posterior surfaces of the earlobe following ear piercing. *B*, Technique of degloving of the keloid prior to its complete excision.

also are the most rapidly growing vascular tumors during infancy. By 1 year of age, approximately 12 per cent of children have one or another type of hemangioma.

The etiology and pathogenesis of hemangiomas and other vascular lesions are poorly understood. There is no hereditary predisposition. According to Batsakis (1979), females are more likely to have vascular lesions than males. Usually, the vascular lesion appears alone. Hemangioma is more common in white infants and rarely occurs in black infants (Mulliken, 1984). The most common types of hemangiomas are capillary and cavernous.

Capillary Hemangioma

Capillary hemangioma usually appears in the newborn immediately after birth or several weeks later. The lesions vary in size and location. They are irregular, pink, intradermal stains and may occupy large areas. The intensity of the color of capillary hemangiomas ranges from light pink to red. Usually the lesion is flat, but it may also be elevated slightly. Sharper demarcation and some elevation may occur when the lesion changes color. This may indicate that elements of a cavernous hemangioma are developing in the dermis. Capillary hemangiomas tend to remain consistent in shape and grow relative to the development of the child.

Treatment of capillary hemangioma may be difficult, especially when the lesion is flat and only slightly discolored. Various treatment techniques have been used for management. It is extremely hard to decide if any of the current treatment techniques will result in the desired improvement to the degree that intervention is justified. Among the various treatment techniques, cryosurgery, surgical tattooing, and laser therapy are used most frequently. Argon laser therapy seems to be most promising. Surgical tattooing and cryosurgery have not been totally successful.

As a rule, surgical treatment for capillary hemangioma is not attempted in infancy or early childhood. Surgical treatment of large, flat lesions with only slight discoloration is also not recommended. Surgical treatment is reserved for adolescents and adults, especially if nodular or cavernous components accompany the existing lesion. Argon laser therapy has become popular; however, in children it is not always successful. Some improvement, though, is usually obtained. Cosmetics are an acceptable way to camouflage the lesions, especially if there are no skin changes besides discoloration.

Cavernous Hemangioma

Cavernous hemangioma in the head and neck area varies in size, shape, and location. This lesion may appear in the newborn or during the first months of life and then may grow rapidly, causing severe deformities that could even be life threatening. Rapid growth usually occurs during the first months of life, with the defect sometimes occupying an enormous area. This intense growth potential is explained differently by investigators. However, the clinical course is not well defined by any of these various hypotheses.

Rapidly growing cavernous hemangiomas are difficult to treat. In most cases the tumor spontaneously involutes. This can complicate the option for surgical intervention. More than 60 per cent of patients with cavernous hemangioma are considered cured after spontaneous involution; the remaining patients definitely require treatment (Fig. 35–10A through C). The most problematic decision is if and when to operate in infancy and early childhood.

Patients with large and so-called invasive cavernous hemangiomas are not good candidates for early surgical management because total excision may be technically life threatening. Periodic observations are needed to monitor the behavior of a cavernous hemangioma for continued growth or signs of involution. Spontaneous ulceration of rapidly growing cavernous hemangiomas occurs frequently and is considered beneficial because of the resulting fibroses that occlude the caverns and inhibit further growth. However, in large cavernous hemangiomas, ulceration can lead to hemorrhage that can be fatal. It is interesting that, despite the large size and rapid growth of a cavernous hemangioma, hemorrhage rarely occurs; if it does, the bleeding can be stopped in most cases by simple pressure.

Special attention should be given to cavernous hemangiomas. Although cavernous hemangiomas are described as benign vascular lesions, they may exhibit invasive growth that may be difficult to control. If rapid growth is observed in an area that may be endangered by invasive growth, early surgical treatment may be indicated to arrest the growth and limit the undesirable consequences. This applies to sites such as the periorbital area, oral cavity, lips, and nasal tip. Cavernous hemangioma located in deep tissue may present a serious treatment problem, as it is difficult to determine the extent of its growth and to attempt total excision.

In the author's experience, early excision of cavernous hemangioma is indicated when the surgeon is sure that the entire tumor can be removed, or when growth

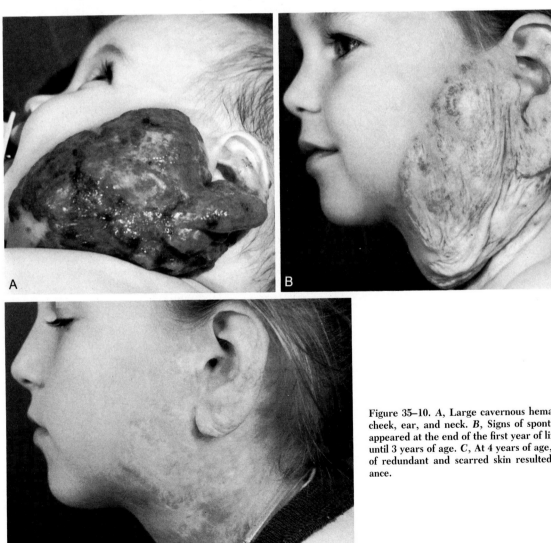

Figure 35–10. *A*, Large cavernous hemangioma involving cheek, ear, and neck. *B*, Signs of spontaneous involution appeared at the end of the first year of life and progressed until 3 years of age. *C*, At 4 years of age, simple reduction of redundant and scarred skin resulted in good appearance.

is rapid and the tumor is located so it causes functional or aesthetic problems. Hemangiomas in the perioral, periorbital, or nasal tip areas (Fig. 35–11A and B) require early surgical intervention.

There are insufficient data to indicate in what percentage of patients and at what age large cavernous hemangiomas of the head and neck spontaneously involute. Spontaneous involution usually is completed by age 4 to 6 years. If by this time there is no sign of involution, treatment may be indicated.

The choice of treatment depends on the size, location, and area of tissue involvement. In small cavernous hemangiomas, a series of injections of sodium morrhuate have been successful. These injections stimulate fibrosis, change of color, decreased size, and complete disappearance of symptoms. For medium-size hemangiomas, sodium morrhuate can be used as a precursor to surgical excision.

Treatment of large cavernous hemangiomas is most difficult. Various treatment techniques have been used (e.g., corticosteroids, cryosurgery, radiation therapy, embolization, sclerotizing agents, laser therapy, and surgical excision). There is no evidence that steroid therapy has a beneficial effect on large cavernous hemangiomas or that it accelerates involution; thus, the author does not use steroids. Cryosurgery or electrosurgery has not been successful and is not recommended. Irradiation therapy should be forbidden because of the detrimental late results such as growth inhibition of the irradiated area. Embolization as a preparation for surgical excision is used by many surgeons; however, great caution is necessary because

an embolus could occur within the brain vessels owing to the vast anastomosis between the hemangioma in the head and neck area and intracranial vessels.

Suture Technique

Observing the beneficial effects of ulceration and sclerotizing agents (i.e., ulceration resulting in fibrosis), Bardach introduced the "suture technique" for treatment of cavernous hemangiomas. He has used this technique successfully for many years in the treatment of large cavernous hemangiomas, even of some that were considered inoperable because of their size and location (Bardach and Panje, 1981). The suture technique is used to isolate the entire hemangioma, or a part of it, as completely as possible by surrounding it with deep 2–0 silk mattress sutures, cutting off the blood supply to the area. On the lips, cheeks, and tongue, through-and-through mattress sutures placed around the hemangioma may be used prior to surgical excision.

In other areas of the head and neck, where through-and-through sutures cannot be used, mattress sutures are placed as deeply as possible to cut off the circulation as completely as possible. With this technique, excision of large areas of cavernous hemangioma can be performed with minimal blood loss. It is important to retain silk sutures for 10 to 14 days after the excision of a hemangioma.

The suture technique also can be used in preparation for surgical procedures in an attempt to decrease the blood supply to the extent that circulation is impaired

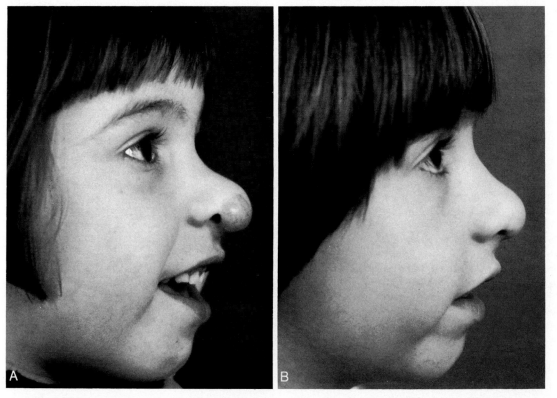

Figure 35–11. A, Profile view of large cavernous hemangioma of the nasal tip. B, One year postoperatively.

and ulceration and necrosis will occur. To do this, multiple horizontal and vertical mattress sutures with 2–0 silk are used and retained for 2 to 3 weeks. Ulceration and partial necrosis is followed by fibrosis and obliteration of the caverns. The same technique is repeated during the final surgery to prevent dangerous blood loss. This technique can be used until the entire hemangioma is gone.

A great many hemangiomas grow on the surface; however, some cavernous hemangiomas develop deep within the tissue. These must be differentiated from lymphangiomas, arteriovenous malformations, and hemifacial hypertrophy.

Port Wine Stains—Mixed Hemangiomas

Port wine stains are a mixed type of hemangioma. They have components of both capillary and cavernous hemangiomas and have proliferative changes in the form of nodules. Port wine stains usually are detected in the newborn and are difficult to distinguish from capillary hemangiomas. The port wine stain has irregular margins and initially is pink or red; however, with age, the color becomes dark red or bluish. As the color changes, other differences in the lesion may occur as well (e.g., the formation of nodules or elevation). All conservative treatment techniques used for capillary hemangiomas should be explored for treatment of port wine stains.

Argon laser treatment seems to promote the best results in management of port wine stains. In severe cases that involve a large area with marked discoloration and multiple nodules, total excision and free skin grafting may be indicated.

Arteriovenous Malformations

Arteriovenous malformations are believed to be lesions with wide communications between the arterial and venous systems. Fistulas of various sizes are embryologic remnants between the arteries and veins. Arteriovenous malformations usually do not appear in infancy, the way hemangiomas do. The literature suggests that clinical appearance of these lesions is usually triggered by an episode of trauma, infection, or surgery. Growth may accelerate owing to hormonal changes at puberty, during pregnancy, or during hormone therapy. Clinically, these malformations present pulsations, bruits, thrills, and increased skin temperature in the area of the lesion.

Continued growth of arteriovenous malformations may cause apparent facial deformities. When located in the oral cavity, the lesions may be easily injured, causing profuse bleeding. Precise diagnosis and localization is achieved by angiography and computed tomography (CT) scans. Angiography helps to determine the dynamics of the malformation and its extent. Mulliken (1984) emphasized that therapy for arterio-

venous malformations is challenging, frustrating, and potentially life threatening.

Total excision is recommended whenever possible. The suture technique enhances fibrosis in the area of the lesion and has been effective, even in cases with no surgical intervention. Selective embolization may be helpful; however, most surgeons use embolization as a preparation for excision.

Syndromes Associated with Vascular Lesions

There are many syndromes that include vascular malformations or hemangiomas. It seems that some are associated with true hemangiomas, whereas others are associated with vascular malformations. This differentiation is important because it guides treatment strategies.

One of the most common syndromes is *Sturge-Weber syndrome* in which a port wine stain appears in the area of distribution of the trigeminal nerve. On the same side of the head, vascular malformations are found in the meninges with or without calcification. Seizures may occur in children and electroencephalography may demonstrate spiked wave patterns characteristic of epilepsy. Port wine stains may also be present on the scalp, neck, trunk, or extremities or intraorally. Each child suspected to have Sturge-Weber syndrome should be examined carefully to rule out or confirm this suspicion.

Facial port wine stains associated with macroglossia and macrosomia are present in *Beckwith-Wiedemann syndrome*. *Klippel-Trenaunay syndrome* includes port wine stains, varicose veins, and venous and lymphatic malformations with associated skeletal hypertrophy. *Maffucci syndrome* presents multiple cavernous hemangiomas and chondromatosis. The involved bones are usually shortened and deformed. Visceral vascular lesions occur, as well as cutaneous lesions. Chondrosarcoma may develop in patients with this syndrome.

Other syndromes associated with vascular lesions are the blue rubber bleb nevus syndrome and the Rendu-Osler-Weber syndrome.

Lymphangioma

Lymphatic malformations, referred to as lymphangiomas, are also known as cystic hygromas. According to Batsakis (1979), these lesions are classified as

1. Lymphangioma simplex—composed of thin walled, capillary-size lymphatic channels.

2. Cavernous lymphangioma—composed of dilated lymphatic spaces, often with fibrous adventitia.

3. Cystic lymphangioma or cystic hygroma—composed of cysts of various sizes (a few millimeters to several centimeters in diameter).

Despite this differentiation, it seems appropriate to discuss lesions of lymphatic origin together because their clinical symptoms and treatment strategies are similar. Between 50 and 60 per cent of lymphangiomas are present at birth. By the end of the second year of life, 80 to 90 per cent are detected. This is the time of greatest lymphatic activity (Batsakis, 1979).

Lymphangiomas in the facial area and oral cavity are relatively common. Usually, the cheeks, lips, floor of the mouth, and tongue are affected (Fig. 35–12A and B). There is always an enlargement of the affected side and asymmetry, which can be easily detected. The skin covering the lymphangioma is stretched with no discoloration or change in skin temperature. On palpation, the lesion may fluctuate; however, the margins of the lesion are hardly detectable. Lymphangiomas are not tender or painful unless infected. The lesions vary in size and grow progressively, relative to the development of the child. Accelerated growth, pain, or both may indicate infection.

One of the most important clinical symptoms of a lymphangioma is a change in the buccal mucosa, tongue, and floor of the mouth, where multiple blebs appear that look like exophytic, rubbery masses with a white or brownish discoloration. The buccal mucosa may have a cloudy appearance.

Differential diagnosis is necessary to distinguish among lymphangiomas, hemangiomas, and hemifacial hypertrophy. Total excision is indicated for small lymphangiomas. Treatment for medium-size and large lymphangiomas is difficult. Spontaneous regression of lymphangiomas has not been observed. Surgery, in the form of serial excisions, may not be adequate; however, no other treatment for this type of lesion is effective.

Melanocytic Nevi and Malignant Melanoma

Melanocytic nevi vary considerably in their appearance. Lever and Schaumburg-Lever (1983) indicate that all melanocytic tumors composed of nevus cells can be divided into junctional nevi, compound nevi, and intradermal nevi. Clinical types of nevi include the following:

1. Flat lesions.
2. Slightly elevated lesions.
3. Papillomatous lesions.
4. Dome-shaped lesions.
5. Pedunculated lesions.

The clinical appearance of the melanocytic nevi corresponds closely to the histologic type. Melanocytic nevi are rarely found in the newborn, only in approximately 1 per cent (Walton et al., 1976). Congenital nevi are usually larger than acquired nevi. Rarely do they represent a giant congenital melanocytic nevi occupying a large area of the head and neck or trunk. Giant congenital nevi are deeply pigmented; however, their pigmentation may vary in different areas of the lesion. Often, there are many scattered satellite lesions with similar appearances. Most of these lesions are covered with hair. Nongiant congenital melanocytic nevi typically are elevated, are of varying pigmentation, and bear hair.

The division of melanocytic nevi into junctional, compound, and intradermal indicates their location within the skin; however, they may invade other layers of the skin as well. Junctional nevi are nevus cell nests within the lower epidermis or between the epidermis and dermis. Frequently, the upper layer of dermis has been infiltrated by this type of lesion. Compound nevi have features of both junctional and intradermal nevi. Nevus cell nests may be found in the epidermis and dermis. Intradermal nevi are limited to the dermis.

When dealing with a melanocytic nevus, excluding giant congenital nevi, there is always the risk of potential malignancy. According to Solomon (1980), the incidence of malignancy in nongiant melanocytic nevi less than 20 cm in diameter is at least 1 per cent. The predicted percentage of malignant melanoma in the general population is 0.4 per cent.

Excision of nongiant melanocytic nevi is advised by some surgeons (Solomon, 1980; Rhodes et al., 1982). Other surgeons (Kopf et al., 1973) do not agree with this idea. The incidence of malignant melanoma arising in giant melanocytic nevi or in one of the many satellite

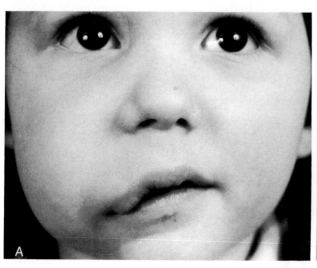
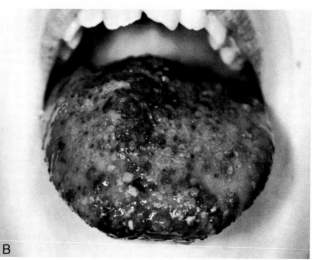

Figure 35–12. Lymphangioma of the right cheek (A) and tongue (B).

lesions is approximately 12 per cent. Clinically, a change of pigmentation or accelerated growth may indicate transformation into a malignant stage. A high incidence of melanoma arising from giant nevi suggests the need for total excision with no consideration of subsequent severe secondary deformities. Congenital, nongiant nevi should be observed closely, as there is always a risk of potential malignancy.

Despite these indications, in many cases it is difficult to decide if a giant pigmented nevus should be excised completely in a child. Each case must be followed closely by a dermatologist who may indicate to a surgeon the timing of and area for excision. Malignant melanoma is described in detail in Chapter 90 and will not be discussed further here.

BASIC PRINCIPLES OF LOCAL SKIN FLAPS

In plastic and reconstructive surgery of the head and neck, local flaps play a major role. Therefore, the basic principles for their use and design will be presented.

Types of Skin Flaps

All skin flaps can be divided into three basic types:
1. Random-pattern flaps—skin flaps whose pedicle does not contain a specific artery that supplies the entire flap area. Examples are S plasty, Z plasty, and V-Y advancement.
2. Axial-pattern flaps—skin flaps whose pedicle contains an artery that supplies the entire flap area. Examples include skin flaps based on the superficial temporal artery and forehead flaps based on the supratrochlear artery or supraorbital artery.
3. Mixed flaps—skin flaps in which only part of the flap area is supplied by a specific artery while the remaining flap area has random blood supply. One example is deltopectoralis flap in which the proximal area represents an axial pattern flap, whereas the distal area represents a random pattern skin flap.

Local skin flaps are frequently used in the head and neck area for closure of defects and reconstructive procedures. There is usually more than one choice for closure of a particular defect or for a specific reconstructive procedure. Therefore, careful analysis of the defect and planning of the surgical procedures are important steps for achieving success. Some guidelines have been established to determine when local skin flaps should be used for reconstruction. The following factors should be considered during preoperative planning to choose the technique for reconstruction: origin of the defect or deformity; time elapsed from the original defect or deformity; location; size; shape; depth; status of the surrounding tissue; age; sex; general health; and specific factors (e.g., use of glasses, hearing aid, and dental prosthesis).

In preoperative planning, the location, size, shape, and depth of the defect must be considered to determine the surgical technique for reconstruction. Creating a secondary deformity that requires further correction is considered a reconstructive failure. For example, large defects near sites such as the lower eyelid, medial or lateral canthus, commissure, or lips present potential problems in regard to secondary deformities resulting from tissue transposition, tension, and scar contracture. Secondary deformities (e.g., ectropion and elevated upper lip) may be more disturbing to the patient than the primary deformity.

The origin of the defect also may be a factor influencing the choice of reconstructive procedures. When considering all possible surgical techniques for a particular case, the simplest method should be examined first; but if it is not the optimal choice, more complex procedures should be considered. Age, sex, general health status, and specific factors should also be considered prior to reconstruction.

If a local flap is planned, it is necessary to design the shape, size, and location of the pedicle to ascertain its viability. Most local flaps in the head and neck area are random pattern flaps and therefore good blood supply is critical for flap survival. Local flaps should be substituted by another surgical technique if the secondary defect or postoperative scars add to the existing deformity. Tension, kinking, and pressure have to be avoided in designing and using local flaps.

In some cases, flap survival can be improved by using the delay procedure. Delay can be used in a variety of ways:
1. Undermining and raising the flap on one pedicle, returning it to its bed.
2. Undermining the whole flap, leaving two pedicles.
3. Two-stage delay procedure with two pedicles. In the second stage, one of the pedicles is detached but the flap is transferred during the next procedure.
To improve flap survival, the delay should be used for at least 4 to 6 days. The length-width ratio and the location and width of the pedicle should be considered in planning. Local flaps provide skin with the same color and texture as that around the defect. Free skin grafts and distant flaps have different color and texture than the surrounding facial skin.

Indications

Local flaps in the head and neck area are the best choice because they have the same color and texture as the skin around the defect. Use of local flaps has to be carefully planned so that there is enough local tissue to close the defect and not add to the existing deformity. In planning local flaps, the basic principles of design are important, especially in transposition and rotation flaps.

Among the various types of transposition flaps, Z plasty enables lengthening, shortening, or movement up or down. Another useful type of local flap is S plasty. Both of these methods are helpful in the reconstruction of defects in the head and neck area.

Rotation skin flaps are often used because a large primary and secondary defect may be closed at the same time. Local advancement flaps and interpolation flaps are not as commonly used in the head and neck area because of the poor aesthetic result. Most local flaps are random-pattern flaps, but in the head and neck area, they do not require delay. One exception may be the use of local flaps in an irradiated area.

In the design of local flaps, attention should be given to the location of the pedicle to assure the best possible blood supply to the area. Tension, kinking, and pressure must be avoided.

Timing of Reconstruction

Every defect should be closed as soon as possible. The primary closure can be temporary or definite. Closure depends on the general status of the patient and on the size, shape, and location of the defect. Final closure is performed when local or free flaps present the best choice. In some cases, delayed reconstruction is indicated. In these cases, closure of the defect with a free skin graft is recommended to aid wound healing.

Advantages and Disadvantages

The following are the advantages of local flaps, including Z plasty, S plasty, rotation, transposition, and advancement: (1) The local flap is of the same texture and color as the surrounding skin, and (2) closure of the defect in many cases is also the final reconstructive procedure. Disadvantages of local flaps include the following: (1) Additional scars may be produced on the face or neck, and (2) sometimes secondary deformities result from use of local flaps (e.g., ectropion and displacement of the commissure).

AESTHETIC CONSIDERATION IN CHILDREN AND ADOLESCENTS

Congenital and acquired facial deformities present definite problems for children and young adults. Psychologic reactions may develop in response to trauma, surgery, or congenital deformities. Defects in the head and neck area may range in severity from small, almost undetectable scars to complicated anomalies, posttraumatic or postsurgical tissue loss, functional impairment, or contracted scarring. A description of the many deformities of the head and neck area and their reconstructive techniques is far beyond the scope of this book.

In general, the following surgical techniques may be applicable for treatment of head and neck deformities:

1. Local flaps, including advancement flaps, Z plasty, S plasty, rotation-advancement flaps, and transposition flaps.
2. Free skin grafts, including full-thickness, split-thickness, and dermal grafts.
3. Regional flaps, including scalp flaps, forehead flaps, cheek flaps, and neck flaps.
4. Distant flaps, including myocutaneous, tube pedicle, and free flaps with microvascular anastomosis.
5. Transposition of sections of the bony skeleton in cases of craniofacial anomalies and subsequent to trauma.
6. Bone grafts and cartilage implants.
7. Alloplastic implants.

The main problem with reconstruction is that in many cases, more than one surgical technique may be considered to achieve successful results. For example, in a young girl, a small skin defect on the cheek after excision of a pigmented nevus can be closed with a free skin graft, with full- or split-thickness graft with simple approximation of the wound edges, or with a transposition flap using S plasty or a rhomboid flap. Given these options, the advantages and disadvantages of each must be weighed to select the most appropriate technique. A free skin graft would be the last choice because the defect is small and could be closed easily with a local flap that would provide skin of the same color and texture. Of the techniques available, S plasty or a rhomboid flap would be best. Simple closure would be a poor choice for this type of defect. The final decision depends on the surgeon's experience and skill.

Another example of the complexity of decision making for reconstruction is the treatment of nasal deformities. Typical nasal deformities include a deviated septum, hypertrophied turbinates, and abnormalities of the cartilaginous or bony skeleton (e.g., long nose, short nose, broad nose, nasal hump, asymmetry of the nasal tip, hanging columella, saddle nose, subtotal nasal deformity, and total absence of nose). These may occur when the child is young. A detailed description of the surgical techniques for reconstruction is addressed in many atlases and books devoted to the problems of aesthetic rhinoplasty.

A variety of nasal deformities can be corrected during childhood; however, surgical intervention for septoplasty or rhinoplasty is not performed during childhood. This is delayed until adolescence because surgery on the nasal septum and cartilaginous or bony skeleton may inhibit midfacial growth. There is little evidence that corrective septoplasty without removal of large segments of the septum adversely affects nasal growth. Moreover, there is no evidence to prove that early tip rhinoplasty or complete rhinoplasty influences growth.

Despite this lack of information, the idea that early septoplasty or rhinoplasty may be detrimental to growth and development of the nasal structures and midfacial complex is so strongly established that surgery is usually delayed until age 13 to 14 years or older. The author has found that corrective rhinoplasty in cleft patients aged 7 to 8 years, involving only the cartilaginous skeleton, does not appear to interfere with growth of the midfacial complex. Complete excision of cavernous hemangioma on the nasal tip, which is done early in some cases, also does not interfere with normal nasal growth.

Proceeding with the example of the nasal deformity, discussion of correction of the alar or nasal tip defect follows: Depending on the size, location, and depth of the defect, reconstructive procedures may be considered: local skin flaps from the nose, cheek, or upper lip; transposition flaps, including all layers of the nasal alae with closure of the secondary defect with a skin flap from the cheek; forehead flaps; scalp flaps; free skin grafts; and composite grafts with skin and cartilage from the ear. In a child or young adult, any surgical technique that leaves a visible secondary deformity is not recommended. Reconstructive procedures must be planned, keeping in mind that correction of the existing deformity cannot be justified by creation of another defect that may be more conspicuous than the primary one.

Of the basic principles that must be considered in aesthetic facial reconstructive surgery, the most important is to assess the existing deformity and have the experience to weigh the many existing options. The most difficult part is to make the best choice for a given patient, and this can only be judged when the final result has been evaluated.

When only aesthetic aspects are considered (e.g., scars, nasal hump, and prominent ears), surgical correction can be performed successfully; however, many factors must be evaluated prior to surgery. When scar revision is planned, the current status of the scar must be assessed, in addition to its cause and the time elapsed since the initial injury. Scar revision, even for small atrophic scars, must always be discussed with the parents so they are aware of the potential danger of scar hypertrophy. For this reason, delaying scar revision in children is fully justified to preclude any secondary recurrence. Corrective rhinoplasty for removal of a nasal hump should be delayed until the patient is aged 13 to 14 years. Otoplasty for prominent ears may be considered when the child is 5 to 7 years of age or possibly earlier, depending on the type and severity of the existing deformity.

There is no justification in any facial defect to use a surgical technique that would repair one site while damaging another. If there is any way to avoid secondary facial deformities of any degree of severity by using an alternative technique, this is recommended, even though the technique may be more complex or of higher risk.

As mentioned previously, aesthetic and functional facial reconstructive surgery may present many challenges. In young patients, it is also important to adjust the timing of surgical intervention so that potential psychologic problems are avoided. Even young children are sensitive to and aware of being different, especially if they are teased by their peers. Fostering a healthy self-image is one of the main goals parents, family, and school personnel should have. Some de-formities, even slight ones that are not readily apparent, may be perceived by a youngster (particularly adolescents) as detrimental to his or her appearance. In some cases, there may be no indication for surgical intervention. In these situations, consultation with a pediatric psychologist may be helpful. However, when there is a possibility that surgery may be beneficial, although totally elective, it should be seriously considered because if successful, the result will have a positive impact on the child's self-image.

REFERENCES

Anderson, R., and Kurtay, M. 1971. Reconstruction of the corner of the mouth. Plast. Reconstr. Surg. 47:463.

Bardach, J. 1967. Rozszczepy wargi gornej i podniebienia. Warszawa, Panstwowy Zaklad Wydawn.

Bardach, J. 1974. Reconstruction of the microtic auricle in a four-stage operation. ORL 78:349.

Bardach, J., and Panje, W. 1981. Surgical management of the large cavernous hemangioma. Otolaryngol. Head Neck Surg. 89:792.

Bardach, J., and Salyer, K. E. 1987. Surgical Techniques in Cleft Lip and Palate. Chicago, Year Book Medical Publishers.

Batsakis, J. G. 1979. Tumors of the Head and Neck: Clinical and Pathological Considerations, 2nd ed. Baltimore, Williams & Wilkins Co.

Batsakis, J. G., and Rice, D. H. 1981. The pathology of head and neck tumors. Part 9A. Vasoformative tumors. Head Neck Surg. 3:231.

Bennett, J. E., and Zook, E. C. 1972. Treatment of arteriovenous fistulae on cavernous hemangiomas of the face by muscle embolization. Plast. Reconstr. Surg. 50:84.

Bingham, H. G. 1979. Predicting the course of a congenital hemangioma. Plast. Reconstr. Surg. 63:161.

Bosse, J. P., Papillon, J., and Aube, M. 1983. Difficult management problems in adult hemangiomas: Possible relationship to trauma. In Williams, H. B. (ed.): Symposium on Vascular Malformations and Melanotic Lesions. St. Louis, C. V. Mosby Co.

Brent, B. 1971. Reconstruction of the microtic ear with autogenous rib cartilage. In Jackson, I. J. (ed.): Recent Advances in Plastic Surgery, Vol. 2. New York, Churchill Livingstone.

Brown, S. H., Neerhaut, R. C., and Fonkalsrud, E. W. 1972. Prednisone therapy in management of large hemangiomas in infants and children. Surgery 71:168.

Clemons, J. E., and Connelly, M.V. 1973. Reattachment of a totally amputated auricle. A.M.A. Arch. Otolaryngol. 97:269.

Clodius, L. 1977. Excision and grafting of extensive facial hemangiomas. Br. J. Plast. Surg. 30:185.

Colclengh, R. G., and Ryan, J. E. 1976. Splinting electrical burns of the mouth in children. Plast. Reconstr. Surg. 48:239.

Conley, J. 1976. Regional Flaps of the Head and Neck. Philadelphia, W. B. Saunders Co.

Converse, J. M., and Brent, B. 1977. Acquired deformities of the auricle. In Converse, J. M. (ed.): Reconstructive Plastic Surgery, 2nd ed., Vol. 3. Philadelphia, W. B. Saunders Co.

Converse, J. M., McCarthy, J. G., Dobrkovsky, M., and Larson, D. L. 1977. Facial burns. In Converse, J. M. (ed.): Reconstructive Plastic Surgery, 2nd ed., Vol. 3. Philadelphia, W. B. Saunders Co.

Cook, T. A. 1986. Reconstruction of facial defects. In Cummings, C., Fredrickson, J., Harker, L., et al. (eds.): Otolaryngology—Head and Neck Surgery, Vol. I. St. Louis, C. V. Mosby Co.

Cosman, B. 1980. Experience in the argon laser therapy of port wine stains. Plast. Reconstr. Surg. 65:119.

Cronin, T. D. 1961. The use of a moulded splint to prevent contracture after split skin grafting on the neck. Plast. Reconstr. Surg. 27:7.

Davidson, T. M. 1986. Lacerations and scar revision. In Cummings, C., Fredrickson, J., Harker, L., et al. (eds.): Otolaryngology—Head and Neck Surgery, Vol. I. St. Louis, C. V. Mosby Co.

Edgerton, M. T., Jr. 1983. Steroid therapy of hemangiomas. *In* Williams, H. B. (ed.): Symposium on Vascular Malformations and Melanotic Lesions. St. Louis, C. V. Mosby Co.

Elliot, R. A. 1982. The lateral scalp flap for anterior hairline reconstruction. Clin. Plast. Surg. 9:241.

Falvey, M. P., and Brody, G. S. 1978. Secondary correction of the burned eyelid deformity. Plast. Reconstr. Surg. 62:564.

Farkas, L. G. 1974. Growth of normal and reconstructed auricles. *In* Tanzer, R. C., and Edgerton, M. T. (eds.): Symposium on Reconstruction of the Auricle, Vol. 10. St. Louis, C. V. Mosby Co.

Feldman, J. J. 1984. Reconstruction of the burned face in children. *In* Serafin, D., and Georgiade, N. (eds.): Pediatric Plastic Surgery, Vol. 1. St. Louis, C. V. Mosby Co.

Gantz, B. J.: Personal communication.

Grabb, W. C., and Myers, M. B. 1975. Skin Flaps. Boston, Little, Brown, and Co.

Grace, S. G., and Brody, G. S. 1978. Surgical correction of burn deformities of the nose. Plast. Reconstr. Surg. 62:848.

Gunter, J. P., Carder, H. M., and Fee, W. E. 1977. Rhomboid flap. Arch. Otolaryngol. 103:206.

Hobby, L. W. 1983. Further evaluation of the potential of the argon laser in treatment of strawberry hemangioma. Plast. Reconstr. Surg. 74:481.

Holmdahl, K. 1955. Cutaneous hemangioma in premature and mature infants. Acta Paediatr. 44:370.

Hoopes, J. E. 1979. Multiple excisions of the face. *In* Feller, I., and Grabb, W. C. (eds.): Reconstruction and Rehabilitation of the Burned Patient. Ann Arbor, MI, National Institute for Burn Medicine.

Hurwitz, D. J., and Futrell, J. W. 1986. Congenital vascular malformations and hemangiomas. *In* Cummings, C., Fredrickson, J., Harker, L., et al. (eds.): Otolaryngology—Head and Neck Surgery, Vol. I. St. Louis, C. V. Mosby Co.

Hurwitz, D. J., and Kerber, C. W. 1981. Hemodynamic considerations in the treatment of arteriovenous malformations of the face and scalp. Plast. Reconstr. Surg. 67:421.

Jabaley, M. E., Cat, N. D., and Lac, N. T. 1971. Use of local flap for burn contracture of the neck. Plast. Reconstr. Surg. 48:288.

Jacobs, A. H., and Walton, R. G. 1976. The incidence of birthmarks in the neonate. Pediatrics. 58:218.

Juri, J., and Juri, C. 1982. Temporo-parieto-occipital flap for the treatment of baldness. Clin. Plast. Surg. 9:255.

Kopf, A. W., Bart, R. S., and Hennessey, P. 1979. Congenital nevocytic nevi and malignant melanomas. J. Am. Acad. Dermatol. 1:123.

Leikensohn, J. R., Epstein, L. I., and Vasconez, L. O. 1981. Superselective embolization and surgery of noninvolving hemangiomas and AV malformations. Plast. Reconstr. Surg. 68:143.

Lever, W. F., and Schaumburg-Lever, G. 1983. Melanocytic nevi and malignant melanoma. *In* Lever, W. F., and Schaumburg-Lever, G. (eds.): Histopathology of the Skin. Philadelphia, J. B. Lippincott Co.

Limberg, A. A. 1984. The Planning of Local Plastic Operations on the Body Surface: Theory and Practice. Lexington, MA, Collamore Press.

McCabe, B. F. Personal communication.

McGrath, M. H., and Ariyan, S. 1978. Immediate reconstruction of full-thickness burns of the ear with an undelayed musculocutaneous flap. Plast. Reconstr. Surg. 62:618.

McGregor, I. A. 1982. Local skin flaps in facial reconstruction. Otolaryngol. Clin. North Am. 15:77.

McGregor, I. A., and Morgan, G. 1973. Axial and random pattern flaps. Br. J. Plast. Surg. 26:202.

Merland, J. J. 1983. The use of superselective arteriography, embolization, and surgery in the current management of cervicocephalic vascular malformations (in 350 cases). *In* Williams, H. B. (ed.): Symposium on Vascular Malformations and Melanotic Lesions. St. Louis, C. V. Mosby Co.

Mulliken, J. B. 1984. Cutaneous vascular lesions of children. *In* Serafin, D., and Georgiade, N. (eds.): Pediatric Plastic Surgery, Vol. 1. St. Louis, C. V. Mosby Co.

Mulliken, J. B., and Glowacki, J. 1982. Hemangiomas and vascular malformations in infants and children: A classification based on endothelial characteristics. Plast. Reconstr. Surg. 69:412.

Mulliken, J. B., Murray, J. E., Castaneda, A. R., et al. 1978. Management of a vascular malformation of the face using total circulatory arrest. Surg. Gynecol. Obstet. 146:168.

Neuman, Z., and Wexler, M. R. 1979. Reconstruction of facial burns. *In* Feller, I., and Grabb, W. C. (eds.): Reconstruction and Rehabilitation of the Burned Patient. Ann Arbor, MI, National Institute for Burn Medicine.

Noordhoff, M. S. 1974. Control and prevention of hypertrophic scarring and contracture. Clin. Plast. Surg. 1:49.

Oldfield, M. C., and Tate, G. T. 1964. Cleft lip and palate. Br. J. Plast. Surg. 17:1.

Paletta, F. X. 1982. Surgical management of the burned scalp. Clin. Plast. Surg. 9:167.

Parks, D. H., Baur, P. S., Jr., and Larson, D. L. 1977. Late problems in burns. Clin. Plast. Surg. 4:556.

Parks, D. H., Larson, D. L., and de la Houssaye, A. J. 1979. Hypertrophic scarring: Pressure dressings. *In* Feller, I., and Grabb, W. C. (eds.): Reconstruction and Rehabilitation of the Burned Patient. Ann Arbor, MI, National Institute for Burn Medicine.

Peacock, E. E., Jr. 1981a. Pharmacologic control of surface scarring in human beings. Ann. Surg. 193:592.

Peacock, E. E., Jr. 1981b. Control of wound healing and scar formation in surgical patients. Arch. Surg. 116:1325.

Peacock, E. E., Jr. 1984. Surgery of scars. *In* Serafin, D., and Georgiade, N. (eds.): Pediatric Plastic Surgery, Vol. 1. St. Louis, C. V. Mosby Co.

Persky, M. S., Berenstein, A., and Cohen, N. L. 1984. Combined treatment of head and neck vascular masses with pre-operative embolization. Laryngoscope 94:20.

Rhodes, A. R., Sober, A. J., Day, C., et al. 1982. The malignant potential of small congenital nevocellular nevi. J. Am. Acad. Dermatol. 6:230.

Solomon, L. M. 1980. The management of congenital melanocytic nevi. Arch. Dermatol. 116:1017.

Swanson, N. A., and Grekin, R. C. 1986. Recognition and treatment of skin lesions. *In* Cummings, C., Fredrickson, J., Harker, L., et al. (eds.): Otolaryngology—Head and Neck Surgery, Vol. I. St. Louis, C. V. Mosby Co.

Tanzer, R. C. 1971. Total reconstruction of the auricle. The evolution of a plan of treatment. Plast. Reconst. Surg. 47:523.

Vallis, C. P. 1982. Surgical treatment of cicatricial alopecia of the scalp. Clin. Plast. Surg. 9:167.

VanDemark, D. 1987. Personal communication.

Vecchione, T. R. 1980. Management of the "skeletonized" nose. Br. J. Plast. Surg. 33:224.

Walton, R. G., Jacobs, A. H., and Cox, A. J. 1976. Pigmented lesions in newborn infants. Br. J. Dermatol. 95:389.

Warpeha, R. L. 1981. Resurfacing the burned face. Clin. Plast. Surg. 8:255.

Chapter 36

CONGENITAL MALFORMATIONS OF THE NOSE AND PARANASAL SINUSES

Arthur S. Hengerer, M.D.   Julie A. Newburg, M.D.

In order to obtain a better understanding of congenital malformations of the nose and paranasal sinuses, it is best to briefly look at normal embryonic development.

Normal nasal development begins with the migration of neural crest cells from their origin in the dorsal neural folds (Fig. 36–1), proceeding laterally around the eye, and traversing the frontonasal process (Fig. 36–2). This occurs during the fourth to twelfth week of embryonic life. During this time, neural crest cells migrate beneath the epithelium, through a meshwork of hyaluronic acid, and attach to collagen filaments within the facial processes. These pluripotential cells undergo rapid proliferation and differentiation into a matrix of mesenchymal tissue that forms muscle, cartilage, and early bone, thus creating the human facial configuration. These changes occur very rapidly and require unbelievable accuracy in mesenchymal migration if normal nasal and paranasal growth is to occur.

ENCEPHALOCELES AND GLIOMAS

Gliomas and encephaloceles are rare lesions of neurogenic origin containing glial tissue. Gliomas have lost their central nervous system (CNS) and subarachnoid attachments, whereas encephaloceles maintain a cerebrospinal fluid (CSF) connection to the subarachnoid space. Approximately 15 per cent of gliomas maintain a fibrous stalk connection with the subarachnoid space without any CSF connection.

Gliomas are locally aggressive lesions noticed at birth or during early childhood. They are not familial but have a gender predilection of males over females (3:1). Gliomas present as follows: extranasal, 60 per cent; intranasal, 30 per cent; and combination, 10 per cent (Fig. 36–3).

Nasal encephaloceles occur in 1 in 35,000 live births in the United States and Europe; however, in southern Asia they occur in 1 in 6000 live births. There is no familial incidence or sex predilection. Approximately 30 to 40 per cent of infants with encephaloceles have other associated abnormalities. Nasal encephaloceles are divided into sincipital and basal encephaloceles. Sincipital encephaloceles present around the nasal dorsum, orbits, and forehead and are associated with

an external mass. Basal encephaloceles are less common, appear in the nasal cavity, nasopharynx, or posterior aspect of the orbits and have no external mass.

Embryology

Most believe encephaloceles and gliomas arise from the same embryonic defect: faulty closure of the fora-

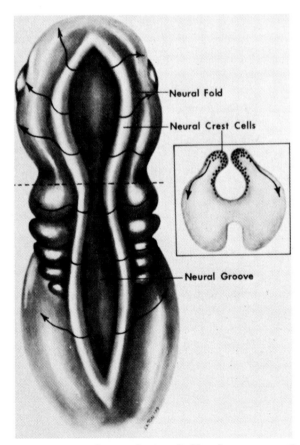

Figure 36–1. Dorsal view of 3½-week-old embryo, representing neural fold. *Insert:* Cross-section locating neural crest cells within folds. (Courtesy of Hengerer, A. S., and Oas, R. 1987. Congenital Anomalies of the Nose: Their Embryology, Diagnosis, and Management. Washington, D.C., The American Academy of Otolaryngology, Head and Neck Surgery Foundation, p. 12.)

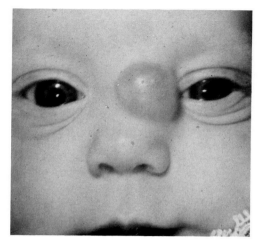

Figure 36–3. Nasal glioma.

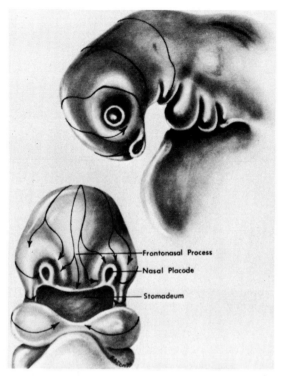

Figure 36–2. Migration patterns of neural crest cells. Arrows indicate routes followed by these cells to reach facial processes. (Courtesy of Hengerer, A. S., and Oas, R. 1987. Congenital Anomalies of the Nose: Their Embryology, Diagnosis, and Management. Washington, D.C., The American Academy of Otolaryngology, Head and Neck Surgery Foundation, p. 15.)

men caecum at about the third week of fetal development, when the anterior neuropore usually closes. In the usual sequence of events, after the foramen caecum closes, the skin becomes separated from the cranium by an ingrowth of mesoderm from each side. If there is an incomplete separation of the epithelial elements at the anterior neuropore, brain tissue will remain attached to the skin. This prevents mesodermal tissue, which will form the bony cartilaginous skeleton of the midface, from migrating between them. Thus, a bony

defect is created that the brain tissue can herniate through (Fig. 36–4). The fact that approximately 15 per cent of gliomas retain a fibrous stalk to the CNS lends support to a common developmental process of the two anomalies.

Diagnosis

Extranasal gliomas usually appear near the root of the nose as smooth, firm, noncompressible lesions that do not transilluminate. The overlying skin may be discolored or telangiectatic (Fig. 36–3).

Intranasal gliomas are less common than extranasal gliomas and appear as reddish, firm, noncompressible polypoid lesions in the nasal cavity. Large gliomas may cause nasal obstruction, septal distortion, and hypertelorism.

Approximately 15 per cent of gliomas have a fibrous stalk connection with the dura. This is more common with intranasal gliomas, and the connection is through the cribriform plate.

Figure 36–4. Pathways taken by neural elements that lead to formation of internal or external encephaloceles. (Courtesy of Hengerer, A. S., and Oas, R. 1987. Congenital Anomalies of the Nose: Their Embryology, Diagnosis, and Management. Washington, D.C., The American Academy of Otolaryngology, Head and Neck Surgery Foundation, p. 56.)

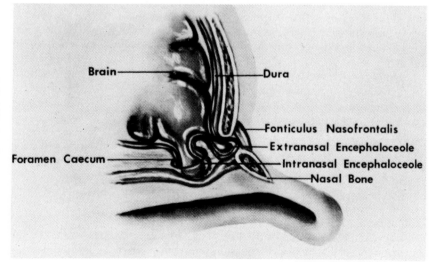

Sincipital and basal encephaloceles appear as soft, bluish, compressible lesions that may transilluminate and pulsate. They usually exhibit a positive (+) Furstenburg sign (expansion of the mass with compression of the jugular veins).

Nasofrontal encephaloceles must be differentiated from gliomas, congenital dermoid cysts of the nose, obstruction of the lacrimal sac apparatus, epidermal inclusion cysts, and other benign neoplasias of the nasofrontal areas.

Congenital dermoid cysts are differentiated by the accompanying pit, which usually contains hair. The pit may be located anywhere between the glabella and the columella of the nose.

Epidermal inclusion cysts are not usually seen until after puberty, whereas meningoencephaloceles are congenital defects. In addition to the conditions just mentioned from which nasofrontal encephaloceles must be differentiated, nasoethmoid meningoencephaloceles must be distinguished from nasal polyposis.

Sincipital Encephaloceles

The bony defect in sincipital encephaloceles occurs between the frontal and ethmoid bones anterior to the crista galli, corresponding to the site of the foramen caecum. In the majority of patients, the defect is in the midline of the nose at the glabella. The osseous defect is constant; however, the location of the overlying facial bones can be variable, forming three types of sincipital encephaloceles: (1) nasofrontal, (2) nasoethmoidal, and (3) nasoorbital. The size of the mass can vary from a slight elevation to an enormous mass larger than the infant's head. Typically, the larger the mass, the greater the degree of hypertelorism.

Basal encephaloceles form a defect in the anterior cranial fossa and appear as internal masses. They form between the anterior border of the cribriform plate and the superior orbital fissure or posterior clinoid fissure. Four types may occur: transethmoidal, sphenoethmoidal, transsphenoidal, and sphenoorbital. The transethmoidal type is the most common and appears as an intranasal mass through a defect in the cribriform plate. This type, as well as the sphenoethmoidal type, usually appears as unilateral intranasal masses that may cause hypertelorism and broadening of the bony nasal vault.

A computed tomography (CT) scan in conjunction with a magnetic resonance imaging (MRI) scan provides excellent detail of bony defects and soft tissue masses. In combination, they are the radiographic studies of choice (Figs. 36–5 and 36–6).

Treatment

Gliomas can be managed by an extracranial approach if radiographic studies fail to reveal a bony defect in the skull. An external glioma requires complete excision through an elliptical or Y incision over the nasal

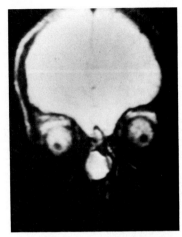

Figure 36–5. MRI of nasal glioma.

dorsum. If a CSF leak is encountered, a bifrontal craniotomy approach may be required. Intranasal gliomas usually arise from the lateral nasal wall and can be approached via a lateral rhinotomy incision. If an intracranial connection is found, a craniotomy or an external ethmoidectomy may be necessary.

Encephaloceles require an intracranial exploration and a CSF-leakproof closure of the dural defect. Early surgical intervention during the first few months of life is advised to alleviate the increased risk of meningitis. Also, the size of the encephalocele increases with time, increasing the cosmetic deformity and the amount of herniated brain tissue that needs to be excised. A frontal craniotomy allows for accurate identification of the intracranial stalk, as well as excellent visualization of the dural defects. Extracranial repair can be performed simultaneously or deferred to a later date. Surgical routes for extracranial excision include later rhinotomy, osteoplastic flap, or sagittal approach over the root of the nose.

DERMOID CYSTS OF THE NOSE

Unlike teratomas, which contain all three embryonal germ layers, congenital dermoid cysts contain only ectodermal and mesodermal embryonic elements. Mesodermal elements, which include hair follicles, adnexal sweat glands, and sebaceous glands in the wall of the dermoid cyst, differentiate it from simple epidermoid cysts. Nasal dermoids account for nearly 10 per cent of the total number of dermoid cysts occurring in the head and neck. Nasal dermoid cysts are benign lesions, with a slight male predominance, usually occurring in a random fashion, although a familial tendency has been reported.

Nasal Dermoid Embryology

Nasal dermoid cysts and sinuses represent an embryonic defect. Between the second and third months

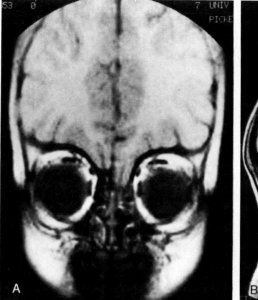
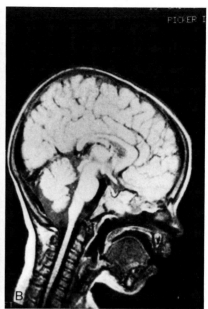

Figure 36–6. *A,* Coronal MRI reveals an encephalocele extending into the right nasal cavity. (Courtesy of Dr. Rodney Lusk of St. Louis, MO.) *B,* Arrows point to brain herniating into the nasal cavity on a sagittal MRI scan. (Courtesy of Dr. Rodney Lusk of St. Louis, MO.)

of fetal life, the nasal and frontal bones begin intramembranous ossification. The fonticulus nasofrontalis is a firm membrane that begins to fill in between the frontal bone superiorly and the nasal bone inferiorly. The prenasal space, a potential space, exists between the nasal bones anteriorly and the cartilaginous capsule posteriorly (Fig. 36–7). The foramen caecum, a bony opening in the cranial vault, allows a herniation of dura to pass through it and form the internal periosteal lining of the nasal bones. In normal fetal development, the foramen caecum and the fonticulus nasofrontalis are obliterated by bony growth.

The two most prominent theories to explain nasal dermoid development are failure of the neuropore to close and abnormal obliteration of the prenasal space. Failure of the fonticulus nasofrontalis or foramen caecum to close allows for dermal elements to invaginate through the frontonasal suture line area or between the developing nasal bones and cartilage (Fig. 36–8).

Luongo (1933) developed the prenasal space theory to explain the development of nasal dermoids. The prenasal space extends from the dura at the base of the skull along the nasal midline to the nasal tip. During embryonic development, this dura develops in close approximation with the skin of the nose. Normally, however, the dura separates from the nasal skin and retracts through the foramen caecum, losing its connection with the skin. If faulty separation or obliteration of the prenasal space occurs, a dermal sinus or cyst may persist anywhere from the foramen caecum to the nasal tip (Fig. 36–8).

Figure 36–7. Anatomy of the base of the anterior cranial fossa and prenasal space during embryologic development. (Courtesy of Hengerer, A. S., and Oas, R. 1987. Congenital Anomalies of the Nose: Their Embryology, Diagnosis, and Management. Washington, D.C., The American Academy of Otolaryngology, Head and Neck Surgery Foundation, p. 45.)

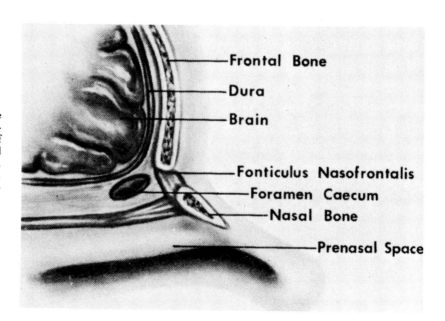

—Frontal Bone
—Dura
—Brain
—Fonticulus Nasofrontalis
—Foramen Caecum
—Nasal Bone
—Prenasal Space

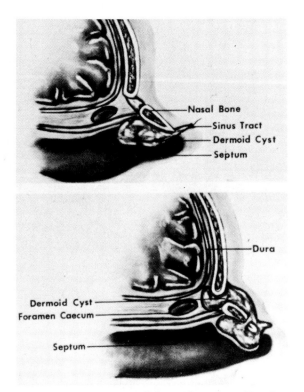

Figure 36–8. *Top*, Location of dermoid cyst extending deep to nasal bones. *Bottom*, Other pathways possible for dermoid cyst and sinus tract development. (Courtesy of Hengerer, A. S., and Oas, R. 1987. Congenital Anomalies of the Nose: Their Embryology, Diagnosis, and Management. Washington, D.C., The American Academy of Otolaryngology, Head and Neck Surgery Foundation, p. 46.)

Sites of Involvement

Nasal dermoids usually present only on the nasal dorsum; the single pit with extruding hair is the most common clinical appearance. However, cystic remnants, either with or without associated infected fistulas, may present in the forehead, glabella, nasal tip, or columella or along the nose to the sphenoid sinus area with varying degrees of involvement.

Diagnosis

Nasal dermoids can present as an external mass, an intranasal mass, a dermoid sinus without a cyst, a dermoid cyst without a fistula, or an extracranial-intracranial mass. A dermoid cyst is a subcutaneous collection on the nasal dorsum superficial to the nasal bones without a cutaneous opening. Thus, only a simple local excision is required. A dermoid sinus is a more involved defect, extending into the deep nasal elements, with a cutaneous opening and often a tuft of hair (Fig. 36–9). Clinically, the dermoid lesion is firm, noncompressible, nonpulsatile, and occasionally lobulated. Intracranial extension is rare, but if it is present, a bony defect can be identified and CSF leakage may occur.

Treatment

Successful management of dermoid lesions requires complete excision to prevent recurrence. A small, superficial cyst can be removed easily via an incision over the nasal dorsum. When a sinus is present, it should be excised with an elliptical incision.

Nasal dermoid cysts must be differentiated from sebaceous cysts, which are also attached to the skin but which are usually not seen prior to puberty. Nasal dermoid cysts may be differentiated from meningoceles by the fact that the latter characteristically transilluminate, whereas dermoids and gliomas do not. Gliomas, in addition, are solid masses.

Other conditions from which nasal dermoid cysts must be differentiated include obstruction of the nasolacrimal system, hemangiomas, and simple lipomas. These last do not transilluminate and are freely movable in the subcutaneous tissue. The CT scan, in conjunction with the MRI scan, is the radiographic study of choice and will provide the surgeon with adequate information about the extent of the lesion. This alleviates any potential surprises such as intracranial extension at the time of surgery (Fig. 36–10A, B, C).

Complete removal of nasal dermoid cysts is necessary, as progressive expansion, infection, and fistula formation have occurred when such conditions have been ignored. Complete surgical removal must include the excision of cystic structures extending through and beneath the nasal bones or along the superior nasal septum posteriorly toward the pituitary. The surgeon must plan for plastic reconstruction of the area of excision before surgery is begun.

Usually, surgery for the removal of nasal dermoid cysts is not performed until the patient is 2 to 5 years old. Such surgery normally requires administration of a general anesthetic, as it is not always possible to determine preoperatively the full extent to which the cyst has invaded the subcribriform plate. Differential diagnosis of congenital midline nasal masses is seen in Table 36–1. Management flowsheets of intranasal and

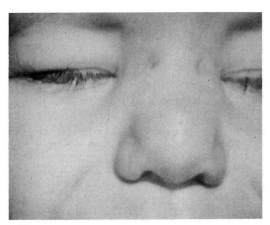

Figure 36–9. Nasal dermoid on dorsum with single fistula on each side.

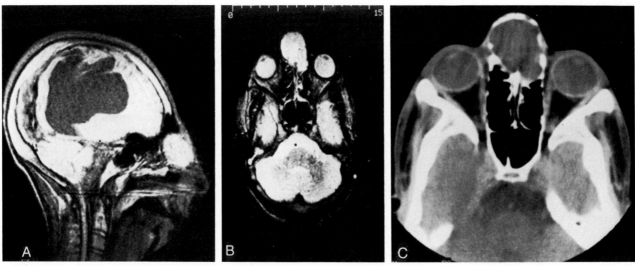

Figure 36–10. *A*, Sagittal MRI showing large glabellar mass found to be a nasal dermoid at the time of surgery. *B*, Axial MRI of the same mass. *C*, CT scan of nasal dermoid. (All courtesy of Dr. Rodney Lusk.)

extranasal masses are shown in Figures 36–11 and 36–12, which provide direction in the treatment of the masses. Although CSF may be encountered in the course of the dissection, this is not the rule.

In summary, congenital dermoid cysts and fistulas of the nose may occur at any point from the glabella to the base of the columella, but the most common site of presentation is at the inferior border of the nasal bone. These cysts may be superficial and may not involve the nasal bone, although many cysts may appear to be superficial but in fact extend through the nasal bone and superior nasal septum toward the region of the pituitary. The cysts probably represent the persistence of ectodermal elements in the line of fusion of the embryonic nose. Treatment of these cysts is complete surgical removal, with the extent of surgery varying according to the individual case.

HEMANGIOMAS

Hemangiomas are commonly occurring benign tumors that present during infancy or childhood. They may occur anywhere in the head and neck, including the nose. They are the single most frequently observed tumor in the region of the head and neck in childhood.

Historically, hemangiomas have been classified histologically as follows: (1) capillary, (2) cavernous, (3) mixed, and (4) hypertrophic or juvenile.

Batsakis (1979) feels that this classification is somewhat artificial and academic, as there is considerable overlap in category in any individual lesion. In addition, the histologic appearance of the tumor seems to have little bearing on the long-term behavior of these lesions. Batsakis (1979) also believes that the most important determinants of the prognosis in cases involving these lesions are (1) the anatomic site of the lesion; (2) the size, extent, and depth of the lesion; and (3) selection of the primary treatment.

While it is well documented that many, if not most, of these hemangiomas will resolve spontaneously, there has been no good way of predicting which lesions will not regress and will thus need surgical intervention. A promising technique is to follow these children through serial Doppler examinations of the lesions at regular intervals. If the number of arteriovenous fistulas increases, the prognosis for spontaneous regression is poor.

Although hemangiomas commonly occur in the head and neck, they only infrequently involve the nose. Generally, conservative management with watchful waiting is the treatment of choice for these lesions. In

TABLE 36–1. Differential Diagnosis of Congenital Midline Nasal Masses

	ENCEPHALOCELE	GLIOMA	DERMOID
Age	Infants, children	Infants, children	Usually children, rarely adults
Location of mass	Intranasal and extranasal	Intranasal and extranasal	Intranasal and extranasal
Appearance	Soft, bluish, compressible	Reddish-blue, solid, noncompressible	Solid, dimple with hair follicle
Pulsation	Yes	No	No
Transillumination	Yes	No	No
CSF leak	Yes	Rarely	Rarely
Furstenburg test	Positive	Negative	Negative
Cranial defect	Yes	Rarely	Rarely
Previous history	Meningitis	Rarely meningitis	Local infection

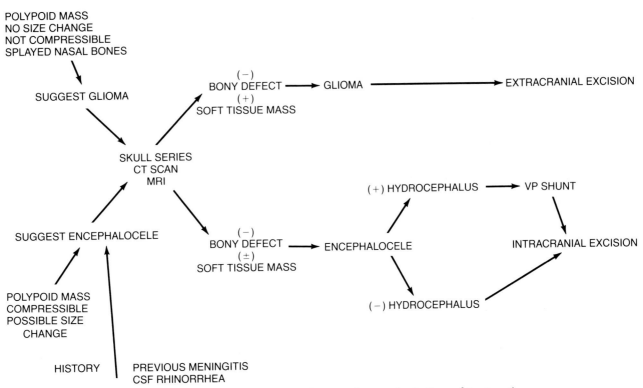

CLINICAL PRESENTATION   LABORATORY EVALUATION   DIAGNOSIS   TREATMENT

Figure 36–11. Management flowsheet of intranasal masses (evaluation and treatment).

a series of 19 patients with hemangiomas of the nasal tip whom Thomson and Lanigan (1979) reviewed, eight had been treated conservatively, and in all eight patients the hemangioma had spontaneously regressed to an aesthetically acceptable degree. In only three of the 11 patients treated surgically were the results attained aesthetically acceptable. Thus, it would appear that when dealing with lesions of the nose (unless the lesion is rapidly invasive or is causing a respiratory situation incompatible with life), the best course is watchful waiting.

COMPLETE AGENESIS OF THE NOSE

The complete absence of the nose and anterior nasopharynx is an exceptionally rare anomaly. Fewer than a dozen cases of such an anomaly have been reported in the literature. These patients had absence of the nasal bones and premaxilla. The soft tissue of the face was intact with no clefting, and there were no nostrils or evidence of any nasal development. In two patients treated by Gifford and MacCollum (1972), the infants had minimal airway and feeding difficulties at birth, in spite of the absence of nasal passages. Establishment of a nasal airway was deferred until age 5 or 6, when removal of several incisor teeth and drilling through the hard palate beneath the oral mucosa created a channel. The passage was then lined with skin but required a permanent Silastic stent to main-

tain the patency. This provided an adequate airway and supported an external nasal prosthesis. Nasal reconstruction can begin when full facial growth has occurred. Prosthetic noses were used until the nasal reconstruction could be carried out.

NASAL CLEFTING—NASAL DYSPLASIA

Actual clefting of the nose is a very rare deformity that is usually associated with some degree of hypertelorism and probably should fall under the broad term "frontonasal dysplasia" or "median cleft-face syndrome." The hallmarks of this disorder are (1) ocular hypertelorism; (2) broad nasal root; (3) lack of formation of the nasal tip; (4) widow's peak scalp bone anomaly; (5) anterior cranium bifidum occultum; (6) median clefting of the nose, lip, and palate; and (7) unilateral orbital clefting or notching of the nasal ala (Gifford and MacCollum, 1972).

MEDIAN NASAL CLEFT

The degree of involvement in median nasal cleft deformity is extremely variable, ranging from a simple median scar at the cephalic end of the nasal dorsum to a completely split nose forming separate halves and creating its own medial wall. The airway is usually adequate despite the cosmetic appearance. Prior to

CLINICAL PRESENTATION   LABORATORY EVALUATION   DIAGNOSIS   TREATMENT

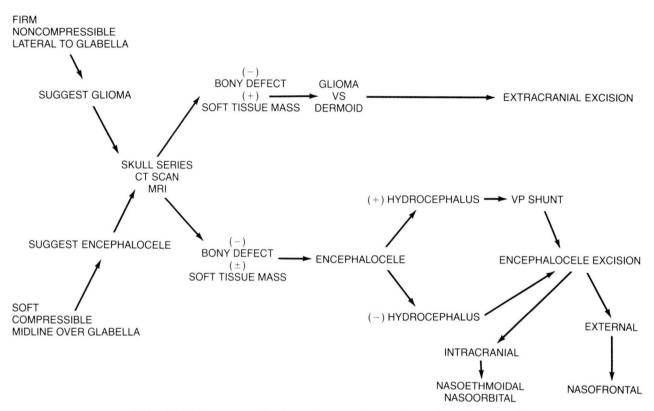

Figure 36–12. Management flowsheet of extranasal masses (evaluation and treatment).

surgical reconstruction of these defects, requiring a multidisciplinary approach in severe defects, it is important to rule out a possible dermoid cyst or encephalocele within the nasal septal area.

LATERAL NASAL CLEFTS

Lateral nasal clefts are rare anomalies involving defects in the nasal alae or lateral nasal wall area. The etiology of lateral nasal clefts involves a mix-up in mesenchymal flow between the medial and the lateral nasal processes. Involvement of the clefts ranges from scarlike lines in the alae to trianglelike defects in the alae that may extend to the inner canthal fold, affecting the nasal lacrimal duct system. If possible, it is best to allow for as much normal nasal development as possible prior to surgical intervention. Reconstruction usually consists of rotation of local flaps or composite grafts of skin and cartilage from the auricle.

DeMyer and colleagues (1963) believe that there are strong associations between the degree of hypertelorism, cephalic anomalies, and the probability of mental deficiency in a given patient. According to their findings, the greater the degree of hypertelorism and the more extracephalic anomalies were present, the more likely the child was to be mentally deficient. If, on the other hand, the degree of hypertelorism was mild and there were no extracephalic anomalies, the chance that normal or nearly normal CNS formation had occurred was good.

The surgical reconstruction of the more severe defects will probably require several procedures and a multidisciplinary approach, thus making it preferable that they be managed in a center where there is a craniofacial team.

MEDIAN FACIAL ANOMALIES

The group of defects lumped into the category of median facial anomalies was classified by DeMyer and colleagues (1963) into five categories of facies (Table 36–2). They found that individuals with these types of facies usually had associated holoprosencephaly.

The hallmarks of median facial anomalies are as follows: (1) ocular (may range from a single eye to orbital hypotelorism); (2) nasal (may range from arrhinia with proboscis to a flat nose); and (3) cleft (there may be no cleft, there may be a median cleft of the lip with no premaxilla prolabium, or a bilateral lateral cleft of the lip with a rudimentary premaxilla prolabium may be present). Diagnostic evaluation of children with such characteristics should include skull radiographs, CT scan, a transillumination, and genetic characterizations.

Embryologically, these defects are formed by a marked reduction in the number of migrating neural crest cells, causing multiple defects in the facial mesenchyme and forebrain derivatives.

Children with median facial anomalies may have physiologic abnormalities, including poikilothermy,

TABLE 36–2. Severe Degrees of Holoprosencephaly (Arrhinencephaly)

TYPE OF FACIES	FACIAL FEATURES	CRANIUM AND BRAIN
I. Cyclopia	Single eye or partially divided eye in single orbit; arrhinia with proboscis	Microcephaly Alobar holoprosencephaly
II. Ethmocephaly	Extreme orbital hypotelorism but separate orbits; arrhinia with proboscis	Microcephaly Alobar holoprosencephaly
III. Cebocephaly	Orbital hypotelorism, proboscislike nose but no median cleft of lip	Microcephaly; usually has alobar holoprosencephaly
IV. With median cleft lip	Orbital hypotelorism, flat nose	Microcephaly and sometimes trigonocephaly; usually has alobar holoprosencephaly
V. With median philtrum-premaxilla anlage	Orbital hypotelorism, bilateral lateral cleft of lip with median process representing philtrum-premaxilla anlage	Microcephaly and sometimes trigonocephaly. Semilobar or lobar holoprosencephaly

This table presents five facies diagnostic of holoprosencephaly. Although transitional cases do occur, the facies of each category are remarkably similar from patient to patient.

spasticity, hyperreflexia, apneic spells, seizures, poor growth, and psychomotor retardation. Because those with the more severe defects generally have a life expectancy of less than one year (Fig. 36–13), surgical treatment of these infants is generally not indicated. Rarely, it may be necessary for the well-being of the family to perform a limited reconstruction. There have been sporadic reports of children with similar facies and normal CNS development (Pashayan, 1983).

If the CNS development is normal, of course, a well thought out plan of reconstruction should be followed. The surgical reconstruction of these types of defects presents a twofold problem of lack of both soft tissue and the underlying skeletal support. Postoperatively, maintaining a nasal airway in these patients is a major problem. For this reason, artificial nasal airways should be left in place for the first 12 to 24 hours postoperatively.

PROBOSCIS LATERALIS

Proboscis lateralis is an unusual deformity in which the medial and lateral nasal processes, as well as the

globular process, are absent. This causes the maxillary process of the affected side to fuse with the opposite nasal and globular processes, forming a tubular structure compound of skin and soft tissue that is attached at the inner canthus. There may be coexistent maldevelopment of the nasal cavity, varying from a normal nose to complete agenesis of the nasal cavity and the paranasal sinuses on that side (Fig. 36–14).

The embryology of this lesion is uncertain. The most commonly accepted theory is that imperfect mesodermal proliferation occurs in the frontonasal and maxillary processes after formation of the olfactory pits. Epidermal breakdown then takes place, leaving the lateral nasal process sequestered as a tube arising in the frontonasal region. Also, as a result of the epidermal breakdown, no nasolacrimal duct is produced.

When these defects are reconstructed, as much of the soft tissue as is needed may be taken from the tube, the remainder being sacrificed. The skeletal deficiency may be corrected by use of bone or radiated costal cartilage.

POLYRHINIA (DOUBLE NOSE)

This is an exceedingly rare anomaly associated with pseudohypertelorism. It is hypothesized that the usual development of the frontonasal process is lessened, allowing separation and thus forming two lateral portions of the nose that develop as usual. However, the medial nasal processes and septal elements are reduplicated, thus forming double noses. Surgical correction involves a transnasal approach to correct the associated choanal atresia, followed by removal of both medial portions of both noses and anastomosis of both lateral halves in the midline.

CLEFT LIP NASAL DEFORMITY

Children with cleft lip and palate usually have a coexistent nasal deformity. With unilateral clefts, the nasal ala on the side of the cleft is laterally based, giving the appearance of a flat, flaring nostril. The

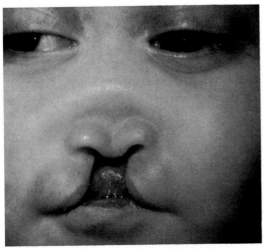

Figure 36–13. Central facial hypoplasia.

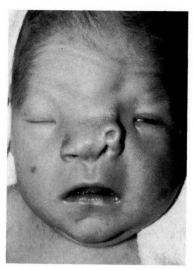

Figure 36–14. Proboscis lateralis.

columella is usually short on the cleft side. The maxilla on the cleft side is frequently hypoplastic, resulting in a relative retropositioning of the ala on that side. The nasal tip may also have a bifid appearance.

The most severe defects are those associated with a bilateral complete cleft. Individuals with such deformity frequently have very short columellas, 1 to 2 mm in length. They also may have bilateral maxillary hypoplasia with relative prognathism.

Children with clefts also may have severe nasal septal deformities, which may cause airway problems. If possible, it is best to wait until they have become teenagers before doing septal surgery, if at all. In some instances, this may not be possible, and a very conservative septal approach should be used. The surgeon should be cautioned that the resultant improvement in the nasal airway may have a deleterious effect on the individual's speech, leaving him or her with a velopharyngeal incompetence that had not been evident prior to surgery.

Many ways of handling cleft nasal deformities have been put forth. We prefer to perform an open tip rhinoplasty in combination with a velopharyngeal lengthening of the columellas as described by Bardach (personal communication). This technique is advantageous in that it allows excellent exposure of the lower lateral cartilages so that they may be aligned and trimmed and adjusted to the proper height, and it also permits lengthening of the columella. This procedure may be carried out any time after the child has reached the age of 8 or 10 years without the fear of impairment of normal growth of the face (Chap. 35).

In the children in whom the degree of unilateral maxillary hypoplasia is so severe that there is obvious depression of the ala on that side, an implant under the ala of Supramid mesh or irradiated costal cartilage has been used to correct this defect. This implant is placed by a peroral route through the buccal sulcus.

CHOANAL ATRESIA

The incidence of choanal atresia is approximately 1 in 7000 live births. The female-to-male ratio is 2:1, and unilateral to bilateral 2:1. Ninety per cent of atresia plates are bony, whereas 10 per cent are membranous. Associated congenital anomalies occur in 50 per cent of patients with choanal atresia, with the anomalies occurring more frequently in bilateral cases. Bergstrom (1984) described the CHARGE association involving the following anomalies with choanal atresia. These include colobomas of the retina, cardiac defects, genitourinary anomalies, mental retardation, and hearing loss.

Embryology

Several theories have been proposed to explain the etiology of choanal atresia. Until recently, the simplest and most widely held theory was persistence of the nasobuccal membrane. A more recent theory by Hengerer and Oas (1987) proposed misdirection of mesodermal flow secondary to local factors. As discussed earlier, neural crest cells migrate through a meshwork of hyaluronic acid and collagen filaments to reach a preordained position in the facial processes. If the flow of these cells is altered with regard to their position or total numbers, the burrowing of the nasal pits may not create the same rotation from the ventrodorsal to the cephalocaudal plane. Thus, the thinning that allows breakthrough at the anterior choana is altered.

Diagnosis

Bilateral choanal atresia causes complete nasal obstruction in the newborn, with immediate onset of respiratory distress and possible death by asphyxia unless immediate intervention is undertaken by inserting an oral airway. This occurs because neonates are obligate nose breathers. The whole length of a neonate's tongue is in close proximity with the hard and soft palate, creating a vacuum and causing airway obstruction in bilateral choanal atresia. Mouth breathing is a learned response by neonates, occurring approximately 4 to 6 weeks after birth.

Unilateral atresia rarely causes any acute respiratory distress, and the most common finding is unilateral mucoid discharge. If a no. 6 French catheter or dilator placed in the nose fails to pass into the oropharynx, choanal atresia is probable. A CT scan is the radiographic study of choice to delineate this anomaly. Harner (1981) divides the anatomic deformities of congenital atresia based on CT scan and clinical observation into four areas: narrow nasal cavities, lateral bony obstruction, medial obstruction secondary to the vomer, and membranous obstruction.

Treatment

Unilateral atresia usually does not cause any acute respiratory distress. A common finding is simply a unilateral nasal discharge, for which no immediate intervention is necessary. Definitive therapy can be carried out at any time during childhood, usually before the patient starts school, to stop the rhinorrhea. The surgical approach can be transnasal or transpalatal, depending on the age, the palate shape, and the makeup of the choanal atresia plate.

In bilateral atresia, immediate treatment in the neonate requires an artificial airway. An anesthesia oral airway is sufficient and rarely is a tracheotomy necessary if no other anomalies exist. The surgical procedures for correction of choanal atresia include those previously listed. They all allow immediate and early correction of the defect.

The first technique, developed by Emmert in 1853, was a transnasal blind puncture through the atretic plate. This technique should be avoided because of potential serious complications: CSF leaks, midbrain trauma, and Gradenigo syndrome. Other transnasal approaches involve microsurgical and endoscopic techniques. The anterior mucoperiosteum is carefully elevated, and the bony plate is drilled out, including the posterior septum and the lateral bony buttress. The preserved mucosal flaps then cover the raw areas. A cavity can be examined with the Storz-Hopkins telescopes or flexible fiberoptic scopes.

Generally, the transnasal approach offers less satisfactory results than those of the transpalatal approach. Patients usually have lesser degrees of long-term nasal patency, require long-term nasal stents, and frequent dilatations. Explanations for the poorer results using the transnasal approach include the difficulty in obtaining access to the bony posterior airway; the fact that mucosal flaps are often insufficiently preserved; and the difficulty in completely removing the thick atretic bony plates.

It is generally agreed that a transpalatal approach for choanal atresia is the preferred method in all age groups. This approach allows direct visualization, with fewer immediate postoperative difficulties such as recurrent stenosis and granulation formation. An adequate choanal passage requires that the posterior septum and the lateral superior nasal walls be removed.

REFERENCES

Bardach, J. 1988. Professor, Dept. of Otolaryngology and Maxillofacial Surgery, University of Iowa Hospital and Clinics. Personal communication.

Batsakis, J. 1979. Tumors of the Head and Neck. Baltimore, Williams & Wilkins Co.

Benjamin, B. 1985. Evaluation of choanal atresia. Ann. Otol. Rhinol. Laryngol. 94:429.

Bergstrom, L., and Owens, O. 1984. Posterior choanal atresia: A syndromal disorder. Laryngoscope 94:1273.

DeMyer, W., Zeman, W., and Palmer, C. G. 1963. Familial alobar holoprosencephaly with median cleft lip and palate. Neurology 13:913.

Gifford, G. H., and MacCollum, D. W. 1972. Congenital malformations. In Ferguson, C. F., and Kendig, E. L. (eds.): Pediatric Otolaryngology. Philadelphia, W. B. Saunders Co.

Harner, S. 1981. The anatomy of congenital choanal atresia. Otolaryngol. Head Neck Surg. 89:7.

Hengerer, A. S., and Oas, R. 1987. Congenital Anomalies of the Nose: Their Embryology, Diagnosis and Management. Washington, D.C., The American Academy of Otolaryngology, Head and Neck Surgery Foundation.

Hengerer, A. S., and Strome, M. 1982. Choanal atresia: A new embryologic theory and its influence on surgical management. Laryngoscope 92:913.

Hughes, G. B. 1980. Management of the congenital midline nasal mass: A review. Head Neck Surg. 1:222.

Luongo, R. A. 1933. Dermoid cyst of the nasal dorsum. Arch. Otolaryngol. 17:755.

Pashayan, H. 1983. Genetics and Birth Defects in Clinical Practice, 1st ed. Boston, Little, Brown and Co.

Theogaraj, T., and Dawson, S. 1981. Practical management of congenital choanal atresia. Plast. Reconstr. Surg. 72:634.

Thomson, H. G., and Lanigan, M. 1979. The cyrano nose: A clinical review of hemangiomas of the nasal tip. Plast. Reconstr. Surg. 63:155.

Chapter 37

RHINITIS AND ACUTE AND CHRONIC SINUSITIS

Ellen R. Wald, M.D.

RHINITIS

Infection of the upper respiratory tract is the single most common organic disease presenting to the primary care practitioner. It is usually characterized by nasal discharge and nasal congestion, with variable components of cough, conjunctivitis, sore throat, and constitutional symptoms. When rhinitis is self-limited, it is almost certainly infectious in origin. When rhinitis is persistent or seasonal, allergic problems must be considered (see Chap. 42).

Viral Rhinitis

Infectious rhinitis is caused by viruses or bacteria; infection with the former is many times more frequent than that with the latter. The common cold is a syndrome caused by more than 100 antigenically different viruses that may intermittently colonize and infect the upper respiratory tract. The viruses can be divided into four groups: (1) the myxovirus and paramyxovirus group of viruses (containing influenza, parainfluenza, and respiratory syncytial viruses), (2) the adenovirus group (containing 35 different human serotypes), (3) the picornavirus group (containing enteroviruses and more than 100 different rhinoviruses), and (4) the coronavirus group (Gwaltney, 1985). The specific etiology of a cold can be identified in 60 to 70 per cent of cases, using sensitive culture techniques. Rhinoviruses account for 30 to 40 per cent of infections, coronaviruses for at least 10 per cent, and respiratory syncytial viruses, influenza viruses, parainfluenza viruses, and adenoviruses together for about 10 to 15 per cent. Many of the remaining as yet unidentified cases are probably caused by coronaviruses that elude current methods of virus isolation (Gwaltney, 1985).

Epidemiology

It is common experience, and several epidemiologic studies show, that colds are much more frequent in children than in adults. The range of reported frequencies for upper respiratory infections in young children is between 6 and 21 per year (Beem, 1969).

The incidence of infection in children varies with age, siblings, and day care arrangements. Most adults experience two to three colds per year; however, this may increase during the years of parenting young children or when occupational exposure provides contact with a large number of youngsters. The respiratory viruses show definite seasonal trends, with least activity seen in the summer months. The rhinovirus is found most frequently during fall and spring, whereas the coronaviruses and influenza and respiratory syncytial viruses are most prevalent in the winter.

The seemingly endless susceptibility of humans to viral infections of the upper respiratory tract is a consequence of (1) incomplete immunity following infection with certain agents (e.g., respiratory syncytial virus), (2) multiple viral serotypes in other groups of viruses to which immunity does develop after infection (e.g., adenovirus, rhinovirus, coronavirus), and (3) antigenic shift and drift for influenza viruses and possibly coronaviruses as well.

Transmission of respiratory viruses from person to person occurs by means of virus-contaminated respiratory secretions. The potential routes for spread are inhalation of small airborne particles, inhalation of large airborne particles (when the transmitter and susceptible individual are physically close), and hand contact with contaminated environmental articles or other hands (Couch, 1984). Although all routes contribute to the spread of infection, the last category seems to be the most important. The susceptible individual can acquire hand colonization with infective virus from contaminated inanimate objects or other hands. Once the susceptible person's hands are colonized, the virus is easily inoculated onto mucosal surfaces through hand-to-eye or hand-to-nose contact (Gwaltney and Hendley, 1982; Hall and Douglas, 1981). Spread of virus is difficult to control, as virus can be shed for a day or two prior to the onset of symptoms and, rarely, by an individual who never develops symptoms.

Pathogenesis

The usual method for inducing experimental rhinovirus infection has been instillation of small amounts of virus suspension into each nasal passage, with the volunteer in a supine position. Recent studies have shown that other effective inoculation sites are the conjunctival sac or the posterior nasopharyngeal wall at the level of the eustachian tube orifices (Winther et al., 1986). Infection may be established first in the nasopharynx and then spread secondarily to the nasal turbinates, but recovery of virus from within the nasal cavity may be spotty. Additionally, destruction of the nasal epithelium during symptomatic rhinovirus infection has not been detected in several studies (Winther et al., 1986). In view of the spottiness of infection and the frequent lack of detectable morphologic change in the nasal mucosa, some have speculated that symptoms may result from the release of chemical mediators that activate the inflammatory cascade (Turner et al., 1982; Gwaltney et al., 1984). Two potent mediators, lysyl-bradykinin and bradykinin, have recently been found in the nasal secretions of volunteers with rhinovirus colds (Naclerio et al., 1985).

In contrast to the absence of morphologic changes in the nasal mucosa of patients infected with rhinoviruses, dramatic but focal cytopathic effect may be seen in the nasal mucosa of children naturally infected with influenza virus. Similarly, dysmorphology of ciliary microtubules of nasal epithelial cells has been observed with adenovirus, influenza virus, parainfluenza virus, and respiratory syncytial virus infections (Carson et al., 1985). In these instances, the viral infection appears to induce direct cellular injury that may lead to impaired mucociliary transport.

Clinical Features

The clinical features of the common cold are variable and may include nasal congestion, nasal discharge (of any quality—serous, mucoid, or purulent), sneezing, cough, conjunctival inflammation, and sore throat with or without the constitutional symptoms of fever, malaise, and myalgias. Appetite and sleep patterns may be disturbed. On physical examination, the nasal and pharyngeal mucosa appear erythematous, and lymphoid hyperplasia may be seen in the posterior pharynx. There may be tonsillar and adenoidal hypertrophy; the cervical lymph nodes may be modestly enlarged and slightly tender. Frequently, irritative skin manifestations become apparent around the alar nasi and the upper lip. Early in the course of a cold, there may be secondary bacterial infection of the middle ears (evidenced by an opaque, immobile tympanic membrane) or paranasal sinuses (evidenced by high fever, purulent nasal discharge, and ill appearance). The duration of most colds is five to seven days; although patients may not be completely asymptomatic by day ten, they are almost always improving.

Diagnosis

In clinical practice, it is rarely necessary to know the precise etiology of the common cold. However, virus may be isolated from the nasopharynx (by direct swabbing) or from the nasal cavity (with nasal washes) by conventional tissue culture techniques. These cultures are expensive, and the results are not usually available for four to seven days. Rapid diagnostic techniques such as enzyme immunoassay and flourescent antibody methods have been developed for detecting respiratory syncytial virus, parainfluenza virus, and influenza virus. Although precise etiologic information is not essential for the practitioner, community surveillance cultures may provide useful epidemiologic information, for example, signaling the onset of influenza season.

Treatment

The availability of specific antiviral chemotherapy for respiratory syncytial virus (ribavirin aerosol) and influenza (amantadine) are primarily intended to treat the lower respiratory component of these infections. Attempts at acute treatment of upper respiratory infection with topical enviroxime, a potent antirhinovirus compound in vitro, (Lilly Research Laboratories, Indianapolis, IN) have been unsuccessful in experimentally induced infections (Hayden and Gwaltney, 1982; Levandowski et al., 1982).

Apart from specific antiviral therapy, treatment of the common cold is largely symptomatic. Normal saline nose drops may be useful to liquify nasal mucus, thereby reducing forceful nose blowing. Nasal irrigation with normal saline may also be soothing, when used with a water pick in the older child or adult. Systemic and topical decongestants are used to decrease nasal secretions and mucosal edema, thereby decreasing nasal resistance and increasing airway patency. Oral phenylpropanolamine and pseudoephedrine have been shown to be effective for this purpose (Aschan, 1974; Roth et al., 1977).

Topical decongestants (sympathomimetic amines), although not tested in clinical trials, usually decrease nasal congestion and provide symptomatic relief. However, if they are used for more than three days, rebound congestion (rhinitis medicamentosa) may result. Patients should be cautioned against protracted use.

Antihistamines or antihistamine-decongestant combinations are also available as common cold remedies. Antihistamines are more likely to be effective in allergic rhinitis. All five classes of antihistamines act by competitively blocking the histamine receptor site and may relieve such symptoms as sneezing, nasal itchiness, and watery rhinorrhea. Whether any of these agents hasten the resolution of the upper respiratory infection or prevent the development of suppurative complications (i.e., otitis media or sinusitis) is unknown.

Other symptomatic remedies include the use of acetaminophen (for fever or myalgias), increased fluid intake (to keep secretions liquified and mucous membranes comfortable), and bed rest, if possible, for comfort.

Prevention

Major efforts to control the common cold have focused on prevention of transmission. Intranasally applied alpha$_2$-interferon has been evaluated for its prophylactic and therapeutic efficacy. Although twice daily use of interferon is effective in the prophylaxis of natural rhinovirus infections, daily use beyond two weeks results in the development of nasal stuffiness, dryness, and blood tinged mucus in 40 per cent of adults. Accordingly, more recent evaluations have assessed the efficacy of interferon for short-term use in the family setting. It has been found to result in about 40 per cent fewer episodes of rhinovirus-associated illness (Hayden et al., 1986; Douglas et al., 1986). The major limitation to the use of alpha$_2$-interferon is its lack of effectiveness against parainfluenza viruses, influenza A, and community coronaviruses, thereby considerably reducing its impact on "all" respiratory illness.

Another preventive strategy in its preliminary stages of development has been the intranasal administration of a monoclonal antibody directed at the cellular receptor site to which the rhinovirus attaches. Although there are numerous rhinoviruses, 88 of 100 clinical isolates attach to one of two cellular receptor sites in tissue culture (Tomassini and Colonno, 1986).

Another strategy to prevent spread of rhinoviruses has been aimed at reducing hand-to-hand transmission of the virus. A highly virucidal paper handkerchief was developed for individuals with colds in order to reduce the likelihood that the rhinovirus would be dispersed into the environment or onto the user's hands. Employing an interesting human volunteer model of virus transmission, it has been shown that these virucidal tissues may prevent dissemination of colds (Dick et al., 1986). Virucidal tissues have not been evaluated in a "field" situation, and their expense has been an unattractive marketing feature.

Bacterial Rhinitis

Group A Streptococcal Infection

The most common clinical expression of infection with *Streptococcus pyogenes* is pharyngitis, often accompanied by fever and tender anterior cervical lymph nodes, in children 5 to 15 years of age. However, persistent rhinitis in infants or young children (younger than 3 years of age) suggests the possibility of streptococcal infection, or streptococcosis (Powers and Boivert, 1944). Streptococcal infection in this age group often fails to localize to the throat and instead causes a clinical picture of a protracted cold with low-grade fever. Occasionally, an older child (above 5 years of age) with streptococcal infection and superimposed sinusitis may present with persistent nasal discharge and cough (Wald et al., 1986).

If streptococcal infection is proved by culture of the nasopharynx or throat, treatment with penicillin for ten days is appropriate. Dosages of phenoxymethyl-

penicillin of 125 mg three or four times daily, for those under 60 pounds, and 250 mg three or four times daily, for those over 60 pounds, are recommended. In penicillin-allergic patients, erythromycin, 40 mg/kg/day in three to four divided doses, is a suitable substitute.

In both infants and older children, paranasal sinusitis should be considered as a cause of persistent nasal discharge (see next section on sinusitis). Purulent rhinorrhea may also be indicative of an intranasal foreign body, especially when fetor oris is prominent or when the discharge is unilateral, bloody, or both.

Whether bacteria other than group A streptococci can cause purulent rhinitis has not been adequately evaluated. Staphylococci, *Haemophilus influenzae*, *Branhamella catarrhalis*, and *Streptococcus pneumoniae* may be normal nasal or nasopharyngeal flora. Therefore, the recovery of these bacteria from superficial cultures of the nose or throat of a child with a cold is not easily interpretable. Antimicrobial preparations are not recommended in the management of uncomplicated upper respiratory infections. However, data suggest that antibiotic prophylaxis (daily or during the course of a cold) may be effective in preventing symptomatic episodes of acute otitis media in otitis-prone children (see section on otitis media prophylaxis).

Pertussis

Early in the catarrhal phase of pertussis, nasal symptoms are prominent (congestion and discharge), and the clinical syndrome is indistinguishable from those of other causes of upper respiratory infection. Only when cough becomes a prominent part of the clinical picture and specific cultures of the nasopharynx yield *Bordetella pertussis* can the clinician retrospectively implicate pertussis as the cause of the early coryza.

Diphtheria

The most characteristic clinical expression of infection with *Corynebacterium diphtheriae* is a membraneous pharyngitis. In some cases, there may be nasal involvement—either actual membrane occurrence or bloody nasal secretions.

The onset of nasal diphtheria is indistinguishable from that of the common cold. In the early stages, the nasal discharge is serous; later, it becomes serosanguineous and occasionally mucopurulent, thereby potentially obscuring the white membrane on the nasal septum. The copious nasal discharge, which is highly contagious, leads to excoriation of the anterior nares and upper lip. Diphtheria toxin is poorly absorbed nasally, consequently the patient lacks constitutional symptoms, including fever.

Chlamydia trachomatis

A syndrome of afebrile pneumonitis affecting infants in the age group of 3 to 16 weeks was described nearly a decade ago (Beem and Saxon, 1977). The clinical picture, which is characterized by protracted cough (for more than seven days), tachypnea, and absence of fever, may be caused by *Chlamydia trachomatis, Ureaplasma urealyticum, Pneumocystis carinii*, or cytomegalovirus (Stagno et al., 1981). In each case, the protracted cough may be preceded by prominent nasal symptoms—congestion, discharge, and sneezing. Again, it is only belatedly that these "colds" can be recognized to be caused by specific microbiologic agents.

Syphilis

Congenital syphilis is characterized by the triad of rash, snuffles, and pseudoparalysis. Usually, the infant is well at birth but develops a persistent nasal discharge that is mucoid and intermittently bloody by the end of the first or second week of life. The nasal discharge is irritating to the nares and the upper lip and leads to excoriation and scarring. The diagnosis of syphilis should be confirmed by serologic tests. Positive results should be obtained with the fluorescent treponemal antibody test and the nontreponemal tests, including the venereal disease research laboratory (VDRL) test, the rapid plasma reagin (RPR) test, and the standard test for syphilis (STS). Treatment should be instituted with benzathine penicillin as long as the central nervous system is not involved.

SINUSITIS

Introduction

When considering a diagnosis of sinusitis in a child or an adult, the major problem is to distinguish, on the one hand, simple upper respiratory tract infection (URI) or allergic inflammation from, on the other hand, secondary bacterial infection of the paranasal sinuses. The former categories of URI and allergy may prompt consideration of symptomatic treatment, whereas patients with sinusitis will benefit from specific antimicrobial therapy. Both URI and allergic inflammation are recognized risk factors for acute sinusitis, with URI being most common.

Epidemiology

It is estimated that 0.5 per cent of upper respiratory infections are complicated by acute sinusitis (Dingle et al., 1964). However, in the absence of a precise definition of sinusitis, that estimate may be inaccurate. It is probable that the number falls somewhere between 0.5 and 5.0 per cent. As adults average two to three colds per year and children six to eight, sinusitis is a very common problem in clinical practice (Gwaltney et al., 1981).

Embryology and Anatomy

All the paranasal sinuses develop as outpouchings of the nasal chamber, with varying extensions into their respective bony vaults. Along the lateral wall of the nasal chamber are three shelflike structures—the inferior, the middle, and the superior turbinates. Beneath each turbinate is the corresponding meatus. The frontal, maxillary, and anterior ethmoid sinuses open into the middle meatus; the sphenoid and the posterior ethmoid cells open high in the nasal vault into the superior meatus.

The maxillary sinus develops early in the second trimester of fetal life as a lateral outpouching in the posterior aspect of the middle meatus. At birth it is a slitlike structure, with its long axis parallel to the attachment of the inferior turbinate and its floor barely below that. The sinus cavity grows in width and height. Ultimately, at full size, the lateral border of the maxillary sinus reaches the lateral orbital rim. The position of the floor of the sinus is determined by the eruption of the dentition. Infrequently, one can find septae in the maxillary sinus, resulting in separate compartments rather than a single large cavity (Karmody et al., 1977). The volume of the fully developed maxillary sinus is approximately 12 to 15 ml.

Of special note is the position of the maxillary ostium in relation to the body of the sinus. The location of this outflow tract, high on the medial wall of the maxillary sinus, impedes gravitational drainage of secretions; ciliary activity is required to move secretions from the body of the maxillary sinus through the ostium to the nose. From there, secretions are carried into the nasopharynx to be either expectorated or swallowed.

The ethmoid sinus develops in the fourth month of gestation. It is not a single large cavity but a grouping of individual cells, 3 to 15 in number, each with its own opening, or ostium. Aeration of the ethmoid cells is variable, leading to a honeycombed radiographic appearance. The cells are small anteriorly and large in the posterior group. The walls of the ethmoid labyrinth are thin, especially in the lateral aspect bordering on the orbit. The lateral wall of the ethmoid sinus is referred to as the lamina papyracea, or paper wall. Purulent infection may spread by direct extension from the ethmoid sinus through natural dehiscences in the bone to involve the orbit (Ritter, 1973).

The variability of frontal sinus development is well known. In adults, 80 per cent have bilateral but often asymmetric frontal sinuses, 1 to 4 per cent have agenesis of the frontal sinuses, and the remainder have unilateral hypoplasia. The position of the frontal sinus is supraorbital after age 4 years but is not distinguishable radiographically from the ethmoid sinus until 6 to 8 years of age. After that, it progresses for another 8 to 10 years before reaching full adult size. Depending on the particular cell in the frontal recess or anterior ethmoid sinus, which develops into the frontal sinus, the conduit between sinus and nasal cavity will be either a short and wide ostium or a long and narrow nasofrontal duct.

Although the sphenoid sinus occupies a strategic position in the base of the skull, its slow growth and relative isolation preserve it from frequent infection. Isolated involvement of the sphenoid sinuses is uncommon; however, they may be involved as part of a pansinusitis. For further reading see Chapter 28.

Pathophysiology and Pathogenesis

Three key elements are important in the normal physiology of the paranasal sinuses: the patency of the ostia, the function of the ciliary apparatus, and, integral to the latter, the quality of secretions (Reimer et al., 1978). Retention of secretions in the paranasal sinuses is due to one or more of the following: obstruction of the ostia, reduction in the number of cilia, impaired function of the cilia, or overproduction or change in viscosity of secretions.

Sinus Ostia

The ostia of the paranasal sinuses are the key to pathology in the sinus area. The ostia of the maxillary sinuses are small, tubular structures with a diameter of 2.5 mm (cross-sectional area approximately 5 mm) and a length of 6 mm (Drettner, 1980). The diameter of the ostium of each of the individual ethmoid air cells that drain independently into the middle meatus are even smaller, measuring 1 to 2 mm; the anterior are smaller than the posterior (Rachelefsky et al., 1982). The narrow caliber of these individual ostia sets the stage for obstruction to occur easily and often.

The factors predisposing to ostial obstruction can be divided into those that cause mucosal swelling and those due to mechanical obstruction (Rachelefsky et al., 1982). The various factors that may cause mucosal swelling, consequent either to systemic illness or to local insults, are shown in Table 37–1. In addition, the conditions that predispose to mechanical obstruction of the sinus ostia are listed. Although many conditions may lead to ostial closure, viral upper respiratory infection and allergic inflammation are by far the most frequent and most important causes of ostial obstruction. In acute rhinitis, a completely patent ostium is present only 20 per cent of the time (Drettner, 1980).

**TABLE 37–1. Factors Predisposing to
Sinus Ostial Obstruction**

MUCOSAL SWELLING	MECHANICAL OBSTRUCTION
Systemic disorder	Choanal atresia
Viral URI	Deviated septum
Allergic inflammation	Nasal polyps
Cystic fibrosis	Foreign body
Immune disorders	Tumor
Immotile cilia	
Local insult	
Facial trauma	
Swimming, diving	
Rhinitis medicamentosa	

When complete obstruction of the sinus ostium occurs, there is a transient increase in intrasinal pressure followed by the development of a negative intrasinal pressure (Aust et al., 1979). When the ostium opens again, the negative pressure within the sinus relative to atmospheric pressure may allow the introduction of bacteria into the usually sterile sinus cavity. Alternatively, sneezing, sniffing, and nose blowing with altered intranasal pressure may facilitate the entry of bacteria from a heavily colonized posterior nasal chamber into the sinus cavity. The mucosa of the paranasal sinus continues to secrete actively even after obstruction occurs. Clearance of secretions is impossible when the ostium is totally obstructed. If the ostium is patent but reduced in size, removal of secretions will be delayed.

Gas exchange within the sinus cavity also will be impaired if the ostium is obstructed. The rapidity and the efficiency of gas exchange is dependent on two factors: (1) ostial patency and (2) nasal breathing (Drettner, 1980). As nasal breathing decreases, as is probable when there is nasal congestion and secondary obstruction, gas exchange in the sinus decreases. A decreased partial pressure of oxygen within the sinus cavity is a local factor that favors the multiplication of certain bacterial species.

The mucociliary apparatus is fairly hardy with regard to alterations in its oxygen supply. Function will not be impaired unless both the oxygen concentration within the sinus cavity and that supplied by the circulation are compromised (Drettner, 1980). While the former is common, on the basis of reduced patency of the sinus ostia, the latter probably occurs only when intrasinal pressure is high enough to impair mucosal blood flow.

Mucociliary Apparatus

Disorders of the mucociliary apparatus in conjunction with reduced patency of the sinus ostia are major pathophysiologic events in acute sinusitis. In the posterior two thirds of the nasal cavity and within the sinuses, the epithelium is pseudostratified columnar, in which most of the cells are ciliated.

The normal motility of the cilia and the adhesive properties of the mucous layer usually protect respiratory epithelium from bacterial invasion. However, certain respiratory viruses may have a direct cytotoxic effect on the cilia. The alteration of cilia number, morphology, and function may facilitate secondary bacterial invasion of the nose and the paranasal sinuses. For further reading see Chapter 29.

Sinus Secretions

Cilia can beat only in a fluid medium. There appears to be a double layer of mucus in the airways: the gel layer (superficial viscid fluid) and the sol layer (underlying serous fluid). The gel layer acts to trap particulate matter such as bacteria and other debris. The tips of the cilia touch the gel layer during forward movement and thereby move the particulate matter along. However, the bodies of the cilia move through the sol layer, a fluid thin enough to allow the cilia to beat.

Alterations in the mucus, as in cystic fibrosis or asthma, may impair ciliary activity. One can easily imagine that the presence of purulent material in the acutely infected sinus may also impair ciliary movement and further compound the effects of ostial closure. Interestingly, in chronic purulent sinusitis, there are conflicting reports regarding the reduction of ciliary activity (Reimer et al., 1978; Ohashi and Nakai, 1983).

Clinical Presentation

Commonly recognized symptoms of sinusitis in adults and adolescents are facial pain, headache, and fever. However, children with acute sinusitis frequently have complaints that are less specific. During the course of apparent viral upper respiratory tract infections, there are two common clinical developments that should alert the clinician to the possibility of bacterial infection of the paranasal sinuses (Table 37–2).

The first, most common, clinical situation in which sinusitis should be suspected is when the signs and symptoms of a cold are persistent. Nasal discharge and daytime cough that continue beyond ten days and are not improving are the principal complaints. The nasal discharge may be of any quality (thin or thick; clear, mucoid, or purulent) and the cough (which may be dry or wet) is usually present in the daytime, although it is often noted to be worse at night. Cough occurring only at night is a common residual symptom of an upper respiratory tract infection. When it is the only residual symptom, it is usually nonspecific and does not suggest a sinus infection. On the other hand, the persistence of day time cough is frequently the symptom that brings a child to medical attention. This child may not appear ill, and, usually, if fever is present, it will be low-grade. Fetid breath is often reported by parents of preschoolers. Facial pain is absent, although intermittent, painless, morning periorbital swelling may have been noted by the parent. In this case, it is not the severity of the clinical symptoms but their persistence that calls for attention.

The second, less common, presentation is a cold

TABLE 37–2. Common Clinical Presentations for Acute Sinusitis

"PERSISTENT" RESPIRATORY SYMPTOMS
  Nasal discharge of any quality and/or
  Daytime cough for 10–30 days without clinical improvement
  Low-grade or no fever
  Eye swelling
  Fetid breath (children younger than 5 yr)
"SEVERE" RESPIRATORY SYMPTOMS
  High fever (> 39°C)
  Purulent nasal discharge with or without
  Eye swelling
  Headache

that seems more severe than usual: the fever is high (greater than 39.0°C), the nasal discharge is purulent and copious, and there are associated periorbital swelling and facial pain. The periorbital swelling may involve the upper or lower lid; it is gradual in onset and most obvious in the early morning shortly after awakening. The swelling may decrease and actually disappear during the day, only to reappear once again the following day. A less common complaint is headache (a feeling of fullness or a dull ache either behind or above the eyes), most often reported in children older than 5 years of age. Occasionally, there may be dental pain, either from infection originating in the teeth or referred from the sinus infection.

Chronic sinusitis should be suspected in children with very protracted respiratory symptoms—nasal discharge, nasal obstruction, or cough that has lasted for more than 30 days. Although the nasal discharge is most often purulent, it may be thin and clear. Once again, the cough should be present during the daytime, although it is usually reported to be worse at night. In addition, the patient may complain of facial pain, headache, or malaise. However, unless these less specific complaints are accompanied by respiratory symptoms, they should not be attributed to sinus infection. Fever is less prominent and found less frequently than in acute sinusitis.

The signs of chronic sinusitis are not specific. They include mucopurulent nasal discharge, hypertrophied nasal turbinates, and, occasionally, intranasal polyps. The latter are seen principally in association with allergy or cystic fibrosis. Some have noted that in children with chronic sinusitis, widening of the nasal bridge develops, producing a pseudohypertelorism.

Diagnosis

Physical Examination

On physical examination, the patient with acute sinusitis may have mucopurulent discharge present in the nose or posterior pharynx. The nasal mucosa is erythematous; the throat may show moderate injection. The cervical lymph nodes are usually not significantly enlarged or tender. None of these characteristics differentiates rhinitis from sinusitis. Occasionally, there will be either tenderness, as the examiner palpates over or percusses the paranasal sinuses, or appreciable periorbital edema—soft, nontender swelling of the upper and lower eyelid, discoloration of the overlying skin, or both. Malodorous breath (in the absence of pharyngitis, poor dental hygiene or a nasal foreign body) may suggest bacterial sinusitis.

Transillumination may be helpful in diagnosing inflammation of the maxillary or frontal sinuses (Fig. 37–1). The patient and the examiner must be in a darkened room. To transilluminate the maxillary sinus, the light source, shielded from the observer, is placed over the midpoint of the inferior orbital rim. The transmission of light through the hard palate is then assessed with

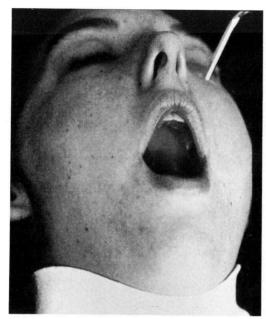

Figure 37–1. Transillumination of the right maxillary sinus.

the patient's mouth open. Light passing through the alveolar ridges should be excluded in judging light transmission. Transillumination of the frontal sinus is accomplished by placing a high-intensity light source beneath the medial border of the supraorbital ridge and evaluating the symmetry of the blush bilaterally. Transillumination is useful in adolescents and adults if light transmission is either normal or absent. "Reduced" transmission or "dull" transillumination are assessments that correlate poorly with clinical disease. The increased thickness of both the soft tissue and the bony vault in children younger than 10 years of age limits the clinical usefulness of transillumination in the younger age group (Wald et al., 1986).

In general, for most children younger than 10 years of age, the physical examination is not very helpful in making a specific diagnosis of acute sinusitis. On the other hand, if the mucopurulent material can be removed from the nose and the nasal mucosa is treated with topical vasoconstrictors, pus may be seen coming from the middle meatus. The latter observation, and periorbital swelling or facial tenderness (when present), are probably the most specific findings in acute sinusitis.

Radiography

Radiography has traditionally been used to determine the presence or absence of sinus disease. Standard radiographic projections include an anteroposterior, a lateral, and an occipitomental view (Waters view). The anteroposterior view is optimal for evaluation of the ethmoid sinuses, and the lateral view is best for the frontal and sphenoid sinuses. The occipitomental view, taken after tilting the chin upward 45 degrees to the horizontal, allows evaluation of the maxillary sinuses. Some radiologists may also add a

submental vertex view to optimize evaluation of the sphenoid sinuses in the older child.

Although much has been written about the frequency of abnormal sinus radiographs in "normal" children, these studies have been flawed either by inattention to the presence of symptoms and signs of respiratory inflammation or by failure to classify abnormal radiographic findings into major (significant) and minor (insignificant) categories (Maresh and Washburn, 1940; Shopfner and Rossi, 1973). A recent report shows that abnormal maxillary sinus radiographs are infrequent in children beyond their first birthday, who are without recent symptoms and signs of respiratory tract inflammation (Kovatch et al., 1984).

The radiographic findings most diagnostic of bacterial sinusitis are the presence of an air-fluid level in, or complete opacification of, the sinus cavities. However, an air-fluid level is an uncommon radiographic finding in children younger than 5 years of age with acute sinusitis. In the absence of an air-fluid level or complete opacification of the sinuses, measuring the degree of mucosal swelling may be useful (Fig. 37–2). If the width of the sinus mucous membrane is at least 5 mm in adults or 4 mm in children, it is probable that the sinus contains pus or will yield a positive bacterial culture (Hamory et al., 1979; Wald et al., 1981). When clinical signs and symptoms suggesting acute sinusitis are accompanied by abnormal maxillary sinus radiographic findings, bacteria will be present in a sinus aspirate 70 per cent of the time (Wald et al., 1981). A normal radiograph suggests but does not prove that a sinus is free from disease.

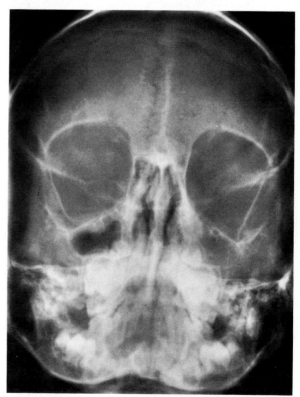

Figure 37–2. Radiograph showing complete opacification of the left maxillary sinus and mucosal thickening of the roof of the right maxillary sinus.

For cases of sinusitis that are complicated by intracranial or intraorbital suppuration, computed tomography (CT) or magnetic resonance imaging (MRI) are helpful procedures. Appropriate coronal and axial scans permit simultaneous evaluation of the central nervous system, orbit, and paranasal sinuses (Fig. 37–3A and B). For patients with allergy to contrast material or those with a vascular occlusion complicating sinusitis, MRI is optimal.

In patients with recurrent or persistent sinusitis, there may be a concern that either a congenital bony defect or a traumatic skeletal deformity is the underlying problem. For these patients, CT imaging procedures are ideal for evaluation of skeletal structures of the paranasal sinuses (Fig. 37–4A and B).

Ultrasonography

Several reports have evaluated ultrasonography as a diagnostic aid in maxillary sinusitis (Revonta, 1979; Mann, 1979). The advantages of ultrasonography as compared with radiography are the use of nonionizing radiation and supposedly better ability to discriminate between mucosal thickening and retained secretions. Conformity between ultrasound findings and those of sinus aspiration has been reported in approximately 90 per cent of patients (Revonta, 1979). To carry out the procedure, an ultrasound probe is held against the cheek in the area of the maxillary sinus. When the

ultrasound beam is reflected from the anterior wall of the sinus, a series of positive deflections is produced, referred to as the anterior wall echo. In an air-filled sinus, only an anterior wall echo is seen (Fig. 37–5A). If the sinus is fluid-filled, the ultrasound beam produces an anterior wall echo and is further transmitted until it hits the posterior or back wall of the sinus cavity, giving rise to a posterior wall echo (Fig. 37–5B). In a study correlating ultrasound and sinus aspiration findings in children, there were occasionally falsely normal ultrasound tracings in children whose sinus aspirates yielded positive cultures and indeterminate patterns in children younger than 4 years of age (Wald et al., 1981).

A recent report, comparing a commercially available A-mode ultrasound and radiographs in a population of allergic children and adults showed a considerable number of sharp discrepancies even when ultrasound tracings and radiographs could be interpreted unambiguously (Shapiro et al., 1986). At present, insufficient experience exists to assess the value of ultrasonography in the diagnosis of sinusitis in children.

Sinus Aspiration

The diagnosis of acute bacterial sinusitis is probably best proved by a biopsy of the sinus mucosa, which demonstrates acute inflammation and invasion by bacteria. In practice, confirmation of the diagnosis is more

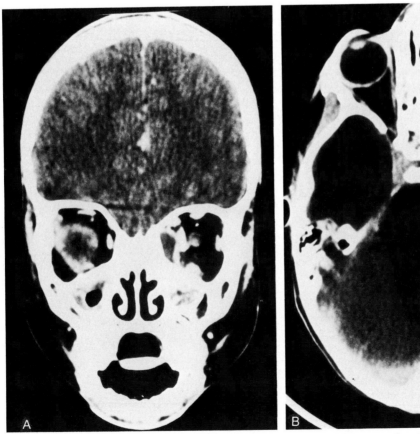

Figure 37–3. Coronal (A) and axial (B) CT scans of the orbit, sinuses, and brain showing a subperiosteal abscess of the right orbit.

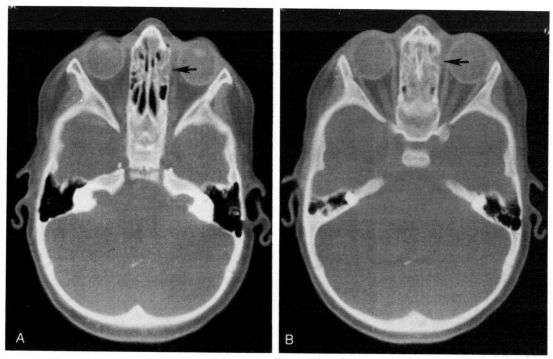

Figure 37–4. *A* and *B*, Axial CT scans in a child with recurrent acute sinusitis and periorbital swelling demonstrating a bony defect in the left ethmoid bone.

often accomplished by culturing an aspirate of sinus secretions. Nonetheless, when simultaneous mucosal biopsies and sinus aspirates are submitted for bacterial cultures, biopsies more often yield positive results.

Although by no means a routine procedure, aspiration of the maxillary sinus (the most accessible of the sinuses) can be accomplished easily in an outpatient setting with minimal discomfort to the patient. Puncture is best performed by the transnasal route, with the needle directed beneath the inferior turbinate through the lateral nasal wall (Fig. 37–6). This route for aspiration is preferred in order to avoid injury to the natural ostium and permanent dentition. If the patient is unusually apprehensive or too young to cooperate, a short-acting narcotic agent can be used for sedation, or the procedure may be performed in the operating room with the patient under general anesthesia.

Careful sterilization of the puncture site is essential to prevent contamination by nasal flora. Four per cent cocaine solution applied intranasally will achieve mucosal anesthesia and antisepsis. Lidocaine should be injected into the submucosa at the site of the actual puncture. Secretions obtained by aspiration should be submitted for Gram stain and quantitative aerobic and anaerobic cultures. Bacterial isolates should be tested for their sensitivity to various antibiotics. A high bacterial colony count assures that the culture results reflect actual sinus infection rather than contamination; counts of greater than 10^4 colony-forming units per milliliter give a high degree of assurance of *in situ* infection. Alternatively, a Gram stain preparation of sinus secretions may be helpful, as bacteria that are

present in low colony count (likely to be contaminants) will usually not be seen on smear.

Indications for sinus aspiration in patients with suspected sinusitis include clinical unresponsiveness to conventional therapy, sinus disease in an immunosuppressed patient, severe symptoms such as headache and facial pain, and life-threatening complications such as intraorbital or intracranial suppuration at the time of clinical presentation.

Microbiology

A knowledge of the bacteriology of secretions obtained directly from the maxillary sinus by needle aspiration (with careful avoidance of contamination from mucosal surfaces) provides essential information to plan antimicrobial therapy.

Whether there is a "normal flora" of the paranasal sinuses is an area of controversy. It is the opinion of some, and there are scant data to support the notion, that the paranasal sinuses are normally sterile. On the other hand, in a study of adults undergoing correction of nasal septal deviation, anaerobic and aerobic bacteria were recovered from all individuals (Brook, 1981). The question here is whether such patients constitute a "normal" population. Septal deviation is a known risk factor for sinusitis, and no radiographs were obtained prior to sinus punctures in these individuals. It will be difficult to resolve this controversy, because the violation of normal sinus cavities can rarely be justified.

The role of anaerobic bacteria as pathogens in sinusitis has only recently been examined with adequate

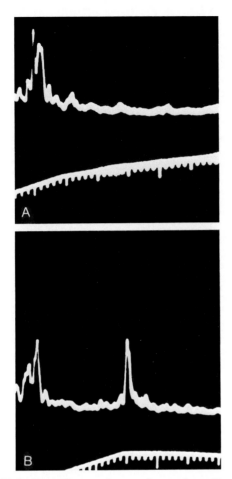

Figure 37–5. *Top,* Ultrasound scan of normal maxillary sinus. *Bottom,* Ultrasound scan of fluid-filled maxillary sinus.

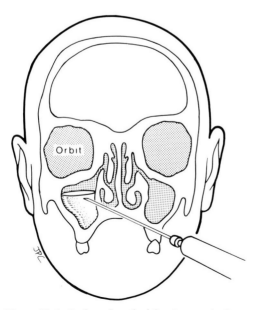

Figure 37–6. Preferred method for sinus aspiration.

attention to anaerobic transport and culture techniques. Poor drainage of the inflamed sinus results in a lower pH and a lower partial pressure of oxygen, thereby providing an excellent environment for the growth of anaerobic bacteria. However, the *in vitro* growth of anaerobic bacteria may be impaired in sinus secretions obtained by irrigation, since this procedure increases the oxygen pressure and dilutes bacterial titers. Finally, few studies have looked for viral agents as a cause of sinus infection, despite evidence that viruses alone may produce acute sinus disease.

Sinus Aspirates

Two elegant studies performed in adults in which careful attention was given to bacteriologic technique, show nontypable *Haemophilus influenzae* and *Streptococcus pneumoniae* to be the most commonly found pathogens, accounting for approximately 74 per cent of all bacterial strains recovered (Hamory et al., 1979; Evans et al., 1975). Anaerobic bacteria accounted for 9 per cent of isolates. Other bacteria implicated include *Branhamella catarrhalis* (formerly *Neisseria catarrhalis*), *Streptococcus pyogenes* (group A *Streptococcus*), and alpha-hemolytic *Streptococcus*. Mixed infection with heavy growth of two bacterial species was occasionally found, although most cultures grew only a single organism. Viruses were recovered from 12 of the 103 positive specimens; there were seven isolates of rhinovirus, three of influenza A, and two of parainfluenza virus. Five of these specimens also had significant growth of bacteria.

A study performed in 50 children with acute maxillary sinusitis has shown the bacteriology of sinus secretions to be similar to that found in adults (Wald et al., 1984). The predominant organisms include *S. pneumoniae, B. catarrhalis,* and nontypable *H. influenzae.* Both *H. influenzae* and *B. catarrhalis* may produce beta-lactamase and, consequently, may be ampicillin-resistant. Of interest, only a single anaerobic isolate, a *Peptostreptococcus* was recovered from sinus secretions during this study. *Staphylococcus aureus* was not isolated from a maxillary sinus aspirate in this series. Several viruses, including adenovirus and parainfluenza, were also recovered (Wald et al., 1981). Summary figures for the incidence of various bacteria in children with acute sinusitis are shown in Table 37–3.

The microbiology of chronic sinusitis has been studied less thoroughly than that of acute sinusitis in both children and adults. Anaerobic bacteria appear to be

TABLE 37–3. Bacteriology of Acute Sinusitis

	INCIDENCE (%)
Streptococcus pneumoniae	25–30
Branhamella catarrhalis	15–20
Haemophilus influenzae	15–20
Streptococcus pyogenes	2–5
Anaerobes	2–5
Sterile	20–35

the predominant pathogens in most studies. The predominant anaerobic organisms are Bacteroides, anaerobic gram-positive cocci, Veillonella, and Fusobacterium (Brook, 1984). The common aerobic organisms isolated include *Streptococcus viridans* and *H. influenzae*. Occasionally, *S. aureus* has been isolated. The discrepancies in the bacterial results of several investigations may be explained by differences in the subjects studied: Some had had chronic sinusitis for many years; others, more probably, had acute exacerbations of a chronic condition.

Surface Cultures

It would be desirable to culture the nose, throat, and nasopharynx in patients with acute sinusitis if the predominant flora isolated from these surface cultures were predictive of the bacterial species recovered from the sinus secretions. It is unfortunate that the results of surface cultures have no predictive value; accordingly, nose, throat, and nasopharyngeal cultures cannot be recommended as guides to the bacteriology and therapy of acute or chronic sinusitis (Wald et al., 1981).

Treatment

Treatment for acute maxillary sinusitis in the preantibiotic era consisted of topical decongestants and analgesics. In severe cases, sinus aspiration was performed. The current availability of numerous antimicrobial agents, to which the bacteria recovered from sinus secretions are susceptible, prompts consideration of antimicrobials as standard treatment of acute sinusitis. The objectives of antimicrobial therapy of acute sinus infection are achievement of a rapid clinical cure, sterilization of the sinus secretions, prevention of suppurative orbital and intracranial complications, and prevention of chronic sinus disease.

Conflicting reports have appeared regarding the efficacy of antimicrobials in the treatment of acute sinus infection in children and adults as judged by radiographic resolution and findings at subsequent irrigation procedures. An array of antimicrobial agents and varying dosage schedules make comparisons between different studies difficult, and discrepancies hard to explain. However, several points emerge:

1. Appropriate antimicrobials eradicate susceptible microorganisms in sinus secretions, whereas inappropriate agents fail to do so (Wald et al., 1984).

2. To accomplish sterilization of the sinus secretions, a level of antimicrobial agent exceeding the minimum inhibitory concentration for the infecting microorganism must be present in the sinus secretions.

3. In some instances in which adequate antimicrobial levels within sinus secretions are reported, sterilization of secretions is still not accomplished. This latter observation points to the importance of local defense mechanisms (such as ciliary activity and phagocytosis) that may be impaired in the altered environ-

ment within purulent sinus secretions (decreased partial pressure of oxygen, increased carbon dioxide pressure, and decreased pH). Accordingly, irrigation and drainage of sinus secretions may be required in some patients.

4. There does appear to be a decreased frequency of serious suppurative orbital and intracranial complications of paranasal sinus disease consequent to the use of systemic antimicrobials.

Antimicrobial Agents

ACUTE AND CHRONIC SINUSITIS. Medical therapy with an antimicrobial agent is recommended in children diagnosed as having acute maxillary sinusitis. The relative frequency of the various bacterial agents suggests that amoxicillin is an appropriate agent for most uncomplicated cases of acute sinusitis (Table 37–4). Amoxicillin is safe, effective, and reasonably priced. Safety is an especially important consideration when treating an infection that has a 40 per cent rate of spontaneous recovery (Wald et al., 1986). The incidence of beta-lactamase–positive, ampicillin-resistant *H. influenzae* and *B. catarrhalis* may vary geographically. In areas where ampicillin-resistant organisms are prevalent, or when the patient is allergic to penicillin, or when the presentation is accompanied by mild periorbital swelling, or when there has been an apparent antibiotic failure, several alternative regimens are available. The combination agent trimethoprim-sulfamethoxazole (Bactrim; Septra) has been shown to be efficacious in acute maxillary sinusitis in adults. However, it is important to remember that this agent may be ineffective in patients with group A streptococcal infections. Cefaclor (Ceclor), and the combination of erythromycin-sulfisoxazole (Pediazole), are also suitable. A combination of amoxicillin and potassium clavulanate (Augmentin) is another potential therapeutic agent for use in patients with beta-lactamase–producing bacterial species in their maxillary sinus secretions. Potassium clavulanate irreversibly binds the beta-lactamase, if present, and thereby restores amoxicillin to its original spectrum of activity.

Patients with acute sinusitis may require hospitalization because of systemic toxicity or inability to take oral antimicrobials. These patients may be treated with cefuroxime at a dosage of 100 to 200 mg/kg/per day, intravenously, in three divided doses.

Clinical improvement is prompt in nearly all chil-

TABLE 37–4. Antimicrobial Agents for Acute Sinusitis

ANTIMICROBIAL	DOSAGE
Amoxicillin	40 mg/kg/day in 3 divided doses
Erythromycin and sulfisoxazole	50/150 mg/kg/day in 4 divided doses
Trimethoprim and sulfamethoxazole	8/40 mg/kg/day in 2 divided doses
Cefaclor	40 mg/kg/day in 3 divided doses
Amoxicillin and potassium clavulanate	40/10 mg/kg/day in 3 divided doses

dren treated with an appropriate antimicrobial agent. Patients febrile at the initial encounter will become afebrile, and there is a remarkable reduction of nasal discharge and cough within 48 hours. If the patient does not improve, or worsens, in 48 hours, clinical reevaluation is appropriate. If the diagnosis is unchanged, sinus aspiration may be considered for precise bacteriologic information. Alternatively, an antimicrobial agent effective against beta-lactamase–producing bacterial species should be prescribed. If the patient fails to respond to a broader-spectrum antimicrobial, a sinus aspiration is necessary to ventilate the sinus cavity and allow specific diagnosis of the etiologic agent.

The antimicrobial regimens recommended to treat acute sinusitis are similar in type and duration to those used to treat acute otitis media. The usual duration of antimicrobial therapy is 10 to 14 days. This recommendation is based on an experience in adults that demonstrated that 20 per cent of sinus aspirates obtained after seven days of antimicrobial treatment still produced positive culture results (Hamory et al., 1979). When the patient's condition has improved but the patient has not completely recovered by 10 or 14 days, it seems reasonable to extend treatment for another one to two weeks.

There are virtually no data available regarding duration of antimicrobial therapy for patients with chronic sinusitis. Many clinicians recommend a minimum course of three to four weeks. Most anaerobes isolated from patients with chronic sinusitis have been penicillin sensitive. All S. viridans and most H. influenzae will be susceptible to amoxicillin. However, there is the potential for the respiratory anaerobes or H. influenzae to produce beta-lactamase and thereby to be amoxicillin resistant. The list of appropriate antimicrobial agents for chronic sinusitis is the same as that for acute sinusitis, unless the patient has already failed to respond to a particular regimen. However, because many patients with chronic sinusitis present with very protracted symptoms, the clinician may wish to initiate therapy with an antimicrobial agent that will be effective against beta-lactamase–producing bacteria from the outset.

RECURRENT ACUTE SINUSITIS. It is not uncommon for some children to have recurrent episodes of acute sinusitis. A definition of recurrent acute sinusitis that may be useful is similar to the one that is used to characterize recurrent acute otitis media, that is, three episodes in six months or four episodes in a year. Most commonly, frequent viral upper respiratory infections, often facilitated by day care arrangements, predispose to such recurrent episodes of acute sinusitis. However, it is appropriate when caring for a child with recurrent acute sinusitis to consider the factors in Table 37–1 that may predispose to ostial obstruction. A careful physical examination will eliminate the mechanical factors that might be etiologic or the presence of an apical tooth abscess. Further evaluation might include a search for upper respiratory allergy, a sweat test for cystic fibrosis, quantitative immunoglobulins including

immunoglobulin G subclasses (and assessment of responsiveness to polysaccharide antigens), and ciliary function tests. If none of these predisposing conditions is present, prophylactic antimicrobials may be helpful. Although this strategy has not been systematically evaluated, extrapolation from experience with recurrent acute otitis media suggests that this therapy might prevent simple upper respiratory infections from becoming complicated by bacterial sinusitis. Appropriate antimicrobials might include amoxicillin or sulfisoxazole as the two principal agents previously assessed for efficacy in recurrent otitis media. The recommended dose is one half the therapeutic dose, given at bedtime. If several clinical episodes occur despite prophylaxis, a broader spectrum antimicrobial such as amoxicillin–potassium clavulanate or erythromycin-sulfisoxazole may be tried. When medical therapy fails to provide control of the problem, a nasal antrostomy should be considered.

Decongestants and Antihistamines

The effectiveness of antihistamines or decongestants or combinations thereof applied topically (by inhalation) or administered by mouth in patients with acute or chronic sinus infection has not been adequately studied. Limited investigation of specific agents in clinical rhinitis has shown that some produce a decrease in nasal resistance. However, a study of patients with sinorhinitis found that oral phenylpropanolamine did not significantly increase the size of the maxillary ostium (Aust et al., 1979).

Topical decongestants such as phenylephrine or oxymetazoline shrink the nasal mucous membrane, improve ostial drainage, and provide symptomatic improvement; however, they may cause ciliostasis. Ciliary motion is an important local defense mechanism; the entire mucous covering of the maxillary antrum is normally cleared every ten minutes. By inhibiting ciliary motion, topical decongestants may delay clearance of infected material. In addition, by decreasing blood flow to the mucosa, topical decongestants may further lower oxygen tension and impair diffusion of antimicrobial agents into the sinuses. The net effect of the various topical preparations on clinical recovery from sinusitis as well as the incidence of complications is unknown.

Irrigation and Drainage

Irrigation and drainage of the infected sinus may result in dramatic relief from pain for patients with acute sinusitis. In addition, with relief of pressure in the sinus, oxygenation and blood flow improve, thus restoring compromised defense mechanisms. Local immunoglobulin and complement levels increase, and proteolytic enzymes decrease in sinus secretions after irrigation procedures. Drainage procedures are usually reserved for those who fail to respond to medical therapy with antimicrobial agents or who have a suppurative intraorbital or intracranial complication. If an episode of acute or chronic sinusitis cannot be effectively treated by medical therapy alone, drainage of the sinus cavity may be required. Several techniques are available. The Proetz displacement method is the simplest of these and can be used when obstruction of the sinus ostium is incomplete (Fig. 37–7). The nose and the nasopharynx are filled with saline while the patient is supine and the head hyperextended. Suction of the nostrils removes the irrigating solution and nasal secretions. As the irrigation is repeated, the sinus ostia are cleaned, and drainage of the sinuses is accomplished. A decongestant solution such as 0.25 per cent phenylephrine in saline may be used as the irrigating solution. When the obstruction of the sinus ostium is complete, then aspiration of the maxillary sinus may be performed as described earlier. In patients with frontal sinusitis who are unresponsive to medical therapy, the frontal sinus may be trephined through the brow or supraorbital rim; isotonic saline may be used for irrigation. If patients do not respond to medical therapy alone or medical therapy with sinus irrigation or aspiration, more radical surgery may become necessary.

Surgical Therapy

The procedure of first choice would be a nasal antrostomy to provide ventilation of the sinus cavity and drainage of maxillary secretions into the nasal chamber (Ritter, 1986). Although the cilia continue to beat toward the natural ostium, when sinus secretions

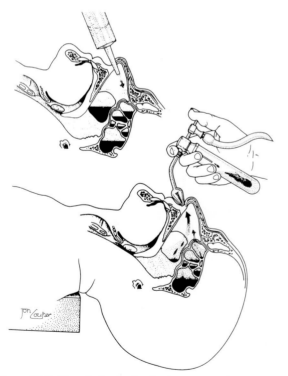

Figure 37–7. Sinus irrigation by the Proetz procedure. *Top,* The nose is first partially filled with normal saline. *Bottom,* The saline is then removed by suction through one nostril while the other nostril is occluded. The intent of the procedure is to irrigate sinuses with partially patent ostia.

are excessive, the presence of the nasal antrostomy facilitates gravitational drainage. This procedure may be helpful in patients with acute sinusitis who fail to respond to antimicrobial treatment and sinus aspiration. Nasal antrostomy may also benefit patients with recurrent acute sinusitis or chronic sinusitis who cannot be successfully managed with antimicrobials and adjunctive medical therapies.

The nasal antrostomy is usually performed with the patient under general anesthesia; submucosal injection of a combination of anesthetic and vasoconstrictor will help control the bleeding. The inferior meatal bone is exposed after elevating a mucosal flap. The bone is penetrated with a punch, and the opening extended to a size of at least 5 × 10 mm. A pack beneath the inferior meatus is used to prevent postoperative bleeding.

In patients with severe and protracted signs and symptoms of sinusitis, a more radical procedure, the Caldwell-Luc procedure, is required to remove the diseased mucosa and create a nasoantral window (Fig. 37–8). Microabscesses beneath the sinus mucosa are presumed to account for the chronic process that is not responsive to more conservative measures (Ritter, 1986). This procedure is contraindicated in children (because of the developing dentition), although it might be performed in late adolescence. The approach is through the anterior wall of the sinus, reached by creating a horizontal incision in the sulcus of the buccal gingiva. In adults, a 2 × 2 cm window is created in the anterior wall of the sinus. All the inflamed mucosa is removed, and a nasal antrostomy is formed. The antrum is usually packed to prevent bleeding. The end of the packing is brought through the antrostomy into the nose, to facilitate removal after a few days.

Ethmoid surgery is rarely indicated in children unless polyposis is present or there is a congenital bony defect between the ethmoid sinuses and the orbit. Frontal sinus surgery is occasionally indicated in adolescents who have developed chronic sinusitis or have had previous facial fractures involving the frontal sinus.

Odontogenic Sinusitis

The floor of the maxillary sinus is formed by the alveolar process of the maxillary bone. After birth, as the alveolar process and the sinus develop, the roots of the teeth and the sinus come into close proximity, at times separated only by paper-thin bone or sinus mucosa. Because of this proximity, periapical abscesses or periodontitis of the upper teeth may extend into the sinus cavity and cause maxillary sinusitis (Chow et al., 1978). Perforation may occur from minor trauma to the area, dental instrumentation, or extraction or displacement of a chronically inflamed tooth. Congenital bony defects or dental cysts may provide a direct channel to the sinus, thus eliminating the need to traverse bone. If perforation of the sinus mucosa is not

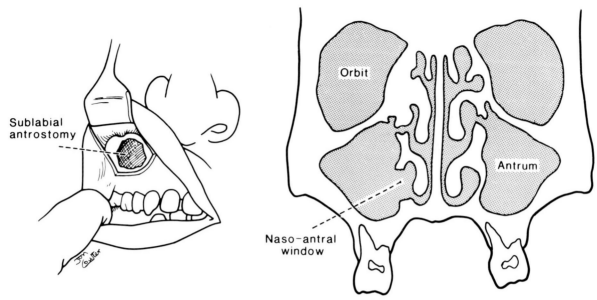

Figure 37–8. Caldwell-Luc procedure.

recognized, the tract may become epithelialized and an oroantral fistula may form.

The incidence of odontogenic sinusitis in children is unknown but is probably significant, particularly in adolescents. In adults, 10 to 15 per cent of all cases of maxillary sinusitis are thought to be of dental origin.

Symptoms are similar to those of primary sinusitis. A fetid odor may be prominent because the infection is often caused by anaerobic organisms. If an oroantral fistula is present, the patient may complain that pus is dripping into the mouth; fluids and air may pass from the oral cavity into the sinus and nose. Treatment consists of drainage of the dental abscess and operative closure of the oroantral fistula, if present, coupled with antimicrobial therapy (Chow et al., 1978).

Allergy and Sinusitis

Individuals with atopic disease, either allergic rhinitis or asthma, have an increased frequency of sinusitis. The nasal and sinus mucosa of these patients are hypersecretory. Histologically, there is mucosal hyperplasia and infiltration with plasma cells and eosinophils. Secondary to this immune-mediated hyperplastic sinusitis, ostial obstruction followed by bacterial infection is common. This may result in acute exacerbations of respiratory symptoms (particularly cough and rhinorrhea) or in difficulty in controlling symptoms (nasal congestion and wheezing) with usual therapy.

Maxillary sinus aspirates obtained from asthmatic children with exacerbations of asthma despite bronchodilator therapy show bacterial isolates similar to those obtained from nonasthmatic children with acute sinusitis (Friedman et al., 1984). Clinical symptoms and pulmonary function improve after antibiotic therapy. Selection of antimicrobial agents in the treatment of an infectious episode in the atopic individual is not different from treatment of the nonallergic child with sinusitis, except that duration of therapy may need to be continued beyond 14 days.

Fungal Sinusitis

Fungal sinusitis can take several different clinical forms and may occur in compromised or otherwise healthy individuals. The compromised subgroup may include immunosuppressed, debilitated, or otherwise impaired patients who have malignancies or diabetes or who are receiving cytotoxic drugs. Depending on the particular fungus involved and the site of infection, this may be a terminal event.

In contrast, previously healthy patients may be infected with fungi and do rather well. The most common example is sinusitis caused by *Aspergillus*. Patients with this infection usually present with unilateral infection of the maxillary sinus after long-standing sinus symptoms (Stevens, 1978). A similar disease process may be caused by *Alternaria, Petriellidium, Paecilomyces,* or *Bipolaris,* all common soil organisms (Shuger et al., 1981; Bryan et al., 1980; Rowley and Strom, 1982; Frankel et al., 1987). Chronic disease and local invasion are the hallmarks of infection. Occasionally, death results from local extension of the infectious process into the central nervous system.

Another form of chronic sinus infection is an allergic sinusitis caused by aspergillosis. This manifestation of infection is similar to allergic bronchopulmonary aspergillosis. The patients usually have asthma or other evidence of atopy. Their sinus symptoms are very protracted, and characteristically more than one sinus is involved. The distinguishing feature, on histologic analysis of the sinus secretions, is degenerated eosinophils, Charcot-Leyden crystals, and an occasional fungal form on a pale amorphous background of mucin

(Katzenstein et al., 1983). Treatment with steroids is speculated to be helpful but has not been carefully studied.

A similar picture of allergylike fungal sinusitis has also recently been reported to be due to *Myriodontium keratinophilum* (Maran et al., 1985). The patient presented with chronic sinusitis, recurrent nasal polyps, and finally proptosis. The latter was due to progressive local invasion of the roof of the orbit and the ethmoid air cells. Treatment was accomplished with amphotericin and drainage.

In cases of long-standing sinus symptoms, fungal infection must be suspected. Appropriate specimens of sinus secretions and mucosal biopsies are required for definitive diagnosis. Surgical débridement is virtually always necessary for treatment and, on occasion, is sufficient, particularly in previously healthy persons. On the other hand, in patients with underlying diseases, systemic antifungals (usually amphotericin) are the recommended adjunct to aggressive local surgical débridement.

ANNOTATED REFERENCES

Rachelefsky, G. S., Katz, R. M., and Siegel, S. C. 1982. Diseases of the paranasal sinuses in children. Curr. Probl. Pediatr. 12:1.
   A very comprehensive review of sinus disease in children, with emphasis on allergic problems.
Carson, J. L., Collier, A. M., and Shi-Chin, S. H. 1985. Acquired ciliary defects in nasal epithelium of children with acute viral upper respiratory infections. N. Engl. J. Med. 312:463.
   An important study demonstrating nasal epithelial injury during uncomplicated viral upper respiratory tract infections. These findings may explain predisposition to secondary bacterial infection in the paranasal sinuses.
Gwaltney, J. M., Jr. 1985. Virology and immunology of the common cold. Rhinology 23:265.
   An extensive review of the etiology and immunology of the common cold.
Wald, E. R., Chiponis, D., and Ledesma-Medina, J. 1986. Comparative effectiveness of amoxicillin and amoxicillin clavulanate potassium in acute paranasal sinus infections in children: A double-blind, placebo-controlled trial. Pediatrics 77:795.
   An important study highlighting the natural history of treated and untreated paranasal sinus infection in children.
Bluestone, C., Wald, E. R., Shapiro, G. G., et al. 1985. The diagnosis and management of sinusitis in children: Proceedings of a closed conference. Pediatr. Infect. Dis. 4:549.
   A comprehensive review and consensus from a multidisciplinary panel.

REFERENCES

Aschan, G. 1974. Decongestion of nasal mucous membranes by oral medication in acute rhinitis. Acta Otolaryngol. 77:433.
Aust, R., Drettner, B., and Falck, B. 1979. Studies of the effect of peroral phenylpropanolamine on the functional size of the human maxillary ostium. Acta Otolaryngol. 88:455.
Beem, M. O. 1969. Acute respiratory illness in nursery school children: A longitudinal study of the occurrence of illness and respiratory viruses. Am. J. Epidemiol. 90:30.
Beem, M. O., and Saxon, E. M. 1977. Respiratory-tract colonization and a distinctive pneumonia syndrome in infants infected with *Chlamydia trachomatis*. N. Engl. J. Med. 296:306.
Brook, I. 1984. Bacteriologic features of chronic sinusitis in children. J.A.M.A. 246:967.

Brook, I. 1981. Aerobic and anaerobic bacterial flora of normal maxillary sinuses. Laryngoscope 91:372.
Bryan, C. S., Disalvo, A. F., Kaufman, L., et al. 1980. *Petriellidium boydii* infection of the sphenoid sinus. Am. J. Clin. Pathol. 74:846.
Carson, J. L., Collier, A. M., and Shi-Chen, S. H. 1985. Acquired ciliary defects in nasal epithelium of children with acute viral upper respiratory infections. N. Engl. J. Med. 312:463.
Chow, A., Roser, S., and Brady, F. 1978. Orofacial odontogenic infections. Ann. Intern. Med. 88:392.
Couch, R. B. 1984. The common cold: Control? J. Infect. Dis. 150:167.
Dick, E. C., Hossain, S. U., Mink, K. A., et al. 1986. Interruption of transmission of rhinovirus colds among human volunteers using virucidal paper handkerchiefs. J. Infect. Dis. 153:352.
Dingle, J. H., Badjer, D. F., and Jordan, W. S., Jr. 1964. Patterns of illness. Illness in the Home. Cleveland, Western Reserve University, p. 347.
Douglas, R. M., Moore, B. W., Miles, H. B., et al. 1986. Prophylactic efficacy of intranasal alpha₂ interferon against rhinovirus infections in the family setting. N. Engl. J. Med. 315:65.
Drettner, B. 1980. Pathophysiology of paranasal sinuses with clinical implications. Clin. Otolaryngol. 5:272.
Evans, R. D., Jr., Sydnor, J. B., Moore, W. E. C., et al. 1975. Sinusitis of the maxillary antrum. N. Engl. J. Med. 293:735.
Frankel, L., Kuhls, T. L., Nitta, K., et al. 1987. Recurrent *Bipolaris* sinusitis following surgical and antifungal therapy. Pediatr. Infect. Dis. 6:1130.
Freidman, R., Ackerman, M., Wald, E., et al. 1984. Asthma and bacterial sinusitis in children. J. Allergy Immunol. 74:185.
Gwaltney, J. M., Jr., Hendley, J. O., and Mygind, N. 1984. Symposium on rhinovirus pathogenesis: Summary. Acta Otolaryngol. 413:43.
Gwaltney, J. M., Jr. 1985. Virology and immunology of the common cold. Rhinology 23:265.
Gwaltney, J. M., Jr., Sydnor, A., Jr., and Sande, M. A. 1981. Etiology and antimicrobial treatment of acute sinusitis. Ann. Otol. Rhinol. Laryngol. 90:68.
Gwaltney, J. B., Jr., and Hendley, J. O. 1982. Transmission of experimental rhinovirus infection by contaminated surfaces. Am. J. Epidemiol. 116:828.
Hall, C. B., and Douglas, R. G., Jr. 1981. Modes of transmission of respiratory syncytial virus. J. Pediatr. 99:100.
Hamory, B. H., Sande, M. A., and Sydnor, A., Jr., et al. 1979. Etiology and antimicrobial therapy of acute maxillary sinusitis. J. Infect. Dis. 39:197.
Hayden, F. G., and Gwaltney, J. M., Jr. 1982. Prophylactic activity of intranasal enviroxime against experimentally induced rhinovirus type 39 infection. Antimicrob. Agents Chemother. 21:892.
Hayden, F. G., Albrecht, J. K., Kaiser, D. L., et al. 1986. Prevention of natural colds by contact prophylaxis with intranasal alpha₂-interferon. N. Engl. J. Med. 314:71.
Karmody, C. S., Carter, B., and Vincent, M. E. 1977. Developmental anomalies of the maxillary sinus. Trans. Am. Acad. Ophthalmol. Otolaryngol. 84:723.
Katzenstein, A., Sale, S. R., and Greenberger, P. A. 1983. Pathologic findings in allergic Aspergillus sinusitis. Am. J. Surg. Pathol. 7:439.
Kovatch, A. L., Wald, E. R., Ledesma-Medina, J., et al. 1984. Maxillary sinus radiographs in children with non-respiratory complaints. Pediatrics 73:306.
Krugman, S., Katz, S. L., Gershon, A. A., et al. 1985. Infectious Diseases of Children, 8th ed. St. Louis, C. V. Mosby Co.
Levandowski, R. A., Pachucki, C. T., Rubenis, M. 1982. Topical enviroxime against rhinovirus infection. Antimicrob. Agents Chemother. 22:1004.
Mann, W. 1979. Diagnostic ultrasonography in paranasal sinus diseases: A 5-year review. ORL 41:168.
Maran, A. G. D., Kwong, K., Mine, L. J. R., et al. 1985. Frontal sinusitis caused by *Myriodontium keratinophilum*. Br. Med. J. 290:207.
Maresh, M., and Washburn, A. H. 1940. Paranasal sinuses from birth to late adolescence. II. Clinical and roentgenographic evidence of infection. Am. J. Dis. Child. 60:841.
Naclerio, R., Gwaltney, J., Hendley, O., et al. 1985. Preliminary observations in rhinovirus-induced colds. *In* Myers, E. N. (ed.):

New Dimensions in Otorhinolaryngology—Head and Neck Surgery, Vol. 2. New York, Elsevier, p. 341.

Ohashi, Y., and Nakai, Y. 1983. Functional and morphological pathology of chronic sinusitis mucous membrane. Acta Otolaryngol. 397:11.

Powers, G. F., and Boivert, P. D. 1944. Age as a factor in streptococcosis. J. Pediatr. 25:481.

Rachelefsky, G. S., Katz, R. M., and Siegel, S. C. 1982. Diseases of paranasal sinuses in children. Curr. Probl. Pediatr. 12:1.

Reimer, A., von Mecklenburg, C., and Tormalm, N. G. 1978. The mucociliary activity of the upper respiratory tract. III: A functional and morphological study of human and animal material with special reference to maxillary sinus disease. Acta Otolaryngol. (Stockh.) 355:3.

Revonta, M. 1979. A-mode ultrasound of maxillary sinusitis in children. Lancet 1:320.

Ritter, F. N. 1973. The Paranasal Sinuses: Anatomy and Surgical Technique. St. Louis, C. V. Mosby Co.

Ritter, F. N. 1986. Surgical management of paranasal sinusitis. Otolaryngol. Head Neck Surg. 1:937.

Roth, R. P., Cantekin, E., Bluestone, C. D., et al. 1977. Nasal decongestant activity of pseudoephedrine. Ann. Otol. Rhinol. Laryngol. 86:235.

Rowley, S. D., and Strom, C. G. 1982. Paecilomyces fungus infection of the maxillary sinus. Laryngoscope 92:332.

Shapiro, G. G., Furukawa, C. T., Person, W. E., et al. 1986. Blinded comparison of maxillary sinus radiography and ultrasound for diagnosis of sinusitis. J. Allergy Clin. Immunol. 77:59.

Shopfner, C. E., and Rossi, J. O. 1973. Roentgen evaluation of the paranasal sinuses in children. A.J.R. 118:176.

Shugar, M. A., Montgomery, W. W., and Hyslop, N. E. 1981. Alternaria sinusitis. Ann. Otol. 90:251.

Stagno, S., Brasfield, D. M., Brown, M. B., et al. 1981. Infant pneumonitis associated with cytomegalovirus, Chlamydia, Pneumocystis, and Ureaplasma: A prospective study. Pediatrics 68:322.

Stevens, M. H. 1978. Aspergillosis of the frontal sinus. Arch. Otolaryngol. 104:153.

Tomassini, J. E., and Colonno, R. J. 1986. Isolation of a receptor protein involved in attachment of human rhinoviruses. J. Virol. 58:290.

Turner, R. B., Hendley, J. O., Gwaltney, J. M., Jr. 1982. Shedding of infected ciliated epithelial cells in rhinovirus colds. J. Infect. Dis. 145:846.

Wald, E. R., Milmoe, G. J., Bowen, A., et al. 1981. Acute maxillary sinusitis in children. N. Engl. J. Med. 304:749.

Wald, E. R., Reilly, J. S., Casselbrant, M., et al. 1984. Treatment of acute maxillary sinusitis in children: A comparative study of amoxicillin and cefaclor. J. Pediatr. 104:297.

Wald, E. R., Chiponis, D., and Ledesma-Medina, J. 1986. Comparative effectiveness of amoxicillin and amoxicillin–clavulanate potassium in acute paranasal sinus infections in children: A double-blind, placebo-controlled trial. Pediatrics 77:795.

Winther, B., Gwaltney, J. M., Jr., Mygind, N., et al. 1986. Sites of rhinovirus recovery after point inoculation of the upper airway. J.A.M.A. 256:1763.

Chapter 38

COMPLICATIONS OF NASAL AND SINUS INFECTIONS

Daniel D. Rabuzzi, M.D.   Arthur S. Hengerer, M.D.

The treatment of complications of nasal and paranasal sinus infections remains a significant portion of the practice of pediatric medicine. This is often true, despite the early and judicious use of antibiotic therapy. However, with the advent of antibiotics, the total number of these complications has been dramatically reduced over the years, and the average practitioner today may not be as well versed as older colleagues in the early recognition of, and therapy for, these problems.

The physician can make the proper diagnosis only if he or she knows the presenting characteristics of these complications and looks for them. It is the purpose of this chapter to provide an overview of such nasal and paranasal sinus infection complications so the reader will be more attuned to their accurate diagnosis and treatment (Table 38–1).

NASAL INFECTION COMPLICATIONS

A child's nose is a prominent structure of facial anatomy, exposed to frequent blunt trauma. Coupling that fact with the known specific nasal diseases, it is then quickly appreciated why the fragile, pseudostratified, ciliated, columnar epithelium of the nasal mucosa is so frequently disturbed and prone to complications of infection.

Synechiae

Physiologic function of the normal nasal mucosa with its cyclic swelling allows opposing surfaces within the nasal cavity to contact one another. If, as a result of inflammatory, traumatic, or iatrogenic causes, a raw surface of granulating tissue exists, a fibroblastic matrix may be laid down along these opposing surfaces. Consequently, bands of scar tissue, so-called synechiae, will then be formed, stretching between any two anatomic structures within the nasal vault.

Once formed, the complications of mechanical blockage from these bands of scar tissue will occur, with altered air currents and interference with the proper physiologic flow of the "mucous blanket." This may result in a chronic rhinorrhea and a change in the viscosity and the amount of postnasal drainage. Posterior pharyngeal irritation and possibly eustachian tube inflammation may be a result of this. Moreover, metaplastic changes in the nasal mucosa can occur with concomitant crusting, ulceration, and bleeding in the area anterior to the synechial formation. Synechiae located in the lateral aspects of the nose, between the turbinates and the floor of the nose, may alter normal sinus drainage from the hiatus semilunaris or from surgically created nasoantral windows. This occurrence could lead to an obstructive sinusitis.

Lysis of the synechial bands is usually corrective, providing the raw surfaces are allowed to heal unopposed. This is best accomplished by the use of Teflon sheets placed within the nasal vault between the lateral wall of the nose and the nasal septum. These sheets are sutured through-and-through to the nasal septum to allow them to stay in position for a 10- to 14-day period.

Septal Hematoma and Abscess

Septal hematoma, abscess, or both from nasal trauma or recurrent nasal and paranasal sinus infection is one of the most feared complications because of the significant cosmetic and functional sequelae that may result. Saddle nose deformity, nasal airway obstruction, nasal septal perforation, and extension of infection into paranasal or even intracranial structures all are problems that have occurred as complications of septal hematoma and abscesses. When the hematoma develops, the septal mucosa is erythematous and swollen, often touching the turbinates or lateral nasal wall. The swelling is doughy in consistency and may be quite tender. Depending on whether or not there is a communication within the cartilaginous septum, the hematoma or abscess cavity may be either unilateral or bilateral. This fact may be determined by direct visual examination and palpation. If only unilateral involvement exists, the likelihood of permanent complications is somewhat lessened because of the persistent nourishment to the cartilage through the opposite nasal mucoperichondrium.

Once recognized, a septal hematoma or abscess must be treated by adequate incision and drainage with

TABLE 38–1. Complications of Nasal and Sinus Infections

LOCAL
Synechiae
Polyps
Osteomyelitis
Septal hematomas
Septal abscesses
Mucoceles
Pyoceles

ORBITAL
Cellulitis
Abscesses

INTRACRANIAL
Meningitis
Brain abscesses
Epidural
Subdural
Cavernous sinus thrombosis

SYSTEMIC
Lower respiratory diseases
Chronic bronchitis
Bronchiectasis

wide opening of the tissue planes. This will require the use of general anesthesia in most children. The cavity should be packed lightly with one quarter inch iodoform gauze, and the patient should be placed on appropriate intravenous antibiotic therapy. High-dose penicillin is the initial drug of choice in these instances and should be given unless culture reports of the abscess drainage indicate the presence of resistant organisms. Recently, there has been a trend toward the use of antibiotics such as nafcillin to protect against penicillinase-resistant organisms. When the treatment is not given early enough or when results are ineffective, additional significant complications can develop.

The interruption of the septal cartilage blood supply by the hematoma or abscess may result in eventual cartilage necrosis and resorption. An anterior septal perforation of varying size often develops in this necrotic area and will usually persist. The margins of these perforations often contain exposed cartilage edges and areas of granulation tissue, which maintain a superficial infection of saprophytic organisms. This, and the dryness caused by the irregular air currents passing through the perforation, will cause mucosal crusting and the subjective sensation of nasal obstruction. These crusts need to be removed frequently, a process often accompanied by bleeding, which at times may be quite significant. The child's annoyance with such crusting will often lead to habitual nose picking, with resulting perforation enlargement. Depending on the size of the perforation, a "whistling" sound may also be created by nasal breathing, which is quite aggravating to child and parent alike. Repairs of such perforations by the use of various mucosal flaps or connective tissue grafts are satisfactory only if the perforation is less than 1 cm in diameter.

Further septal cartilage necrosis can cause collapse of all septal support, with concomitant airway obstruction. Such collapse will alter the shape of the nasal vault, specifically in the so-called "valve" area between the septum and the upper lateral cartilage, which is considered so important to the patient's awareness of nasal airflow. Similarly, the same collapse will also create the cosmetic deformity known as saddle nose. This external collapse may appear immediately if the cartilage loss is severe, or it may develop gradually with increasing age as a result of the loss or possibly from the alteration in the growth centers with maturity. Conservative repair of such a functional and cosmetic deformity need not wait until the child reaches maturity, but should be instituted 6 to 12 months after the active disease process has been controlled.

More serious complications secondary to septal cartilage infection are the effects of intracranial extension and abscesses. Since the angular veins between the nose and the midportion of the face are without intraluminal valves, direct extension of infection into them may allow early development of septicemia and involvement of the cavernous sinus, meninges, and bony cranial vault. These complications will be surveyed later.

PARANASAL SINUS INFECTION COMPLICATIONS

Aside from the children suffering from generalized metabolic or inherited defects such as diabetes, cystic fibrosis, and aplastic anemias, chronic sinus infections are relatively rare in children younger than 16 years of age. This is in marked contrast to statistics for adults, in whom acute and chronic infections occur without associated systemic disease (Table 38–2). In children, complications of acute sinus infections seem to occur more frequently than among the general adult population. These complications can be divided into those with local spread, those with intracranial involvement, and those with systemic symptoms.

The complications that do ensue from acute and chronic sinus disease in children are linked directly to the anatomic relationship of the paranasal sinuses to other structures of the head, neck, and chest. These relationships are surprisingly constant (see Chapters 28 and 36). Most commonly involved are the structures of the orbit, cranial vault, chest, and nares.

Orbital Complications

The discussion of this topic at this time in medical history has been radically changed by the advent of antibiotics. For this reason, the previously defined classifications of the step-by-step development of the spread of sinus infections to other areas is no longer classic. The recent classification by Schramm and colleagues (1982) seems most practical (Table 38–3). The local, direct extension of disease causing the orbital complications is the result of several distinct factors limited to the facial structures of childhood. These influencing tendencies are the thinner bony septa of

TABLE 38–2. General Trends in Sinusitis

	ASSOCIATED ILLNESS	ACUTE INFECTION	CHRONIC INFECTION	COMPLICATIONS
Children	+	+ + +	+/−	+
Adults	−	+/−	+ + +	+/−

the sinus walls, larger vascular foramina, more porous bones, and open suture lines.

The paper-thin bony plates separating the ethmoid and maxillary sinuses from the orbit allow infection to spread to the orbit in this age group particularly (Bernstein, 1971). With ethmoid sinusitis, the thickened, inflamed mucosa obstructs drainage into the nose, and when pus under pressure develops, this leads to necrosis of the lamina papyracea by interrupting the periosteal blood supply. Contiguous and vascular spread of infection from the ethmoid labyrinth into the orbit will first produce edema and erythema of the eyelids, especially in their upper medial quadrants. Similarly, spread of infection from the maxillary antra will particularly cause lower lid swelling. From this stage, unless it is aggressively treated, it can rapidly progress to an orbital cellulitis. When that occurs, there is usually an increase in body temperature, tenderness over the lids increases markedly, and the globe itself may show some forward protrusion. Usually, extraocular mobility is present but limited, and some chemosis of the conjunctiva may be seen. Even at this stage, hospitalization and intravenous antibiotic therapy, along with topical nasal decongestants, will often abort any further progression of symptoms. Since the most virulent pathogens tend to be *Haemophilus influenzae* and penicillinase-resistant *Staphylococcus*, ampicillin or chloramphenicol and nafcillin would be the combined drugs of choice (Haynes and Cramblett, 1967; Watters et al., 1976). However, as this therapy is instituted, investigations must commence to rule out either a subperiosteal abscess or an intraorbital abscess. At the time of admission, a clinical evaluation permits the classification of the child into one of the six groups listed in Table 38–3. If the patient falls in group 1 or 2, periorbital cellulitis with or without chemosis, and has no proptosis or decreased eye movements, then antibiotics without an immediate CT scan are appropriate. If there is a lack of clinical improvement or progression of the infection, a CT scan is necessary by 24 hours after initiating treatment. When the patient presents with significant proptosis, limitation of eye movements, or vision change, a CT

TABLE 38–3. Classification of Orbital Complications

Periorbital cellulitis (PC)
Periorbital cellulitis with chemosis (PCC)
Orbital cellulitis (OC)
Subperiosteal abscess (SPA)
Orbital abscess (OA)
Cavernous sinus thrombosis (CST)

From Schramm, V. V., Carter, H. D., and Kennerdell, J. S. 1982. Evaluation of orbital cellulitis and results of treatment. Laryngoscope 92:732.

scan should be obtained immediately. The CT scan cuts should include the brain to rule out an early frontal lobe abscess, as well as the ethmoid and maxillary sinuses.

The new generation of CT scanners offer high-resolution images of the orbit and greatly assist the clinician in monitoring and deciding the appropriate therapy. Magnetic resonance imaging (MRI) provides even further detail of the orbit with coronal images, but whether MRI surpasses the information obtained from the CT scans remains to be seen. One of the drawbacks of MRI is the absence of bone detail.

Studies have shown that the most difficult differentiation in these cases is between orbital cellulitis and a subperiosteal abscess (Table 38–4). The significance of this is that the former group usually responds to medical therapy, whereas the latter requires surgical drainage. If the necessary surgical drainage is deferred, dire consequences, including possible permanent vision loss, can ensue.

Should such radiologic innovations not be available to the clinician, the progressive symptoms that suggest purulent abscess formation are increasing edema and lid erythema with the inability to close the eye completely, marked orbital chemosis, proptosis of the eye either straight forward or in the down-and-out position (depending on the site of abscess), further diminution of extraocular motion, and loss of visual acuity. These findings should, of course, be verified by a consulting ophthalmologist. Whatever the set of diagnostic circumstances, be they purely radiologic, purely clinical, or a combination of both, once the diagnosis of periorbital abscess is decided on, surgical intervention must be carried out (Maniglia et al., 1984).

The proper method of draining a periorbital abscess is through an external ethmoidectomy skin incision midway between the inner canthus of the eye and the midnasal dorsum. The procedure is performed with the patient under general anesthesia with the use of a local anesthetic, with epinephrine (1:200,000) infiltrated into the skin for its vasoconstrictor effect. A layer dissection should be carried out down to and through the periosteum, as this will aid immeasurably in precluding inadvertent cutting of the angular vein and concomitant heavy bleeding. The elevation of the periosteum over the nasal projection of the maxillary bone and lamina papyracea of the medial wall of the orbit may expose the ethmoid sinus through a necrotic bony defect. If a subperiosteal abscess is present, it is rapidly drained. In addition to the abscess drainage, a partial ethmoidectomy should then be performed to remove diseased tissue, although without attempting a complete and meticulous dissection of all mucosa. Should a subperiosteal abscess not be found or should

TABLE 38–4. Accuracy of Diagnostic Modalities in Determining Treatment of Orbital Complications

		FALSE (−)	FALSE (+)	ACCURACY (%)
CLINICAL CLASSIFICATION	**AGREEMENT**			
PCC	10	0	0	100
OC	13	11	0	54
SPA	2	0	2	50
OA	1	0	0	100
Totals: 39	26	11	2	67
CT SCAN CLASSIFICATION				
PCC	9	0	0	100
OC	9	5	0	65
SPA	6	0	0	100
OA	2	0	0	100
Totals: 31	26	5	0	84

Data from Gutowski, M., Mulbury, P. E., and Hengerer, A. S. 1988. The use of CT scanning in the management of orbital cellulitis. Int. J. Pediatr. Otol. 15:117–128.

the CT scan have shown an orbital abscess, the periorbita must be incised and the intraorbital abscess found and drained. The wound is then closed in layers with one small drain from the incision line and another placed intranasally through the middle meatus into the cleaned ethmoid sinus. If the maxillary sinus is the source of the orbital complication, drainage should be done either through the inferior meatus or via the anterior maxillary bony wall with a spinal needle. This technique is discussed elsewhere in this chapter. Once the drainage has been accomplished and adequate chemotherapy is continued, resolution of the fever and associated symptoms is usually dramatic.

Unhalted infection and retrograde venous thrombophlebitis via the nasal and angular veins that surround the ethmoid labyrinth and orbital structures can ultimately spread to cause cavernous sinus thrombosis (Price et al., 1971) (Fig. 38–1). This devastating complication is diagnosed mainly by its orbital signs consisting of lid edema, erythema, and chemosis (which is most often present bilaterally). In addition, the paresis of the extraocular muscles innervated by the oculomotor, abducens, or trochlear nerve may be present, which eventually leads to a complete ophthalmoplegia. The body temperature is usually quite high from the marked toxicity and septic emboli, which cause the "picket fence" fever spikes. Massive antibiotic therapy, and more recently the adjunctive use of anticoagulants such as heparin, have improved the survival rates for these children.

A special comment should be made here regarding the sequelae of facial pain and headache that occur from the orbital complications and their further progression to intracranial areas. From the onset of sinus infection, some degree of discomfort is noted by all patients. Initially, it is the sense of congestion and pressure within the nasal region that can create the associated complaint of facial pressure and temporal region headache. As the step-by-step progression of the infection occurs, there is a shifting in location and intensity of pain. Once the orbital structures become involved, a severe, deep-seated pain behind the eyes develops, and with attempted eye movement aggravation of this pain occurs. If only the orbit is involved, the pain remains unilateral and is associated with headache, which may be localized or diffuse. The headache is due to the pus under pressure as well as to the localized vascular changes. With cavernous sinus involvement, the pain becomes more deeply placed in the center of the head. The headache is also severe, as the sinus thrombosis and the venous pressure increase throughout the intracranial vessels.

Clinically, patients' responses to this worsening pain are likely to be altered by the obtunded state that frequently accompanies the condition. Therefore, if the patient is severely toxic, there may be no real awareness of headache or facial pain.

Intracranial Complications

Intracranial spread of infection from the frontal, ethmoid, or sphenoid sinuses can produce further complications, such as meningeal irritation and infection, brain abscess, and peridural abscess. As mentioned earlier in the chapter, one of the most important benefits of the CT scan in evaluating sinus complications is the ability to detect early central nervous system (CNS) complications. These include epidural abscess, cerebritis, or a brain abscess in the silent areas of the frontal lobes. As experts gain more information and experience with MRI, further strides in early diagnosis are probable. However, clinical experience and interpretation will still be required to determine which of these studies and treatments are indicated and when. These problems should be managed by a multidisciplinary team composed of a pediatrician, a neurologist or a neurosurgeon, and an otolaryngologist.

The early and widespread use of antibiotics has caused osteomyelitis of the frontal or maxillary bones to become quite a rare entity, but it still may be seen

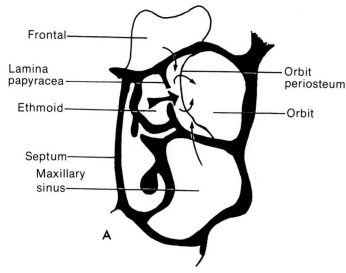

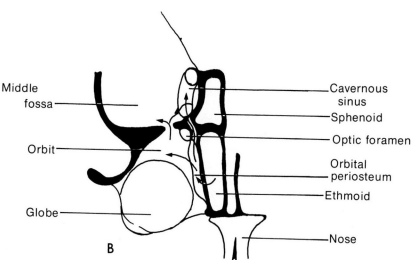

Figure 38–1. *A*, Spread of infection from sinuses to the orbit. *B*, Spread of infection from orbit to cavernous sinus.

in neglected patients or, more commonly, in under-treated patients. In infants and children, it is the spongy bone over the anterior wall of the maxilla that is usually infected, producing erythema, edema, and marked tenderness with swelling. Since the frontal sinus does not develop until the age of 6 years or older, complications of bony spread of sinus infection over the frontal area will not occur except in the older age group. The signs are similar in that swelling over the sinus, particularly with periosteal edema, is present. This often produces a "doughy" feeling to the skin over the affected area ("Pott's puffy tumor"). The patient should be treated with intravenous antibiotics and opening of the periosteum over the affected area to evacuate any collection of pus with insertion of drains. When surgery is performed, removal of only the obviously unhealthy and irreversibly diseased bone should be done. Long-term postoperative intravenous antibiotic therapy of two to three weeks' duration, followed by another six weeks of oral medication, has been found to allow resorption and regeneration of infected bone to the point that the surgeon can afford to be somewhat more conservative in his or her

management than previously (Small and Dale, 1984). The best possible surgical approach is through a non-infected area; thus, a coronal incision and elevation of a scalp flap are ideal procedures for frontal sinus work. However, one is obliged to use a buccal incision for the maxilla, despite the obviously contaminated field. It is fortunate that this has not seemed to have been a deterrent to rapid healing.

Meningeal inflammation secondary to the spread of infection from the nasal regions into the cranial vault will cause pain in the head and neck region, lethargy, fever, and nuchal rigidity. The pain in these patients is most often a diffuse, intense headache due to involvement of the meninges. The pain increases when the head is lowered to a dependent position or when the venous pressure is increased by coughing, crying, or straining. The same pathologic changes in the meninges are responsible for the pain created by head movement, especially neck flexion when done to demonstrate the rigidity. This occurs because of the stretching of the inflamed meninges and nerve roots, and is known as a positive Kernig sign.

If this is suspected, a spinal tap for examination of

cerebrospinal fluid must be done, and the patient must be hospitalized for administration of high doses of intravenous antibiotics (Brook and Kriedman, 1982). The response to this therapy is usually quite satisfactory once the offending organism has been identified and adequately treated. Brain and peridural abscesses tend to produce a somewhat more chronic and quiet symptom complex, which causes their diagnosis to be made relatively late in their course. This is especially true when the lesion is in the frontal lobe, where clinical findings are minimal. Therefore, in anyone complaining of deep headaches, difficulty in concentrating, and general lethargy who also has an unresolved sinus problem, the clinician's responsibility is to rule out an intracranial problem (Blumenfeld and Skolnik, 1966). In these patients, the CT scan has been an invaluable diagnostic tool, for it allows a noninvasive technique to be used for intracranial diagnostic purposes. If a brain abscess is discovered, it should be managed by a neurosurgeon. Later sinus surgery may be necessary for removal of residual intrasinus disease, but this is very rare in children.

Polyps and Mucoceles

The finding of nasal polyps in the prepubescent child is quite unusual and rarely secondary to chronic sinus disease. It is more probable that they would arise from a metabolic or immunologic problem, especially cystic fibrosis. For this reason, all these children deserve testing for immunoglobulin levels and low sweat chlorides. The treatment can then be directed to the basic underlying systemic problem.

Nasal polyps secondary to allergic-inflammatory causes are seen in the older pediatric age group about as frequently as in adults. This nonneoplastic polyp tissue consists of thickened, edematous mucosal stroma, infiltrated with both eosinophils and polymorphonuclear leukocytes. Most often, the polyps project from the ethmoid sinuses via the middle meatus but may also be found in the superior meatus, where they extend from both the posterior ethmoid air cells and the sphenoid sinus. The primary treatment of these polyps consists of strenuous antibiotic therapy and decongestants, with surgical excision being reserved only for those obstructive polyps that have become recalcitrant to this treatment. The smaller, nonobstructive polyps are usually not removed unless chronic sinus infection continues behind them. In many cases, the combination of a course of antibiotics and allergic desensitization will result in their complete resorption. In the event that surgery becomes necessary, a simple nasal polypectomy is the procedure of choice, since recurrence of these lesions without resolution of the basic medical problem is very common. In this age group, it is also obvious that any major intrasinus surgery must not be done until full facial growth has occurred.

In the discussion of nasal polyps, there is a distinct clinical entity known as the antrochoanal polyp. This polyp is almost always unilateral and tends to cause posterior choanal obstruction. It is a very pedunculated mass with a small stalk being present, extending from one of the maxillary sinus ostia through the nose into the posterior choana. The site of attachment of the stalk is in the sinus itself, most frequently on the lateral wall. These lesions do not respond to decongestants or antibiotic therapy and therefore must be removed surgically in every instance. The Caldwell-Luc approach with conservative removal of the bony anterior sinus wall and excision of only that mucosa around the site of the stalk is indicated. The polyp may then be removed through the nose or mouth. The important step is to remove the entire stalk; otherwise, recurrence is frequent, especially if a simple avulsion technique is used.

Chronic sinus disease can, on occasion, produce complete obstruction of the ostia or ducts of the major paranasal sinuses. When this occurs, the mucous lining of the sinus continues to produce secretions, only now there is no effective egress available, and a mucocele is formed. Over a period of years, the sinus walls may flatten and bow to accommodate the steadily increasing pressure created by the trapped mucus. When this process occurs from an obstructed nasofrontal duct, there will be a downward bulging of the orbital roof, producing an upper inner canthal swelling of the orbit with downward and outward deviation of the eye. On the other hand, mucoceles of the ethmoid and sphenoid sinuses are quite difficult to diagnose without radiographic evaluation because of the paucity of physical findings except for headache and a feeling of frontal pressure or impaired ocular muscle function. Therefore, diagnosis must be by radiograph, with both plane radiographs and CT scans, or more recently MRI. By and large, since mucoceles or their infected equivalent, pyoceles, takes years rather than months to develop to any significant size, it is very unusual to see these problems in the pediatric age group. However, if discovered, treatment must be by surgical intervention. A frontal sinus mucocele can be handled by use of an osteoplastic frontal sinusotomy with fat obliteration of the sinus and its nasofrontal duct. Ethmoid and sphenoid mucoceles are best treated by the external ethmoidectomy approach and drainage.

Lower Respiratory Tract Diseases

The spread of infection between the upper and the lower respiratory tracts has been the subject of controversy and conjecture for many years (Farrell, 1936). In children with chronic nasal and paranasal sinus infection, there seems to be an increased incidence of cough and recurrent pneumonitis over and above what would be expected on a purely incidental basis. This is most easily seen in the asthmatic child or the child with Kartagener syndrome in whom the immunologic and hereditary dysfunctions are readily apparent. However, there are many other children without any known metabolic or immunologic deficit who exhibit similar symptoms of malaise, low-grade fevers, chronic sinus mucosal disease, and recurrent tracheobronchitis or pneumonitis. It is in reference to these children that the term sinobronchial syndrome has been used.

The pathways of infection in this syndrome are probably twofold: (1) by direct extension along the mucosa from the sinuses, via the pharynx with some laryngeal aspiration leading to intratracheal and bronchial disease, and (2) by lymphatic spread from the sinuses via the mediastinum to the tracheobronchial tree. Studies have been done by several investigators to promote each concept (Sasaki and Kirchner, 1967). In the first instance, the mucosal spread could logically be seen to promote a chronic cough and recurrent tracheobronchial infection. On the other hand, it seems apparent that the repeated bouts of interstitial pneumonitis might be more readily explained when attributed to spread along known lymphatic pathways from the sinuses, through the mediastinum, and to the lungs themselves. The rare retropharyngeal or deep neck abscess seen without evidence of Waldeyer ring infection may also be attributed to such spread.

Having discovered this systemic connection, when children have recurrent pulmonary disease, the physician should search for associated chronic sinus infection via direct nasal examination and sinus radiographs. If the sinobronchial syndrome is diagnosed, then fairly aggressive antibiotic therapy and nasal decongestant therapy should be instituted. Cultures should be taken in the middle meati, even if no specific purulence is noted, to give some guidance as to the proper chemotherapeutic agent. Most commonly, either penicillin or one of its derivatives turns out to be the drug of choice in controlling the usual gram-positive infections. The maxillary sinuses seem to become secondarily infected. If good resolution of intrasinus disease does not occur after three weeks of therapy, an antral irrigation should be done, and repeat cultures should be taken. This is classically performed by a puncture with a sharp, curved trocar or spinal needle through the inferior meatus. In older children, the authors have preferred to perform irrigation by direct puncture through the anterior sinus wall with the patient under local anesthesia. It is hoped that this will resolve the sinusitis and eventually permit resolution of the pulmonary complications.

REFERENCES

Bernstein, L. 1971. Pediatric sinus problems. Otolaryngol. Clin. North Am. 4:127.

Blumenfeld, R. J., and Skolnik, E. M. 1966. Intracranial complications of sinus disease. Trans. Am. Acad. Ophthalmol. Otolaryngol. 70:899.

Brook, I., and Kriedman E. M. 1982. Intracranial complications of sinusitis in children. Ann. Otol. Rhinol. Laryngol. 91:41.

Chandler, J. R., Langenbrunner, D. J., and Stevens E. R. 1970. The pathogenesis of orbital complications in acute sinusitis. Laryngoscope 80:1414.

Farrell, J. T. 1936. The connection of bronchiectasis and sinusitis. J.A.M.A. 106:92.

Gutowski, M., Mulbury, P. E., and Hengerer, A. S. 1988. The use of CT scanning in the management of orbital cellulitis. Int. J. Pediatr. Otol. 15:117.

Haynes, R. E., and Cramblett, H. G. 1967. Acute ethmoiditis: Its relationship to orbital cellulitis. Am. J. Dis. Child. 114:261.

Maniglia, A. J., Kronberg, F. G., and Culbertson, W. 1984. Visual loss associated with orbital and sinus disease. Laryngoscope 94:1050.

Price, D. D., Hameroff, S. B., and Richards, R. D. 1971. Cavernous sinus thrombosis and orbital cellulitis. South. Med. J. 64:1243.

Sasaki, C. T., and Kirchner, J. A. 1967. A lymphatic pathway from the sinuses to the mediastinum. Arch. Otolaryngol. 85:432.

Schramm, V. V., Carter, H. D., and Kennerdell, J. S. 1982. Evaluation of orbital cellulitis and results of treatment. Laryngoscope 92:732.

Small, M., and Dale, B. A. 1984. Intracranial suppuration 1968–1982. A 15-year review. Clin. Otolaryngol. 9:315.

Watters, E. C., Waller, P. H., Hiles, D. A., et al. 1976. Acute orbital cellulitis. Arch. Ophthalmol. 94:785.

Chapter 39

FOREIGN BODIES OF THE NOSE

Robert S. Shapiro, M.D.

The otorhinolaryngologic, pediatric, radiologic, and general medical literature contains reports of unusual foreign bodies in the nose but few comprehensive discussions of this problem. This is understandable, since nasal foreign bodies are commonly seen by the otolaryngologist and pediatrician and are usually removed quite easily. However, frequently there is a delay in referral to the otolaryngologist because a foreign body is not suspected to be present. Furthermore, certain foreign bodies can be quite difficult to remove and present a challenge in management. Removal of some of the animate foreign bodies (such as maggots) can prove to be quite difficult. A foreign body in the nasal cavity may accidentally be pushed backward and may be aspirated during an attempt at removal. This can result in acute respiratory obstruction. Nasal foreign bodies are more common in children than in adults, as children are more likely to put objects into the nose or to have objects placed there by other children.

ETIOLOGY

The foreign body may enter the nose by itself, or it may be placed there by the child or another person. Children are prone to making a game of placing objects into their nasal cavities and other body orifices. Children also tend to put objects into the noses of friends or younger siblings. This is especially common in retarded children. Some foreign bodies are iatrogenic, having accidentally been left in the nose following intranasal manipulation or surgery. Retrograde lodgement from coughing, regurgitation, and vomiting has been reported. Reports exist of teeth entering the nose during dental extractions.

Flies, insects, and fungi may enter the nose and may lead to an odorous discharge. This is more common in warmer climates. Predisposing factors include diabetes, syphilis, ozena, poor hygiene, and working with animals.

TYPES OF FOREIGN BODIES OF THE NOSE

Inanimate Foreign Bodies

The number of different objects that have been removed from the nose is virtually endless. Common foreign bodies include beans, nuts, peas, beads, chalk, eyelets, erasers, buttons, studs, pieces of sponge rubber, Plasticine, pieces of wood, bones, sticks, paper, chewing gum, crayons, meat, pits (fruit stones), paper clips, jewelry, pieces of plastic, bread, small toys, and seeds. Essentially any object that can be placed in the nose has probably been found there (Fig. 39–1), and the literature contains numerous reports of unusual foreign bodies.

Marrone and colleagues (1968) reported on a patient with a tooth in the nose as the result of evulsion during endotracheal intubation for a surgical procedure. McAndrew (1976) reported the displacement of a lower wisdom tooth into the posterior nasal aperture during dental extractions. The tooth was located by radiograph. Wood and Case (1973) reported finding an apparent splinter of bone in the nasal cavity. This proved to be the fractured end of a dental root tip fragment. Another foreign body of dental origin was described by Nazif (1971): a rubber dam clamp disappeared during a dental procedure; radiographs revealed the presence of the clamp in the nasal cavity.

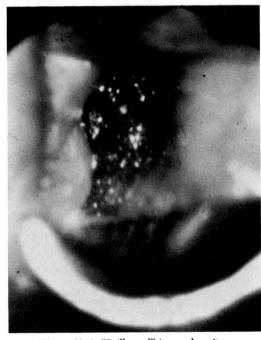

Figure 39–1. "Brillo pad" in nasal cavity.

Malhotra and associates (1970) described a very unusual foreign body in a man who was struck by the door of an Army vehicle. The patient subsequently noted inability to open his mouth, nasal obstruction, and pain and swelling on the side of his nose. Twenty-four days later he presented for examination and was found to have a 3.5 inch long piece of a door handle from the vehicle in his nose. Dayal and Singh (1970) reported two cases of inanimate foreign bodies of the nasopharynx. One was a toy whistle, and the second was a large metallic foreign body that entered the nasopharynx through the ethmoid and frontal sinuses after an explosion. Awty (1972) described the removal of a large metal fragment lodged in the posterior nares and nasopharynx. This was a shell fragment from a gunshot injury. Tolhurst (1974) reported finding three foreign bodies in the nose at the time of repair of a cleft palate; there were two pieces of rolled paper and a small piece of wood.

Utrata (1977) reported on a safety pin that had probably been present in the nose of a young child for two years. The object was found perforated through the soft palate while the child was undergoing anesthesia for eye surgery. The child had been asymptomatic except for one episode of epistaxis six months before discovery of the foreign body. The safety pin had opened while in the nose, but it was removed with an alligator forceps with the patient under general anesthesia, and the palatal wound healed smoothly. Sharma and coworkers (1978) reported on a 14-month-old boy with an eight-month history of right nasal discharge who presented with swelling of the right eye for four months. The child had orbital cellulitis and meningitis. The middle of the hard palate was found to be sloughed and irregularly perforated. Two small pieces of wood found in the right nasal cavity were removed, and the child was treated with parenteral antibiotics. The child's general condition improved, and the orbital swelling subsided. Since the child was lost to further follow-up, it is not known if the palate perforation healed.

In a retrospective review of patients requiring admission to The Montreal Children's Hospital for removal of nasal foreign bodies under general anesthesia, the author found that 29 children were admitted for this reason between 1970 and 1977. The ages of the children ranged between 1.5 and 17 years. There were 16 girls and 13 boys. In one child, the foreign body (a stone) passed into the stomach prior to the child going to the operating room, and surgery was canceled. In four of the other children, no foreign body was actually found. The foreign bodies found in the other 24 children are listed in Table 39–1. Three children had bilateral foreign bodies: two of these were sponges, and the others were magnets. Eighteen children had foreign bodies or suspected foreign bodies in the right nasal cavity, and eight children had foreign bodies in the left nasal cavity (one passing spontaneously into the stomach). Of the children whose parents could be reached by telephone, 14 were right-handed, and 2 were left-handed. No relation could be established

TABLE 39–1. Foreign Bodies of the Nose Removed with the Patient Under General Anesthesia at the Montreal Children's Hospital between 1970 and 1977

TYPE OF OBJECT	NUMBER
Plastic objects	5
Buttons	4
Sponges	4 (2 bilateral)
Metal objects	2
Food	2
Paper clip	1
Magnet	1 (bilateral)
Eraser	1
Nut	1
Pit	1
Leather	1
Seed	1

between handedness and the particular nasal cavity in which the foreign body was placed. All foreign bodies were easily removed, and there were no complications. These were only foreign bodies that required removal under general anesthesia. The majority of foreign bodies were removed in the outpatient department without using general anesthesia.

Das (1984) reported on 156 patients with foreign bodies in the nose presenting to the E.N.T. service of his hospital over a four-year period. Close to 44 per cent were found to have irritative nasal disease, such as acute rhinitis, chronic rhinitis, and chronic vestibulitis. The author emphasized the need to treat irritative conditions after removal of foreign bodies from the nose.

A button battery found in the nasal cavity was first reported in 1981 by Babu. A 5-year-old boy had been admitted with a history of facial swelling for five days. Necrosis of the left inferior turbinate was found. The battery was removed, and the patient treated with intramuscular penicillin. Follow-up after one and a half years revealed a saddle nose deformity with loss of most of the septal cartilage, stenosis of the left nostril, and a small septal perforation. Kavanagh and Litovitz (1986) reported on two cases of button batteries in the nasal cavities. One was easily removed, leaving only a 2- to 3-mm superficial burn on the inferior turbinate with bloody drainage, whereas the second case produced a large septal perforation. Their recommendation was immediate removal of button batteries from the nasal cavity. Skinner and Chui (1986) reported on a 5-year-old child with a three-day history of left-sided, offensive, purulent rhinorrhea. For 12 hours prior to admission a tender swelling had been noted over the left side of the face. The child wore a hearing aid for severe bilateral congenital sensorineural deafness, powered by a button battery. The battery, whose casing was corroded, was removed from the nasal cavity with the patient under general anesthesia. Burns of the inferior turbinate, nasal septum, nasal floor, and nasal vestibule were present. Oral ampicillin was given, and the burns healed. One year postoperatively, no evidence of external nasal deformity or intranasal adhesions was present. However, there was persistent crusting within the left nasal cavity that was felt to be consistent with a degree of local atrophic rhinitis.

Capo and Lucente (1986) reported one case of a button battery in the nasal cavity requiring general anesthesia for its removal. Examination demonstrated extensive excoriation and burns in the region where the battery had been lodged. Maxillary and ethmoid sinusitis developed on the side of the foreign body but healed following intravenous antibiotic therapy without further sequelae. They pointed out that the moist environment of the nasal cavity causes leakage of battery contents. Furthermore, tissue electrolysis may occur, owing to low-voltage direct current set up between the anode and cathode. A third mechanism of injury involves pressure necrosis resulting from the presence of a foreign body. (A general review of the subject of burns resulting from ingestion of button batteries is found in the article by Kost and Shapiro [1987].)

Rhinoliths

Rhinoliths are formed from intranasal foreign bodies that become encrusted with mineral salts, usually calcium and magnesium (Fig. 39–2). The vast majority are thought to arise from exogenous foreign bodies. These are frequently fruit stones (pits). The theoretic possibility of endogenous nuclei such as blood clots and dried pus has been hypothesized, but most authors doubt this origin. Most reports show a preponderance of females among the patients with rhinoliths.

Animate Foreign Bodies

A wide variety of insects, maggots, intestinal worms, and leeches have been reported to be found in the nose. In hot climates, flies may deposit their ova in the nose, with maggots resulting. This is rare in the healthy nose but is more common in patients with ozena or syphilis. Epistaxis, headache, lacrimation, and sneezing develop and are soon followed by a bloody discharge that becomes purulent. Ulceration and destruction of the nasal structures may occur. Death may result from meningitis (Smith, 1968). Maggots represent the larval stage of certain flies, such as the screw worm fly and the blow fly; a single screw worm fly may deposit as many as 300 eggs in five minutes (Hunter et al., 1976).

Rhinosporidium seeberi infestation is a fungal infection found mainly in India and Sri Lanka. Nasal polyps are formed and contain the spores in all stages of development. The masses appear as slender filiform or narrow leaflike processes of a dull pink or reddish tint, with the surface studded with many minute, pale spots owing to the presence of the sporangia in the tissue (Smith, 1968). The growths are very friable and bleed easily when touched.

Ascaris lumbricoides, a nematode or intestinal round worm, is one of the most common helminthic parasites of humans. Ascariasis has a world-wide distribution and is particularly common in regions with poor sanitation. Endemic regions exist in the United States, especially in southeastern parts of the Appalachian range. Humans are infected by ingestion of the mature eggs in fecally contaminated food or drink. These eggs hatch in the intestine, liberating minute larvae, which penetrate blood or lymph vessels in the intestinal wall. Some larvae reach the portal circulation and are carried to the liver, while others pass through the thoracic duct. By either route, they finally reach the lungs, where they are filtered out of the blood stream, and in a few days many perforate the alveoli. After increas-

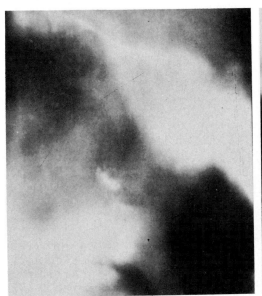
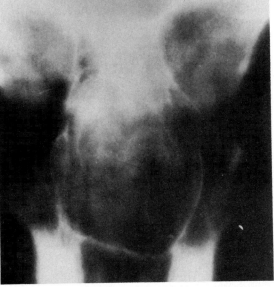

Figure 39–2. Lateral tomogram and anteroposterior tomogram showing large rhinolith filling the nasal cavity. This 15-year-old girl had nasal obstruction for three years but no history of insertion of a foreign body into the nose. The rhinolith had displaced the septum. It was removed transnasally, and there was considerable bleeding, which was controlled with packing. The postoperative course was uneventful. (From Children's Hospital of Pittsburgh.)

ing in size, the larvae migrate up the respiratory passages to the epiglottis and then down the esophagus (Hunter et al., 1976). The parasite may lodge in the nose when regurgitated.

Leeches may cause epistaxis when present as foreign bodies in the nose. Alavi (1969) reported on 54 patients with leeches in the upper respiratory tract, 35 per cent of them presenting with epistaxis. Dayal and Singh (1970) reported on an 18-year-old boy with a history of a leech entering the nose two months before examination. He complained of recurrent epistaxis. The leech was found hanging from the nasopharynx and was easily removed.

Aspergillus infections of the nose cause sneezing, rhinorrhea, headache, and the discharge of pieces of tough, greenish membrane, which may coexist with polyps and granulation tissue (Smith, 1968).

PATHOLOGY

The inanimate foreign bodies tend to cause edema and inflammation of the nasal mucous membrane. Ulceration and epistaxis may result. Granulation tissue may be produced. Sinusitis may also occur.

Baluyot (1973) reported that maggots in the nose cause varying degrees of inflammatory reaction, from a mild localized infection to massive destruction of the cartilaginous and bony nasal walls, with formation of deep, odorous, suppurating areas. The *Ascaris* worms cause a varying degree of irritation by their presence and constant motion.

CLINICAL MANIFESTATIONS

The child with a foreign body in the nose may not bring this to the attention of his or her parents. It may remain asymptomatic and stay in the nose for a great length of time. Eventually, a rhinolith may form around the foreign body. More frequently, however, a nasal discharge develops on the side of the nose with the foreign body. A unilateral rhinorrhea, particularly if purulent or odorous, should alert one to the possibility of a foreign body. There may be pain, nasal obstruction, epistaxis, and sneezing. Examination usually shows edema with inflammation of the nasal mucosa. Ulceration may have occurred. The foreign body may also pass posteriorly and may be swallowed or aspirated. An ipsilateral serous otitis media may be present when the foreign material has been present for a long time.

A very common nasal foreign body that is particularly prone to causing infection is foam rubber. With foam rubber, the nasal cavity very quickly develops a foul-smelling discharge. Seeds are common foreign bodies, and they may swell and become impacted. Stool and McConnel (1973) reported that special problems have arisen in recent years because of plastic toys. They cause little odor because of their low

reactivity, and yet granulation tissue forms around them to give the gross appearance of a tumor.

Oh and Gaudet (1977) reported on a 30-month-old girl with acute epiglottitis. At the time of intubation, it was noted that the right side of the supraglottic larynx was more inflamed than the left. She had had rhinorrhea and fever for two days. Two foreign bodies were found in the nostril, one a piece of plastic, and the other a portion of yarn. These were removed, and cultures from the foreign bodies as well as from the throat and the blood grew *Haemophilus influenzae,* type B. She was extubated after 24 hours without complication.

Leiberman and coworkers (1985) reported on a 2-year-old child admitted with sudden onset of sleep apnea. Her tonsils were only slightly hypertrophic, but she had had 150 apneic episodes of the obstructive type documented during eight hours of night sleep. At the time of tonsillectomy and adenoidectomy, a 1 cm × 3.5 cm piece of cellophane was found in the nasopharynx. When the foreign body was removed, the sleep apnea was totally resolved.

With a rhinolith, nasal discharge is frequent, usually unilateral, and often foul-smelling. It may be purulent and tinged with blood. Epistaxis may occur, as may anosmia, headache, and sinusitis. The septum may be deviated. Bicknell (1970) reported perforation of the hard palate resulting from a rhinolith. Carder and Hill (1966) reported on an asymptomatic rhinolith. They found only two other asymptomatic rhinoliths in the literature. Smith (1968) reported that rhinoliths are more common in cases of cleft palate.

The diagnosis of the presence of a rhinolith can usually be made by visual inspection and palpation with a probe. Rhinoliths also show up well on radiographs. The films reveal a dense, irregular, but not necessarily homogeneous mass lying within the nasal passage. There may be local bone absorption or distortion resulting from pressure on the turbinates, with deflection of the septum. The medial wall of the antrum may be similarly indented (Harrison and Lamming, 1969).

Brown (1945) reported that nasal occlusion, headaches, and sneezing with serosanguineous discharge usually begin two or three days after parasitic infestation of the nose. The patient usually complains of intense pain and a sensation of "crawling." Delirium is not uncommon (Hunter et al., 1976). A septic temperature accompanies the reaction to the larvae, and the nose has a disagreeable fetid odor. Leukocytosis results from the accompanying secondary infection. Examination reveals marked swelling of the mucous membrane, with obliteration of the cavity. The mucosa is fragile and bleeds easily. The worms are firmly attached and difficult to extract. The late stage of the infestation shows marked cartilaginous and bony destruction. Infestation with *Ascaris* worms results in severe congestion and large amounts of mucopurulent discharge with absence of erosion of the cartilaginous and bony walls (Baluyot, 1973). The worms are easily recognized because of their size, measuring 6 to 10 inches.

Kecht (1969) reported a case of localized tetanus with facial paralysis resulting from a wooden foreign body in the nasal cavity opposite the facial paralysis. Sarnaik and Venkat (1981) reported on a 2-year-old girl with unilateral nasal discharge for two days. A match stick was removed from the nasal cavity; however the child returned the following day with fever, irritability, trismus, and opisthotonos. She had received no immunizations. The diagnosis of cephalic tetanus was made, and she was treated with human tetanus immune globulin and penicillin G. She required positive-pressure ventilation and subsequent nasotracheal intubation. Tracheotomy was performed after seven days. She improved over the next two weeks and was decannulated.

Waldman (1979) reported on a 28-year-old woman with facial cellulitis. There was granulation tissue in the nose, and radiographs revealed what appeared to be a supernumerary tooth or odontoma in the maxilla. At surgery, one of a pair of dice was removed. She was treated with penicillin, and healing was complete. In retrospect, it was felt that the woman may have placed the die in her nose when she was a young child.

Golding (1965) reported on an 18-month-old child with a history of an unbearably foul odor emanating from his entire body for four weeks. No part of his body appeared to be free of the fetid odor. Bathing brought relief for only 15 minutes. His clothes had the same odor as his body. There was no evidence of illness otherwise, except for slight coryza. The child was found to have a piece of blanket in the right nasal cavity. One hour after removal of the foreign body, the odor was gone. The odor did not recur. This was felt to be a case of bromidrosis or osmidrosis, which denotes a malodorous condition of human perspiration. Golding could find no other reports in the literature of a nasal foreign body being the cause of generalized bromidrosis. He did report that a colleague of his had a similar case, the etiology being a nasal foreign body. Three similar cases were reported by Katz and colleagues (1979) and two by Stegman (1987). Individual cases of a similar nature were reported by Feinstein (1979) and Eun and associates (1984).

DIAGNOSIS AND DIFFERENTIAL DIAGNOSIS

Diagnosis of the presence of an inanimate foreign body may be difficult. The first step is inspection of the nasal cavities with adequate illumination and a nasal speculum. An uncooperative child may require general anesthesia for proper examination. The diagnosis of a foreign body may be helped by vasoconstriction of the nasal mucosa with a nasal spray such as 1 per cent phenylephrine hydrochloride. Posterior rhinoscopy with a nasopharyngeal mirror is helpful in ruling out the presence of a foreign body in the nose far posteriorly. Radiographs may be of help in verifying the presence of a radiopaque foreign body (Fig. 39–

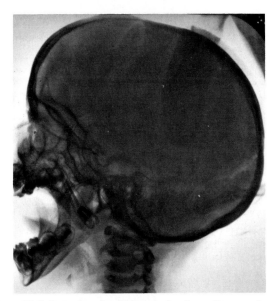

Figure 39–3. Lateral neck radiograph showing radiopaque foreign body (hair clip) in the nasopharynx of a 2-year-old child. The presenting symptom had been bilateral nasal discharge. (From Children's Hospital of Pittsburgh.)

3). Furthermore, sinus radiographs are useful in ruling out an accompanying sinusitis. Radiopaque media studies are occasionally helpful with nonradiopaque foreign bodies. In any child with a nasal foreign body, both ear canals should be thoroughly checked, as the child who puts a foreign body into the nose is also likely to put things into the ears.

The diagnosis of parasitic and larval infestation of the nose is by anterior rhinoscopy with adequate illumination and a nasal speculum, as well as by posterior rhinoscopy with a nasopharyngeal mirror. The diagnosis of fungal infection is established by culture and microscopic demonstration of the hyphae and spores. However, *Rhinosporidium seeberi* cannot be cultured (Hunter et al., 1976).

In the differential diagnosis, such things as unilateral choanal atresia, polyps, sinusitis, and tumors should be considered. The radiologic differential diagnosis of a rhinolith includes calcified polyp, opaque foreign body of similar density (teeth or bone), osteoma, odontoma, and sequestration following local osteomyelitis (Harrison and Lamming, 1969).

MANAGEMENT

Stool and McConnel (1973) stated that "Any attempt at removal of a foreign body which does not succeed will make a bad situation worse. The child is usually apprehensive and the parents are aggravated. The physician, therefore, should be wary of falling into the trap of trying to do a removal without adequate instruments or good control of the patient." They also pointed out that removal of a foreign body is rarely an emergency. Time should be taken to obtain the proper instruments and illumination. If necessary, sedation or anesthesia can be provided.

The first step in attempting to remove a nasal foreign body without sedation or general anesthesia is to fully explain the situation and the procedure to the parents and the child. Adequate restraint is necessary in most young children. One very good method of restraint is for the child to sit on the parent's lap with the parent's arms around the child's arms and body. An assistant stabilizes the head. In the absence of an assistant, the parent can use one arm to hold the child's body and the other arm to stabilize the head by holding the forehead. The legs can be stabilized by an assistant or can be held between the parent's legs. Another method of restraint is to have the child lying on the back, immobilized by wrapping in a sheet or with a commercial restraint apparatus such as a Papoose Board.* An assistant is still required for stabilization of the head.

Adequate illumination should be provided with a head mirror or headlight. The use of the headlight by the pediatrician allows both hands to be free. A nasal speculum should be used for visualization of the nasal cavity. Most objects can be grasped with a Hartman forceps (Fig. 39–4A). Another useful instrument is the alligator forceps. Some objects are best removed by passing a wire loop or a right-angled hook behind them before withdrawing (Fig. 39–4B). If necessary, a topical nasal vasoconstrictor, such as 1 per cent phenylephrine hydrochloride, can be used prior to removing the foreign body. Topical anesthesia, such as with 4 per cent lidocaine hydrochloride or dilute cocaine, may also be of help.

Many techniques of foreign body removal have been described. Irvine (1973) recommended the use of a small curved oval ring. McMaster (1970) recommended the use of a fine wire loop ear curette. He bent the wire loop into an arc to form a shallow scoop. After

*Olympic Medical Corp., 4400 Seventh South, Seattle, Washington.

using a topical vasoconstrictor, and a topical anesthetic if necessary, he passed the wire loop alongside the foreign body, following the curve of the scoop. Virnig (1972) recommended the use of a Fogarty biliary catheter for removal of foreign bodies. The catheter is passed along the floor of the nose, and the balloon is inflated when it is beyond the foreign body. The catheter and the foreign body are then withdrawn. A similar technique was described by Fox (1980), using a Fogarty catheter; however, in his technique, the catheter is passed above the foreign body into the nasopharynx. Henry and Chamberlain (1972) recommended the use of a Foley catheter after spraying the nasal cavity with cocaine and epinephrine. They used a number 8 Foley catheter, passed into the nasopharynx along the inferior turbinate, passing beneath the foreign body. The balloon was inflated with 2 to 3 ml of saline, and the object was then removed as the catheter was withdrawn. Stool and McConnel (1973) reported on a method that does not require instrumentation. The child is placed in the supine position after the application of a nasal vasoconstrictor. The child's uninvolved nasal cavity is compressed with a finger, and the physician's mouth is placed over the child's as in applying mouth-to-mouth resuscitation. A sudden, strong blast of air is used to force the foreign body out through the anterior naris. Edmunds (1971) recommended spraying the involved nasal cavity with a vasoconstrictor and then immobilizing the child. A blower was then applied to the unobstructed naris. He timed the short, quick application of air blown into the unobstructed side with one of the child's cries. Messervy (1973) recommended that the child be placed in a sitting position, leaning slightly forward. The physician occludes the opening of the free nostril with a finger, and the child takes a deep breath through the mouth and exhales forcibly through the nose. He recommended that this be tried at least 15 times before giving up. He also recommended that for children

Figure 39–4. Removal of foreign body. *A,* Object grasped with a Hartman forceps. *B,* Wire loop passed behind foreign body prior to withdrawing.

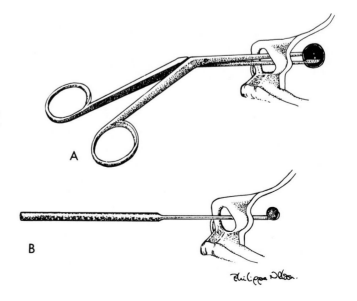

unwilling or unable to play this "game," sneezing while occluding the free nostril can be tried instead, pepper being utilized to initiate the reflex.

Stool and McConnel (1973) pointed out that pushing the object posteriorly into the nasopharynx should be avoided because of the possibility of the foreign body entering the trachea or esophagus. Occasionally, general anesthesia is required for the removal of an inanimate foreign body, especially with an uncooperative child or with an impacted foreign body. Lowering the head during the procedure helps prevent the foreign body from entering the larynx, trachea, or esophagus. An endotracheal tube is helpful. Lateral rhinotomy is occasionally necessary for the removal of severely impacted foreign bodies.

The treatment of rhinoliths consists of removal. If the rhinolith is too large to be removed in one piece, it can be broken with a strong forceps and removed in small pieces. If removal of the rhinolith requires displacing it posteriorly and recovering it from the nasopharynx, this should be done with the patient under general anesthesia with the head lowered. Occasionally, lateral rhinotomy is required for a massive rhinolith.

Hunter and coworkers (1976) recommended that larvae in the nose be anesthetized by applying benzol, ether, or chloroform, either on a cotton pledget or with an atomizer. An alternative method recommended by the same authors is irrigation with 20 per cent chloroform in sweet milk or 15 per cent chloroform in light mineral or vegetable oil. Following anesthesia of the larvae, they are removed with forceps and by having the patient blow the nose. If the patient is under general anesthesia, the larvae are removed by forceps or suction.

Ascaris worms are removed by forceps extraction. They need not be killed prior to removal. The intestinal infestation, however, must also be treated to prevent recurrence of worms in the nose.

Rhinosporidium seeberi infestation is treated by surgical removal of the infected areas. Oral treatment with diaminodiphenylsulfone (DDS, dapsone) has recently been found to be effective in controlling nasal and nasopharyngeal rhinosporidiosis (Nair, 1979). Treatment of *Aspergillus* in the nose consists of thorough removal of all the fungus (Smith, 1968).

CONCLUSION

Because a child may not admit to placing a foreign body in the nose, the physician must be alert to suspect a foreign body in the presence of a persistent unilateral nasal discharge, especially when the discharge is odorous, mucopurulent, or sanguineous. The removal of the foreign body should be done in a carefully planned manner with all appropriate instruments and illumination available. Precautions should be taken to prevent the foreign body from entering the larynx, trachea, or esophagus. General anesthesia should be utilized if necessary, rather than repeated, traumatic,

unsuccessful attempts at removal in the uncooperative child. The ear canals should be checked for foreign bodies, as the child who is prone to placing things into the nose may very well have one in the ear canal as well.

SELECTED REFERENCES

Harrison, B. B., and Lamming, R. L. 1969. Case reports. Exogenous nasal rhinolith. Br. J. Radiol. 42:838.
  This article reviews the problem of rhinoliths in general and has in particular some detail concerning the radiologic aspects of rhinoliths.
Kavanagh, K. T., and Litovitz, T. 1986. Miniature battery foreign bodies in auditory and nasal cavities. J.A.M.A. 255:1470.
  This article discusses the mechanisms of tissue injury, patient management, and method of foreign body removal for button batteries in the ear and in the nasal cavity.
Stool, S. E., and McConnel, C. S., Jr. 1973. Foreign bodies in pediatric otolaryngology. Some diagnostic and therapeutic pointers. Clin. Pediatr. (Phila.) 12:113.
  This article describes a practical approach to the diagnosis and management of foreign bodies in the ear, nose, and throat.

REFERENCES

Alavi, K. 1969. Epistaxis and hemoptysis due to *Hirudo medicinalis* (medical leech). Arch. Otolaryngol. 90:178.
Awty, M. D. 1972. Removal of a large shell fragment from the nasopharynx. Oral Surg. 33:513.
Babu, K. N. 1981. An unusual foreign body in the nose. J. Laryngol. Otol. 95:961.
Baluyot, S. T., Jr. 1973. Foreign bodies in the nasal cavity. *In* Paparella, M. M., and Shumrick, D. A. (eds.): Otolaryngology. Philadelphia, W. B. Saunders Co., pp. 62–68.
Bicknell, P. G. 1970. Rhinolith perforating the hard palate. J. Laryngol. Otol. 84:1161.
Brown, E. H. 1945. Screwworm infestation in the nasal passages and paranasal sinuses. Laryngoscope 55:371.
Capo, J. M., and Lucente, F. E. 1986. Alkaline battery foreign bodies of the ear and nose. Arch. Otolaryngol. Head Neck Surg. 112:562.
Carder, H. M., and Hill, J. J. 1966. Asymptomatic rhinolith: A brief review of the literature and case report. Laryngoscope 76:524.
Das, S. K. 1984. Aetiological evaluation of foreign bodies in the ear and nose. J. Laryngol. Otol. 98:989.
Dayal, D., and Singh, A. P. 1970. Foreign body nasopharynx. J. Laryngol. Otol. 84:1157.
Edmunds, P. K. 1971. Removal of nasal foreign body. J.A.M.A. 217:212.
Eun, H. C., Kim, K. H., and Lee, Y. S. 1984. Unusual body odour due to a nasal foreign body in a child. J. Dermatol. (Tokyo) 11:501.
Feinstein, R. J. 1979. Nasal foreign bodies and bromidrosis (letter). J.A.M.A. 242:1031.
Fox, J. R. 1980. Fogarty catheter removal of nasal foreign bodies. Ann. Emerg. Med. 9:37.
Golding, I. M. 1965. An unusual cause of bromidrosis. Pediatrics 36:791.
Harrison, B. B., and Lamming, R. L. 1969. Case reports. Exogenous nasal rhinolith. Br. J. Radiol. 42:838.
Henry, L. N., and Chamberlain, J. W. 1972. Removal of foreign bodies from esophagus and nose with the use of a Foley catheter. Surgery 71:918.
Hunter, G. W., Swartzwelder, J. C., and Clyde, D. F. 1976. Tropical Medicine, 5th ed. Philadelphia, W. B. Saunders Co.
Irvine, G. C. 1973. Foreign bodies in the ear and nose. A method of removal. East Afr. Med. J. 50:116.
Katz, H. P., Katz, J. R., Bernstein, M., et al. 1979. Unusual

presentation of nasal foreign bodies in children. J.A.M.A. 241:1496.

Kavanagh, K. T., and Litovitz, T. 1986. Miniature battery foreign bodies in auditory and nasal cavities. J.A.M.A. 255:1470.

Kecht, B. 1969. Tetanus facialis durch Nasenfremdkörper. Monatsschr Ohrenheilkd Laryngorhinol. 103:204.

Kost, K. M., and Shapiro, R. S. 1987. Button battery ingestion: A case report and review of the literature. J. Otolaryngol. 16:252.

Leiberman, A., Yagupsky, P., and Lavie, P. 1985. Obstructive sleep apnoea probably related to a foreign body. Eur. J. Pediatr. 144:205.

Malhotra, C., Arora, M. M. L., and Mehra, Y. N. 1970. An unusual foreign body in the nose. J. Laryngol. Otol. 84:539.

Marrone, M. P., Goodwin, M., and Genovese, M. 1968. A unique foreign body in the nose. Case report. Ann. Dent. 27:156.

McAndrew, P. G. 1976. The lost tooth. J. Dent. 4:144.

McMaster, W. C. 1970. Removal of foreign body from the nose. J.A.M.A. 213:1905.

Messervy, M. 1973. Forced expiration in treatment of nasal foreign bodies. Practitioner 210:242.

Nair, K. K. 1979. Clinical trial of diaminodiphenylsulfone (DDS) in nasal and nasopharyngeal rhinosporidiosis. Laryngoscope 89:291.

Nazif, M. 1971. A rubber dam clamp in the nasal cavity: Report of case. J. Am. Dent. Assoc. 82:1099.

Oh, T. H., and Gaudet T. 1977. Acute epiglottis associated with nasal foreign body: Occurrence in a 30-month-old girl. Clin. Pediatr. (Phila.) 16:1067.

Sarnaik, A. P., and Venkat, G. 1981. Cephalic tetanus as a complication of nasal foreign body. Am. J. Dis. Child. 135:571.

Sharma, D. B., Lahori, U. S., and Singh, G. 1978. Foreign body nose perforating the hard palate in an infant. Indian Pediatr. 15:353.

Skinner, D. W., and Chui, P. 1986. The hazards of "button-sized" batteries as foreign bodies in the nose and ear. J. Laryngol. Otol. 100:1315.

Smith, A. B. 1968. Epistaxis, foreign bodies, and parasites. In Stewart, J. P. (ed.): Logan Turner's Diseases of the Nose, Throat and Ear, 7th ed. Bristol, John Wright & Sons, Ltd., pp. 60–62.

Stegman, J. C. 1987. Unusual presentation of nasal foreign bodies (letter). Am. J. Dis. Child. 141:239.

Stool, S. E., and McConnel, C. S., Jr. 1973. Foreign bodies in pediatric otolaryngology. Some diagnostic and therapeutic pointers. Clin. Pediatr. (Phila.) 12:113.

Tolhurst, D. E. 1974. The ubiquitous foreign body. Cleft Palate J. 11:237.

Utrata, J. 1977. Erosion of the soft palate by a foreign body in the nose. Ear Nose Throat J. 56:403.

Virnig, R. P. 1972. Nontraumatic removal of foreign bodies from the nose and ears of infants and children. Minn. Med. 55:1123.

Waldman, L. A. 1979. Facial cellulitis caused by unrecognized foreign body. Oral Surg. Oral Med. Oral Pathol. 48:408.

Wood, G. L., and Case, J. H. 1973. A nasal splinter of dental origin. Dent. Surv. 49:87.

Chapter 40

INJURIES OF THE NOSE, FACIAL BONES, AND PARANASAL SINUSES

Frank I. Marlowe, M.D.

GENERAL CONSIDERATIONS

Since entire textbooks have been written on the subject of facial injuries, it becomes obvious that the material to be presented in this chapter cannot be exhaustive or all-inclusive, but an attempt will be made to deal particularly with those aspects of each problem most peculiar to these injuries in children. In so doing, the basic principles that are of importance in children, as well as in adults, will be emphasized.

Children's exuberance, lack of fine physical control, and desire to explore their environments make them more susceptible to injuries involving the facial structures, especially during the early years. Offsetting this tendency to facial injury are the relative elasticity of the young child's facial bones and the somewhat lesser chance of exposure to the common causes of fractures in adults, such as high-velocity impacts and violent assault. In general, children suffer a surprisingly low incidence of severe facial fractures (Hall, 1972).

Despite the infrequency of facial fractures in children, the problem should not be construed as one of little magnitude. Of every ten deaths in children, four are the result of accidents; the highest incidence of these trauma-related deaths is in children between the ages of 2 and 3 years. In addition to these fatalities, 50,000 children are permanently crippled, and 2 million are temporarily incapacitated each year as a result of trauma.

Evaluation and treatment of the injured child present special challenges, and it cannot be reiterated too often that the child is not a small adult, but differs greatly from adults in terms of the type of injury sustained and his or her general physiologic response to the injury.

Attention to the ABCs of care of the adult trauma patient—airway, bleeding and shock, and cerebral and spinal cord injuries—is even more critical in caring for children who suffer trauma (Schultz, 1970).

Airway

The smaller anatomic dimensions and different tissue make-up of the child's airway predisposes the child to obstruction with very little mucosal edema or hematoma. Thus, these potential problems must be recognized early and managed rapidly. Blood, vomitus, or foreign bodies can fully or partially obstruct the airway, and in many cases, these obstructions can be cleared quickly by sweeping a finger deep into the mouth and pharynx. Airway problems stemming from uncontrolled facial bleeding or grossly displaced facial tissues can often be alleviated rapidly and simply by moving the child to an upright position. Fractures of the mandible with severe posterior displacement may allow the tongue to drop posteriorly and occlude the airway. In such cases, the tongue may be pulled forward and sutured in this position, or an appropriate nasopharyngeal tube may be placed to maintain the airway. In all but very unusual and exceptional instances, immediate management of upper airway obstruction is most effectively handled by some form of intubation rather than by tracheostomy. Intubation is more rapidly accomplished, and usually personnel skilled in its use are more apt to be immediately available at the appropriate time. If the nature of the obstruction is temporary, endotracheal intubation may preclude the necessity for tracheostomy entirely. Even if the obstruction will probably require a long time to manage adequately, intermediate intubation will allow the physician time to perform the tracheostomy later under controlled conditions with good light, suction, and control of the patient's airway, making it a much safer procedure.

Since manipulation of the neck during intubation or tracheostomy may produce permanent neurologic damage, the possibility of a coexistent cervical spine injury must be kept in mind in the patient with airway obstruction.

Bleeding

The next important consideration is control of bleeding, which usually can be checked without too great difficulty in facial wounds by direct pressure. It must be borne in mind, however, that blood loss in cases of pediatric trauma is a critical factor, since the child has

760

a much smaller circulating blood volume, and shock may follow the loss of as little as 100 to 200 cc of blood. Any readily apparent arterial bleeding should be clamped and ligated directly through the wound.

Shock is rarely the result of facial injury alone, but many factors predispose a child suffering from apparently minor facial trauma to shock. The critical nature of blood loss has already been mentioned. In addition, loss of body heat is an important consideration, as the child's relatively greater ratio of body surface to body volume makes him or her more prone to heat loss and to the development of hypothermia. Also, the child's ability to maintain homeostasis is much more endangered than the adult's by changes in blood volume, fluid volume, and blood pH. Because of this, children become ill faster than do adults, and there is much less time in which to recognize and treat these threats to homeostasis before they cause death.

The treatment for shock is dependent upon reestablishing an appropriate intravascular fluid volume (which may be done with crystalloids or blood products), controlling pain, conserving body heat, and controlling the patient's apprehension.

Central Nervous System

Once a clear airway has been ensured, and hemorrhage and shock have been controlled, consideration is given to the possible presence of associated injuries before definitive treatment of the facial trauma is undertaken. It has been said that patients do not die of facial injuries, but patients with facial injuries do die of associated injuries.

Injury to the central nervous system in instances of significant facial trauma is not uncommon; central nervous system injury may be intracranial or may involve an injury to the spinal cord. A careful evaluation of the child's level of consciousness, vital signs, and pupillary reactions is necessary to detect an intracranial injury, such as concussion, contusion, or hemorrhage. Nausea, vomiting, headache, or cerebrospinal fluid leakage from the nose or ear are also signs of cervical involvement. Localized pain or tenderness over the cervical spine, any alterations of mobility of the limbs, or changes in sensation in the limbs should also alert the physician to the possibility of an injury to the cervical spine. These symptoms and signs are particularly important to remember when manipulating the head and neck for placement of an endotracheal tube.

Radiographs of the cervical spine should be obtained, as should skull radiographs, in all instances of significant head trauma. If a neck injury is suspected, the head should be immobilized until radiographic evaluation can be carried out.

Attention may be drawn to thoracic injuries by the presence of pain, shortness of breath, or the presence of an obvious lag on one side of the chest, which may herald a pneumothorax. Localized tenderness or ecchymoses over the thoracic cage may indicate underlying rib fracture, a possible etiologic factor in pneumothorax.

Localized pain, tenderness, or obvious distention may call attention to an intraabdominal injury. Changes in bowel sounds or the presence of "rebound" or of free blood in the abdominal cavity may also be noted in cases of severe abdominal injury.

Pain, swelling, or obvious deformity of any of the extremities or joint areas is presumptive evidence of a musculoskeletal injury, and precautions must be taken so as not to aggravate the injury further.

Immediate consultation with the appropriate specialist, should any of the aforementioned findings be noted, is necessary to avoid serious consequences. Generally, the possible need for a thoracotomy or laparotomy takes priority over definitive care of the facial injury. In addition, evaluations of special organs, such as the eye and the ear, must be made prior to institution of definitive care of a facial injury. For instance, a hematoma overlying the mastoid process, a hemotympanum, or frank bleeding or loss of cerebrospinal fluid from the ear canal indicates a basilar skull fracture. Although injuries to the eye may often seem "trivial," and swelling and discoloration of the eyelids, as well as subconjunctival hemorrhage, are commonly seen in association with other facial fractures, the possibility of ocular trauma must be borne in mind if disastrous results are to be avoided. Direct injury to the globe with leakage of fluid and possible iris prolapse is generally quite obvious, and the need for immediate ophthalmologic consultation is readily apparent. However, in some instances, the eye may appear to be normal, but a detached retina or hemorrhage into the vitreous may have occurred. In addition, a small intraocular foreign body may easily escape detection, even upon relatively close examination of the eyes. Assessment of visual acuity, even grossly, in each eye in turn, is absolutely essential.

Once the patient's general status is determined to be satisfactory and stable, and the absence of any serious associated injury has been determined, evaluation of the facial injury may be undertaken.

Maxillofacial trauma in children differs from that seen in adults in many ways. Good historical information is often more difficult to obtain in the child, and clinical and radiologic examinations are certainly more difficult, to the point where anesthesia may have to be utilized to allow adequate evaluation. In addition, the small size and poorly developed pneumatization of the sinus cavities make interpretation of radiographic studies more difficult, and false-negative findings are not uncommon. Intracranial and cervical spine injuries appear to accompany maxillofacial trauma in children more frequently than they do in adults. This has been attributed in part to the fact that it takes a greater force to break the more elastic and stable bones of the child than it does to break an adult's bones. Thus, if the force is sufficient to break the bones of the face, it is usually sufficient to damage the child's central nervous system as well. These same developmental factors, plus the presence of unerupted teeth or mixed dentition in the mandible of the child, make internal fixation or fixation by interdental means more difficult. This problem is further compounded by the need for stabilization at an earlier time owing to the rapid healing of the facial bones in the child. Finally, unwarranted surgical treatment of the child may alter growth patterns and may lead to greater long-term functional losses and deformities than in the adult (Yarrington, 1977).

SOFT TISSUE INJURIES

The importance of early and proper wound care cannot be overemphasized, as it may eliminate totally or certainly minimize the need for future scar revision (McGregor, 1969).

Certain types of wounds deserve special consideration on the basis of the inflicting agent. For example, the treatment of dog bites is controversial. In general, if cleansing has been thorough, these may be closed primarily within eight hours of the bite. Of course, proper attention must be given to tetanus and rabies preventive measures. With regard to human bites, it is generally agreed that no primary closure of these wounds should be carried out, but rather, routine cleansing and wound care should be performed, followed by delayed closure if no infection supervenes. Electrical burns usually involve the lips and oral tissues, and the extent of injury to the tissues is often difficult to evaluate. For this reason, one mode of acceptable treatment has been to allow spontaneous demarcation between living and dead tissue to occur, with spontaneous separation of the necrotic tissue. The defect is then allowed to heal for 6 to 12 months before reconstruction is begun. One alternative is immediate excision of damaged tissues and reconstruction; another is using mucosal flaps to cover the injured tissues, possibly minimizing the tissue loss, with healing for 6 to 12 months followed by reconstruction as necessary.

Contusions of the soft tissues almost invariably heal spontaneously without a need for any more active treatment than cleansing and observation. A hematoma may accompany a contusion, but if the former is small, it usually will resorb spontaneously without treatment. On occasion, however, a hematoma may become encapsulated, producing a subcutaneous scar with a visible deformity. If this appears to be probable, the hematoma may be evacuated by incision when in the "gel" state, or by aspiration when liquefaction has occurred.

Abrasions require meticulous cleansing of the wound, which may necessitate anesthetizing the child in some way. All debris or foreign material must be removed by irrigation, mechanical débridement (sponge, brush, scalpel, dermabrader), or excision to preclude permanent "tattooing," which is difficult to treat secondarily (Fig. 40–1). Solvents, such as ether, may be necessary for the removal of oily or greasy,

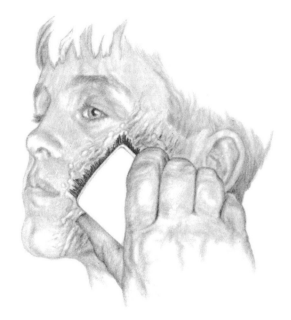

Figure 40–1. Accidental tattoo. (With permission from Grabb, W. C., Kleinert, H. E., and Puckett, C. L. 1976. Technics in Surgery: Facial and Hand Injuries. Somerville, N.J., Ethicon, Inc.)

tarlike substances. Use of a nonadherent dressing allows good healing to take place.

With deeper wounds, such as lacerations and avulsions, in the absence of infection and with accurate approximation of the skin, healing of the epidermal wound occurs quite rapidly. Healing in the dermis takes considerably longer and may be more important from the standpoint of the ultimate appearance of the wound. The progression from a fibrin clot to a quiescent, avascular scar may take several months to several years, and clinically consists of a gradual change from a red, sometimes elevated scar with a surrounding area of induration to a pale, sometimes flat, soft scar. In unusual instances, this orderly progression is disrupted by the appearance of overabundant fibrous tissue in the dermis, which results clinically in a hypertrophic scar, or keloid. The aphorism that "children heal well" may be entirely true, but a corollary is that the progression through the various phases of healing may be quite prolonged, and the likelihood of development of a hypertrophic scar and subsequent enlargement of this scar with future growth and development is greater. Wounds in the child can often retain signs of redness and elevation for several years after the initial wounding. Therefore, the physician must be particularly careful to avoid excessive skin tension in wound closure in children. Similarly, the surgeon must give more consideration to techniques such as Z-plasty that will reorder the lines of tension on the wound repair. In some instances, it is necessary to consider the effect of an extensive scar upon the future growth of the child. At times, the presence of a dense band of scar tissue over a growing bony prominence may actually produce limitation of bone growth in that area. The factors of concern in wound care are (1) placement of the scar, (2) preparation of the wound, (3) stitch craft, and (4) postoperative care.

Scar Placement

In traumatic injuries, the scar has already been placed at the time of the wounding; however, an intimate knowledge of the tissue tension lines of the face, variously referred to as "relaxed skin tension lines" (RSTL), "lines of election," or erroneously as "Langer lines," is still of great importance. This knowledge allows the surgeon to predict the quality of the ultimate healing and to choose the best incision for initial or later rearrangements of the wound or surrounding tissues. Scars placed in a "wrinkle line" or parallel to it tend to heal well, as do those placed in a line of election in nonwrinkled areas. Scars may also be "hidden" by placement in hair-bearing tissues, such as the scalp or eyebrow, or behind the ear in the postauricular sulcus. In addition, scars placed at natural junction zones of various facial features, such as the nasofacial sulcus or the nasolabial crease, tend to be less conspicuous to the casual observer.

Wound Preparation

Initial care of the wound is directed toward meticulous cleansing, as has been outlined in the care of abrasions. The excellent blood supply of the face allows excision of "damaged" tissue in the wound to be extremely conservative, and only obviously nonvital tissue should be sacrificed. This same excellent blood supply minimizes the problem of infection and allows primary closure of many facial wounds several hours after the injury. In the case of a clean wound, with little or no traumatized tissue, primary closure, or excision of the wound edges followed by primary closure, may be used, and the final result will be quite satisfactory (Fig. 40–2). In more extensive wounds, the more conservative approach dictates only thorough cleansing and removal of obviously nonviable tissue, with salvage of all remaining tissue, which is replaced in its normal position and sutured. Since in extensive

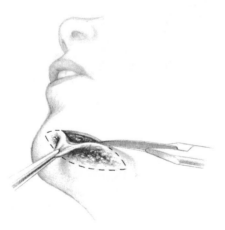

Figure 40–2. Trimming skin wounds with irregular edges. (With permission from Grabb, W. C., Kleinert, H. E., and Puckett, C. L. 1976. Technics in Surgery: Facial and Hand Injuries. Somerville, N.J., Ethicon, Inc.)

wounds it is seldom possible to achieve final reconstruction at the time of the primary treatment, the aim is to preserve as much tissue as possible for use in subsequent reconstruction. Irregular wounds are usually effectively closed by first approximating normal landmarks (eyebrow, eyelid, vermilion of the lip), distinctive portions of the wound itself that "mate" or "fit," or both landmarks and wound portions (Fig. 40–3). Where tissue has been lost, as in avulsion injuries, suturing of mucosa to skin or use of split skin grafts may be necessary.

The wound edges must be vertical, and the faces of these edges should be of the same thickness for the best scar. This usually requires undercutting or undermining of the skin edges. In wounds being sutured without tension, 3 to 5 mm of undermining will suffice to allow the proper amount of (slight) eversion of the wound edges. Where tension is a problem, undermining must be more extensive to allow for advancement of the skin to relieve the tension. The plane of undermining in the face is just deep to the dermis to avoid injury to the branches of the facial nerve, but this may be altered somewhat in the scalp and neck.

Finally, it is good to consider what is beneath the wound before embarking on closure. A beautifully executed wound closure over a nonrepaired transection of the parotid duct or a facial nerve branch is hardly a tribute to the surgeon's skills. In the same vein, it hardly seems worthwhile to use great care to close a soft tissue wound over multiple, severe bony injuries without first considering what subsequent treatment may be required. Often, the reduction and fixation of the bony injuries may best be done through the original wound. However, at other times, the manipulation of the bones takes place at just about the time of suture removal, and the wound is disrupted by traction and must be closed secondarily. If either of these situations appears likely to occur, it is often advisable to approximate the wound loosely with tape strips rather than to perform a suture closure.

Stitch Craft

Suture materials should be selected on the basis of the particular properties of the material and the specific application intended. In general, braided silk is easy to tie, and the knots hold well. However, it has relatively low tensile strength. Synthetics, such as Nylon, Dacron, and polyethylene, are available as monofilaments or braided. They have good tensile strength and cause little tissue reaction; however, they do not "handle" like silk and require a more meticulous knot-tying technique and more knot "throws." Catgut is the standard absorbable suture and may be chromicized to reduce tissue reaction and retard the rate of resorption; it is primarily employed as a buried suture to obliterate dead space and thus to help prevent hematoma. Some of the newer synthetics, such as the polyglycolic acid derivatives, Dexon and Vicryl, combine the absorbable properties of catgut

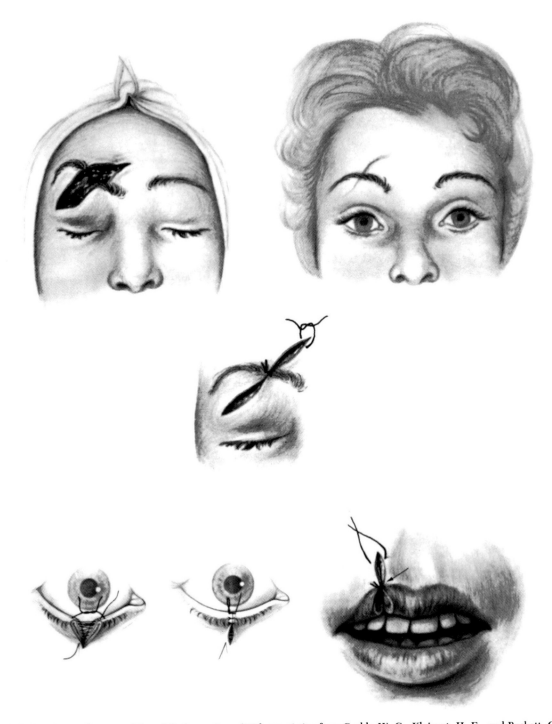

Figure 40–3. Suturing eyebrow, eyelid, and lip lacerations. (With permission from Grabb, W. C., Kleinert, H. E., and Puckett, C. L. 1976. Technics in Surgery: Facial and Hand Injuries. Somerville, N.J., Ethicon, Inc.)

with the tissue tolerance qualities of the synthetic fibers.

Instruments should be selected carefully to minimize tissue trauma. Skin hooks and needle holders must be fine, tissue forceps atraumatic, and scissors sharp. Atraumatic needles with swaged-on sutures are generally best for plastic repairs.

Suture techniques vary widely and must be tailored to coaptation of the specific wound. Interrupted sutures provide accurate approximation with minimal

chances of tissue strangulation. Continuous sutures are speedy to place and provide good hemostasis along the wound edge when interlocked. It should be remembered that the best scars result with the least tension on each suture; thus, for any given wound, the more sutures that are made the less the tension on each suture. However, this concept must be balanced against the risk of tissue strangulation, which would lead to the unsatisfactory result illustrated in Figure 40–4. Small bites of tissue, with care not to tie the suture overly tight or to place undo tension on the wound edges, will lead to the satisfactory result illustrated in Figure 40–4.

Hematoma is the absolute nemesis of good wound healing as it (1) creates tension on the wound, (2) is a good culture medium for infecting organisms, and (3) contributes to failure of flaps and grafts by interfering with neovascularization. Careful suturing to obliterate dead space and the appropriate use of drains or suction will minimize this problem.

Postoperative Care

The aim of proper postoperative care is to preserve the status of the repair in such a manner as to ensure optimal healing. This includes immobilization of the wound for healing, prevention of hematoma, and prevention of suture marks and requires careful dressing, with pressure if appropriate, care in suture removal, and continued wound support.

Suture removal is a particularly significant consideration in children. When appropriate, the surgeon should select the subcuticular closure method or place adhesive paper strips over the wound closure.

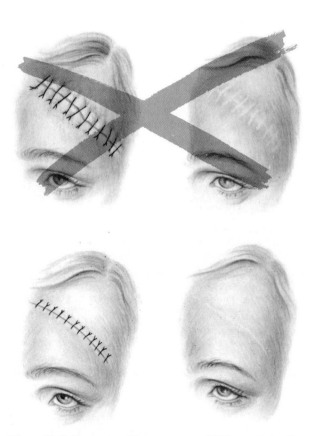

Figure 40–4. Preventing skin suture scars. (With permission from Grabb, W. C., Kleinert, H. E., and Puckett, C. L. 1976. Technics in Surgery: Facial and Hand Injuries. Somerville, N.J., Ethicon, Inc.)

Scar Revision

While it is often difficult to resist the demands of a concerned patient and anxious parents for immediate revisional surgery, such surgery is usually ill-advised before a year or longer has elapsed. This may be modified, based on the appearance of the wound and estimates of its maturity (Chap. 35).

Some scars may be highly visible because of differences in color or level from surrounding tissues and in the regularity of pattern of the scar, which tends to lead the eye along the entire length of the scar. Small discrepancies in level are often more significant than they might initially appear to be, owing to the shadowing effect of light falling on the skin surface. While little can be done surgically to alter color differences, many procedures can be employed to minimize level differences.

Scar revision may take the form of local revision, limited to the scar itself, or revision requiring rearrangements of adjacent tissues. One local revision might be simple excision and resuturing of a scar that was the result of a technically poor primary closure. This may be done repeatedly, as in serial excision for burn scars or to replace split-skin grafts. Epithelial shaving for larger elevations and dermabrasion for smaller elevations may be used to correct disparities in level within a scar or between a scar and the surrounding tissue. Running W-plasties and geometric broken-line closures are both attempts to fool the eye by changing the linear scar to an irregular or random scar, which is more difficult to follow and thus less noticeable.

Revisions involving adjacent tissue rearrangements include basic advancement, rotation, and transposition flaps, and variations of these flaps, such as the frequently mentioned but less frequently understood Z-plasty and the rhomboid flap. A detailed discussion of the construction and mechanics of transfer of these regional flaps is beyond the scope of this chapter, but some general remarks regarding their applicability are appropriate.

Z-plasty may be used for breaking a long, straight scar line; for lengthening a scar, such as to relieve a contracture or to revise a linear scar crossing a hollow (bridle deformity); or in a curvilinear scar that has produced a trap-door deformity (Fig. 40–5). In addition, it may be used to correct abnormal positioning of facial features, such as the outer canthus or oral commissure. It must be borne in mind, however, that the gains in length obtained by performing a Z-plasty are at the expense of losses in width and that the transpositions may result in tension changes in the surrounding tissues, which lead to areas of bunching and hollowing. The advantages of the revision must be balanced against these undesirable possibilities.

Rhomboid flaps are versatile variations of the transposition flap in which the transposition of the flap actually closes the donor defect. These flaps can also be modified or used in series to close larger defects, as in the flaps of Limberg and Dufourmentel (Fee, 1976).

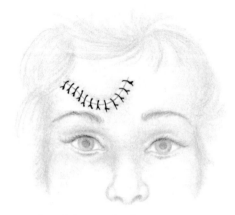
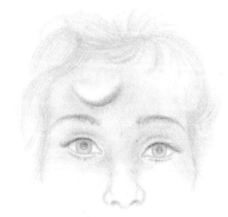

Figure 40–5. Trap-door deformity. (With permission from Grabb, W. C., Kleinert, H. E., and Puckett, C. L. 1976. Technics in Surgery: Facial and Hand Injuries. Somerville, N.J., Ethicon, Inc.)

Another useful variant of the transposition flap is the bilobed, or Zimany, flap, which is in essence a double transposition in a single step. This flap is used when the initial donor site does not lend itself to easy primary closure, so a further transposition is used to obliterate this site, and the second donor site is then repaired primarily (Tardy, 1972).

In the use of these and all other local or regional flaps, it is good to bear in mind that the closer the donor site is to the recipient site, the better will be the match as regards skin color and texture of the ultimate repair. This is also true of free grafts, with full or with partial-thickness skin.

In spite of all the aforementioned recommendations, it must be realized that there is great, uncontrollable individual variation in healing characteristics, and this sets a limit to what can be achieved by pure surgical technique. It is impossible always to get a perfect scar, but to produce the best result in a given set of circumstances, meticulous technique is essential, and failure in a single element is enough to give a poor result, however careful the attention may be to all other aspects of the repair.

EVALUATION OF FACIAL INJURY

The extent of facial injury may be assessed by three techniques: observation, palpation, and radiographic examination (Converse and Dingman, 1977).

Observation

Careful observation of all facial surfaces for indications of soft tissue injury is the starting point. Any erythema or ecchymosis should be carefully noted. Any apparent facial asymmetry, either at rest or with movement of the face, should be noted carefully. It should be remembered that many people have some small degree of facial asymmetry on a developmental basis, so that the findings of the physical examination must be correlated with the patient's history. The

eyelids should be opened to check for associated ocular injury, and examination of the mucosal surfaces of the oral cavity and pharynx must not be neglected.

Palpation

Palpation of the bony prominences of the face is next carried out, and this examination may be hampered somewhat by hematoma or edema, depending on the length of time that has elapsed since the injury. Tenderness at any site may indicate an underlying facial bone fracture, and comparison of the relative heights of the malar eminences (zygoma) is helpful in determining whether or not a fracture of the midfacial bones has occurred. A systematic and orderly palpation of the facial skeleton, even in the absence of obvious injury, may detect subtle deformities. A suggested plan of organization and the observations to be made as attention is focused on each of these areas appears in Table 40–1.

Radiographic Examination

Although radiographic examination of the facial bones is an important part of the overall evaluation of the facial injury, it cannot be relied on exclusively. Often, gross facial bone displacements will not be readily apparent on radiographs, and at other times apparent displacements of facial bones noted on radiography are not confirmed by clinical evaluation. The most informative radiographic views of the face are (1) Waters (occipitomental) views, (2) posteroanterior view, (3) lateral view, (4) lateral view of the nasal bones, (5) occlusive view of the nasal bones, (6) posteroanterior view of the mandible, (7) oblique view of the mandible, (8) occlusive view of the mandible, (9) Towne view (for ascending mandibular rami and condyles), and (10) tangential views of the zygomatic arch.

Additional and sometimes more precise information regarding a particular area may be obtained by the use of special radiographic techniques, including tomog-

TABLE 40–1. Orderly and Systematic Examination of the Face

AREAS TO EXAMINE
Supraorbital and lateral orbital rims
Infraorbital rims
Malar eminences (zygoma)
Zygomatic arches
Nasal bones
Maxilla
Mandible
As attention is focused on each of these areas, certain observations should be noted.

SUPRAORBITAL AND LATERAL ORBITAL RIMS
a) Bony depression or angulation
b) Tenderness
c) Eyebrow irregularity
d) Ocular proptosis or enophthalmos
e) Periorbital ecchymosis
f) Scleral ecchymosis
g) Swelling or ecchymosis of the upper eyelids
h) Limitation or lag in ocular movements
i) Diplopia (subjective)
j) Anesthesia of forehead
k) Muscular activity of forehead

INFRAORBITAL RIMS
a) Depression or angulation
b) Tenderness
c) Periorbital ecchymosis
d) Scleral ecchymosis
e) Limitation or lag in ocular movements
f) Diplopia in various directions of gaze (subjective)
g) Anesthesia of nasolabial fold and upper lip
h) Anesthesia of maxillary teeth

MALAR EMINENCES
a) Comparison of height (unilateral depression)
b) Periorbital ecchymosis
c) Crepitus
d) Angulation

ZYGOMATIC ARCHES
a) Depression or angulation
b) Periorbital ecchymosis
c) Tenderness
d) Limitation of mandibular excursion

NASAL BONES
a) Depression or angulation
b) Periorbital ecchymosis
c) Epistaxis
d) Tenderness
e) Crepitus
f) Loss of pyramidal support
g) Septal obstruction or deviation
h) Tenderness at base of columella

MAXILLA
a) Dental malocclusion
b) Periorbital ecchymosis
c) Motion of maxilla
d) Asymmetry or collapse of dental arch form
e) Misplaced or damaged teeth
f) Tear of upper buccal sulcus or mucoperiosteum of palate

MANDIBLE
a) Tenderness and pain (subjective)
b) Asymmetry of mandibular contour and lower lip
c) Asymmetry or collapse of dental arch
d) Dental malocclusion
e) Limitation of mandibular excursion
f) Abnormal motion
g) Misplaced or damaged teeth
h) Tear of lower buccal sulcus
i) Anesthesia of lower lip or teeth
j) Injury to tongue

Data from Facial Injuries, 3rd edition, by Richard Carlton Schultz. Copyright © 1988 by Year Book Medical Publishers, Inc., Chicago. Reproduced with permission.

---

raphy, polytomography, and xeroradiography (Fig. 40–6), which tend to give better delineation of the bony outlines. In addition, panoramic scanning radiographs are of particular value in visualizing fractures of the lower third of the face, including the lower portions of the maxilla and the mandible. A further radiographic

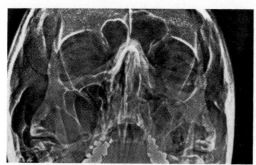

Figure 40–6. Xeroradiograph. (With permission from Marshall, K. A., Sadowsky, N. L., and Sigman, D. Xeroradiography in the diagnosis of facial fractures. Plast. Reconstr. Surg. 62:207–211, 1978.)

technique of value, often neglected, is the use of stereo views, particularly the stereo Waters view. Recently, widespread use of computed tomography (CT) scanning has further enhanced our ability to clearly define bony injuries of the facial skeleton (Rowe and Brandt-Zawadzki, 1982) (Fig. 40–7). Several very specialized techniques that are only now coming into use include three-dimensional image reconstruction of computed tomograms in the pediatric age group (Armstrong et al., 1985) and moire topography, a form of biostereometric contour analysis (Karlan and Madden, 1979) (Fig. 40–8).

INJURIES OF SPECIFIC SITES

Nose

The primary difference between the child's nose and that of the adult, other than the obvious ones of size and configuration, consists of the proportionally smaller part of the nose of the child contributed by

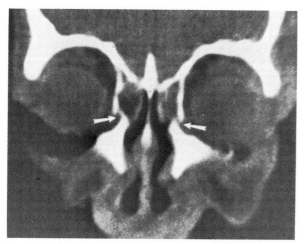

Figure 40–7. CT scan of fracture. (With permission from Rowe, L. D., and Brandt-Zawadzki, M. 1982. Spatial analysis of midfacial fractures with multidirectional and computed tomography: Clinicopathologic correlates in 44 cases. Otolaryngol. Head Neck Surg. 90:651.)

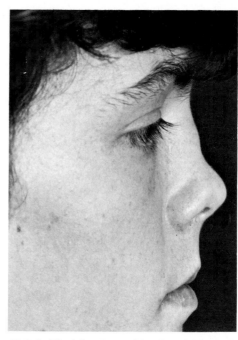

Figure 40–9. Saddle deformity resulting from injury to the nose.

the bony nasal pyramid and the relatively greater elasticity of the bones and the immaturity of the suture lines. Because of these factors, injuries to the nasal bones of a child may not be as obvious as in an adult, and the overall elasticity and compliance of the structures may allow a significant cartilaginous injury, with subsequent septal hematoma to coexist with unharmed bony structures. In addition, a relatively "minor" injury may result in arrested development and maturation of the nasal structures, with a resultant infantile nasal configuration (Fig. 40–9). Soft tissue injuries of the nose are usually easily diagnosed by inspection, and repair, in the absence of tissue loss such as avulsion or amputation, is readily accomplished. Meticulous

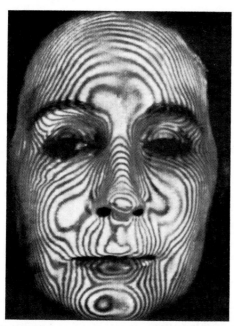

Figure 40–8. Moire topograph. (With permission from Karlan, M. S., and Madden, M. 1979. Moire topography in facial plastic surgery. Otolaryngol. Head Neck Surg. 87:533.)

reapproximation of all tissue layers of the nose begins with the mucosa, including that of the nasal septum and turbinates. This is commonly accomplished with absorbable catgut sutures, and these may be placed to include the perichondrium and thus approximate the cartilaginous structures, such as the upper and lower lateral cartilages or the septal cartilage. Sutures may also be placed directly in the cartilage for accurate approximation as long as these are carefully placed to avoid strangulation or deformity of the cartilage. The superficial muscle tissues of the nose are generally adherent to the skin, and they need not be repaired separately. Accurate approximation of the skin edges with appropriate regard to important anatomic features, such as the rim of the nasal ala, is the final stage in the soft tissue repair, although it is often advisable to splint the repair with an intranasal dressing of an appropriately lubricated packing material, such as adaptic gauze, and an external dressing of appropriate tape and a malleable or moldable splint.

In cases of tissue loss, avulsed segments of the lower nasal vault, if small, may be used as autografts and may be carefully sutured in place with a good chance of satisfactory survival. If the avulsed segments are not available, the use of composite grafts of skin and cartilage from the ear may be employed in the primary repair with a fair degree of success.

Cartilaginous and bony injuries to the nose are not diagnosed as easily as are soft tissue injuries but are nonetheless important and may even occur in the newborn. A dislocated nasal septum as a result of the trauma of delivery is readily reduced by gentle traction on the nose to effect realignment. Radiographs are generally of little value for demonstrating cartilaginous injuries and, in the case of children, are often of little value in demonstrating bony injuries. This, coupled with the difficulties of satisfactorily examining the interior and exterior of the nasal structures in the child, contributes toward these injuries being considered "insignificant" and remaining untreated. Although displacement of these structures may not be great at the time of injury, gross deformity may result from continued growth and development of unaligned structures. For instance, hematomas of the septum must be evacuated immediately if a saddle deformity is to be prevented. This requires satisfactory incision and appropriate placement of dressings to prevent reaccumulation of blood, and this may require a general anesthetic. Infection of a hematoma, leading to a septal abscess, can cause rapid and disastrous loss of cartilage and requires immediate incision and drainage and vigorous antibiotic therapy. If the possibility of a septal hematoma or serious intranasal injury can be excluded, it is often better to wait several days to allow most of the edema and ecchymosis to resolve before attempting a definitive repair of the bony derangement. Bleeding from the nose of the child who has been struck suggests the presence of a fracture, and this is especially true if the bleeding is accompanied by edema and ecchymosis of the overlying tissues. Nasal bleeding may be the result of displaced nasal bones that have penetrated the nasal mucosa. In a study of nasal injury, seven signs suggestive of nasal fracture were noted to occur in this order of frequency: epistaxis, swelling of the nasal dorsum, ecchymosis of the eyes, tenderness of the nasal dorsum, radiographic evidence of fracture, nasal deformity, and crepitus of the nasal bones. This last finding is felt by some to be diagnostic of nasal fracture (Moran, 1977).

Immediate treatment of a nasal fracture is the same in children as in adults and begins with control of any epistaxis, which usually ceases spontaneously. If epistaxis fails to stop spontaneously, the soft tissue portions of the nose may be grasped between the thumb and forefinger and pressure maintained for several minutes. Should no significant swelling be noted at this point, evaluation of the external nose by inspection and palpation may be advisable. This applies also to examination of the intranasal structures, which requires satisfactory illumination, restraint, and vasoconstriction, along with a satisfactory source of suction. If there is doubt at this point as to the extent of the injury, one has the choice of carrying out further examination, including manipulation of the nasal cartilages and bones with appropriate instruments and with the patient under general anesthesia, or of allowing time to pass in hopes that the tissue reaction will subside adequately enough to allow better clinical evaluation. However, it must be remembered that the nasal tissues heal rapidly and that fixation with malposition may occur unless the fractures are properly reduced within a period of a few days.

Treatment of bony injuries in the young child revolves about satisfactory digital and instrument manipulation of the fractured fragments into appropriate positions, and then splinting to maintain the alignment. Comminuted nasal fractures are especially difficult to stabilize in children and may require splinting by means of external plates and fixation wires. Open reduction of nasal fractures in the young child is seldom justified, although it may occasionally be helpful in treating older children.

It should be remembered that, in spite of apparently satisfactory reduction of nasal fractures and correction of cartilaginous or soft tissue injuries, there is no assurance that a deformity will not develop with progressive growth and development. The parents of these patients should be advised of the possible necessity for further treatment at some later date.

Some nasal fractures that require special consideration include the so-called "open-book" type of fracture, in which the fractured segments splay out to involve the frontal processes of the maxillae (Zaydon and Brown, 1964). This may be associated with fragmentation of the entire bony nasal bridge and its displacement into the ethmoid or frontal region (Fig. 40–10). These fractures of the nasofrontal and nasoethmoid regions may result in injuries to the nasofrontal ducts, the nasolacrimal apparatus, and the medial canthal ligaments with resultant later formation of a frontal mucocele, pseudohypertelorism and rounding of the medial canthus region, or epiphora and dacryocystitis. The treatment of these injuries is complex and largely surgical and may involve exploration of the frontal sinus or exploration of the medial portions of each orbit with direct wire fixation of the canthal ligaments to the repositioned bony structures of the lateral nasal wall and medial orbital wall (Weber and Cohn, 1977).

Midface

There are several special features to be considered in evaluating injuries to the midfacial region in the child (McCoy et al., 1966). In the very young, the size of the face relative to that of the cranial vault is quite small, so that injuries to this area are relatively infrequent. At approximately 6 years of age, the midfacial skeleton has achieved most of its ultimate growth, but there remain some anatomic differences between the midface skeleton of the 6-year-old child and that of an adult. The sinuses of the child are quite small and poorly pneumatized, and the bones are still quite resilient and tend to fracture in a greenstick manner. In addition, the mixed dentition of children is such that the decision to perform intermaxillary fixation must be considered carefully: At this age the roots of the deciduous teeth are gradually being resorbed, and there is frequent absence of teeth and a poor retentive shape to the crowns of some teeth. In addition, indiscriminate use of interdental wiring may damage the tooth buds and may result in losses or distortions of the permanent dentition.

SOFT TISSUE INJURIES. These are particularly important in children, as injuries that damage a child's appearance inflict great damage on his or her self-esteem. This is a distinct possibility in the case of facial lacerations, and adequate attention must be paid to

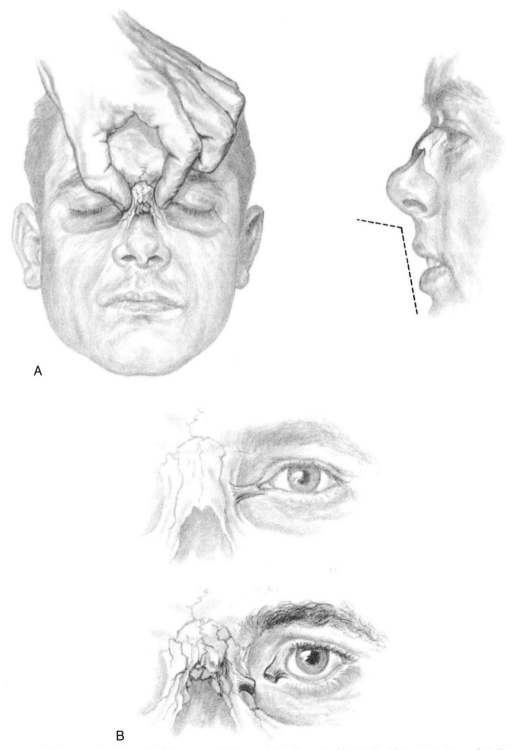

A

B

Figure 40–10. *A*, Nasal fractures. *B*, Nasoorbital fractures. (With permission from Grabb, W. C., Kleinert, H. E., and Puckett, C. L. 1976. Technics in Surgery: Facial and Hand Injuries. Somerville, N.J., Ethicon, Inc.)

possible injuries to branches of the facial nerve. Proper management of such injuries must include careful preanesthetic evaluation of facial motion, and any injuries to a nerve must be repaired using microtechniques and the binocular operating microscope, possibly with the aid of a nerve stimulator, during the

first 72 hours after injury if optimal results are to be obtained.

Soft tissue injuries to specific sites may require slightly different approaches (Bailey, 1977). Laceration of the cheek is probably the most commonly encountered soft tissue injury in children. While the superficial aspects of the repair are relatively simple, several structures deserve special consideration. Included among these are the branches of the facial nerve, the parotid gland and duct (Stensen duct), and the muscles of mastication and expression. A good guideline in the evaluation of these injuries is that those occupying an area posterior to a line dropped vertically from the lateral canthus and inferior to a line drawn from the external auditory canal to the nasal tip are most apt to involve significant injuries to the aforementioned structures (Fig. 40–11). Lacerations extending into the parotid gland may result in the development of a salivary fistula, which may be avoided by careful closure of the capsule of the gland and a meticulous, layered closure of the overlying soft tissue.

Injury to the parotid duct should be suspected when clear fluid is seen leaking from the wound surface. Patency of the duct is essential and may be obtained by suture closure over a fine polyethylene catheter. An alternative treatment is fistulization of the glandular segment of the duct into the oral cavity at some point other than the normal orifice. In very unusual circumstances, such as when extensive damage to the duct has occurred or it has been lost at its insertion into the gland, the identifiable portion may be ligated to produce atrophy of the gland. Injuries to facial nerve branches anterior to the region of the parotid duct do not usually result in significant loss of muscle function because the superficial facial muscles are innervated in their posterior portions, and, therefore, repair of these small anterior branches, which have multiple anastomoses in most cases, is unnecessary. Clean divisions of the identifiable nerve branches require careful approximation of the nerve sheaths, with fine

sutures and with the aid of magnification and appropriate microinstruments. In cases in which a significant portion of the nerve has been lost, the ends of the remaining portions can be marked for later use in free grafting or crossed anastomosis, as this type of sophisticated repair is rarely indicated at the time of primary treatment.

Wounds of the chin are somewhat unique in that the bulk of the subcutaneous tissue of the area is comprised of a somewhat avascular fat pad, and the tissues are therefore more prone to infection and subsequent resorption. Careful approximation of the injured tissues in layers, however, will usually ensure satisfactory healing. Repair of lacerations of the lip requires careful attention to the alignment of the tissues, the most important landmark being the vermilion border. The vermilion-cutaneous junction should therefore be marked with an appropriate solution prior to the injection of any local anesthetic agent to avoid distortion of the tissue and to ensure accurate reapproximation. In lacerations that are through and through, the muscular closure of the orbicularis oris fibers is of great importance for ensuring good physiologic function. When areas of tissue loss are less than 20 per cent, repair by direct closure is usually readily accomplished. In losses involving greater amounts of tissue, the use of regional transposition flaps from the remaining uninvolved areas of the lip is in order.

Intraoral soft tissue wounds are often neglected under the erroneous assumption that these will always heal satisfactorily spontaneously. While this may be true of small punctate wounds, such as those inflicted by the other oral structures (teeth and alveolar fragments), it does not apply to more extensive injuries. On the other hand, however, too meticulous a closure without adequate consideration of drainage requirements for these injuries is equally undesirable and can result in the development of large hematomas of the buccal space or other undesirable sequelae. Intraoral wounds should be closed primarily whenever possible, avoiding distortion of natural landmarks and compromises of physiologic function just as is done in closures of cutaneous wounds. Suture closure can be carried out with permanent materials such as silk, although the use of absorbable materials such as chromic catgut is quite acceptable and may be preferred in areas in which suture removal presents a problem. Large, raw surfaces may require coverage by adjacent flaps (tongue flaps, regional mucosal flaps) or dermal grafts. In general, when patients have fractures that are compounded into the oral cavity and for which repair must be delayed, the intraoral soft tissue injury should be closed to reduce the incidence of infection and to convert the open to a closed fracture. Small or incomplete lacerations of the tongue may be left unsutured, especially in the uncooperative child who would have to be anesthetized to accomplish the suturing satisfactorily. In the case of more extensive lacerations in which the possibility of extensive scarring or the development of a permanent cleft of the tongue exists, careful suturing should be done. In addition, suturing

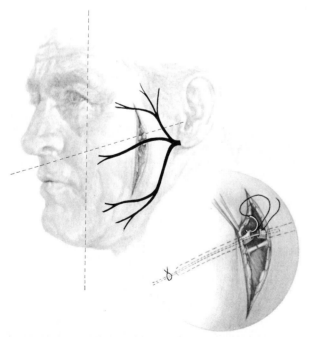

Figure 40–11. Suturing severed facial nerve and parotid duct. (With permission from Grabb, W. C., Kleinert, H. E., and Puckett, C. L. 1976. Technics in Surgery: Facial and Hand Injuries. Somerville, N.J., Ethicon, Inc.)

of the tongue may be required as the method of choice for obtaining hemostasis in such a wound.

Lacerations involving the forehead and brow require careful attention to facial landmarks to reconstitute the hairline and eyebrow adequately. It should be realized that it is never necessary or advisable to shave the eyebrow in performing such repairs. In making secondary incisions or local tissue rearrangements, careful attention must be paid to the natural forehead lines. One of the more important anatomic structures of the midface from both a functional and an aesthetic standpoint is the eyelids, and this dictates extremely meticulous attention to repair. Since this tissue is quite delicate and separates readily, it is not unusual to gain the false impression that tissue loss has occurred. The preferred repair of through-and-through lacerations involving the lid margin is careful approximation of conjunctiva, tarsus, and lid skin in layers, without using staggering methods or Z-plasty. While it is often recommended that the orbital septum be repaired with fine catgut sutures to prevent herniation of orbital fat, the septum is often left widely open following cosmetic blepharoplasty without any untoward result. Careful attention must be paid to appropriate repositioning of displaced lateral and medial canthal ligaments and to the integrity of the lacrimal duct system. Extensive injuries in this area warrant ophthalmologic consultation to evaluate the possibilities for restoration of function of the tear duct system and any associated intraocular injury. When tissue loss does occur in the lids, a graft may be obtained from the skin of an uninvolved upper lid in older children if some excess of this tissue exists, or thinned-out postauricular skin may be used.

In soft tissue injuries to the auricle, the presence of contusions and hematomas takes on more significance than it might in other specific anatomic sites. Contusions may predispose the underlying tissues to the development of perichondritis and possible loss of cartilage support. Hematomas must be drained adequately and conforming dressings applied so as to prevent any reaccumulation of the fluid if severe distortion from loss of cartilage or fibrous organization of the clot (cauliflower ear) is to be avoided. In the case of lacerations, initial efforts should be toward reconstruction of the external auditory canal and external meatus. The canal must be approximated meticulously or anastamosed and stented to maintain the patency of the canal and to prevent subsequent stenosis or obliteration. The next step in orderly repair of the auricle is accurate reapproximation of the helical rim. Following this, the remaining cartilage and skin areas are sutured. Tissue loss in cases of auricular trauma is of particular importance, since there is no truly satisfactory donor site for secondary reconstruction except composite grafts from the opposite ear. Since the blood supply of the ear is abundant and the metabolic demands of the tissues are relatively low, the use of avulsed flaps of tissue with even extremely small pedicles carries a high rate of success. Even amputated composite tissue segments, if of a limited size (less

than 25 per cent), often survive when relocated primarily. Case reports show that even when auricles have been totally avulsed, replantation has been occasionally successful. On occasion, it is necessary to preserve the cartilaginous skeleton of the ear by removing damaged skin covering it and burying the segment beneath the postauricular skin. This may be done by making a small incision some distance superiorly or posteriorly in the scalp, so as not to interfere with the blood supply of the covering flap. The uniquely convoluted cartilage segment thus preserved becomes the keystone for subsequent reconstruction.

Bony injuries to the midface include those of the zygoma and orbital confines, those of the maxilla proper (including Le Fort fractures), and those involving the alveolar process. Fractures of the bones of the face differ from fractures of bones of the remainder of the body in several respects. Because of their exposed position and minimal soft tissue cover, they may be fractured in spite of a relatively insignificant-appearing injury to the overlying tissues. In addition, injuries of a single isolated bone are the exception, whereas combined injuries to several bones constituting a segment of the facial skeleton are the rule. When displacement occurs, it is invariably determined by the direction of the injuring force rather than by any effect of muscle pulls. The latter accounts for the tendency for reduced facial fractures to remain reduced and stable without unduly elaborate apparatus for traction and fixation. Fractures of the midfacial bones are usually readily apparent on physical examination, and attention is often drawn to the possibility of facial fracture by the presence of contused or abraded overlying soft tissues. In fractures of the maxilla, inspection may reveal flattening, shortening, or elongation of the face. The alignment of the teeth may be abnormal, with the upper teeth overlapping the lower or with the presence of an open bite. Abnormal mobility may be observed by grasping the anterior upper teeth or alveolus and attempting to move the maxilla up and down or in and out. In fractures of the zygoma or orbital rim, subconjunctival hemorrhage or ecchymosis of the eyelids may be noted, and the patient may complain of numbness of the upper lip and gums. Careful palpation of the bony margins of the orbit may reveal separations or misalignments, which may be confirmed by comparing both sides of the face. Placement of the index fingers on the high points of the cheeks or malar bones when viewed from above and behind the patient's head helps the physician detect fractures by measuring and comparing the levels of the fingers (and thus the bones). Variations in the level of the pupils or lateral canthi of the eyes may indicate depressions of the orbital rim (Fig. 40–12), another sign of fracture.

Emphysema of the cheek or periorbital tissues may result from a fracture that extends into the antrum or ethmoid complex and that allows air to pass into the soft tissues. Sneezing or blowing the nose may forcibly increase this emphysema.

The second most common fracture of the facial bones, the most common being fracture of the nasal

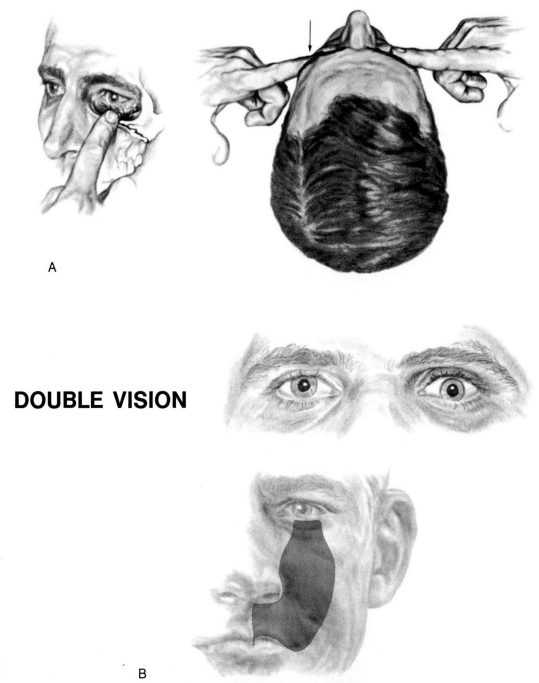

DOUBLE VISION

Figure 40–12. *A*, Zygomatic fracture. *B*, Diplopia and hypesthesia of the cheek often accompany a zygomatic fracture. (With permission from Grabb, W. C., Kleinert, H. E., and Puckett, C. L. 1976. Technics in Surgery: Facial and Hand Injuries. Somerville, N.J., Ethicon, Inc.)

bones, is a fracture of the zygomatic complex. The signs of this fracture found on examination include periorbital ecchymoses, flattening of the malar eminence, depression of the inferior rim of the orbit, and hypesthesia of the distribution of the infraorbital nerve. There may be tenderness at the infraorbital and lateral orbital rims and, on occasion, diplopia secondary to displacement of the lateral canthal tendon attached to the depressed bone. Displacement of the zygoma is most often associated with fracture separation at three points: along the infraorbital rim at the zygomatico-

maxillary suture, along the lateral orbital rim at the zygomaticofrontal suture, and in the midportion of the zygomatic arch, at the junction of its temporal and zygomatic portions. Although isolated fractures of the zygoma do occur, they are much less frequent than are injuries associated with extension into the orbital floor along the orbital rim at the infraorbital foramen. Plane radiographs usually demonstrate these fractures well in the Waters view, and often show opacification of the maxillary antrum or the presence of an air or fluid level in the antrum on the side of the injury, which indicates bleeding into the antrum from torn mucosal lining. In cases of severe comminution of the orbital floor or dehiscence of orbital soft tissue through the floor, laminographic studies may be necessary to demonstrate the pathologic condition. In addition, stereoradiographic views and, more recently, xeroradiographic studies, have been found to be extremely helpful in evaluating such injuries.

Displaced fractures of the zygoma usually require open reduction and internal fixation to avoid the development of deformities, a depression, and possible enophthalmos or diplopia. Multiple surgical approaches to the treatment of these fractures exist, and their application must be based on a careful consideration of the individual requirements of each patient (Lore, 1973). In general, the simplest and most direct approaches are preferred in children. Fractures of the zygoma may be reduced by direct traction or by approaches through the oral cavity or maxillary antrum or both. Fixation is then accomplished by direct wiring or internal splinting.

Fractures of the zygomatic arch proper are occasioned by direct, medially applied force, and the fracture most often consists of a central fracture, fracture at the origin of the zygoma, and fracture at the temporal insertion accompanying depression of the middle segment. Swelling may be noted over the arch initially, but this is superseded by a definite depression or flatness following resorption of the edema and hematoma. Ecchymosis over the involved periorbital areas and associated tenderness with occasional depression may be noted. Mandibular excursions may be limited from impingement of the depressed fragments on the coronoid process of the mandible.

Fracture displacements of the zygomatic arch are usually readily demonstrated radiographically, and the best views are generally the tangential views, such as the submentovertex or the so-called "jug-handle views" (Fig. 40–13). A patient and skillful technician may be required to obtain these views in the anxious

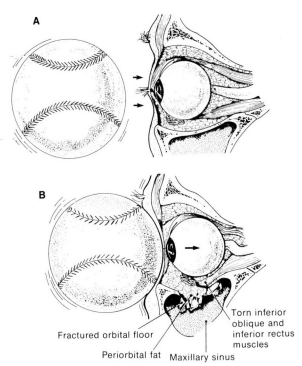

Figure 40–14. Blowout fracture of the orbit. (With permission from Dodd, G. D. 1977. Radiology of the nose, paranasal sinuses, and nasopharynx. *In* Golden, R., et al. [eds.]: Golden's Diagnostic Radiology. © 1977, The Williams & Wilkins Co., Baltimore.)

and frightened child. Reduction of these fractures is usually not difficult, and the structural nature of the arch and its cantileverlike arrangement make support or fixation unnecessary.

True *"blowout" fractures of the orbit* (Fig. 40–14) are probably quite rare in children owing to the lack of pneumatization of the developing maxillary antrum and the thickness of the bones of the inferior and medial walls of the orbit. The suggested mechanism of a blowout fracture is based on hydraulic pressures. Anterior pressure on the globe forces the orbital contents posteriorly. This results in increased hydraulic pressure and increased pressure on the surrounding bony frame. It is postulated that the thin areas fracture, and the orbital contents are forced through the opening into the surrounding sinus. The most common point of involvement is the floor and antrum. This theory is not without controversy, and a recent study has suggested a different mechanism. In this study, the orbital floor could consistently be fractured by pressure applied only to the orbital rim, and it was suspected that the forces on the rim alone caused a "buckling" of the floor. In this study, the hydraulic pressure effect was not part of the blowout mechanism. Orbital fractures are similar to fractures of the malar and zygomatic areas previously described and share many of the presenting symptoms and radiographic findings. Arbitrarily, they have been categorized as either "pure," in which no associated fracture of the orbital rim exists, or "impure," in which an associated fracture of one of the bony confines of the orbital rim does exist. Initially, ecchymoses involving the lids and periorbita may be

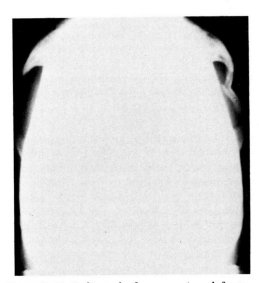

Figure 40–13. Radiograph of a zygomatic arch fracture.

noted without any significant displacement of the involved eye because of compensatory hematoma and edema within the orbit. This may be noted even though a significant amount of periorbital fat has herniated into the maxillary antrum. It has been stated that hypesthesia of the nasolabial area and upper lip is uncommon in blowout fractures and is more characteristic of zygomatic fractures. This has been attributed to the fact that, in the former case, the infraorbital rim remains intact and tends to protect the infraorbital foramen. In the author's experience, hypesthesia of the infraorbital nerve may be *more* characteristic of a blowout fracture, since the nerve is injured in its traverse through the infraorbital canal, contained in the thin bone of the orbital floor. This hypesthesia is usually of limited duration and probably represents contusion of the nerve rather than true disruption. Diplopia is an inconstant finding and has usually been attributed to actual muscle entrapment in the fracture site. This is probably most often *not* the case, as diplopia may be secondary to either or both bleeding within the orbital soft tissues with consequent displacement of the globe and hematoma within the muscle sheath itself, or the nerve sheath, with attendant limitation of range of motion on a neuromuscular basis. Ironically, the diplopia may be masked by the presence of edema and hematoma, which compensate for the depression of the orbital floor. Probably, the pathogenesis of most forms of persistent, and clinically significant, diplopia is atrophy and resorption of traumatized periorbital fat, whether actually entrapped in a fracture site or merely contused. With the accompanying decrease in the volume of the orbital contents, the globe tends to settle into an enophthalmic position. Late enophthalmos and diplopia may occur even following apparently successful and technically excellent reductions of orbital fractures.

Orbital blowout fractures may be difficult to demonstrate radiographically, although an air or fluid level or partial opacification of the involved antrum on plane views is suggestive of this injury. Tomograms may reveal the so-called "teardrop" or "bomb-bay" signs (Fig. 40–15), which have been thought to be due to dehiscence of periorbital fat through the fracture site in the roof of the antrum. However, this can be misleading, and when on occasion, these radiographic signs have been present, a small fracture of the orbital floor without dehiscence has been discovered at the time of surgery, and the radiographic finding was attributed to the presence of a submucoperiosteal hematoma of the antral roof. The decision as to whether or not these fractures should be treated is often a very difficult one and must be an individual one based on the particular findings in, and requirements of, each patient. Previously, the presence of diplopia, when associated with limitation of movement in a cardinal direction of gaze and infraorbital hypesthesia, and especially when accompanied by suggestive radiographic findings, was an absolute indication for surgical exploration. However, the trend has been away from exploration except in those cases in which true herniation of intraorbital contents or entrapment of muscles is clearly evident. Even in cases where true diplopia exists and limitation of range of motion of the eye can be demonstrated readily, it has become acceptable to observe the patient over a period of 7 to 14 days and to assess the resolution or progression of symptoms as the acute tissue reaction subsides. It has commonly been found that no intervention will be necessary after this period of time, and this concept of watchful waiting has partially been justified on the basis that surgical intervention immediately may not provide any assurance of normal function without diplopia or enophthalmos. The general criteria for surgical intervention are persistent diplopia and enophthalmos. Diplopia lasting longer than two weeks indicates a definite functional abnormality and a strong possibility of entrapment of muscle, whereas early enophthalmos suggests a significant loss of orbital tissues. Patients with these findings are considered candidates for surgical exploration and repair.

Fractures of the orbital rim with palpable step-offs must be corrected. Downward displacement of the globe may at first not be noticeable owing to the compensation by periorbital edema. Unlike the situation in the adult, after this type of fracture has healed in a child it is not as amenable to correction by refracturing or by bone grafting. Accurate reduction must therefore be done within the first five to seven days after injury. These same principles apply to the typical tripod fracture of the malar-zygomatic complex in which there is obvious asymmetry with a palpable step-off type of displacement and flattening of the malar eminence.

Approaches to the operative treatment of these fractures are largely similar to those used in fractures of the zygoma and consist of replacing herniated orbital tissues in their normal position and repositioning displaced bony fragments (Dingman and Natvig, 1964).

Maxillary fractures may occur in many forms, varying even between opposite sides of the same maxilla. An understanding of these fractures is possible if one considers them as Le Fort originally described them: Type I (transverse), Type II (pyramidal), and Type III (craniofacial dysjunction) (Fig. 40–16). The most consistent symptom in these fractures is malocclusion, and

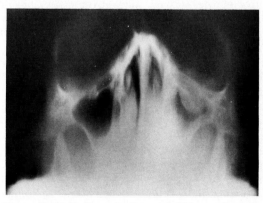

Figure 40–15. Radiograph of an orbital blowout fracture.

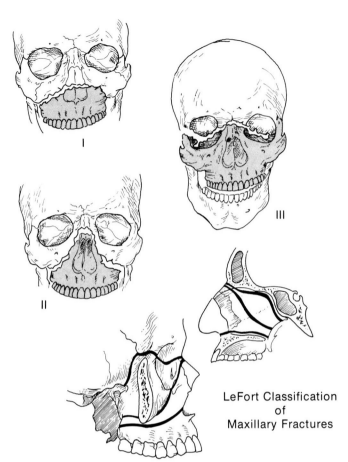

Figure 40–16. Maxillary fractures. (Reproduced with permission from Schultz, R. C. Facial Injuries, 2nd ed. Copyright 1977 by Year Book Medical Publishers, Inc., Chicago.)

LeFort Classification
of
Maxillary Fractures

the most common accompanying finding is elongation of the midface area. There is almost invariably periorbital swelling and ecchymosis, and palpation reveals mobility of the upper dental arch and surrounding maxilla. An anterior open bite is not an absolute indication of a maxillary fracture but is certainly presumptive evidence for one. The radiographic evaluation for suspected injury of the maxilla is similar to that for suspected injury to the zygomatic and malar complex.

Consideration of the Le Fort classification system may be helpful in planning treatment, but variations of these fractures are so common as to demand even more individualized treatment than for other facial fractures (Mustarde, 1971). The need for access to the midfacial and dental arch areas means that techniques for maintaining the airway during anesthesia and postoperatively must be considered carefully. A tracheostomy is frequently performed in these cases, although its use should be predicated on firmer indications than the mere need for convenient access to the face. Nasotracheal intubation allows excellent access to the midface and teeth for application of arch bars, and even orotracheal intubation allows satisfactory access to these regions, although it requires that intermaxillary fixation be delayed until extubation has been accomplished. Commonly, extubation occurs after 24 hours and is accomplished without anesthesia in adults. However, in children, this is a much less practical

method, since although it does offer the benefit of leaving the mouth open in the immediate postoperative period, thereby reducing the danger of aspiration should the patient vomit while recovering from the anesthesia, extubation is more difficult.

In low transverse maxillary fractures (Guérin fracture or Le Fort I Type fracture), when vertical displacement is minimal, interdental elastic fixation is usually sufficient. In children, a firm, fibrous union is usually evident three to four weeks after fixation.

Pyramidal fractures (Le Fort Type II) are central, midfacial fractures in the subzygomatic area and extend through the nasal bones and maxilla, usually at the zygomaticomaxillary suture areas. In common with fractures of the zygoma, they involve the maxillary antrum, inferior orbital rims, and the orbital floors but, in addition, involve the central segment, which is displaced posteriorly with upward angulation to produce an open bite. The apex of this fracture commonly involves the nasal bones and the bones of the medial aspect of the orbital floor. Surgical treatment is similar to that for open reduction of fractures of the zygoma and may require suspension of the maxilla from the intact frontal bone.

The Le Fort Type III, or high-level, fracture is suprazygomatic and extends through the orbit and nasofrontal regions, constituting a separation of the midface from the cranium, as the term "craniofacial dysjunction" implies. The entire middle third of the face is fractured, with involvement of both zygomas, the nose, and the maxilla, presenting the characteristic appearance of a "bloated" edematous midface. Malocclusion, with an open, anterior open bite, is a characteristic of this type of fracture, and a "free-floating" maxilla is usually detectable by palpation. Once again, the cornerstone of surgical treatment is suspension of the fractured and displaced fragments from the adjacent stable cranial fragments by appropriate incisions and direct wiring through these incisions. Recently, the use of minicompression plates of various configurations has found increasing favor, although extensive experience with their use in children is still lacking at this time (Fig. 40–17).

Various types of dental and alveolar injuries may be associated with fractures of the middle third of the face. A loosened tooth usually will solidify spontaneously; however, wire fixation to an adjacent tooth helps ensure its position and retention. A fractured segment of alveolus may be stabilized and alignment restored by wiring a tooth of the flail segment to an adjacent solid tooth or to an arch bar. Intermaxillary wire fixation will further secure the fracture and help restore normal occlusion. Extensive alveolar fractures and avulsions, especially those having any periosteal or mucosal attachment, should be replaced and immobilized very securely. Most often, these segments will heal solidly in position.

Mandible

The management of fractures of the mandible in children is similar to their management in adults, with some notable exceptions (Freid and Baden, 1954).

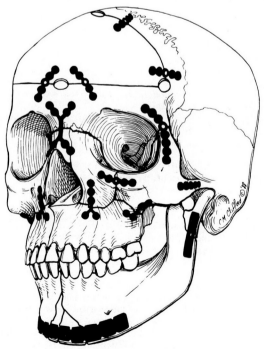

Figure 40–17. Minifixation plate system.

Initially, the deciduous teeth may not provide adequate support for intermaxillary fixation. In children between the ages of 6 and 12 years, the mixed dentition may prove to be inadequate for ligation of arch bars or intermaxillary fixation owing to the fact that the roots of the temporary teeth are undergoing resorption, and the teeth are exfoliating as the permanent teeth erupt to replace them. In addition, the rapid healing of fractures in children makes it mandatory that treatment be carried out within five to seven days if malunion is to be avoided. As in the case of other facial fractures, general anesthesia may more frequently be required for the management of fractures of the mandible in children, as fear and immaturity may limit the child's ability to cooperate. Finally, since many fractures of the body and ramus of the mandible are of the greenstick variety in children, early but relatively short-term fixation may provide for adequate and functional healing. Special consideration must be given to fractures of the condylar process, as possible interference with the growth center of this bone may result in developmental arrest and possible ankylosis of the joint.

As in fractures of the upper jaw, the most consistent physical finding in fractures of the mandible is malocclusion. While in fractures of the upper dental arch this is apt to be represented by an anterior open bite, a lateral crossbite is probably more common in fractures of the lower dental arch. Where the jaw is subluxed or dislocated, there may be severe restriction of motion, with the jaw open and locked. Other common findings in fractures of the mandible are deformity, mobility of the fracture fragments, swelling, ecchymosis, and lingual deviation of the teeth, with associated tenderness to palpation of the involved area. The most useful radiographic views are the lateral or oblique, the posteroanterior, the Towne, and the occlusive. Panoramic views (Panorex) have given a useful, wide view of the dental arches, which is often helpful. Finally, for diagnosing injuries to the temporomandibular joint area, tomograms may be useful.

In general, treatment of fractures of the mandible in the child should include early reduction and fixation for the shortest possible time consistent with good healing and stability, by the most conservative means available, but this must of necessity vary with the site of the injury. In young children, fractures usually occur in the anterior region of the mandible (mental or paramental) where the mandible is thin and contains many tooth buds. In addition, the cuspid region is particularly susceptible to trauma, as it is located at the anterior angle of the body of the mandible.

Following the diagnosis of a fracture, a treatment plan designed to be simple and effective and to require the least amount of cooperation from the child must be formulated. It must also be practical, permit easy feeding, and cause no unusual discomfort. Reduction must correct the displacement, and immobilization must ensure adequate surgical rest for the injured parts. In certain instances in which displacement is minimal and there is no significant discomfort or motion of the fracture line, simple rest and a soft diet, with perhaps the use of a Barton bandage, is adequate. For treatment of extensive fractures, interdental wiring in conjunction with acrylic splints may be required (Bernstein, 1969).

Special consideration must be given to fractures at special sites. Fractures at the precise midline of the mandible, the symphysis, are quite rare and, when found, are commonly associated with a fracture of one or both condyles. These fractures, both vertical and oblique, and often greenstick in nature, are exceedingly difficult to treat. The distracting forces acting on the fragments because of the attachment of multiple powerful muscles in this region compounds the problem.

Treatment of fractures of the body of the mandible spans the spectrum of simple immobilization with a Barton bandage for nondisplaced fractures, to reduction by either open or closed methods and fixation with splints or arch bars, with or without intermaxillary fixation. In general, prolonged fixation, beyond four to six weeks, is not required in children (Kaban et al., 1977).

Fractures of the coronoid process are exceedingly uncommon and may require no treatment if malocclusion is not present or if there is no significant pain. Lateral crossbite may be seen in this injury initially, secondary to muscle spasm rather than to any fracture displacement.

Condylar fracture treatment is somewhat controversial but recently has tended toward a short period on a liquid diet or only very brief immobilization. Feared growth disturbances do not seem to materialize when normal temporomandibular joint function is maintained. Those few patients with residual deviation on opening the jaw may do special exercises to correct the deviation. While some authorities have suggested that "selected" fracture dislocations of the condyle be managed by open reduction of the fragments, the risks in this approach are significant, and possibly unwarranted, when one considers the extreme amount of remodeling that occurs in the condylar stump when jaw motion is constantly maintained. In addition, some recent evidence suggests that the condylar head, per se, is not as critical for growth as is normal function of the joint. Overzealous therapy for mandibular fractures in children, including prolonged intermaxillary fixation or interosseous wiring, may indeed be more apt to result in complications than would more conservative therapy.

Complications

Complications of facial injury in children are fortunately rare but can be devastating. Facial deformity may result from soft tissue injuries or from bony injuries with malunion or interference with growth and development of the facial bones. Functional losses secondary to ankylosis of the mandible may occur with aseptic necrosis of the articular surface of the condyle as a consequence of complete separation of the condyle from the ramus. Permanent diplopia secondary to fracture of the zygoma and orbital floor may require corrections in the position of the orbital floor, eye muscle surgery, or both. A saddle nose deformity may result from unreduced nasal bone fractures or unrecognized septal hematoma or abscess. Fractures with displacement of the nasal and lacrimal bones and detachment of the palpebral ligaments may result in traumatic pseudohypertelorism. Cerebrospinal fluid rhinorrhea, with its ever-present risk of meningitis, may be a consequence of craniofacial disjunction.

Summary

In summary, the care of facial injuries in the child requires, in addition to the usual knowledge and understanding of these injuries in the adult, special consideration for the many significant differences between children and adults. One must also recognize that these special considerations are such that, occasionally, even with the most meticulously proper treatment, the results can be less than optimal. It is hoped that careful attention to the many details outlined in this section will minimize the number of such instances.

SELECTED REFERENCES

Converse, J. M., and Dingman, R. O. 1977. Facial injuries in children. *In* Reconstructive Plastic Surgery. Vol. 2, Chap. 26. Philadelphia, W. B. Saunders Co.
    This excellent chapter is part of the second edition of Dr. Converse's definitive multivolume text on reconstructive surgery and emphasizes child-adult differences in diagnosis and treatment. Other volumes in this series provide more detailed discussion and illustration of the numerous treatment methods available.
Dingman, R. O., and Natvig, P. 1964. Surgery of Facial Fractures. Philadelphia, W. B. Saunders Co.
    Although this highly regarded standard text does contain a chapter on facial fractures in children (Chapter 11), its outstanding feature is the clear linedrawing depiction of the types of injuries and the beautifully illustrated operative techniques employed for their correction.
Lore, J. M., Jr. 1973. An Atlas of Head and Neck Surgery. Philadelphia, W. B. Saunders Co.
    As indicated by the title, this work is an atlas of operative procedures and, as such, contains a number of excellent plates dealing with facial fractures. Its organization is unusually clear and concise, and it points out indications for each procedure as well as pitfalls to avoid. The illustrations are particularly accurate and realistic.
McGregor, I. A. 1969. Fundamental Techniques of Plastic Surgery. Baltimore, Williams & Wilkins Co.
    A small, concise book with particular attention to basic soft tissue handling techniques in facial injuries.
Mustarde, J. C. 1971. Plastic Surgery in Infancy and Childhood, Chaps. V, VII, IX, XIV. Philadelphia, W. B. Saunders Co.
    The chapters noted, especially Chapter VII, Traumatic Injuries of the Jaws and Teeth by Drs. Rowe and Winter, provide excellently detailed accounts of the surgical management of various injuries in children of different ages.
Otolaryngologic Clinics of North America. 1982. Plastic Surgery of the Face, Vol. 15, No. 1. Philadelphia, W. B. Saunders Co.
Otolaryngologic Clinics of North America. 1983. Trauma to the

Head and Neck, Vol. 16, No. 3. Philadelphia, W. B. Saunders Co.

The above-noted issues provide a good update on the management of soft tissue injuries and bony injuries, with particular reference to the pediatric patient in certain chapters.

REFERENCES

Armstrong, E. A., Smith, T. H., and Salyer, K. E. 1985. Three-dimensional image reconstruction of computed tomograms of the head and neck in the pediatric age group. Ann. Radiol. (Paris) 28:241.

Bailey, B. J. 1977. Management of soft tissue trauma of the head and neck in children. Otolaryngol. Clin. North Am. 10:193.

Bernstein, L. 1969. Maxillofacial injuries in children. Otolaryngol. Clin. North Am. 2:397.

Converse, J. M., and Dingman, R. O. 1977. Facial injuries in children. *In* Reconstructive Plastic Surgery, Vol. 2, Chap. 26. Philadelphia, W. B. Saunders Co.

Dingman, R. O., and Natvig, P. 1964. Surgery of Facial Fractures. Philadelphia, W. B. Saunders Co.

Fee, W. E., Jr. 1976. Rhomboid flap principles and common variations. Laryngoscope 86:1706.

Freid, M. G., and Baden, E. 1954. Management of fractures in children. J. Oral Surg. 12:129.

Hall, R. K. 1972. Injuries of the face and jaws in children. J. Oral Surg. 1:65.

Kaban, L. B., Mulliken, J. B., and Murray, J. E. 1977. Facial fractures in children. Plast. Reconstr. Surg. 59:15.

Karlan, M. S., Madden, M. 1979. Moire topography in facial plastic surgery. Otolaryngol. Head Neck Surg. 87:533.

Lore, J. M., Jr. 1973. An Atlas of Head and Neck Surgery. Philadelphia, W. B. Saunders Co.

Marshall, K. A., Sadowsky, N. L., and Sigman, D. 1978. Xeroradiography in the diagnosis of facial fractures. Plast. Reconstr. Surg. 62:207.

McCoy, F. J., Chandler, R. A., and Crow, M. L. 1966. Facial fractures in children. Plast. Reconstr. Surg. 37:209.

McGregor, I. A. 1969. Fundamental Techniques of Plastic Surgery. Baltimore, Williams & Wilkins Co.

Moran, W. B., Jr. 1977. Nasal trauma in children. Otolaryngol. Clin. North Am. 10:95.

Mustarde, J. C. 1971. Plastic Surgery in Infancy and Childhood, Chaps. V, VII, IX, XIV. Philadelphia, W. B. Saunders Co.

Rowe, L. D., Brandt-Zawadzki, M. 1982. Spatial analysis of midfacial fractures with multidirectional and computed tomography. Otolaryngol. Head Neck Surg. 90:651.

Schultz, R. C. 1970. Facial Injuries. Chicago, Yearbook Medical Publishers.

Tardy, M. E., Jr. 1972. The bilobed flap in nasal repair. Arch. Otolaryngol. 95:1.

Weber, S. C., and Cohn, A. M. 1977. Fracture of the frontal sinus in children. Arch. Otolaryngol. 103:241.

Yarrington, C. T., Jr. 1977. Maxillofacial trauma in children. Otolaryngol. Clin. North Am. 10:25.

Zaydon, T. J., and Brown, J. B. 1964. Early Treatment of Facial Injuries. Philadelphia, Lea & Febiger.

Chapter 41

TUMORS OF THE NOSE, PARANASAL SINUSES, AND NASOPHARYNX

John F. Stanievich, M.D.   **John M. Lore, Jr., M.D.**

Since the first edition of this textbook, important advances in imaging techniques, as well as the emergence of cranial base surgery, have improved the incidence of resectability and the subsequent survival rate in many cases of nasal and paranasal sinus tumors. However, one should not be lulled into a false sense of security, since improved survival rates correlate best with early diagnosis and timely effective therapy.

PRESENTING SYMPTOMS AND SIGNS

In their early stages, most nasal tumors present with nasal obstruction, occasional epistaxis, and nasal discharge. However, in the young child, unilateral foul nasal discharge and obstruction are usually associated with an intranasal foreign body. In this instance, a careful history from a parent is usually helpful in distinguishing a benign condition from a more serious problem. Most infectious rhinosinal conditions are characterized by the acute onset of a serous or mucoid rhinorrhea with obstruction very often accompanied by systemic symptoms and signs such as malaise, muscle aches, and fever. These symptoms and signs are usually self-limited and resolve with brief courses of antimicrobial therapy and decongestants. Allergic nasal symptoms may be related to the particular season of the year: "rose fever" in the spring, and "hay fever" in the fall. After appropriate allergy testing, elimination of the offending environmental antigen, immunotherapy, or topical intranasal steroids usually bring relief of symptoms. The remaining group of children with persistent nasal obstruction, nasal discharge, and bleeding resistant to the previously mentioned common nasal therapies are those in whom rhinosinal tumor should be suspected (see Chaps. 31, 37, and 42).

Progressive facial numbness, pain, otalgia, hearing loss, and visual disturbances are usually symptoms of a tumor of the nose, nasopharynx, or paranasal sinus.

CLINICAL SIGNS

Inspection of the child's face may reveal expansion of the nasal dorsum associated with a nasal dermoid tumor or nasal glioma. Widening of the intercanthal distance may be associated with ethmoid disease. Proptosis or strabismus is often associated with periorbital disease affecting the ethmoid, the maxillary, and, rarely, the frontal sinuses. Epiphora is caused by obstruction of the lacrimal canal in the lateral wall of the nose. Other serious clinical signs of rhinosinal disease include reduced visual acuity, hypesthesia of the cheek, trismus, and swelling of the nose, cheek, or periorbita. The intranasal examination often reveals an obstructing mass. In young children, anterior rhinoscopy or flexible fiberoptic rhinoscopy using a 1.7-mm nasopharyngoscope is routinely performed. In older, cooperative children, the nasopharynx and the larynx can be well visualized using the traditional headlight and mirror examination. In the case of maxillary sinus disease, intraoral examination may reveal ulceration and distortion of the palate and gingival buccal sulcus or an oroantral fistula.

Even in young children complete head and neck examinations can still be accomplished if examiners take their time in a friendly, nonthreatening fashion. In addition, all regional and distant lymph node groups as well as the liver and spleen should be examined, insofar as lymphoma is the most prevalent tumor of the pediatric age group (Stanievich et al., 1987). (For a complete listing of the various types of benign and malignant rhinosinal tumors see Table 41–1.)

NASAL TUMORS

Benign Nasal Tumors

In children, most nasal tumors are benign, in contrast to adults, in whom basal cell carcinomas or squamous cell carcinomas are frequently seen. The most common benign nasal tumors in children are hemangiomas, nasal polyps, and squamous papillomas.

Hemangiomas

Hemangiomas can be classified according to depth, level of tissue involvement, or histologic features. A *cutaneous hemangioma* (nevus flammeus) is a dermal

TABLE 41–1. Benign and Malignant Tumors of the Nose, Paranasal Sinuses, and Nasopharynx

NASAL TUMORS

Benign	Malignant
Hemangiomas	Rhabdomyosarcomas
Nasal polyps	Carcinomas
Squamous papillomas	Olfactory neuroblastomas
Dermoid tumors	Lymphomas
Nasal gliomas	Leukemia
Teratomas	
Pyogenic granulomas	
Rhinoliths	
Fibromas	
Chondromas	
Mixed tumors	
Ectopic lacrimal gland	

PARANASAL SINUS TUMORS

Benign	Malignant
Polyps	Rhabdomyosarcomas
Mucoceles	Carcinomas
Dental cysts	Sarcomas
Fibrous dysplasia	Lymphomas
Ossifying fibromas	
Giant cell tumors	
Hemangiomas	

NASOPHARYNGEAL TUMORS

Benign	Malignant
Angiofibromas	Carcinomas
Teratomas	Rhabdomyosarcomas
Hemangiomas	Lymphomas
Gliomas	
Chondromas	
Chordomas	
Rhabdomyomas	

lesion consisting primarily of capillaries. *Nevi flammeus* and *strawberry nevus* (subcutaneous hypertrophic capillary hemangioma) usually present at birth and grow rapidly during the first year of life. They slowly resolve during the next 5 years of life. Hemangiomas of the nose are very often bulbous, and have soft, compressible texture. They are not mobile and are poorly demarcated. A reddish tinge of the overlying skin is often present. Treatment usually consists of waiting for spontaneous regression. In the past, intralesional or systemic steroids have been utilized, with varying degrees of success. Systemic therapy for large hemangiomas is best handled in conjunction with a pediatric endocrinologist, or oncologist, since they often treat children with high doses of corticosteroids and are thus experienced in managing the side effects of these powerful medicines. At times, the child's condition may become frankly cushingoid for several months before tumor regression is noted. Cavernous hemangiomas are characterized by deep invasion of muscular layers and fascial planes. They may form large vascular lakes and are generally refractory to drug therapy.

Smaller, superficial vascular lesions are now being successfully managed with the yttrium aluminum garnet (YAG), or tunable dye, laser (Simpson, 1988). Radiation therapy, cryotherapy, injection of sclerosing solutions, and radon seed implantation historically have not been very effective. At times, in the smaller or medium-sized lesions, it is very difficult to resist the parents' desire to "do something," rather than wait for spontaneous regression of the lesion. Careful observation of the lesion and a thorough discussion with the parents regarding the natural history of hemangiomas are of major importance in the conservative management of these tumors.

Hereditary Hemorrhagic Telangiectasia (Osler-Weber-Rendu Disease)

Although hereditary hemorrhagic telangiectasia is not in the same category as a large nasal hemangioma, the pediatric otolaryngologist will occasionally be called upon to treat children with this disorder. Recurrent epistaxis is a common presenting complaint. Diagnosis is made on the basis of characteristic telangiectasia of the oral mucosa, facial skin, and intranasal mucosa. The disease is transmitted in a non–sex-linked, autosomal dominant fashion. Affected children have bleeding diatheses early in life. The mucocutaneous lesions may be spider like, punctate, or nodular and may be quite large.

Intranasal lesions have been managed by intranasal excision, cautery, or dermal overgrafting of the nasal septum. Since none of these treatment methods are totally successful, these patients often become quite well-known to several generations of otolaryngology house officers during their training programs.

Nasal Polyps

Nasal polyps are semitransparent, wet-appearing herniations of respiratory mucosa and are usually found in the nasal chamber (Fig. 41–1). Nasal polyps may originate in the mucosa of the maxillary sinus and ultimately protrude through the middle meatus into the nose posteriorly, thus forming the well-known antral choanal polyp. Polyps originating primarily in the ethmoid sinus tend to be smaller and multiple and also tend to be found high in the nose. If a child with nasal polyps is younger than 12 years of age, the possibility of cystic fibrosis should be investigated. A sweat chloride test is usually a sufficient screening test for cystic fibrosis.

In the older child, allergy and chronic infection are the major factors associated with nasal polyp formation (Johnson et al., 1982). Apparently, respiratory mucosa has a limited physiologic response to either allergy or chronic infection, namely, the production of more goblet cells and a watery edema of the mucosa, hence, the wet glistening, boggy appearance of nasal polyps. The treatment of nasal polyposis is surgical excision (intranasal polypectomy). X-ray films should be obtained, since the polyps very often originate in the mucosa of the sinus. If so, adequate excision involves intranasal polypectomy and, also, removal of the affected sinus mucosa. To enter the maxillary sinus of the young child, care must be taken not to disturb the tooth buds in the anterior maxillary wall. A sublabial incision, with a small keyhole opening superior to the

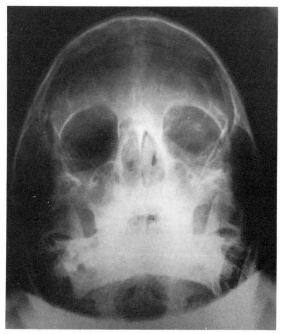

Figure 41–1. Widening of the nasal bridge from extensive intranasal benign polyps in a 4-year-old child. Over the years, this child had multiple polypectomies and eventually required an external ethmoidectomy.

tooth buds, will often give adequate access to the sinus through which endoscopic instruments may be used to excise the diseased mucosa. In children with ethmoid polyps, intranasal ethmoidectomy is a difficult procedure for even an experienced operator because of the small size of the sinus, the proximity of the cribriform plate, and generally poor visualization. A safer, more conservative approach is external ethmoidectomy using the operating microscope. For children with allergic rhinitis and polypoid degeneration of the turbinates, allergy immunotherapy or corticosteroid nasal sprays have been used with varying degrees of success. If these therapies fail, electrocautery of the inferior turbinates sometimes is effective. Freezing of the inferior turbinates with a cryogenic probe has also been tried.

Nasal Papillomas

Papillomas of the nasal vestibule are common lesions seen in a pediatric practice (Fig. 41–2). Most vestibular papillomas present as exophytic, 1- to 3-mm, cauliflowerlike, pedunculated growths arising medially from the septum or laterally from the mucosa of the vestibule or nasal alae. Successful treatment consists of total surgical excision, utilizing a cold knife, carbon dioxide (CO_2) laser (Crockett et al., 1985), Bovie electrocautery, or cryotherapy. Applications of podophyllin directly to the papillomas have also been successful (Dedo and Jackler, 1982; Bennett and Grist, 1985). However, extreme care must be taken to limit the systemic absorption of the drug, since fatalities have

been reported due to podophyllin toxicity (Cassidy et al., 1982).

Since vestibular papillomas may recur despite adequate surgical excision, frequent follow-up is recommended for at least the first year. Other types of nasal papillomas include *fungiform* and *cylindric cell papillomas* (Lucente and Hyams, 1987). Fungiform papillomas are confined to the nasal septum and are exophytic, with a wide base. Surgical excision is the treatment of choice. Cylindric cell papillomas arise from the lateral wall of the nasal vestibule and appear as irregular, red, papillary growths. Surgical excision is also the treatment of choice. Their proclivity for recurrence is similar to that of the inverted papilloma, and close follow-up is advised.

Inverted nasal papillomas (Fig. 41–3) are probably the most difficult type of nasal papillomas to cure. Despite adequate surgical excision, they often recur, and associated squamous cell malignancies have been reported, although usually in adult patients.

Typical intranasal, inverting papillomas usually present as unilateral, red, granular, polypoid masses attached to the lateral nasal wall. Histologically, they appear as endophytic growths of multilayered squamous epithelium, involving the stroma of the surrounding tissues. The basement membrane is intact, and histologic evidence of malignancy is absent. The normal amount of mitoses are seen, and keratin pearl formation is absent. This benign histologic picture is at odds with the aggressive clinical nature of this tumor. Recurrence rates of 25 to 75 per cent have been reported (Weissler et al., 1986; Stanley et al., 1984), probably due to inadequate surgical exposure and excision. Since this tumor has a propensity for

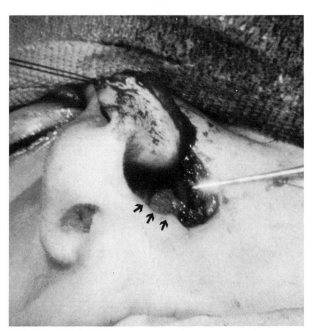

Figure 41–2. A large mass of benign intranasal squamous papillomas found along the inferior septum and the floor of the nose. This photograph demonstrates the excellent intranasal exposure afforded by the lateral rhinotomy incision.

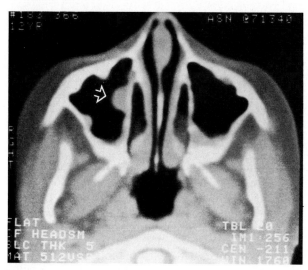

Figure 41–3. An inverting papilloma involving the medial wall of the maxillary sinus in a 12-year-old male. It was excised using a lateral rhinotomy approach. Portions of the medial wall of the maxillary sinus were removed.

invading the maxillary or ethmoid sinuses, computed tomography (CT) scans should be obtained for bone detail prior to definitive surgical excision. A lateral rhinotomy gives the best exposure of this tumor and permits easier inspection of the maxillary sinus to rule out local extension. Affected patients should have continuing, close postsurgical examinations for recurrent or persistent tumor.

Nasal Gliomas

Nasal gliomas (Fig. 41–4), dermoid tumors, and encephaloceles represent anomalies of nasofrontal de-velopment in the area of the embryonic foramen caecum and fonticulus frontalis. Many of these anomalies may be present as firm, prominent masses over the dorsum of the nose. During embryonic development, there exists an evagination of embryonic neu-roectodermal tissue through a patent nasofrontal fontanelle, the foramen caecum. During normal development, this neuroectodermal tissue is retracted by the dura during the period of differential growth rates of the anterior base of the skull as compared with the nasofrontal process. Normally, the foramen caecum closes, and nasofrontal tissues become separated from the intracranial contents. An encephalocele is formed when the foramen caecum remains patent and dura-covered intracranial contents herniate into the nasal cavity. Encephaloceles other than the nasofrontal type are the *nasoethmoid encephalocele*, with herniation between the foramen caecum and the ethmoid process, and the *nasoorbital encephalocele*, which protrudes through the medial wall of the orbit and may involve the frontal, ethmoid, and lacrimal bones. Encephalo-celes herniating through the base of the skull may be *transethmoid*, *sphenoethmoid*, *transsphenoid*, and *sphenomaxillary*. They usually present as compressi-ble, smooth, intranasal masses that transilluminate and get larger when the child cries.

Partial or incomplete closure of the foramen caecum leads to a trapping of heterotopic neuroglial tissue above and beneath the nasal bones, that is, a *nasal glioma*. Nasal gliomas may be intranasal, extranasal, or a combination of both. Extranasal gliomas are firm and somewhat movable and usually do not increase in size when the child cries. Intracranial connections in the case of extranasal gliomas are rare. *Intranasal gliomas*, however, represent a greater degree of difficulty in management and diagnosis, since they are

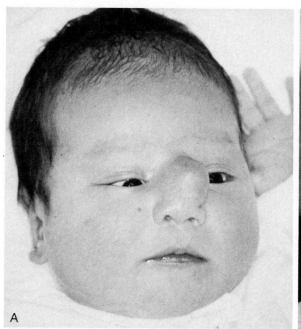
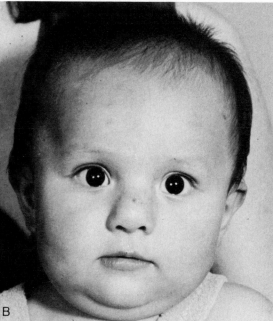

Figure 41–4. A, A congenital extranasal glioma, excised using a horizontal incision. B, The postoperative result one year later.

more like nasal encephaloceles. At surgery, 20 per cent of intranasal gliomas have demonstrable connections with the intracranial contents. They often present as glistening, distensible, polyplike lesions that increase in size on Valsalva maneuver. Diagnosis of both intranasal and extranasal gliomas involves a detailed CT study of the nasofrontal area and anterior cranial fossa to rule out intracranial connections. Needle aspiration of these masses is to be avoided, because of the danger of iatrogenic meningitis. In the case of an intranasal glioma, if connections with the central nervous system (CNS) are demonstrated, a combined craniotomy and external incision should be planned. If no CNS connection is demonstrated, the external lateral rhinotomy approach may be used to expose the cribriform-ethmoid area if necessary during the resection of this congenital mass.

Extranasal gliomas with no obvious CNS connection may be excised externally, using either an elliptic vertical midline incision or a horizontal incision over the dorsum of the nose. In the authors' experience, both types of incisions have yielded equally good cosmetic results. In external nasal gliomas, care must be taken to track the stalk of neuroglial tissue superiorly for a complete excision. Very often, the stalk extends superiorly under the nasal bone toward the cribriform plate area. Postsurgical defects of the nasal bones may spontaneously fill in over time or may require bone grafting at a later date. Cerebrospinal fluid rhinorrhea in the perioperative period is an ominous sign and requires immediate neurosurgical consultation, since meningitis is a definite risk. Other intranasal neural tumors include neurofibromas and neurilemomas. They may be indistinguishable from the intranasal glioma. Diagnosis is usually made by biopsy after the integrity of the anterior base of the skull has been determined. Treatment is also by surgical excision.

Nasal Dermoid Tumors

Nasal dermoid tumors are formed by processes converse to those that form encephaloceles. Rather than an outpouching of the CNS, the nasal dermoid tumor consists of an area of surface ectodermal tissue that is caught in the nasofrontal fontanelle area during early development. The nose and the frontal bone develop and extend around this trapped tissue, not unlike the formation of a branchial cleft sinus. As a result, a deep, ectoderm-lined tract may extend all the way from the anterior cranial fossa to the tip or the dorsum of the nose. Since this tract is of ectodermal origin, sebaceous secretions, as well as hair, may be seen at the opening of the fistula on the dorsum or the tip of the nose. The tract, or fistula, is usually noticed during the first year of life and is most commonly found at the dorsum or the root of the nose. Other areas for the opening of the fistula can be at the tip of the nose, and also midline in the columella. The parents of such patients often state that whitish, mucoid material drains from these fistulas. Often, the fistulas become infected, and large cysts or abscesses become evident over the dorsum of the nose.

Anterior skull base and cribriform plate involvement has been reported in as many as 26 per cent of children in some series (Clark et al., 1985). For this reason, preoperative, high-resolution CT scanning of the nasofrontal area and neurosurgical consultation are valuable in preparing these patients for surgery. A bifid crista galli, a wide or bifid nasal septum, and a dehiscent anterior skull base all are indications of CNS involvement in this lesion.

Total surgical excision is the treatment of choice. If it is known that the anterior skull base is involved, a combined frontal craniotomy and external nasal procedure should be planned to remove the fistulous tract *en bloc*. For less complicated cases with external nasal involvement only, a vertical or horizontal excision is cosmetically acceptable. Care must be taken to follow the ectodermal tract as high as possible. Temporary mobilization of the nasal bones via medial and lateral osteotomies has been described, in order to obtain better visualization of the superior portions of the tract (Kelly and Strome, 1982). As in nasal glioma, perioperative cerebrospinal fluid leaks are troublesome and demand immediate neurosurgical consultation as well as vigorous full-spectrum antibiotic therapy.

Pyogenic Granulomas and Rhinoliths

Pyogenic granulomas are friable, red, soft, sessile, broad-based vascular lesions usually seen on the anterior septum. Histologically, they are composed of fibroblasts and capillaries. They often arise from insignificant trauma or are associated with retained intranasal foreign bodies. Recently, several adolescent patients, admitting to frequent intranasal cocaine use, have been seen with these lesions. Treatment is usually accomplished by curettage of the lesion, removal of the offending foreign body, or cessation of stimuli noxious to the nasal mucosa.

Rhinoliths are calcareous encrustations usually associated with long-standing intranasal foreign bodies. Total resolution and healing of the mucosa is obtained by removal of the rhinolith and curettage of the surrounding granulation tissue.

Other Tumors

Other sporadic reports of benign pediatric nasal tumors include pleomorphic adenoma of the inferior turbinate (Baraka et al., 1984), congenital monomorphic adenoma of the nasal septum (Vaze, 1983), ectopic lacrimal gland under the nasal mucosa (Pê'êr and Ilsar, 1982), and a benign osteoblastoma of the nasal bones (Fig. 41–5) (Sooknundun et al., 1986).

Childhood Malignant Tumors

In general, malignant tumors of the head and neck in children are statistically rare. A retrospective review

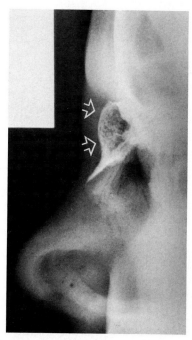

Figure 41–5. A benign osteoma of the nasal bones in a 4-year-old child. The arrows point to the lesion that was excised using an external incision.

of 2835 head and neck lesions either excised or biopsied at Buffalo Children's Hospital revealed malignancies in fewer than 2 per cent of patients. Of these children, almost half (43 per cent) had Hodgkin disease. The remaining 57 per cent of tumors were distributed more or less evenly in various sites around the head and neck.

Malignant Nasal Tumors

Malignant tumors of the nose are rare in pediatric age groups, since children have not lived long enough to receive damaging doses of solar radiation, which make cutaneous squamous cell and basal cell carcinomas so common in adults. Rather, the most common malignant nasal tumor in children is rhabdomyosarcoma (Fig. 41–6), both the embryonal cell type and the alveolar cell type. Often, these are congenital lesions and grow rapidly during the first year of life. Usually, a friable, ulcerating mass is present. Facial swelling and cranial nerve palsies are unfavorable signs, indicating regional spread with destruction of contiguous structures. Therapy consists of wide local excision and multiple-drug chemotherapy, including actinomycin D, vincristine, cyclophosphamide (Cytoxan), and, more recently, cisplatinum. Radiotherapy has been helpful, although later deformities and asymmetric facial growth problems are common.

Diagnosis is made by open biopsy. Specimens should be taken for light microscopy, electron microscopy, and special stains to show banding of the rhabdomyocytes. The extent of the tumor is mapped using computed tomography with three-dimensional recon-

structions and using magnetic resonance imaging (MRI).

Intranasal Carcinomas

Carcinomas of the nose may be mistaken for nasal polyps, septal abscesses, or septal hematomas. Diagnostic treatment principles are the same as those for rhabdomyosarcoma, although the patients with undifferentiated carcinoma do not survive as long as those with sarcoma.

Lymphomas and Leukemia

Several children with nasopharyngeal and intranasal non-Hodgkin lymphoma of the large cell types and the lymphoblastic types have been reported (Yamanaka et al., 1985). Extranodal non-Hodgkin lymphoma arising from a nasal cavity has a poor prognosis, in contrast with Hodgkin lymphoma arising from Waldeyer ring. In obtaining tissue for biopsy, the specimen should be sent to the laboratory wrapped in a wet saline gauze, since immunohistochemical studies, B-cell and T-cell studies, cell cultures, and light and electron microscopy need to be performed in order completely to characterize the tumor. Treatment usually consists of a combination of chemotherapy and radiation therapy after diagnostic staging procedures such as technetium-99m (^{99m}Tc) and gallium-67m (^{67m}Ga) scintiscans; computed tomography of the head, chest, and abdomen; lymphangiograms; bone marrow biopsies; and radiographic examinations of the gastrointestinal tract.

A report has described a pediatric patient with acute myeloid leukemia whose presenting sign was a solitary leukemic skin nodule on the tip of the nose (Brama et al., 1982).

Other Tumors

Other pediatric malignant nasal tumors described are malignant teratoma (Heffner and Hyams, 1984), malignant histiocytosis (Aozasa, 1982), and olfactory neuroblastoma (Olsen and DeSanto, 1983).

Surgical Approaches to Nasal Tumors

The mainstay of intranasal exposure is the lateral rhinotomy incision. It begins inferiorly at the base of the ala nasi and can be extended superiorly in the nasoalar groove to explore even the ethmoid and cribriform areas. By including the nasal bones in the skin flap and by retracting the orbital contents laterally, complete exposure of the roof of the nasal vault, the ethmoid sinuses, and the sphenoid is possible. In addition, disease in the roof of the nose can be dealt with under direct visualization. Full thickness, *en bloc* resections of the cribriform plate, ethmoid sinus, and sphenoid sinus can be accomplished in conjunction with a frontal craniotomy, with the osteotomies being

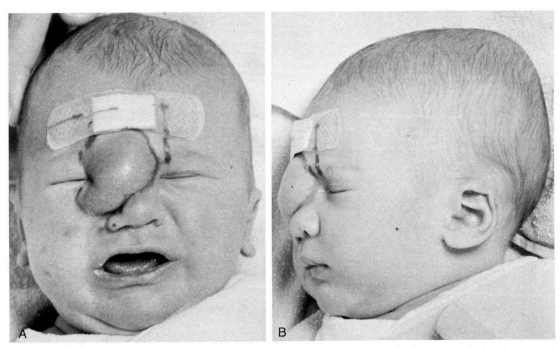

Figure 41–6. *A* and *B*, A congenital rhabdomyosarcoma of the nasofrontal area in a neonate. The child succumbed to this aggressive tumor within a year despite radiation therapy, combination chemotherapy, and surgical excision.

made from above as the tumor margins are visualized simultaneously from below. Posterior septal and nasopharyngeal lesions can be approached via a palate-splitting incision.

At present, patients with carcinomas and sarcomas of the nasal cavity all are enrolled in modern, multiinstitutional treatment protocols, which include multiple chemotherapeutic agents, radiation therapy, and surgery when the tumor is resectable.

SINUS TUMORS

Benign Sinus Tumors

As mentioned previously, antral choanal polyps are the most common benign sinus tumors in children.

Mucoceles

Mucoceles of the paranasal sinuses and retention cysts located in their respiratory epithelial lining are also common. Mucous retention cysts arise from blockage of microscopic secretory ducts in the respiratory epithelium. However, the term "mucocele" as it is generally used denotes a greatly enlarged retention cyst within a paranasal sinus that may expand and cause bony erosion. Strictly speaking, all mucoceles were once mucous retention cysts, since histologically they all are lined with secretory epithelium. Sinus retention cysts and mucoceles are usually asymptomatic until they reach a critical size when sinus ostia become blocked. Purulent nasal discharge, facial pain, and pressure symptoms ensue, and most often sinus

x-ray films are obtained that demonstrate the presence of a retention cyst or mucocele. Clinical decisions sometimes are difficult, since facial pain may be due to other causes (e.g., migraine variants, facial vascular pain, and pain of dental origin), and the sinus retention cyst may be an innocent radiographic finding. If the cyst or mucocele is large enough to obstruct the sinus ostia, surgical removal is justified. Removal of a maxillary sinus cyst through an intranasal endoscopic approach may be used in older children, otherwise a keyhole sublabial antrostomy, taking care to avoid the tooth buds, is commonly used. The cyst should be at least uncapped, if not totally removed, and a nasoantral window should be performed for continued drainage. Mucoceles of the ethmoid and sphenoid sinuses are rare and should be drained using the external approach in conjunction with the operating microscope.

Odontogenic Tumors and Dentigerous Cysts

These tumors were very common in some reviews of maxillary tumors (Schramm, 1979). This incidence probably reflects a close working relationship with the oral surgeons at a specific institution. The *adenomatoid odontogenic tumor* (adenomeloblastoma) probably is a hamartoma or overgrowth of odontogenic tissue. It is common in females aged 10 to 20 years and is usually found in the maxillary incisor-cuspid area in association with an impacted tooth. Simple enucleation of the tumor with a free margin usually suffices.

The *dentigerous cyst* arises from a developing enamel organ and surrounds the crown of an unerupted tooth. Marsupialization or careful enucleation with the tooth of origin is the treatment of choice (McClatchey, 1981).

Fibroosseous Lesions

Fibroosseous lesions of the maxilla and midface constitute a group of histologically benign but clinically aggressive lesions that demand surgical treatment. In a classic description of benign tumors of the mandible and the maxilla, Dehner (1973) reported 15 cases of fibroosseous lesions. They were divided into three categories: fibrous dysplasia, ossifying fibroma, and cementifying fibroma. *Fibrous dysplasia* is probably the most aggressive of these dysplastic disorders. This disease can be monostotic or polyostotic. Polyostotic disease carries a poorer prognosis and may be part of the Albright-McCune-Sternberg syndrome, with multiple café au lait spots on the back, precocious puberty, and multiple radiolucent defects in the bones of the lower extremities. Histologically, fibrous dysplasia is ill-defined and merges with the surrounding bone. The bony trabeculae are immature, and osteoblastic and osteoclastic activity is minimal. *Ossifying fibroma* shows greater mineral deposition and birefringence under the microscope. In addition, radiologically, the lesion tends to be better defined and well-circumscribed histologically from normal bone. The cementifying fibroma reacts strongly with the PAS stain. The ossifying fibroma is clinically the most benign lesion, responding well to excision and curettage. Fibrous dysplasia and cementifying fibroma are more difficult to manage clinically. In fibrous dysplasia, curettage alone results in a 50 per cent treatment failure rate. Children treated with curettage alone usually go on to partial maxillectomies or die of persistent disease. Cementifying fibroma is characterized by multiple local recurrences.

Giant Cell Granuloma and Giant Cell Tumor (Osteoclastoma)

Fifteen giant cell granulomas were reported by Dehner in his 1973 review of benign tumors of the mandible and maxilla in children. This number represented about one third (15 of 46) of all the benign tumors in this series. In 1979, Schramm reported a lesser incidence (11 per cent), but this may have been due to the individual referral patterns at their respective institutions. Dehner originally described painless swelling in the upper or lower jaws as the most frequent initial sign. Facial asymmetry and palpable maxillary and palatal masses were described, as well as the typical "cherubic facies" in one child. Radiologically, large, well-circumscribed osteolytic lesions are seen, with a fine rim of calcification at the margin of the tumors. Histologically, these lesions are characterized by multinucleated giant cells, stroma formed from elongated spindle-shaped cells, and erythrocytes located prominently in the stroma. Handler (1982), in a case report on a giant cell tumor of the ethmoid sinuses, makes a fine distinction between a giant cell

tumor (osteoclastoma) and the previously reported reparative giant cell granuloma, although clinically these lesions act the same. They grow slowly and destroy bone locally. They have a tendency to recur after simple curettage or incomplete excision. Effective treatment involves complete surgical removal, with a margin of normal tissue. The differential diagnosis includes the previously mentioned fibroosseous lesions such as fibrous dysplasia and ossifying fibroma. In addition, the "brown tumor" of hyperparathyroidism is similar radiographically and may be clinically differentiated by elevated serum calcium levels.

Myxofibromas and Hemangiomas of the Sinuses

Myxofibromas and hemangiomas can occur in the paranasal sinus area. Hemangiomas are especially troublesome, since they intermittently hemorrhage and destroy bone by local invasion. In addition, depending on the size of the lesion, a significant percentage of the cardiac output may be shunted through these lesions if there are numerous arteriovenous fistulas in this tumor or if the internal carotid system is feeding the tumor. Multiple surgical excisions as well as a partial maxillectomy may be required for ablation of this tumor.

Malignant Sinus Tumors

The most frequent primary malignant neoplasms of the paranasal sinuses are undifferentiated carcinoma and rhabdomyosarcoma. Other reports of tumors include adenocarcinomas, osteogenic sarcomas of the maxilla, chondrosarcomas, fibrosarcomas, and lymphoma. In addition, in children, secondary malignancies may develop in irradiated fields. A child in the authors' care developed an osteogenic sarcoma of the maxilla in a field postoperatively irradiated for a retinoblastoma that required enucleation (Stanievich et al., 1987).

Tumors of the sinuses usually present as facial swellings that are red, tender, and associated with infection. Clinically, these lesions can be confused with acute sinusitis, although on radiographic studies the bone destruction is immediately evident. Biopsy and CT staging of the lesion determines the desirability of a surgical attempt for a cure.

For maxillary sinus disease, a radical maxillectomy may yield deep margins that are free of tumor. A transfrontal ethmoidectomy and craniofacial resection can be employed for malignant ethmoid sinus disease if the tumor involved is primarily anterior. Resection of posterior ethmoid and sphenoid sinus malignancies is complicated by the proximity of the optic chiasm and the cavernous sinus. Patients with paranasal sinus malignancy currently do best with combined radiation therapy, chemotherapy, and complete tumor excision for intended cure when surgically possible. In those patients with tumors judged to be surgically nonresectable, surgical drainage of the affected sinuses and debulking of the tumors by curettage may be beneficial for pain relief and control of sepsis.

NASOPHARYNGEAL TUMORS

Benign Nasopharyngeal Tumors

Nasopharyngeal Angiofibroma

Nasopharyngeal angiofibromas are the most common type of benign nasopharyngeal tumors (Fig. 41–7). They occur mostly in prepubescent males. These patients present with nasal obstruction and recurrent epistaxis. As the symptoms progress, rhinolalia, deformity of the soft and hard palate, and swelling of the cheek may become evident. The tumor appears as a red, smooth, mucosa-covered compressible mass in the nasopharynx. Varying degrees of tumor vascularity may be seen. Depending on the superior extension of the tumor, orbital proptosis may be present. Cheek or zygomatic swelling is indicative of tumor spread into the infratemporal fossa. Magnetic resonance imaging is excellent for visualizing the extent of the tumor and also has the advantage of minimizing the patient's exposure to ionizing radiation. Computed tomography scanning is excellent for bony detail and three-dimensional reconstructions in the sagittal and coronal planes may aid in planning the surgical approach. Rarely should biopsy be necessary to establish the diagnosis.

Treatment consists of complete surgical excision, very often easier to recommend than to actually accomplish. Once the definitive, noninvasive radiographic studies have been obtained, angiography is then used to define the vascular anatomy of the tumor. Embolization of the tumor via the external carotid artery has recently become popular; however, this procedure is not without risk. This author has personally seen an

inadvertent flow of Gelfoam into the internal carotid and vertebral-basilar system because of a failure of an occluding balloon, with a resultant transient blindness and hemiplegia. These potential risks should be considered, especially in the case of small, pedunculated angiofibromas. If tumor embolization is desired, Gelfoam or implantable occluding balloons can be used. The surgical approach to the tumor should be via an extended lateral rhinotomy, with extension intraorally, over the gingivobuccal sulcus, and behind the maxillary tuberosity. The palate may be split to give access to the vault of the nasopharynx. An approach to the infratemporal fossa includes the aforementioned incisions, with the addition of a total parotidectomy and retraction of the facial nerve superiorly. At this point, the holes for a minicompression plate may be drilled on the ascending ramus of the mandible, 2 cm inferior to the condylar head. The mandibulotomy is then performed. This approach gives wide exposure to the troublesome tumors that fill the infratemporal fossa. The tumor may then be palpated and mobilized from both its lateral and its medial aspects. Since the holes for the mandibular plate had been drilled prior to the mandibulotomy, installation of the plate is easier, and the difficulties of trying to drill an unstable condylar segment are eliminated. In addition, the need for postoperative intermaxillary fixation is obviated.

Despite adequate surgical exposure, some of these tumors recur or persist. This is probably due to the multilobular nature of the tumor and its ability to invade adjacent sinuses and insinuate itself into potential fascial spaces and suture lines. It is currently recommended that recurrent tumors receive low-dose radiation therapy (3600 Rad).

It may take up to one year for the effects of radiation therapy to become evident. If radiation therapy is successful, these tumors involute and lose much of their vascularity. Radiation failures and large tumors demonstrating intracranial spread are best handled in

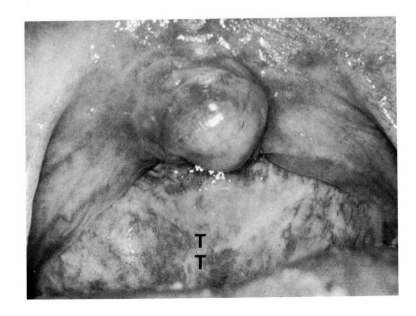

Figure 41–7. A large nasopharyngeal angiofibroma hanging down below the level of the soft palate. ("T" indicates the tumor.) This extensive lesion went unnoticed for several months by the child's physician, who thought his nasal obstruction was caused by "allergies."

conjunction with a neurosurgical team experienced in surgery directed at the base of the skull. Especially troublesome are recurrent tumors with large feeding vessels coming off the internal carotid artery at its siphon. The angiofibroma is composed of fibrous tissue with blood vessels and occasional large lakes and is histologically benign but quite aggressive clinically. Complete excision of this tumor is best carried out at a medical center where expert neurosurgical consultation is available and where the anesthesia department is experienced in managing large and sudden fluid shifts during surgery.

Other Benign Nasopharyngeal Tumors

Benign nasopharyngeal tumors also include teratomas, nasopharyngeal dermoid tumors ("hairy polyps"), base of the skull encephaloceles, fibrous dysplasia, hemangiomas, gliomas, chondromas, chordomas, and hamartomas (Heffner, 1983) (Fig. 41–8). These tumors are usually covered with mucosa and have a broad, sessile base. Total excision of these tumors from this area can be quite complicated.

Malignant Nasopharyngeal Tumors

In the authors' series, nasopharyngeal rhabdomyosarcoma and nasopharyngeal carcinoma (Fig. 41–9) occurred equally as frequently in this area. Fewer than 20 per cent of affected children survive five years, most dying of distant metastases and sepsis. Patients with lymphoma fared better, with 50 per cent survival. Nasopharyngeal malignancy often presents with a firm, posterior triangle node, unilateral eustachian tube dysfunction, and nasal obstruction. Horner syndrome, torticollis, and cranial nerve palsies are late signs

indicative of regional invasion. Radiation therapy and chemotherapy are instituted once immunohistologic and microscopic examinations of the tumor are accomplished and the disease has been clinically staged. Heroic, combined craniofacial resections of nasopharyngeal tumors have proved futile in the face of a rapidly growing, aggressive undifferentiated tumor (Fig. 41–10).

IMAGING TECHNIQUES

Since the first edition of this textbook, MRI has rapidly evolved into a clinically useful tool, because of the development of newer surface coils with high resolution, newer pulse sequences permitting more rapid scanning, and use of paramagnetic contrast agents. In a study comparing CT scanning and MRI (Mafee et al., 1988), it was found that MRI could often accurately image cystic, hypovascular, hypervascular, and most solid tumors. However, necrotic lymph nodes and some cystic lesions at times were not well-distinguished from solid tumors. CT scanning remains the study of choice for dense cortical bone and studies of fine bony details. At present, three-dimensional CT scanning is best used for the imaging of bony profiles and contours rather than soft tissue masses and, therefore, may be helpful in the assessment of patients who need reconstruction of large postsurgical defects. Other well-established imaging techniques include fluoroscopy, barium swallow, radionuclide scanning for thyroid disease, gallium and technetium scanning for infections and bony metastases, and Doppler ultrasonography to assess regional blood flow patterns.

GENERAL PRINCIPLES

From the aforementioned discussions, the pediatric otolaryngologist can formulate some general principles

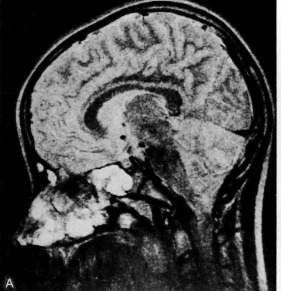
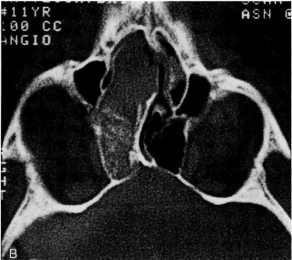

Figure 41–8. *A* and *B*, A large congenital hamartoma in an 11-year-old boy. The tumor filled the entire nasal cavity and displaced the right orbit laterally. Excision was via a facial degloving approach.

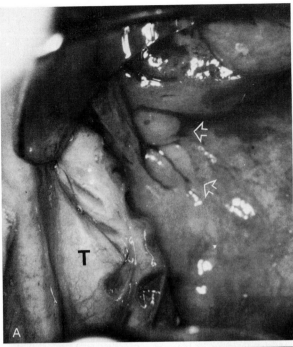

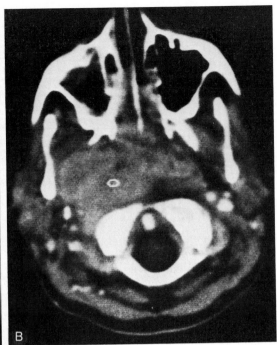

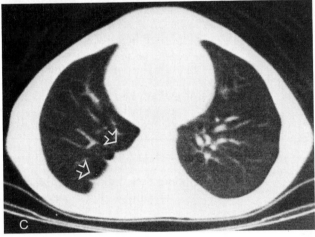

Figure 41–9. *A*, A poorly differentiated nasopharyngeal carcinoma in a 12-year-old boy. The arrows point to the tumor. The right tonsil is marked with the letter "T." *B*, The CT scan shows extensive tumor spread into the infratemporal fossa. Treatment was with high-dose radiation therapy and multiple-agent chemotherapy. *C*, The child eventually died from intrathoracic metastases and cardiac constriction by the tumor.

regarding tumors of the nose, paranasal sinuses, and nasopharynx.

1. Accurate taking of the patient's history and a good head and neck examination in the office are essential in the early diagnosis of potentially life-threatening malignancy. In the authors' series, the long-term survival of the child was best correlated with the stage at which the disease was diagnosed and the speed with which treatment regimens were instituted.

2. An exact knowledge of the embryology, anatomy, and clinical behavior of tumors and congenital lesions in the nasofrontal area is essential for a surgeon entrusted with the care of these children.

3. A firm histologic diagnosis and proper imaging techniques are required to accurately stage and determine the resectability of tumors in the nasofrontal and the maxillary areas. A child with a malignancy in these areas deserves the talents of the pediatric head and neck surgeon, pediatric oncologist, radiotherapist, diagnostic radiologist and pathologist, since multiple-therapy regimens are currently yielding the best results.

4. Should a complex tumor be considered resecta-

ble, a surgical team consisting of a pediatric head and neck surgeon, a neurosurgeon, a plastic and reconstructive surgeon, and a pediatric anesthesiologist should formulate a surgical plan prior to the procedure. They should try to anticipate blood-component requirements as well as surgical equipment needs in order to keep the operating time to the absolute minimum. Staged regional flap delays may need to be performed days prior to the definitive ablative procedure.

5. Enthusiasm for complex and heroic surgical procedures must be tempered with realistic expectations of obtaining a free surgical margin. A 1-mm surgically free margin in a histologically uncontrolled aggressive tumor does the patient a disservice, since previously intact fascial planes are violated and tumor may be seeded into the field. Perhaps future therapies may be directed toward the stereotaxic ablation of unresectable tumor via radiofrequency thermocoagulation, use of the gamma knife, or radionuclide implantation with the preservation of natural fascial and bony barriers against tumor spread.

6. Recognizing the oftentimes poor prognosis of

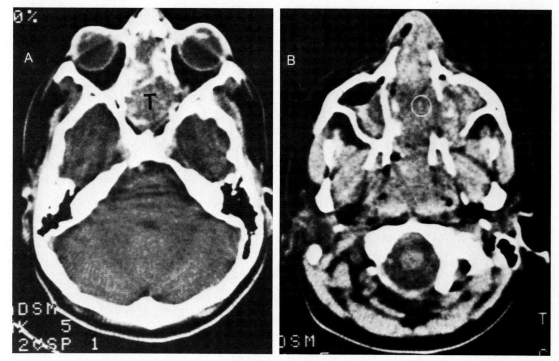

Figure 41–10. *A,* A large, poorly differentiated carcinoma located in the roof of the nasal vault. This teenaged girl was originally thought to have a nasoseptal abscess. Tumor was found at the time of the drainage procedure. The letter "T" indicates the tumor mass. *B,* Extensive involvement of the base of the skull.

pediatric nasal and sinus malignancies, the team entrusted with the care of these children should be familiar with the newer techniques of pain control. There is no excuse for inadequate use of analgesics and mood elevators in children with postsurgical terminal head and neck malignancy.

Pharmacologic agents include intravenous meperidine, morphine, and newer synthetic narcotics. When appropriate, these agents may be administered by a patient-controlled intravenous infusion pump. Small, incremental doses are given until the patient obtains pain relief and becomes slightly somnolent. Naloxone is sometimes added to this mixture in order to counteract undesirable narcotic side effects such as pruritus, nausea, vomiting, urinary retention, and respiratory depression. The mood elevator, desipramine, is frequently used to counteract depression caused by chronic illness, pain, and impending death. It is also thought to alter pain thresholds in the CNS. Long-acting (24 to 36 hours) narcotics such as methadone have been used to establish baseline levels of analgesia, and pulsed shorter-acting narcotics are used to control acute exacerbations of pain. Physicians treating these children should adopt a therapeutic approach that recognizes that the pain threshold of each individual is different and varies with the course of each person's disease and the site of the lesion. Fear of drug dependency is not a valid consideration for withholding narcotics in a child with a terminal malignancy (Moore, 1988).

Neurosurgical approaches to controlling pain in the head and neck include transcutaneous electric nerve stimulation (TENS), stereotactic trigeminal thermocoagulation, and trigeminal sensory tractotomy, an intracranial procedure. Newer procedures include deep brain electrode implantation into pain centers and the installation of an infusion pump directly into the ventricular system for pulsed or continuous administration of opiates (Soloniuk, 1988).

SELECTED REFERENCES

Dehner, L. P. 1973. Tumors of the mandible and maxilla in children. I. Clinicopathologic study of 46 histologically benign lesions. Cancer 31:364.
    One of the largest and earliest reports of rare pediatric head and neck tumors.
Heffner, D. K. 1983. Problems in pediatric otorhinolaryngic pathology. III. Teratoid and neural tumors of the nose, sinonasal tract, and nasopharynx. Int. J. Pediatr. Otorhinolaryngol. 6:1.
    A large compendium of rare tumors reported from a pathologist's viewpoint.
Schramm, V. L. 1979. Inflammatory and neoplastic masses of the nose and paranasal sinus in children. Laryngoscope 89:1887.
    The original series of tumors on which the first edition of this chapter was based.

REFERENCES

Aozasa, K. 1982. Biopsy findings in malignant histiocytosis presenting as lethal midline granuloma. J. Clin. Pathol. 35:599.
Baraka, M. E., Sadek, S. A. A., and Salem, M. H. 1984. Pleomorphic adenoma of the inferior turbinate. J. Laryngol. Otol. 98:925.
Bennett, R. G., and Grist, W. J. 1985. Nasal papillomas: Successful treatment with podophyllin. South. Med. J. 78:224.

Brama, I., Goldfarb, A., Shalev, O., et al. 1982. Tumour of the nose as a presenting feature of leukaemia. J. Laryngol. Otol. 96:83.

Cassidy, D. E., Drewry, J., and Fanning, J. P. 1982. Podophyllum toxicity: A report of a fatal case and a review of the literature. J. Toxicol. Clin. Toxicol. 19:35.

Clark, W. D., Bailey, B. J., and Stiernberg, C. M. 1985. Nasal dermoid with intracranial involvement. Otolaryngol. Head Neck Surg. 93:102.

Crockett, D. M., Healy, G. B., McGill, T. J. I., et al. 1985. Benign lesions of the nose, oral cavity, and oropharynx in children: Excision by carbon dioxide laser. Ann. Otol. Rhinol. Laryngol. 94:489.

Dedo, H. D., and Jackler, R. K. 1982. Laryngeal papillomas: Results of treatment with the CO_2 laser and podophyllum. Ann. Otol. Rhinol. Laryngol. 91:425.

Dehner, L. P. 1973. Tumors of the mandible and maxilla in children. I. Clinicopathologic study of 46 histologically benign lesions. Cancer 31:364.

Handler, S. D., Savino, P. J., Peyster, R. G., et al. 1982. Giant cell tumor of the ethmoid sinus: An unusual cause of proptosis in a child. Otolaryngol. Head Neck Surg. 90:513.

Heffner, D. K. 1983. Problems in pediatric otorhinolaryngic pathology. III. Teratoid and neural tumors of the nose, sinonasal tract, and nasopharynx. Int. J. Pediatr. Otorhinolaryngol. 6:1.

Heffner, D. K., and Hyams, V. J. 1984. Teratocarcinosarcoma (malignant teratoma?) of the nasal cavity and paranasal sinuses: A clinicopathologic study of 20 cases. Cancer 53:2140.

Johnson, J. T., Effron, M. Z., and Schramm, V. L. 1982. Nasal masses in children. Postgrad. Med. 72:87.

Kelly, J. H., and Strome, M. 1982. Surgical update on nasal dermoids. Arch. Otolaryngol. 108:239.

Lucente, F. E., and Hyams, V. J. 1987. Inflammatory and neoplastic disorders of the nasal mucosa. Clin. Dermatol. 5:35.

Mafee, M. F., Campos, M., Raju, S., et al. 1988. Head and neck: High field magnetic resonance imaging versus computed tomography. In Otolaryngologic Clinics of North America, Vol. 21 (3), Diagnostic Imaging in Otolaryngology II: Sinuses,

Neck, and Temporomandibular Joint. Philadelphia, W. B. Saunders Co.

McClatchy, K. 1981. Odontogenic lesions: Tumors and cysts. In Batsakis, J. G. (ed).: Tumors of the Head and Neck. Baltimore, Williams & Wilkins, pp. 531–561.

Moore, B. 1988. Personal communication. Department of Pediatric Anesthesiology, Children's Hospital of Buffalo, School of Human Medicine, State University of New York at Buffalo.

Olsen, K. D., and DeSanto, L. W. 1983. Olfactory neuroblastoma. Arch. Otolaryngol. 109:797.

Pê'êr, J., and Ilsar, M. 1982. Ectopic lacrimal gland under the nasal mucosa. Letter to the Editor. Am. J. Ophthalmol., 94:418.

Rockley, T. J., and Liu, K. D. 1986. Fibrosarcoma of the nose and paranasal sinuses. J. Laryngol. Otol. 100:1417.

Schramm, V. L. 1979. Inflammatory and neoplastic masses of the nose and paranasal sinus in children. Laryngoscope 89:1887.

Simpson, G. 1988. Personal communication. Department of Otolaryngology, Boston University Laser Center, Boston, MA.

Soloniuk, D. 1988. Personal communication. Department of Neurosurgery, School of Human Medicine, State University of New York at Buffalo.

Sooknundun, M., Kacker, S. K., and Kapila, K. 1986. Benign osteoblastoma of the nasal bones. A case report. J. Laryngol. Otol. 100:229.

Stanievich, J. F., Hafezi, B., Brodsky, L., et al. 1987. The incidence of head and neck tumors in the pediatric age group: A 10-year experience at Buffalo Children's Hospital and Roswell Park Memorial Institute. Proceedings of the Second International Congress of Head and Neck Oncology, Arlington, VA.

Stanley, R. J., Kelly, J. A., Matta, I. I., et al. 1984. Inverted papilloma in a 10-year-old boy. Arch. Otolaryngol. 110:813.

Vaze, P., Aterman, K., Hutton, C., et al. 1983. Monomorphic adenoma of the nasal septum in a newborn. J. Laryngol. Otol. 97:251.

Weissler, M. D., Montgomery, W. W., Montgomery, S. K., et al. 1986. Inverted papilloma. Ann. Otol. Rhinol. Laryngol. 95:215.

Yamanaka, N., Harabuchi, Y., Sambe, S., et al. 1985. Non-Hodgkin's lymphoma of Waldeyer's ring and nasal cavity. Clinical and immunologic aspects. Cancer 56:768.

Chapter 42

ALLERGIC RHINITIS

Philip Fireman, M.D.

Allergic rhinitis is the most common of all the allergic disorders, affecting over 20 million people in the United States. Because it is not a fatal disease and its symptoms may not be incapacitating, allergic rhinitis may at times be slighted or ignored by the surgical and medical community. Yet this frequent illness causes significant morbidity, which results in the expenditure of many millions of dollars in health care and the loss of millions of working and school days. Allergic rhinitis has a familial tendency and is induced by exposure to antigenic environmental factors, called allergens, with resultant sneezing, nasal pruritus, watery rhinorrhea, nasal mucosal edema, and subsequent nasal obstruction. The symptoms can be episodic or perennial; when symptoms recur annually during certain months, the syndrome is called seasonal allergic rhinitis. Typically, seasonal allergic rhinitis does not develop until after the patient has been sensitized by two or more pollen seasons. Seasonal allergic rhinitis is frequently referred to as "hay fever" or a "summer cold." These descriptive terms are misleading and should be discarded because fever is not a symptom associated with allergic rhinitis and neither hay nor the common cold virus is incriminated in the etiology of this syndrome.

The prevalence of allergic rhinitis in the general population is considered to be about 10 per cent, with the peak incidence in the postadolescent teenage child. Broder and colleagues (1974), in a study of a well-defined population in Tecumseh, Michigan, found the incidence of allergic rhinitis to increase during childhood from less than 1 per cent during infancy to an incidence of 4 to 5 per cent from ages 5 to 9 years to 9 per cent during adolescence to 15 to 16 per cent after adolescence. The incidence of allergic rhinitis remains constant in the young adult but gradually declines during the middle years and in the elderly. Even though seasonal allergic rhinitis is infrequent in the very young child, perennial allergic rhinitis has been recognized in infancy and even in the neonate (Ingall et al., 1965). For reasons that are not clear, more male than female children are affected with allergic rhinitis prior to adolescence, whereas females are more often affected with nasal allergy after adolescence. Race and socioeconomic factors are not thought to be important factors in the expression of allergic

rhinitis. The Tecumseh study also showed seasonal allergic rhinitis to be almost twice as common as perennial allergic rhinitis (Broder et al., 1974).

Even though syndromes identical to what we now classify as allergic rhinitis have been described for centuries, the concept of an immuologic pathogenesis dates to the beginning of the 20th century. At first, allergy diagnosis and therapy developed empirically, because the criteria for documentation of allergic disease and allergen-antibody interaction were difficult to quantify and were mostly subjective. The past 20 years have seen many advances in the elucidation of immunologic phenomena and have enabled the clinician to understand allergic diseases better. These discoveries have had considerable impact on the clinical practice of allergy and have provided a more scientific basis for many of the diagnostic and therapeutic procedures that developed without well-controlled documentation of efficacy over the past 75 years.

It is necessary to define the terms used by the allergist because the manner in which the words "immunology," "immunity," "allergy," "hypersensitivity," and "atopy" are used, and at times abused, indicates confusion as to their meaning. Medical dictionaries define *immunology* as the study of an antigen-antibody interaction that induces *immunity* and implies a beneficial protective response induced by the specific antigen. This definition of immunity is appropriate for the study of infectious diseases because the body will develop serum antibodies and sensitized lymphocytes to control the infectious agents upon reexposure; however, it is not appropriate to use this limited definition of immunity to describe the response to noninfectious environmental factors such as pollens, animal products, and drugs. As used in this chapter, immunology means the study of antigens, antibodies, and their interaction, whether beneficial or not.

The term *allergy* was introduced by a pediatrician, Clemens von Pirquet, in 1906 to designate the host's altered reactivity to an antigen (allergen) that develops after previous experience with the same material; the end result could be helpful or harmful to the host (von Pirquet, 1906). This all-inclusive immunologic concept of allergy has been popularized by Coombs and Gell (1975) and may have merit in permitting an organized and systematic approach to understanding the pathogenesis of immune mechanisms. Nevertheless, the terms *allergy* and *allergic* as commonly used in clinical practice indicate an adverse reaction, and allergic rhinitis is best defined as that adverse pathophysiologic response of the nose and adjacent organs that results from the interaction of antigen (allergen) with antibody in a host sensitized by prior exposure to that allergen. Almost 50 per cent of allergic rhinitis patients have immediate symptoms within minutes after allergen exposure (the early phase response), followed several hours later by a recurrence of symptoms (the late phase response). This immunologic definition of allergic rhinitis is accepted by most but not all clinical allergists and otolaryngologists because nonimmune processes can, on occasion, participate as additional contributory factors in the clinical expression of allergic diseases. *Hypersensitivity* indicates a heightened or exaggerated immune response that develops after more than one exposure to an allergen. Hypersensitivity will be considered synonymous with allergy. The terms *atopy* and *atopic* are also frequently used by allergists. These terms were introduced by Coca and Cooke in 1923 to classify those allergic diseases such as allergic rhinitis, asthma, and infantile eczema (atopic dermatitis) that had a familial predilection and implied genetic predisposition (Coca and Cooke, 1923). Other allergic diseases, such as contact dermatitis (poison ivy) or serum sickness, have no familial tendency and are referred to as nonatopic. It was also recognized that serum from these atopic individuals contained a factor identified as a reagin or skin-sensitizing antibody. This serum factor had the capacity to sensitize passively the skin of a nonsensitive individual, and after intradermal challenge of the passively sensitized skin site with specific allergen, a wheal and flare reaction developed within 20 minutes. This passive transfer test, also known as the Prausnitz-Kustner test (PK test), had been described only several years earlier and was the first documentation of the specific serum and tissue antibody important in the pathogenesis of allergic diseases (Prausnitz and Kustner, 1921). As will be discussed later, more than 90 per cent of these reaginic antibodies are of the IgE immunoglobulin class (Yunginger and Gleich, 1975). Even though some allergists and clinical immunologists, including this author, frequently use the term *atopic* to identify these allergic patients and their families, the term *atopy* has never gained universal acceptance.

ETIOLOGY

The development of allergic rhinitis requires two conditions: the atopic familial predisposition to develop allergy and exposure of the sensitized patient to the allergen. Patients are not born with allergies but do have the capacity to develop symptoms spontaneously through repeated exposure to allergens in their environment. Inhalants are the principal allergens responsible for allergic rhinitis and may be present outdoors and indoors. These microscopic airborne particles in-

clude the pollens from weeds, grasses, and trees, mold spores, animal products and environmental dusts, either house or occupational (Solomon and Mathews, 1978). Seasonal allergic rhinitis is primarily induced by pollens from the germination of "nonflowering" vegetation. In the temperate climates, the most important are tree pollens in the spring, grass pollens in the late spring and early summer, and ragweed in the late summer and early fall. Since there is variation from one geographic area to another, it is necessary for each clinician to become familiar with the pollination patterns in his or her region. "Flowering" vegetation, such as roses and fruit blossoms, rarely causes allergic rhinitis because these pollens are too heavy to be airborne and germination is facilitated by the action of bees and other insects. In warm climates, mold spores may be airborne year round, but in climates in which snow and freezing occur in the winter months, airborne mold spores are present intermittently during the spring, summer, and fall until there is significant frost. In patients with perennial allergic rhinitis, mold spores may be a significant inhalant allergen indoors along with house dust. The principal allergen in house dust can vary, but a major portion can be due to the house dust mite, *Dermatophagoides* (Voorhorst et al., 1967). Animal epidermal danders, as well as salivary proteins, urinary proteins, feces, and feathers, especially from pets such as cats, dogs, and birds, are potential inhalant allergens. Most allergens, including the pollens, have not been chemically characterized, and each consists of multiple antigenic determinants. Food allergens are of lesser importance in the etiology of allergic rhinitis but cannot be ignored, especially in young children (Johnstone, 1957). Patients can be sensitive to one or multiple allergens. Although it is a well-established fact that exposure to an allergen is necessary to develop sensitivity and symptoms, it is not known why allergic individuals with the same exposure become sensitive to certain allergens but not to others. The threshold of reactivity to each allergen varies greatly from one patient to another; certain individuals react to small allergenic challenges, and others tolerate a large allergen dose before developing symptoms. In addition to allergens, other nonallergenic factors can contribute to the development of nasal symptoms. These include aerosolized cosmetics, cigarette smoke, industrial fumes, and changes in temperature, humidity, and barometric pressure (Brown and Ipsen, 1968). Psychologic and social stresses and anxiety can also induce nasal congestion (Wolf et al., 1950). The importance of these additional contributory factors varies greatly from patient to patient and should not be neglected in patient management.

Even though it is not possible to predict with certainty the potentially atopic patient, the familial nature of allergic rhinitis has been recognized for years, and a positive family history of atopy has been noted in 50 to 75 per cent of allergic patients (Cohen, 1974). Despite several extensive retrospective family and twin studies, there is no agreement as to the hereditary pattern in atopic diseases. Most investigators feel that several genetic loci are involved in the expression of allergic disease, and inheritance is multifactorial. Immunologic studies have isolated some of these genetic influences. Elevated serum levels of IgE are sometimes associated with certain allergic diseases, and a recessive genetic influence has been suggested (Marsh et al., 1974). Animal studies have shown that synthesis of specific antibodies to well-characterized antigens is controlled in part by immune response (Ir) genes, which are linked to the major tissue histocompatibility locus (HLA). The studies by Levine and coworkers (1972) have suggested that ragweed allergic rhinitis and immune responses to purified ragweed antigen E were linked to a particular HLA haplotype in successive generations of allergic families. Marsh and colleagues (1973) reported a significant correlation between haplotype HL-A7 and increased IgE antibodies to a low molecular weight purified ragweed antigen (Ra5) in a group of allergic rhinitis patients sensitive to this small portion of the ragweed allergen. Similar studies of other purified allergens are indicated in allergic rhinitis patients because the responses to the more complex allergens, such as those used in clinical practice, may or may not be controlled by similar or different genetic influences.

IMMUNOPATHOPHYSIOLOGY

Allergic rhinitis, along with allergic asthma and allergic urticaria, are described immunologically as immediate hypersensitivity syndromes and are mediated in large part by immunoglobulin E (IgE) antibodies (Ishizaka et al., 1966). The properties of IgE as compared to the other serum and secretory immunoglobulins are shown in Table 42–1. Normally, IgE is present in minute quantities as compared to the serum immunoglobulins IgG, IgA, and IgM. Because of their ability to fix to primate tissues, IgE antibodies are called homocytotropic. In a few patients, a small subset of IgG antibodies of IgG Subclass 4 may fix to mast cells. Specific IgE antibodies have been demonstrated both in secretions and in sera. Unlike IgG, IgE antibodies do not cross the placenta, and the fetus will not be passively sensitized by maternal IgE antibodies.

However, the fetus is capable of synthesizing IgE (Miller et al., 1973). The IgE antibodies are synthesized after allergen challenge in large part by plasma cells located in lymphoid tissues adjacent to mucosal membranes. These IgE antibodies passively sensitize the membranes of tissue mast cells and circulating blood basophils at unique high affinity receptor sites for the Fc portion of the IgE antibody (Coleman and Godfrey, 1981). During this sensitization phase, there may not be any apparent deleterious host reaction. Upon subsequent challenge, the allergen combines with its specific IgE antibody at the cell membrane of the sensitized tissue mast cell and blood basophil with resulting cell activation (Fig. 42–1). The interaction of IgE antibodies and allergen at the mast cell membrane does not appear to be capable of activating the complement sequence by the classic pathway, but studies have suggested that IgE antibodies may initiate complement activation by the alternate pathway (Ishizaka, 1976).

The combination of allergen and IgE antibody results in a sequence of calcium- and energy-dependent enzyme reactions, with alteration of the mast cell membrane, which initiates the release of preformed mediators, especially histamine, eosinophil chemotactic factor (ECF-A), and neutrophil chemotactic factor (NCF) of the classic early phase allergic reaction. The synthesis of additional pharmacologic mediators of the IgE hypersensitivity reaction, especially leukotrienes and prostaglandins, is generated from the phospholipid constituents of the mast cell membrane via arachidonic acid metabolism. The interaction of antigen (allergen) and antibody (IgE) at the mast cell membrane, releasing as well as generating mediators of inflammation and manifestations of the early and later phase allergic reactions, is diagrammed in Figure 42–1. The mediators listed in Table 42–2 cause the increased vascular permeability, local edema, and increased eosinophil-laden secretions seen in allergic rhinitis. The early phase of the allergic reaction occurs in seconds or minutes after exposure to the allergens. In contrast, patients who manifest the late phase IgE allergic reaction show prolonged tissue inflammation. The tissue injury in this reaction can subside rapidly in minutes but may persist for hours or days, depending on the extent and the duration of allergen exposure.

Table 42–1. **Properties of Human Serum and Secretory Immunoglobulins**

	IgG	IgA	S-IgA*	IgM	IgD	IgE
Adult serum concentration (mg/ml)	10	2	–	1.5	0.03	0.0002
Antibody activity	+	+	+	+	?	+
Neutralization (antiviral, antitoxin)	+	±	+	+	–	–
Anaphylactic (histamine release)	±	–	–	–	–	+
Blocking antibody	+	±(?)	±(?)	–	–	–
Maternal-fetal transfer	+	–	–	–	–	–
Present in secretions	±	+	+ +	–	–	+
Fix to mast cell (homocytotropic)	±†	–	–	–	–	+
Classic complement activation	+	–	–	+	–	–
Alternate complement pathway	–	+	+	–	–	+

*S-IgA is secretory IgA.

†Subclass 4 IgG antibodies may fix to mast cells.

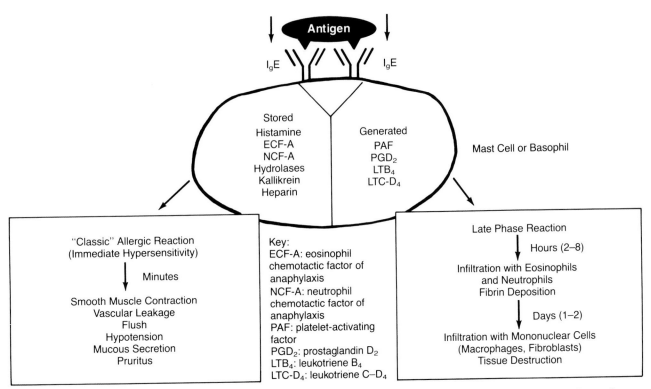

Figure 42–1. Mechanism of antigen-IgE reaction and indirect mediator release from mast cell or basophil in patients with allergic rhinitis. Note that both an early (classic) and a late-phase reaction follow the antigen-IgE reaction. (With permission from Skoner, D. P., Stillwagon, P. K., Friedman, R., et al. 1987. Pediatric allergy and immunology. *In* Zitelli, B. J., and Davis, H. W. [eds.]: Atlas of Pediatric Physical Diagnosis. New York, Gower Medical Publishing, p. 4.2.)

Histamine from mast cells as well as basophils appears to be a major chemical mediator in nasal allergy. The mechanism by which histamine produces tissue edema is based on its ability to produce vasodilation and to increase capillary permeability (Riley and West, 1953). Intranasal challenge with histamine produces immediate pruritus, sneezing, rhinorrhea, and congestion but without eosinophilia. Increased levels of histamine can be formed in nasal secretions during both the immediate and the late phase nasal reactions (Naclerio et al., 1983, 1985). Histamine stimulates both H and H_2 receptors in the nose, although the H_2 effect in the nose is probably minimal. The increased vascular permeability generated by histamine indirectly leads to the production of kinins, including bradykinin, which require kallikrein for their formation. TAME esterases, which include kallikrein along with kinins, are elevated in nasal washings during the early and the late phase allergic reactions. The leukotrienes, formerly designated as slow-reacting substance of anaphylaxis (SRS-A), are very potent mediators. Leukotrienes Cy, Dy, and Ey are formed in nasal secretions after both allergen and cold air challenges. Topical nasal challenge with leukotriene D_4 (LTD_4) increases nasal blood flow and congestion but not apparent hypersecretion. Prostaglandin Dz is the only currently studied mediator to be found elevated during the immediate nasal reaction but not during the late

TABLE 42–2. Mediators Released During Intranasal Allergen Challenges

MEDIATOR	CHALLENGE	IMMEDIATE REACTION	LATE PHASE REACTION	TISSUE EFFECTS
Histamine (H_1)	Allergen; cold, dry air	+	+	Vasodilation, plasma protein leakage; mucus hypersecretion; itching and sneezing
Leukotrienes C_4, D_4, E_4, B_4, (SRS-A)	Allergen; cold, dry air	+	?	Mucus hypersecretion; vasodilation; neutrophil chemotaxis
PGD_2	Allergen; cold, dry air	+	–	Basophil medical release; vasodilation; neutrophil chemotaxis
TAME esterases (kallikreins)	Allergen; cold, dry air	+	+	Produce kinins; vasodilation
Kinins	Allergen	+	+	Vasodilation

phase (Naclerio et al., 1985). Since this prostaglandin is produced by mast cells and not basophils, it has been suggested that mast cells are involved primarily in the early allergic reaction, whereas basophils and mast cells contribute to the late reaction. The function of the eosinophil that is attracted to nasal tissue by ECF-A has yet to be defined clearly. A regulatory or modulatory role for the eosinophil has been suggested because the enzymes histaminase and arylsulfatase, which effectively inactivate histamine and leukotrienes, respectively, are more abundant in eosinophils than in other leukocytes (Wasserman et al., 1975). In addition, phospholipase, which inactivates platelet-activating factor (PAF) released from mast cells, is located primarily in the eosinophil. A product of eosinophils, major basic protein (MBP), may participate in the inflammation that accompanies the allergic reaction (Frigas and Gleich, 1986). The mediators of inflammation, including histamine, leukotriene, and prostaglandins (see Table 42–2), have been demonstrated in nasal secretions following specific allergen intranasal provocative challenge in patients with allergic rhinitis (Naclerio et al., 1983, 1985). These mediators can directly affect the vascular bed of the nose, and the edema and congestion of the nasal tissues can disturb the balance of autonomic nervous control of nasal functions. Since patients with allergic disease overreact to cholinergic stimuli, it may be that vascular dilatation and hypersecretion are aggravated by the disturbance and resulting imbalance of autonomic control. The participation of neurohumors and vasoactive peptides, including factors such as substance P and vasoactive intestinal peptide (VIP), has been suggested, but their role needs definition. The immunologic effectors of the immediate hypersensitivity allergic reaction have been shown to be IgE antibodies in most situations. However, it should be emphasized that it is the mediators, such as histamine, leukotrienes, prostaglandins, and ECF-A, that are responsible for the pathophysiology of the immediate hypersensitivity reaction.

Examination of the nasal mucosa after allergen challenge demonstrates distended goblet cells in the presence of enlarged, congested mucous glands, as well as impaired ciliary beating and some epithelial exfoliation. The tissues are infiltrated with eosinophils and lymphoid cells with a paucity of neutrophils. The intracellular spaces are enlarged, and the basement membrane is thickened. Mast cells are present in both the nasal epithelium and the lamina propria and represent more than 80 per cent of the metachromatic cells (mast cells and basophils) seen in nasal biopsies, with degranulated mast cells significantly increased by 20 minutes after a provocative allergen challenge. Heterogeneity of mast cells has been proposed, with mucosal mast cells in the epithelium and connective tissue mast cells in the lamina propria. Basophils are the predominant metachromatic cell type found in nasal secretion and may be increased during the late phase reactions (Otsuka et al., 1985, 1986). Connell (1969a) found increased numbers of mast cells in nonspecific and vasomotor rhinitis without any evidence of allergy. It appears that the number of mast cells cannot be utilized in discriminating the pathologic features of different types of rhinitis. The ground substance surrounding the cells and blood vessels changes during allergic rhinitis from its normal semisolid state to a relatively fluid state (Rappaport et al., 1953). This change may account for the boggy appearance of the nasal mucosa frequently seen in allergic rhinitis.

Allergic rhinitis adversely affects nasal function, which, besides the role as an airway, includes filtration of particulate matter from inspired air, humidification of air, olfaction, and phonation. The testing of nasal resistance to air flow, that is, rhinomanometry, is being widely used in clinical investigation of allergic rhinitis but has not yet been widely accepted or standardized for routine clinical practice. There are two approaches to the measurement of pressure and flow relationships in the nose, anterior and posterior rhinomanometry. Anterior rhinomanometry requires minimum patient cooperation but is compromised by the normal nasal cycling phenomenon in which air flow is predominant on one side of the nose for 2 to 3 hours and then alternates to the contralateral side. This requires measurement of nasal resistance on both sides of the nose, or total nasal airway resistance. Alternatively, posterior rhinomanometry monitors posterior pharyngeal pressure via an oral tube as nasal air flow is being monitored, but 10 per cent of adults cannot perform this test. The methodology requires a storage oscilloscope because it is necessary to establish that an artifact-free pressure-flow curve has been achieved before nasal resistance measurements can be made. The development of computer-assisted rhinomanometry has now made this a fast and accurate test when used in conjunction with specific allergen intranasal provocation and has provided obstructive measurements of allergic rhinitis (Stillwagon et al., 1987). It seems probable that in the not too distant future computer-assisted rhinomanometry will be utilized more widely in clinical practice.

It has been shown that posture can affect airway resistance, since the supine position was found to increase nasal resistance in allergic rhinitis threefold over that experienced in a sitting position (Rundcrantz, 1969). Exercise and increased activity can also temporarily reverse the nasal obstruction seen in allergic rhinitis (Richerson and Seebohn, 1968). These effects may contribute to the patient's interpretation of increased symptoms when in bed, resulting not only from allergenic contents of the furniture but also from the change in posture and activity.

Following an intranasal challenge with a specific allergen, the patient with allergic rhinitis will not only develop symptoms of allergic rhinitis associated with increased mediators of inflammation in nasal washings and increased nasal resistance as measured by rhinomanometry (Naclerio, 1985) but also manifest eustachian tube dysfunction (Friedman et al., 1983). The allergen-provoked functional eustachian tube obstruction as detected by tympanometry using the nine-step procedure swallow test or, more recently, by sonotubometry was allergen dose dependent, inversely related to serum IgE antibody titer and partially preventable with antihistamines (Fireman, 1985). During seasonal natural pollen exposure, eustachian tube obstruction as well as allergic rhinitis develops and correlates with atmosphere pollen counts (Stillwagon et al., 1985). Intranasal challenge with histamine provoked eustachian tube obstruction in allergic rhinitis patients but not in normal subjects, whereas there were similar degrees of nasal obstruction as assessed by rhinomanometry in both allergic rhinitis patients and normal subjects (Skoner et al., 1987). Since eustachian tube obstruction is considered a risk factor for the development of otitis media with effusion, allergic rhinitis–induced eustachian tube obstruction may also be a risk factor. As yet, intranasal allergen challenge in both humans and laboratory animals has not provoked otitis media in allergic subjects (Fireman, 1987). Allergic rhinitis is also considered a risk factor for the expression of bronchial obstruction, that is, asthma. Histamine or allergen bronchial challenge provokes bronchial obstruction and increases forced expiratory volume (FEV) during pulmonary function testings in 30 per cent of patients with allergic rhinitis but no history of asthma. The possibility that allergic rhinitis contributes to the pathogenesis of sinusitis has also been suggested but lacks documentation.

Using airway resistance studies and quantitative pollen challenges, Connell (1969b) has shown that a larger dose of allergen was required to increase resistance in the nasal mucosa that had remained unchallenged than was required to obtain the same effect after a week of daily exposures. He also demonstrated, in patients sensitized to several pollens, that repeated challenges with one allergen conditioned the nasal mucosa to react to a lower dose of the second allergen than would have been needed if the allergen were given singly. This priming phenomenon could well account for the persistence of symptoms experienced in many patients toward the end of the pollen season in spite of decreased allergen exposure. It is also thought that this priming effect favors an increase in responsiveness to nonspecific stimuli such as changes in humidity and temperature. It has been suggested that a defect exists in the nasal mucous membrane in patients with allergic rhinitis that permits inhaled allergen macromolecules an easier access to the immune recognition system than in nonatopic subjects. Salvaggio and colleagues (1964) found atopic subjects to have increased permeability to specific allergens instilled in the nose, but other more recent studies were unable to detect any differences in permeability between atopic and nonatopic subjects (Konton-Karakitsos et al., 1975).

SYMPTOMS AND SIGNS

Initial symptoms in seasonal allergic rhinitis progress from frequent sneezing and nasal pruritus to rhinorrhea and finally to nasal obstruction. Patients with perennial allergic rhinitis have more nasal stuffiness and obstruction than sneezing and pruritus. These symptoms not only vary considerably from season to season but also differ markedly at various times of night and day. Patients will complain of early morning and late evening symptoms, and sleep can frequently be interrupted because of nasal obstruction. Patients complain of not only nasal pruritus but also itching of the eyes, throat, and ears. Many children constantly rub the nose with the hand or arm in an effort to relieve the nasal itch and perhaps to improve the nasal obstruction. Other children may press the palm of the hand upward against the nose in an "allergic salute." Constant rubbing of the nose often leads to the development of a transverse nasal crease, a horizontal groove across the lower third of the nose.

With nasal obstruction the patient will be a constant mouth breather and snoring will be a prominent nighttime symptom. It has been suggested that constant mouth breathing may contribute to the development of orofacial dental abnormalities requiring orthodontic procedures, but this has not been established definitively. Seasonal allergic rhinitis is frequently accompanied by allergic conjunctivitis with lacrimation, bilateral ocular pruritus, bilateral watery ocular secretions, and photophobia. Symptoms involving the adjacent sinuses may also be evident, especially maxillary discomfort or headaches when the symptoms of nasal obstruction are severe. In patients with eustachian tube dysfunction, allergic rhinitis may contribute to the development of otitis media with effusion. Patients may complain of a feeling of fullness or a popping sound in their ears. A hearing loss in a child with chronic or perennial allergic rhinitis should raise the suspicion of a conductive hearing deficit associated with otitis media with effusion. Loss of sense of smell and taste may also be described. Patients may also complain of generalized malaise, irritability, and fatigue; these symptoms are often difficult to differentiate from the side effects of the frequently used antihistamine therapy. Patients with seasonal pollinosis describe a gradual increase in the severity of symptoms as the season progresses, especially on dry, windy days. At times, patients relate a history of continuation of the symptoms beyond the pollen season, and many clinicians feel that repeated exposure to allergens increases the reactivity of the nasal mucosa so that ordinarily inocuous allergens and environmental factors can produce symptoms. The pattern of the patient's symptoms frequently distinguishes those with seasonal from those with perennial allergic rhinitis, especially in temperate climates with obvious seasonal climatic changes. In the warmer subtropical climates, the seasonal pollen pattern may not be obvious, since the grass pollen season extends over many months and mold spores can remain in the air throughout the year. In much of the United States, trees pollinate in the spring, primarily in March and April; grasses in late spring and summer, especially May, June, and July; and ragweed during the last two weeks of August until the first frost. The arid southwestern United States was traditionally pollen free, but the advent of irrigation and increased vegetation has changed that clinical impression. Ragweed tends to grow at the edges of cultivated fields and along highways and tends to cause increased symptoms during automobile trips. Even though airborne pollens spread for miles, increased concentrations of pollens are noted in areas of high plant density, and patients frequently complain of more symptoms in areas of high pollen density. If there is direct contact with a substantial quantity of pollen, patients may have very significant symptoms including angioedema, especially of the eyes and throat and, on occasion, urticaria.

As mentioned earlier, ingested foods are rarely the cause of allergic rhinitis in the young child. It behooves the clinician to take a very careful environmental history and survey in all patients who complain of intermittent or year-round symptoms that do not fit the usual seasonal pattern previously outlined. In general, these patients with year-round symptoms are much more of a diagnostic challenge than those with only intermittent complaints. The almost continuous exposure to house or industrial factors may induce perennial symptoms because congestion of the mucosal tissues may not have the opportunity to subside or return to normal during the few hours free of allergen exposure. It is also in these patients that the nonallergenic environmental factors tend to contribute to the symptoms: these additional nonallergenic factors include changes in barometric pressure, temperature, and humidity and aerosolized irritants such as cigarette smoke, automobile fumes, industrial pollutants, and aerosolized cosmetics and drugs.

With development of the allergic reaction, clear nasal secretions will be evident, and the nasal mucous membranes will become edematous without much erythema. The mucosa appears boggy and blue-gray. With continued exposure to the allergen, the turbinates will appear to be not only congested but also swollen, and they will obstruct the nasal airway. If nasal obstruction is present, it may be necessary to shrink the mucosa with a vasoconstrictor to document the absence of nasal polyps, which may complicate allergic rhinitis but are relatively uncommon in allergic rhinitis, occurring in less than 0.5 per cent of patients (Caplin et al., 1971). Conjunctival edema and hyperemia are frequent findings in patients with associated conjunctivitis. Allergic rhinitis patients with significant nasal obstruction and venous congestion, particularly children, may also demonstrate edema and darkening of the tissues beneath the eyes. These so-called "allergic shiners" are not pathognomonic for allergic rhinitis; they also can be seen in patients with recurrent nasal congestion and venous stasis of any other cause. The conjunctiva may also demonstrate a lymphoid follicular pattern with a cobblestone appearance. Pallor of the palatine and pharyngeal tissues is also evident, and on occasion small follicular lymphoid hyperplasia is evident on the posterior pharyngeal surface without regional cervical lymphadenopathy or tonsillar hypertrophy. Purulent secretions are only seen in the presence of secondary infections.

LABORATORY STUDIES

The nasal secretions of patients with allergic rhinitis usually contain increased numbers of eosinophils. Eosinophilia may not be present in patients not recently exposed to specific allergens or in the presence of a superimposed infection. Steroids can significantly reduce eosinophilia, but antihistamine therapy has no significant effect on nasal eosinophils. The usefulness of nasal eosinophilia is, in large part, dependent on the technique used to obtain the specimens and preparation of the slides for examination. It is difficult to quantify nasal eosinophilia accurately, and more than 3 per cent eosinophils seen on stained smear of expelled nasal secretions is considered an increase. Analysis of the nasal cytology obtained by gently pressing down on the mucosal surface of the inferior turbinate with a flexible plastic nasal probe can be helpful in the differential diagnosis of selected patients with recurrent rhinitis (Meltzer et al., 1983). Increased mucosal basophils, mast cells, or both are found in varying proportions in allergic rhinitis, nonallergic eosinophilic rhinitis, and primary nasal mastocytosis. Infection is usually evidenced by a predominance of polymorphonuclear leukocytes on the nasal smear. Although several methods of measuring nasal airway resistance by rhinomanometry have been developed in the past few years, the diagnostic usefulness of quantifying this parameter in children is yet to be established and documented.

Laboratory confirmation of specific IgE antibody synthesis to specific allergens is not mandatory in every patient with seasonal allergic rhinitis. These laboratory tests should be considered in those patients in whom the presence of a seasonal pattern is not clear-cut. In other patients, it can be helpful to confirm the clinical impression with documentation of specific IgE antibodies by in vivo skin testing or in vitro serum immunoassay testing in order to reinforce the importance of environmental control. Skin testing with the suspected allergens is mandatory in all patients prior to initiation of immunotherapy with allergy extracts because the intensity of the local wheal and flare skin reaction will be utilized as a guide in determining the initial dose of allergen. Clinicians should be selective in the use of allergens for skin testing and should employ only common allergens of potential clinical importance in their patient. The most useful allergens in the study of allergic rhinitis are the pollens, molds, house dust, and epidermal danders. Allergens used for skin testing should be selected on the basis of prevalence in the patient's area of the country and the environment in which he or she lives and works.

There is no need to test for allergy to foods in patients with clear-cut seasonal allergic rhinitis; food testing should be reserved for those patients whose conditions are diagnostic problems, with intermittent or perennial symptoms. The major problem with skin testing, especially for food allergens, has been the lack of potency, stability, and purity of the allergen solutions. The crude, undefined composition of allergens often produces false-positive reactions secondary to an irritating effect on the skin. It is well known that great care must be used in interpreting the results of food skin testing because there is often a discrepancy between the production of clinical symptoms and positive skin reactions to foods. If allergy testing is indicated, there is no need to test with a multitude of allergens. To avoid false-negative skin tests, antihistamine drugs should be withheld for 24 hours before skin tests are performed. Prick skin testing may be more reliable than intradermal skin testing; the specifics of skin testing are outlined in standard allergy textbooks (Norman, 1978). As mentioned earlier, the *in vitro* serum immunoassay (RAST, FAST, ELISA) tests for assessing the presence of serum IgE antibodies to various allergens has recently been employed as a diagnostic aid in allergic rhinitis. For certain allergens, this test has been shown to be as reliable as skin tests; however, its cost has been its major disadvantage. In addition, skin testing is 10 to 20 per cent more sensitive than the serum immunoassays. Table 42–3 compares the usefulness of skin testing as compared to serum testing.

On occasion, a nasal provocation test is useful in assessing a patient who has had negative results on skin testing and who is suspected of reacting to a particular allergen because of the recent observations that IgE antibodies may be present in nasal secretions but not evident by skin testing or the presence of serum IgE antibodies (Huggins and Brostoff, 1975). Provocation testing is performed by introducing the allergen into the nostril after its suspension or dilution in saline. A positive reaction is manifested by local pruritus, sneezing, and watery rhinorrhea and edema. It is always necessary to place a diluent control in the opposite nostril for comparison. The sublingual challenge with allergen is not a useful diagnostic tool for allergic rhinitis, in the opinion of this author. The *in vitro* cytotoxic leukocyte test with foods and other allergens is not useful as a laboratory test in controlled studies and is not recommended (Lieberman et al., 1974).

TABLE 42–3. Comparison of Skin Testing Vs. Serum Immunoassay in Allergic Diagnosis

SKIN TEST	SERUM IMMUNOASSAY
Less expensive	No patient risk
Greater sensitivity	Patient convenience
Wide allergen selection	Not influenced by drugs
Results available immediately	Results are quantitative
Will detect non–IgE-mediated allergic reactions	Preferable to skin testing in certain patients: Patients with dermographism Patients with widespread dermatitis Uncooperative children

DIFFERENTIAL DIAGNOSIS

Children who present to the clinician with complaints of rhinorrhea and nasal obstruction may have symptoms not only of allergy but also of infections, foreign bodies, structural changes, drug reactions, or neoplasms. Allergic rhinitis can be associated with or preceded by a history of atopic dermatitis, allergic asthma, or both. Nasal infections are usually characterized by burning and redness of the nasal mucosa and a purulent discharge. Without a doubt, the common cold virus is the most frequent cause of upper respiratory infection, and at its outset a viral upper respiratory infection with its clear watery rhinorrhea and sneezing resembles allergic rhinitis. Redness of the nasal mucosa is characteristic of an upper respiratory infection and distinguishes it from allergic rhinitis. After several days, the purulent nature of the nasal discharge clearly identifies the presence of infection, or in a confusing clinical situation, demonstration of the predominance of neutrophils on a smear of nasal secretions will confirm that impression. One must realize that nasal infections can be superimposed on allergic rhinitis.

Nasal obstruction and rhinorrhea, usually purulent, can also occur with foreign objects in the nares. However, usually the symptoms are unilateral, and this differentiates the presence of foreign objects from allergic or infectious rhinitis. Nasal obstruction can also occur because of nasal polyps, which may not be associated with allergic disease but can be associated with cystic fibrosis or, rarely, with aspirin therapy. Polyps can usually be demonstrated by inspection and the use of a vasoconstrictor to reduce the local edema that may obscure the nasal polyps. Another cause of unilateral nasal obstruction may be deviation of the nasal septum or a neoplasm; both conditions are detectable on visual examination of the nasal airway. Drugs administered systemically can simulate allergic rhinitis. Reserpine treatment of hypertension can produce nasal congestion, and a similar syndrome can be associated with the use of methantheline in the treatment of gastrointestinal disease and ulcers. The cessation of symptoms on withdrawal of the drug will establish this diagnosis. The most common drug rhinopathy is rhinitis medicamentosa following topical administration of vasoconstrictors for more than three to five days. The mucosa becomes pale and edematous, quite similar to the situation seen in allergic rhinitis. It is important to question patients carefully to diagnose this condition, because some patients will consider the use of nose drops insignificant in their medical history. Frequently, the seasonal allergic rhinitis or the upper respiratory infection for which the topical vasoconstrictor was initially applied has subsided by the time it is recognized that the problem is being perpetuated by the topical therapy. Another cause for nasal congestion is pregnancy, which may be considered in appropriate adolescent patients.

The aforementioned conditions can usually be differentiated from allergic rhinitis, but the separation of allergic from nonallergic perennial rhinitis (see Table 42–4) is often complicated. Nonallergic rhinitis may occur during childhood but more often is seen in adults. It simulates the perennial type of allergic rhinitis, but no immunologic etiology can be implicated. In nonallergic rhinitis, the edematous mucous membranes are often pale. Eosinophilia may occasionally be present, but the usual methods of detecting a specific allergen and its mediating antibodies are unable to suggest a specific cause. When eosinophilia is present, the syndrome is diagnosed as nonallergic rhinitis with eosinophilia (NARES). Vasomotor rhinitis is a nonallergic form of persistent nasal disease also manifested by watery rhinorrhea and nasal obstruction. Vasomotor rhinitis is a vague category of chronic or intermittent nasal disease usually seen in older children and adults that does not lend itself to a specific definition. The patient complains of overresponsiveness of the nose to minimal changes of air temperature, obnoxious odors, and often change in position of the head. Eosinophils are not seen in nasal secretions, and mast cells and basophils are not detected in the nasal mucosa or submucosa. These patients seem to have unusual awareness of their symptoms and complain disproportionally to their magnitude. It is important to differentiate these patients with nonspecific, nonallergic rhinitis and vasomotor rhinitis from patients with allergic disease because of their different responses to therapy. Immunotherapy is not to be used in these diseases, and drug therapy with antihistamine decongestants controls their symptoms inconsistently. As expected, these patients do not have historical or *in vivo* or *in vitro* tests to confirm allergic disease, and eosinophilia is not as common a laboratory feature with this problem. A comparison of these different types of rhinitis is made in Table 42–4.

THERAPY

Successful therapy of allergic rhinitis involves three primary considerations: (1) identification and avoidance of the specific allergens and other contributory factors, (2) pharmacologic management, and (3) immunotherapy to alter the patient's immune response to the allergen.

IDENTIFICATION AND AVOIDANCE. Complete avoidance of the allergens is the best therapy for allergic disease because without exposure to allergens the allergic reaction will not take place. Once the specific allergens that are responsible for the symptoms are identified, each patient should make some effort to reduce the exposure to these allergens. Elimination of exposure to an animal dander by elimination of a feather pillow or removal of a pet from the house or elimination of a food allergen from the diet may provide complete or partial relief of symptoms. Avoidance of more ubiquitous allergens such as pollens, dust, and molds may be more difficult. Patients who are sensitive to grass pollens should avoid increased exposure through gardening and grass cutting during the grass pollen season. Camping trips and picnics in the countryside should be postponed by ragweed-sensitive patients during the ragweed pollen seasons until another time of the year. Pollen rubbed into the nose and eyes can produce severe local edema, a point particularly important to remember in dealing with children, who often play outdoors in close contact with pollinating plants; patients should avoid direct contact with pollinating plants. House dust control measures, especially in the bedroom, can be a quite effective treatment for certain patients. These measures include providing rubberized or plastic airtight enclosures for mattresses and box springs; the use of synthetic bedding fabrics; and the removal of stuffed toys or stuffed furniture, heavy drapery, and dust catchers, such as bookshelves and record cabinets, from the bedroom.

Environmental control measures should also include removal of hair carpet underpads and if feasible, sealing of the forced-air heating ducts and vents in the bedroom. Thorough weekly cleaning and vacuuming of the bedding and rugs in the bedroom effectively reduces the house dust allergen concentration. Electrostatic precipitrons can be installed in central forced-air heating and cooling systems, and these can substantially reduce not only house dust but also pollens and other airborne particles. Single-room air conditioners, which recirculate the air, can also effectively reduce pollen in the bedroom. Because single-room electrostatic precipitron units are less effective and may generate irritating ozone, they are not recommended. Mold-sensitive patients should be advised against raking leaves, since the outdoor molds, especially *Alternaria* and *Hormodendrum*, thrive on dead leaves and cut vegetation. Damp basements and wallpaper, as well as glass-enclosed shower stalls, are often sources of molds in the home, and removal of the source of moisture will eliminate mold proliferation. If the moisture cannot be eliminated, mold retardants can be incorporated into the house paints or used in washing the walls. Molds in damp basements can be reduced by aerosolized paraformaldehyde or other antifungal agents. It is unfortunate that many patients do not have sufficient motivation to carry out adequate avoidance procedures in order to control their symptoms.

PHARMACOLOGIC MANAGEMENT. If the patient cannot completely avoid the allergen, the symptoms can be controlled with drugs in many cases. Antihistamines are preferred for treating mild to moderate allergic rhinitis. The antihistamines function by competing with histamine, the principal mediator of allergic rhinitis, for the H_1 cell receptor on endothelial and smooth muscle cells (Paton, 1973). There are several groups of antihistamines, which differ in chemical structure and in action (Table 42–5). Since the effectiveness of one group may diminish after several months or years of use, an antihistamine of another group may then be clinically efficacious. Therefore, the clinician should become familiar with the use of one or more antihistamines in each of the listed groupings. Chlorpheniramine or any of the several

TABLE 42–4. Comparison of Allergic and Nonallergic Rhinitis

| | ALLERGIC | NONALLERGIC | |
		NARES*	Vasomotor
Usual onset	Child	Child	Adult
Family history of allergy	Usual	Coincidental	Coincidental
Collateral allergy	Common	Unusual	Unusual
Symptoms			
Sneezing	Frequent	Occasional	Occasional
Itching	Common	Unusual	Unusual
Rhinorrhea	Profuse	Profuse	Profuse
Congestion	Moderate	Moderate to marked	Moderate to marked
Physical examination			
Edema	Moderate to marked	Moderate	Moderate
Secretions	Watery	Watery	Mucoid to watery
Nasal eosinophilia	Common	Common	Occasional
Allergic evaluation			
Skin tests	Positive	Coincidental	Coincidental
IgE antibodies	Positive	Coincidental	Coincidental
Therapeutic response			
Antihistamines	Good	Fair	Poor to fair
Decongestants	Fair	Fair	Poor to fair
Corticosteroids	Good	Good	Poor to fair
Cromolyn	Fair	Unknown	Poor
Immunotherapy	Good	None	None

*NARES, Nonallergic rhinitis with eosinophilia syndrome.

equivalents given early in the morning and at bedtime should provide good symptomatic control with the least number of side effects. Additional doses may be taken at four- to six-hour intervals. The effectiveness of antihistamines is sometimes interfered with by their side effects, which include drowsiness, headache, restlessness, nausea, and vomiting. These can sometimes be alleviated by switching to another group of antihistamines. Patients who become drowsy should be warned against driving an automobile or operating machinery after taking the medication and are candidates for Terfenadine, which does not cross the blood-brain barrier into the CNS and is less sedating than the other antihistamines. When nasal obstruction by secretions is a prominent symptom, an alpha-adrenergic decongestant, such as phenylephrine, phenylpro-

TABLE 42–5. Representative Antihistamines for Therapy for Allergic Rhinitis

GENERIC NAME	BRAND NAME	SEDATIVE EFFECT
Alkylamines		
Chlorpheniramine	Chlor-Trimeton	Mild
Dexchlorpheniramine	Polaramine	Mild
Brompheniramine	Dimetane	Mild
Triprolidine	Actidil	Mild
Ethylenediamines		
Tripelennamine	Pyribenzamine	Moderate
Methapyrilene	Histadyl	Moderate
Ethanolamines		
Diphenhydramine	Benadryl	Marked
Carbinoxamine	Clistin	Moderate
Doxylamine	Decapryn	Moderate
Terfenadine	Seldane	Slight
Astemizole	Histamol	Slight

panolamine, and cyclopentamine, should be used individually or in combination with an antihistamine to alleviate nasal mucosal engorgment, to decrease the nasal obstruction, and to improve the upper airway ventilation. Sometimes, it is necessary to employ one or more trials of an antihistamine or antihistamine-decongestant combination in order to ascertain the most effective preparation for each patient. Topical nasal alpha-adrenergic vasoconstrictors usually provide prompt symptomatic relief but should not be used for more than several days. Many patients, after 7 to 10 days of using a topical decongestant, will develop so-called rebound vasodilatation and at times habituation. It is necessary to discontinue nose drops to relieve this "rhinitis medicamentosa."

If symptoms cannot be controlled with antihistamines, decongestants, and avoidance, clinicians utilize intranasal topical corticosteroid therapy. For pediatrics, the risk-to-benefit ratio of treating even severe allergic rhinitis with oral or parenteral corticosteroids is so high that we feel that those routes of administration are usually contraindicated. However, aerosol topical corticosteroids, especially for short-term seasonal use, have proved useful in older children and adolescents. Beclomethasone, a poorly absorbed and rapidly metabolized topical corticosteroid, has been shown to be efficacious for the treatment of allergic rhinitis without apparent systemic corticosteroid side effects (Mygind, 1973). Funisolide is another topical steriod that can control symptoms of allergic rhinitis. These topical agents achieve better compliance in adults than in children, perhaps because adults tolerate the inconvenience or discomfort associated with the delivery systems better than children. Another topical aerosol pharmacologic agent that has gained widespread acceptance for the treatment of allergic rhinitis is cromolyn sodium, which inhibits the release of mediators from mast cells. Although European investigators have found the drug to be effective in 75 per cent of patients treated, such high efficacy has not been reported in a study of allergic rhinitis patients in the United States (Handelman et al., 1977). Since there are minimal potential or deleterious side effects associated with the use of intranasal topical cromolyn as compared with corticosteroids, cromolyn should be considered in patients who require continuous long-term therapy.

IMMUNOTHERAPY. If symptomatic drug therapy and avoidance cannot adequately control symptoms or inadvertently provoke significant side effects, immunotherapy (hyposensitization) with allergen solutions should be considered. Before proceeding with immunotherapy, the physician should institute a comprehensive investigation of the causative factors, and the patient's history of symptoms should be closely correlated with the presence of specific IgE antibodies, determined either by skin test results or by an *in vitro* immunoassay. Positive results of skin or blood tests that do not confirm the clinical presentation are considered as false-positive reactions and are not used as criteria for immunotherapy. The abuse and the use of these false-positive test results contribute to unnecessary and unsuccessful immunotherapy. In several double-blind studies, immunotherapy or hyposensitization injections with solutions of pollen have been shown to be effective in reducing the symptoms of allergic rhinitis (Sadan et al., 1969). More recently, immunotherapy has been known to decrease the mediators of inflammation in nasal secretions following intranasal allergen provocation challenge in patients with allergic rhinitis. Studies of the clinical efficacy of nonpollen immunotherapy with house dust, molds, and animal dander allergens in perennial allergic rhinitis are not as conclusive as those reported for seasonal allergy (Norman, 1974). There is no place for immunotherapy with allergens that can be removed or avoided. This is especially true for food allergens. The use of animal danders for immunotherapy should be limited to those individuals, such as veterinarians and farmers, who cannot avoid exposure to animal products. Even though it is not known precisely how immunotherapy promotes clinical improvement in allergic rhinitis, studies have shown a reasonable relationship between the higher doses of allergens administered, a decrease in specific IgE antibodies as measured by RAST over a period of months, an increase in IgG blocking antibodies, an increase in the number of allergen-specific suppression T-lymphocytes, and a reduction in the release of leukocyte histamine *in vitro* (Patterson et al., 1978). After the decision is made to initiate immunotherapy, the clinician should carefully select the allergens to be employed. The clinical history should be correlated with skin test results, and the magnitude of the local skin reaction should be a guide to the dose of allergen to initiate injection therapy. This author does not agree with the suggestion that

immunotherapy be initiated based only on the results of *in vitro* serum immunoassay. Not only does this hypothesis lack adequate documentation and clinical confirmation, but also it contributes to remote provision of clinical care by nonphysician health providers who do not see or examine the patient. End-point titration skin testing has also been recommended as a guide for initiation of immunotherapy, but this suggestion adds significantly to the cost of skin testing and also requires better documentation as well as confirmation prior to widespread acceptance.

The clinician begins with relatively weak subcutaneous injections of aqueous- or alum-precipitated solutions of allergens. These are gradually increased in volume and concentration to the maximally tolerated dose as indicated by a moderate local reaction. It is imperative that the clinician not induce systemic symptoms that provoke exacerbation of allergic rhinitis. After reaching the maximally tolerated dose, allergy injection therapy may be given on a perennial or year-round basis, during which the time interval between injections is increased from weekly to biweekly to monthly and given usually for several years. Another mode of immunotherapy is preseasonal weekly injections for several months prior to the season. Most patients with multiple seasonal sensitivities, certainly those with perennial allergic rhinitis, will more conveniently and practically be treated with a perennial schedule of injections approximately every four weeks. Immunotherapy may be expected to provide significant clinical improvement in 80 to 90 per cent of patients with pollen-induced allergic rhinitis. If improvement is not obtained after a two-year trial with immunotherapy, the patient should be reevaluated, and discontinuation of immunotherapy should be considered. Duration of immunotherapy injections in patients who achieve clinical benefits is dependent on the patient's overall clinical response. In the presence of clinical improvement, the patient should be given the opportunity to see if the clinical benefits are sustained after discontinuing the allergy immunotherapy. These patients should be given the opportunity to stop their immunotherapy after approximately five years of injections. Many children with allergic rhinitis tend to improve with time, but they are not "growing out" of the allergy because improvement is not related to physical growth but to an as yet undefined cause. It has been claimed that immunotherapy in children for seasonal allergic rhinitis may reduce their chances of developing pollen-induced asthma, but this report is open to many questions and has never been confirmed (Johnstone, 1957). In general, patients with seasonal allergic rhinitis are more responsive to immunotherapy than those with perennial allergic rhinitis. The factors responsible for clinical improvement are multiple. Certain patients have exacerbations of symptoms after a spontaneous or induced remission for several seasons, and immunotherapy can be reinstituted without complication. Overall, the prognosis of allergic rhinitis, with or without therapy, is better than that for nonallergic and vasomotor rhinitis.

REFERENCES

Broder, I., Higgins, M. W., Mathews, K. P., et al. 1974. Epidemiology of asthma and allergic rhinitis in a total community, Tecumseh, Michigan. III. Second survey of community. J. Allergy Clin. Immunol. 53:127.

Brown, E. B., and Ipsen, J. 1968. Changes in severity of symptoms of asthma and allergic rhinitis due to air pollutants. J. Allergy 41:254.

Caplin, I., Haynes, J. T., and Spohn, J. 1971. Are nasal polyps an allergic phenomenon? Ann. Allergy 29:631.

Coca, A. F., and Cooke, R. A. 1923. On the classification of the phenomena of hypersensitiveness. J. Immunol. 8:163.

Cohen, C. 1974. Genetic aspects of allergy. Med. Clin. North Am. 58:25.

Coleman, J. W., and Godfrey, R. C. 1981. The number and affinity of IgE receptors on dispersed human lung mast cells. Immunology 44:859.

Connell, J. T. 1969a. Nasal mastocytosis. J. Allergy 43:182.

Connell, J. T. 1969b. Quantitative intranasal pollen challenges. III. Priming effect in allergic rhinitis. J. Allergy 43:33.

Coombs, R. R. A., and Gell, P. G. H. 1975. The classification of allergic reactions underlying disease. In Gell, P. G. H., Coombs, R. R. A., and Lachman, P. H. (eds.): Clinical Aspects of Immunology, 3rd ed. Oxford, Blackwell Pub., p. 761.

Fireman, P. 1985. Eustachian tube obstruction and allergy: A role in otitis media with effusion. J. Allergy Clin. Immunol. 76:137.

Fireman, P. 1987. New concepts of the pathogenesis of otitis media with effusion. Immunol. Allergy Clin. North Am. 7:133.

Friedman, R. A., Doyle, W. J., Casselbrant, M. L., et al. 1983. Immunologic-mediated eustachian tube obstruction: a double-blind crossover study. J. Allergy Clin. Immunol. 71:442.

Frigas, E., and Gleich, G. J. 1986. The eosinophil and the pathophysiology of allergy. J. Allergy Clin. Immunol. 77:527.

Handelman, N. I., Friday, G. A., Schwartz, H. J., et al. 1977. Cromolyn sodium nasal solution in the prophylactic treatment of pollen-induced seasonal allergic rhinitis. J. Allergy Clin. Immunol. 59:237.

Huggins, K. G., and Brostoff, J. 1975. Local production of specific IgE antibodies in allergic rhinitis patients with negative skin tests. Lancet 2:148.

Ingall, M., Glaser, J., Meltzer, R. S., et al. 1965. Allergic rhinitis in early infancy: Review of the literature and report of a case in a newborn. Pediatrics 35:108.

Ishizaka, K. 1976. Cellular events in the IgE antibody response. Adv. Immunol. 23:1.

Ishizaka, K., Ishizaka, T., and Hornbrook, M. M. 1966. Physicochemical properties of reaginic antibody. V. Correlation of reaginic activity with IgE globulin antibody. J. Immunol. 97:840.

Johnstone, D. E. 1957. Study of the role of antigen dosage in the treatment of pollinosis and pollen asthma. Am. J. Dis. Child. 94:1.

Johnstone, D. E. 1969. Food allergy in children under two years of age. Pediatr. Clin. North Am. 16:211.

Kaliner, M. A., Wasserman, S. I., and Austen, K. F. 1973. Immunologic release of mediators from human nasal polyps. N. Engl. J. Med. 289:277.

Konton-Karakitsos, K., Salvaggio, J. E., and Mathews, K. P. 1975. Comparative nasal absorption of allergens in atopic and non-atopic subjects. J. Allergy Clin. Immunol. 55:241.

Levine, B. B., Strembas, R. H., and Fotino, M. 1972. Ragweed hayfever, genetic control and linkage to HL-A haplotypes. Science 178:1201.

Lieberman, P., Crawford, L., Bjelland, J., et al. 1974. Controlled study of the cytotoxic food test. J. Allergy Clin. Immunol. 53:89.

Marsh, D. G., Bias, W. B., and Ishizaka, K. 1974. Genetic control of basal immunoglobulin E level and its effect on specific reaginic sensitivity. Proc. Nat. Acad. Sci. USA 71:3588.

Marsh, D. G., Bias, W. B., and Hsu, S. H. 1973. Association of the HL-A7 cross-reacting group with a specific reaginic antibody response in allergic man. Science 179:691.

Meltzer, E. O., Zeiger, R. S., Schatz, M., et al. 1983. Chronic rhinitis in infants and children. Pediatr. Clin. North Am. 30:847.

Miller, D. L., Hirvonen, T., and Gitlin, D. 1973. Synthesis of IgE by the human conceptus. J. Allergy Clin. Immunol. 52:182.

Mygind, N. 1973. Local effect of intranasal beclomethasone aerosol in hay-fever. Br. Med. J. 4:464.

Naclerio, R. M., Meier, H. L., Kagey-Sobotka, A., et al. 1983. Mediator release after nasal antigen challenge with allergen. Am. Rev. Respir. Dis. 128:597.

Naclerio, R. M., Proud, D., Togias, A. G., et al. 1985. Inflammatory mediators in late antigen-induced rhinitis. N. Engl. J. Med. 313:65.

Norman, P. S. 1974. Specific therapy in allergy. Pro (with reservations). Med. Clin. North Am. 58:111.

Norman, P. S. 1978. In vivo methods of study of allergy: skin and mucosal tests, techniques and interpretation. In Middleton, E., Reed, C. E., and Ellis, E. F. (eds.): Allergy: Principles and Practice, Vol. 1. St. Louis, The C. V. Mosby Co., p. 256.

Otsuka, H., Denburg, J., Dolovich, J., et al. 1985. Heterogeneity of the metachromatic cells in the human nose. Significance of mucosal mast cells. J. Allergy Clin. Immunol. 76:695.

Otsuka, H., Dolovich, J., Befus, A. D., et al. 1986. Basophilic cell progenitors, nasal metachromatic cells, and peripheral blood basophils in ragweed-allergic patients. J. Allergy Clin. Immunol. 78:365.

Paton, W. D. M. 1973. Receptors for histamine. In Schacter, M. (ed.): Histamine and antihistamines, Vol. 1, International Encyclopedia of Pharmacology and Therapeutics. Oxford, Pergamon Press.

Patterson, R., Lieberman, P., Irons, J. S., et al. 1978. Immunotherapy. In Middleton, E., Reed, C. E., and Ellis, E. F. (eds.): Allergy: Principles and Practice, Vol. 2. St. Louis, The C. V. Mosby Co., p. 877.

Prausnitz, C., and Kustner, H. 1921. Studies uber Uberemphfindlichkeit, Centralbl. f. Baktinol. Abt. Orig. 86:160.

Rappaport, B. F., Sampter, M., Catchpole, H. R., et al. 1953. The mucoproteins of the nasal mucosa of allergic patients before and after treatment with corticotropin. J. Allergy 24:35.

Richerson, H. B., and Seebohn, P. M. 1968. Nasal airway response to exercise. J. Allergy 41:269.

Riley, J. F., and West, G. B. 1953. The presence of histamine in mast cells. J. Physiol. (Lond.) 120:528.

Rundcrantz, A. 1969. Postural variations of nasal patency. Acta Otolaryngol. 68:1.

Sadan, N., Rhyne, M. B., Mellitis, E. D., et al. 1969. Immunotherapy of pollinosis in children. N. Engl. J. Med. 280:623.

Salvaggio, J. E., Cavanaugh, J. J. A., Lowell, F. C., et al. 1964. A comparison of immunologic responses of normal and atopic individuals to intranasally administered antigen. J. Allergy 35:62.

Skoner, D. P., Doyle, W. P., and Fireman, P. 1987. Eustachian tube obstruction (ETO) after histamine nasal provocation: With double-blind dose regimen study. J. Allergy Clin. Immunol. 79:27.

Solomon, W. R., and Mathews, K. P. 1978. Aerobiology and inhalant allergens. In Middleton, E., Reed, C. E., and Ellis, E. F. (eds.): Allergy: Principles and Practice, Vol. 2. St. Louis, The C. V. Mosby Co., p. 899.

Stillwagon, P. K., Doyle, W. J., and Fireman, P. 1987. Effect of an antihistamine/decongestant on nasal and eustachian tube function following intranasal pollen challenge. Ann. Allergy 58:442.

Stillwagon, P. K., Skoner, D. P., Chamiritz, A., et al. 1985. Eustachian tube function and allergic rhinitis during pollen season (abstract). J. Allergy Clin. Immunol. 75:197.

von Pirquet, C. 1906. Allergie. Munch Med. Wochenschr. 53:1457.

Voorhorst, R., Spieksma, F. T. M., Varekamp, H., et al. 1967. The house dust mite (Dermatophagoides pteronyssinus) and the allergens it produces, identity with the house dust allergen. J. Allergy 39:325.

Wasserman, S. I., Goetzl, E. J., and Austen, K. F. 1975. Inactivation of human SRS-A by intact human eosinophiles and by eosinophil arylsulfatase. J. Allergy Clin. Immunol. 55:72.

Wolf, S., Holmes, T. H., Treuting, T., et al. 1950. An experimental approach to psychosomatic phenomenon in rhinitis and asthma. J. Allergy 21:1.

Yunginger, J. W., and Gleich, G. 1975. Impact and discovery of IgE in practice of allergy. Pediatr. Clin. North Am. 22:3.

Index

Note: Page numbers in *italics* refer to figures;
page numbers followed by t refer to tables.